BSAVA M:
Canine and Feline
Neurology
Fourth edition

Editors:

Simon R. Platt
BVM&S DipACVIM (Neurology) DipECVN MRCVS
Department of Small Animal Medicine, College of Veterinary Medicine,
University of Georgia, Athens, GA 30602-7371, USA

and

Natasha J. Olby
BA VetMB PhD DipACVIM (Neurology) MRCVS
Department of Clinical Sciences, College of Veterinary Medicine,
North Carolina State University, Raleigh, NC 27607, USA

Published by:

British Small Animal Veterinary Association
Woodrow House, 1 Telford Way,
Waterwells Business Park, Quedgeley,
Gloucester GL2 2AB

A Company Limited by Guarantee in England
Registered Company No. 2837793
Registered as a Charity

Copyright © 2024 BSAVA
First edition 1989
Second edition 1995
Third edition 2004
Fourth edition 2012
Reprinted 2014, 2015, 2017, 2019, 2020, 2022 twice, 2024

All rights reserved. No part of this publication may be reproduced, stored in a retrieval system, or transmitted,
in form or by any means, electronic, mechanical, photocopying, recording or otherwise without prior written
permission of the copyright holder.

The following illustrations were created by Allison L. Wright, MS, CMI, Athens, Georgia, USA:

Figures 1.14, 1.24, 1.29, 1.35, 1.37 2.1, 2.2, 2.7, 2.8, 2.9, 2.15, 2.16, 3.9, 3.12, 3.14, 4.3, 4.6, 4.12, 4.13, 4.17,
4.19, 4.20, 4.21, 6.10, 8.2, 8.3, 8.4, 8.5, 8.6, 8.9, 9.2, 9.3, 9.4, 9.5, 9.25, 10.2, 11.2, 11.4, 12.1, 12.2, 12.4, 12.6,
12.7, 12.9, 12.10, 12.12, 12.13, 12.14, 12.27, 13.1, 13.2, 13.3, 14.2, 14.5, 14.15, 14.19, 15.2, 15.4, 15.5, 15.6,
15.11, 15.15, 15.19, 15.20, 16.4, 16.40, 17.1, 17.2, 17.6, 17.7, 17.17, 18.3, 18.5, 18.16, 19.4, 19.6, 19.24, 19.25,
19.26, 20.22, 26.4

A catalogue record for this book is available from the British Library.

ISBN 978-1-905319-34-3

The publishers, editors and contributors cannot take responsibility for information provided on dosages and
methods of application of drugs mentioned or referred to in this publication. Details of this kind must be verified
in each case by individual users from up to date literature published by the manufacturers or suppliers of those
drugs. Veterinary surgeons are reminded that in each case they must follow all appropriate national legislation and
regulations (for example, in the United Kingdom, the prescribing cascade) from time to time in force.

Printed in the UK by Hobbs the Printers Ltd, Totton SO40 3WX
Printed on paper made from FSC® certified timber supporting sustainable forestry/forest management.

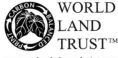

WORLD LAND TRUST™
www.carbonbalancedprint.com
CBP2250

Carbon Balancing is delivered by World Land Trust,
an international conservation charity, who protects the
world's most biologically important and threatened
habitats acre by acre. Their Carbon Balanced
Programme offsets emissions through the purchase
and preservation of high conservation value forests.

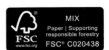

MIX
Paper | Supporting
responsible forestry
FSC® C020438

19877PUBS24

Other titles in the BSAVA Manuals series:

Manual of Avian Practice: A Foundation Manual
Manual of Backyard Poultry Medicine and Surgery
Manual of Canine & Feline Abdominal Imaging
Manual of Canine & Feline Abdominal Surgery
Manual of Canine & Feline Advanced Veterinary Nursing
Manual of Canine & Feline Anaesthesia and Analgesia
Manual of Canine & Feline Behavioural Medicine
Manual of Canine & Feline Cardiorespiratory Medicine
Manual of Canine & Feline Clinical Pathology
Manual of Canine & Feline Dentistry and Oral Surgery
Manual of Canine & Feline Dermatology
Manual of Canine & Feline Emergency and Critical Care
Manual of Canine & Feline Endocrinology
Manual of Canine & Feline Endoscopy and Endosurgery
Manual of Canine & Feline Fracture Repair and Management
Manual of Canine & Feline Gastroenterology
Manual of Canine & Feline Haematology and Transfusion Medicine
Manual of Canine & Feline Head, Neck and Thoracic Surgery
Manual of Canine & Feline Musculoskeletal Disorders
Manual of Canine & Feline Musculoskeletal Imaging
Manual of Canine & Feline Nephrology and Urology
Manual of Canine & Feline Neurology
Manual of Canine & Feline Oncology
Manual of Canine & Feline Ophthalmology
Manual of Canine & Feline Radiography and Radiology: A Foundation Manual
Manual of Canine & Feline Rehabilitation, Supportive and Palliative Care: Case Studies in Patient Management
Manual of Canine & Feline Reproduction and Neonatology
Manual of Canine & Feline Shelter Medicine: Principles of Health and Welfare in a Multi-animal Environment
Manual of Canine & Feline Surgical Principles: A Foundation Manual
Manual of Canine & Feline Thoracic Imaging
Manual of Canine & Feline Ultrasonography
Manual of Canine & Feline Wound Management and Reconstruction
Manual of Canine Practice: A Foundation Manual
Manual of Exotic Pet and Wildlife Nursing
Manual of Exotic Pets: A Foundation Manual
Manual of Feline Practice: A Foundation Manual
Manual of Practical Animal Care
Manual of Practical Veterinary Nursing
Manual of Psittacine Birds
Manual of Rabbit Medicine
Manual of Rabbit Surgery, Dentistry and Imaging
Manual of Raptors, Pigeons and Passerine Birds
Manual of Reptiles
Manual of Rodents and Ferrets
Manual of Small Animal Practice Management and Development
Manual of Wildlife Casualties

For further information on these and all BSAVA publications, please visit our website:
www.bsava.com

Contents

Video access
Previous printings of this edition included a DVD containing videos, but as most computers no longer have a DVD drive, the videos are now available via the BSAVA Library. The videos can be accessed by typing **bsavalibrary.com/neurology4e_videos** into a browser, then navigating to the relevant chapter and clicking on the videos tab. All references to the DVD within this manual relate to the videos that are now available via the BSAVA Library.

DVD Contents

Contributors

T. James Anderson BVM&S MVM PhD DSAO
DipECVN FHEA MRCVS
Associate Head of School (Learning and
Teaching), Professor of Veterinary Neurology and
Neurosurgery, School of Veterinary Medicine,
College of Medical, Veterinary and Life Sciences,
University of Glasgow,
464 Bearsden Road, Glasgow G61 1QH

Sònia Añor DVM PhD DipECVN
DipACVIM(Neurology)
Hospital Clínic Veterinari, Edifici Hcv, Campus UAB,
Universitat Autònoma de Barcelona, 08193, Spain

Rodney S. Bagley DVM DipACVIM(Neurology and
Internal Medicine)
Professor and Chair, Veterinary Clinical Sciences,
Iowa State University, College of Veterinary
Medicine, Ames, IA 50011, USA

Cheryl L. Chrisman DVM MS EdS
DipACVIM(Neurology) CVA
Professor Emeritus Small Animal Clinical Sciences,
College of Veterinary Medicine,
University of Florida, Gainesville, FL 32610;
Editor-in-Chief of the *American Journal
of Traditional Chinese Veterinary Medicine*;
Faculty of the Chi Institute of Chinese Medicine,
9700 West Highway 318, Reddick, FL 32686, USA

Joan R. Coates DVM MS DipACVIM(Neurology)
Professor, Veterinary Neurology/Neurosurgery,
Department of Veterinary Medicine and Surgery,
College of Veterinary Medicine, University of
Missouri, Columbia, MO 65211, USA

Peter J. Dickinson BVSc PhD
DipACVIM(Neurology)
Professor of Neurology/Neurosurgery,
Department of Surgical and Radiological Sciences,
University of California Davis, School of Veterinary
Medicine, Davis, CA 95616, USA

A. Courtenay Freeman DVM
DipACVIM(Neurology)
South East Veterinary Neurology and Neurosurgery,
11774 SW 88th Street, Miami, FL 33186, USA

Laurent Garosi DVM DipECVN MRCVS
*RCVS and European Recognized Specialist in
Veterinary Neurology*
Davies Veterinary Specialists,
Manor Farm Business Park, Higham Gobion,
Hertfordshire SG5 3HR

Carley J. Giovanella DVM DipACVIM(Neurology)
Gulf Coast Veterinary Neurology
and Neurosurgery, 3800 Southwest Freeway,
Suite 136, Houston, TX 77027, USA

Nicolas Granger DVM DipECVN MRCVS
Senior Lecturer in Veterinary Neurology,
School of Veterinary Sciences,
University of Bristol, Langford House,
Langford, North Somerset BS40 5DU

Krista B. Halling DVM CCRP DipACVS
Mississauga-Oakville Veterinary Emergency
Hospital and Referral Group, 2285 Bristol Circle,
Oakville, Ontario, L6H 6P8, Canada

Nick Jeffery BVSc PhD DipECVS DipECVN
DSAS FRCVS
Iowa State University, College of Veterinary
Medicine, Ames, IA 50011, USA

Sam Long BVSc PhD DipECVN
Senior Lecturer, Veterinary Neurology and
Neurosurgery, University of Melbourne
Faculty of Veterinary Science, 250 Princes Hwy,
Werribee, Vic 3030, Australia

Mark Lowrie MA VetMB MVM DipECVN MRCVS
*RCVS and European Recognized Specialist in
Veterinary Neurology*
Davies Veterinary Specialists, Manor Farm
Business Park, Higham Gobion,
Hertfordshire SG5 3HR

Karen R. Muñana DVM MS DipACVIM(Neurology)
Professor of Neurology, Department of Clinical
Sciences, College of Veterinary Medicine,
North Carolina State University, Raleigh,
NC 27607, USA

Gabrielle C. Musk BSc BVMS PhD Cert VA
DipECVAA
Senior Lecturer, Veterinary Anaesthesia,
School of Veterinary and Biomedical Sciences,
Murdoch University, South Street, Murdoch,
WA 6150, Australia

Dennis O'Brien DVM PhD DipACVIM(Neurology)
Professor of Neurology, College of Veterinary
Medicine, University of Missouri, Columbia,
MO 65211, USA

Natasha J. Olby BA VetMB PhD
DipACVIM(Neurology) MRCVS
Professor of Neurology, Department of Clinical
Sciences, College of Veterinary Medicine,
North Carolina State University, Raleigh,
NC 27607, USA

Mark G. Papich DVM MS DipACVP
Professor of Clinical Pharmacology,
Department of Molecular Biomedical Sciences,
North Carolina State University, College of
Veterinary Medicine, Raleigh, NC 27607, USA

Jacques Penderis BVSc MVM PhD CertVR
DipECVN MRCVS
*RCVS and European Recognized Specialist in
Veterinary Neurology*
Professor of Comparative Neurology/Head of
Clinical Neurology, School of Veterinary Medicine,
College of Medical, Veterinary and Life Sciences,
University of Glasgow, Bearsden Road,
Glasgow G61 1QH

Simon R. Platt BVM&S DipACVIM (Neurology)
DipECVN MRCVS
Professor of Neurology, Department of Small Animal
Medicine, College of Veterinary Medicine, University
of Georgia, Athens, GA 30602-7371, USA

Michael Podell MSc DVM DipACVIM(Neurology)
Chicago Veterinary Neurology and Neurosurgery
Group, Chicago Veterinary Emergency and
Specialty Center, 3123 N. Clybourn Avenue,
Chicago, IL 60618

Roberto Poma[†] DMV DVSc DipACVIM(Neurology)
Department of Clinical Studies,
Ontario Veterinary College, University of Guelph,
Guelph, Ontario, N1G2W1, Canada

Luc Poncelet DMV DScV DipECVN
Faculty of Medicine, Université Libre de Bruxelles,
Route de Lennik 808, B-1070, Brussels, Belgium

Amy F. Pruitt DVM PhD
DipACVR(Radiation Oncology)
14 Castleknock Drive, Asheville,
NC 28803, USA

Anthea L. Raisis PhD DVA BVSc MANZCVSc
MVetClinSt
Senior Lecturer Veterinary Anaesthesia,
School of Veterinary and Biomedical Sciences,
Murdoch University, South Street, Murdoch,
WA 6150, Australia

G. Diane Shelton DVM PhD
DipACVIM(Internal Medicine)
Professor, Department of Pathology, School of
Medicine, University of California San Diego,
La Jolla, CA 92093-0709, USA

John Sherman[†] DVM
Vethab Rehabilitation Office, 6300 Limousine Drive,
Raleigh, NC 27617, USA

Beverly K. Sturges DVM MS DipACVIM(Neurology)
Associate Professor of Clinical Neurology/
Neurosurgery, Department of Surgical and
Radiological Sciences, University of California Davis,
School of Veterinary Medicine, Davis,
CA 95616, USA

Donald E. Thrall DVM PhD DipACVR(Radiology
and Radiation Oncology)
Ross University School of Veterinary Medicine, Box
334, Basseterre, St. Kitts, West Indies

Heather L. Wamsley DVM PhD
DipACVP(Clinical Pathology)
Assistant Professor, Department of Physiological
Sciences, College of Veterinary Medicine,
University of Florida, 2015 SW 16th Ave,
Gainesville, FL 32610-0103, USA

Foreword

The Editors have asked me to write the Foreword for this new edition of the *BSAVA Manual of Canine and Feline Neurology*. I am happy to do so and feel it is a great honour. The fact that this Manual is now in its fourth edition indicates how knowledge has changed rapidly in this area since the first edition was produced in 1989.

Many veterinary practitioners consider neurology to be one of the more difficult specialties, yet it is an area that simply requires a logical and systematic approach.

Part 1, Diagnostic procedures, describes the increasing availability of additional diagnostic tests such as MRI, which has greatly advanced this discipline; but this does not devalue the importance of 'the neurological examination', which is well covered and revised and updated in Chapter 1. The requirement to consider lesion location within the nervous system is very important in diagnosis, as highlighted in Chapter 2. It is worth purchasing this Manual for chapters 1 and 2 alone!

Part 2, Neurological presentations, provides an excellent resource and will be well thumbed – as the previous edition has been in my practice. These chapters cover the diverse signs and symptoms of neurological conditions exceptionally well.

Part 3, Therapeutics, provides a wide range of up-to-date material for all levels of veterinary surgeons.

The Editors and BSAVA team have expanded beyond the usual text-based method of learning, and the video clips in the accompanying DVD will be invaluable.

I thank the Editors, their authors and the BSAVA team assisting them from behind the scenes for all their work, and I congratulate them on an excellent publication.

Mark Johnston BVetMed MRCVS
BSAVA President 2012–13

Preface

Neurology cases in veterinary medicine are still some of the most challenging and frustrating cases that are seen. The availability of MRI and the advances in this diagnostic technique's capabilities have made neurology more accessible, though unfortunately more expensive and potentially more complicated. As other specialties have also advanced, the effects of long-term systemic diseases, ongoing cancer control and new drugs for many diseases of the nervous system create novel problems for us to deal with. However, the neurological examination has remained the mainstay of patient evaluation and monitoring. It is from this basis that we can keep neurology as straightforward as it should be, with advances only making the diagnostics and treatments more successful.

In compiling this new edition we have retained the original broad sections of the third edition, dealing with diagnostic procedures and the clinical presentations and therapeutics of neurological diseases. We have added a new chapter addressing the genetic aspect of neurological diseases, which reflects the advances made in molecular biology over the last decade and the need for us to identify breed associations and counsel pet owners on breeding policies. We have also added a new chapter in the therapeutics section of the Manual, which details the science behind the traditional Chinese approach to adjunctive medicine for neurological conditions. Adjunctive treatment approaches to diseases of the nervous system are being requested by a greater proportion of owners but unfortunately it is not an area that we are especially knowledgeable in. This new chapter serves as an introduction to one area of adjunctive medicine, which includes acupuncture and focuses on what we know and what benefits such treatment could offer in the future. This chapter serves to remind us that multimodal therapy should be considered whenever possible.

Any updated neurology text would be incomplete without describing the advances made in the use of MRI. The neuroimaging chapter now contains more examples of the use of MRI in neurodiagnostics and provides an explanation of specialized imaging techniques now used in veterinary medicine. Each clinical presentation chapter contains expanded descriptions of MRI findings, reflecting the value of this modality in the field of neurology. Throughout the book, each chapter contains updated reviews of the diseases we see affecting dogs and cats and the treatments that are currently available. The latter is seen most prominently in the seizure chapter, which details the new anticonvulsant drugs that we now use routinely in our epilepsy cases.

The major addition for the fourth edition is the accompanying DVD, which contains many movies of the neurological examination and examples of lesion localization. In addition, many chapters have videos to complement the descriptions of the neurological diseases given in the text. This is a truly valuable bonus to the text given the fact that neurology is such a visual subject.

Given all the advances, it would be easy to over-complicate the approach to the neurological case in practice. However, throughout the compilation of the Manual we have always remained aware that the focus should be on the practicalities of diagnosis and treatment that veterinarians in practice and students need to know. At the same time, this book should provide useful information for those specializing in neurology as well as imaging, critical care and internal medicine through up-to-date disease descriptions and extensive referencing. Many of the contributors from the third edition have returned to update their chapters and we are very grateful for their time and expertise in helping us compile what we believe to be an exciting new addition to everyone's library of references.

We are truly grateful to everyone who has helped make this new edition possible. It goes without saying that this includes all of our authors, who are experts in their field; their knowledge and experience have been invaluable. However, there are those behind the scenes that we would also like to thank; these include the BSAVA publications team and Allison Wright, our wonderful illustrator.

Simon Platt
Natasha Olby
September 2012

Dedication

Simon: For my parents, Ron and Jackie – your love, support and inspiration have made this all possible.

Natasha: For Erik and Izzy, whose love keeps me grounded.

The neurological examination

Laurent Garosi and Mark Lowrie

Aims of the neurological examination

The aims of the neurological evaluation of a patient are to answer the following questions:

1. Do the clinical signs observed refer to a nervous system lesion?
2. What is the location of this lesion within the nervous system?
3. What are the main types of disease process that can explain the clinical signs?
4. How severe is the disease?

The first two questions are answered by the neurological examination and aim to determine the anatomical diagnosis (location and distribution of the lesion within the nervous system). The third question is answered by compiling information on the patient's signalment and history, together with the anatomical diagnosis, to determine the differential diagnosis. Disease severity can help the clinician to determine the eventual prognosis of the conditions considered in the differential diagnosis. Diagnostic tests are then carried out. The choice and interpretation of these tests must rely on a clear knowledge of the lesion localization within the nervous system and the expected disease processes.

History

Taking an accurate and complete history is the first step in the neurological evaluation (Figure 1.1). A detailed neurological examination form is presented in Figure 1.2.

Signalment
The signalment includes species, age, breed, sex and coat colour. Many neurological disorders have an age and breed predilection that should be considered when forming a differential diagnosis for a particular problem (see Appendix 1). Similarly, genetic neurological disorders can be related to coat colour.

Chief complaint
The chief complaint is the reason the owners sought medical assistance. The owners must be encouraged to give a clear and concise description

---

General information

- Confirmed age of patient
- Sibling numbers and health
- How long the owner has cared for the pet
- Vaccination status (diseases vaccinated for and time since last vaccination)
- Travel history
- Parasite treatments (including fleas and worms)
- Access to toxins
- History of trauma
- Environment
- Health of other animals in the same household
- Diet, including supplementary therapies
- Current or recent medication
- Medical or surgical history
- Drug allergies

Specific complaint

Detailed description of the chief complaint:
- When did it start?
- How did it start?
- How has it altered since onset?
- Is pain a feature?
- Has medication been associated with a change in the condition?

Systemic health

- Appetite and thirst
- Vomiting/regurgitation/diarrhoea/coughing/sneezing
- Urinary and faecal incontinence
- Bodyweight change
- Exercise tolerance
- Assessment of vision

1.1 Important information to obtain from the owner of a neurological patient.

---

of their concern. The precise meaning of the words used to refer to the chief complaint must be clarified to prevent any ambiguity and, ultimately, misdiagnosis. This is particularly important when the chief complaint is a paroxysmal event such as an epileptic seizure, loss of balance or collapse. In the absence of clinical findings, the owners' description of the event might be the sole basis for establishing an anatomical and differential diagnosis. Video footage of such an event could offer valuable information and clarify many ambiguities. The onset, evolution and course of the illness are of paramount importance and may provide insight into specific differential diagnoses (see Chapter 2).

Chief complaint

Historical background

Onset
Duration
Evolution   Static/Progressive/Regressive
                   Wax and wane/Episodic
Lateralization of signs

Animal background

Previous medical problems

Previous surgical problems

Previous travel

Vaccination status

Diet

Family history

Treatment

Neurological findings

Neurological exam   Normal/Abnormal

Abnormalities   Neurolocalization
-
-
-
-
-
-
-
-

Is the lesion?:

Focal   Multifocal   Diffuse

Symmetrical   Asymmetrical

Anatomical diagnosis   Focal   Multifocal   Diffuse

- ☐ Forebrain
- ☐ Brainstem
- ☐ Cerebellar
- ☐ Vestibular: peripheral/central
- ☐ C1–C5
- ☐ C6–T2
- ☐ T3–L3

- ☐ L4–L6
- ☐ L6–S3
- ☐ Neuromuscular
- ☐ Mononeuropathy
- ☐ Polyneuropathy
- ☐ Junctionopathy
- ☐ Myopathy

Suspected aetiological diagnosis

- ☐ Degenerative
- ☐ Anomalous
- ☐ Metabolic
- ☐ Neoplastic
- ☐ Nutritional

- ☐ Inflammatory/infectious
- ☐ Idiopathic
- ☐ Trauma
- ☐ Toxic
- ☐ Vascular

Recommended diagnostic tests

1.2   Comprehensive neurological examination form. (continues)   ▶

Observation

Mental status   Normal/Abnormal
Confusion/Depressed/Stuporous/Comatose

Behaviour   Normal/Abnormal

Body posture   Normal/Abnormal
Head tilt/Head turn/Spinal curvature/
Wide-based stance/Decerebrate/
Decerebellate/Schiff–Sherrington

Gait   Normal/Abnormal
Ataxia   Symmetrical/Asymmetrical
                       Thoracic/Pelvic limbs
Paresis/plegia   Tetra/Para/Mono/Hemi
Circling   Left/Right
Lameness

Involuntary movement

Cranial nerves

Left		Right
	Facial symmetry	
	Palpebral	
	(V + VII)	
	Corneal	
	(V + VI, VII)	
	Oculovestibular	
	(VIII + III, IV, VI)	
	Jaw tone	
	(V)	
	Gag reflex	
	(IX, X)	
	Tongue	
	(XII)	
	Menace	
	(Retina, II, forebrain + cerebellum, VII)	
	Nasal stimulation	
	(V, forebrain)	
	Pupil size	
	(Retina, II + III)	
S M L	In light	S M L
S M L	In dark	S M L
	(Sympathetic)	
	Pupillary light reflex	
	(Retina, II + III)	
	Left eye	
	Right eye	
	Nystagmus	
H V R	Spontaneous	H V R
	(VIII)	
H V R	Positional	H V R
	Strabismus	
	Permanent	
	(III or IV or VI)	
	Positional	
	(VIII)	

Postural reactions

Left		Right
	Proprioceptive positioning	
	Thoracic	
	Pelvic	
	Hopping	
	Thoracic	
	Pelvic	
	Wheelbarrowing	
	Extensor postural thrust	
	Visual placing	
	Tactile placing	

Spinal reflexes

Left		Right
	Withdrawal thoracic	
	(C6–T2)	
	Extensor carpi radialis	
	(C7–T2)	
	Withdrawal pelvic	
	(L6–S2)	
	Patellar	
	(L4–L6)	
	Gastrocnemius	
	(L6–S1)	
	Perineal	
	(S1–S3)	
	Tail movement?	
	Y/N	

Urinary function

Evidence of voluntary urination?	Y/N
Bladder distended?	Y/N
Easy bladder expression?	Y/N

Sensory evaluation

Left	Nociception	Right
	Thoracic	
	Pelvic	
	Perineal	
	Cutaneous trunci reflex	
	Cutaneous sensation	
	Thoracic	
	Pelvic	
	Specific nerve affected?	

Palpation/manipulation

Spinal pain?	Cerv/Thor/Lumb/Sacral
Joint pain?	Y/N
Muscle pain?	Y/N
Neck movement	Normal/Abnormal

1.2 (continued) Comprehensive neurological examination form. Cranial nerves: H = horizontal; L = large; M = mid-range; R = rotary; S = small; V = vertical.

Through careful questioning, the onset should be defined as:

- Acute (onset over minutes to hours)
- Subacute (onset over days)
- Chronic (onset over several days, weeks or months)
- Episodic (animal returns to normal between episodes).

The evolution of the condition should be recognized as progressive, static, improving or waxing and waning. It is also important to identify factors that trigger or improve the signs, and previous therapy and its effect on disease course.

Animal's background

After determining the chief complaint, collecting the history should end with general information regarding any previous medical or surgical conditions, family history, vaccination status, diet, previous travel history, concurrent drug use and drug reactions, and the animal's environment (i.e. access to toxins).

General physical examination

In all patients, the neurological examination should be preceded by a thorough general physical examination of all other body systems. This is essential in detecting an abnormality in other body systems that: might also affect the nervous system (e.g. animals with liver disease presented for epileptic seizures and abnormal mentation); mimics a primary neurological disorder (e.g. bilateral cranial cruciate ligament rupture in an animal presented for a pelvic limb gait abnormality); or could influence the prognosis (e.g. bladder rupture in an animal with a traumatic spinal fracture). A thorough orthopaedic examination is particularly important in animals with gait disturbances.

Neurological examination

A general overview of the neurological examination is presented in Figure 1.3 (see Figure 1.2 for a comprehensive examination form). Sedation, analgesia or neurological conditions such as epileptic seizures can transiently influence the results of this neurological evaluation.

Part I: hands-off examination
• Mental status and behaviour • Posture and body position at rest • Evaluation of gait • Identification of abnormal involuntary movements
Part II: hands-on examination
• Cranial nerve assessment • Postural reaction testing • Spinal reflexes; muscle tone and size • Sensory evaluation

1.3 Overview of the neurological examination.

Part I: hands-off examination

Consciousness, awareness and behaviour

Anatomy and function

Two anatomical structures are involved in maintaining wakefulness (a state in which the individual is fully aware of its environment). These are the ascending reticular activating system (ARAS) within the brainstem, and the cerebral cortex. The ARAS receives input from all sensory modalities (except muscle and joint proprioception) at both the level of the spinal cord and brainstem. It then projects stimulatory input diffusely to all areas of the cerebral cortex via the thalamus to maintain a state of consciousness. The portion of the forebrain commonly associated with behaviour is the limbic system, which consists of portions of the cerebrum and diencephalon (see Chapter 9).

Clinical signs

The state of consciousness, awareness and behaviour of the patient can be observed initially whilst collecting historical information from the owners. Disturbances in the state of consciousness are classified, in order of severity, as depressed/obtunded, stuporous (semi-coma) and comatose (Figure 1.4). As a rule, altered states of consciousness relate either to a diffuse lesion or widespread multifocal lesions of both cerebral hemispheres, or a focal lesion affecting the ARAS within the brainstem.

Status	Clinical signs
Confused and disoriented	Responding to environmental stimuli in an inappropriate manner
Normal	Alert; normal response to environmental stimuli
Depressed	Drowsiness, inattention and less responsive to environmental stimuli
Stuporous	State of unconsciousness with reduced responses to external stimuli, but can be roused by painful stimulus
Comatose	State of unconsciousness with absence of response to any environmental stimuli, including pain

1.4 Classification of consciousness.

Common changes in the animal's level of awareness and behaviour include disorientation, delirium, aggression, compulsive walking, loss of learned behaviour (e.g. loss of toilet training), vocalizing and head pressing (Figure 1.5). Hemi-neglect syndrome, also known as hemi-inattention syndrome, refers to an abnormal behaviour in which animals with structural forebrain disease ignore sensory input from one half of their environment (e.g. eating from one half of the bowl, turning in the wrong direction in response to sound). This syndrome indicates a forebrain lesion on the side contralateral to the side apparently 'ignored' by the animal.

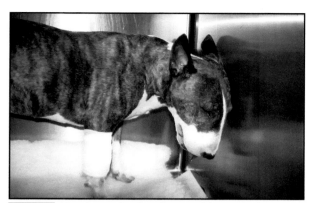

1.5 Head pressing in a 9-year-old neutered Staffordshire Bull Terrier bitch with a thalamic brain tumour.

Posture and body position at rest

The posture and body position at rest should be evaluated and determined as being normal or abnormal. Common abnormalities encountered include:

- Head tilt
- Head turn
- Ventroflexion of the neck
- Spinal curvature
- Decerebrate rigidity
- Decerebellate rigidity
- Schiff–Sherrington posture
- Wide-based stance.

Head tilt

This abnormal head posture is characterized by a rotation of the median plane of the head (one ear is held lower than the other) (Figure 1.6). A head tilt often indicates a vestibular disorder (peripheral or central). The head is usually tilted toward the same side as the lesion. Lesions affecting the cerebellar portion of the vestibular apparatus (cerebellar peduncle or flocculonodular lobe) can cause a central vestibular syndrome with a paradoxical head tilt (i.e. head tilted to the contralateral side to the lesion).

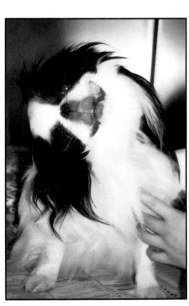

1.6 Severe head tilt in a 3-year-old neutered Japanese Chin bitch with a vestibular syndrome caused by granulomatous meningoencephalitis.

Head turn

In contrast to a head tilt, the median plane of the head remains perpendicular to the ground but the nose is turned to one side. A head turn is often associated with body turn (pleurothotonus) (Figure 1.7) and circling. These signs (called aversion syndrome) are usually toward the side of a forebrain lesion.

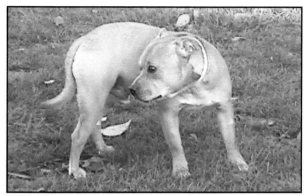

1.7 Right-sided head and body turn (pleurothotonus) in a 10-year-old male Staffordshire Bull Terrier with a right-sided forebrain tumour.

Ventroflexion of the neck

This abnormal head and neck posture is usually associated with either a neuromuscular disorder or a severe cervical spinal cord grey matter lesion.

Spinal curvature

This can be congenital or acquired, and permanent or intermittent. The aetiology is not always discernible. Common lesions include:

- Malformed vertebrae (e.g. hemivertebrae)
- Intraparenchymal spinal cord disease (e.g. syringohydromyelia) causing denervation of the associated paraspinal musculature, producing asymmetrical muscle tension and subsequent vertebral deviation
- Spinal pain (e.g. disc herniation) (Figure 1.8).

Spinal curvatures are commonly classified as:

- Scoliosis (lateral deviation of the spine)
- Lordosis (ventral curvature of the spine)

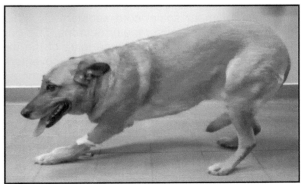

1.8 Low head carriage and severe neck pain caused by cervical intervertebral disc herniation in a 6-year-old neutered mixed-breed bitch.

- Kyphosis (dorsal curvature of the spine)
- Torticollis (twisting of the neck).

These are not specific for disease aetiology.

Decerebrate rigidity
This posture is observed as a result of a rostral brainstem lesion (between the colliculi of the midbrain). It is characterized by extension of all limbs and opisthotonus (extension of the head and neck) associated with a stuporous or comatose mental status (Figure 1.9).

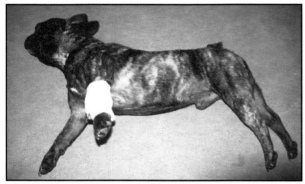

1.9 Decerebrate rigidity in a 4-year-old male French Bulldog with caudal subtentorial brain herniation associated with a large frontal lobe brain tumour.

Decerebellate rigidity
The rostral part of the cerebellum inhibits the stretch reflex mechanism of antigravity muscles (extensor muscle tone). Lesions at this level can result in opisthotonus with the thoracic limbs extended (decerebellate posture). Compared with decerebrate posture, the hips may be flexed by the increased tone in the iliopsoas muscles and mentation remains normal. This posture is often caused by an acute cerebellar lesion and can sometimes be episodic.

Schiff–Sherrington posture
This posture is observed with an acute severe thoracic or cranial lumbar spinal cord lesion in dogs. Such a lesion may interfere with the inhibitory ascending neurons (also known as border cells) that project cranially from the lateral grey matter of the cranial lumbar spinal cord segments to inhibit the thoracic limb extensor motor neurons. This posture consists of an extensor hypertonia of the thoracic limbs, with retention of voluntary movements and normal proprioceptive placing in these limbs, in addition to paralysis of the pelvic limbs (Figure 1.10). Classically, pelvic limb paralysis is hypotonic, despite the fact that the paralysis is caused by direct interference with the upper motor neuron system; however, the reflexes are intact in these limbs. In practice, this decrease in tone is transient and by the time the animal is presented to the veterinary surgeon, pelvic limb tone has returned. This sign is present only in acute lesions and does not have any prognostic significance.

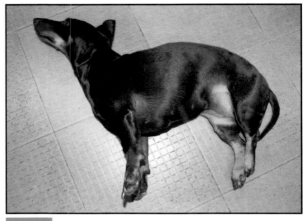

1.10 Schiff–Sherrington posture. (Courtesy of S Platt)

Wide-based stance
This posture is characteristic of a balance disorder with diseases particularly affecting the cerebellum.

Evaluation of gait
Gait disturbances are one of the most common neurological presentations. One of the first stages of the neurological examination involves assessing the animal's ability to generate and make coordinated movements. Examination of gait should be performed in a place where the patient can be allowed to move freely. This is best accomplished by having the owner walk the animal over a non-slip surface. If the animal is not making any attempt to walk, body support (such as a sling or harness) should be provided, so that any subtle voluntary movement can be detected. Normal gait requires intact function of the brainstem, cerebellum, spinal cord and sensory and motor peripheral nerves, neuromuscular junctions and muscles. The contribution of the cerebrum to gait is less important in dogs and cats than in primates. Evaluation of gait should aim to determine whether the animal is presenting with an abnormality of coordination (ataxia), an abnormality in the strength of the voluntary movement (paresis) or lameness (from either peripheral nerve disease or an orthopaedic disorder) and which limb(s) are involved.

Gait generation

Gait generation requires interaction between two motor systems: the upper motor neuron (UMN) and lower motor neuron (LMN).

UMN system
The UMN system refers to any efferent neuron originating within the brain and synapsing indirectly (i.e. via an interneuron) with a LMN to modify its activity. UMNs are responsible for the initiation and maintenance of normal movements and for the maintenance of tone in the extensor muscles to support the body against gravity. UMNs also have an inhibitory effect on myotatic reflexes. The cell body of an UMN lies within the cerebral cortex, basal nuclei or brainstem.

Lesions of the UMN system typically result in loss of motor function and release of the inhibitory effect (disinhibition) that the UMN system has on LMNs located caudal to the level of the injury. This disinhibition is usually more apparent in the extensor muscles.

▶

Gait generation

LMN system
The LMN system connects the central nervous system (CNS) with the muscles of an effector organ. The cell body of a LMN lies within the ventral horn of the spinal cord grey matter or within the cranial nerve (CN) nucleus of the brainstem. The axon of a LMN leaves the CNS as a ventral nerve root, becomes a spinal nerve and then a peripheral nerve, before finally synapsing with an effector organ (muscle or gland). The LMN is the last neuron in a chain of neurons that produce the muscular contraction necessary to maintain posture, support bodyweight and provide gait (i.e. the final common pathway to the effector organ).

Ataxia
Ataxia is defined as uncoordinated gait. This deficit can arise from:

- Lack of information reaching the CNS, which is responsible for the awareness of the movement and position of the neck, trunk and limbs in space (general proprioceptive ataxia; see **General proprioceptive ataxia** clip on DVD)
- A vestibular disorder (vestibular ataxia; see **Vestibular ataxia** clip on DVD)
- A cerebellar disorder (cerebellar ataxia; see Figure 1.11 and **Cerebellar ataxia** clip on DVD).

Ataxia can be further described based on the following characteristics of limb movement:

- Hypometria (shorter protraction phase of gait)
- Hypermetria (longer protraction phase of gait)
- Dysmetria (ability to control the distance, power and speed of an action is impaired – when applied to limb movements, it may describe a combination of both hypometria and hypermetria; see **Dysmetria** clip on DVD).

Paresis
Paresis is defined as a loss of ability to support weight (LMN disorder) or an inability to generate gait (UMN disorder). The term paresis implies that some voluntary movement is still present; paralysis (-plegia) refers to a more severe paresis with complete loss of voluntary movement. The severity of gait impairment depends somewhat on the lesion localization in the CNS. Brainstem or spinal cord lesions result in an obvious gait abnormality, whilst forebrain lesions usually cause only subtle gait abnormalities. Depending on which limbs are affected, the terms can be further defined:

- Tetraparesis/tetraplegia: paresis/paralysis of all four limbs, resulting from a lesion cranial to T3 or from a generalized LMN disorder
- Paraparesis/paraplegia: paresis/paralysis of the pelvic limbs caused by a lesion caudal to T2
- Monoparesis/monoplegia: paresis/paralysis of one limb, usually caused by a lesion of the LMN innervating the affected limb; very lateralized lesions caudal to T2 can also result in monoparesis
- Hemiparesis/hemiplegia: paresis/paralysis of the limbs on one side due to a lesion cranial to T2. This hemiparesis/plegia is ipsilateral to a lesion located between T2 and the caudal midbrain, and contralateral to a lesion located in the rostral midbrain or cerebrum.

Based on whether a lesion affects the UMN or LMN system, two different types of paresis can be distinguished:

- UMN paresis causes a delay in the onset of protraction (swing phase of gait) with the resultant stride being longer than normal with a stiff quality of movement. UMN lesions typically result in the release of the inhibitory effect that the UMN system has on LMNs (disinhibition) located caudal to the level of the injury. This disinhibition is usually more apparent in extensor muscles and results clinically in spastic paresis/paralysis. Lesions at many different levels of the CNS can produce the same set of UMN clinical signs. Due to their close anatomical relationship within the brainstem and spinal cord, most gait abnormalities involving the UMN pathways

Type of ataxia	Neurolocalization	Clinical signs
Proprioceptive	General proprioceptive pathways: • Peripheral nerve • Dorsal root • Spinal cord • Brainstem • Cerebral cortex	Abnormal postural reactions with limb paresis
Vestibular	Vestibular apparatus: • Vestibular nuclei (central) • Vestibular portion of CN VIII or vestibular receptors (peripheral)	Head tilt, leaning, falling or rolling to one side, abnormal nystagmus, strabismus, normal (peripheral) or abnormal (central) postural reactions. Crouched posture, reluctance to move and wide head excursion in case of bilateral dysfunction
Cerebellar	Cerebellum	Wide-based stance, intention tremors of the head, loss of balance and truncal sway, dysmetric gait, pendular nystagmus, delayed onset and dysmetric hopping reactions, ipsilateral menace deficit with normal vision, absence of limb paresis and proprioception placement deficits, and normal mentation (pure cerebellar disease)

1.11 Classification and criteria for differentiation of ataxia.

necessary for gait generation are also associated with some degree of general proprioceptive ataxia. In terms of lesion localization, UMN paresis and general proprioceptive ataxia visible in gait can occur as a consequence of lesions affecting the brainstem or spinal cord. With the exception of lesions caused by peracute disease processes (i.e. infarct, haemorrhage and head trauma), lesions affecting the forebrain can cause such a mild contralateral paresis that it is usually not apparent in the gait

- LMN paresis causes difficulty in weight bearing, with results varying from a short-strided, choppy gait, to a complete inability to support weight (i.e. the limb collapses whenever weight is placed upon it). When standing, the affected limb(s) may exhibit a tremor in the muscles. LMN paresis visible in gait can occur with lesions affecting the peripheral nerves, neuromuscular junction and muscles. Motor deficits observed are ipsilateral to the lesion. Compared with UMN paresis, disorders of the LMN system only cause paresis and not ataxia.

Circling

Circling can be caused by lesions in the vestibular system or by an asymmetrical/focal lesion in the forebrain. Tight circles are usually, but not exclusively, associated with a vestibular disorder, whilst wide circles are often associated with a forebrain lesion. With vestibular disease, circling is associated with other signs of vestibular involvement (head tilt, nystagmus, strabismus or falling) and is usually ipsilateral to the lesion (with the exception of lesions affecting the caudal cerebellar peduncle, fastigial nucleus and flocculonodular lobes of the cerebellum). Circling is usually toward the side of an asymmetrical/focal forebrain lesion.

Lameness

Lameness usually presents with a short stride of the affected limb and a long stride of the contralateral limb, and is typically associated with pain from orthopaedic disease. In addition, it can be associated with nervous system dysfunction referred to as 'nerve root signature' (referred pain down a limb, causing lameness or elevation of the limb, as a result of entrapment of the spinal nerve, usually by a lateralized disc extrusion or nerve root tumour).

Identification of abnormal involuntary movements

Epileptic seizure

An epileptic seizure (see Chapter 8) is the clinical manifestation of excessive or hypersynchronous electrical activity in the cerebral cortex. It can be focal or generalized. An epileptic seizure implies a forebrain disorder. Its cause may originate from outside or inside the brain.

Myoclonus

Myoclonus (see Chapters 9 and 18) is the sudden contraction followed by immediate relaxation of a specific muscle group. It can be sporadic or repetitive.

- Sporadic myoclonus can be benign and idiopathic or a form of simple partial seizure due to a forebrain disorder.
- Repetitive myoclonus can be:
  - Constant: often as a result of encephalitis or myelitis caused by canine distemper virus
  - Action-related: congenital (most commonly caused by a diffuse abnormality of CNS myelination) or acquired (e.g. idiopathic generalized tremor syndrome)
  - Postural: head 'bobbing'.

With rapid and repeated cycles, repetitive myoclonus manifests as a tremor.

Tremors

Tremors (see Chapter 13) are defined as synchronous involuntary oscillating contractions of antagonistic muscle groups. They can affect all or part of the body and can be classified as:

- Resting tremors (only present during rest)
- Intention tremors (occur as the animal intends to move)
- Action tremors (can be classified as postural or kinetic): occur following initiation of voluntary movement and worsen with increasing levels of activity. They disappear when the animal is at rest.

Myotonia

Myotonia (Myotonia clip on DVD and Chapter 18) is the sustained irregular contraction with delayed relaxation of a muscle or group of muscles following voluntary contraction. It occurs in certain congenital and acquired muscle disorders and is often asynchronous and asymmetrical.

Myokymia

Myokymia is the undulating vermiform movement of the overlying skin due to the contraction of small bands of muscle fibres.

Cataplexy

Cataplexy (see Chapter 13) is the paroxysmal onset of flaccid paralysis (muscle atonia) with preservation of consciousness, lasting for a few seconds to a few minutes. The attacks are frequently induced by excitement (such as eating, playing or the presence of the owner/another dog) and can be reversed by an external stimulus. Cataplexy can be accompanied by narcolepsy.

Movement disorders

Movement disorders are defined as episodic sudden involuntary contractions of a group of skeletal muscles in a conscious patient with normal sensorium during rest or activity. Various terms have been used to describe clinical observations in affected animals, including dyskinesia, dystonia, chorea, athetosis and ballism.

Head 'bobbing'

Intermittent head 'bobbing' is a common complaint often seen in Bulldogs and Dobermanns. It can occur as an idiopathic disorder or as a consequence of structural brain disease (especially with pathology affecting the thalamus).

Part II: hands-on examination

Cranial nerve assessment

CN function tests are summarized in Figure 1.12. The following is an overview of the function, clinical evaluation and signs of dysfunction for each CN. Testing of these nerves should be performed in conjunction with the assessment of proprioceptive placing and mentation to determine whether there is brainstem disease or peripheral nerve disease.

CN I – olfactory nerve

Anatomy and function: CN I is involved in the conscious perception of smell. It is a unique sensory CN, in that the cell bodies lie in the olfactory epithelium on the ethmoturbinate bones rather than in a ganglion. Axons pass through the cribriform plate to synapse with secondary neurons in the olfactory bulb. These secondary neurons pass successively into the olfactory peduncle and olfactory tracts before synapsing with third order neurons in the olfactory tubercle. These final neurons project to the piriform lobe in the olfactory region of the brain.

Clinical evaluation: Evaluation of smell is difficult in animals and remains a subjective assessment. This sensory function can be assessed by testing the response of the animal (sniffing or licking of the nose, aversion of the head) to aromatic sub-stances whilst blindfolded. Care should be taken not to use irritating substances that could stimulate the trigeminal nerve (CN V) and cause a similar response.

Clinical signs of dysfunction: Decreased or absent sense of smell is defined as hyposmia or anosmia, respectively. Detecting deficits in smell is difficult and often based on historical findings (e.g. decreased appetite). Non-neurological causes (such as rhinitis) are more common causes than CNS disease.

CN II – optic nerve

Anatomy and function: The optic nerve is not a 'true' nerve but an extension of the brain. It is part of the central visual pathway (involved in sensory visual perception) and the afferent component of the menace response and pupillary light reflex (PLR).

The visual pathway (see Chapter 10) involves three consecutive neurons:

- The first neuron represents the bipolar cells of the retina and receives visual information from the neuroepithelial cells of the retina (i.e. rods and cones)
- The second neuron corresponds to the ganglion cell of the retina. Its axon lies in the optic nerve and continues through the optic chiasm and proximal part of the optic tract on the opposite side (55% decussation in humans, 66% in cats and 75% in dogs)
- The cell body of the third neuron is located in the lateral geniculate nucleus in the diencephalon. Its axon projects to the visual cortex (mostly contralateral occipital cortex) in a band of fibres called the optic radiations.

Test	Afferent CN	Intermediate brain region	Efferent CN	Principal effect
Palpebral reflex	CN V – trigeminal (ophthalmic or maxillary)	Brainstem	CN VII – facial	Blink elicited by touching the medial or lateral canthus of the eye
Corneal sensation	CN V – trigeminal (ophthalmic)	Brainstem	CN VII – facial CN VI – abducent	Blink and globe retraction elicited by touching the cornea
Vestibulo-ocular reflex	CN VIII – vestibulocochlear	Brainstem	CN III – oculomotor CN IV – trochlear CN VI – abducent	Nystagmus induced by moving the head
Menace response	CN II – optic	Forebrain; cerebellum; brainstem	CN VII – facial	Blink elicited by a menacing gesture
Response to stimulation of nasal mucosa	CN V – trigeminal (ophthalmic)	Forebrain; brainstem	None	Withdrawal of the head elicited by touching the nasal mucosa
Pupillary light reflex	CN II – optic	Brainstem	CN III – oculomotor	Pupillary constriction elicited by shining a light in the eye
Gag reflex	CN IX – glossopharyngeal CN X – vagus	Brainstem	CN IX – glossopharyngeal CN X – vagus	Contraction of the pharynx elicited by its palpation

1.12   Important cranial nerve tests.

The menace response (Figure 1.13; see also **Menace response** clip on DVD) is a cortically mediated blink produced by a threatening or unexpected image suddenly appearing in the near visual field. It is present from about 10–12 weeks of age in dogs and cats. The afferent part of this response involves the same structures as the visual pathway. The efferent part of the response is not well understood. The information generated in the visual cortex is forwarded to the motor cortex to initiate a motor response. The corticobulbar pathways to the facial nerve (CN VII) nucleus then transmit the motor information. This response requires intact facial nerve function as well as an intact cerebellum (ipsilateral function). The neuronal pathways through the cerebellum are not known.

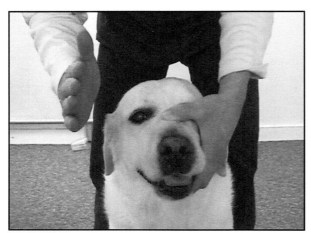

1.13 The menace response is elicited by making a threatening gesture at the eye. The afferent pathway is in the retina, optic nerve, contralateral optic tract and visual cortex. The efferent pathway involves the contralateral motor cortex, the ipsilateral cerebellar cortex and the facial nerve (CN VII). The expected response is closure of the eyelid. The contralateral eye must be blindfolded with the other hand to assess each eye separately. Care must be taken not to touch the eyelashes or to create air currents that might stimulate sensation of the face (CN V, trigeminal nerve) and elicit a palpebral or corneal reflex.

The afferent part of the PLR shares some common pathways (up to the level of the optic tract) with the visual pathway (see **Pupillary light reflex** clip on DVD). Whilst the axons involved in vision reach the conscious level after synapsing with the lateral geniculate nucleus, the axons involved in the PLR synapse with a third neuron in the pretectal nucleus. Most of the axons arising from this nucleus decussate again and synapse in the parasympathetic component of the oculomotor nucleus (ipsilateral to the stimulated eye) in the mesencephalon. Those axons that do not decussate project to the oculomotor nucleus on the contralateral side to the stimulated eye. As the majority of axons decussate, this explains why the direct response (constriction in the eye receiving the light stimulus) is greater than the consensual response (constriction in the eye not receiving the light stimulus). The efferent arm of the PLR involves parasympathetic axons in the oculomotor nerve (CN III), causing constriction of the pupil.

Clinical evaluation: The optic nerve is the common component of the afferent pathways involved in vision, menace response, visual placing and the PLR. These tests use different integration centres within the brain and different efferent pathways. The integrity of the optic nerve can be determined by combining the results of these tests. Vision in animals is evaluated by observing the animal navigate an obstacle course (animal walking into or avoiding obstacles) and by testing the menace response. If unilateral visual loss is suspected, each eye can be blindfolded in turn prior to completion of the obstacle course. The PLR tests the integrity of the optic nerve to the level of the lateral geniculate nucleus, but does not test the animal's vision. The PLR should therefore be performed in all blind animals to determine the location of the lesion. Fundic examination and evaluation of the appearance of the optic disc are also important parts of the evaluation of the optic nerve (see the *BSAVA Manual of Canine and Feline Ophthalmology* for further information).

Clinical signs of dysfunction: Lesions of the optic nerve can be manifest as partial or complete loss of vision and/or dilated and unresponsive pupils (see Chapter 10).

CN III – oculomotor nerve

Anatomy and function: CN III innervates the ipsilateral dorsal, ventral and medial recti (extraocular) muscles as well as the ventral oblique muscle. The oculomotor nerve also plays an important role in the efferent arm of the PLR and eyelid movement. It is involved in the elevation of the upper eyelid (levator palpebrae superioris) and controls pupillary constriction via its parasympathetic component. The oculomotor nuclei are located in the rostral mesencephalon. The axons exit the brainstem and traverse the middle cranial fossa lateral to the hypophysis before exiting the skull through the orbital fissure (Figure 1.14).

Clinical evaluation: CN III function can be assessed by observing eye position and movements at rest, and by testing for normal physiological nystagmus (vestibulo-ocular reflex; see **Physiological nystagmus** clip on DVD); this is achieved by moving the head from side to side as well as up and down (see CN VIII – vestibulocochlear nerve). The parasympathetic function of CN III can be assessed by observation of pupil size (Figure 1.15) and evaluation of the PLR (see **Pupillary light reflex** clip on DVD).

Clinical signs of dysfunction: Lesions of the oculomotor nerve result in a ventrolateral strabismus and an inability to rotate the eye dorsally, ventrally or medially during oculovestibular testing (external ophthalmoplegia) (Figure 1.16). This type of strabismus must be differentiated from a vestibular strabismus, which only occurs in certain head positions and is termed positional strabismus. These signs

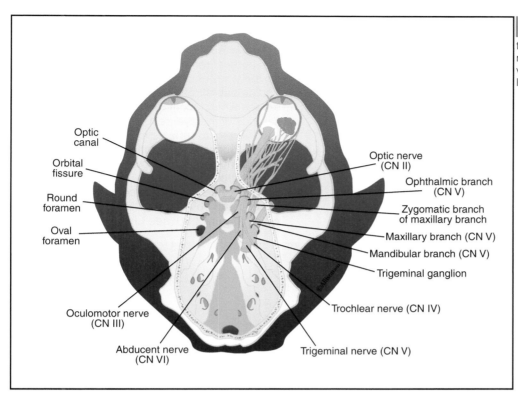

1.14 Ventral aspect of the skull and cranial nerves that exit the various foramina after leaving the brainstem.

Optic canal

Orbital fissure

Round foramen

Oval foramen

Oculomotor nerve (CN III)

Abducent nerve (CN VI)

Trigeminal nerve (CN V)

Trochlear nerve (CN IV)

Trigeminal ganglion

Mandibular branch (CN V)

Maxillary branch (CN V)

Zygomatic branch of maxillary branch

Ophthalmic branch (CN V)

Optic nerve (CN II)

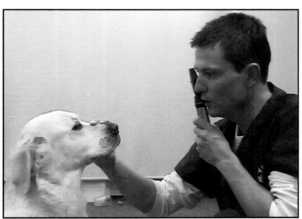

1.15 Pupil symmetry can be assessed using the indirect ophthalmoscope. The animal should be examined in room light as well as in darkness to evaluate the ability of the pupils to constrict (parasympathetic function) and to dilate (sympathetic function), respectively.

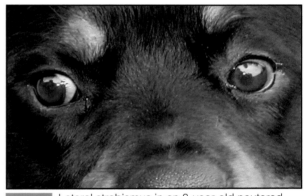

1.16 Lateral strabismus in an 8-year-old neutered Rottweiler bitch with a cavernous sinus meningioma. The compression of the oculomotor nerve (CN III) by this tumour is causing paralysis of the medial, dorsal and ventral recti and ventral oblique muscles. The result is a lateral deviation of the eyeball. The eyeball failed to adduct when testing the normal physiological nystagmus. Compared with a vestibular strabismus (which depends on head position), this type of strabismus is visible whatever the position of the head.

can also be associated with a dilated unresponsive pupil (referred to as internal ophthalmoplegia) and/or narrowing of the palpebral fissure (ptosis of the upper eyelid). However, any of these signs can exist on their own.

CN IV – trochlear nerve

Anatomy and function: CN IV innervates the contralateral dorsal oblique muscle. This muscle is responsible for inward rotation of the eyeball. The trochlear nucleus is located in the caudal mesencephalon. After leaving the brainstem, the axons decussate on the dorsal surface of the brainstem and course rostrally through the middle cranial fossa before exiting the skull via the orbital fissure.

Clinical evaluation: As for CN III, CN IV can be assessed by observation of eye position at rest and by testing for normal physiological nystagmus (see **Physiological nystagmus** clip on DVD).

Clinical signs of dysfunction: Lesions of the trochlear nerve result in a dorsolateral strabismus (extorsion) of the contralateral eye. In dogs this is best evaluated by fundoscopic examination, observing temporal deviation of the dorsal retinal vessels. In cats, it can be seen as an alteration in pupil orientation. This is a very rare isolated finding: lesions of this nerve usually occur in combination with lesions of CN III and CN VI, producing complete internal and external ophthalmoplegia.

CN V – trigeminal nerve

Anatomy and function: CN V provides sensory innervation of the face (cutaneous elements of the face as well as the cornea, mucosa of the nasal septum and mucosa of the oral cavity) and motor innervation of the masticatory muscles (temporalis, masseter, medial and lateral pterygoid and rostral part of the digastric muscles). The cell body of the sensory part of CN V lies in the trigeminal ganglion. The sensory nuclei form a large separate continuous and elongated nuclear column extending along the brainstem. The motor nuclei are located in the pons. CN V consists of three branches: ophthalmic, maxillary and mandibular. Each branch provides sensation to specific areas of the face:

- Ophthalmic branch – innervates the cornea, medial canthus of the eye, nasal septal mucosa and skin on the dorsum of the nose
- Maxillary branch – innervates the lateral canthus of the eye, skin of the cheek, side of the nose, muzzle, palates, mucous membrane of the nasopharynx, teeth and gingiva of the upper jaw
- Mandibular branch – innervates the mandibular portion of the face and oral cavity.

The ophthalmic and maxillary branches are located in close proximity to the cavernous sinus before exiting the skull through the orbital fissure and round foramen, respectively. These two branches have only a sensory function. The mandibular branch exits the skull through the oval foramen and serves both a motor and sensory function.

Clinical evaluation: The motor function of CN V is assessed by evaluating the size and symmetry of the masticatory muscles and testing the resistance of the jaw to opening of the mouth (Figure 1.17).

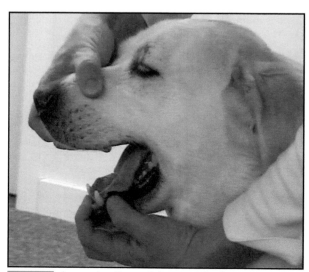

1.17 Assessing the resistance of the jaw on opening of the mouth (jaw tone) tests the motor function of the trigeminal nerve (CN V).

The sensory function (sensation of the face) can be tested by:

- The corneal reflex (ophthalmic branch) (see **Corneal reflex** clip on DVD)
- The palpebral reflex (ophthalmic or maxillary branch when touching the medial or lateral canthus of the eye, respectively) (Figure 1.18; see **Palpebral reflex** clip on DVD)
- The response to stimulation of the nasal mucosa (ophthalmic branch) (Figure 1.19; see **Nasal stimulation** clip on DVD)
- Pinching the skin of the face with haemostat forceps and observing an ipsilateral blink or facial twitch (Figure 1.20; see **Lip pinch** clip on DVD).

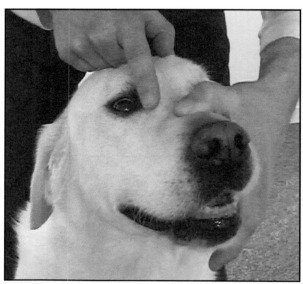

1.18 Touching the medial or lateral canthus of the eye and observing for a blink test (the palpebral reflex). The afferent arm of this reflex is mediated by the trigeminal nerve (CN V; facial sensation) whilst the efferent arm is mediated by the facial nerve (CN VII; closure of the eyelid).

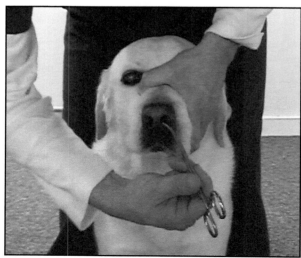

1.19 The response to stimulation of the nasal mucosa is a cortically mediated withdrawal of the head. The afferent arm is mediated by the trigeminal nerve (CN V). The integration of this response occurs in the contralateral forebrain. Both sides should be carefully assessed to evaluate possible asymmetry.

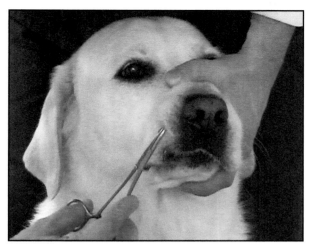

1.20 Observing a curl of the lip as it is pinched indicates that the afferent arm (CN V – trigeminal nerve) and efferent arm (CN VII – facial nerve) of this reflex are intact. Depending on the intensity of the stimulation, a behavioural response (vocalization, turning of the head) may also be observed (cortically mediated response). Both sides must be assessed to evaluate possible asymmetry. Occasionally, decreased perception of facial sensation (hypoalgesia) can be observed in animals with contralateral forebrain disease. In such cases, the animal curls its lip (normal reflex arc) but fails to show a behavioural response after stimulation of the lip contralateral to the lesion (abnormal response).

A reflex response is best distinguished from a conscious response by stimulating the nasal mucosa: the normal animal will pull its head away, whilst the animal with forebrain disease may blink or show a facial twitch, but not show a conscious reaction.

Clinical signs of dysfunction: Unilateral involvement of the motor part of CN V causes ipsilateral masticatory muscle atrophy (Figure 1.21) and decreased jaw tone. Enophthalmia and protrusion of the third eyelid can be observed in the ipsilateral eye (passive retraction of the eyeball due to the loss of the temporalis muscle mass). Bilateral involvement of the motor branches results in a dropped jaw and an inability to close the mouth voluntarily (Figure 1.22), which is associated with various degrees of

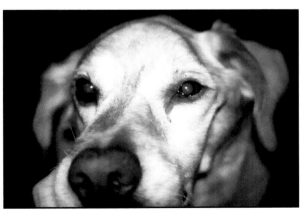

1.21 Unilateral temporalis and masseter muscle atrophy in a 9-year-old male Labrador with a trigeminal nerve sheath tumour. The ipsilateral enophthalmia is caused by loss of the temporalis muscle bulk and therefore passive retraction of the eyeball.

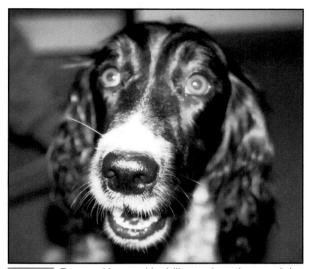

1.22 Dropped jaw and inability to close the mouth in a 5-year-old neutered Cocker Spaniel bitch with idiopathic trigeminal neuritis.

masticatory muscle atrophy depending on the duration of the signs. Decreased or complete loss of facial sensation is defined as facial hypoaesthesia or anaesthesia. Involvement of the ophthalmic branch of CN V can result in decreased tear secretion and neurotropic keratitis secondary to the loss of afferent stimulation to the lacrimal reflex (see Chapter 10).

CN VI – abducent nerve

Anatomy and function: CN VI innervates the ipsilateral lateral rectus and retractor bulbi muscles. The CN VI nucleus is located in the rostral medulla oblongata. The axons follow the same pathway as the axons of CN III and CN IV. The abducent nerve exits the cranial cavity through the orbital fissure.

Clinical evaluation: The function of CN VI can be assessed by:

* Observation of eye position and movement at rest
* Testing for normal physiological nystagmus (see **Physiological nystagmus** clip on DVD)
* Testing for normal eyeball retraction during the corneal reflex (see **Corneal reflex** clip on DVD).

Clinical signs of dysfunction: Lesions of the abducent nerve result in: an ipsilateral convergent strabismus; an inability of the eye to cross the midline when evaluating the horizontal physiological nystagmus; and an inability to retract the eyeball. Isolated lesions are rare, as for CN IV.

CN VII – facial nerve

Anatomy and function: CN VII provides motor function to the muscles of facial expression and sensory function to the rostral two-thirds of the tongue and palate (providing the sense of taste). The parasympathetic component innervates the lacrimal glands and the mandibular and sublingual salivary glands.

Neurons innervating the muscles of facial expression are located in the facial nucleus in the rostral medulla oblongata. The axons pass through the internal acoustic meatus of the petrosal bone on the dorsal surface of the vestibulocochlear nerve and exit the skull through the stylomastoid foramen. The facial nerve courses through the middle ear before branching to the muscles of facial expression (ear, eyelids, nose, cheeks, lips) and caudal portion of the digastric muscle. The parasympathetic fibres (which produce lacrimal gland secretion) leave the facial nerve as it courses through the middle ear.

Clinical evaluation: The motor function of CN VII is primarily assessed by observation of the face for symmetry (position of the ears and lip commissure on each side within the same plane, symmetry of the palpebral fissure), spontaneous blinking and movement of the nostrils. The facial nerve also provides the motor response (efferent part) of the following tests:

- Palpebral reflex (CN V and CN VII; see **Palpebral reflex** clip on DVD)
- Corneal reflex (CN V and CN VII; see **Corneal reflex** clip on DVD)
- Menace response (CN II and CN VII; see **Menace response** clip on DVD)
- Pinching of the face (CN V and CN VII; see **Lip pinch** clip on DVD).

The Schirmer tear test can evaluate the parasympathetic supply of the lacrimal gland associated with CN VII. Examining the moistness of the oral mucosa can subjectively assess salivation.

Clinical signs of dysfunction: Motor dysfunction of CN VII results in: an ipsilateral drooping of and inability to move the ear and lip; a widened palpebral fissure and absent spontaneous and provoked blinking; absent abduction of the nostril during inspiration; and deviation of the nose toward the normal side due to unopposed muscle tone on the unaffected side (Figure 1.23) (see Chapter 12). With chronic denervation, the lips are retracted further than normal and the nostril is deviated to the affected side as a result of muscle fibrosis. Facial spasm can also be seen, causing retraction of the lips and nostril to the affected side, and narrowing of the palpebral fissure on the affected side. This can be distinguished from chronic denervation by performing the palpebral test: with facial spasms the eye can blink.

Unilateral involvement can be seen in the asymmetry of the ears, eyelids, lips and nose. Lesions of the individual branches of the facial nerve result in paresis or paralysis of the specific muscles they innervate. Dysfunction of the parasympathetic supply of the lacrimal gland results in keratoconjunctivitis sicca (KCS). This is mainly seen with lesions of the facial nerve located between the medulla and the middle ear. Lesions distal to the facial canal in the temporal bone do not affect the parasympathetic neurons.

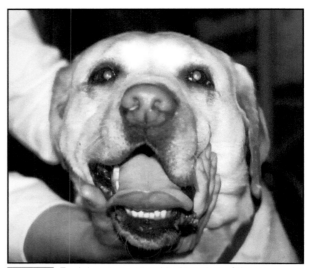

1.23 Facial asymmetry with drooping of the ear, drooping of the lip and deviation of the nostril to the unaffected side in a 7-year-old male Labrador with acute idiopathic facial nerve (CN VII) paralysis.

CN VIII – vestibulocochlear nerve

Anatomy and function: The vestibulocochlear nerve is involved in hearing and vestibular function (adaptation of the position of the eye and body with respect to the position and movement of the head). The vestibular system consists of special proprioreceptors within the petrous temporal bone (inner ear), the vestibular nerve and four brainstem nuclei located in the rostral medulla oblongata on each side of the fourth ventricle (see Chapter 12).

The receptor organs (saccule, utricle and semicircular canals) detect the position and movement of the head. The neurons of the vestibular ganglia receive impulses from these receptors and project into the vestibular nuclei via the internal acoustic meatus, where this special proprioceptive information is integrated. The vestibular nuclei connect to the nuclei of the CNs responsible for eye movement (CNs III, IV and VI) via the medial longitudinal fasciculus. They also project to the ipsilateral extensor muscles of the limb via the vestibulospinal tract. In addition, these neurons project to the ipsilateral flocculonodular lobe of the cerebellum via the caudal cerebellar peduncles. Through these pathways, the vestibular system controls the position of the eyes, trunk and limbs depending on the position and movement of the head.

The hearing system involves the sensory receptor organ (organ of Corti) within the cochlea of the inner ear. The neurons forming the cochlear branch of CN VIII have cell bodies in the spiral ganglion of CN VIII. Impulses received from the neuroepithelial hair cells of the organ of Corti enter the brainstem and synapse with the cochlear nuclei. The auditory information is then transmitted to the contralateral medial geniculate nucleus of the diencephalon via the lateral lemniscus. From this nucleus, a third neuron projects via the auditory radiation to the contralateral auditory cortex.

Clinical evaluation: Observation of the body and head posture at rest, along with evaluation of gait, can provide a lot of information about the vestibular function of CN VIII. This function can also be more specifically assessed by testing the vestibulo-ocular reflex (see **Physiological nystagmus** clip on DVD). This type of nystagmus (also called 'jerk' nystagmus) is an involuntary rhythmic movement of the eyes, which typically presents with a slow phase in one direction and a quick phase in the other direction. It can occur in normal animals (physiological or vestibular nystagmus) or may be associated with an underlying abnormality (pathological nystagmus; see Chapter 12). The direction of the nystagmus is classically described by the fast-phase movement.

A physiological nystagmus can be induced in normal individuals by lateral rotation of the head (Figure 1.24; see **Physiological nystagmus** clip on DVD). With a cat, this is best achieved by holding the animal at arm's length and rotating it from side to side. The physiological nystagmus stabilizes images on the retina during head movement. It is always observed in the plane of rotation of the head and consists of a slow phase in the direction opposite to that of the head rotation and a fast phase in the same direction as the head rotation. In the absence of any head movement, nystagmus should never be present in a normal animal.

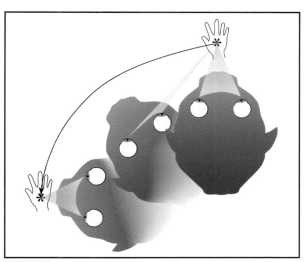

1.24 Vestibular eye movements are triggered by movement of the head in a lateral direction. The eye movements are seen to be slower than the head movement, but the eyes eventually return to the centre of the palpebral fissure.

The auditory function of CN VIII is difficult to assess clinically. The startle reaction consists of observing the animal's response to noise (e.g. handclap or whistle). Unilateral or partial deafness is virtually impossible to detect using this test. The best assessment is the animal's response to noise when asleep: most owners can report whether they have to touch their animal in order to wake them. Electrophysiological assessment (such as the brainstem auditory evoked potential (BAEP) test; see Chapter 4) is necessary to confirm and assess the severity of hearing loss.

Clinical signs of dysfunction: Vestibular dysfunction may result in any or all of the following clinical signs:

- Head tilt
- Falling
- Leaning
- Rolling
- Circling
- Abnormal and/or positional nystagmus (Figure 1.25)
- Positional strabismus (Figure 1.26)
- Asymmetrical ataxia (see Chapter 12).

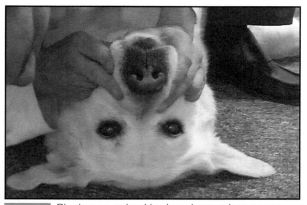

1.25 Placing an animal in dorsal recumbency can help detect a positional nystagmus or strabismus by 'challenging' the vestibular system.

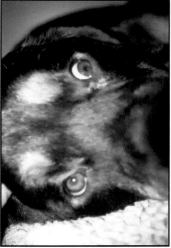

1.26 Ventrolateral positional strabismus in a Rottweiller with a central vestibular syndrome. This strabismus was only visible when the head was placed in a certain position, indicating a sensory dysfunction (vestibular apparatus) rather than a motor dysfunction (CN III – oculomotor disorder).

The clinical signs may be the result of lesions involving the receptor organs in the inner ear or the vestibular portion of CN VIII (e.g. peripheral vestibular dysfunction), or of lesions involving the brainstem vestibular nuclei (e.g. central vestibular dysfunction). Less frequently, lesions affecting the caudal cerebellar peduncle, the fastigial nucleus and the flocculonodular lobes of the cerebellum can cause central vestibular dysfunction with a resulting paradoxical head tilt (see **Paradoxical vestibular disease** clip on DVD). Bilateral vestibular disease is characterized by head sway from side to side, loss of balance on both sides and symmetrical ataxia with a wide-based stance (see **Bilateral vestibular disease** clip on DVD). A physiological nystagmus cannot be elicited.

The presence of spontaneous or positional jerk nystagmus indicates vestibular dysfunction, but does not further localize the lesion to the peripheral or central vestibular system. Some exceptions are worth mentioning:

- Positional, spontaneous and physiological nystagmus are usually absent with bilateral lesions
- Vertical nystagmus and nystagmus that changes direction with different head positions are most commonly seen with central lesions.

CN IX and CN X – glossopharyngeal and vagus nerves

Anatomy and function: The glossopharyngeal and vagus nerves share sensory (nucleus solitarius) and motor (nucleus ambiguous) nuclei. CN IX innervates the musculature of the pharynx and palatine structures. It provides sensory innervation to the caudal third of the tongue and pharyngeal mucosa (providing the sense of taste). The parasympathetic component innervates the parotid and zygomatic salivary glands. CN X controls motor function of the larynx (recurrent laryngeal branch), pharynx and oesophagus (the cervical oesophagus is innervated by the pharyngeal and recurrent laryngeal branches; the thoracic oesophagus is innervated by the vagal branches). It provides sensory function to the larynx, pharynx and thoracic and abdominal viscera. The parasympathetic component provides innervation to all thoracic and abdominal viscera, except those of the pelvic region. The nerve enters and exits the skull through the tympano-occipital fissure located behind the osseous bulla on each side.

Clinical evaluation: The pharyngeal (swallowing or gag) reflex can assess the function of CN IX and CN X (see **Gag/swallow reflex** clip on DVD). It is evaluated by applying external pressure to the hyoid bones to stimulate swallowing (Figure 1.27) or by stimulating the pharynx with a finger to elicit a gag reflex. It can also be evaluated by observing the animal eat or drink or by opening its mouth wide; the animal will usually close its mouth, swallow and lick its nose, allowing simultaneous evaluation of the tongue. The parasympathetic portion of CN X can be evaluated by testing the oculocardiac reflex. This is achieved by applying digital pressure to both eyeballs and observing simultaneously a reflex bradycardia (also mediated by CN V).

Clinical signs of dysfunction: CN IX dysfunction results in dysphagia, absent gag reflex and reduced pharyngeal tone. Animals frequently cough after drinking and swallow repeatedly due to an accumulation of saliva in the pharynx. CN X dysfunction results in dysphagia, inspiratory dyspnoea (due to laryngeal paralysis), voice changes (dysphonia) and

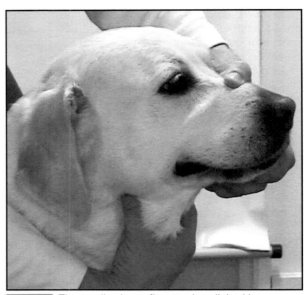

1.27 The swallowing reflex can be elicited by applying gentle pressure on the hyoid bones and thyroid cartilage.

regurgitation (due to megaoesophagus in the case of bilateral vagal disorder). The pharyngeal and oculocardiac reflexes are absent.

CN XI – accessory nerve

Anatomy and function: CN XI provides motor innervation to the trapezius and part of the sternocephalicus and brachiocephalicus muscles.

Clinical signs of dysfunction: Lesions of this nerve result in trapezius muscle atrophy. The neck may be deviated toward the affected side in chronic cases. Isolated lesions of the accessory nerve are an extremely rare finding.

CN XII – hypoglossal nerve

Anatomy and function: CN XII provides motor innervation to the muscles of the tongue. The nucleus is in the caudal medulla and can therefore be affected by high cervical lesions. The hypoglossal nerve exits the skull via the hypoglossal canal.

Clinical evaluation: CN XII function can be evaluated by inspecting the tongue for atrophy, asymmetry or deviation to one side. Tone can be assessed by manually stretching the tongue and observing a voluntary retraction. Tongue movement can be examined by applying food paste to the nose and observing the animal licking.

Clinical signs of dysfunction: Lesions affecting CN XII can result in problems with prehension, mastication and deglutition. With unilateral and recent lesions, the tongue tends to deviate toward the contralateral side (Figure 1.28). With unilateral and chronic lesions, the tongue protrudes toward the side of the lesion and atrophy is observed ipsilaterally. Muscle fasciculations may be obvious on the affected side of the denervated tongue.

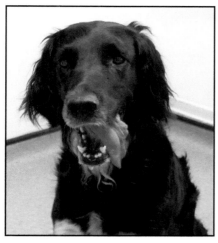

1.28 Deviation and atrophy of the tongue caused by a left-sided hypoglossal nerve paralysis. (Courtesy of S Platt)

Postural reaction testing

Anatomy and function
The sense of kinaesthesia is the awareness of the precise position and movements of the body, especially the limbs. Proprioreceptors are specific receptors sensitive to these movements. They are located in joints, tendons and muscles (general proprioception) as well as in the inner ear (special proprioception). The information collected by these receptors is transmitted to the cerebral cortex, where it is consciously perceived (proprioception placement). This sensory function can be tested using the following postural reactions:

- Proprioceptive placing (paw position or 'knuckling' response; see **Proprioceptive placing** clip on DVD)
- Hopping, wheelbarrowing, extensor postural thrusting and hemi-walking (see **Hopping, Wheelbarrowing, Extensor postural thrusting** and **Hemi-walking** clips on DVD)
- Visual or tactile placing response.

These responses have complex pathways, but generally involve:

- In the afferent arc – a proprioceptive receptor, a peripheral sensory nerve, the spinothalamic ascending pathways and the contralateral somatic sensory area of the cerebral cortex (integration centre)
- In the efferent arc – the contralateral motor cortex, the descending motor pathways within the brainstem and spinal cord (UMN), the peripheral motor nerve (LMN) and the skeletal effector muscles (Figure 1.29).

The entire nervous system is needed to be able to perform postural reactions. Testing them is a very important tool for detecting subtle dysfunction and asymmetry and confirming that a neurological disease is present. Lesions affecting any of the above anatomical sensory and/or motor components could result in abnormal postural reactions. Although these reactions detect neurological dysfunction, they do not provide specific information for lesion localization. In general, postural reactions remain normal in postsynaptic junctional and muscular diseases, as long as the animal has the strength to support its own bodyweight.

Clinical evaluation
The primary aim of postural reaction testing is to detect any subtle deficits that are not obvious on gait evaluation.

Proprioceptive placing: This test is designed to evaluate the conscious awareness of limb position and movement in space. It is the most commonly used postural reaction test in the dog. It is particularly difficult to perform in cats, which resent having their feet handled during proprioceptive positioning.
Proprioceptive placing is evaluated by placing the paw in an abnormal position (turned over so that

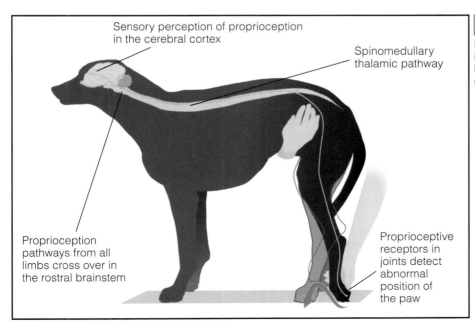

Sensory perception of proprioception in the cerebral cortex

Spinomedullary thalamic pathway

Proprioception pathways from all limbs cross over in the rostral brainstem

Proprioceptive receptors in joints detect abnormal position of the paw

1.29 Proprioceptive positioning response in the pelvic limb. Note: it is important to support the bodyweight of the animal (as shown).

the dorsal surface is in contact with the ground) and determining how quickly the animal corrects the paw position (Figure 1.30; see **Proprioceptive placing** clip on DVD). When performing this test, the animal should be standing squarely on all four limbs. It is fundamental that the majority of the animal's bodyweight is supported in order to improve test sensitivity. Failure to do so causes flexion of the limb, which results in the stimulation of proprioreceptors within the flexed joints. Supporting the patient's bodyweight is also helpful for animals that are reluctant to bear weight because of a painful limb (as seen with some orthopaedic diseases). The test should be repeated until the examiner is confident with the result. Proprioceptive placing deficits are seen in many neurological conditions and are sensitive but non-specific indicators of nervous system disease.

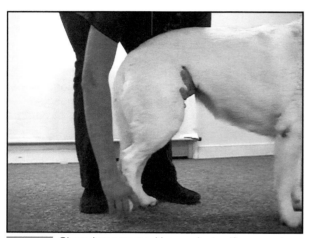

1.30 Changing paw position evaluates the conscious awareness of limb position by the animal (proprioceptive placement function). This cortically mediated response is elicited by gently placing the dorsal surface of the foot of the animal on the floor. Care should be taken to support the animal's bodyweight. The animal should immediately replace its foot in a normal position.

The 'sliding paper' test is another proprioceptive positioning test. A piece of paper is placed under the weight-bearing foot of the animal and slowly pulled laterally. A normal animal will pick up the limb and replace it in the correct position. This sliding paper test mainly evaluates proprioception in the proximal part of the limb.

Hopping reaction: This is the preferred postural reaction test in cats. It can be particularly difficult to perform in large-breed dogs. The hopping reaction is tested by holding the patient so that the majority of its bodyweight is placed on one limb whilst the animal is moved laterally (Figure 1.31; see **Hopping clip** on DVD). Normal animals hop on the tested limb to accommodate a new body position as their centre of gravity is displaced laterally. An equal response should be seen on both sides. Subtle ataxia or weakness of one limb may be detected. Animals with severe orthopaedic disease will have difficulty performing this test unless their bodyweight is supported adequately.

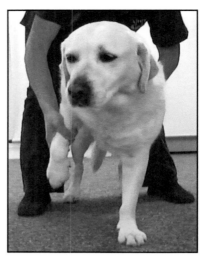

1.31 The hopping response is tested in the left thoracic limb of this dog. The right thoracic limb is held off the ground and the hind end is supported to put the majority of the bodyweight on the left thoracic limb. The dog is then pushed to the left.

Placing response: Visual and tactile placing are, in principle, much more complex postural reaction tests. They are mainly used when proprioceptive positioning or hopping reactions do not confirm a disorder. Visual placing can also be useful in assessing visual function in an animal where the menace response or obstacle course testing is difficult to interpret. Tactile placing is tested with the eyes of the animal covered. The animal is lifted and the distal part of the thoracic limb is brought into contact with the edge of a table. When the dorsal surface of the paw makes contact with the edge of the table, the animal should immediately place its foot on the surface. Visual placing is tested by allowing the animal to see the table surface. Normal animals will reach for the surface before the paw touches the table.

Hemi-walking, extensor postural thrusting and wheelbarrowing: These are also more complex postural reaction tests.

- Wheelbarrowing tests the thoracic limbs – the pelvic limbs are lifted off the ground by supporting the animal under the abdomen and forcing it to walk forwards. This test highlights subtle thoracic limb weakness and ataxia (see **Wheelbarrowing** clip on DVD). Subtle vestibular dysfunction can be detected by extending the head and neck of the animal whilst testing.
- Extensor postural thrusting tests the pelvic limbs – the animal is supported by the chest caudal to the thoracic limbs and the pelvic limbs are lowered to the floor, forcing the animal to walk backwards. This test highlights pelvic limb weakness and ataxia (see **Extensor postural thrusting** clip on DVD).
- Hemi-walking tests the ability of the animal to walk on the thoracic and pelvic limbs on one side whilst holding the limbs on the other side. The animal should be pushed away from the side on which its limbs are supported and the speed and coordination of the movements assessed. This is best performed on a non-slip surface (see **Hemi-walking** clip on DVD).

Spinal reflex examination

Spinal reflex evaluation should be considered as a continuation of gait evaluation and postural reaction testing and not as a sole entity. Following gait and postural reaction testing, the clinician should be in a position to narrow down the lesion localization to:

- Cranial to T3 spinal cord segment
- Caudal to T3 spinal cord segment
- Within the peripheral nervous system (PNS: peripheral nerve, neuromuscular junction or muscles).

Spinal reflex evaluation is performed to help classify the neurological disorder as either an UMN or LMN type (Figure 1.32). This allows the examiner to localize the lesion to specific spinal cord segments or peripheral nerves (Figure 1.33). In dogs, spinal reflexes and muscle tone are evaluated with the patient in lateral recumbency. In cats, spinal reflexes are best evaluated with the animal in dorsal recumbency, held between the thighs of the examiner. This examination does not require the patient to be conscious. Spinal reflexes are segmental: they only evaluate the spinal segment(s) within the intumescences corresponding to the stimulated nerve. Functionally, the spinal cord can be divided into four regions:

- Cranial cervical (C1–C5)
- Cervicothoracic (C6–T2)
- Thoracolumbar (T3–L3)
- Lumbosacral (L4–S3).

LMN cell bodies are located within the grey matter of the cervicothoracic intumescence (segments C6 to T2) for the thoracic limbs and within

Criterion	UMN paresis	LMN paresis
Posture	Often normal (unless the animal is paralysed); abnormal limb position (knuckling, abducted, adducted or crossed over)	Difficulty in supporting bodyweight; crouched stance as a result of overflexion of the joints
Gait	Stiff and ataxic strides; delayed protraction	Short strides; tendency to collapse
Motor function	Spastic paresis/paralysis	Flaccid paresis/paralysis
Segmental reflexes	Normal to increased	Decreased to absent
Resting muscle tone	Normal to increased	Decreased to absent
Passive limb flexion and extension	Slight resistance	Decreased resistance
Muscle atrophy	Late and mild disuse atrophy	Early and severe neurogenic atrophy

1.32 Criteria for differentiating between UMN and LMN paresis.

Location of lesion	Thoracic limbs	Pelvic limbs
Brain	UMN	UMN
C1–C5	UMN	UMN
C6–T2	LMN	UMN
T3–L3	Normal	UMN
L4–S3	Normal	LMN
Polyradiculopathy; polyneuropathy	LMN	LMN

1.33 Neurolocalization based on the presence of UMN or LMN paresis.

the lumbosacral intumescence (segments L4 to S3) for the pelvic limbs. Lesions at these intumescences result in LMN signs in the corresponding limb(s). Lesions at the level of these intumescences or affecting the PNS also result in loss of segmental spinal reflexes as well as reduced muscle tone and mass. Lesions cranial to the intumescence (UMN dysfunction) result in normal to increased segmental spinal reflexes (due to the release of the inhibitory modulatory effect of the UMN system on LMNs).

One exception to this rule is worth mentioning in the context of the emergency patient. Animals with severe peracute transverse thoracolumbar spinal cord lesions usually show severe pelvic limb hypotonia and depressed spinal reflexes for a few days following onset. Although it has been compared with a similar condition in humans called spinal shock, the reasons why an UMN pathway interruption causes LMN-like pelvic limb signs are poorly understood.

Despite many spinal reflexes being described, the most reliable are the withdrawal reflex in the thoracic limb and the patellar and withdrawal reflexes in the pelvic limb. Other spinal reflexes (triceps, biceps, extensor carpi radialis, cranial tibial and gastrocnemius) are more difficult to perform and to interpret.

Evaluation of the thoracic limbs

Withdrawal (flexor) reflex: In the thoracic limb, this reflex evaluates the integrity of spinal cord segments C6–T2 (and associated nerve roots) as well as the brachial plexus and peripheral nerves (axillary, musculocutaneous, median and ulnar nerves) (see **Withdrawal reflex: thoracic limb** clip on DVD). A noxious stimulus is applied to the tested limb by pinching the nail bed or digit with the fingers or a haemostat. This stimulus causes a reflex contraction of the flexor muscles and withdrawal of the tested limb. Sensory input is through the median, ulnar and radial nerves, and motor output is through C6–T2 spinal cord segments and the nerve roots of the axillary, musculocutaneous, median and ulnar nerves. If this withdrawal reflex is absent, individual toes should be tested to detect whether specific nerve deficits are present. When testing the flexor reflex, the contralateral limb should be observed for extension (crossed-extensor reflex), indicating an UMN lesion cranial to the C6 spinal cord segment. It should be stressed that the withdrawal reflex in the thoracic or pelvic limbs does not depend on the animal's conscious perception of the noxious stimuli (nociceptive function). The withdrawal reflex is a segmental spinal cord reflex that only depends on the function of the local spinal cord segments.

Extensor carpi radialis reflex: This is tested by striking the extensor carpi radialis muscle belly with a reflex hammer at the proximal region of the ante-brachium whilst the carpus is slightly flexed (Figure 1.34). The desired reaction is a slight extension of the carpus. This reflex evaluates the integrity of spinal cord segments C7–T2 (and associated nerve roots) as well as the radial nerve.

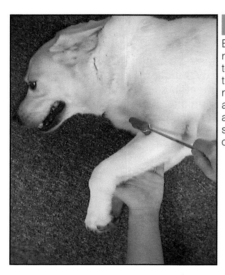

1.34

Extensor carpi radialis reflex is tested by hitting the proximal region of the antebrachium and observing a slight extension of the carpus.

Biceps brachii and triceps reflexes: These are less reliable than the withdrawal and extensor carpi radialis reflexes and are not always present in the normal animal. A finger is placed over the distal end of the biceps brachii and brachialis muscle at the level of the elbow. Striking the finger with a reflex hammer can elicit the biceps reflex; a normal reaction is flexion of the elbow or at least contraction of the biceps muscle. The triceps reflex is elicited by striking the triceps tendon proximal to its insertion on the olecranon. The desired reaction is extension of the elbow or carpus. These reflexes evaluate the integrity of spinal cord segments C6–C8 (biceps) and C7–T1 (triceps) (and associated nerve roots), as well as the musculocutaneous (biceps) and radial (triceps) nerves.

Evaluation of the pelvic limbs

Withdrawal (flexor) reflex: In the pelvic limb, this reflex evaluates the integrity of spinal cord segments L4–S2 (and associated nerve roots) as well as the femoral and sciatic nerves. A normal reflex constitutes flexion of the hip (femoral nerve function), stifle and hock (sciatic nerve function) (Figures 1.35 and 1.36; see also **Withdrawal reflex: pelvic limb** clip on DVD). Sensory input is through the tibial and peroneal branches of the sciatic nerve (lateral, dorsal and ventral aspect of the foot) and the saphenous branch of the femoral nerve (medial aspect of the foot including the second digit). Motor output is through L4–S2 spinal cord segments and nerve roots, femoral nerves, sciatic nerves and associated tibial and peroneal branches. The hock must be extended in order to evaluate sciatic function (i.e. hock flexion). A crossed-extensor reflex in the pelvic limb indicates an UMN lesion cranial to the L4 spinal cord segment.

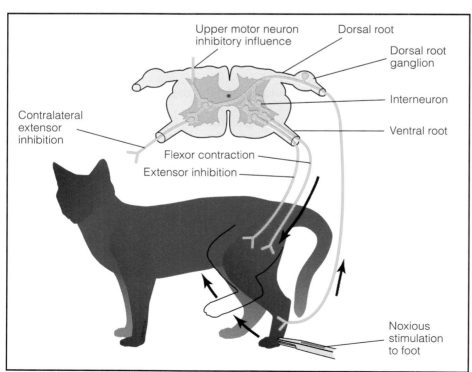

1.35 Withdrawal (flexor) reflex. When a noxious stimulus is applied to a digit, the limb should be withdrawn towards the body. Sensory input enters the spinal cord through the dorsal root to activate ipsilateral flexor motor neurons via interneurons and simultaneously inhibit the antagonistic extensor muscles. Contralateral stimulation of extensor muscles is inhibited by the descending UMN influence on the contralateral LMNs.

Upper motor neuron inhibitory influence

Dorsal root

Dorsal root ganglion

Interneuron

Ventral root

Contralateral extensor inhibition

Flexor contraction

Extensor inhibition

Noxious stimulation to foot

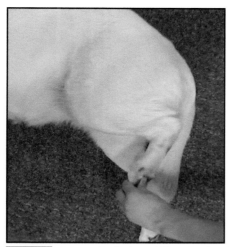

1.36 A normal withdrawal (flexor) reflex in the pelvic limb implies flexion of the hock, stifle and hip. Whilst the withdrawal is evoked, the contralateral limb should be observed for reflex extension (crossed-extensor reflex).

Patellar reflex: This monosynaptic myotatic (or stretch) reflex involves the following anatomical components: muscle spindles (fusus neuromuscularis sensitive to stretch); sensory neuron; spinal cord segment; efferent motor neuron; and muscle effector (Figure 1.37; see **Patellar reflex** clip on DVD).

This reflex evaluates the integrity of spinal cord segments L4–L6 (and associated nerve roots) as well as the femoral nerve. It is performed with the animal in lateral recumbency and the stifle slightly flexed. The limb being tested is supported by placing one hand under the thigh. Striking the patellar tendon with a reflex hammer induces extension of the limb due to a reflex contraction of the quadriceps femoris muscle (Figure 1.38). A weak or absent reflex indicates a lesion of the L4–L6 spinal cord segments or the femoral nerve. A similarly weak or absent reflex can occasionally be seen with previous stifle disease or as an age-related change. A lesion cranial to the L4 spinal cord segment can cause a normal or exaggerated reflex. In the absence of other neurological deficits, an exaggerated patellar reflex means little and can be observed in an excited or nervous animal. In addition, the patellar reflex can appear hyperreflexic with a sciatic nerve or L6–S2 spinal cord segment lesion. This pseudo-hyperreflexia is a result of decreased tone in the muscles that flex the stifle and normally counteract stifle extension during the patellar reflex.

Cranial tibial and gastrocnemius reflexes: These are less reliable than the patellar reflex. The cranial tibial reflex is elicited by striking the proximal part

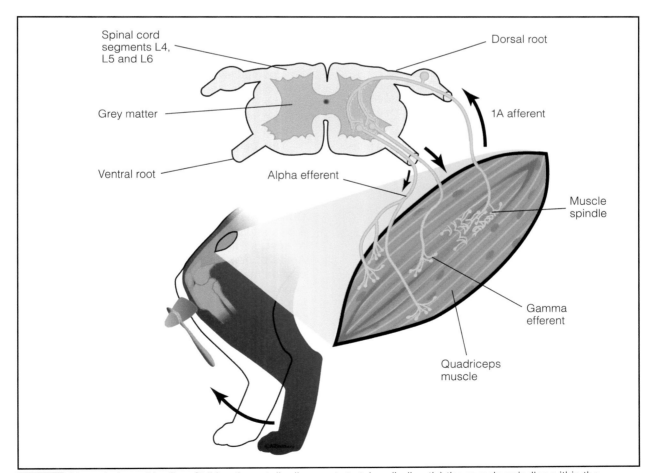

1.37 Myotatic (stretch) reflex. Striking the patellar ligament stretches (indirectly) the muscle spindles within the quadriceps muscle, which activates the 1A afferent fibres. The sensory fibres synapse directly on to motor neurons to the quadriceps femoris.

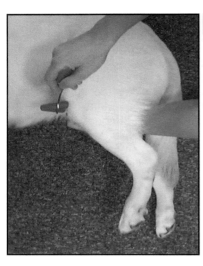

1.38

The patellar reflex is elicited by hitting the patellar ligament and observing a reflex extension of the stifle joint.

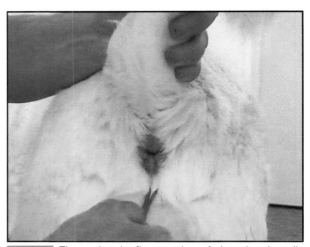

1.40 The perineal reflex consists of clamping the tail and contraction of the anal sphincter as a result of stimulation of the perineum.

of the cranial tibial muscle with a reflex hammer and observing for flexion of the tarsus (Figure 1.39; see **Cranial tibial reflex** clip on DVD). The gastrocnemius reflex is elicited by placing a finger over the gastrocnemius muscle and striking it with a hammer. The normal reaction is extension of the hock (see **Gastrocnemius reflex** clip on DVD). These reflexes evaluate the integrity of spinal cord segments L6–S1 (cranial tibial) and L7–S1 (gastrocnemius) (and associated nerve roots), as well as the peroneal (cranial tibial) and tibial (gastrocnemius) peripheral nerves.

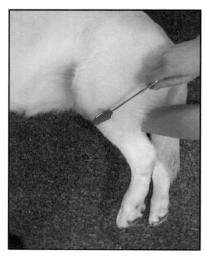

1.39

The cranial tibial reflex is elicited by hitting the proximal part of the cranial tibial muscle and observing a reflex flexion of the tarsus.

Evaluation of the tail and anus

Examination of the tail and anus is an essential part of the evaluation of spinal reflexes, which is often overlooked by the clinician. Bladder function and evaluation are described in Chapter 19.

Perineal reflex: Stimulation of the perineum with a haemostat results in contraction of the anal sphincter and flexion of the tail (Figure 1.40; see **Perineal reflex** clip on DVD). This reflex tests the integrity of the caudal nerves of the tail, the pudendal nerve and spinal cord segments S1–Cd5 (and associated nerve roots).

Sensory evaluation

Apart from proprioception placing (see above), evaluation of the sensory system in animals largely depends on tests for pain perception (nociception). Touch, pressure and temperature sensation are extremely difficult to assess objectively in animals.

- Anaesthesia refers to a complete loss of all forms of sensation.
- Hypoaesthesia refers to a diminution of sensation.
- Hyperaesthesia refers to increased sensitivity to a normal level of stimulation.
- Analgesia, hypoalgesia and hyperalgesia refer to loss, impairment and increased sensitivity to pain, respectively.

The purpose of testing pain perception is to detect and map out any areas of sensory loss. Assessment of pain sensation requires a noxious stimulus and evaluation of the animal's response.

Cutaneous sensory testing

A dermatome is an area of skin that corresponds to a specific nerve root and spinal cord segment. Areas of decreased or absent cutaneous pain perception may aid in identifying the specific peripheral nerves, nerve roots and spinal cord segments involved in the disease process. Dermatomal mapping of clinical use in the dog is summarized in Figure 1.41. Cutaneous sensation is evaluated by pinching the skin with a haemostat. The response elicited may be a behavioural response or a withdrawal reflex. The presence of either response indicates functional integrity of the particular sensory nerve tested. Conscious perception of the stimulus (e.g. behavioural response such as turning the head or vocalization) indicates that the cutaneous nerve being tested, the afferent nociceptive pathways within the spinal cord and brain, and the appropriate portions of the cerebral cortex are functional. A withdrawal reflex simply indicates that the cutaneous nerve tested, the spinal cord segments and the

Nerve	Spinal cord segment	Cutaneous sensory distribution
Musculocutaneous	C6, C7, C8	Medial antebrachium
Radial	C7, C8, T1, T2	Cranial aspect of the antebrachium and foot, except the fifth digit
Median and ulnar	C8, T1, T2	Caudal aspect of the antebrachium and foot (including fifth digit)
Femoral	L4, L5, L6	Medial aspect of the limb and first digit (saphenous branch)
Sciatic: Peroneal branch Tibial branch	L6, L7, S1, S2	Craniolateral aspect of limb distal to stifle Caudal aspect of limb distal to stifle

1.41 Dermatomal mapping of clinical use in dogs.

efferent motor neuron of the withdrawal reflex are functional. If an area of diminished or absent pain sensation is encountered, its boundaries should be demarcated to see whether it has a segmental or peripheral nerve distribution and whether it is absent below a certain level of the trunk.

Evaluation of the cutaneous trunci (panniculus) reflex

This reflex is evaluated by pinching the skin on the dorsal trunk between T2 and L4–L5 and observing the contraction of the cutaneous trunci muscles bilaterally, which produces a twitch in the overlying skin (Figure 1.42; see **Cutaneous trunci reflex** clip on DVD). This reflex is present in the thoracolumbar region and absent in the neck and sacral region. From the dermatome tested, the sensory nerve from the skin enters the spinal cord at the level of the segment(s) corresponding to that dermatome (approximately two vertebrae cranial to the level tested). Afferent sensory information ascends the spinal cord and synapses bilaterally at the C8–T1 spinal cord segments with the motor neurons of the lateral thoracic nerve, which courses through the brachial plexus and innervates the cutaneous trunci muscle. The cutaneous trunci reflex can be decreased or lost caudal to a lesion anywhere in this pathway.

Testing begins at the level of the ilial wings: if the reflex is present at this level the entire pathway is intact and further testing is not necessary. With spinal cord lesions, this reflex is lost caudal to the spinal cord segment affected, indicating the presence of a transverse myelopathy. Pinching the skin cranial to the lesion results in a normal reflex, whilst stimulation of the skin caudal to the lesion does not elicit any reflex. Such findings help to further localize lesions between T3 and L3. This reflex can also be lost ipsilaterally (with a normal contralateral reflex) with disease affecting the brachial plexus (and hence the motor lateral thoracic nerve) regardless of the level at which the skin is stimulated. In the absence of other neurological deficits, the lack of a cutaneous trunci reflex means very little.

Nociception testing

For pain to be perceived consciously, the sensory component of the peripheral nerves and the associated spinal cord segments, the spinal cord and brainstem and the related thalamocortical system must all be intact and functional. The nociceptive fibres are located deep in the spinal cord white matter and project to both sides of the spinal cord, forming a multisynaptic bilateral network. Thus, only a severe bilateral spinal cord lesion impairs nociception. For this reason, testing of nociception (Figure 1.43; see **Nociception response** clip on DVD) is a useful prognostic indicator in cases of spinal cord

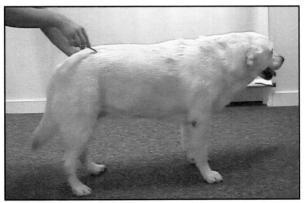

1.42 The cutaneous trunci (panniculus) reflex is elicited by pinching the skin over the lumbar spine with forceps. It should be tested from caudal to cranial on each side of the spine, starting at the level of the wings of ilium. Bilateral contraction of the cutaneous trunci muscle indicates a normal reflex. In the absence of muscle contraction, the point of skin stimulation should be moved cranially until a normal reflex is observed.

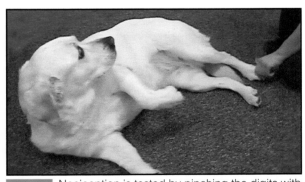

1.43 Nociception is tested by pinching the digits with fingers or haemostats. Only a behavioural response to the noxious stimulus (turning of the head, vocalization or attempting to bite) indicates conscious pain perception. If no response is elicited when using fingers, the test should be repeated with haemostats to ensure that the response is absent.

disease. This conscious pain perception must be assessed in all four limbs, the tail and the perineal region. The expected reaction is a behavioural response such as turning the head, trying to bite or vocalization (Figure 1.43).

The animal is placed on its side, ideally with a second person talking to it or stroking it to distract its attention. A gentle squeeze is applied initially to the digits to elicit the withdrawal reflex. If the animal does not manifest any behavioural response following a gentle squeeze, heavier pressure is applied. Withdrawal of the limb is only due to the flexor reflex and should not be taken as evidence of pain sensation.

Palpation

Palpation and manipulation to detect painful areas and/or restricted movement (Figures 1.44 and 1.45) are usually performed last to avoid losing the cooperation of the patient.

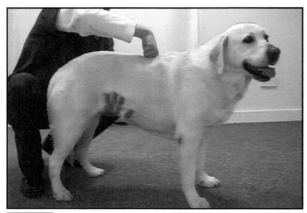

1.44 The spine can be palpated whilst the animal is standing or recumbent. Spinal hyperaesthesia is detected by applying gentle pressure on the dorsal spinal processes and transverse processes of the spine. Simultaneous palpation of the abdomen can help to detect the focus of hyperpathia.

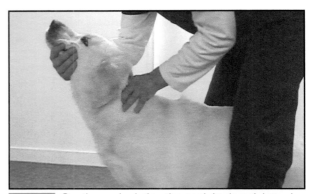

1.45 Gently manipulating the neck in dorsal, lateral and ventral flexion can help to detect pain and a reduced range of movement.

Head: The head must be palpated to detect any asymmetry, focus of pain or persistence of the bregmatic fontanelles.

Spine: Palpation of the spine is started by applying gentle downward pressure on the spinous process and then along the transverse processes. The degree of pressure applied should be increased progressively. The presence of spinal hyperaesthesia or deformity should be noted.

Limbs: Palpation of the limbs is indicated to evaluate the animal for musculoskeletal conditions that could mimic a neurological disorder. The joints should be palpated carefully for evidence of swelling, pain or instability. Palpation of the muscular system can help detect focal muscle atrophy. Such findings could indicate disease in the spinal cord segment, nerve root or peripheral nerve that innervates that muscle, or could be related to disuse atrophy associated with an orthopaedic condition.

References and further reading

Available on accompanying DVD

DVD extras
- Bilateral vestibular disease
- Cerebellar ataxia
- Corneal reflex
- Cranial tibial reflex
- Cutaneous trunci reflex
- Dysmetria
- Extensor postural thrusting
- Gag/swallow reflex
- Gastrocnemius reflex
- General proprioceptive ataxia
- Hemi-walking
- Hopping
- Lip pinch
- Menace response
- Myotonia
- Nasal stimulation
- Nociception response
- Palpebral reflex
- Paradoxical vestibular disease
- Patellar reflex
- Perineal reflex
- Physiological nystagmus
- Proprioceptive placing
- Pupillary light reflex
- Vestibular ataxia
- Wheelbarrowing
- Withdrawal reflex: pelvic limb
- Withdrawal reflex: thoracic limb

2

Lesion localization and differential diagnosis

Laurent Garosi

Precise localization of the causative disorder within the nervous system (neuroanatomical diagnosis) and an understanding of the suspected disease processes (differential diagnosis) are key to an accurate neurological diagnosis.

The past decade has seen a dramatic increase in the availability of sophisticated neurodiagnostic tests (e.g. electrodiagnosis, computed tomography and magnetic resonance imaging). The advantages of using such technology are undeniable when considering diagnostic capability and progress in the understanding of complex neurological problems. Unfortunately, despite the relatively high sensitivity, these diagnostic tests often lack specificity in identifying the exact nature of the disease process. The clinician must therefore still rely on clinical acumen to choose and interpret the appropriate diagnostic test. Accurate determination of the neurolocalization is essential in the choice and interpretation of any diagnostic tests. Furthermore, valuable information can be obtained from the suspected lesion distribution to establish a differential diagnosis list.

Functional neuroanatomy and anatomical diagnosis

Based on the history and neurological examination, the clinician can determine whether an animal suffers from a neurological disease. If so, attempts should be made to localize the lesion within the nervous system (neuroanatomical diagnosis) prior to establishing a differential diagnosis list.

The major anatomical regions of the nervous system include intracranial and extracranial structures (Figures 2.1 and 2.2).

Intracranial structures

- Forebrain (prosencephalon):
  - Cerebrum (telencephalon)
  - Diencephalon (which includes the thalamus and hypothalamus).
- Brainstem:
  - Midbrain (mesencephalon)
  - Pons (ventral metencephalon)
  - Medulla oblongata (myelencephalon).
- Cerebellum (dorsal metencephalon).

Extracranial structures

- Spinal cord:
  - C1–C5 spinal cord segments
  - C6–T2 spinal cord segments (cervicothoracic intumescence)
  - T3–L3 spinal cord segments
  - L4–S3 spinal cord segments (lumbosacral intumescence).
- Peripheral nervous system (PNS):
  - Peripheral nerve
  - Neuromuscular junction
  - Muscle.

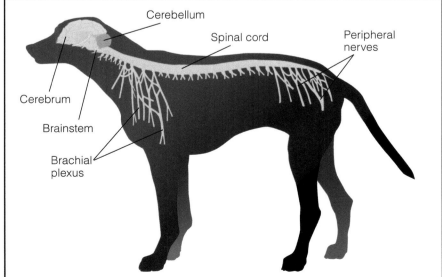

2.1 General overview of the topographical anatomy of the central and peripheral nervous systems. This overview can be seen throughout the manual, highlighting the specific section(s) of the nervous system relevant to the particular clinical signs under discussion.

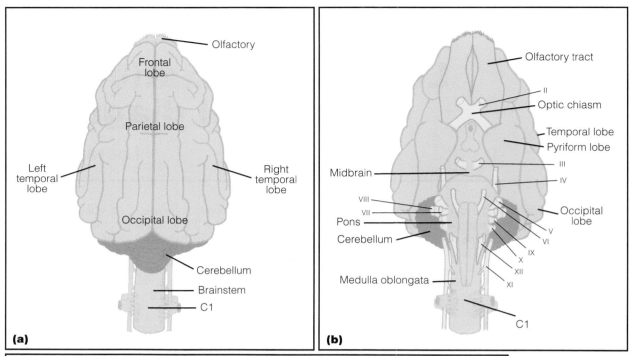

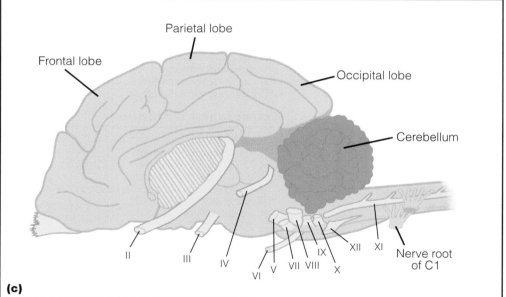

2.2 The brain. **(a)** Dorsal view showing the lobes of the cerebral hemispheres. **(b)** Ventral view. **(c)** Lateral view. C1 = cervical 1 segment of the spinal cord. Cranial nerves: I = olfactory; II = optic; III = oculomotor; IV = trochlear; V = trigeminal; VI = abducent; VII = facial; VIII = vestibulocochlear; IX = glossopharyngeal; X = vagus; XI = accessory; XII = hypoglossal.

A basic knowledge of the function of each of these anatomical regions is essential in the interpretation of neurological examination findings. The neurological examination aims to test the integrity of the various components of the nervous system and to detect any functional deficits. Normal results are as important as abnormal in establishing the anatomical diagnosis.

Interpretation of the neurological evaluation begins with making a list of the abnormal results collected from the history and examination. Each of these abnormal findings should then be correlated to a specific region or to specific pathways within the PNS and/or central nervous system (CNS; Figure 2.3). An attempt should always be made to explain all the abnormal findings by a single lesion within one of the regions of the nervous system. Lesions within these regions result in predictable and specific neurological signs. It should be noted that in localizing a lesion, it is not necessary that all of the clinical signs referable to one location are present. If a single lesion cannot explain all the listed abnormal findings, the anatomical diagnosis is considered as multifocal or diffuse.

Clinical signs	Neurolocalization
Seizures [8]	Forebrain
Narcolepsy–cataplexy [18]	Diencephalon
Hemi-neglect syndrome [9]	Forebrain
Abnormal behaviour [9]	Forebrain
Visual dysfunction [10]	Eye, optic nerve, optic chiasm, forebrain
Head pressing [9]	Forebrain
Circling: With loss of balance [11] Without loss of balance [9]	Vestibular apparatus Forebrain
Head tilt, nystagmus, falling, rolling [11]	Vestibular apparatus
Strabismus [10]	Vestibular apparatus, CNs III, IV and VI
Depression, stupor, coma [9]	Brainstem or forebrain
Abnormal prehension [12]	CNs V and XII, caudal brainstem
Dysphagia [12]	CNs IX and X, caudal brainstem
Dropped jaw [12]	Bilateral CN V
Paralysis of eyelids, lips, nostrils and/or ears [12]	CN VII
Megaoesophagus [12]	CN X
Laryngeal paralysis [12]	CN X
Tongue paralysis [12]	CN XII
Deafness [12]	Auditory apparatus

2.3 Clinical signs and localization of the disorder causing them. The numbers in square brackets denote the chapters in this manual where these conditions are discussed in detail. CN = cranial nerve.

Forebrain

Anatomy and function
The forebrain is the area of the brain located rostral to the tentorium cerebelli (rostrotentorial region). It includes the cerebrum or telencephalon (cerebro-cortical grey matter, cerebral white matter and basal nuclei) and diencephalon (divided into the epithalamus, thalamus, subthalamus, metathalamus and hypothalamus).

Cerebrum
The cerebral cortex is important for behaviour, vision, hearing, fine motor activity and conscious perception of touch, pain (nociception), temperature and body position (proprioception). The cerebral white matter mainly conveys ascending and descending sensory and motor function instructions. The basal nuclei are involved in muscle tone, and initiation and control of voluntary motor activity.

Diencephalon
The diencephalon is the chief sensory integrating system of the CNS. It is responsible for:

- Control of autonomic and endocrine functions (appetite, thirst, temperature, electrolyte and water balance), sleep and consciousness or wakefulness
- Olfactory function – via cranial nerve (CN) I, the olfactory nerve, which projects to the hypothalamus and other parts of the limbic system
- Vision and the pupillary light reflex – via CN II, the optic nerve and optic chiasm, which are located on the ventral surface of the hypothalamus
- A visual (via the lateral geniculate nucleus), auditory (via the medial geniculate nucleus), nociceptive and proprioceptive sensory relay system to the cerebral cortex
- Emotional behavioural patterns via connections with the limbic system.

The cell bodies of upper motor neurons (UMNs) are located in the motor cortex (pyramidal system) and the diencephalon, as well as the motor centres of the brainstem (extrapyramidal system).

Clinical signs of dysfunction
Figure 2.4 details the neurological abnormalities seen with lesions in the forebrain.

Function	Abnormalities
Mental status	Altered (depression, delirium, dementia (confusion), stupor, coma); behavioural changes
Cranial nerves	Contralateral blindness and decreased/absent menace reaction with normal pupillary light reflex
Posture/gait	Normal gait; abnormal movements and posture: pleurothotonus (body turn towards lesion), head turn, head pressing, pacing, wandering aimlessly and/or circling (usually ipsilateral)
Postural reactions	Postural reaction deficits in contralateral limbs
Spinal reflexes	Unaltered to increased in contralateral limbs
Muscle tone	Unaltered to increased in contralateral limbs
Sensation	Facial hypoalgesia; hypoaesthesia to contralateral half of body
Other findings	Seizures; cervical hyperaesthesia; hemi-neglect syndrome (see Chapter 9); rarely, narcolepsy–cataplexy (see Chapter 18); rarely, movement disorders such as dyskinesias (see Chapter 13)

2.4 Clinical signs caused by lesions in the forebrain.

Brainstem

Anatomy and function
Embryologically, the brainstem consists of all of the brain apart from the forebrain and cerebellum. It includes the midbrain (mesencephalon), the pons (metencephalon), the medulla oblongata

(myelencephalon) and the cerebellar peduncles. The brainstem contains the regulatory centres for consciousness (ascending reticular activating system), the cardiovascular system and breathing (medullary reticular formation). It links the cerebral cortex to the spinal cord through ascending sensory and descending motor pathways, via what are often known as 'long tracts'. In addition, the brainstem has ten pairs of CNs (III to XII), which are involved in a variety of motor and sensory functions (see Chapter 1), including equilibrium and hearing.

Clinical signs of dysfunction

Figure 2.5 details the neurological abnormalities seen with lesions in the brainstem. The typical order of appearance of signs with progressive brainstem disease is:

1. CN deficits.
2. Proprioceptive deficits.
3. Hemi/tetraparesis.
4. Stupor/coma.
5. Abnormalities in respiratory and cardiovascular function.

Function	Abnormalities
Mental status	Altered (depression, stupor, coma)
Cranial nerves	Abnormalities in CNs III to XII
Posture/gait	Paresis/paralysis of all four limbs (tetraparesis/plegia) or of ipsilateral thoracic and pelvic limbs (hemiparesis/plegia); possibly opisthotonus; possibly decerebrate rigidity
Postural reactions	Postural reaction deficits in all four limbs or in ipsilateral thoracic and pelvic limbs
Spinal reflexes	Normal to increased spinal reflexes in all four limbs or in ipsilateral thoracic and pelvic limbs
Muscle tone	Normal to increased tone in all four limbs or in ipsilateral thoracic and pelvic limbs
Sensation	Unaltered but can have cervical hyperaesthesia
Other findings	Respiratory and cardiac abnormalities

2.5 Clinical signs caused by lesions in the brainstem.

Cerebellum

Anatomy and function

The cerebellum controls the rate, range and force of movements, without actually initiating motor activity. The cerebellum coordinates muscle activity and 'smoothes' movements induced by the UMNs. Due to its close association with the brainstem vestibular nuclei, the cerebellum also plays a role in the maintenance of equilibrium and the regulation of muscle tone when the body is at rest or during motion. In addition, the cerebellum normally has an inhibitory influence on urination.

Clinical signs of dysfunction

Figure 2.6 details the neurological abnormalities seen in patients with cerebellar disease.

Function	Abnormalities
Mental status	Unaltered
Cranial nerves	Ipsilateral menace deficit with normal vision and normal facial motor function; possibly vestibular signs; possibly anisocoria
Posture/gait	Intention tremors of head and eyes; hypermetria with preservation of strength; truncal ataxia; broad-based stance; possibly decerebellate rigidity
Postural reactions	Delayed initiation and then (exaggerated) dysmetric response
Spinal reflexes	Unaltered
Muscle tone/mass	Normal to increased
Sensation	Unaltered
Other findings	Possibly increased frequency of urination

2.6 Clinical signs caused by lesions in the cerebellum.

Spinal cord

Anatomy and function

The spinal cord lies within the vertebral canal. It arises at the level of the foramen magnum and extends to the level of the sixth lumbar vertebra in most dogs and the seventh lumbar vertebra in cats, where it tapers to form the conus medullaris. The spinal cord comprises central grey matter and peripheral white matter. The diameter of the spinal cord is not constant throughout its length. In the caudal part of the cervical region and the lumbar region it widens to form the cervical and lumbar intumescences, respectively, from which the lower motor neurons (LMNs) to the thoracic and pelvic limbs arise.

Grey matter

The spinal cord comprises a central core of grey matter containing cell bodies of sensory neurons, interneurons and LMNs (Figure 2.7). The cell bodies of the efferent neurons are present in the ventral grey columns (somatic motor neurons responsible for innervation of striated muscles) and lateral grey columns (cell bodies of preganglionic sympathetic neurons in the thoracic and lumbar segments and preganglionic parasympathetic neurons in the sacral segments). The cell bodies of afferent (sensory) neurons are present in the dorsal root ganglions.

White matter

The outer portion of the spinal cord comprises white matter divided into three columns or funiculi (Figure 2.8):

- The dorsal funiculus – consists essentially of ascending tracts mainly involved in proprioception

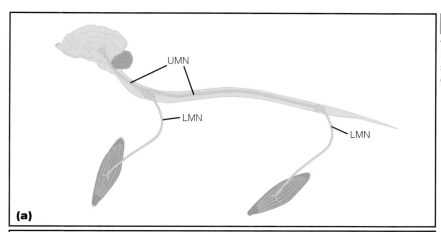

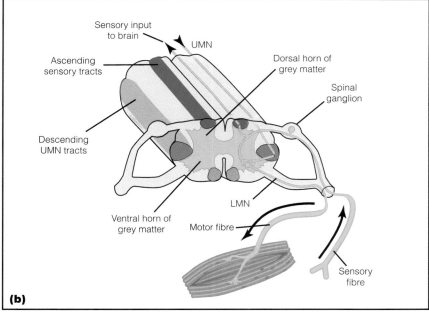

2.7 The spinal cord. **(a)** Lateral view of the whole cord showing UMNs and LMNs. **(b)** Cross-section of the cord showing the grey matter and spinal ganglia.

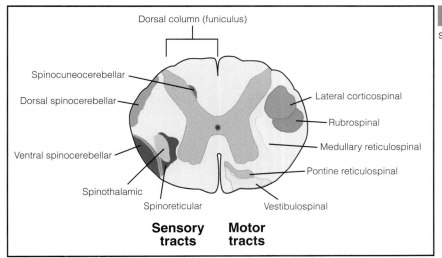

2.8 Cross-section through the spinal cord showing the sensory and motor tracts.

- The lateral funiculus – contains both ascending (proprioception, touch, pressure, temperature and pain pathways) and descending (motor pathways) tracts
- The ventral funiculus – contains only descending motor tracts.

Segmentation
A spinal cord segment is defined as a portion of the spinal cord that gives rise to one pair of spinal nerves. There are 8 cervical, 13 thoracic, 7 lumbar, 3 sacral and at least 2 caudal spinal cord segments in the dog and cat. Some spinal cord segments lie

in the vertebra of the same annotation, whilst others lie cranial to the corresponding vertebra and the spinal nerves course caudally in the vertebral canal to exit at the correct intervertebral foramen (Figure 2.9). Spinal lesion localization refers to the spinal cord segments rather than the vertebral bodies.

Innervation in the body is organized in a segmental pattern. Each cutaneous region of the body (dermatome) and group of muscle fibres (myotome) is innervated by one spinal cord segment. Functionally, the spinal cord can be divided into four regions:

- Cranial cervical (C1–C5)
- Cervicothoracic (C6–T2)
- Thoracolumbar (T3–L3)
- Lumbosacral (L4–S3).

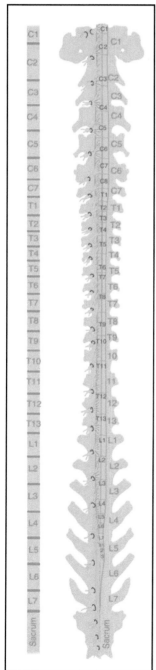

2.9 Spinal cord segments and their location relative to vertebral levels in the dog. With the exception of the first one or two cervical segments and segments L1 and L2, most spinal cord segments are positioned in the vertebral canal cranial to the vertebra of the same number. The disparity between the location of the spinal cord segments and their respective vertebrae is a result of the extra number of spinal cord segments in the cervical region (8 segments for 7 vertebrae) and the differential growth of skeletal and neural structures during embryological development. The cervical intumescence (C6–T2) lies within vertebrae C5–T1 and the lumbar intumescence (L4–S3) lies within vertebrae L3–L6. The C1 spinal nerves exit through the lateral foramina in the C1 vertebra. The other cervical spinal nerves exit the vertebral canal cranial to the vertebrae of the same annotation, except the C8 nerves, which exit between C7 and T1. All the other spinal nerves exit behind the same-named vertebrae.

Lower motor neurons

LMNs are efferent neurons connecting the CNS to somatic or visceral muscle. The cell bodies of LMNs are located within the grey matter of the cervicothoracic intumescence (spinal cord segments C6–T2) for the thoracic limbs and the lumbosacral intumescence (spinal cord segments L4–S3) for the pelvic limbs. Lesions at the level of these intumescences result in LMN signs in the corresponding limb(s).

Clinical signs of dysfunction

Figures 2.10 to 2.14 detail the neurological abnormalities seen in patients with spinal cord disease. The typical order in which functions are lost with progressive spinal cord disease is:

1. Conscious proprioception.
2. Motor function.
3. Bladder function.
4. Nociception.

Function	Abnormalities
Mental status	Unaltered
Cranial nerves	May be ipsilateral Horner's syndrome
Posture/gait	Paresis/paralysis of all four limbs (tetraparesis/plegia) or of ipsilateral thoracic and pelvic limbs (hemiparesis/plegia); may be torticollis or scoliosis from asymmetrical paraspinal muscle weakness
Postural reactions	Postural reaction deficits in all four limbs or in ipsilateral thoracic and pelvic limbs
Spinal reflexes	Normal to increased spinal reflexes in all four limbs
Muscle tone/mass	Normal to increased tone in all four limbs; no muscle atrophy in any of the limbs
Sensation	May be hyperaesthesia of the cervical spine
Other findings	Respiratory difficulty in tetraplegic patients; urinary retention

2.10 Clinical signs caused by lesions in the C1–C5 spinal cord segments.

Function	Abnormalities
Mental status	Unaltered
Cranial nerves	May be ipsilateral Horner's syndrome
Posture/gait	Paresis/paralysis of all four limbs (tetraparesis/plegia) or of ipsilateral thoracic and pelvic limbs (hemiparesis/plegia) or of one thoracic limb (monoparesis); may be torticollis from asymmetrical paraspinal muscle weakness
Postural reactions	Postural reaction deficits in all four limbs, in ipsilateral thoracic and pelvic limbs or in one thoracic limb

2.11 Clinical signs caused by lesions in the C6–T2 spinal cord segments. (continues) ▶

Function	Abnormalities
Spinal reflexes	Normal to increased spinal reflexes in the pelvic limbs; decreased to absent spinal reflexes in the thoracic limb(s)
Muscle tone/ mass	Normal to increased tone in pelvic limbs; decreased to absent tone in thoracic limb(s); muscle atrophy in thoracic limb(s); no muscle atrophy in the pelvic limbs
Sensation	Reduced/absent ipsilateral cutaneous trunci reflex if C8–T1 spinal cord segments involved; may be hyperaesthesia over caudal cervical/ cranial thoracic spine
Other findings	Respiratory difficulty in tetraplegic patients; urinary retention

2.11 (continued) Clinical signs caused by lesions in the C6–T2 spinal cord segments.

Function	Abnormalities
Mental status	Unaltered
Cranial nerves	Unaltered
Posture/gait	Paresis/paralysis of both pelvic limbs (paraparesis/plegia) or of one pelvic limb (monoparesis/plegia); Schiff–Sherrington phenomenon possible in acute and severe lesions
Postural reactions	Normal in thoracic limbs; postural reaction deficits in one or both pelvic limbs
Spinal reflexes	Normal in thoracic limbs; normal to increased spinal reflexes in pelvic limbs
Muscle tone/ mass	Normal to increased tone in pelvic limbs; no muscle atrophy in the pelvic limbs
Sensation	Reduced/absent cutaneous trunci reflex caudal to the level of the last intact dermatome; hypo/anaesthesia of the pelvic limbs; may be hyperaesthesia of thoracolumbar spine
Other findings	Urinary retention (UMN bladder)

2.12 Clinical signs caused by lesions in the T3–L3 spinal cord segments.

Function	Abnormalities
Mental status	Unaltered
Cranial nerves	Unaltered
Posture/gait	Paresis/paralysis of both pelvic limbs (paraparesis/plegia) or of one pelvic limb (monoparesis)
Postural reactions	Normal in the thoracic limbs; postural reaction deficits in both or one pelvic limb
Spinal reflexes	Normal in the thoracic limbs; decreased to absent patellar reflex (unilateral or bilateral); intact pelvic limb withdrawal reflex

2.13 Clinical signs caused by lesions in the L4–L6 spinal cord segments. (continues)

Function	Abnormalities
Muscle tone/ mass	Decreased to absent pelvic limb extensor muscle tone; muscle atrophy in the quadriceps femoris muscle
Sensation	Hypo/anaesthesia restricted to dermatomal distribution over limbs; may be hyperaesthesia over lumbar spine
Other findings	Urinary retention (UMN bladder)

2.13 (continued) Clinical signs caused by lesions in the L4–L6 spinal cord segments.

Function	Abnormalities
Mental status	Unaltered
Cranial nerves	Unaltered
Posture/gait	Paresis of both pelvic limbs (paraparesis) or one pelvic limb (monoparesis) characterized by difficulty rising and plantigrade stance; ability to walk remains intact; paresis/paralysis of tail
Postural reactions	Normal in the thoracic limbs; postural reaction deficits in both or one pelvic limb
Spinal reflexes	Normal in the thoracic limbs; decreased to absent pelvic limb withdrawal reflex (unilateral or bilateral); decreased to absent perianal and/or perineal reflex
Muscle tone and mass	Flaccid/decreased pelvic limb and tail muscle tone; dilated anal sphincter; muscle atrophy in the caudal thigh, hip and/or distal pelvic limb muscles
Sensation	Hypoaesthesia in the pelvic limb, perineal area and tail; may be hyperaesthesia in the lumbosacral spine/rectal palpation
Other findings	Urinary retention (LMN bladder); faecal incontinence

2.14 Clinical signs caused by lesions in the L6–S3 spinal cord segments (cauda equina; correlates to L3–S3 vertebrae).

Peripheral nerves

Anatomy and function

The PNS consists of 12 pairs of cranial nerves and 36 pairs of spinal nerves, which extend from or to the spinal cord and brainstem. Peripheral nerves contain both motor and sensory axons. The motor axons extend from neurons located in the ventral horn of the spinal cord or grey matter of the brainstem. The sensory axons have their cell bodies in the dorsal root ganglion or homologous ganglia of the cranial nerves. Most spinal nerves leave the vertebral canal through intervertebral foramina formed between the pedicles of adjacent vertebrae.

- A cutaneous region innervated by afferent nerve fibres from a single spinal nerve is called a dermatome.
- The musculature innervated by a single spinal nerve is termed a myotome.

Individual muscles are innervated by multiple spinal nerves. In the limbs, muscles are supplied by nerves arising from either the brachial or lumbosacral plexi, which consist of intermingled nerve fibres from the ventral branches of the spinal nerves. The brachial plexus (formed by the ventral branches of the sixth, seventh and eighth cervical and the first two thoracic spinal nerves) serves the thoracic limb (Figure 2.15), whilst the lumbosacral plexus (formed by the last five lumbar and the three sacral spinal nerves) serves the pelvic limb (Figure 2.16). The lumbosacral trunk is the largest and most important part of the plexus, and arises from the sixth and seventh lumbar and the first and second sacral spinal nerves.

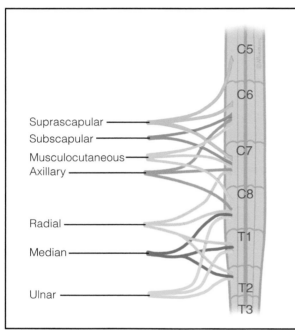

2.15 Cervicothoracic spinal cord segments, indicating nerve origins.

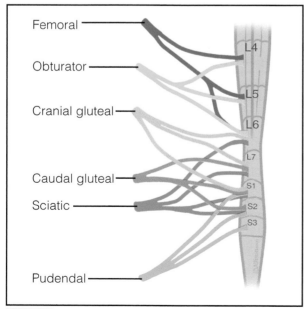

2.16 Lumbosacral spinal cord segments, indicating nerve origins.

Clinical signs of dysfunction

Figure 2.17 details the neurological abnormalities seen in patients with peripheral nerve disease.

Function	Abnormalities
Mental status	Unaltered
Cranial nerves	Variable involvement, dependent on disease. CNs VII, IX and X commonly affected in generalized neuropathies (see Chapter 12)
Posture/gait	Flaccid paresis/paralysis of affected limb(s)
Postural reactions	Postural reaction deficits in affected limb(s) (sensory)
Spinal reflexes	Decreased to absent spinal reflexes in affected limb(s)
Muscle tone	Decreased to absent tone in affected limb(s) (motor); muscle atrophy in affected limb(s) (motor)
Sensation	Decreased to absent nociception and sensation; paraesthesia
Other findings	Self-mutilation

2.17 Clinical signs caused by lesions of the peripheral nerves.

Neuromuscular junction

Anatomy and function

The neuromuscular junction consists of an axon terminal, a synaptic cleft and the endplate region of a skeletal muscle fibre (see Chapter 18). This junction is a transducer, converting electrical signals (nerve impulses) to chemical signals then back to electrical signals (muscle action potentials). The action potential in the nerve terminal depolarizes the distal region of the axon, causing calcium channels on the axolemma to open. The influx of calcium leads to a discharge of acetylcholine (ACh) vesicles via exocytosis into the synaptic cleft, and the released ACh binds to the receptors located in the endplate region of the skeletal muscle fibres. This binding mechanism opens sodium and potassium channels, generating a local depolarization, which then triggers the action potential and subsequent muscle fibre contraction.

Clinical signs of dysfunction

Transmission of the electrical impulse from the axon to the muscle fibre may be disturbed at a number of locations. Disorders of the neuromuscular junction are classified as presynaptic (e.g. botulism or tick paralysis; see Chapter 15), postsynaptic (e.g. congenital or acquired myasthenia gravis; see Chapter 18) or enzymatic (e.g. organophosphate and carbamate toxicity; see Chapter 18).

- Presynaptic disorders result in a decrease in the quantity of ACh released. Clinically, affected animals present with LMN-type deficits in all four limbs (severe hypotonia and hyporeflexia). Cranial nerves may be involved, leading to dysphagia, dysphonia and facial weakness (see Chapters 12 and 14).

- Postsynaptic disorders are due to interference with the ACh receptor activation mechanism. Typically, affected animals present with exercise-induced weakness which improves following rest. The neurological examination is normal during periods of inactivity following rest.
- Enzymatic disorders: chemical compounds can interfere with acetylcholinesterase, the enzyme that inactivates ACh in the synapse. Clinical signs manifest as autonomic nervous system overstimulation and neuromuscular dysfunction, and are often similar to those of postsynaptic disorders (stiff, rigid gait with muscle tremors and exercise intolerance).

Muscle

Anatomy and function

Skeletal muscle functions to maintain body posture, produce movement and provide a reservoir source of energy. It is an integral part of the motor unit, which comprises the LMN (cranial nerve nucleus or ventral horn cell body and axon extending along a peripheral nerve), the neuromuscular junction and the muscle fibres innervated. The motor unit is the final common pathway for motor activity and the muscle is the final effector of this motor unit. The functional cellular unit is the muscle fibre or myofibre. Each muscle fibre is composed of several hundred myofibrils, which in turn contain several hundred myofilaments (actin and myosin proteins). The number of myofibres innervated by one motor neuron varies according to the muscle group: muscles responsible for coarse movement (e.g. antigravity muscles) have large motor units, whereas those responsible for fine movements (e.g. extraocular muscles) have small motor units.

Clinical signs of dysfunction

Figure 2.18 details the neurological abnormalities seen in patients with muscle disease.

Function	Abnormalities
Mental status	Unaltered
Cranial nerves	Reflexes may be altered by involvement of facial muscles or muscles of mastication and swallowing
Posture/gait	Stiff and stilted gait (tetraparesis); exercise-induced weakness/stiffness
Postural reactions	Unaltered to altered if severe weakness
Spinal reflexes	Unaltered (unless severe muscle atrophy/fibrosis)
Muscle tone/ mass	Normal, increased or decreased tone; muscle atrophy or hypertrophy; limited joint movement due to muscle contractures
Sensation	Usually unaltered but can have hyperaesthesia of muscles

2.18 Clinical signs caused by lesions in skeletal muscle.

Differential diagnosis

The formation of a differential diagnosis list is essential in choosing and interpreting any diagnostic test, however sophisticated the test may be. The aim of performing such diagnostic tests should only be to confirm or rule out the differential diagnoses in the list and not to replace the clinical evaluation. The list of differential diagnoses should be developed taking into account:

- Signalment (see Appendix 1: breed-specific disorders)
- History – questioning the owner should be aimed at defining the onset and progression of the condition. In addition, the history can give clues as to how widespread or focal the disease process is in the nervous system, whether there is evidence of asymmetry and how severe the signs have been
- Neurological findings – the aim of the neurological evaluation is to define the lesion localization (forebrain, brainstem, cerebellum, spinal cord segments, peripheral nerves, neuromuscular junction and muscles) and distribution of the disease (focal, multifocal, diffuse) within the nervous system.

Disease processes

Disease processes that can affect the nervous system can be classified according to the cause, using the mnemonic DAMNITV:

D Degenerative
A Anomalous
M Metabolic
N Neoplastic, Nutritional
I Inflammatory, Infectious, Idiopathic
T Traumatic, Toxic
V Vascular

Each of these disease processes has a typical signalment, onset and progression, as well as distribution within the nervous system (Figures 2.19 and 2.20).

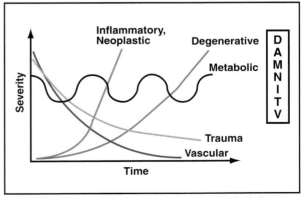

2.19 Onset and progression of neurological diseases of differing causes.

Acute, progressive with asymmetrical signs
• Degenerative (e.g. intervertebral disc disease) • Neoplastic • Inflammatory/infectious disease
Acute, progressive with symmetrical signs
• Metabolic disorders • Nutritional disorders • Neoplastic • Inflammatory/infectious disease • Toxicity
Acute, non-progressive (often asymmetrical)
• Idiopathic • Trauma • Vascular disorders
Chronic, progressive with symmetrical signs
• Degenerative disorders • Anomalous disorders • Metabolic disorders • Neoplastic disorders • Nutritional disorders • Inflammatory/infectious disease • Toxicity
Chronic, progressive with asymmetrical signs
• Degenerative (e.g. intervertebral disc disease) • Neoplastic disease • Inflammatory/infectious disease

2.20 Disease categories based on onset and progression of signs. These guidelines are based on the most common disease course.

Degenerative diseases

Degenerative diseases, which involve morphological degeneration of the nervous tissue, can affect any part of the nervous system and many are familial or hereditary. They typically have an insidious onset and slow progression. The age of onset is variable: some diseases may affect young mainly purebred animals shortly after birth (e.g. most cerebellar abiotrophies); these diseases often affect the nervous system in a symmetrical fashion. Less frequently, adult animals may be affected (e.g. degenerative myelopathy, degenerative disc disease) and these can be asymmetrical in presentation.

Anomalous diseases

Neurological signs can result from malformations that directly involve the nervous tissue (e.g. hydrocephalus) or that involve the tissue surrounding the neuraxis (cranium and vertebral column). However, it should be noted that malformations of the cranium and vertebral column do not always affect the nervous system and are often incidental findings on imaging.

Neurological disease caused by cranium or vertebral malformation is usually recognized early in life and signs tend to be non-progressive or slowly progressive. Occasionally, vertebral malformations do not result in neurological signs until adulthood, as a result of stenosis of the vertebral canal, progressive

deformity, instability or disc disease. Such malformations can cause an acute onset of signs if, for example, stability is suddenly lost, as in the case of atlantoaxial subluxation.

Metabolic disorders

Metabolic disorders can affect animals of any age. Clinical onset of neurological signs is variable but is most often acute, even though accompanying signs of systemic disease are often subacute to chronic. Diffuse non-specific signs, bilaterally symmetrical deficits referable to the forebrain, or symmetrical peripheral neuropathies are the most common signs. Most of these conditions tend to wax and wane with time.

Neoplastic disorders

Neoplasia is more common in animals >5 years old but can occur at any age. Neurological signs are usually chronic and progressive in nature, although acute deterioration can be seen (especially if associated with spontaneous haemorrhage, impairment of vascular supply or loss of a compensatory mechanism to the normal surrounding tissue). Other factors determining the clinical expression of neoplasia are lesion size, histological nature, growth rate, associated inflammatory response and location within the CNS *versus* PNS. Neurological deficits can be asymmetrical or symmetrical, and often suggest a focal lesion. Paraneoplastic neurological syndromes can be seen, although these are classically inflammatory in nature.

Nutritional diseases

Nutritional diseases affecting the nervous tissue are rare in dogs and cats nowadays, as a result of the excellent balanced diets available. As with metabolic disease, neurological signs are typically bilaterally symmetrical. The onset of signs is variable (acute or insidious) and they are often slowly progressive. The distribution of signs can be diffuse or multifocal, as some nutritional diseases can affect selective areas of the CNS.

Inflammatory and infectious diseases

Sterile inflammatory (immune-mediated) or infectious diseases can have an acute, subacute or a more insidious onset, depending on the cause. Signs usually progress without treatment, although they may wax and wane in some cases early after onset. Neurological deficits can refer to a focal or multifocal lesion and can be asymmetrical or symmetrical.

Idiopathic disorders

Idiopathic disorders tend to result in acute onset of non-progressive or regressive signs. Neurological deficits vary with each syndrome. The term should be reserved for specific documented conditions or syndromes of unknown aetiology rather than for cases where a diagnosis could not, or has not, been confirmed. These disorders most often affect the PNS, including the cranial nerves, with epilepsy being the stand-out exception. They are rarely accompanied by other signs of neurological disease.

Trauma

Traumatic disorders often have a peracute or acute onset. Signs usually remain static or improve over time. Neurological deficits can be symmetrical or asymmetrical, and often refer to a focal lesion; however, multiple lesions can frequently exist. Worsening of oedema (associated with secondary injury phenomena; see Chapter 20) can result in the progression of neurological signs for a short period of 24–72 hours, and undetected spinal instability can cause delayed deterioration in signs.

Toxic disorders

Numerous toxins can affect the nervous system, either primarily or secondarily. Toxicities often result in acute onset disease and diffuse or bilaterally symmetrical signs from the time of the onset and are non-progressive.

Vascular disorders

Vascular disorders can result from loss of blood supply (ischaemia) or from haemorrhage into the nervous system. They are characterized clinically by peracute or acute onset of non-progressive or regressive signs. Deficits are usually initially focal and often asymmetrical. Worsening of oedema (associated with secondary injury phenomena) can result in the progression of neurological signs for a short period of 24–72 hours. Haemorrhage may be an exception, and can be responsible for a more progressive onset over a very short period of time. Clinical signs usually regress after 24–72 hours; this is attributable to diminution of the mass effect secondary to haemorrhage and reorganization or oedema resolution.

References and further reading

Available on accompanying DVD

3

Clinical pathology

Heather Wamsley

Laboratory evaluation of patients presenting with neurological diseases can be challenging due to the numerous assays that may be performed and the non-specific results that are often obtained from routinely performed laboratory tests. However, when coupled with signalment, clinical findings and other ancillary diagnostic tests (e.g. imaging techniques), laboratory tests can be extremely valuable in the accurate identification of a number of conditions that affect neurological and neuromuscular function.

Standard minimum database

Performing the standard minimum database of tests is always indicated in cases of neurological and neuromuscular disease:

- Complete blood cell count (CBC) and examination of peripheral blood films

- Serum biochemistry
- Urinalysis.

Although patients that have disease restricted to the central nervous system (CNS) often do not exhibit specific minimum database findings, these tests can be useful in detecting systemic diseases that may have neurological manifestations. In addition, specific findings in the minimum database may direct further diagnostic testing. Figure 3.1 provides a detailed list of diseases that may manifest concurrent neurological signs and minimum database abnormalities.

Specific minimum database findings are not observed in most cases of degenerative and anomalous neurological diseases with one exception: leucocyte inclusions are identified uncommonly in the peripheral blood and cerebrospinal fluid (CSF) of patients with certain lysosomal storage diseases (Figures 3.2 and 3.3).

Disorder	Haematology abnormalities	Biochemistry abnormalities	Urinalysis abnormalities
Degenerative			
Lysosomal storage disease	Inclusions within WBCs		
Metabolic			
Diabetes mellitus	Mild normocytic, normochromic, non-regenerative anaemia	Hyperglycaemia; hypercholesterolaemia; hypertriglyceridaemia; ↑ hepatocellular enzymes (e.g. ALT); ↑ cholestatic markers (e.g. ALP)	Glucosuria; ketonuria; bacteruria ± pyuria
Hepatic failure/hepatic encephalopathy (e.g. portovascular anomaly, cirrhosis)	Microcytosis (reduced mean cell volume of erythrocytes), usually without anaemia	↑ ALT and other hepatocellular enzymes; ↑ ALP and other cholestatic markers; hypoalbuminaemia; ↓ BUN; hypoglycaemia; hyopcholesterolaemia	Ammonium urate crystalluria
Hyperadrenocorticism/hypercortisolaemia	Stress leucogram shows mature neutrophilia, monocytosis, lymphopenia and eosinopenia	↑ ALT; ↑ ALP; hypercholesterolaemia; lipaemia; hyperglycaemia; normal or ↓ BUN; hypernatraemia; hypokalaemia; hypophosphataemia	Isosthenuria; bacteruria ± pyuria
Hypoadrenocorticism	Variable anaemia (typically mild normocytic, normochromic, non-regenerative anaemia; severe anaemia with chronic disease or severe gastrointestinal haemorrhage); normal to ↑ eosinophil count; normal to ↑ lymphocyte count	Hyponatraemia; hyperkalaemia; hypochloraemia; hypercalcaemia; Na:K ratio <27; hypoglycaemia; azotaemia; metabolic acidosis	Inappropriately low urine specific gravity

3.1 Diseases that may manifest concurrent neurological signs and minimum database abnormalities. ALP = alkaline phosphatase; ALT = alanine aminotransferase; AST = aspartate aminotransferase; BUN = blood urea nitrogen; CK = creatine kinase; RBC = red blood cell; WBC = white blood cell. (continues) ▶

Disorder	Haematology abnormalities	Biochemistry abnormalities	Urinalysis abnormalities
Metabolic (continued)			
Hypercalcaemia		Neurological signs usually apparent when total calcium >3.5–4.0 mmol/l (>14–16 mg/dl), depending on ionized calcium levels	
Hypocalcaemia		Neurological signs usually apparent when total calcium <1.9 mmol/l (<7.5 mg/dl), depending on ionized calcium levels	
Hyperglycaemia		Neurological signs usually apparent when >55.5 mmol/l (>1000 mg/dl)	
Hypoglycaemia		Neurological signs usually apparent when <2.5 mmol/l (<45 mg/dl)	
Hyperkalaemia		Neurological signs usually apparent when >6.5 mmol/l	
Hypokalaemia		Neurological signs usually apparent in cats when <3.0–3.5 mmol/l and in dogs when <2.5 mmol/l	
Hypermagnesaemia (severe)		Neurological signs usually apparent when >4.1 mmol/l (>10.0 mg/dl)	
Hypomagnesaemia		Neurological signs usually apparent when <0.4 mmol/l (<1.0 mg/dl)	
Hypernatraemia		Neurological signs usually apparent when >170 mmol/l	
Hyponatraemia		Neurological signs usually apparent when <125 mmol/l	
Hyperosmolality		Neurological signs usually apparent when >350–360 mmol/kg (>350–360 mOsm/kg), depending on rate of change	
Hypo-osmolality		Neurological signs usually apparent when <250 mmol/kg (<250 mOsm/kg), depending on rate of change	
Hypophosphataemia		Neurological signs usually apparent in cats when 0.6–0.8 mmol/l (<2.0–2.5 mg/dl) and in dogs <0.5 mmol/l (<1.5 mg/dl)	
Hyperthyroidism	↑ Heinz bodies	↑ hepatocellular enzymes (e.g. ALT); ↑ ALP (bone isoenzyme)	
Hypothyroidism	Mild normocytic, normochromic, non-regenerative anaemia	Hypercholesterolaemia	
Hypoxia	Anaemia; methaemoglobinaemia; carboxyhaemoglobinaemia		
Renal failure/uraemic encephalopathy	Normocytic, normochromic, non-regenerative anaemia	Azotaemia; hyperkalaemia; hyperphosphataemia; hypo/hypercalcaemia; hypernatraemia; ↑ anion gap metabolic acidosis	Inappropriately low urine specific gravity
Neoplastic			
CNS lymphoma or multicentric lymphoma with paraneoplastic polyneuropathy	Atypical lymphocytosis or lymphocytic leukaemia		

3.1 (continued) Diseases that may manifest concurrent neurological signs and minimum database abnormalities. ALP = alkaline phosphatase; ALT = alanine aminotransferase; AST = aspartate aminotransferase; BUN = blood urea nitrogen; CK = creatine kinase; RBC = red blood cell; WBC = white blood cell. (continues) ▶

Disorder	Haematology abnormalities	Biochemistry abnormalities	Urinalysis abnormalities
Neoplastic (continued)			
Hyperviscosity syndrome	Increased rouleaux formation; absolute polycythaemia (primary, e.g. polycythaemia vera; secondary, e.g. renal neoplasia)	Hyperproteinaemia due to monoclonal gammopathy	
Insulinoma		Hypoglycaemia	
Immune			
Immune myositis of masticatory muscles	Mild normocytic, normochromic, non-regenerative anaemia; neutrophilia; eosinophilia	↑ CK; ↑ AST; hyperglobulinaemia	Proteinuria
Myasthenia gravis with pneumonia	Inflammatory leucogram with toxic change		
Infectious			
Acute canine distemper viraemia	Round eosinophilic RBC and/or WBC inclusions; lymphopenia		
Discospondylitis	Inflammatory leucogram	Hyperglobulinaemia, usually polyclonal gammopathy	Bacteruria; pyuria
Feline immunodeficiency virus	Normocytic, normochromic, non-regenerative anaemia; neutropenia; thrombocytopenia	↑ hepatocellular enzymes (e.g. ALT); azotaemia; gammopathy, usually polyclonal	Proteinuria
Feline infectious peritonitis	Inflammatory leucogram	Hyperglobulinaemia, usually polyclonal gammopathy	
Feline leukaemia virus	Macrocytic (often) or normocytic, normochromic, non-regenerative anaemia; neutropenia; lymphopenia; thrombocytopenia	↑ hepatocellular enzymes (e.g. ALT); hyperbilirubinaemia; azotaemia; gammopathy, usually polyclonal	Proteinuria
Infectious meningoencephalitis (e.g. bacterial, fungal)	Inflammatory leucogram		
Tick-borne infections	Thrombocytopenia; mild normocytic, normochromic, non-regenerative anaemia; inflammatory leucogram; leucocytes containing morulae (_Ehrlichia_ spp., _Anaplasma phagocytophilum_); rare spirochaetaemia (Lyme disease – _Borrelia burgdorferi_)	Gammopathy, usually polyclonal	
Inflammatory			
Myositis/myopathy	Eosinophilia, if secondary to protozoal infection	↑ CK; ↑ AST	
Steroid-responsive meningitis	Often neutrophilia, rarely neutropenic		
Inherited			
Hyperchylomicronaemia-associated neuropathy in cats	Fasting lipaemic plasma	Persistent fasting hypertriglyceridaemia	
Hyperoxaluric peripheral neuropathy		Renal azotaemia and other findings supportive of renal failure	Inappropriately low urine specific gravity; recurrent calcium oxalate mono-hydrate crystalluria, oxaluria and L-glyceric aciduria
Muscular dystrophy		↑ CK; ↑ AST	

3.1 (continued) Diseases that may manifest concurrent neurological signs and minimum database abnormalities. ALP = alkaline phosphatase; ALT = alanine aminotransferase; AST = aspartate aminotransferase; BUN = blood urea nitrogen; CK = creatine kinase; RBC = red blood cell; WBC = white blood cell. (continues) ▶

Disorder	Haematology abnormalities	Biochemistry abnormalities	Urinalysis abnormalities
Toxic			
Ethylene glycol toxicity		Azotaemia; hypocalcaemia; hyperkalaemia; hyperphosphataemia; hypernatraemia; marked hyperglycaemia in cats (>19.4 mmol/l ≡ >350 mg/dl); severely increased anion gap metabolic acidosis; hyperosmolality with increased osmolal gap	Inappropriately low urine specific gravity; calcium oxalate monohydrate crystalluria (early)
Lead toxicity	Aberrant metarubricytosis (nucleated RBCs); basophilic stippling; normal haematocrit or mild normocytic, normochromic, non-regenerative anaemia		
Metaldehyde toxicity		Increased anion gap metabolic acidosis	
Strychnine toxicity		↑ CK; ↑ AST; metabolic acidosis due to lactic acidaemia	Myoglobinuria

3.1 (continued) Diseases that may manifest concurrent neurological signs and minimum database abnormalities. ALP = alkaline phosphatase; ALT = alanine aminotransferase; AST = aspartate aminotransferase; BUN = blood urea nitrogen; CK = creatine kinase; RBC = red blood cell; WBC = white blood cell.

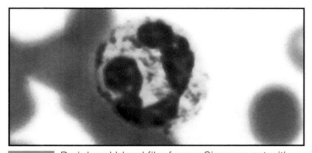

3.2 Peripheral blood film from a Siamese cat with lysosomal storage disease (mucopolysaccharidosis VI). The cytoplasm of the neutrophil contains several irregularly shaped magenta inclusions, which are present due to an abnormal accumulation of substrate material that would normally be degraded by the deficient lysosomal enzyme. The cytoplasm in normal neutrophils should be virtually colourless or very pale basophilic. (Wright–Giemsa stain; original magnification X50)

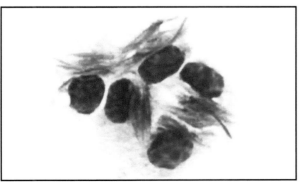

3.3 Spinal fluid from a Muntjac deer with lysosomal storage disease (GM2 gangliosidosis). The mononuclear phagocytes contain linear, eosinophilic cytoplasmic inclusions, which are present due to an abnormal accumulation of substrate material that would normally be degraded by the deficient lysosomal enzyme. (Wright–Giemsa stain; original magnification X50)

Many systemic metabolic diseases (see Figure 3.1) manifest concurrent neurological and minimum database abnormalities. Neurological signs can be the result of a single electrolyte abnormality (such as hypocalcaemia) that has multiple underlying causes. These causes are not presented here; the reader is referred to an internal medicine or clinical pathology text for an in-depth discussion of this topic. Identification of specific serum biochemical abnormalities may prompt additional clinical pathology testing (e.g. bile acids).

A few neoplasms uncommonly demonstrate concurrent neurological and haematological abnormalities, including:

- CNS lymphoma associated with leukaemia
- Polycythaemia vera or renal neoplasia associated with absolute erythrocytosis
- Multiple myeloma associated with hyperviscosity due to monoclonal gammopathy
- Insulinoma in older adult large-breed dogs that are hypoglycaemic.

Specific minimum database findings are not observed in most cases of infectious, inflammatory, immune-mediated and ischaemic neurological diseases, with some rare exceptions. *Ehrlichia* or *Anaplasma* morulae (Figure 3.4) or, very rarely, *Borrelia* spirochaetes may be identified during examination of peripheral blood films from infected animals. These animals are often also thrombocytopenic and hyperglobulinaemic; however, these findings are non-specific. Erythrocyte and leucocyte inclusions are identified uncommonly in the peripheral blood and CSF of dogs that have acute canine distemper viraemia (Figures 3.5 and 3.6). The intensity and colour of the inclusions depends upon the type of stain used to prepare the peripheral blood film. Variably sized and rounded inclusions

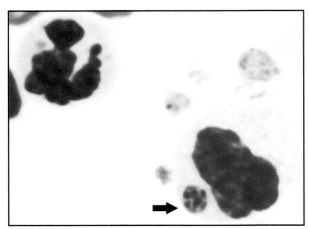

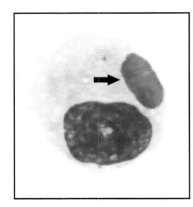

3.6 Spinal fluid from a dog with acute canine distemper virus. The large mononuclear cell contains a pink, oval inclusion of viral capsid proteins (arrowed). (Wright–Giemsa stain; original magnification X100)

3.4 Buffy coat film from a dog with acute anaplasmosis. The neutrophil on the right contains a round, basophilic, stippled *Anaplasma phagocytophilum* morula (arrowed). (Wright–Giemsa stain; original magnification X100)

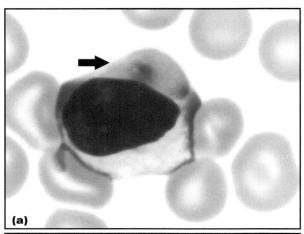

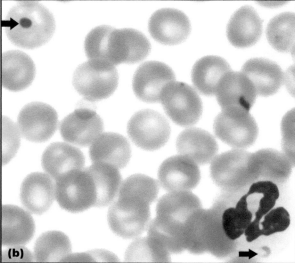

3.5 Peripheral blood films from a dog with acute canine distemper virus infection showing cytoplasmic viral inclusions. Eosinophilic inclusions are visible in the cytoplasm of **(a)** a reactive lymphocyte (arrowed) and **(b)** an erythrocyte (top; arrowed) and a neutrophil (bottom; arrowed). These blood films have been stained with Diff-Quik®. If they had been stained with Wright–Giemsa, the inclusions would have been expected to be pale aqua. (Original magnification X100)

are more easily identified when an aqueous Wright's stain is used (e.g. Diff-Quik®), which stains the inclusions intensely eosinophilic. When stained with Wright–Giemsa, the inclusions are pale blue-green.

The severity and specificity of minimum database changes that occur with different intoxications are variable. The most dramatic example is ethylene glycol toxicity, which can cause marked changes in the serum biochemical profile. Minimum database changes suggestive of secondary acute renal failure are seen (e.g. azotaemia, hyperkalaemia and hyperphosphataemia). These observations, coupled with the more specific findings of moderate to marked hypocalcaemia, increased osmolal gap (detailed below) and calcium oxalate monohydrate crystalluria (which occurs early during the intoxication), are strongly suggestive of ethylene glycol intoxication.

With chronic lead intoxication, marked aberrant metarubricytosis (i.e. severely increased nucleated red blood cells (RBCs) in the absence of polychromasia) can be seen in approximately 50% of cases, and basophilic stippling can be seen in approximately 25% of cases. Increased circulating nucleated RBCs is also a common finding in dogs with heat stroke, the severity of which is inversely proportional to the likelihood of survival and correlates well with other predictors of outcome (e.g. presence of acute renal injury and hypoglyaecemia) (Aroch *et al.*, 2009).

Other biochemical assays

Specific analytes can be measured in the serum of neurological patients, either if indicated by abnormalities identified by the minimum database tests or for therapeutic monitoring (e.g. thyroid hormone level). Commercial laboratories can perform many of these tests; however, test availability and sample handling needs may vary with each laboratory. Local commercial laboratories should be contacted for their specific sample handling requirements.

Anticonvulsant serum concentration
Since seizure control correlates with serum drug concentration and not the dosage, serum anticonvulsant monitoring is indicated for patients receiving such therapy. Samples for measurement of the serum phenobarbital concentration should be collected into plain

red topped tubes (without serum separator gel). Samples should be obtained 2 weeks after initiation of therapy or a dosage alteration (Levitski and Trepanier, 2000). If an initial loading dose is used, the serum concentration should be measured 1 week later and then again in 3–4 weeks. During therapy for a controlled epileptic patient, the serum phenobarbital concentration should be reassessed every 6–12 months. Peak and trough phenobarbital concentrations do not vary significantly in most epileptic dogs; samples intended for phenobarbital measurement can be collected randomly during the daily dosing interval, rather than during the anticipated trough period. However, in refractory cases, it may be advisable to measure peak and trough levels (Levitski and Trepanier, 2000).

The serum concentration of potassium bromide should be measured 3–4 months after initiation of therapy or a dosage alteration in dogs (use of potassium bromide is not recommended in cats). If an initial loading dose is used, the serum concentration should be measured 1 week later and then again in 4 weeks. In a controlled epileptic patient, the serum bromide concentration should be reassessed every 6–12 months. Patients receiving potassium bromide may have spuriously elevated serum chloride concentrations (i.e. pseudohyperchloraemia) because the reagents used in most commercially available tests for chloride detect total halides without discrimination between chloride, bromide and other halides. In humans, pseudohyperchloraemia may be used as an indirect gauge of the serum bromide concentration; however, in dogs pseudohyperchloremia should not be used as a sole substitute for direct bromide measurement when monitoring an individual's therapeutic dose (Rossmeisl et al., 2006).

Less commonly used anticonvulsants, such as gabapentin, levetiracetam, zonisamide and felbamate, can also be assayed in the serum. Not all of the newer anticonvulsants have established canine therapeutic ranges and the optimal timing of sample collection in each case has not been determined. If necessary, advice can be sought from a neurologist or local diagnostic laboratory. Chapter 8 gives further information on anticonvulsants.

Bile acids and ammonia

Pre- and postprandial bile acids measurement are indicated in cases of suspected hepatic dysfunction and for any patient that is to be given an antiepileptic drug which is potentially hepatotoxic and/or metabolized by the liver, such as phenobarbital. In cirrhosis, the serum bile acids concentration is typically moderately to markedly elevated in both the pre- and postprandial samples. In patients with portovascular anomalies, the preprandial serum bile acids concentration is typically normal or mildly elevated and the postprandial sample is typically moderately to markedly elevated.

Hepatic function can also be assessed by measuring the resting ammonia concentration. This test is less sensitive than measurement of pre- and postprandial bile acids concentration, but can be useful in patients with hepatic encephalopathy since feeding is not required. In addition, hyperammonaemia is implied if ammonium biurate crystalluria is observed. Provocative ammonia tolerance testing is contraindicated in patients exhibiting hepatoencephalopathic signs. In Maltese dogs that are not hepatoencephalopathic, ammonia tolerance testing may be useful to confirm suspected portovascular anomalies, since healthy Maltese dogs may have elevated postprandial bile acids in the absence of a portovascular anomaly (Tisdall et al., 1995). Samples intended for ammonia measurement must be collected in anticoagulant (ethylenediamine tetraacetic acid (EDTA) or heparin) and put on ice for transportation to the laboratory. Plasma should be harvested and refrigerated within 30 minutes of collection, and the test should be completed within 60 minutes of collection. Samples intended for ammonia measurement should not be frozen, as ammonia will degrade with freezing.

Cholinesterase

In cases of suspected organophosphate or carbamate intoxication, exposure is confirmed by identification of blood cholinesterase activity decreased to <25% of the control activity level (cholinesterase activity is greatest in erythrocytes in most domestic animals). Blood cholinesterase activity does not necessarily correlate with the severity of the clinical signs. Organophosphate inhibition of cholinesterase activity is stable. However, since carbamates reversibly bind cholinesterase, reactivation of carbamate-inhibited cholinesterase activity can occur during transport for laboratory determination of activity. Therefore, cholinesterase activity may spontaneously return to normal in cases of carbamate intoxication. Results should be interpreted in light of the history of potential toxicant exposure, the clinical signs and appropriate response to therapy. In addition, cholinesterase activity in tissues such as the brain (particularly the caudate nucleus), retina, liver, kidney, fat or hair can be measured post-mortem. Organophosphates can also induce a delayed-onset, dying-back peripheral neuropathy with demyelination 1–6 weeks after exposure (Jokanovi et al., 2011). Suspicion of this condition may be raised by toxicant exposure history and the results of a nerve biopsy. As with acute intoxication, identification of decreased blood cholinesterase activity is confirmatory. Anecdotal clinical experience indicates that CSF cholinesterase may be elevated above 300 IU/l during inflammatory CNS disease.

Congenital disease testing

Dogs with von Willebrand's disease (vWD) may uncommonly present with neurological signs due to CNS haemorrhage secondary to thrombopathia, which can be screened for by determining the buccal mucosal bleeding time (BMBT; see Tests of haemostasis). The diagnosis of vWD is substantiated by enzyme-linked immunosorbent assay (ELISA) quantitation of the amount of circulating von Willebrand factor (vWF) in the plasma. Plasma samples should be harvested from unclotted, non-haemolysed blood collected into EDTA or citrate anticoagulant (clotting and haemolysis decrease the concentration of vWF). Samples should be analysed by a commercial laboratory that uses assays that have been validated for dogs and cats, since canine and feline vWF are antigenically different from human vWF.

Diagnosis of lysosomal storage diseases has been thoroughly reviewed elsewhere (Skelly and Franklin, 2002) and may include genetic testing, specific enzyme assays, specialized urine staining techniques or electron microscopy of biopsy material. Urine organic acid and amino acid screening may be useful to document rare inborn errors of metabolism (e.g. L-2-hydroxyglutaric aciduria in dogs, hyperoxaluric peripheral neuropathy in cats; Nyhan et al., 1995; Abramson et al., 2003; De Lorenzi et al., 2005; Sewell, 2006). A neurologist or local diagnostic laboratory should be consulted for availability of tests to diagnose these rare diseases. For further information on lysosomal storage diseases, see Chapter 7; Appendix 1 provides details on specific breed-related disorders.

Endocrine testing

A brief summary of endocrine testing is presented here. For further information the reader is referred to the *BSAVA Manual of Canine and Feline Endocrinology* (2012).

Total serum calcium abnormalities that are suspected of being clinically significant should be confirmed by measuring the ionized calcium concentration, which can be performed using either an in-house analyser or a commercial laboratory. Based upon the ionized calcium concentration and other clinical findings, assays for parathyroid hormone, parathyroid hormone-related protein and vitamin D concentrations may be indicated.

Hypothyroidism may be associated with disorders of muscle, the peripheral nervous system (PNS) or the CNS. In dogs with appropriate clinical signs or moderate to marked hypercholesterolaemia, evaluation of thyroid function is indicated, such as the measurement of total thyroxine (T4), free T4 by equilibrium dialysis or thyroid-stimulating hormone (TSH). Feline hyperthyroidism may be associated with CNS or neuromuscular signs. Evaluation of thyroid function is indicated (e.g. total T4) in cats with appropriate clinical signs and/or hepatocellular enzyme and alkaline phosphatase elevations without other evidence to support the diagnosis of cholestasis.

Hypoadrenocorticism is a differential diagnosis for dogs with an episodic history of muscular cramping, neuromuscular weakness, collapse and consistent clinicopathological findings (e.g. hypoglycaemia, hyponatraemia, hyperkalaemia), which can be investigated with an adrenocorticotropic hormone (ACTH) stimulation test. Animals with hyperadrenocorticism may present with neuromuscular or CNS signs due to myopathy or the space-occupying effects of an expanding pituitary gland macroadenoma, respectively. Diagnostic evaluation of hyperadrenocorticism may involve an ACTH stimulation test, dexamethasone suppression test, measurement of endogenous ACTH, urine cortisol:creatinine ratio determination and abdominal ultrasonography. The ACTH stimulation test and urine cortisol:creatinine ratio can be used to monitor dogs treated with trilostane. The urine cortisol:creatinine ratio may aid in recognition of hypocortisolism during trilostane treatment (Galac et al., 2009).

A presumptive diagnosis of insulinoma is based on recognition of clinical signs, laboratory evidence and imaging. Definitive diagnosis requires histopathological analysis of samples obtained from the primary tumour and/or metastatic lesions. Clinical diagnosis of insulinoma is supported by identifying an inappropriately high serum insulin concentration (>140 pmol/l) in a middle-aged to older animal that exhibits persistent fasting hypoglycaemia with glucose levels <3.9 mmol/l (<70 mg/dl) and a history of episodic weakness or seizures associated with fasting, excitement, exercise or the postprandial period (2–6 hours after feeding). In some cases, insulin concentrations may be within the normal range but are considered inappropriate in the presence of hypoglycaemia. The blood sample for insulin measurement should be taken whilst the animal's glucose concentration is below normal. This method of diagnosing beta-cell neoplasia is preferred; use of the insulin:glucose and amended insulin:glucose ratios is no longer recommended as dogs with other causes of hypoglycaemia can have abnormal ratios.

As beta-cell tumours are typically very small, failure to detect a pancreatic mass using abdominal ultrasonography (as occurs in approximately 25–72% of dogs with an insulinoma) does not exclude an insulinoma. The diagnosis is often made on the basis of appropriate signalment, history, clinical signs and laboratory findings (Goutal et al., 2012). During the diagnosis and management of patients with diabetes mellitus, measurement of serum fructosamine (a glycosylated protein) is occasionally indicated. The serum concentration of fructosamine is directly proportional to the serum glucose concentration over the preceding 2–3 weeks. However, fructosamine can be elevated after 3–5 days with severe hyperglycaemia, and after 7 days with moderate hyperglycaemia. It is useful in cats to distinguish diabetic hyperglycaemia from transient stress-induced hyperglycaemia and can be used as an indicator of glycaemic control during the medical management of diabetic patients, which may develop a diabetic neuropathy.

Tests of haemostasis

Animals with haemorrhagic diatheses may present with neurological signs due to CNS haemorrhage. Coagulation cascade function can be assessed by determining the prothrombin time (extrinsic and common pathways), the activated partial thromboplastin time (intrinsic and common pathways) or the activated clotting time (intrinsic and common pathways). The platelet count (per microlitre) can be rapidly estimated during examination of a stained peripheral blood film by determining the average number of platelets in at least ten X100 high-power fields, which is then multiplied by

15,000. The platelet count can also be determined using a haemocytometer or automated CBC machine. Counts obtained from automated haematology analysers should always be verified by examination of the peripheral blood film. This is because falsely decreased platelet counts are extremely common due to platelet clumping associated with blood sample collection. Once coagulopathy and thrombocytopenia have been excluded as the cause of the haemorrhagic diathesis, platelet function may be assessed by determining the BMBT. Identification of a coagulopathy, thrombocytopenia or thrombopathia should prompt further diagnostic testing (e.g. specific coagulation factor assay, tick-borne disease titres, bone marrow cytology, vWF assay) to determine the underlying aetiology of the haemostatic defect.

Thromboelastography (TEG) may be useful to evaluate the potential of a patient for inappropriate clot formation (hypercoagulability) or bleeding (hypocoagulability). It is a promising adjunct to other traditional haemostatic tests and may be of benefit in predicting hypercoagulability; this is of particular use in critical care patients with conditions that predispose to hypercoagulability (e.g. malignant neoplasia, immune-mediated disease and canine parvovirus infection). TEG (a whole blood test of haemostasis) has been validated in dogs, cats and horses. However, results of prospective research and veterinary publications that characterize the sensitivity and specificity of the test are currently limited. TEG determines the strength of the clot (graphical data) and the time taken for a clot to form (numerical data). The test involves recording and interpreting data obtained from a torsion wire that oscillates within the blood sample, which has been mixed with reagents in a cup, as it clots (Figure 3.7). When considering TEG, care should be taken to select a laboratory with its own established reference ranges and personnel experienced in performing and interpreting the test, with particular reference to the factors

that influence the assay (e.g. time between collection and analysis, and the fibrinogen, platelet and erythrocyte concentrations in the patient samples). For further information, the reader is referred to Kol and Borjesson (2010) and McMichael and Smith (2011).

Blood lead concentration

In cases of suspected lead toxicity, identification of a blood lead concentration >40 µg/ml is confirmatory. Half of these patients may exhibit aberrant metarubricytosis (nucleated RBCs without appropriate polychromasia) and one quarter may have basophilic stippling.

Markers of muscular injury

Evaluation of serum creatine kinase (CK) may be useful in suspected cases of myopathy or myositis. Since CK has a short half-life and is highly sensitive and specific for skeletal and cardiac muscle injury, single measurements >10,000 IU/l or persistent elevation >2000 IU/l are considered clinically significant. However, with degenerative myopathies, CK levels may be normal or only mildly increased. The serum concentration of aspartate aminotransferase (AST) is also elevated with muscular injury, and alanine aminotransferase (ALT) may be elevated with severe skeletal muscle necrosis. However, since these enzymes are also present in hepatocytes (ALT and AST), cardiac myocytes (AST) and erythrocytes (AST), they lack the tissue specificity of CK.

Plasma or blood lactate measurement is indicated for patients with suspected metabolic myopathy (e.g. pyruvate dehydrogenase deficiency in Sussex Spaniels). The lactate concentration is measured both before and after exercise. Typically, the animal is exercised until signs are induced prior to taking the post-exercise sample. A lactate concentration in the sample collected after exercise that is dramatically increased above the reference range is suggestive of a metabolic myopathy (see Chapter 18). In addition to myopathy, lactate levels may be

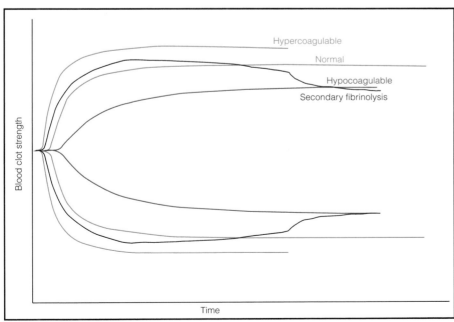

3.7 Thromboelastography tracings: normal (green); hypercoagulable (red); hypocoagulable (blue); and secondary fibrinolysis (black). Time is shown on the x-axis; blood clot strength is shown on the y-axis. Hypocoagulable sample: it has taken longer for the blood clot to establish than normal, which is evident by the increased length of the tracing before it bifurcates. In addition, the clot is weaker than normal, which is evident by the smaller distance between the two arms of the tracing following birfurcation, which corresponds with the force required of the torsion wire as it oscillates in the clotting blood sample (modified from Kol and Borjesson, 2010).

elevated with an increased anion gap metabolic acidosis due to lactic acidosis, as occurs with hypoperfusion (e.g. hypovolaemia) or decreased oxygen delivery to the tissues (e.g. severe anaemia).

With significant muscle injury, myoglobinuria may occur and can be detected as a positive urine dipstick haem reaction. Once haematuria has been excluded by examination of the urine sediment, pigmenturia due to myoglobinuria may be distinguished from that due to haemoglobinuria by an ammonium sulphate precipitation test, which is available through most commercial laboratories or may be performed in-house. Mixing ammonium sulphate with urine followed by centrifugation causes haemoglobin to precipitate and myoglobin to remain in solution. Possible results that may be seen with this test include: only red-brown precipitate (indicating haemoglobinuria), only red-brown supernatant (indicating myoglobinuria) or both red-brown precipitate and supernatant (indicating both haemoglobinuria and myoglobinuria). If haemoglobinuria is suspected, pale red plasma due to haemoglobinaemia should also be present.

Serum osmolality and osmolal gap

Measurement of serum osmolality may be indicated in cases of suspected ethylene glycol intoxication or other hyperosmolar states (e.g. diabetic hyperosmolar non-ketotic syndrome). In addition to abnormalities consistent with acute renal failure, ethylene glycol intoxication is associated with a markedly increased anion gap (often 40–50 mmol/l) metabolic acidosis. The osmolal gap, which is determined by subtracting the calculated serum osmolality from the actual measured serum osmolality, is normally 10–15 mmol/kg. Values >25 mmol/kg are suggestive of intoxication with osmotically active agents, such as ethylene glycol, mannitol or ethanol. Low osmolal gap values are essentially artefactual. The formula for calculation of serum osmolality (expressed as mmol/kg) is:

$$(1.86 \times ([Na^+]\,mEq/l + [K^+]\,mEq/l)) + ([Glucose]\,mg/dl \div 18) + ([BUN]\,mg/dl \div 2.8) + 9$$

Where: BUN = blood urea nitrogen.

Serum protein electrophoresis

Serum protein electrophoresis (SPE) is indicated when an increased serum globulin concentration has been identified. This test identifies whether there is polyclonal immunoglobulin production, as seen with infectious, autoimmune and inflammatory diseases, or whether there is monoclonal immunoglobulin production, as seen with lymphoid neoplasia. With chronic infectious diseases (e.g. ehrlichiosis, leishmaniosis and feline coronavirus), an oligoclonal immune response may rarely occur, which is difficult to distinguish from monoclonal immunoglobulin production using SPE.

Urine protein:creatinine ratio

Measurement of the urine protein:creatinine (UPC) ratio is indicated in proteinuric animals when the urine sediment is inactive (i.e. no cells or bacteria).

The UPC ratio should be <1; values >1 raise concern for glomerular disease (glomerulonephritis, glomerulosclerosis, canine amyloidosis), Bence Jones proteinuria or, less commonly, tubular proteinuria. However, some clinicians favour the use of lower UPC ratio reference values: <0.5 in non-azotaemic animals; <0.5 in azotaemic dogs; and <0.4 in azotaemic cats. A UPC ratio >1 indicates the need for increased frequency of monitoring and a ratio >2 suggests that therapeutic intervention may be required (Lees *et al.*, 2005).

A screening test for microalbuminuria is available; however, controlled clinical studies correlating the identification of microalbuminuria in apparently healthy animals with the subsequent development of renal disease have not yet been published. In addition, to date, no controlled studies to establish reference ranges for clinically normal animals, animals with non-renal disease and animals with early renal disease have been performed. Currently, this test provides little additional value to UPC ratio determination.

Serology and microbiology

Serological and microbiological testing are frequently indicated during the evaluation of patients with neurological and neuromuscular disease, especially when inflammatory or autoimmune disease is suspected. Commercial laboratories typically perform many of these tests. Local laboratories should be checked for availability and sample handling requirements.

In suspected cases of myasthenia gravis, measurement of serum acetylcholine receptor antibody titre is indicated. In addition to blood and urine culture, measurement of serum *Brucella canis* titre is indicated in cases of discospondylitis. For patients that exhibit an unexplained neutrophilic pleocytosis, bacterial meningitis should be considered, and CSF bacterial culture is indicated, especially if degenerative changes are present in the neutrophils. In addition, blood and urine cultures may aid in diagnosis. When fungal infection is suspected, serum and CSF fungal titres (e.g. *Aspergillus*), careful examination of the urine sediment for fungal elements and fungal culture of the urine may be useful.

In cases of inflammatory CNS disease, peripheral neuropathy or polymyositis, it may be useful to measure infectious disease and antinuclear antibody (ANA) titres. Figure 3.8 provides a list of infectious organisms that may be tested for during assessment of these patients. Factors such as history and clinical signs, likelihood of exposure to infectious agents based upon geography, vaccination status and client finances often dictate which titres are most useful and affordable.

In order to establish exposure to an infectious agent that may be the cause of disease, antibody titres are routinely measured to show that an immune response against a given organism has occurred. While antibody titres are extremely useful

Arthropod-borne

- *Ehrlichia* spp.
- *Anaplasma phagocytophilum* [a]
- Rocky Mountain spotted fever (*Rickettsia rickettsii*)
- Lyme disease (*Borrelia burgdorferi*)
- *Bartonella* spp.

Viral

- Canine distemper virus (CDV) [b]
- Rabies virus
- Feline leukaemia virus
- Feline immunodeficiency virus
- Feline infectious peritonitis (FIP) virus [c]

Protozoal

- *Toxoplasma gondii*
- *Neospora caninum*
- *Babesia* spp.
- *Encephalitozoon cuniculi* (rare)
- *Leishmania* spp. (rare)

Fungal

- *Blastomyces dermatitidis*
- *Crytococcus* spp.
- *Histoplasma capsulatum*
- *Coccidioides immitis*
- *Aspergillus* spp.

Parasitic helminth

- *Dirofilaria immitis*

Bacterial

- *Brucella canis* (discospondylitis)

3.8 Infectious organisms that may be detected serologically in patients with neurological and neuromuscular disease. [a] *A. phagocytophilum* may uncommonly be associated with neurological disease (Grieg *et al.*, 1996; Ravnik *et al.*, 2011). [b] PCR may be more useful to diagnose CDV. [c] Serum and/or fluid protein electrophoresis or PCR may be more useful to diagnose FIP.

as supportive evidence of infection, problems such as previous natural exposure to the agent (e.g. *Toxoplasma gondii*), previous vaccination against the agent, or assay cross-reactivity with antibodies formed against other infectious agents (e.g. feline coronavirus (also called feline infectious peritonitis virus (FIPV)) and other coronavirides) may result in misleading information about the diagnosis of an active infection as the cause of current neurological signs. In certain circumstances, polymerase chain reaction (PCR) analysis may be available and can be used for specific identification of active infection by a given agent. When optimized, this technique identifies an active infection by detecting minuscule amounts of organism-specific DNA in tissues or body fluids.

A thorough review of conventional and molecular (DNA- or RNA-based) diagnostic tests for neurological patients is available elsewhere (Nghiem and Schatzberg, 2010). Results from immunological and molecular tests for infectious diseases should be considered in conjunction with the clinical presentation, history, diagnostic imaging studies and clinical pathology when attempting to determine the specific aetiology in some cases of meningoencephalitis. However, even with advanced immunological and/or molecular testing, the aetiology may remain undefined. The sensitivity and specificity of these tests have only been published for a limited number of agents (e.g. canine distemper virus immunohistochemistry, FIPV reverse transcriptase-PCR, *T. gondii* serology and PCR, *Cryptococcus* and *Aspergillus* immunological tests, and fungal urinary antigen screening) (Spector *et al.*, 2008; Garcia *et al.*, 2012). In some instances the sensitivity of the test is low (e.g. FIPV reverse transcriptase-PCR) or there may be problems with cross-reactivity (immunological assays), leading to either false–positive results or an inability to distinguish between pathogens of the same class, as seen with *T. gondii* and *B. dermatitidis*, respectively (Connolly *et al.*, 2012). The data supporting direct causation of neurological disease are equivocal for some arthropod-borne infections (e.g. *Rickettsia*, *Ehrlichia*, *Anaplasma*, *Borrelia* and *Bartonella* species) since DNA is rarely (if ever) detected in the CNS tissue or CSF from patients with clinical signs and positive serum immunological tests (Carrade *et al.*, 2009; Jäderlund *et al.*, 2009; Barber *et al.*, 2010; Krimer *et al.*, 2011). This may reflect the true nature of the diseases, a low concentration of organisms in the sample, the presence of PCR inhibitors in the specimens, diagnostic insensitivity of the currently available molecular tests or other factors.

Molecular testing is evolving and novel assays (which, in some cases, screen concurrently for multiple agents) are actively being developed. In the UK, the Wellcome Trust may be a useful resource. In the USA, the Vector Borne Disease Diagnostic Laboratory (VBDDL) at North Carolina State University and the Real-time PCR Research and Diagnostic Core Facility at the University of California, Davis maintain an online request form for currently available tests along with sample and shipping requirements. Consultation with a laboratory in your area may provide additional information.

Cerebrospinal fluid analysis

CSF is an ultrafiltrate of plasma that is produced predominantly by the choroid plexi within the ventricular system. CSF flows caudally through the ventricular system to the central canal of the spinal cord toward the cauda equina. It passes from the ventricular system through the CNS parenchyma to the subarachnoid space, where it is resorbed into the venous system via the arachnoid villi (Figure 3.9); a small portion exits along the spinal nerve roots. CNS disease does not consistently cause alterations in the CSF; abnormalities depend on the location and extent of the CNS lesion. Parenchymal, extradural and non-exfoliative lesions may cause minimal (e.g. only microprotein elevation) or no changes in the CSF. In addition, the CSF leucocyte count does not correlate with CNS disease severity or prognosis; it simply reflects the

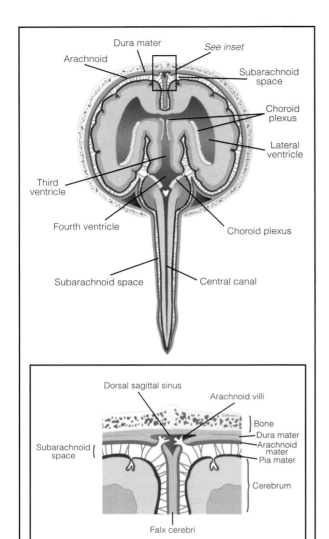

Risks

- General anaesthesia (e.g. hypotension, hypothermia, apnoea, bradycardia, arrhythmia)
- Loss of airway patency during atlanto-occipital collection due to patient positioning and use of unguarded endotracheal tube (see Chapter 21)
- Cerebral and/or cerebellar herniation due to intracranial pressure change
- CNS haemorrhage
- Brainstem trauma due to needle puncture at atlanto-occipital site
- Spinal cord trauma due to needle puncture at lumbar site

Contraindications

- High risk of anaesthetic complications
- Suspected increased intracranial pressure (e.g. progressive obtundation, papilloedema, miosis with responsive pupillary light reflex, intermittent extensor rigidity or opisthotonus)
- Suspected active intracranial haemorrhage
- Radiographic evidence of very large intracranial space-occupying masses
- Severe hydrocephalus
- Severe cerebral oedema on magnetic resonance imaging (MRI)
- Haemorrhagic diathesis as a predisposition for iatrogenic CNS haemorrhage
- Atlanto-occipital collection is contraindicated in cases of suspected atlantoaxial luxation or other causes of cervical vertebral instability
- MRI indicated absence of the atlanto-occipital cistern

3.10 Risks and contraindications associated with CSF collection.

3.9 The ventricular system depicting the neuroanatomical origins of CSF production and sites of absorption (modified from deLahunta, 1983).

degree of meningeal or ependymal cell involvement in the disease process.

CSF analysis is an ancillary diagnostic test that is indicated when a patient has neurological signs that are referable to the CNS. Ideally, CSF analysis should be performed prior to myelography to exclude meningitis, since clinical signs may be exacerbated by radiopaque contrast medium-induced meningeal irritation. CSF collection requires general anaesthesia and is associated with uncommon but significant risks (Figure 3.10). These risks are minimized by employing proper anaesthetic and collection techniques and by excluding patients that have an increased risk of complications (e.g. those with increased intracranial pressure, ICP). For information on the treatment that can be employed for patients with elevated ICP, see Chapters 9 and 20. To minimize the risks of CSF collection, the anaesthetic protocol can be manipulated in an attempt to decrease ICP. Drugs such as ketamine should be avoided in

these patients. Patients with suspected increased ICP may be given mannitol and ventilated to achieve and maintain a P_aCO_2 of approximately 30–35 mmHg to reduce the ICP. Further details on the anaesthetic management of such patients can be found in Chapter 21.

During collection, CSF should not be aspirated using negative pressure applied via a syringe attached directly to a needle hub. Aspiration can cause a rapid decrease in CSF pressure, which may trigger intracranial haemorrhage or herniation (transtentorial and/or transforamen magnum). Similarly, removal of an excessive volume of CSF can potentiate haemorrhage or herniation, but 1 ml per 5 kg bodyweight can be safely collected from most patients.

CSF is collected aseptically from the atlanto-occipital (AO) site (also referred to as the cerebellomedullary cistern (CMC) or cisterna magna) and/or from the caudal lumbar site, using the equipment listed in Figure 3.11. Collection from both sites is detailed below, although in small animals CSF is more commonly collected from the AO site. Collection from the AO site is less difficult, usually results in a larger sample volume, and is typically associated with less iatrogenic blood contamination. In cases of focal CNS disease, CSF samples are more likely to be abnormal or representative of the lesion when they are collected caudal to the lesion. Therefore, in animals with lesions involving the spinal cord or canal, lumbar CSF samples are more consistently abnormal than AO samples. In this situation, it is preferable to collect CSF from both sites.

- Hair clippers
- Surgical scrub
- Sterile gloves
- Spinal needle (20- or 22-gauge; 1.5 inch for AO; 2.5 or 3.5 inch for lumbar)
- Sterile collection container: 3 ml syringe, conical centrifuge tube, plain tube (free of anticoagulant) and/or an EDTA tube

3.11 Equipment required for CSF collection.

Atlanto-occipital CSF collection

The procedure for AO CSF collection is illustrated in Figures 3.12 and 3.13 (see also **Atlanto-occipital CSF collection** clip on DVD). The patient is placed in lateral recumbency with the dorsum near the edge of the table and the nose elevated to place the sagittal plane of the muzzle parallel to the table. The neck is then fully flexed and the ears pulled rostrally. It is important to be aware that with full neck flexion there is a risk of the endotracheal tube kinking and interference with anaesthesia. There are two ways to identify the AO space properly, using anatomical landmarks:

- Palpate a triangle of landmarks formed by the occipital protuberance and the most prominent points of the lateral wings of the atlas (Figure 3.12). The location for needle insertion is on the dorsal midline between the wings of the atlas, one-third to one-half of the way caudal to the occipital protuberance (the most cranial point of the triangle formed by the landmarks)
- Alternatively, use the occipital protuberance to identify the midline and use the most cranial margins of the wings of the atlas to identify the location of the AO space, which should be at the same level along the neck.

The needle is positioned directly on the midline, perpendicular to the neck, at the level of the AO space and advanced slowly 1–2 mm at a time. Once the skin has been penetrated, the stylet can be removed. One or two slight 'pops' may be felt as the needle is advanced through the muscle layers and meninges into the cisterna magna. Resistance will decrease when the dura is penetrated. When the subarachnoid space has been entered, CSF will appear in the needle hub. If blood is obtained, a few drops of CSF should be allowed to flow. If the fluid clears, it can be collected for analysis; if it remains bloody, the needle should be removed and the procedure started again. If the needle hits bone whilst being advanced, it may be redirected caudally, moving the needle off the bone and into the AO space. If this is not possible, the needle may be removed and collection attempted again after reassessment of anatomical landmarks.

Once the needle is in place, fluid is collected either by allowing it to drip into a sterile collection tube or by suctioning the drops into a sterile syringe as they form at the spinal needle hub. *Do not attach the syringe to the spinal needle hub and aspirate.* The rate of CSF flow out of the needle may be

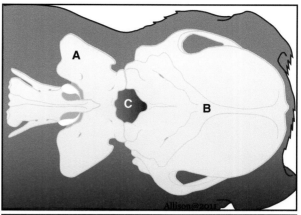
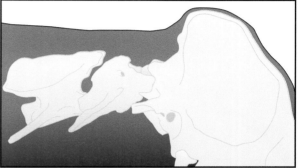
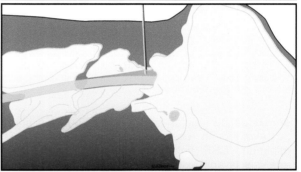
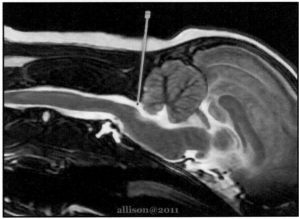

3.12 Anatomical landmarks for AO CSF collection. The dog is placed in lateral recumbency with the head flexed at 90 degrees to the neck. This flexion opens up the cerebellomedullary cistern (C) accessible via the AO space. With the head flexed at 90 degrees to the cervical spine the AO joint opens up so that the tap can be performed. The spinal needle is placed perpendicular to the cord and advanced into the cistern situated above the cord. A = wing of the atlas vertebra; B = occipital protuberance.

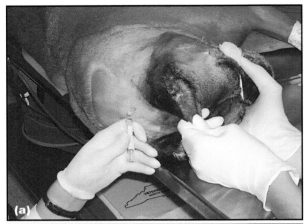

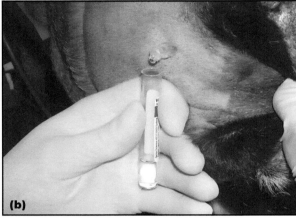

3.13 AO CSF collection. **(a)** Proper positioning. **(b)** Close-up demonstrating CSF dripping from the hub of the spinal needle into the collection tube.

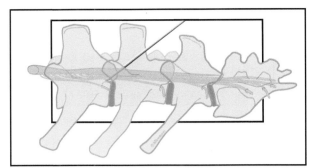

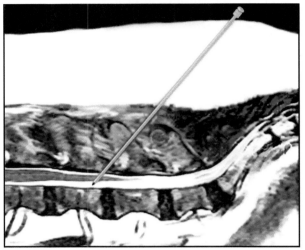

3.14 Anatomical landmarks for lumbar CSF collection. The spinal needle is inserted over the spinous process of L6 and angled forward to access the CSF via the interarcuate space of L5–L6. The dorsal or ventral subarachnoid space at this site can be used to obtain samples.

enhanced by jugular compression, but this should be avoided in cases with increased ICP. The minimum CSF volume required for a complete analysis is approximately 0.5 ml. Once a sufficient volume has been collected or the CSF flow stops, the spinal needle is removed from the cisterna. Several drops of CSF typically remain within the spinal needle; they can be forced out of the needle into the collection tube by replacing the stylet, whilst holding the end of the needle over the tube.

Ideally, CSF should be collected into a sterile syringe or plastic tube, because cells may adhere to glass containers. If the sample is haemorrhagic, it should be placed in an EDTA tube to prevent clotting. Samples intended for bacterial culture should be free of anticoagulant. For optimal preservation of cytological details, CSF samples should be analysed or preserved within 1 hour of collection.

Lumbar CSF collection

Anatomical landmarks for lumbar CSF collection are shown in Figure 3.14. With the patient in lateral recumbency, the lumbar spine is flexed. The appropriate intervertebral space is identified, which is L4–L5 or L5–L6 (preferred) in dogs and L6–L7 in cats. This is achieved by palpating the ilial crests; the spinous process found immediately cranial to the ilial crests is that of L6. The needle is positioned on the midline, just cranial to the appropriate spinous

process, at a 45 degree angle with the needlepoint directed cranially. The needle is advanced as described for AO collection, but the stylet may be left within the spinal needle. When correctly positioned, the needle typically passes through or alongside the cauda equina/caudal spinal cord, which often elicits a tail or leg twitch. The fluid is frequently collected from the ventral subarachnoid space. Beyond a tail or leg twitch or minor spinal cord haemorrhage with potential sample contamination, persistent untoward effects are not typically manifested as a result of this collection method, although complications have been reported (Platt *et al.*, 2005). The risk of iatrogenic neurological damage is minimized if CSF can be obtained from the dorsal rather than the ventral subarachnoid space.

Sample handling

CSF contains very little protein; this causes the leucocytes that are present to deteriorate rapidly. Ideally, CSF samples should be analysed or preserved as soon as possible after collection, preferably within 1 hour, to minimize cellular degradation. However, if the sample is refrigerated after collection, a delay of up to 8 hours in processing is unlikely to affect the diagnostic interpretation, particularly of those samples that contain ≥50 mg/dl microprotein and an elevated leucocyte count (Fry *et al.*, 2006).

If a commercial laboratory is used for CSF analysis and there is only a 1-hour transport delay, then refrigeration of the sample is adequate. If the anticipated delay is longer than 1 hour, the CSF sample should be preserved by refrigeration and the addition of either serum or hetastarch to carefully labelled aliquots. When serum is used, care should be taken to use pristine serum from the patient or commercially available fetal bovine serum. Three drops of serum should be added per 0.25 ml of CSF (Bienzle *et al.*, 2000; Fry *at al.*, 2006). The addition of serum to the CSF sample raises the protein concentration and dilutes the aliquot. The aliquot containing serum should be clearly labelled. A separate aliquot that does not contain serum should also be submitted to the laboratory for microprotein measurement.

Hetastarch is a useful preservative when pure serum is not available or when the CSF sample volume is low (Figure 3.15). A 1:1 mixture of CSF and hetastarch preserves the cells for analysis (Fry *et al.*, 2006). When hetastarch is used, it is not necessary to send two aliquots for analysis, since hetastarch does not increase the protein concentration of the CSF sample. However, it is necessary to label the sample, indicating that it has been diluted by half, as the dilution will affect the inter-

pretation of the results. Alternatively, one or two drops of 10% buffered formalin can be used to preserve the total number of cells; this does not increase the protein concentration. However, the differential leucocyte count and other microscopic assessments are very unreliable as formalin dramatically alters cytomorphology (Figure 3.16). For this reason, formalin is no longer recommended.

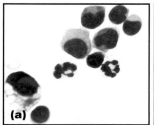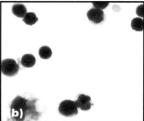

3.16 Cytomorphology of a CSF sample collected from a horse with Eastern equine encephalitis virus. **(a)** Aliquot with no preservative. **(b)** Aliquot with formalin preservative. The cells in the formalin aliquot are compressed making it difficult to distinguish neutrophils from lymphocytes and to fully observe cellular details. (Wright–Giemsa stain; original magnification X50)

If desired, many components of the CSF analysis can be performed in-house, including:

* Determining the cell count
* Estimating the microprotein concentration
* Microscopic examination of a stained slide.

Most CSF samples, even abnormal ones, contain a relatively low concentration of leucocytes; therefore, the samples must be concentrated prior to microscopic examination. Commercial laboratories use a cytocentrifuge to concentrate the cells from a drop or two of CSF on to a small area of a microscope slide. If in-house CSF evaluation is required, or if sample analysis at the commercial laboratory must be delayed for more than 1 hour and sample preservatives cannot be used, a sedimentation chamber can be constructed (Figures 3.17 and 3.18).

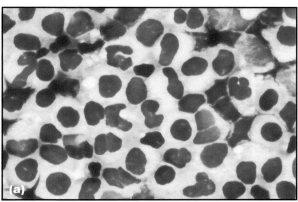
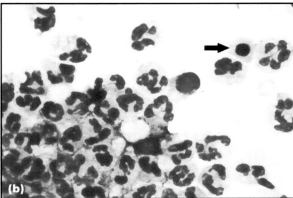

3.15 Comparison of leucocyte morphology in 3-day-old canine CSF samples. **(a)** Aliquot with no preservative. **(b)** Aliquot with hetastarch preservative. The cells in the unpreserved aliquot are swollen and karyolytic, preventing accurate cell identification and differential leucocyte count. The leucocytes in the aliquot with hetastarch are adequately preserved and recognizable as predominately mature, non-degenerative neutrophils. A single pyknotic neutrophil is also present (arrowed). (Wright–Giemsa stain; original magnification X50)

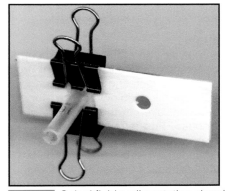

3.17 Spinal fluid sedimentation chamber. The chamber was constructed from a microscope slide, a piece of filter paper with a hole punched in the centre, the barrel of a 1 ml syringe and two binder clips. The second hole in the filter paper is present for illustration. In the functioning chamber, only the hole directly under the barrel of the syringe is needed.

Equipment
• Standard hole punch • 2 binder type paper clips • Filter paper • Clean, glass microscope slide • 1 ml syringe, plunger removed, cut in half

Method
1. Make a hole in the filter paper using the hole punch. 2. Place the filter paper on top of the microscope slide. 3. Cut a 1 ml syringe in half; discard the tip. 4. Centre the flanged end of the syringe barrel (the end where the plunger would be inserted) directly over the hole in the filter paper. 5. Clamp the flanges of the syringe barrel on to the microscope slide using the two binder paper clips. 6. Place the assembled chamber on a flat counter with the microscope slide parallel to the counter. 7. Load 0.25–0.5 ml of CSF into the open end of the barrel. The fluid will diffuse out of the bottom of the syringe into the filter paper, leaving the cells stuck to the glass underneath the hole in the filter paper. 8. Allow the fluid to diffuse for at least 30 minutes. 9. Air-dry the slide; heat-fixing is unnecessary and may damage the cells causing poor preservation for cytological examination. 10. Stain the slide with a Romanowsky-type stain (e.g. Diff-Quik®) or send it to a clinical pathologist for staining and interpretation if required.

3.18 Equipment and method for in-house sedimentation chamber assembly.

A pilot study showed that processing samples using this type of sedimentation chamber yielded 33% of the total cells observed on slides prepared from the same sample using a cytocentrifuge. There was good correlation between the sedimentation chamber and the cytocentrifuge for granulocyte percentages, but moderate to poor correlation for mononuclear cell percentages (i.e. mononuclear phagocytes and lymphocytes). Better correlation was found in samples that had elevated leucocyte counts compared with those that had normal counts (Stacey and Wamsley, unpublished data). Slides made using a sedimentation chamber can be either examined in-house or submitted to a commercial laboratory for microscopic evaluation. Other tests, such as protein measurement or microbial culture, can be performed upon the remaining CSF.

Sample analysis

Results of CSF analysis can rapidly provide information that may be useful in selecting treatment protocols, prognostication or dictating further diagnostic tests (e.g. serology, microbiology). However, the results may be normal even in the presence of significant CNS disease. Furthermore, only occasionally will CSF analysis alone yield a definitive clinical diagnosis. CSF findings need to be interpreted in light of the history, clinical signs and other diagnostic tests. Figure 3.19 gives an overview of the components of CSF analysis and normal findings.

Gross physical characteristics

Normal CSF is colourless. CSF may be coloured by the addition of cells or cellular breakdown products (Figure 3.20). When the CSF is discoloured, it is

Characteristic	Normal findings
Assessment of gross physical characteristics: colour and clarity	Colourless and transparent
Microprotein determination	Atlanto-occipital site: <25 mg/dl Lumbar site: <40 mg/dl
Cell counts	Red blood cells: 0/µl (excluding iatrogenic blood contamination) White blood cells: <5/µl
Microscopic examination with differential leucocyte count	Lymphocytes: 60–70% Monocytes: 30–40% Neutrophils: <1% (excluding iatrogenic blood contamination) Eosinophils: <1% Ependymal lining cells: rare

3.19 Components of CSF analysis and normal findings.

Sample colour	Cause
Red	Iatrogenic haemorrhage (blood contamination) Pathological haemorrhage
Yellow-orange (xanthochromia)	Bilirubin associated with chronic pathological haemorrhage (red blood cell breakdown) Bilirubin associated with hyperbilirubinaemia or disrupted blood–brain barrier
Yellow-green	Markedly increased nucleated cell concentration (e.g. purulent inflammation, neoplasia – rare)
Grey-black	Presence of melanin granules or melanocytes

3.20 Causes of abnormally coloured CSF samples.

often either red or yellow-orange (xanthochromic). When it is red, it is necessary to determine whether iatrogenic or pathological haemorrhage has occurred. This distinction is made possible by gross and microscopic observation. Pathological haemorrhage may be suspected if the sample is uniformly red during collection, whereas blood contamination due to iatrogenic haemorrhage is suggested if the sample is initially colourless but becomes red-tinged during collection. When placed in a tube that does not contain anticoagulant, a moderately to severely blood-contaminated sample is likely to clot. In addition, an aliquot of red CSF can be centrifuged. A xanthochromic supernatant indicates that pathological haemorrhage has probably occurred; a colourless supernatant suggests that contamination due to iatrogenic haemorrhage has occurred.

The presence of bilirubin in the CSF results in xanthochromia. When present, xanthochromia is most commonly due to chronic haemorrhage. Erythrocytes that enter the CSF due to haemorrhage are metabolized, resulting in bilirubin formation. Less commonly, when the serum concentration is markedly increased, conjugated bilirubin may cross the blood–brain barrier. In addition, conjugated and unconjugated bilirubin can cross a damaged blood–brain barrier. Thus, xanthochromia is not pathognomonic for chronic CNS haemorrhage.

Yellow-green and grey-black CSF is observed uncommonly. Yellow-green discoloration can be caused by a high nucleated cell count, as seen with purulent inflammation (e.g. septic meningitis) or a neoplastic infiltration. Melanin granules or melanocytes are a rare abnormal finding in the CSF. If present at a sufficient concentration, as occasionally seen with CNS melanoma, they may result in a grey discoloration.

Normal CSF is transparent (or clear). It becomes cloudy when the number of leucocytes markedly increase above 500 white blood cells (WBCs)/μl. Since the cell count must be substantially increased before the CSF becomes cloudy, estimation of the cell count based on gross examination is of minimal use. It is necessary to perform a manual cell count using a haemocytometer to detect mild or moderate leucocyte elevations above the normal leucocyte count of <5 WBCs/μl.

Microprotein determination
The cranial-to-caudal flow of CSF normally causes a protein concentration differential between samples collected from the AO and lumbar sites. The protein concentration is normally higher in samples collected from the lumbar site than those collected from the AO site. This difference can be increased when CNS disease is present, especially when the spinal cord is involved. The CSF protein concentration is far lower than that in other body fluids and cannot be measured with a refractometer. Precise microprotein quantitation is performed spectrophotometrically using reagents that are typically found only in commercial laboratories. The normal protein concentration varies depending on the species, the site of sample collection and the method used to measure the protein. Results are best interpreted using reference values established by the individual laboratory reporting the microprotein concentration. In general, canine and feline CSF collected from the AO site contains <25 mg protein/dl or from the lumbar site contains <40 mg protein/dl. The microprotein concentration can be estimated using a protein dipstick or the protein pad of a urine dipstick. The protein dipstick reaction results in a colour change that is interpreted in ranges (Figure 3.21).

<30 mg/dl	30 mg/dl	100 mg/dl	300 mg/dl	>2000 mg/dl
Trace	1+	2+	3+	4+

3.21 Protein dipstick interpretation ranges.

Total erythrocyte and leucocyte counts
Normal CSF should contain no erythrocytes. However, a number of erythrocytes may be seen in a sample due to iatrogenic blood contamination or with pathological haemorrhage. Most clinical pathologists consider <5 WBCs/μl to be normal for dogs and cats. An increased number of leucocytes in a CSF sample is referred to as pleocytosis. Pleocytosis can be further characterized during the microscopic examination and differential cell count based upon the predominant leucocyte type(s).

Erythrocyte and leucocyte counts are measured by placing undiluted CSF into both chambers of a haemocytometer. The cell counts are performed after the cells have settled within the haemocytometer chambers, which is accomplished by allowing the haemocytometer to sit within a humidified Petri dish for 5 minutes before counting the cells (Figure 3.22). Each chamber has a grid which comprises nine large squares (Figure 3.23). The number of leucocytes and erythrocytes in the centre large square and the four corner large squares of both chambers (five squares per chamber x two chambers = 10 squares) are counted to determine the total leucocyte and erythrocyte counts per microlitre. If an excessive number of erythrocytes are present, only one large square should be counted and the number multiplied by 10 to get the total erythrocyte count per microlitre. Care must be taken to distinguish leucocytes from any erythrocytes present (Figure 3.24).

- Erythrocytes are small, biconcave, light orange and very translucent; they may also be crenated.
- Leucocytes are larger, stippled, greyish and less translucent than erythrocytes.

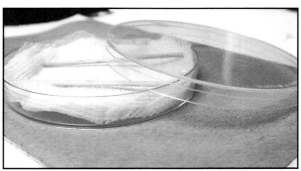

3.22 Humidified Petri dish and haemocytometer. The Petri dish is humidified by placing damp, absorbent material (e.g. thin gauze or filter paper) at the bottom of the dish. The handle of a cotton tipped applicator is broken in half and placed on top of the absorbent material. The haemocytometer is loaded with CSF and placed on the two halves of the applicator handle. The lid is then closed. This prevents the CSF sample from evaporating whilst the cells settle into the grid that is etched in the haemocytometer.

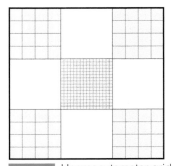

3.23 Haemocytometer grid found in the counting chambers. The cells in the centre large square and the four corner large squares from both chambers are counted (10 large squares in total). The total number of cells in the 10 large squares is equivalent to the number of cells per microlitre.

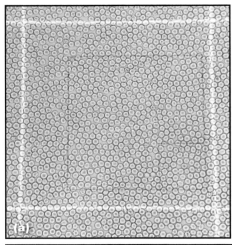

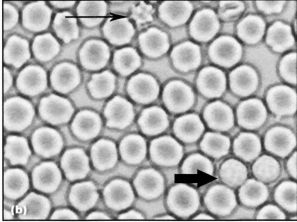

3.24 Erythrocytes and leucocytes in a haemodilute CSF sample in one small square within a large corner square of a haemocytometer counting chamber grid. **(a)** The lines etched in the haemocytometer appear white. Darker squares etched in the ocular Miller's disc for performing reticulocyte counts are also present.
(b) Close-up image showing numerous erythrocytes and two leucocytes. The leucocytes (thick arrow) are stippled and do not transmit as much light as the erythrocytes, which typically appear as biconcave discs. Based on size, the leucocytes are likely to be lymphocytes (mononuclear phagocytes and macrophages are typically larger). A severely crenated erythrocyte (echinocyte; thin arrow) is also present. (Original magnification X20)

Cytology and differential leucocyte count

Microscopic examination is usually performed on concentrated CSF samples stained with a Romanowsky-type stain. In normal CSF, mononuclear cells predominate (Figure 3.25). Small, well differentiated lymphocytes typically comprise 60–70% of the differential cell count; minimally vacuolated, large mononuclear phagocytes frequently comprise 30–40%. The background is usually colourless and may contain a low number of erythrocytes, a small amount of stain precipitate and rare keratinized, squamous epithelial cell contaminants. Ependymal lining cells may occasionally be found in small clusters (Figure 3.26). Mature non-degenerate neutrophils and eosinophils are rarely seen and should represent <2% of the leucocytes in samples that are free of blood contamination.

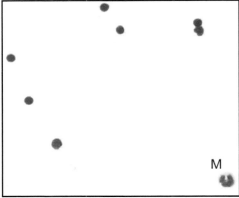

3.25 Spinal fluid from a dog. Small, well differentiated lymphocytes and a minimally vacuolated, large mononuclear phagocyte (M) are visible in this sample. (Wright–Giemsa stain; original magnification X20)

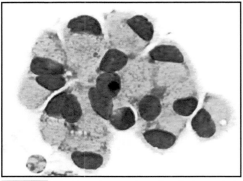

3.26 Cluster of ependymal cells in a canine spinal fluid sample. Note the eccentric nuclei and accumulation of eosinophilic, granular material in the basophilic cytoplasm. (Wright–Giemsa stain; original magnification X20)

Distinction between pathological and iatrogenic haemorrhage

If erythrophagia, haemosiderophages or haematoidin crystals are observed during microscopic examination, pathological haemorrhage is suggested (Figure 3.27).

- Erythrophagia denotes reactive mononuclear phagocyte ingestion of erythrocytes, which are visible within the cytoplasm of the phagocyte.
- Haemosiderophages are reactive mononuclear phagocytes that contain variably sized, round to oval particles of dark blue–green haemosiderin pigment, which stain positively for iron with Prussian blue. The iron is derived from metabolized haemoglobin.
- Bilirubin is another product of haemoglobin metabolism; it forms golden, rhomboid or rectangular haematoidin crystals.

Iatrogenic blood contamination is indicated by the presence of platelets and/or the absence of erythrophagia or erythrocyte breakdown pigments (haemosiderin, haematoidin).

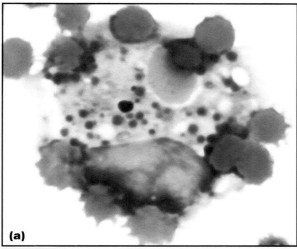

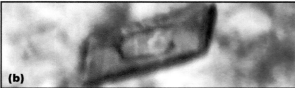

3.27 Spinal fluid sample from a dog demonstrating pathological haemorrhage. **(a)** A large mononuclear phagocyte containing multiple phagocytosed erythrocytes (indicative of acute haemorrhage) is visible. The dark blue–green granules above the nucleus are consistent with haemosiderin pigment and suggest chronic haemorrhage. **(b)** The golden rhomboid crystal is consistent with haematoidin and also indicates chronic haemorrhage. (Wright–Giemsa stain; original magnification X100)

Interpretation

Effects of blood contamination
When blood is present in the CSF, it is commonly due to contamination at the time of collection, rather than pathological haemorrhage. Iatrogenic contamination of the CSF sample with peripheral blood may falsely increase the protein concentration, leucocyte count and relative percentage of neutrophils and eosinophils, particularly when the leucocyte count is <500 cells/μl (Doyle and Solano-Gallego, 2009). Even when samples are contaminated with blood, analysis may still be useful as certain cellular abnormalities may be detected during microscopic examination (e.g. highly vacuolated mononuclear phagocytes, infectious agents and neoplastic cells). When the blood contamination is mild (<5000 RBCs/μl), two correction formulae have been proposed to calculate a very rough estimate of what the protein concentration and leucocyte count would be if the contamination were absent.

- Protein concentration correction formula: for every 1000 RBCs/μl, the protein concentration can be adjusted down by 1 mg/dl.
- Leucocyte count correction formula: for every 500 RBCs/μl, the leucocyte count can be adjusted down by 1 WBC/μl.

Information derived from these formulae is interpreted most effectively when the clinical signs and results of the microscopic examination are also considered (i.e. findings indicative of pathological haemorrhage, infection or neoplasia).

Abnormal findings
Figure 3.28 lists the potential abnormal CSF analysis findings.

Increased microprotein concentration with normal total leucocyte count (albuminocytological dissociation)
• Normal differential leucocyte count • Increased neutrophil percentage
Pleocytosis (usually occurs concurrently with increased protein concentration)
• Lymphocytic • Mixed cell • Neutrophilic • Eosinophilic
Other microscopic findings
• Sample contamination • Myelin • Pathological haemorrhage • Infectious agents • Neoplasia • Degenerative disease

3.28 Potential abnormal CSF analysis findings.

Increased microprotein concentration with normal total cell count: Albuminocytological dissociation occurs with various diseases that alter the blood–brain barrier and allow protein from the blood circulation to enter the CNS, increase the production of protein within the CNS or obstruct the flow of fluid and therefore protein within the CNS. Considerations include:

- An extradural compressive lesion (intervertebral disc disease (IVDD), cervical stenotic myelopathy, spinal synovial cyst, vertebral osseous lesions, neoplasia)
- An intramedullary mass effect (neoplasia, syringomyelia, hydromyelia, protozoal granulomas)
- Degenerative myelopathy
- Ischaemic CNS necrosis (due to fibrocartilaginous embolus)
- Trauma
- Vasculitis
- Intrathecal globulin production (due to infection or neoplasia).

Patients with polyradiculoneuritis may also exhibit albuminocytological dissociation.

Even though the total leucocyte count may be normal, an increased microprotein concentration may be associated with an abnormal cell population, such as an increased percentage of neutrophils. This can occur with CNS disease that does not involve the meninges or ependymal cells (e.g. verte-bral fractures, cervical stenotic myelopathy, IVDD and severe seizure activity) or with CNS necrosis. In cases of acute thoracolumbar IVDD, pleocytosis is directly associated with the severity of the spinal cord injury and, in dogs lacking nociception on pres-entation, a high percentage of macrophages is associated with a negative clinical outcome (Srugo *et al.*, 2011).

An increased percentage of neutrophils with a normal total cell concentration may be seen with inflammatory CNS diseases, if the total CSF leuco-cyte count has been reduced as a result of treat-ment with glucocorticoids or antimicrobials prior to sample collection. Previous glucocorticoid adminis-tration may be suspected if hypersegmented neutro-phils (more than five nuclear lobulations) are visible in the CSF sample (Figure 3.29). In addition, hyper-segmented neutrophils are also occasionally found in cases of long-standing inflammation or in sam-ples which have been subject to a processing delay.

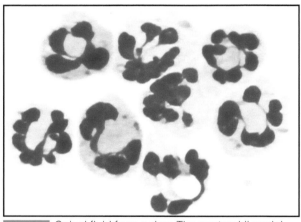

3.29 Spinal fluid from a dog. The neutrophil nuclei are hyperchromic and have >5 lobulations, which is consistent with hypersegmentation. (Diff-Quik stain®; original magnification X50)

Lymphocytic pleocytosis: With lymphocytic ple-ocytosis (Figure 3.30), the CSF protein concentra-tion is typically increased and the leucocyte count is >5 WBCs/μl with >50% lymphocytes. This finding may be seen with a number of different disease con-ditions but is most commonly associated with viral meningitis, including that caused by rabies and canine distemper virus. Pugs, Maltese dogs, Yorkshire Terriers, Chihuahuas and other toy breeds may develop a severe necrotizing, non-suppurative meningoencephalitis, originally called Pug dog encephalitis (Higgins *et al.*, 2008). This type of dis-ease is associated with a moderate to marked ple-ocytosis, which is typically lymphocytic, although a mixed cell pleocytosis can be seen. Feline polioen-cephalomyelitis, an uncommon disease in 2- to 3-month-old cats, may also be associated with lym-phocytic meningitis and pleocytosis. CNS lymphoma can cause lymphocytic pleocytosis in any species. The lymphocytes may appear well differentiated (small lymphocytes) or atypical (lymphoblasts) (see Figures 3.31 and 3.38). Well differentiated lympho-

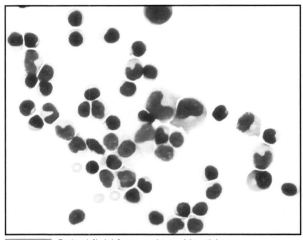

3.30 Spinal fluid from a dog with rabies demonstrating lymphocytic pleocytosis. Several small, well differentiated lymphocytes are present along with a few large mononuclear cells. (Wright–Giesma stain; original magnification X20)

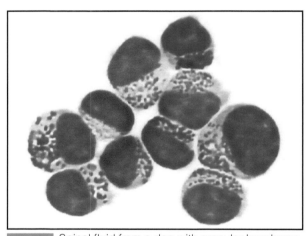

3.31 Spinal fluid from a dog with granular lymphoma. Large lymphoblasts with eccentric magenta granules are visible. (Wright–Giemsa stain; original magnification X50)

cytic pleocytosis occurs more frequently in cats than dogs with lymphoma, since feline lymphoma is usu-ally extradural and, thus, neoplastic cells may not be found in the CSF. Although typically associated with mixed cell pleocytosis, animals with toxoplas-mosis, neosporosis, ehrlichiosis or granulomatous meningoencephalitis (GME) may present with lympho-cytic pleocytosis. Steroid-responsive meningitis also should be considered if the clinical presentation is consistent with this disease, although it typically causes neutrophilic pleocytosis.

Mixed cell pleocytosis: With mixed cell pleocyto-sis the CSF protein concentration is typically increased and the leucocyte count is >5 WBCs/μl. The predominant population of nucleated cells is a mixture of lymphocytes and large mononuclear phagocytes, with a variable number of neutrophils. A lesser number of plasma cells and rarely eosino-phils may also be present. The classic example of mixed cell pleocytosis occurs with canine GME (Figure 3.32). Other diseases that can cause mixed cell pleocytosis include:

- Fungal infections (cryptococcosis, blastomycosis and aspergillosis)
- Rickettsial infections (ehrlichiosis and Rocky Mountain spotted fever)
- Protozoal or algal infections (toxoplasmosis, neosporosis and protothecosis).

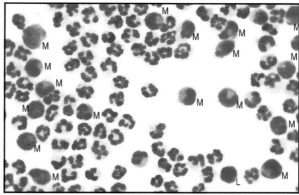

3.33 Spinal fluid from a dog with steroid-responsive meningoencephalomyelitis and neutrophilic pleocytosis. Mature non-degenerative neutrophils are present along with a lesser number of larger mononuclear phagocytes (M) and a lymphocyte (L). (Wright–Giemsa stain; original magnification X20)

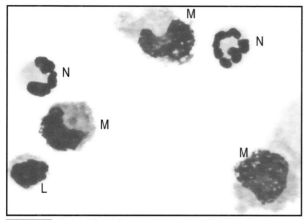

3.32 Spinal fluid from a dog with mixed cell pleocytosis. Three large mononuclear phagocytes (M), two mature non-degenerative neutrophils (N) and one small well differentiated lymphocyte (L) are visible. (Wright–Giemsa stain; original magnification X50)

In addition, when other possibilities have been eliminated, steroid-responsive meningitis should be considered in dogs, due to the variable cytological appearance associated with this disease. In cats, neurological disease associated with chronic FIP may present with mixed cell pleocytosis, although in many cases there is neutrophilic pleocytosis. Most of the above conditions typically cause a moderate to severe pleocytosis (50–500 WBCs/µl). Mild mixed cell pleocytosis (<50 WBCs/µl) can also be seen with any condition that results in CNS infarction or myelomalacia (e.g. acute intervertebral disc herniation).

Neutrophilic pleocytosis: With neutrophilic pleocytosis (Figure 3.33) the CSF protein concentration is typically increased and the leucocyte count is >5 WBCs/µl with a predominant neutrophil population. In dogs, the classic example and most common cause of neutrophilic pleocytosis is steroid-responsive meningitis (see Chapter 14); Beagles, Bernese Mountain Dogs, Boxers and German Wirehaired Pointers as well as other medium and large-breed dogs are typically affected. With this disease, the leucocyte count is usually >50 WBCs/µl, the neutrophils are non-degenerate and bacterial cultures are negative. Other causes of neutrophilic pleocytosis in dogs include Rocky Mountain spotted fever. In cats, FIP is highly likely in those animals <4 years old with >200 mg protein/dl, >100 WBCs/µl and >50% neutrophils in their CSF (Rand et al., 1994). In both cats and dogs, severe seizures, or any disease that

produces an area of CNS necrosis, can cause mild neutrophilic pleocytosis or an increased neutrophil percentage with a normal cell count. Contrast medium injected during myelography may also induce a transient neutrophilic pleocytosis. However, contrary to previously thought, meningiomas are not typically associated with neutrophilic pleocytosis. In one study, nearly 75% of dogs with a meningioma did not have neutrophilic pleocytosis (Dickinson et al., 2006).

The presence of neutrophilic pleocytosis should alert the clinician to the uncommon possibility of bacterial or, less commonly, fungal meningitis. Culture of CSF samples should be considered for animals with neutrophilic pleocytosis, especially if other signs suggestive of bacterial meningitis, such as pyrexia, peripheral neutrophilia with or without a left shift and/or toxic change, and degenerative changes in CSF neutrophils, are present. Degenerative changes are not present in all cases of bacterial meningitis (e.g. due to prior antimicrobial administration or infection by a bacterium producing few cytotoxic substances). The presence or absence of degenerative changes in CSF neutrophils should not be used as the sole criterion to determine whether a CSF sample should be cultured; it is prudent to integrate other clinical information when making this decision. Cytologically, a definitive diagnosis of sepsis can be made by identifying bacteria within the cytoplasm of degenerative neutrophils (Figure 3.34).

Eosinophilic pleocytosis: With eosinophilic pleocytosis (Figure 3.35) the CSF protein concentration is typically increased and the leucocyte count is >5 WBCs/µl with a predominant eosinophil (>20%) population. Steroid-responsive inflammatory CNS disease associated with a large number of eosinophils (e.g. eosinophilic meningitis, meningoencephalitis and meningoencephalomyelitis) has been reported in both dogs (Windsor et al., 2009) and cats. Golden Retrievers are over-represented. This is an uncommon disease, which is associated with severe pleocytosis and >80% eosinophils.

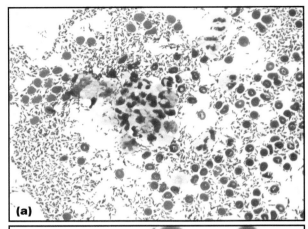

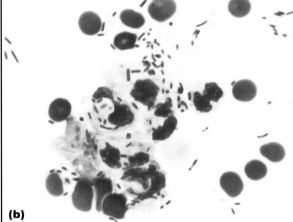

3.34 Spinal fluid from a dog with bacterial meningitis. **(a)** Numerous rod-shaped bacteria are present in both the cytoplasm of the neutrophils and the extracellular background. **(b)** Close-up view. (Wright–Giemsa stain; original magnification X50 and X100, respectively)

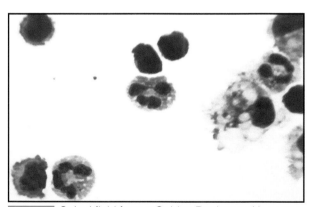

3.35 Spinal fluid from a Golden Retriever with a very marked eosinophilic pleocytosis (21,000 WBCs/μl). Three eosinophils along with a number of small well differentiated lymphocytes and a highly vacuolated macrophage (right) are present in this non-concentrated sample. (Wright–Giemsa stain; original magnification X50)

Eosinophilic pleocytosis has also been reported with aberrant parasitic migration, toxoplasmosis, neosporosis, cryptococcosis, prototheccosis and neoplasia (e.g. T-cell lymphoma). Therefore, these diseases should be excluded using serum or CSF serology prior to glucocorticoid administration.

Other microscopic findings: Infectious agents such as bacteria, fungi and protozoa (rare) may be identified (see Figures 3.34, 3.36 and 3.37). With acute distemper viraemia, round to oval inclusions may occasionally be seen in CSF leucocytes (see Figure 3.6). Pathological haemorrhage (see Figure 3.27)

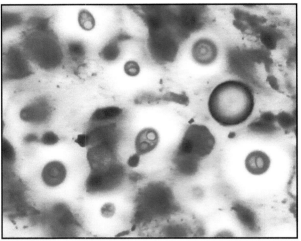

3.36 Spinal fluid from a dog with cryptococcal meningitis. Large *Cryptococcus neoformans* organisms with thick, non-staining capsules are visible. Note that the organism in the centre is exhibiting narrow-based budding. (Diff-Quik® stain; original magnification X50)

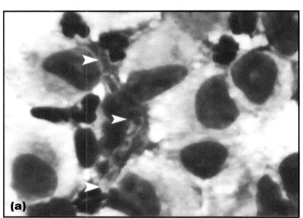

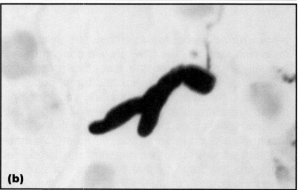

3.37 Spinal fluid from a dog with fungal meningitis due to aspergillosis. **(a)** A septate fungal hypha (arrowheads) is surrounded by large mononuclear phagocytes and neutrophils. (Wright–Giemsa stain; original magnification X100) **(b)** When stained with a special silver stain, the branching fungal hyphae appear black. (Gomori methenamine silver stain; original magnification X100)

may be associated with infectious, inflammatory, traumatic and neoplastic diseases. Most CNS neoplasms are typically poorly exfoliative; therefore, neoplastic cells are rarely identified in the CSF. An exception is CNS lymphoma, which can be associated with moderate to severe lymphocytic pleocytosis. Typically, a significant proportion of the lymphocytes are immature blasts (see Figure 3.31). However, blasts are not visible when neoplastic lymphocytes are well differentiated or when the tumour is extradural, as often occurs in feline lymphoma (Figure 3.38). With lysosomal storage diseases, large round, oval or linear inclusions may be identified uncommonly in CSF mononuclear cells (see Figure 3.3). Sample contaminants may also be observed, including:

- Keratinized, squamous epithelial cells
- Myelin (Zabolotzky *et al.*, 2010)
- Meningeal cells
- Ependymal cells (see Figure 3.26)
- Haemopoietic cells from the bone marrow
- Neuron cell bodies (rare).

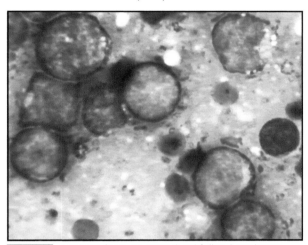

3.38 Aspirate from an extradural feline lymphoma. Large lymphoblasts with subtly indented nuclei, smooth chromatin, indistinct nucleoli and punctate cytoplasmic vacuoles are visible along with a single well differentiated lymphocyte (right). (Wright–Giemsa stain; original magnification X100)

Free myelin may be seen with diseases that are associated with myelin degeneration or damage (e.g. canine degenerative myelopathy), but, more commonly, is a contaminant encountered during CSF collection, particularly in lumbar samples, and is not associated with a more negative prognosis (Figure 3.39a; Zabolotzky *et al.*, 2010). Diseases that cause myelin degeneration or damage are more likely if the myelin has been phagocytosed by macrophages (Figure 3.39b).

Fine-needle aspiration and imprint cytology

Fine-needle aspiration and biopsy imprint cytology can be used to evaluate masses within the CNS (Vernau *et al.*, 2001; see Chapter 6). Fine-needle aspiration cytology is most effective when samples are collected using ultrasonography or computed

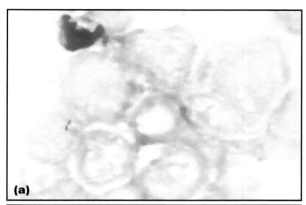

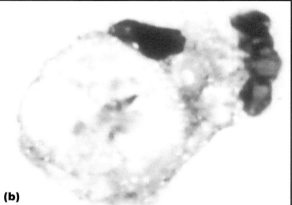

3.39 Spinal fluid samples containing myelin. **(a)** Free myelin is visible as a loose aggregate of circular, pink, moth-eaten material. **(b)** Curvilinear, pink, moth-eaten material is present within a phagocytic vacuole of a macrophage; darker red erythrocytes are visible to the right of the macrophage. (Diff-Quik® stain; original magnification X50)

tomography (CT) guidance. CNS cytology can provide a rapid, economical and (when samples are obtained by aspiration) minimally invasive technique to distinguish inflammatory lesions (Figure 3.40) from neoplastic lesions (see Figures 3.38 and 3.41). In one study (Platt *et al.*, 2002), cytology correctly identified lesions as neoplastic with 100% accuracy but histology was required to determine the specific tumour type. Cytology identified the cell origin of the tumour with 90% accuracy. The

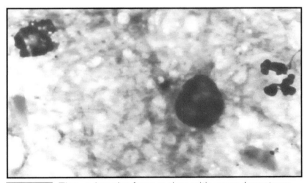

3.40 Tissue imprint from a dog with granulomatous meningoencephalomyelitis. A large neuron cell body with ill defined borders is visible with a single mature, non-degenerative neutrophil (left) and macrophage (right). (Wright–Giemsa stain; original magnification X50)

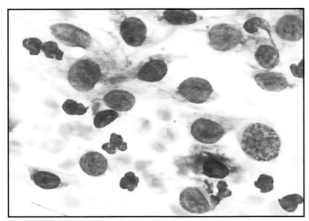

3.41 Tissue imprint from a dog with a meningioma. The cytoplasm of the neoplastic meningeal cells is fusiform and basophilic with ill defined, wispy borders. The oval nuclei exhibit malignant features, such as anisokaryosis (variable nuclear size), open, coarse chromatin and a few prominent nucleoli. (Wright–Giemsa stain; original magnification X50)

cytological diagnosis of the exact tumour type correlated with 50% of the histological diagnoses for samples obtained by needle biopsy and with 60% of those obtained from necropsy specimens.

Other specialized tests

Polymerase chain reaction

PCR for lymphocyte antigen receptor rearrangement (PARR) may be useful when:

- A questionable lymphocyte population has been identified on cytology (i.e. it is not possible based on cytomorphology alone to determine whether the lymphocytes are a mixed, reactive population or a clonal, neoplastic population)
- Staging lymphoma (Burnett et al., 2003; Keller et al., 2004; Lana et al., 2006; Avery, 2009)
- Clinical suspicion of CNS lymphoma is high but cytology of CSF samples is equivocal (Taylor et al., 2002; Scrideli et al., 2003; Pine et al., 2005).

PARR should not be used as a general screening test for lymphoma. In addition, immunodiagnostics (e.g. flow cytometry and immunostaining) are preferred to PARR to determine the phenotype of the lymphoma (i.e. whether it is a B cell or T cell). The sensitivity of PARR to detect lymphoma in dogs and cats is estimated at 75% and 65%, respectively. However, a negative result does not conclusively exclude lymphoma (Avery, 2009). Care should be taken when interpreting test results since other types of neoplasia (e.g. acute myeloid leukaemia) and non-neoplastic infectious conditions (e.g. ehrlichiosis) may yield a false-positive result (Burnett et al., 2003).

In general, suitable samples for PARR include blood, highly cellular fluid samples, fine-needle aspirates either in liquid transport medium or air-dried on a glass slide, and unfixed surgical biopsy specimens. CSF is not currently suitable for PARR because a minimum of 50,000 leucocytes is required and, even when pleocytosis is present, CSF samples typically do not contain this number of cells. Although this test is available for dogs and cats, publications describing PARR for CSF samples are limited to the human literature (Qin et al., 1998; Panzara et al., 1999; Taylor et al., 2002; Scrideli et al., 2003; Mattu et al., 2004; Pine et al., 2005).

Example

A sample of CSF from a patient with mild lymphocytic pleocytosis contains 25 leucocytes/microlitre.
A minimum of 50,000 lymphocytes are required for PARR.

Sample volume required for PARR: 50,000 / 25 = 2000 microlitres
2000 / 1000 = 2 millilitres

Electrophoresis

Protein electrophoresis, high-resolution protein electrophoresis, immunoelectrophoresis with or without isoelectric focusing, and ELISA of CSF samples are active areas of investigation. Without immunostaining (only available in human medicine), routine and high-resolution protein electrophoresis of paired serum and CSF samples cannot be used to determine the aetiology or general category of neurological diseases (Behr et al., 2006). Immunodiagnostics focused upon identifying unique diagnostic markers of disease or potential targets for future therapy are under development and their use may become more widespread as this area of knowledge expands (e.g. lysosomal storage disease markers, glial fibrillary acidic protein (GFAP) and anti-GFAP autoantibodies in necrotizing meningoencephalitis, and oligoclonal bands and myelin basic protein in degenerative myelopathy) (Yamato et al., 2004; Behr et al., 2006; Oji et al., 2007; Shibuya et al., 2007; Toda et al., 2007; Kamishina et al., 2008).

Acute phase proteins

Measurement of positive acute phase proteins (APPs; for example, C-reactive protein, alpha-2 macroglobulin, serum amyloid A, haptoglobin, alpha-1 acid glycoprotein) in serum and CSF has been applied to the diagnosis and management of steroid-responsive meningitis–arteritis (SRMA) in dogs (Bathen-Noethen et al., 2008; Lowrie et al., 2009ab). C-reactive protein concentration and that of other positive APPs may be useful when evaluating suspected SRMA cases, but the results should be interpreted judiciously since positive APP elevations are non-specific and routinely detected with most inflammatory, infectious, autoimmune, neoplastic and some metabolic diseases or, in the case of haptoglobin, with endogenous or exogenous hypercortisolaemia.

References and further reading

Available on accompanying DVD

DVD extras

- **Atlanto-occipital CSF collection**

4

Electrophysiology

Luc Poncelet and Roberto Poma[†]

Electrophysiological studies record the electrical activity of muscles or neural structures as a function of time. This activity can be spontaneous as in electroencephalography (EEG) and electromyography (EMG), or it may be the consequence of stimulation as in nerve conduction velocity (NCV) measurements and evoked potential studies.

Electrophysiological studies evaluate neural tissue, the neuromuscular junction and muscle function. They are minimally invasive but require sedation and frequently anaesthesia. The cost of the equipment and the experience needed for conducting these studies limit their use to academic and referral clinics.

Electrophysiological studies provide immediate and objective data but are rarely diagnostic of a specific disorder. Confirming the nature of lesions requires other diagnostic modalities such as imaging or tissue biopsy (see Chapters 5 and 6). Nevertheless, just as the functional information gathered from the neurological examination allows broad localization of the lesion and estimation of its severity (see Chapter 2), electrophysiological studies can confirm and refine this lesion localization and quantify its severity. In addition, indirect conclusions about the lesion type can often be drawn. For example, the results of motor nerve conduction studies provide information on whether the pathology is primarily affecting the myelin sheath or the axon. EEG patterns can also suggest a lesion type.

Electrophysiological investigations can address the efferent or afferent nervous system and can focus on either the peripheral or central components (Figure 4.1). In addition, the special senses and the cerebral cortex can be evaluated. From a functional point of view, the peripheral components include the neuronal cell bodies in the spinal cord intumescences, brainstem and ganglia, and the nerve roots of the respective peripheral nerves.

Afferent nervous system

The somatic afferent (sensory) nervous system pathways can be investigated by stimulating the peripheral nerves.

- The peripheral afferent system is evaluated using sensory and mixed NCV studies, where recordings are obtained from nerves rather than muscles. Provided that the efferent (motor) arm is normal, H-reflex testing can be used to investigate the peripheral afferent fibres.
- The central nervous system (CNS) is evaluated through somatosensory evoked potentials (SSEPs) that can be recorded at the level of the spine or skull.

Efferent nervous system

Somatic efferent (motor) system investigation involves recording the electrical activity of the effectors (muscles) after stimulation of the nervous tissue at various points in the peripheral nervous system (PNS) and CNS.

- The peripheral components are investigated by stimulating peripheral nerves for motor NCV, repetitive stimulation (RS) and F wave studies.
- Spontaneous electrical activity in muscles is recorded during EMG and forms an important adjunct. Single fibre EMG is a specialized test used to evaluate single myofibres in neuromuscular junctional disease.
- Magnetic and electrical stimulation of the brain and spinal cord has been used to investigate the central efferent pathways (Sylvester *et al.*, 1992;

Somatic afferent (sensory)		Somatic efferent (motor)		Special senses
Peripheral	*Central (+ peripheral)* [a]	*Peripheral*	*Central (+ peripheral)* [a]	
Sensory NCV Mixed NCV (+ motor fibres) [a] Reflex studies (+ efferent arm) [a]	SSEP	Motor NCV F wave studies RS EMG (+ muscles) [a]	Magnetic brain stimulation	BAEP ERG [b] VEP [b]

4.1 Overview of electrophysiological tests. Note that EEG reflects input–output activity of the cerebral cortex and thus cannot be included here. [a] May need to assess separately. [b] Not discussed in this chapter. BAEP = brainstem auditory evoked potential; EEG = electroencephalography; EMG = electromyography; ERG = electroretinogram; NCV = nerve conduction velocity; RS = repetitive stimulation; SSEP = somatosensory evoked potential; VEP = visual evoked potential.

Van Ham *et al.*, 1996). Magnetic brain stimulation and recording of evoked potentials in the extensor carpi radialis and tibialis cranialis muscles has been found useful in screening Dobermanns with clinically relevant spondylomyelopathy (da Costa *et al.*, 2006; De Decker *et al.*, 2011).

Special sensory systems

The special sensory systems can be studied by evoked potentials. The most widely used method is the brainstem auditory evoked potentials (BAEPs) recording (also known as the brainstem auditory evoked responses, BAERs) obtained in response to auditory stimuli. This test is used to investigate auditory function and to assess the functional integrity of the brainstem.

Cerebral cortex

The cerebral cortex can be evaluated with EEG. This technique records spontaneous activity originating mostly from the grouped activity (in the apical dendrites) of cortical neurons.

Types of recorded potential

Two types of potential may contribute to the recorded potentials: the compound action potential and the field potential. Field potentials can be further divided into near and far field potentials (Figure 4.2).

Compound action potentials

Compound action potentials represent the summation of action potentials travelling along muscle or nerve fibres. Each contribution to the potential originates from an action potential (depolarization followed by repolarization) approaching, passing by, and running distant to the recording electrode. In contrast, spontaneous muscle activity is most often a single fibre action potential. Examples of compound action potentials include:

- Voluntary and evoked muscle potentials
- Evoked nerve potentials
- Somatosensory evoked ascending potentials.

Compound action potentials in the normal patient display a variable latency, depending on the distance between the stimulation and recording points, but a relatively constant amplitude and waveform. Pathology alters the latency, amplitude and waveform.

Field potentials

Near field potentials

Near field potentials originate from potentials within cell bodies and processes of neuron groups in close proximity to the recording needle. They result from the synchronous activity of synapses. Each contribution is small and its amplitude diminishes quickly with distance. Being locally generated, near field potentials characteristically display a constant latency independent of the location of the recording electrode and an exponentially decreasing amplitude when the recording electrode is moved away from the potential generating structure. The neuron processes involved in the generation of such potentials should all run toward or away from the recording electrode to record a potential from a distance. Should the neuron processes run in a perpendicular direction or radiate in all directions, no potential would be recorded. Somatosensory cord dorsum potentials, medullary potentials and EEG potentials mostly comprise near field potentials.

Far field potentials

Far field potentials result from the lack of homogeneity of the nervous tissue in which the action potentials are travelling. Changes in the conductivity of the medium, the volume conductor size or the direction of the nerve fibres are the most common causes of far field potentials. For example, at the point where a nerve root enters the spinal cord, the surrounding tissue conductivity changes (i.e. due to epidural fat/cerebrospinal fluid), the volume conductor size changes (root/spinal cord) and the direction of the fibres change (ascending branches of the primary afferents). Far field potentials also display a constant latency but can sometimes be recorded from surprisingly long distances. Most BAEP waves comprise far field potentials.

Type of potential		Amplitude range	Origin	Source	Amplitude fct of distance [a]	Latency fct of distance [a]	Examples
Compound action potential	Muscle	mV	Travelling action potentials	Moving	Almost constant	Increases	CMAP
	Nerve fibre	μV	Travelling action potentials	Moving	Almost constant	Increases	CNAP AEP
Field potential	Near	μV	Currents caused by synaptic activity	Fixed	Exponential decrease	Constant	CDP EEG
	Far	μV	Anisotropy of the volume conductor	Fixed	Recordable from long distances	Constant	Some peaks of BAEP

4.2 Characteristics of recorded potentials. [a] Fct of distance = as a function of the distance from the generator (fixed source) or stimulation point (moving source). AEP = ascending (somatosensory) evoked potential; BAEP = brainstem auditory evoked potential; CDP = cord dorsum potential; CMAP = compound muscle action potential; CNAP = compound nerve action potential; EEG = electroencephalography.

Evaluation of the peripheral motor system

Neuromuscular weakness is the main indication for evaluation of the peripheral motor system, once circulatory, respiratory and metabolic aetiologies have been ruled out (see Chapter 18). Weakness may be of neural, neuromuscular junction or muscular origin. Hypotonia and hyporeflexia are usually observed clinically. Five procedures are of use for the evalu-ation of the peripheral motor system:

- EMG
- Motor NCV
- F wave evaluation
- Repetitive motor nerve stimulation
- Single fibre EMG.

These tests are usually conducted under general anaesthesia because nerve stimulation is painful and because the muscles of the animal must be relaxed in order to detect spontaneous activity. For example, it can be difficult to differentiate fibrillation potentials (spontaneous activity), which represent the coordinated firing of a group of muscle fibres, from voluntarily triggered motor unit activity on EMG without the use of anaesthesia. Voluntary motor activity can also be investigated, but since this requires the collaboration of conscious patients it is seldom used in dogs and cats.

Electromyography

Indications
EMG is used to identify denervated muscles and to identify and characterize myopathies.

Technique
With EMG, muscles are explored using a concentric needle electrode, which measures the electrical activity in a small muscle volume at its tip (Figure 4.3). Nearly all striated muscles can be probed including limb, masticatory, facial, laryngeal, pharyngeal, paraspinal, tail and anal sphincter muscles. A fairly extensive and accurate map of abnormal muscles can be built within a reasonable time (Griffiths and Duncan, 1978; Brown and Zaki, 1979; Farnbach, 1980; Van Ness, 1986a).

Normal findings
A normal relaxed muscle is electrically silent except in the endplate region; this is where endplate noise due to miniature endplate potentials and endplate spikes, thought to be caused by the presence of the electrode near the endplate, are recorded (Figure 4.4). During concentric needle electrode movements, mechanical triggering of muscle fibre potentials generates insertion potentials. The examiner should be familiar with these normal findings, which are related to random neurotransmitter release at the level of the neuromuscular junction and mechanical stimulation of the muscle fibres. By inserting the needle electrode to different depths and in different places a large volume of muscle can be explored.

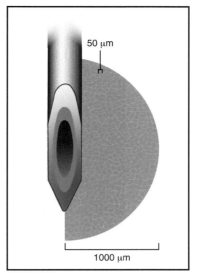

4.3 Relative sizes of the concentric needle electrode and the muscle fibre. The amplitude of the electrode potential decreases exponentially with distance; the electrode is not influenced by muscle fibres more than 1000 μm from its tip. The larger the recording electrode surface, the smaller the potential decay as a function of the distance – non-insulated needles or surface electrodes (alligator clips) give a more comprehensive picture of the underlying muscle activity.

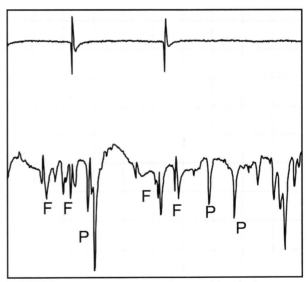

4.4 Spontaneous muscle fibre activity. An intact relaxed normal muscle is electrically silent, except in the endplate region where endplate noise and spikes are found (top tracing). In a denervated muscle, spontaneous electrical activity, such as fibrillation potentials (F) and positive sharp waves (P), may be recorded at various locations (bottom tracing). Vertical = 100 μV/div; horizontal = 10 ms/div; positivity downwards. (Courtesy of N Olby)

Abnormal findings
Five to ten days after the development of a peripheral motor nerve lesion (the time needed for degeneration of the distal axonal segment), denervated muscle fibres exhibit spontaneous depolarization, which is most often recorded in the form of fibrillation potentials and positive sharp waves (see Figure 4.4).

Multifocal muscle disease can result in the isolation of parts of the muscle fibres from the endplate region, and these isolated parts may exhibit spontaneous electrical activity. In cases of severe and long-standing neuromuscular junction blockade, such as is sometimes seen with myasthenia gravis, spontaneous activity may occasionally be recorded.

More complex spontaneous activity, called 'complex repetitive discharges' and characterized by an abrupt start and finish, is sometimes recorded and can be present with both neuropathic and myopathic disease (Figure 4.5). Myotonic discharges, characterized by a waxing and waning amplitude and frequency, are associated with myotonia in dogs.

Spontaneous activity objectively confirms a peripheral nerve or muscular problem and can also infrequently be recorded in junctional problems. EMG alone is unable to discriminate between these possible localizations and poorly correlates to the severity of the problem. Follow-up nerve conduction studies and frequently muscle and/or nerve biopsy are therefore indicated. Concurrent nerve and muscle lesions can also be encountered.

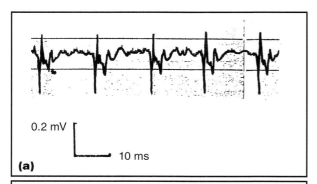

0.2 mV

10 ms

(a)

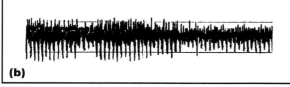

(b)

4.5 Spontaneous activities detected in a dog suffering from muscle disease associated with hyperadrenocorticism. **(a)** Complex repetitive discharges. **(b)** Slowly waxing activity sometimes called 'pseudomyotonia' (positivity downwards). (Reproduced from Poncelet *et al.*, 1992b with permission from the *Journal of Small Animal Practice*)

Maximum motor nerve conduction velocity

Indications
Motor nerve conduction studies are used to investigate suspected peripheral neuropathies.

Technique and findings
Motor NCV is obtained by stimulating a motor nerve at a minimum of two sites (Figure 4.6) and recording the evoked electrical activity, the compound muscle action potential (CMAP), in one of the target muscles each time (Figure 4.7).

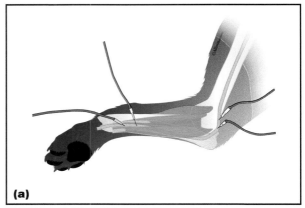

(a)

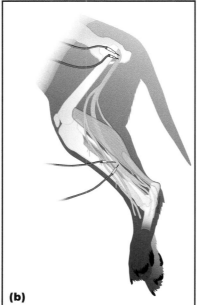

(b)

4.6 Two sites of placement for the stimulating electrodes for maximum motor NCV measurement at proximal and distal locations along **(a)** the ulnar nerve and **(b)** the sciatic–tibial nerve.

- For the thoracic limb, responses in the palmar interosseous muscles to ulnar nerve stimulation are used.
- For the pelvic limb, responses in the plantar interosseous muscles to sciatic–tibial nerve stimulation and responses in the short digital extensor muscles to sciatic–peroneal nerve stimulation are most often used.
- A two site stimulation procedure is also used to evaluate the recurrent laryngeal nerve.

Expected normal ranges for conduction velocity, CMAP amplitude and duration for each nerve have been established. However, it should be noted that the age of the patient and limb temperature can have an effect on the motor NCV of specific nerves. Target muscle responses to single location stimulation of radial, facial and pudendal nerves are also often recorded.

The stimulus is a square electrical pulse, 0.1 ms in duration, with a chosen intensity. It is delivered with a slow repetition rate of 1 or 1.5 Hz. The difference in

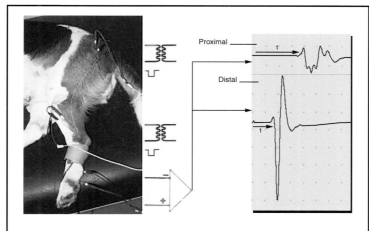

4.7 Maximum motor NCV. The sciatic–tibial nerve is stimulated at a proximal and a distal location and the resulting CMAPs from the plantar interosseous muscles are recorded (left). The onset latency (1) of the evoked muscle potential measured with the distal stimulation (lower tracing) is subtracted from the onset latency (1) measured with the proximal stimulation (upper tracing). The distance (mm) between the two stimulus locations (yellow pathway on photograph) is divided by the latency difference (ms) to give the maximum motor NCV (m/s) between the two stimulation points. The tracings on the right show a normal muscle response to distal stimulation but a low amplitude, polyphasic potential with proximal stimulation, suggesting conduction changes in the proximal part of the nerve. Vertical = 2 mV/div; horizontal = 2 ms/div; positivity downwards.

latency of the CMAP when the nerve is stimulated at two different sites is determined. The resulting latency difference (in ms) is divided by the distance between the two stimulating electrodes (in mm) (see Figure 4.7) and represents the maximum conduction velocity of the motor fibres in the nerve segment between the two stimulating electrodes (in m/s). The amplitude, duration and waveform of the CMAP are also recorded.

Three different types of change may be observed (Figure 4.8):

- CMAP amplitude is severely diminished and the conduction velocity slightly decreased with motor axon loss
- The conduction velocity is severely diminished and CMAP components dispersed with disorders of the myelin sheath
- CMAP to distal stimulation is normal but CMAP to proximal stimulation is altered or suppressed in conduction block as a result of focal demyelination.

With severe lesions CMAP recording becomes impossible. Mixed patterns of lesions, including nerve fibre loss, myelin sheath changes and demyelination are not uncommon. Consequently, clear-cut results only allow reasonable speculation about the lesion type and nerve biopsy is usually performed to characterize the pathology further.

F waves

Indications
With motor NCV studies, the nerve segment between the recording electrodes is directly addressed. Although lesions located either at root level or in nerve fibre terminals will affect CMAP recording, other methods are needed to confirm such lesions.

Technique and findings
When motor fibres are stimulated, action potentials travel along the fibres in an *orthodromic* way toward the target muscle and give rise to the CMAP. They also travel in an *antidromic* way toward the nerve cell bodies, causing subsequent depolarization. From time to time, another action potential can be triggered from the axon hillock of the depolarized neuron. These 'backfirings' give rise to the F waves, which have a longer latency and much lower amplitude and duration than the direct CMAP (Figure 4.9). F wave latencies vary somewhat depending on the conduction velocity of the backfiring motor fibre. The shortest F wave latency out of at least ten repetitions can be used for nerve root conduction evaluation.

The latency of the direct muscle response represents the conduction time in the distal part of the nerve fibre and in its slower conducting intramuscular branches, in addition to the time needed

Change	Distal stimulation			Proximal stimulation			Motor NCV
	Amplitude	*Duration*	*Latency*	*Amplitude*	*Duration*	*Latency*	
Neuron and motor fibre loss	↓	N	↑ or N	↓	N	↑ or N	↓ or N
Myelin sheath changes	↓	↑	↑	↓↓	↑↑	↑↑	↓↓
Segmental demyelination	N	N	N	↓	↑ or N	↑ or N	↓ or N

4.8 Expected evoked muscle potential changes in peripheral nerve diseases. Note that during the first 10 days after nerve damage, conditions involving neuron and motor fibre loss are similar to segmental demyelination. These broad indications may also be used for interpreting changes in nerve evoked potentials. N = within normal range.

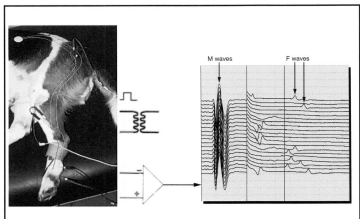

4.9 F wave study. When a motor nerve is stimulated, action potentials travel orthodromically (distal conduction time; green pathway on photograph) and trigger the direct muscle response. The action potentials also travel antidromically toward the spinal cord and may induce a backfiring in some motor neurons from the ventral horn cell. A successful backfiring takes 1 ms. These secondary action potentials travel to the target muscle and evoke F waves. The F wave latency represents the conduction time along the yellow pathway on the photograph and includes the 1 ms backfiring delay. In the tracings on the right, an F wave is not observed on each stimulation and those that are present are dispersed, indicating conduction blocks and conduction slowing at the level of the motor root. Vertical = 0.2 mV/div; horizontal = 5 ms/div; positivity downwards.

for neuromuscular transmission. Two variables can be calculated:

- F wave latency
- F ratio.

F wave latency: The F wave latency (F) represents the conduction time in the proximal part of the nerve fibre in two directions, the time needed for a successful reflection (1 ms) and the latency of the direct muscle response (M). Thus, the conduction time in the proximal part of the nerve can be calculated as (F-M-1)/2. Normal values for the ratio of conduction time to limb length are published elsewhere (Steiss, 1984).

F ratio: The ratio of conduction time in the proximal part of the nerve to conduction time in the distal part of the nerve is known as the F ratio and can be calculated as (F-M-1)/2M. This ratio increases above normal values in diseases that cause proximal conduction slowing, whilst it decreases below normal values in diseases that cause distal conduction slowing. The F ratio is independent of limb length measurements. Not only does the F ratio explore the proximal part of the nerve, but at the same time it is able to detect distal conduction problems (Poncelet and Balligand, 1991). The F ratio is also useful for investigating dogs with acute polyradiculoneuritis (Cuddon, 1998).

Repetitive stimulation

Indications
To investigate patients with suspected myasthenia gravis.

Technique and findings
The neuromuscular junction can be assessed by repetitive motor nerve stimulations with a repetition rate greater than that used for motor NCV measurements (usually 3–5 per second). The quantity of neurotransmitter delivered at the nerve fibre terminals normally decreases during repeated stimulation; however, it always remains above what is needed to efficiently trigger all muscle fibres in a

normal animal. This neurotransmitter excess is called the 'safety factor'. Should the number of functional motor plate receptors diminish, such as in myasthenia, the neurotransmitter quantity becomes relatively insufficient. Consequently, action potentials are not triggered in some muscle fibres, which then do not contribute to the CMAP after several stimuli. The amplitude of the CMAP therefore diminishes as the train of stimuli proceeds. A consistent ≥10% decrease in the CMAP amplitude during a train of 10 stimulations at a rate of 3 Hz is suggestive of myasthenia (Figure 4.10) (Malik *et al.*, 1989; Godde and Jaggy, 1993).

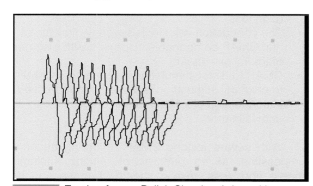

4.10 Tracing from a Polish Shepherd dog with myasthenia gravis using repetitive stimulation of the distal tibial nerve at 3 Hz. The amplitude of the responses diminishes rapidly as the train of stimuli proceeds. The amplitude of the tenth response is 24% less than that of the first response.

Single fibre electromyography

Indications
Single fibre EMG is the most sensitive and specific electrodiagnostic test for myasthenia gravis in humans.

Technique and findings
A fine concentric needle with a side-port close to its tip is used to measure the latency of action potentials following nerve stimulation in individual myofibres. The variation in this latency is called 'jitter' and is usually small. However, this variation

increases with disorders of neuromuscular transmission. Due to the technical difficulty of this test it is rarely performed in veterinary medicine, but its use in dogs (Hopkins *et al.*, 1993) and cats has been reported, as have normal values in dogs (Añor *et al.*, 2003).

Evaluation of the peripheral sensory system

Evaluation of the afferent component of peripheral nerves is indicated to comprehensively evaluate peripheral neuropathies. It is particularly important when investigating cases with suspected altered or diminished peripheral sensation.

Maximum sensory nerve conduction velocity

Indications
Measuring sensory NCV evaluates the peripheral afferent fibres and should be completed whenever a peripheral neuropathy is suspected.

Techniques and findings
Stimuli are delivered to the skin or to a sensory nerve branch and action potentials are recorded proximally from the nerve itself. The conduction velocity is determined by dividing the response latency by the distance between the stimulating and recording points (Figure 4.11), or by dividing the latency difference by the distance between the two recording points. Two recording points are not essential for sensory NCV measurement because the delay that occurs at the neuromuscular junction does not have to be accounted for as with motor NCV measurement.

This method is demanding because the amplitude of a compound action potential in a nerve is approximately 10^3 smaller than that in a muscle. Digitization of the response and an electronic average of 200–500 repetitions are needed to extract the compound action potential from the background electronic and physiological noise (see Figure 4.11). In addition, this method is prone to contamination by reflexively triggered muscle potentials; therefore, administration of a non-polarizing muscle relaxant (atracurium at a rate of 0.2 mg/kg i.v.) may be necessary. Correct placement of the stimulating and recording electrodes, and proper tuning of the stimulus intensity, is not as straightforward as in motor NCV studies (Holliday *et al.*, 1977; Redding *et al.*, 1982; Van Ness, 1985). Sensory nerves, such as the superficial branches of the radial nerve and the saphenous nerve, can be precisely investigated because they are associated with visible or palpable vascular structures (the accessory cephalic vein and the saphenous artery, respectively). Changes in sensory NCV are interpreted in the same way as motor NCV changes. However, amplitude and waveform changes should be interpreted with more caution since they are highly sensitive to procedure conditions.

However, considering that the fastest fibres are primarily involved in conduction velocity measure-

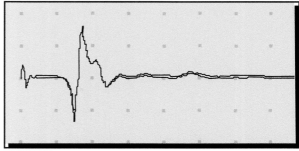

4.11 Sensory NCV. The skin on the dorsal aspect of the paw is stimulated (cathode proximal) and the action potential recorded in the radial nerve at the level of the humeral epicondylar crest. The latency is measured at the tip of the first peak and is divided by the distance between the stimulating cathode and the recording electrode. Vertical = 20 µV/div; horizontal = 1 ms/div; positivity downwards; average of 256 responses; two recordings superimposed.

ments, and that the fastest sensory fibres conduct at a higher speed than the fastest motor fibres, a mixed nerve study is a reasonable substitute to evaluation of a pure sensory nerve in most instances. A mixed nerve study has the advantage of allowing electrode placement and stimulus intensity to be checked by recording the M wave in the target muscle.

H-reflex evaluation

Indications
Evaluation of the H-reflex allows the afferent nerve root to be tested.

Technique
Whilst stimulating a peripheral mixed nerve, action potentials are also elicited in sensory fibres. IA fibres forming the afferent arm of the stretch reflex (see Chapter 1) are recruited and may trigger their target alpha-motor neurons, giving rise to the H-reflex (H refers to Hoffman – the name of the investigator who first described such a reflex in the calf muscle of humans). However, the antidromic volley in the motor neuron fibres cancels the reflex-elicited orthodromic action potentials by collision or by inducing a refractory period at the axon hillock level (Figure 4.12). To address this, the stimulus intensity is reduced to a low enough level to recruit IA afferent fibres (in principle more sensitive) without recruiting motor neuron axons, resulting in the elicitation of a pure H-reflex. However, such a situation is observed inconsistently in normal anaesthetized dogs. With increasing stimulus intensity, F waves are superimposed and eventually largely replace the H-reflex (Poncelet and Balligand, 1991). A technique that takes advantage of the double innervation of the plantar interosseous muscles (through the caudal cutaneous sural nerve and tibial nerve) may favour H-reflex recording in the hindlimb (Malik and Ho, 1991).

Cranial nerves
Cranial nerve reflexes can be recorded consistently (Figure 4.13). Stimulation of a branch of the trigeminal nerve (e.g. the infraorbital nerve) and

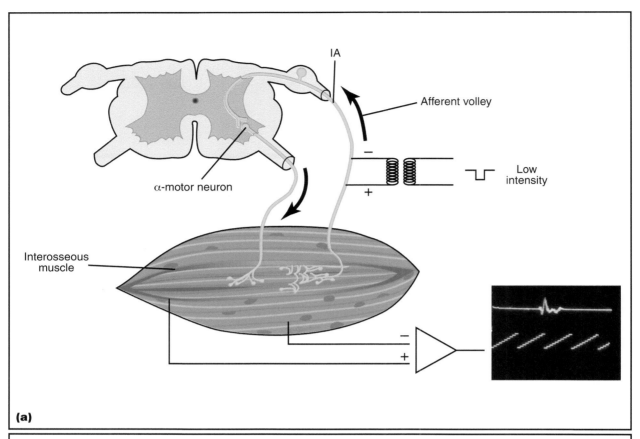

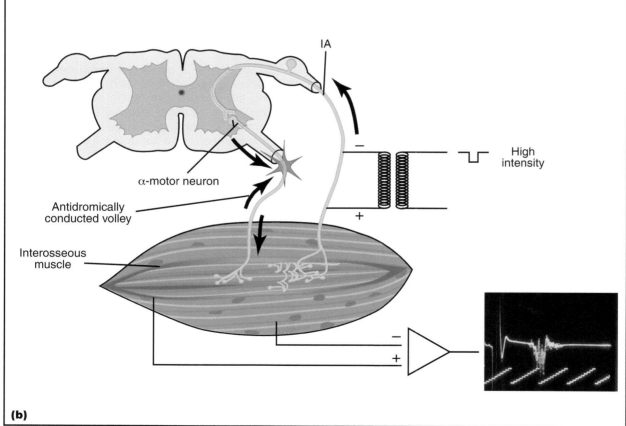

4.12 **(a)** At low stimulus intensity, IA fibres, which are the largest afferents coming from the muscle spindles, may be stimulated in isolation in some dogs to give a pure H-reflex. **(b)** At higher stimulus intensity, antidromically conducted action potentials are elicited in the alpha-motor neurons and cancel the reflexively triggered potentials (tibial nerve, plantar interosseous; positivity downwards).

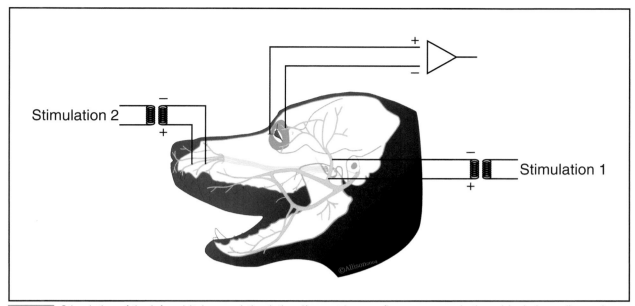

4.13 Stimulation of the infraorbital nerve (stimulation 2) may trigger reflex responses in the orbicularis oculi muscle (CN V–VII reflex) innervated by the facial nerve. The efferent branch of the reflex should first be assessed by stimulating the auriculopalpebral branch of the facial nerve (stimulation 1). (Modified from Whalen, 1985)

recording a facial nerve-innervated muscle (e.g. the orbicularis oculi) can be used to investigate the trigeminofacial reflex. If the efferent arm is found to be normal (assessed by stimulating the auriculo-palpebral branch of the facial nerve), the afferent maxillary nerve can be investigated through reflex testing. The trigemino-trigeminal reflex can be explored by recording the rostral belly of the digastric muscle whilst stimulating the infraorbital nerve (Whalen, 1985).

Perineal reflex
The perineal reflex can be investigated through stimulation of the perineal skin whilst recording from the anal sphincter (Cook *et al.*, 1991).

Evaluation of central afferent pathways

Somatosensory evoked potentials
Indications
Recording the electrical activity at the level of the spine or skull in response to stimulation of a peripheral sensory or mixed nerve allows the central (spinal cord and brain) afferent pathways and the dorsal nerve root to be investigated, provided the peripheral components are intact. Such potentials form SSEPs. These techniques are not commonly performed as they usually provide little diagnostic or prognostic information. However, as techniques become more sophisticated SSEPs may play an important role in the diagnosis and treatment of spinal cord disease.

Technique
The appropriate sensory or mixed nerve is stimulated as for nerve conduction studies. Stimulus frequency should be kept at <4 Hz and its intensity should be

monitored. The recording electrode can be seated in the interarcuate ligament at several different intervertebral spaces, up to the atlanto-occipital membrane. Averaging is needed to faithfully record these low amplitude potentials, as for sensory NCV. Most central conduction velocity measurements are performed with two recording electrodes positioned on either side of the spinal cord region to be evaluated. The reference electrode is seated in the paraspinal muscles at least 3 cm from the midline. Evoked potentials can also be recorded from electrodes positioned over the cranium (Holliday, 1992).

Four types of potential can be recorded over the spine:

- The nerve root component
- The cord dorsum potential
- The ascending evoked potential
- The medullary component.

Nerve root component: The nerve root component is recorded over the L6–L7 intervertebral space (with pelvic limb nerve stimulation; Figure 4.14). It represents the afferent volley in the dorsal roots and antidromically conducted potentials in the ventral roots. It is similar to a mixed nerve compound action potential (CAP).

Cord dorsum potential: The cord dorsum potential is essentially a near field potential best recorded over the lumbosacral spinal cord intumescence with pelvic limb nerve stimulation, or over the cervical spinal cord intumescence with thoracic limb nerve stimulation. It comprises small early deflections (attributed to the intramedullary path of the afferent fibres) and a large negative deflection (result of the activity of interneurons), followed by a long duration blunted wave (caused by the primary afferent depolarization phenomenon; see Figure 4.14).

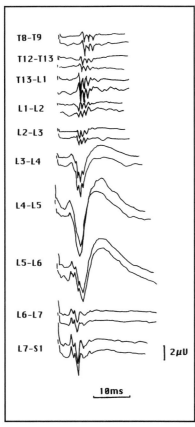

T8-T9

T12-T13

T13-L1

L1-L2

L2-L3

L3-L4

L4-L5

L5-L6

L6-L7

L7-S1

2µV

10ms

4.14

SSEPs recorded along the lumbar and thoracic spine in response to tibial nerve stimulation (two repetitions are superimposed). Caudocranially, the root component (L7–S1 and L6–L7), the large interneuronal component (from L5–L6 to L3–L4) and the ascending evoked potential (from L2–L3) can be recognized. Note that positivity is up in these tracings. (See text for details about waveforms.) (Reproduced from Poncelet *et al.*, 1992a with permission from the *American Journal of Veterinary Research*)

Ascending evoked potential: The ascending evoked potential can be followed over the thoracolumbar and cervical spine. This is typically a CAP. Its latency increases as the recording site moves cranially. A CAP is a small amplitude potential displaying at least three successive positive/negative deflections (see Figure 4.14). Dorsal funiculi and the dorsal part of the lateral funiculi produce the majority of the potential.

Medullary component: The medullary component is recorded at the atlanto-occipital junction. It has the characteristics of a near field potential and is thought to result from the activation of the medullary somatosensory relay nuclei, followed by a recurrent inhibition. It comprises a negative wave followed by a blunted positive wave, corresponding to interneuron relaying and recurrent inhibition, respectively.

Scalp-recorded SSEPs display a positive/negative deflection with many characteristics of near field potentials. Later waves can be recorded, but are usually cancelled by most anaesthesia protocols. Waveform and amplitude may change dramatically depending on the location of the recording electrode on the head. The precise neural generators have not been defined in dogs or cats.

SSEPs in spinal cord lesions
Two main goals of the neurological examination are localization of the lesion and evaluation of its severity. Several efforts have been made to use SSEPs to confirm, refine and quantify observations

drawn from the neurological investigation, especially with the frequent complaint of acute, focal spinal cord damage. With increasing severity of spinal cord injury, SSEPs remain recordable at the level of the scalp whilst being undetectable at the level of the spine cranial to the lesion. However, both types of SSEP recording disappear before the subjective conscious pain perception (nociception) test becomes markedly reduced or absent (Poncelet *et al.*, 1993). Consequently, whilst recording SSEPs cranial to the site of spinal cord compression confirms a mild lesion, SSEP disappearance does not carry the same poor functional prognosis as does the absence of nociception (Holliday, 1992).

However, SSEP recording may be of help in several situations, including:

- Where imaging is unable to delineate a focal cord lesion
- Where more than one lesion is visible on imaging
- In cases of inflammatory, infectious and degenerative diseases where no macroscopic lesion is present.

If more than one site of spinal cord compression is present, desynchronization of the ascending evoked potential components is evident cranial to an old clinically silent lesion (Poncelet *et al.*, 1993). In addition, a reduced SSEP medullary component amplitude has been found in Cavalier King Charles Spaniels with syringomyelia, providing a tool to objectively evaluate the functional damage (Harcourt-Brown *et al.*, 2011).

Evoked injury potentials
When an ascending volley of the SSEP action potential is blocked before reaching the recording electrode, a monophasic positive potential is recorded. If it is blocked just after the recording electrode, a biphasic positive–negative potential is recorded. This transition makes it possible to precisely identify the location of the conduction block along the spinal cord (Figure 4.15). Contrary to ascending evoked potentials or scalp-recorded potentials, the amplitude of the evoked injury potential (EIP) has a tendency to increase with lesion severity (Poncelet *et al.*, 1998). Unfortunately, the relationship between EIP amplitude and clinical severity grading is too loose to be used as an objective measurement of lesion severity.

The EIP can also be used to discriminate between focal and diffuse lesions. With focal lesions an EIP can be recorded, whilst with diffuse lesions a progressive caudocranial decrement of the ascending evoked potential is expected.

SSEPs in brain lesions
With brain lesions the scalp-recorded SSEP is often abnormal. A normal medullary component excludes concurrent spinal cord or peripheral lesions. The use of SSEP to diagnose brain lesions has not been evaluated in veterinary medicine.

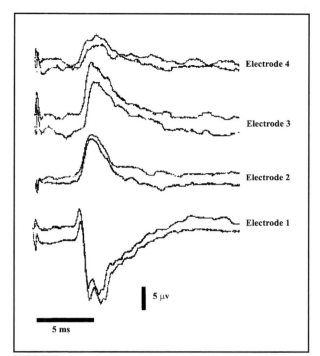

4.15 EIPs in the vicinity of a severe disc herniation. Caudocranial recordings (from bottom to top) over a distance of 2 cm, demonstrating the EIP waveform change from a biphasic to a monophasic character that takes place at the conduction block location. Note that positivity is up in these tracings. (Reproduced from Poncelet *et al.*, 1998 with permission from the *American Journal of Veterinary Research*)

Special senses

Brainstem auditory evoked potentials

BAEP is probably the most widely used electro-physiological test in veterinary medicine. Sounds are used to stimulate the auditory system and the resultant electrical activity is recorded by electrodes placed at strategic sites on the skull. As auditory stimuli are used for this test the functional integrity of the structures of the outer, middle and inner ear is evaluated in addition to the nervous system.

Technique

The most widely used stimulus is the click, which is obtained by feeding a 0.1 ms rectangular electrical pulse to an ear phone. The sound stimulus reaches the ear canal via tubal inserts. The stimulus can include frequencies up to 10 kHz (large band stimulus) and consequently has poor frequency specificity. The ear phone transducer reacts to this electrical stimulus by generating a short duration damped sine pressure wave. By reversing the polarity of the electrical pulse, the polarity of the pressure wave is also reversed (Figure 4.16). Most investigators work with alternating polarity click stimuli as this cancels the electromagnetic artefact from the transducer. Unfortunately, this also cancels the diagnostically relevant cochlear microphonic potentials resulting from cochlear hair cell electrical activity. Each ear is tested in turn, but attenuated stimuli are

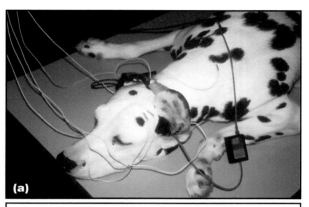

(a)

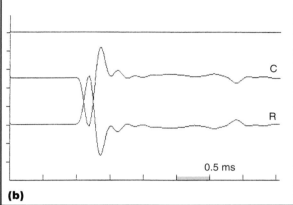

(b)

4.16 **(a)** Set up for recording BAEPs. The recording electrodes are seated at the vertex, the reference electrode in the mastoid area and the ground electrode in the neck area. The transducers are connected to silicone tubing ending with a polyurethane foam cylinder fitted in the external auditory meatus. **(b)** A 0.1 ms rectangular electrical pulse generates a complex pressure wave that may begin with a pressure rise (condensation click, C) or a pressure drop (rarefaction click, R) according to its polarity. The upper tracing is the electronic sum of the two pressure tracings (a zero line), proving that the transducer faithfully reverses the signal.

transmitted to the untested ear through bony conduction. To address this, a wide band continuous masking noise (with an intensity lower than that of the click) is delivered to the untested ear.

The current information available regarding tone evoked auditory potentials in dogs (used to assess hearing at different frequencies) has been obtained under a wide range of different technical conditions and cannot be effectively compared. Exploring the brainstem response in the frequency domain rather than the time domain relies on long duration stimuli with a specific frequency and avoids most of the difficulties associated with the use of short duration tone bursts. In the future, this method might become the way of exploring auditory function at a specific frequency (Markessis *et al.*, 2006).

Findings

In response to click stimuli, the skull electrodes record a succession of positive/negative deflections, which are divided into short, middle and long latency responses. Middle and long latency responses are extremely sensitive to arousal status and, as such, middle latency auditory evoked potentials have been investigated as a tool to monitor anaesthetic depth in sedated patients (Pijpendop *et al.*, 1999). Short latency responses are evaluated when testing hearing.

Short latency responses are usually obtained in dogs and cats under sedation or anaesthesia due to poor tolerance of the skull electrodes and tubal inserts placed in the ears. They comprise five successive positive/negative deflections (numbered with Roman numerals). Some of the deflections, usually IV and V, may be fused and in some individuals further later deflections may be recognized. There has been much speculation about the neural generators responsible for these deflection peaks. Peak I most commonly results from the afferent volley in the auditory nerve. For the subsequent deflections no simple relationship can be established between the relay nuclei and peaks. It seems that all the waves (I–V) are generated by structures caudal to the caudal colliculi (Figure 4.17). Most of the afferent fibres cross the midline and may do so at different levels in the brainstem.

BAEPs in deafness

BAEP recording is widely used as a screening test to identify complete deafness in individuals of breeds prone to hereditary hearing losses, such as the Dalmatian (see Chapter 12). It has proven an invaluable tool in the investigation and control of congenital deafness in numerous dog breeds. The method is objective and identifies unilateral abnormalities that subjective observation of behavioural responses to loud noise cannot do. Regardless of the methodological differences among investigators, BAEP to high intensity click stimuli (60–90 dB normal hearing level) has proved very efficient (Holliday *et al.*, 1992; Strain *et al.*, 1992) with a very low occurrence of equivocal results in puppies. Puppies are usually tested around 45 days of age. A second test can be performed a few weeks later if the results are unclear.

Findings: The presence of waveforms, their latency and amplitude are all considered; although, identification of congenitally deaf animals is simply based on the presence or absence of waveforms.

- The latency of the different peaks increases and amplitude diminishes when the stimulus intensity is lowered in normal animals. Wave V is the last wave to disappear as the stimulus intensity is reduced.
- An increase in the latency of all peaks when using high intensity stimuli suggests external and middle ear transmission problems since the stimulus reaching the cochlea is attenuated by

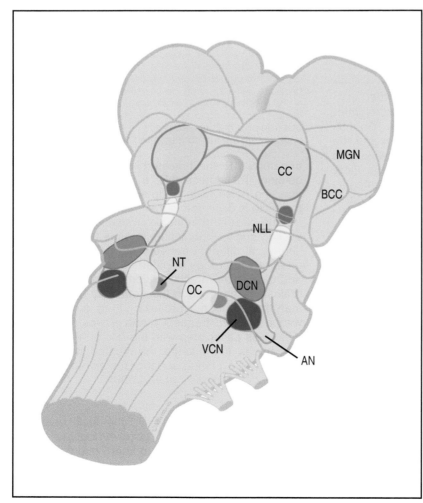

4.17 Auditory nuclei and pathways in the brainstem. All deflection peaks (I–V) of the short latency auditory evoked potentials are generated by structures distal to the caudal colliculi (Moore, 1987). Except for peak I, which mostly originates from the auditory nerve, no simple relationship exists between a given peak and a structure. All information eventually crosses the midline, although it can do so at different levels. AN = auditory nerve; BCC = brachium of the caudal colliculus; CC = caudal colliculus; DCN = dorsal cochlear nucleus; MGN = medial geniculate nucleus; NLL = nuclei of the lateral lemniscus; NT = nucleus of the trapezoid body; OC = olivary complex; VCN = ventral cochlear nucleus.

pathology. The interpeak latency differences are unchanged as the cochlea and brainstem are normal.

- Near normal peak I latency suggests normal cochlear and cranial nerve (CN) VIII function, whilst altered later peak latencies suggest brainstem involvement. Exploring the whole range of stimulus intensity may identify 'partial' hearing loss.
- The click intensity required for threshold response recording increases in the presence of transmission problems in the outer and middle ear as well as with endocochlear and retrocochlear lesions.
- Although relatively infrequently performed, partial hearing loss can be identified and investigated further by repeating the BAEP at progressively lower stimulus intensities. To do this the latency of wave V is recorded as a function of the click stimulus intensity (Figure 4.18). The slope of the curve generated from these data in the low intensity range (threshold to threshold plus 40–50 dB; defined as the regression line) is normal with conductive hearing loss (i.e. disease of the outer or middle ear), whilst it may be steeper with sensory hearing loss (i.e. disease of the sensory apparatus of the inner ear) (Shiu *et al.*, 1997; Poncelet *et al.*, 2000). Further anatomical–functional association studies in dogs and cats are needed before definitive guidelines for interpretation can be established.

BAEPs in brainstem lesions
Changes in waves II–V of the BAEP have been reported in association with various brain lesions

(Fisher and Obermaier, 1994; Steiss *et al.*, 1994). A common measurement taken is the time elapsed from the peak of wave I to the peak of wave V. This is called the central conduction time and believed to represent the time taken for conduction through the brainstem. As expected, caudal fossa lesions can profoundly affect the BAEP, but cerebral disease can also influence the recordings by causing a caudal brain shift or herniation that affects the brainstem. BAEPs are therefore not useful for the precise localization of a brainstem lesion, but could potentially be useful in anticipating life-threatening conditions such as intracranial pressure elevation, cerebellar herniation and brainstem compression.

BAEPs may be of special interest in vestibular syndrome where the differentiation between central and peripheral localization is of paramount prognostic significance (see Chapter 11). The intimate anatomical association between the vestibular and auditory systems makes BAEP testing a worthwhile investigation. Frequently in peripheral vestibular disease the ipsilateral BAEP is abnormal. With central lesions, such as cerebellomedullary pontine angle tumours, BAEPs to both ipsilateral and contralateral stimulations may be affected since most of the contralateral afferent fibres cross the midline. In central disease, wave I may be expected to be normal as the nerve is external to the lesion, but in practice large compressive extra-axial masses can sometimes compress the peripheral nerve as it enters the brain. Such testing may improve the discrimination between central and peripheral vestibular syndrome. Confirming bilateral deafness is additional vital evidence in the diagnosis of bilateral symmetrical vestibular disease. Although behaviourally hearing, Jack Russell Terriers with

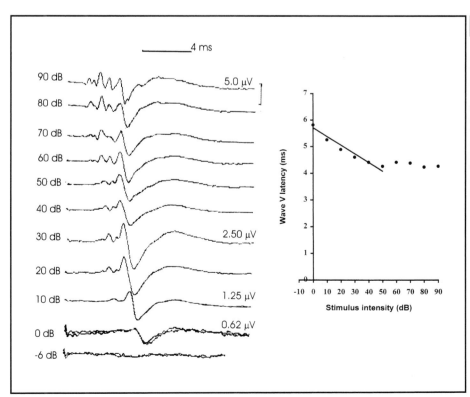

4.18 Short latency auditory evoked potentials in response to click stimuli of decreasing intensity from 90 to –6 dB normal hearing level (left panel). The right panel records the latency of wave V as a function of the stimulus intensity. The slope of the regression line fitting the points in the lower intensity range may have diagnostic value in detecting partial deafness. (Reproduced from Poncelet *et al.*, 2000 with permission from the *Journal of Veterinary Internal Medicine*)

hereditary ataxia often display abnormal BAEP tracings with prominent waves I and II, and dampened or absent following waves (Wessmann *et al.*, 2004). These specific changes may contribute to the diagnosis.

Ophthalmological electrophysiological testing

Two diagnostic modalities exist to evaluate the function of the visual pathways:

- Electroretinogram (ERG) – evaluates the retina
- Visual evoked potentials (VEPs) – evaluate the central visual pathways.

Discussion of these tests is outwith the scope of this Manual and the reader is referred to the *BSAVA Manual of Canine and Feline Ophthalmology* for further information (see also Chapter 10 for specific indications for these tests).

Electroencephalography

With the advent of digital EEG and video-synchronized EEG systems (where available), veterinary EEG is once again becoming a crucial diagnostic tool for the detection of seizure activity, determination of focal cerebral lesions and the management of the refractory epileptic patient.

Neurophysiology

EEG is the recording of spontaneous electrical activity in the cerebral cortex and represents the difference in voltage between two different but specific cerebral locations over time (Fisch, 1999). The EEG signal is generated by cerebral neurons (pyramidal neurons) located in different layers of the neocortex. Pyramidal neurons are constantly influenced by synaptic activity (excitatory and inhibitory postsynaptic potentials): an excitatory synapse acts like a battery, driving current into the pyramidal cell and then outward to the extracellular space, and the reverse holds true for an inhibitory synapse. This generates a variation in potential difference between the intracellular and extracellular space.

The EEG signal represents the sum of the electrical activity generated by large populations of pyramidal neurons (10^5 or more). The process of current flow between the electrical generator (pyramidal neuron) and the recording electrode is called volume conduction (Figure 4.19) (Fisch, 1999; Buzsaki *et al.*, 2003). The EEG signal is modified by multiple factors, including:

- The electrical conductive properties of the tissues
- The distance between the electrical source and the recording electrode on the scalp (Figure 4.20)
- The conductive properties of the electrode itself
- The orientation of the cortical generator to the recording electrode. The source area for a given electrode is maximized when the orientation of the active cortical region is face-on (radial dipole).

Recording technique

The basic functional units of an EEG circuit include recording electrodes, amplifiers and a computer (including monitor). Recording electrodes conduct electrical potentials from the patient to the EEG machine. The most common types of EEG electrodes

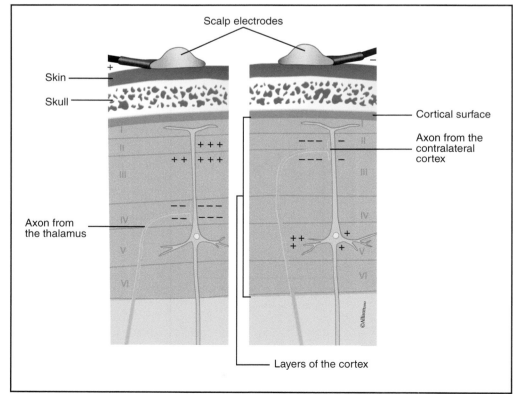

4.19 Generation of extracellular voltage fields from excitatory and inhibitory synaptic activity. The relationship between surface polarity and the site of dendritic postsynaptic potentials is also shown.

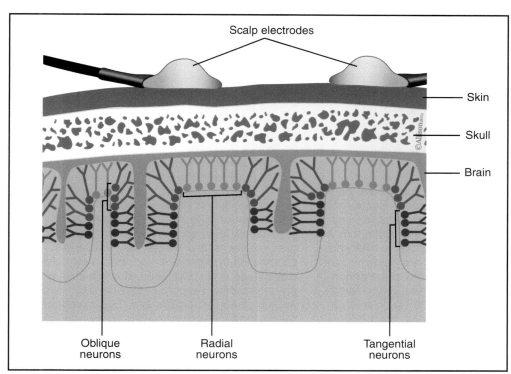

4.20 Position of EEG scalp electrodes in relation to the cortical pyramidal neurons. Note that the EEG signal is modified by the electrical conductive properties of the tissues between the electrical source and the recording electrode, the orientation of the cortical generator to the recording electrode, and the conductive properties of the recording electrode. Only radially oriented neurons closest to the skull significantly influence the recording electrodes.

Scalp electrodes

Skin

Skull

Brain

Oblique neurons

Radial neurons

Tangential neurons

are scalp electrodes, subdermal electrodes, sphenoidal electrodes, subdural electrodes and depth electrodes. In veterinary EEG, scalp electrodes (cup/disc) and subdermal electrodes (needle/wiring) are the most commonly used for clinical applications.

The placement of the electrodes ('electrode array') is adapted from the widely recognized human international system (the 'ten-twenty system'). Nomenclature of the electrodes follows the conventional method adopted by the International Federation of Societies for EEG and Clinical Neurophysiology. Each electrode is denoted by a letter, which corresponds to the cortical lobe from which the EEG signal originates (e.g. F = frontal), and by a number, which represents the 'site' and 'side'. Odd numbers refer to the left side of the head (e.g. F3) whilst even numbers refer to the right side (e.g. F4). EEG electrodes positioned along the midline are expressed with the letter 'z' (e.g. Fz) (Jasper, 1958).

The number of electrodes mounted on the scalp varies according to the patient's head size and shape. Generally, a minimum of 5 to a maximum of 12 active electrodes are used, in addition to a reference and a ground electrode located in neutral positions. The active electrodes are placed on each half of the head and along the midline over the corresponding cortical lobe (frontal, temporal, parietal and occipital; Figure 4.21).

The process of recording from a pair of electrodes in an EEG channel is called 'derivation'. EEG amplifiers have a predefined number of channels, each comprising two inputs (input 1 and input 2), which represent the location where the EEG signal is sent to be amplified. By convention, input 1 is the first of a pair of recording electrodes, and input 2 is the second. Polarity convention for display of the

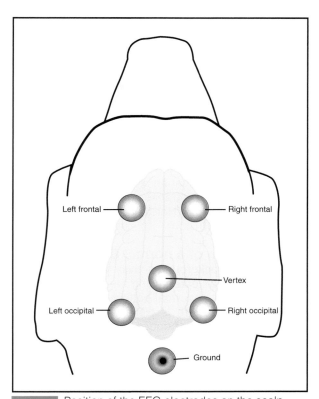

Left frontal

Right frontal

Vertex

Left occipital

Right occipital

Ground

4.21 Position of the EEG electrodes on the scalp. Reference and ground electrodes are located in neutral positions.

EEG signal is negative-up and is expressed by the following rule:

- When input 1 is more negative than input 2, the waveform shows upward deflection

- When input 2 is more negative than input 1, the waveform shows downward deflection.

The particular arrangement by which a number of derivations are displayed simultaneously in an EEG recording is called an electrode montage. Common types of electrode montage include:

- Bipolar montages (longitudinal and transverse)
- Referential montages (reference in a neutral place or linked ear electrodes).

In bipolar montages, input 1 and input 2 are connected to active recording electrodes. Sequential pairs of electrodes are linked in longitudinal or transverse lines. The site of maximum voltage within a field appears as a phase reversal (i.e. waveforms amplified by input 1 and input 2 are facing each other). Bipolar montages eliminate the effect of contaminated references and localize relatively discrete focal abnormalities (Niedermeyer, 2004). In referential montages, a common reference electrode is connected to input 2 of each amplifier and is usually placed 2 cm distal to the last midline electrode (e.g. Pz). This type of montage allows clear characterization of widespread or complex potential fields by recognizing the location of maximum potential on the head.

For reliable recording and interpretation of EEG traces, cortical electrical activity should be recorded during all stages of consciousness, including full arousal, drowsiness, non-REM (rapid eye movement) sleep and REM sleep. Conventional short-term EEG recordings usually last 20–40 minutes, often precluding the observation of all different stages of consciousness and detection of pathological activity. Long-term EEG recording, lasting from a few hours to several days, is now feasible and allows monitoring of the different stages of consciousness. General anaesthesia should be avoided when recording EEG traces since it can significantly affect the readings (Holliday and Williams, 1998; Itamoto *et al.*, 2001).

Interpretation of a normal EEG

By definition, background activity is characterized as any EEG activity representing the setting in which a given normal or abnormal pattern appears and from which such a pattern is distinguished (Chatrian *et al.*, 1999). Numerous frequency bands are observed during an EEG recording, depending on the state of arousal and activity of the patient. The most common EEG frequency bands are characterized by the following ranges:

- Delta: <4 Hz
- Theta: 4–<8 Hz
- Alpha: 8–≤13 Hz
- Beta: 13–30 Hz
- Gamma: 30–60 Hz.

Since age and state of arousal influence EEG analysis, clinicians should be given the required information prior to interpretation. Physiological state of arousal is correlated to specific frequency bands and can be subdivided as follows:

- Awake (eyes open): beta (18–25 Hz)
- Relaxed (eyes closed): alpha (8–13 Hz)
- Stage 1 sleep: theta (4–8 Hz)
- Stage 2 sleep: 12–14 Hz (with the presence of sleep transients)
- Stages 3 and 4 sleep: delta waves (or slow wave sleep) (1–4 Hz)
- REM sleep: 3–7 Hz (equivalent to theta and/or stage 1 sleep).

Activity during sleep is characterized by specific waveforms of differing morphology. The most common sleep features include sleep transients (spindles, vertex sharp waves, K complexes), positive occipital sharp transients, occipital slow waves, slow wave sleep and REM sleep. K complexes constitute an impressive response to arousing stimuli and appear during stage 2 sleep. The maximum occurrence appears over the vertex area and they consist of an initial sharp component followed by a slow component (Niedermeyer, 2004; Figure 4.22).

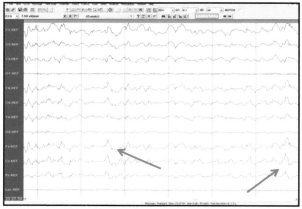

4.22 Diffuse K complexes (arrowed) observed in a dog during sleep. Note the initial negative peak followed by a slow positive component. Referential montage; timescale = 50 mm/s; time line interval = 1.0 s.

Physiological artefacts (e.g. eye movements, blinking, masticatory muscle activity, heartbeat and panting; Figure 4.23) and non-physiological artefacts (e.g. instrumental, environmental and electrode-related) often obscure and interfere with the recordings. The examiner must be aware of and recognize these artefacts when examining the tracings, and should interpret with caution abnormal waveforms displayed on the computer screen.

Clinical applications

The clinical applications of EEG include:

- Detection of epileptic activity (is it a seizure or not?)
- Detection of epileptic syndromes (does the patient suffer from a specific epileptic syndrome?) (Figure 4.24)
- Localization of the seizure focus (where does the seizure originate from?) (Figure 4.25)

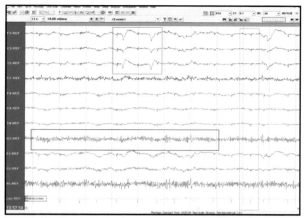

4.23 Physiological artefacts recorded in a dog: eye blink (red box), muscle activity (black box) and heartbeat (green box). Referential montage; timescale = 10 s/page; time line interval = 1.0 s.

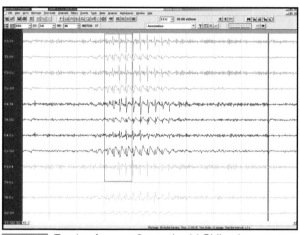

4.24 Tracing from an 8-month-old Chihuahua presented with transient episodes of abnormal demeanour associated with myoclonic twitching of the head and nose. Note the 4 Hz spike and generalized wave discharges (black box), suggestive of absence seizures. Bipolar montage; timescale = 30 mm/s; time line interval = 1.0 s.

- Monitoring the response to antiepileptic drugs (does pathological cortical electrical activity respond to short and/or long-term treatment?) (Figure 4.26)
- Recognition of focal and diffuse disturbances in cerebral functioning (are the EEG abnormalities suggestive of a bilaterally symmetrical encephalopathy or a focal brain lesion?) (Figure 4.27)
- Brain death (is cortical electrical activity still present?).

When interpreting an EEG tracing, clinicians should be able to differentiate normal from abnormal activity, state of arousal (awake or asleep), epileptiform from non-epileptiform activity, and ictal from interictal activity. An abnormal EEG is classified as having either specific or non-specific abnormalities.

- Specific EEG abnormalities include epileptiform and paroxysmal activity characterized by

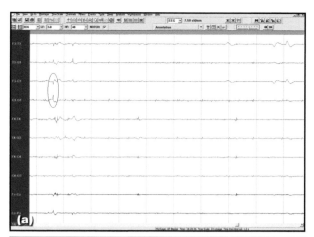

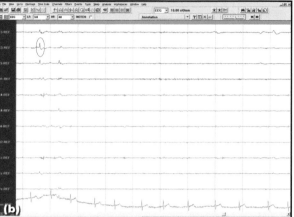

4.25 Tracings from a 3-year-old mixed-breed dog presented with focal seizures secondary to an intracranial meningioma located in the left cerebral hemisphere. **(a)** Interictal focal epileptiform activity (spikes) on the left cerebral hemisphere characterized by true phase reversal. Bipolar montage; timescale = 10 s/page; time line interval = 1.0 s. **(b)** The site of maximum negativity is circled. Referential montage; timescale = 10 s/page; time line interval = 1.0 s.

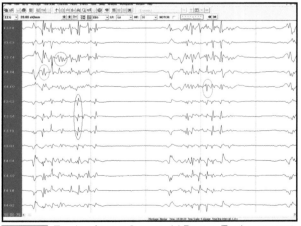

4.26 Tracing from a 3-year-old Boston Terrier presented in status epilepticus. The recording was obtained during treatment with a constant rate infusion of propofol, which was used in an attempt to suppress pathological cortical electrical activity. The tracing shows epileptiform activity, characterized by a burst of polyphasic waveforms (purple oval), spikes (black oval), sharp waves (red oval) and spike and waves (green oval). Bipolar montage; timescale = 5 s/page; time line interval = 1.0 s.

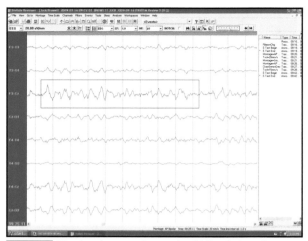

4.27 Tracing from an 8-month-old Dachshund diagnosed with hepatic encephalopathy secondary to a portosystemic shunt. The patient was awake. Note the diffuse, bilaterally symmetrical slow (delta) waves (black box). The EEG waveforms returned to normal frequency and morphology after successful correction of the portosystemic shunt. Bipolar montage; timescale = 20 mm/s; time line interval = 1.0 s.

interictal or ictal discharges. Epileptiform activity is represented by:
- Spikes (single or random)
- Sharp waves
- Polyspikes of multiple spikes
- Spike and wave complexes.
• Non-specific EEG abnormalities include:

- Slowing of the background activity (often in the delta frequency), which is not consistent with the behavioural state. The abnormalities can be localized (focal brain lesions) or diffuse (encephalopathy)
- Generalized periodic sharp waves with triphasic morphology (triphasic waves). Classically associated with metabolic encephalopathies, particularly hepatic encephalopathy. The wave typically displays a negative–positive–negative polarity and is difficult to distinguish from epileptiform activity.

Numerous studies and case reports have been published in the veterinary literature regarding the presence and suspected significance of abnormal EEG activity; although, major limitations were encountered with equipment, length of recording and patient cooperation (Holliday *et al.,* 1970; Holliday and Williams, 1998; Jaggy and Bernardini, 1998; Berendt *et al.*, 1999; Poma *et al.*, 2010; Raith *et al.*, 2010). The advent of digital EEG and video-synchronization of recordings allows better determination of clinical abnormalities and scientific rationality in decision-making for the management of critically ill patients.

References and further reading

Available on accompanying DVD

5

Neuroimaging

Natasha Olby and Donald E. Thrall

The central nervous system (CNS) is encased in the bones of the skull and the spine. Consequently, CNS, and to a certain extent peripheral nervous system (PNS) disease can result both from disorders of the nervous system itself (e.g. inflammatory, neoplastic and degenerative diseases) and from disorders of the bones and soft tissues that encase and protect the nervous system. Therefore, when imaging the nervous system, the ability of the modality to depict lesions in bone and/or soft tissue must be appreciated. Imaging of osseous lesions can be achieved with radiography and computed tomography (CT), whilst imaging of the soft tissues is optimized with techniques that provide greater soft tissue contrast resolution, such as ultrasonography, myelography, contrast-enhanced CT, CT myelography and magnetic resonance imaging (MRI). It is important to understand that the results of nervous system imaging can only be interpreted in the context of the clinical findings of each individual animal. Many dramatic anatomical abnormalities, such as hemivertebrae and hydrocephalus, can be clinically insignificant.

Radiography

Survey radiography is a useful first-line modality for the evaluation of bone, and to a lesser extent, soft tissue. Spinal radiographs can be used to identify fractures and luxations, discospondylitis, some vertebral tumours, congenital abnormalities and degenerative changes, and can provide circumstantial evidence of disc herniation. Bone lesions visible on survey radiographs can be delineated much more accurately using CT. Skull radiographs are not sensitive or useful in the diagnosis of intracranial disease, but are beneficial for the diagnosis of skull fractures, cranial tumours and some meningiomas (particularly in cats) and may be helpful in the diagnosis of otitis media.

Spinal radiography

Technique
The correct positioning for spinal radiography is shown in Figure 5.1.

- Radiographs need to be made under sedation or general anaesthesia in order to achieve adequate patient positioning.

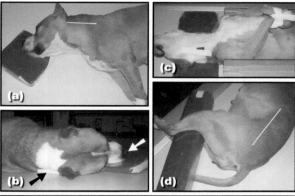

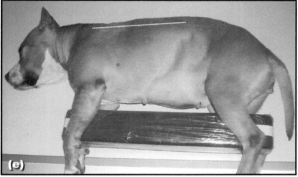

5.1 Correct positioning to obtain spinal radiographs. The white lines indicate the level at which the beam should be centred. **(a–c)** The correct positioning for cervical radiography. Note that there are foam pads placed under the nose and neck of the animal (arrowed) to ensure that a true lateral view is obtained. **(d–e)** The correct positioning for thoracolumbar radiography. Note that here the foam pads have been placed between the limbs to ensure that the thoracolumbar spine is lateral.

- If spinal instability is suspected, as may arise from atlantoaxial subluxation or a vertebral fracture, only lateral views should be acquired initially in order to avoid iatrogenic neural injury that may occur when positioning the patient for ventrodorsal (VD) views. Based on the findings from the lateral views:
  - The examination can be terminated if the diagnosis is obvious (e.g. atlantoaxial subluxation)
  - Conventional VD views can be acquired
  - VD views can be obtained using a horizontal X-ray beam.

- To interpret spinal radiographs accurately, it is important that the spine is not rotated. Padding, ties and troughs (see Figure 5.1) should be used to achieve this.
- It is important to avoid radiographic distortion of the vertebrae and intervertebral disc spaces due to divergence of the X-ray beam. To minimize distortion, multiple radiographs are required so that more vertebrae and disc spaces can be imaged with the centre of the X-ray beam.

Interpretation

Accurate interpretation of spinal radiographs requires good quality images and knowledge of the normal radiographic anatomy of the spine (Figure 5.2). The cranial aspect of the cervical spine is a particularly difficult area to interpret, especially in young animals, as a result of the numerous growth plates in C1 and C2 (Figures 5.3 and 5.4). A full description of normal variants of vertebral anatomy is provided elsewhere (Thrall and Robertson, 2011).

Radiographs should be evaluated for the following:

- Basic anatomy, including the number of vertebrae and the presence of processes and ribs. There should be 7 cervical, 13 thoracic, 7 lumbar and 3 fused sacral vertebrae in both dogs and cats
- Alignment of the vertebrae in two planes
- Width of the intervertebral disc space. Each space should be compared with the disc space immediately cranial and caudal. Only if the disc space being evaluated is not as wide as both adjacent disc spaces should it be considered narrowed
- Shape and opacity of the intervertebral foramina
- Integrity of the vertebral endplates. They should be examined for lysis and sclerosis indicative of infection

- Evidence of vertebral neoplasia in the form of lysis, sclerosis and distortion of the bone outline. It should be noted that a large amount of cancellous bone (up to 50%) must be lost from the vertebral body before bone lysis can be detected radiographically
- Degenerative changes of the vertebrae (e.g. spondylosis deformans) or articular processes.

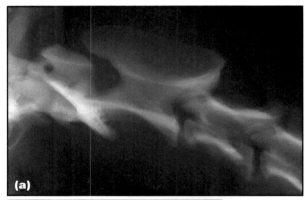
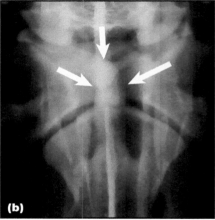

5.3 **(a)** Lateral and **(b)** VD view of the normal adult atlantoaxial junction. The dens is visible in (b) (arrowed).

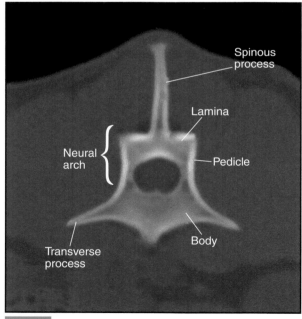

5.2 Anatomy of a vertebra.

Spinous process
Lamina
Neural arch
Pedicle
Neural arch
Transverse process
Body

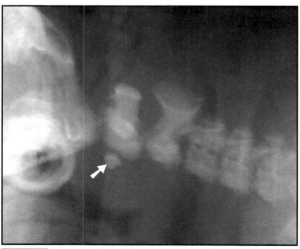

5.4 Lateral view of the atlantoaxial junction in a normal 6-week-old Boston Terrier. The apparently separate fragment of bone (arrowed) ventral to the atlas is part of the developing body of the vertebra.

Characteristics of specific diseases

Congenital malformations: Common congenital malformations (Westworth and Sturges, 2010) include:

- Atlantoaxial subluxation as a result of ligamentous abnormalities and/or aplasia/ hypoplasia of the dens (see Chapter 15)
- Transitional vertebrae, particularly of the lumbosacral junction (see Chapter 19)
- Unusual numbers of vertebrae
- Block vertebrae
- Hemivertebrae and butterfly vertebrae
- Spina bifida (see Chapter 16).

Atlantoaxial subluxation: The examination should begin with lateral views only. VD views may be acquired if judged necessary from the lateral views and the risk of iatrogenic injury from malalignment and/or instability is deemed to be low. An open-mouth rostrocaudal view of the cranial aspect of C2 can be obtained to evaluate the dens, but this carries additional risk and is usually not necessary (see Figure 5.3). The key to diagnosing atlanto-axial subluxation from a lateral radiograph is not the degree of overlap of C1 and C2, but rather the alignment of the dorsal lamina of C1 *versus* C2. In animals without subluxation the alignment is essentially continuous or linear, whereas with sub-luxation the alignment is angular. However, if the lateral radiograph is not truly lateral, accurate assessment of the alignment of the lamina is not possible. More rarely, there can be anomalies of the occipito-atlantal junction with fusion or over-lapping of these two bones, associated with hypo-plasia of the occipital bone, the occipital condyles and the atlas (see Chapter 14).

Transitional vertebrae: It is common to find vertebrae at the thoracolumbar and lumbosacral junctions that have characteristics of vertebrae from both sections, such as an extra rib at the thoracolumbar junction (Figure 5.5), or lack of a transverse process and anomalous sacral fusion at the lumbosacral junction. These anomalies may be incidental, but not always. Asymmetrical rib devel-opment associated with the last thoracic vertebra can result in spinal decompressive surgery being performed at the incorrect location if the last rib is used as an anatomical landmark. In addition, in German Shepherd Dogs with lumbosacral spondy-losis, 78% of the dogs with transitional lumbosacral vertebrae had protrusion of the lumbosacral disc causing cauda equina syndrome. It was therefore hypothesized that lumbosacral transitional verte-brae decreased the stability of the lumbosacral junction, predisposing to degenerative lumbosacral disease (Morgan *et al.*, 1993).

Block vertebrae: Block vertebrae result from a fail-ure of segmentation in the developing vertebrae (Figure 5.6). This can involve fusion of the vertebral bodies, arches or entire vertebrae. They are often

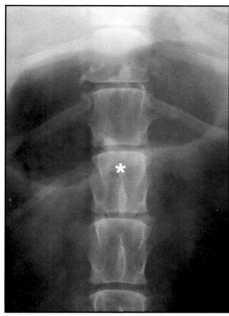

5.5 VD view of the thoracolumbar junction in a Cocker Spaniel. Note that the 13th vertebra (✱) only has one rib.

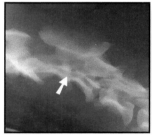 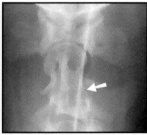

5.6 Lateral and VD views showing a block vertebra at C2–C3 and complete absence of the dens in a 10-year-old Poodle. The point at which the two vertebrae are fused is visible (arrowed).

an incidental finding, but there may be instability and an increased likelihood of intervertebral disc herniation at the site adjacent to the block vertebrae (Bailey and Morgan, 1992).

Hemivertebrae: Hemivertebrae result from the fail-ure of formation of part of the vertebra and most commonly affect vertebrae T7–T9. If the central portion of the vertebra fails to develop, right and left hemivertebrae result, producing a butterfly vertebra. The name derives from its butterfly-like appearance on VD radiographs. Hemivertebrae are particularly common in Bulldogs and other screw tail breeds. Hemivertebrae may be incidental, but are more likely to be associated with clinical signs than most other vertebral anomalies. Typically, hemivertebrae are associated with kyphosis (Figure 5.7) and occa-sionally scoliosis. Neurological deficits are the result of a combination of stenosis of the vertebral canal and instability. However, spinal cord abnormalities such as intra-arachnoid cysts/diverticula and syrin-gomyelia can accompany hemivertebrae. MRI is therefore recommended for animals with clinical signs suspected to arise from hemivertebrae.

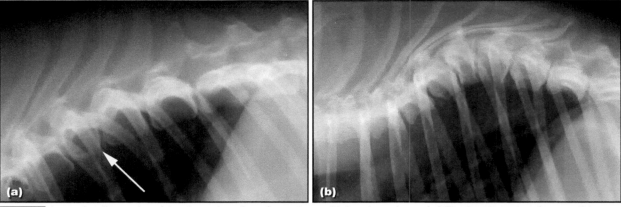

5.7 Lateral radiographs of the thoracic spine of two dogs with hemivertebrae. **(a)** The hemivertebra (arrowed) is not causing clinical problems. **(b)** The vertebral anomalies are causing severe kyphosis and the dog was paraplegic. Note the abnormal shape of the spinous processes of the affected vertebrae.

Spina bifida: Spina bifida results from a failure of fusion of the neural tube and overlying tissues, and is identified most easily on VD views by the split spinous process (Figure 5.8). This may be an incidental finding, but can be associated with severe neurological deficits, particularly in Manx cats with sacrocaudal dysgenesis (see Chapter 19).

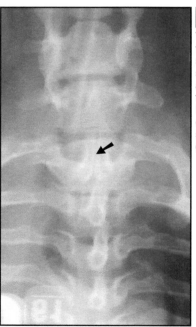

5.8

VD radiograph of the cranial thoracic spine. There is spina bifida affecting the first thoracic vertebra. Note the duplication of the spinous process (arrowed).

Discospondylitis: Discospondylitis describes bacterial or fungal infection of the intervertebral disc and adjacent endplates. The hallmark radiographic sign of discospondylitis is endplate lysis, which may be accompanied by sub-endplate sclerosis and malalignment (Figure 5.9). Multiple sites can be affected, especially with fungal infections, thus survey radiographs of the entire spine are recommended if discospondylitis is suspected (see Chapter 14). As spinal MRI becomes more commonplace, it is apparent that radiography is relatively insensitive for the detection of discospondylitis and negative survey radiographs do not rule out this condition (Carrera *et al.*, 2011).

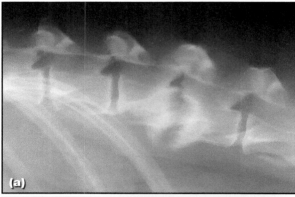

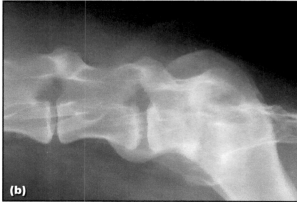

5.9 Lateral radiographs of the lumbar spine and lumbosacral junction in two dogs with discospondylitis. In both dogs there is obvious destruction of the endplates of the affected vertebrae. **(a)** Sclerosis, ventral spondylosis and degenerative changes of the articular processes are also present. **(b)** Mild ventral subluxation of the sacrum and ventral spondylosis are visible.

Neoplasia: Common vertebral tumours include primary mesenchymal and reticuloendothelial tumours (e.g. plasma cell tumour). Meningiomas may also cause spinal cord compression. More rarely, carcinomas may metastasize to the spine, spinal cord or subarachnoid space, and primary tumours of the spinal cord such as ependymomas, gliomas and nephroblastomas can occur (see Chapters 14 to 18). Primary vertebral tumours can be mainly lytic or sclerotic, but should have radiographic signs typical of an aggressive bone process (Figure 5.10a). The intervertebral foramina and vertebral canal can be expanded by pressure from a soft tissue mass (Figure 5.10b). With multifocal reticuloendothelial tumours, such as multiple myeloma, there may be multiple punctate, lytic lesions (Morgan *et al.*, 1980; see Chapter 16).

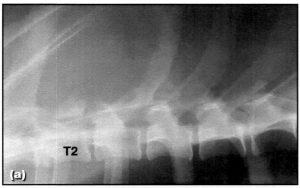

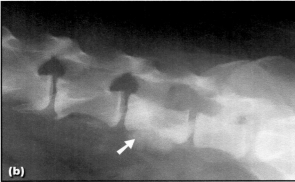

5.10 Lateral radiographs showing vertebral neoplasia. **(a)** There is almost total destruction of the spinous process of T2 by a poorly differentiated sarcoma. **(b)** The vertebral canal and intervertebral foramen at L6–L7 are expanded and there is new bone ventral to the body of L6 (arrowed). The cause was a poorly differentiated sarcoma.

Fractures and luxations: Spinal fractures and luxations occur with greatest frequency at the thoracolumbar junction, the lumbar and lumbosacral spine, and the atlantoaxial junction, but can occur anywhere along the vertebral column. In animals in which trauma is suspected or known to have occurred, lateral views of the spine should be obtained first. If unstable fractures are visible on the lateral views, a horizontal beam should be used to obtain a VD view. If this is not possible, great care should be taken in positioning the animal on its back for the VD view, or the VD view omitted. The radiographs should be examined for alignment, and the vertebral bodies, disc spaces and articular processes carefully evaluated (Figure 5.11; see Chapters 15, 16 and 21).

Disc disease: Radiographs are only 60–70% accurate for diagnosing the site of Hansen type 1 intervertebral disc herniations (Kirberger *et al.*, 1992; Olby *et al.*, 1994). Radiographic features of acute intervertebral disc herniation (Figure 5.12) include:

- Uniform or asymmetrical (wedging) narrowing of the disc space
- Mineralized disc material within the vertebral canal
- A change in shape and opacity of the intervertebral foramina
- Narrowing of the articular process joint space
- Vacuum phenomenon (rare).

However, these findings are not specific and spinal decompressive surgery for disc herniation should never be performed based on survey radiographic findings alone. More sophisticated imaging studies (see below) are needed prior to invasive surgery.

Degenerative changes: Various degenerative changes are commonly seen in spinal radiographs of older dogs and cats and are often clinically unimportant (Figure 5.13). They include degenerative joint disease of the articular processes, ventral spondylosis, dural ossification and mineralization of the nucleus pulposus (Morgan and Miyabayashi, 1988; Hardie *et al.*, 2002; Levine *et al.*, 2006) (see

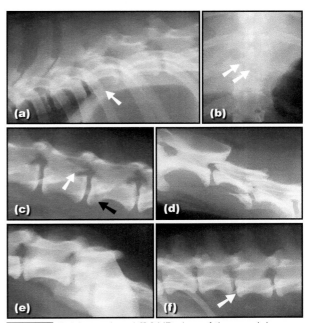

5.11 **(a)** Lateral and **(b)** VD view of the caudal thoracic spine in a dog that had been hit by a car. (a) The body of T11 appears shorter than usual and a fracture line is faintly visible (arrowed). (b) A dramatic fracture of T11 with craniolateral displacement of the caudal fragment is evident, emphasizing the importance of obtaining orthogonal views. **(c)** Lateral view of the lumbar spine of a dog that had fallen from a height. There are fractures of the lateral pedicle (white arrow) and cranial endplate of the caudal vertebra (black arrow). This is an unusual fracture that is stable. **(d)** Lateral view of the cervical spine of a Greyhound that had run into a tree. There is collapse of the C3–C4 intervertebral disc space and cranial displacement of the fractured caudoventral body of C3. **(e–f)** Common fractures and luxations of the lumbosacral articulation and cranial lumbar spine. Flexion of the spine combined with caudal impact results in fractures of the caudoventral aspect of the cranial vertebral body and malalignment in the region of the lumbosacral and thoracolumbar junctions (arrowed).

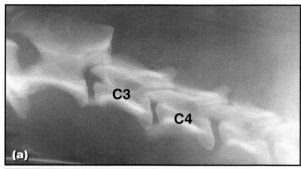

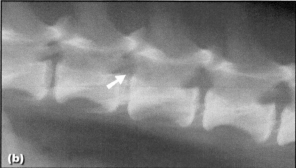

5.12 Lateral views of the **(a)** cervical and **(b)** lumbar spine in two dogs with acute intervertebral disc herniations. (a) There is obvious narrowing of the C3–C4 disc space. Although there is no radiographic evidence of mineralized disc material at this site, a large amount was visible in the canal on CT images. (b) Mineralized disc material is present within the L2–L3 disc space, projecting into the vertebral canal and causing opacification of the intervertebral foramen (arrowed).

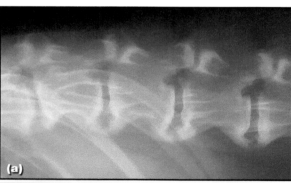

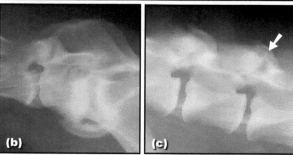

5.13 Degenerative changes commonly identified on spinal radiographs. These changes are often of no clinical significance. **(a)** Ventral spondylosis and sclerosis of the endplates in the thoracolumbar spine of an 8-year-old German Shepherd Dog. **(b)** Marked ventral spondylosis and endplate sclerosis in an old Boxer. **(c)** Degenerative joint disease of the articular processes in the lumbar spine of a 4-year-old Rhodesian Ridgeback (arrowed).

Chapter 14). Articular process hyperostosis, resulting from cervical instability, can be clinically significant if the proliferative new bone encroaches on the vertebral canal causing spinal cord or nerve root compression. Sacral osteochondrosis is an important degenerative condition reported in German Shepherd Dogs, which is associated with degenerative lumbosacral disc disease (see Chapter 19).

Developmental disorders:
Calcinosis circumscripta (tumoral calcinosis): This is a disease in which there is mineralization of the soft tissues of the spine, usually dorsal to C1–C2 or the cranial thoracic spine (see Chapter 15).

Multiple cartilaginous exostoses: This is a disorder of growing dogs (also known as osteochondromatosis; see Chapter 16). Multiple protuberances capped by cartilage develop from the cortical bone of the ribs and vertebrae (Figure 5.14). These protuberances stop growing and undergo endochondral ossification at the time of growth plate closure, but may encroach upon the vertebral canal, causing spinal cord compression. Malignant transformation is also possible.

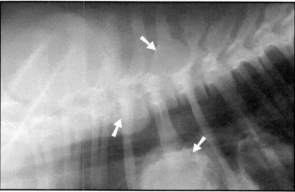

5.14 Multiple cartilaginous exostoses in a 4-month-old Golden Retriever. The exostoses are present on the ribs and the bodies and spinous processes of the thoracic vertebrae (arrowed).

Diffuse idiopathic skeletal hyperostosis:
Diffuse idiopathic skeletal hyperostosis (DISH; Figure 5.15) is a disorder in which there is calcification and ossification of the soft tissues, most notably in the spine. This idiopathic disease was first reported in dogs in the 1990s (Morgan and Stavenborn, 1991) and has recently been described in more detail (Kranenburg *et al.*, 2010, 2011). The changes seen include calcification of the ventral longitudinal ligament, the ventral aspect of the annulus and the paravertebral soft tissues, resulting in an appearance similar to that of spondylosis deformans. A number of radiographic criteria must be met to confirm DISH including the presence of calcification along the ventrolateral aspect of at least four contiguous vertebral bodies (Kranenburg *et al.*, 2011). Boxers are over-represented with 41% of dogs having radiographic evidence of the disease, but clinical signs associated with this condition are rare.

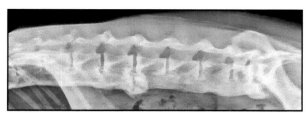

5.15 Lateral view of the lumbar spine of a Boxer with disseminated idiopathic skeletal hyperostosis (DISH). Note the nearly continuous new bone along the ventral margin of the visible vertebrae. This new bone continued cranially throughout the thoracic spine.

Advanced imaging

If survey radiographs do not provide a diagnosis, or adequate information to determine treatment and prognosis, other imaging studies are needed. The three main modalities used are myelography, CT and MRI; the advantages and disadvantages of these imaging modalities are discussed below (da Costa and Samii, 2010). Comparisons of the use of these different imaging modalities to diagnose spinal diseases have started to appear in the veterinary literature (Hecht *et al.*, 2009; Israel *et al.*, 2009; Shimizu *et al.*, 2009; Dennison *et al.*, 2010; Parry *et al.*, 2010; Robertson and Thrall, 2011).

Epidurography and discography are two outdated contrast techniques that were used to evaluate the lumbosacral junction. For a full review of these techniques the reader is referred to Ramirez and Thrall (1998).

Myelography

Myelography can be used to identify compressive and expansile lesions of the spinal cord. The benefits of myelography include its relative inexpense and availability. The disadvantages include the technical difficulty of the imaging study and contrast medium toxicity, leading to seizures and neurological deterioration. Myelograms are also insensitive with regard to the detection of some important intraparenchymal conditions such as infarction, oedema and syringomyelia.

Myelography-induced seizures occur in 10–20% of patients and are more likely in large animals that require a larger volume of contrast medium and in patients in which the contrast medium is injected at the atlanto-occipital junction (Butterworth and Gibbs, 1992; Lewis and Hosgood, 1992; Barone *et al.*, 2002; da Costa *et al.*, 2011). Myelography is a satisfactory imaging study for patients with myelopathy if CT and MRI are not available, and the owner understands all the risks. However, myelography should not be performed in a setting where subsequent spinal surgery is not feasible. Cerebrospinal fluid (CSF) analysis should always be completed prior to performing a myelogram as the contrast medium induces a mild meningitis that complicates interpretation of CSF samples within a week of the imaging study.

Technique

Myelography is performed by intrathecal injection of a non-ionic contrast medium (iohexol or iopamidol)

via the atlanto-occipital or lumbar (preferably L5–L6) interarcuate space. Injection of contrast medium into the lumbar spine has the advantages of a decreased risk of iatrogenic trauma and improved delineation of compressive lesions, as the contrast medium can be forced around the site of severe compression. Disadvantages include the increased likelihood of performing an epidural injection and the technical difficulty of introducing a needle into the lumbar subarachnoid space, especially in overweight dogs with pronounced degenerative joint disease of the articular processes. It is easier to introduce the needle into the atlanto-occipital subarachnoid space, but there is an increased risk of iatrogenic, potentially fatal trauma to the cervical spinal cord/brainstem. It is also difficult to delineate compressive lesions completely as the contrast medium follows the route of least resistance, which usually results in its accumulation in the ventricular system of the brain rather than coursing caudal to the lesion.

To perform a myelogram the animal is anaesthetized, CSF is collected for analysis and survey spinal radiographs are obtained. The contrast medium (approximately 0.3–0.5 ml/kg of iohexol 240) is drawn up into a sterile syringe, which is connected to an extension set. The extension set is then filled with contrast medium (Figure 5.16). The animal is placed in lateral recumbency and the site of injection is clipped and prepared as for surgery. A spinal needle (gauge and length depending on site) is introduced aseptically as if performing a CSF tap. The filled extension set is attached carefully to the needle once CSF appears in the needle hub, and the contrast medium is injected slowly. With a cervical injection, the contrast medium is injected over approximately 1–2 minutes; the needle is then withdrawn and images are taken. With a lumbar injection, the contrast medium can either be followed using fluoroscopy, or a small test injection can be made, followed by a radiograph to ensure that the contrast medium is being injected into the subarachnoid space, prior to injecting the remaining dose.

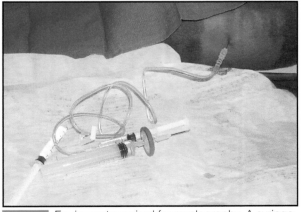

5.16 Equipment required for myelography. A syringe is attached to an extension set and filled with contrast medium. The entire field should be kept sterile. The contrast medium was passed through a 0.22 μm filter when drawn up from the bottle (note the syringe with filter attachment in the foreground).

Once the contrast medium has been injected, lateral and VD images should be acquired as soon as possible (Matteucci *et al.*, 1999; Bos *et al.*, 2007). In addition, oblique views (especially in the cervical region) may be indicated. In some instances, dynamic views (traction, extension and flexion) may be required (e.g. cervical spondylomyelopathy), but any spinal flexion/extension should be undertaken with extreme caution because of the potential for causing an acute concussion or compression of the spinal cord (see Chapter 15). Finally, obtaining a contralateral view often aids in the identification of compressive lesions (Matteucci *et al.*, 1999).

If adequate contrast medium filling is not achieved in certain areas, the animal can be tilted and its spine flexed to allow pooling of contrast medium by gravity. However, care should be taken to keep the head elevated so that the excess contrast medium does not pool in the cranial cavity, as this increases the risk of seizures.

Interpretation

Normal myelograms are shown in Figure 5.17. Three basic pathological patterns are recognized: intramedullary, intradural/extramedullary and extradural (Figure 5.18). Myelographic artefacts resulting from the injection of contrast medium into either the epidural or subdural (a potential space between the dura and arachnoid mater) space will complicate interpretation (Figure 5.19). Inadvertent injection into the central canal can also occur. In unusual instances where there is myelomalacia and loss of integrity of the pia mater, contrast medium may been seen within the spinal cord parenchyma (Lu *et al.*, 2002) (Figure 5.20).

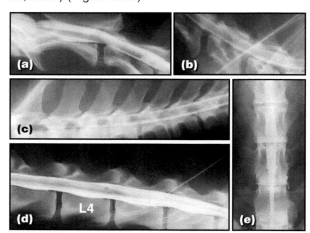

5.17 Normal myelographic appearance of the canine spinal cord with the contrast medium injection made at L5–L6. **(a)** The normal appearance of the cranial cervical spinal cord. **(b)** The normal appearance of the caudal cervical spinal cord. **(c)** The cranial thoracic spine never fills well when the injection is first made, giving the appearance of thinning or even loss of the contrast medium column. **(d)** The small circular filling defect over the caudal aspect of L4 is most likely an air bubble accidently introduced with the contrast medium. **(e)** The spinal cord tapers in the caudal lumbar spine: the level depends on species and breed, but in general the spinal cord terminates more cranially in larger dogs. Therefore, myelography is not useful for delineating the contents of the vertebral column at the lumbosacral junction in dogs.

It is common for myelographic findings to be equivocal with regard to the presence or absence of a lesion. If available, the use of CT following myelography can be quite informative as it allows more precise anatomical lesion localization. In addition, due to the enhanced contrast resolution of CT, contrast medium in the subarachnoid space, which is not visible on radiographs, can be detected with CT images. This is especially useful if spinal cord swelling results in an extensive region of poor subarachnoid space filling with contrast medium and thus no diagnosis with myelography. Subsequent CT images may allow detection of a herniated disc that would account for the spinal cord swelling.

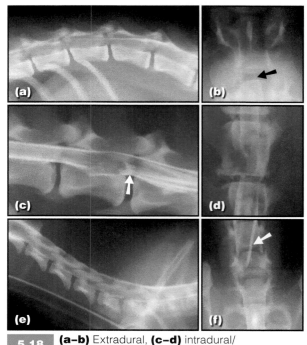

5.18 **(a–b)** Extradural, **(c–d)** intradural/extramedullary and **(e–f)** intramedullary myelographic patterns. (a) Lateral view of a 1-year-old cat with lymphosarcoma. The dorsal aspect of the contrast medium column is clearly deviated ventrally by an extradural mass. (b) VD view of the cat in (a). Note that the left lateral aspect of the contrast medium column is deviated to the right (arrowed). (c) Lateral and (d) VD views of the lumbar spine of a Labrador with a meningioma. On the lateral view, both the dorsal and ventral aspects of the contrast medium column are thinned and deviate abaxially over the caudal aspect of the third lumbar vertebra as if around an intramedullary lesion. However, there is an accumulation of contrast medium in the subarachnoid space delineating an oval filling defect (the classic golf tee sign) just dorsal to the caudal L3 endplate (arrowed). This appearance is most consistent with an intradural/extramedullary lesion. The deviation and splitting of the contrast medium on the right are clearly evident on the VD view. (e) Lateral and (f) VD view of a 1-year-old Yorkshire Terrier that had suffered a fibrocartilaginous embolism. There is expansion of the spinal cord in the caudal cervical region causing thinning and abaxial deviation of both lateral aspects of the contrast medium column. The endotracheal tube (arrowed) is visible on the VD view. If the tube prevents interpretation of the image it should be repositioned or even briefly removed to obtain a diagnostic view.

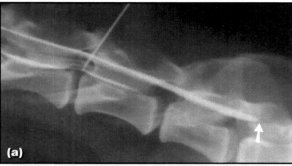

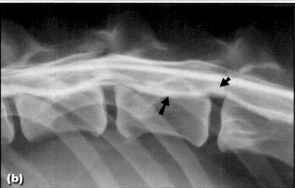

5.19 Myelographic artefacts. **(a)** An L5–L6 injection in which the contrast medium has entered the subdural space, causing a characteristic spindle-shaped end to the contrast medium column caudally (arrowed). **(b)** The contrast medium has been injected into the epidural space, causing opacification of the intervertebral foramina (short arrow) and an undulating appearance to the contrast column due to opacification of the venous sinuses (long arrow).

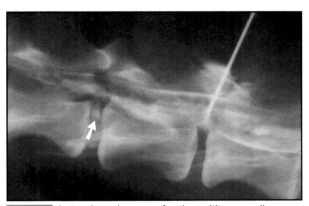

5.20 Lateral myelogram of a dog with ascending myelomalacia precipitated by an intervertebral disc herniation (arrowed). There is contrast medium within the subarachnoid space and spinal cord parenchyma.

Computed tomography

Indications for the use of CT in neurological patients include imaging of the brain and skull, the tympanic bullae, the bones of the cervical and thoracolumbar spine, the cauda equina and, in combination with myelography, the spinal cord. It can also be used to evaluate the soft tissues of the brachial plexus and to identify acute herniation of mineralized disc material.

CT is a tomographic imaging modality (i.e. image slices are created). Image slices overcome the problems associated with superimposition of structures, which prevents accurate spatial localization

(as seen with radiographs). CT also has better contrast resolution than radiography, resulting in enhanced distinction between tissues of different types. For example, extradural haemorrhage can be detected by CT, but not by radiography, due to the slightly greater X-ray absorption by the blood than the spinal cord and CSF. In addition, undertaking a CT study where myelography is inconclusive can be diagnostic due to the enhanced conspicuity of small lesions on CT images, which are not visible on radiographs and myelograms. CT images can also be reformatted in other planes, which can help in spatial localization of lesions, and into 3D volume renderings, which can be helpful for the assessment of complex fractures and other malformations (Figure 5.21). Unfortunately, intraparenchymal detail of the brain and spinal cord is relatively poor with CT and CT-myelography compared with MRI.

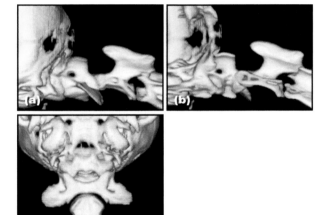

5.21 3D CT surface renderings of a dog with atlantoaxial subluxation. **(a)** The axis is angled slightly with respect to the atlas. **(b)** Approximately 50% of the anatomical structures on the left have been removed. The malalignment of the axis is now more obvious as is the dorsal displacement of the cranial aspect of the axis and the absence of the dens. **(c)** Ventral aspect of the atlantoaxial junction. The anatomical relationships can be evaluated for planning the surgical stabilization. 3D renderings can be very useful for assessing complex anomalies and fractures.

Principles

CT uses the principle that the internal structure of an object can be reconstructed from multiple views of that object. X-rays projected through the animal are measured by detectors. The X-ray tube moves in a circular direction around the patient to obtain multiple views and an image is reconstructed from the data measured by the detectors. There are several generations of CT scanners and the most recent have multiple detectors, which allow the generation of multiple image slices (e.g. 16 or 64) for each rotation of the X-ray tube around the patient. This results in an extremely short scan time (i.e. just a few minutes) for coverage of a body region, such as the brain or T3–L3 spinal segment.

The detectors are actually measuring the extent of X-ray attenuation by the tissues. This attenuation information is used by sophisticated software to generate images consisting of pixels. Each pixel has a grey shade assigned by the computer and an X and Y dimension that depends on the size of the field of view and the number of pixels. CT images usually have an image matrix of 512 x 512 pixels, and having X and Y dimensions in the submillimetre range is common. Pixels also have a Z dimension, which is determined by the thickness of the image slice (typical range: 1–5 mm). With the Z dimension included, the image element becomes a volume element, or voxel.

The shade of grey assigned to the pixel by the computer is normalized to the absorption characteristics of water and given a number called a CT number or Hounsfield unit (HU). Water is assigned a HU value of 0. This results in air having a HU value of –1024 (black) and metallic objects and contrast medium having a HU value up to +3000 (white). Figure 5.22 details the range of HU values for different tissues. CT images can contain up to 4096 shades of grey, many more than can be distinguished by the human eye. Post-processing of the images is undertaken to make use of all the grey shades, and involves adjusting the window and level of the CT image so that only certain parts of the greyscale are within the visible range. The window represents the range of HU values depicted in the visible greyscale and the level represents the specific HU value at the centre of the window.

Tissue	Hounsfield unit (HU) value
Brain and/or spinal cord	25–50
Cerebrospinal fluid	0–15
Recent haemorrhage (<24 hours)	55–95
Fat	–50 to –100
Bone	600–1000
Recently herniated mineralized disc	100–500 [a]
Chronically herniated mineralized disc	450–1000 [a]

5.22 HU values for different tissues. [a] Data from Olby *et al.* (2000).

By adjusting the window and level, CT images that have very high or very low contrast can be generated, with specific tissues and/or substances having a particular grey shade. CT images of any body part must be evaluated at a variety of window and level combinations to ensure that lesions are not overlooked; this is especially true for the CNS. For example, vasogenic brain oedema is not visible in a CT image with a wide window width (i.e. low contrast), but is visible in a CT image with a narrow window width (i.e. high contrast) and a level set for water (i.e. 0) (Figure 5.23).

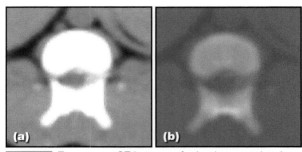

5.23 Transverse CT images of a lumbar vertebra in a Dachshund. **(a)** The image is being viewed in a soft tissue window (high contrast) and the presence of mineralized disc material in the vertebral canal is obvious. **(b)** The same image being viewed in a bone window (low contrast). Note that the herniated disc material is more difficult to identify.

Contrast studies: Contrast studies are a vital part of a CT imaging protocol. Contrast enhancement (a visual change in the appearance of a structure or tissue) will occur in any region where iodinated contrast medium is present in the CT image. This typically includes blood vessels, as well as some lesions, such as tumours or inflammatory lesions, that have an increased number of vessels or leaky vasculature, which results in more contrast medium being present per unit mass of tissue than would normally be encountered. This increase in contrast medium concentration leads to increased X-ray attenuation, which is detected by the computer and assigned a 'white' shade of grey. By comparing a series of pre-contrast images with images acquired following contrast medium administration, lesions that have similar inherent X-ray attenuation to normal tissue but different vasculature can be detected (Figures 5.24 and 5.25). Water-soluble contrast media are used at a dosage of 2 ml/kg, up to a max-

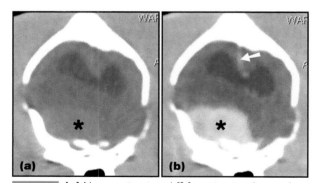

5.24 **(a)** Non-contrast and **(b)** contrast-enhanced transverse CT images of the brain of a 2-year-old Boxer. On the non-contrast image there is clear loss of symmetry in the brain, with dorsal deviation of the right lateral ventricle and expansion of the sutures in the skull, suggesting a pressure effect. A broad-based mass can just be identified on the floor of the skull (∗) to the right of the clinoid process. This mass strongly enhances following intravenous administration of contrast medium. The blood vessels on the midline also enhance (arrowed), clearly showing the mass effect. The location of the mass to the periphery of the brain (i.e. extra-axial) and the strong contrast enhancement make a meningioma the most likely diagnosis, and this was confirmed at necropsy. The skull sutures probably opened as a result of increased intracranial pressure in this young dog.

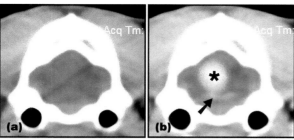

5.25 **(a)** Non-contrast and **(b)** contrast-enhanced CT images of an 8-year-old cat with paradoxical vestibular signs. The non-contrast image is unremarkable, but on the image obtained post-contrast medium administration there is a region of marked contrast enhancement (*) within the cerebellum. This intra-axial lesion was caused by fungal encephalitis. Note the (normal) enhancement of the choroid plexus (arrowed).

imum total dose of 60 ml. Ionic contrast media (Conray, Urografin and Hypaque) can be used, but non-ionic contrast media (iohexol 240) should be used in patients that are seriously systemically compromised or have renal disease. Contrast-enhanced CT images should never be acquired unless a series of plain images have been obtained. It is the comparison of the pre-contrast with the post-contrast images that allows a diagnosis to be reached.

Interpretation
Evaluation of a CT study includes assessment for normal anatomy and symmetry (George and Smallwood, 1992), identification of areas of contrast enhancement, and examination for artefacts (Figure 5.26). Unilateral intracranial mass lesions can cause a midline shift (a so-called mass effect) that can usually be detected on post-contrast images (see Figure 5.24). In addition, oedema causes hypoattenuation and recent haemorrhage causes hyperattenuation.

There are three main sources of artefact:

- Motion – motion artefacts are not problematic in veterinary neuroimaging as patients are under general anaesthesia
- Beam hardening – absorption of lower energy X-rays passing through regions of thick bone increases the average energy (hardening) of the polyenergetic X-ray beam. After passing through a particularly dense bone (e.g. petrous temporal bone) from a variety of angles, the reconstruction algorithm does not allow for the unpredicted increase in energy, resulting in the formation of white and black lines superimposed on the image (Figure 5.27). The anatomy of the caudal fossa predisposes to beam hardening and therefore CT is not accurate for imaging the brainstem
- Partial volume effect – each pixel represents an average of the tissue voxel and so, if there are adjacent fields of very different attenuation, the average may be unexpectedly high or low. This is usually seen with images of a curved object. The preceding and following image slices should be evaluated to determine whether a suspected lesion is present. Decreasing the slice thickness helps to decrease this type of artefact.

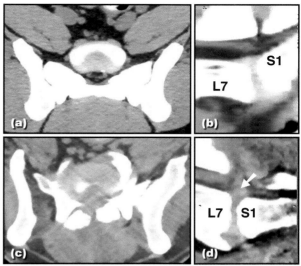

5.26 CT images of **(a–b)** a normal and **(c–d)** an abnormal lumbosacral junction in a dog. The images were taken with the animal in dorsal recumbency. (a) and (c) are transverse images and (b) and (d) are sagittal reconstructions. (a–b) The epidural fat (black) surrounds the cauda equina. (c–d) There is a lumbosacral malformation with a transitional lumbar vertebra. The intervertebral disc has protruded dorsally, obliterating the vertebral canal and displacing the epidural fat, making it impossible to see the cauda equina on the transverse image. The protruding disc material is clearly evident on the sagittal reconstruction (arrowed).

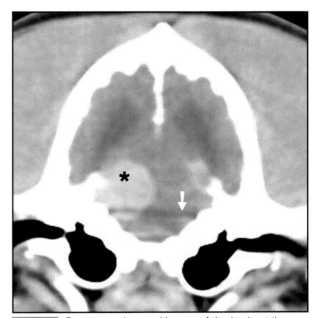

5.27 Contrast-enhanced image of the brain at the level of the cerebellum demonstrating a beam-hardening artefact (arrowed). Note also the large contrast-enhancing mass at the right cerebellopontine angle (*).

Magnetic resonance imaging
The advent of MRI has revolutionized clinical neurology. MRI provides excellent soft tissue contrast resolution, allows imaging in any plane, and does not require the use of ionizing radiation. MRI is the modality of choice for imaging the brain, spinal cord, peripheral nerves and associated plexi. The

disadvantages of MRI include the relatively high cost and limited access. Care must be taken to ensure the elimination of metallic objects from the magnetic field because they can cause pronounced artefacts on MR images and ferrous objects carried into the room can become lethal projectiles due to the extremely high field strength of some magnets.

Principles

Like CT, MRI provides cross-sectional images, but unlike CT these can be acquired in any anatomical plane without repositioning the patient. This means that computer reformatting of images is not necessary; computer reformatted CT images can be of very high quality, but primary image acquisitions have the best detail. MR images are generated by the effect of radiofrequency currents and magnetic fields on protons. The strength of clinical magnets used in veterinary medicine ranges from 0.2–3 Tesla (T); although, some institutions have access to larger magnets for research purposes and imaging smaller animals. Low field magnets are less expensive but the image quality is affected by the lower signal to noise and scan times can be prolonged.

The physics of MR image generation are highly complex and specific details are beyond the scope of this chapter. Simply, the basis of MRI is the alignment of protons in the body into a position that is parallel with the main magnetic field. This occurs as soon as the patient is placed into the strong magnetic field of the MRI scanner. The aligned protons are then knocked out of alignment by a transiently applied radiofrequency current. The realigned protons then generate their own radiofrequency signal which is measured by a coil. The kinetics of radiofrequency signal decay in the coil is then analysed by a computer and used to build an image. The timing of the magnetic field gradients and radiofrequency pulses can be used to emphasize or dampen the signal from various tissue types. This means that the basis of contrast in an MR image is due to the physiochemistry of the tissue, not its physical properties.

The combination of magnetic fields and radiofrequency pulses used to create an MR image is called a pulse sequence. Commonly used imaging sequences are listed in Figure 5.28.

Spin-echo pulse sequences: Spin-echo pulse sequences are the mainstay of MRI and are designed to emphasize various types of proton relaxation. Images generated using spin-echo pulse sequences are either T1-weighted or T2-weighted, depending on whether T1 or T2 relaxation is what controls tissue contrast.

- T1 relaxation relates to the protons in the patient that are perturbed by a radiofrequency pulse realigning into their normal position parallel with the main magnetic field.
- T2 relaxation relates to the relative position of the protons immediately after being perturbed by the radiofrequency pulse.

Various tissues have different T1 and T2 relaxation times, and these differences in relaxation time can be used to influence tissue contrast. For example, fluid has very long T1 and T2 relaxation times; therefore, no signal will be created (fluid appears black) on a T1-weighted image, whereas a high signal will be created (fluid appears white) on a T2-weighted image (Figure 5.29). Thus, because most CNS lesions are associated with increased fluid due to oedema, they are conspicuous as regions of increased signal on T2-weighted images (Figure 5.30). However, some substances, such as proteinaceous exudates and methaemoglobin, have short T1 relaxation times and a high signal on T1-weighted images (Figure 5.31). Thus, the signal characteristics of a lesion on T1-weighted and T2-weighted images can be used to assess its composition.

Contrast studies: As with CT, contrast enhancement is an important feature of MRI. However, the mechanism of action of CT compared with MRI contrast media is quite different. CT contrast media are iodinated and alter X-ray attenuation by the patient; whereas, MRI contrast media are paramagnetic and function by changing the relaxation rate of protons. MRI contrast media accumulate in regions of hypervascularity or altered vascular permeability, and the resulting increased concentration of contrast medium changes the relaxation time of the protons in the immediate area, leading to a signal change in the image. Most MR contrast studies are based on changes in T1 relaxation, where increased relaxation leads to increased signal in T1-weighted images coming from regions of increased contrast medium concentration (see Figure 5.31b).

Inversion recovery sequences: Sequences other than spin-echo pulse sequences can be helpful for CNS imaging. It is possible to suppress the signal from fat. This is beneficial because the high signal emitted by fat in many pulse sequences can hide smaller, adjacent lesions or be misinterpreted as disease (D'Anjou *et al.*, 2011). The signal from fat can be suppressed in a spin-echo pulse sequence by the addition of a radiofrequency saturation

Tissue	T1 ± contrast	T2 (fast spin-echo)	T2 FLAIR	STIR	Gradient-echo (T2)
Fat	Hyperintense	Hyperintense	Hyperintense	Hypointense	Hyperintense
CSF	Hypointense	Hyperintense	Hypointense	Hyperintense	Hyperintense
Tissue oedema	Hypointense	Hyperintense	Hyperintense	Hyperintense	Hyperintense

5.28 The appearance of fat, CSF and tissue oedema on commonly used imaging sequences. Intensity is described relative to normal CNS parenchyma.

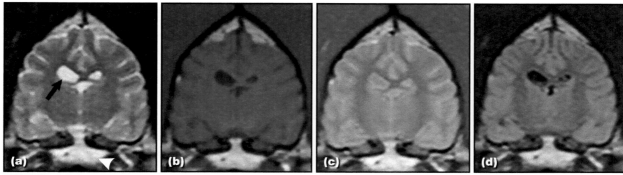

5.29 **(a)** T2-weighed spin-echo brain image. Substances with a long T2 relaxation time (such as pure fluids) have a high signal in this image sequence. Note the high signal of the CSF within the lateral ventricles (arrowed). In modern spin-echo sequences, fat will also have a high signal. Note the high signal of the marrow fat in the bones at the base of the skull (arrowhead). **(b)** T1-weighted spin-echo brain image. Substances with a short T1 relaxation time (such as fat) have a high signal in this image sequence. Note the high signal of the marrow fat in the bones at the base of the skull. Fluid has a long T1 relaxation time and, therefore, a low signal in this image sequence. Note the black signal from the lateral ventricles, which relates to the location of the fluid. **(c)** Proton density-weighted spin-echo brain image. In this sequence, tissue signal is primarily dependent upon the spatial distribution of protons, or the absolute proton density per unit area. Note the lower signal of white versus grey matter due to the differences in proton density. The proton density sequence is the preferred sequence to assess white and grey matter distribution. **(d)** T2-weighted fluid attenuated inversion recovery (FLAIR) brain image. This is a special sequence used to null the signal from free fluid and is useful for detecting hydrated lesions that would otherwise be obscured by the signal from normal fluid. Note the lack of signal from the CSF in the lateral ventricles, which has been nullified in this special sequence. This image is of a normal brain.

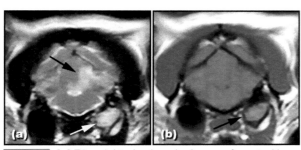

5.30 **(a)** T2-weighted spin-echo image of a cat with cerebellar infarction (black arrow). The cytotoxic oedema has led to an increase in water concentration in the lesion, which creates a region of high signal on T2-weighted images. There is exudate in the left tympanic bulla (white arrow). **(b)** T1-weighted spin-echo image of the cat in (a). As fluid has a low signal in T1-weighted images, the cerebellar lesion is not conspicuous. However, the exudate in the left tympanic bulla (arrowed) can be seen. Some proteinaceous fluids have a shorter T1 relaxation time than more pure fluids and thus become visible on T1-weighted images.

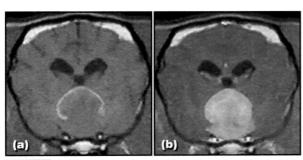

5.31 **(a)** Pre-contrast and **(b)** post-contrast T1-weighted spin-echo brain images of a dog with a pituitary macroadenoma. (a) There is a peripheral rim of high signal due to chronic haemorrhage. The magnetic effects of this chronic haemorrhage, which likely contains methaemoglobin, leads to a shortening of the T1 relaxation time and a high signal. (b) The contrast medium has leaked into the tumour, causing shortening of the T1 relaxation time and a high signal. Without obtaining the pre-contrast image, the peripheral haemorrhage would not have been detected.

band, which prevents the fat signal from appearing on the image. In addition, a special type of sequence called an inversion recovery sequence can be used. For fat, it is the short tau inversion recovery (STIR) sequence that greatly reduces its signal on the image (Figure 5.32). An inversion recovery se-quence can also be used to eliminate the signal from free fluid. In this instance it is the FLAIR sequence (see Figure 5.29d), which allows discrimination between free fluid and oedema. Suppression of the signal from free fluid with a FLAIR sequence makes it possible to distinguish between cystic and oedematous parenchymal lesions, and to assess for periventricular oedema where the high signal from the ventricular CSF may otherwise obscure nearby oedema (Figure 5.33).

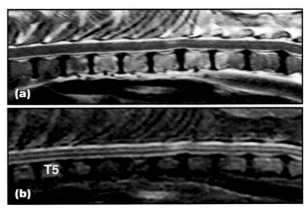

5.32 **(a)** Sagittal T2-weighted spin-echo image of the thoracic spine. The bodies of vertebrae T7–T10 have an increased signal, as may been seen with an infiltrative tumour or infection. **(b)** Sagittal STIR image of the same region. The signal from the fat is reduced, revealing that the signal from vertebrae T7–T10 is no different to any other vertebra. This indicates that the high signal seen in (a) was due to fat in the medullary cavity and not an infiltrative disease.

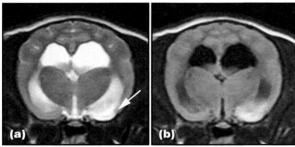

5.33 **(a)** T2-weighted spin-echo brain image. It is difficult to know whether the increased signal at the ventral aspect of the left lateral ventricle (arrowed) is due to CSF in the ventricle or to a lesion of the neuropil. **(b)** T2-weighted FLAIR image of the same area. The signal from the free fluid (such as CSF) has been nullified in this sequence. The presence and extent of the lesion in the left piriform lobe is much more obvious without the superimposed signal from the CSF in the ventricle.

Gradient-echo pulse sequences: Certain types of haemorrhage have paramagnetic effects that can be visualized with MRI. A very effective way of detecting these paramagnetic effects is with a gradient-echo pulse sequence. In this sequence, magnetic gradients are used during a critical step of proton re-phasing, which is needed for image formation. This is very different from the more commonly used spin-echo pulse sequence where refocusing magnetic gradients are not used. Due to the fact that the para-magnetic effects of haemorrhage (especially those of haemosiderin) interfere with the magnetic gradient used for proton re-phasing and image formation, a conspicuous artefact, called a magnetic suscepti-bility artefact, is created. This artefact essentially destroys the image in the region of the haemorrhage and creates a region of signal void (Figure 5.34).

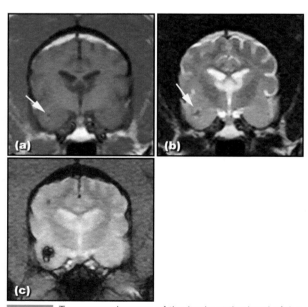

5.34 Transverse images of the brain at the level of the thalamus using **(a)** T1-weighted, **(b)** T2-weighted and **(c)** gradient-echo sequences. The arrows in (a) and (b) indicate a small, hypointense vascular lesion, which is difficult to detect. The same lesion is apparent on the gradient-echo image as a region of signal void due to the paramagnetic effects of haemoglobin.

Inclusion of a gradient-echo pulse sequence can be very useful for ruling haemorrhage in or out. The MRI effects of haemorrhage are quite complex and depend upon the age of the haemorrhage and pulse sequence used. A discussion on the MRI appear-ance of haemorrhage is beyond the scope of this chapter, but explanatory references are available (Bradley, 1993).

Emerging techniques: The field of MRI is moving rapidly and many new techniques have been deve-loped or are under development to better evaluate parameters, including:

- CSF flow using cine MRI (Cerda-Gonzalez *et al.*, 2010)
- Injury severity
- Enhanced diagnosis and anatomical study of tracts using diffusion-weighted imaging (DWI) and perfusion-weighted imaging (PWI) techniques (Mascalchi *et al.*, 2005; Tidwell and Robertson, 2011)
- Functional studies of neuronal activity (functional MRI) (Cheng, 2011)
- Metabolic characteristics of the CNS using MR spectroscopy (Alger, 2010).

Reports of these uses are starting to emerge in veterinary medicine and will likely continue to revo-lutionize our ability to evaluate patients with dys-function of the nervous system.

Interpretation
The philosophy of interpretation of MR images is diametrically opposed to that of most other imaging modalities. CT and radiography, for the most part, produce purely anatomical images. MR images on the other hand do contain anatomical information, but it is the physiochemistry of the tissue that cre-ates the signal, and thus contrast, on the image. Observers new to MR image interpretation often fail to realize that cortical bone has no signal and thus appears black on images. In addition, on radio-graphs and CT images bone is one of the most dominant features, whereas on MR images it is one of the most inconspicuous portions.

Many lesions are also much more conspicuous on MR images compared with radiographs and CT images, but it is the neuroanatomical localization of the lesion and the related neurophysiology that is necessary to correctly interpret its significance. Thus, it is not simply seeing a lesion on an MR image that is important, it is being able to relate the anomaly to the clinical signs and recognize the neuro-anatomical and neurophysiological relationships. MRI is also associated with a complex series of artefacts, such as flow and chemical shift artefacts, that can greatly complicate interpretation (Cooper *et al.*, 2010). It is therefore important to have MR images of the brain and spinal cord interpreted by experienced specialists and to ensure that the find-ings are complementary to the clinical findings.

MRI has provided an opportunity for the definitive diagnosis of many conditions that could not be diagnosed before this modality became available, including Chiari-like malformations, brain and spinal cord infarcts and poorly enhancing masses (e.g. gliomas). In addition, some conditions (such as discospondylitis) are apparent on MR images before any survey radiographic evidence of their presence can be seen. Typical imaging characteristics of different disease processes are given in Figure 5.35, but more details are provided in the relevant chapters.

Ultrasonography

Ultrasonography is a non-invasive and accessible modality, but is of limited use for evaluation of the nervous system because of sound attenuation by the surrounding bone. However, there are specific indications for ultrasonographic evaluation of the nervous system (Hudson *et al.*, 1998), including:

- Assessing the liver for portosystemic shunts (Lamb, 1998)
- Assessing the brain to identify hydrocephalus and other congenital anomalies (Figure 5.36)
- Examination of soft tissue masses (e.g. within the brachial plexus) to aid with biopsy (Platt *et al.*, 1999)
- Intraoperatively to identify and aid with the biopsy of intraparenchymal lesions (Thomas *et al.*, 1993).

A skilled ultrasonographer is needed to address these indications adequately.

The brain can be imaged most reliably via the persistent fontanelles. However, other windows are useful in young animals with thin calvaria, including the foramen magnum, the temporal fossa and the eye. The ultrasonographic anatomy of the brain has been described (see Figure 5.36) and its utility for identifying hydrocephalus and other congenital malformations, such as Dandy–Walker syndrome and cerebellar herniation associated with Chiari-like malformations, has been reported (Hudson *et al.*, 1990; Saito *et al.*, 2003; Schmidt *et al.*, 2008).

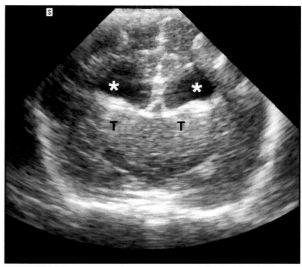

5.36 Transverse ultrasonogram of the brain via the bregmatic fontanelle at the level of the interthalamic adhesion. The lateral ventricles (*) and the thalamus (T) can be seen.

Disease process	T1 pre-contrast	T1 post-contrast	T2 (fast spin-echo)	Comments
Encephalitis and myelitis	Isointense or hypointense	Usually hyperintense; meninges may be enhanced	Hyperintense	Often multifocal; CSF analysis should be performed
Herniated disc material	Isointense or hypointense	Peripheral enhancement possible	Hypointense, isointense or hyperintense, depending on hydration of material	Acute disc herniations are commonly associated with very mixed signal
Infarction	Isointense or hypointense	Slight peripheral enhancement possible after latent period	Hyperintense	Can be wedge-shaped; little mass effect
Meningitis	Isointense to brain	Hyperintense meninges	Isointense	
Neoplasia: glioma	Isointense or hypointense	Classically hyperintense; low grade tumours may not be enhanced	Hyperintense; variably hyperintense beyond the area of the tumour due to vasogenic oedema	Mass effect expected
Neoplasia: meningioma	Isointense or hypointense; rarely hyperintense	Hyperintense, usually homogeneous unless cystic	Sometimes hyperintense; often hyperintense beyond the area of the tumour due to vasogenic oedema	May be cystic; may have dural enhancement (tail sign); may have hyperostosis of overlying skull
Neoplasia: other	Isointense or hypointense	Hyperintense	Hyperintense; variably hyperintense beyond the area of the tumour due to vasogenic oedema	Mass effect expected

5.35 MRI characteristics of different lesions.

Doppler ultrasonography is also useful to evaluate blood flow in the CNS. Transcranial Doppler ultrasonography can be used to evaluate the blood flow in the basilar artery via the foramen magnum in most patients, and the cerebral arteries can be evaluated in animals with a persistent fontanelle. The resistance index, a measure of resistance to blood flow, can be calculated for the basilar artery and has been shown to be related to intracranial pressure and neurological status in dogs (Fukishimi *et al.*, 2000; Saito *et al.*, 2003). The ultrasonographic and Doppler imaging characteristics of the spinal cord have also been described via a laminectomy window (Finn-Bodner *et al.*, 1995; Hudson *et al.*, 1995; Nanai *et al.*, 2007). In addition, ultrasonography has been used to guide lumbar puncture (Etienne *et al.*, 2010).

References and further reading

Available on accompanying DVD

6

Tissue biopsy

Sam Long and T. James Anderson

Obtaining tissue to establish a pathological diagnosis is a valuable tool in the investigation of disease. However, it should be remembered that the first duty of the clinician is to minimize harm to the patient in the process of obtaining a diagnosis. This applies particularly when performing a biopsy on the central nervous and neuromuscular systems, as even minimal damage to these tissues can cause significant and irreversible loss of function. It is therefore important that the clinician understands which parts of the nervous and neuromuscular systems can be sampled safely.

A biopsy may not provide a definitive diagnosis but rather may indicate the nature of the pathological process involved. Although identification of the process may not specify an aetiology, understanding the nature of the disease can help with therapy and prognosis. In this situation it is important that any changes observed by the pathologist are interpreted in conjunction with other information about the patient to refine the diagnosis. Therefore, the better informed the pathologist is by the veterinary surgeon, the more specific the investigation of the tissue can be.

This is particularly important if the sample has been obtained by either fine-needle aspiration or stereotactic needle biopsy (see Brain biopsy) as the number of cells collected is likely to be fewer than with conventional biopsy. However, it should be remembered that even conventional biopsy will sample only a proportion of the entire lesion and may not represent the entire pathological process. Thus, if biopsy findings are not compatible with the clinical picture and other information (such as history, likely differential diagnoses and response to treatment), an attempt should be made to determine whether the tissue sampled is from a representative area of the lesion.

Sample submission

Careful planning is necessary and ideally the clinician should communicate with the pathologist who will be examining the sample prior to submission. This is important firstly to ensure that the biopsy targets the most appropriate area of the tissue, and secondly because of the specific considerations that apply to processing and transporting biopsy samples of muscle, nerve and brain.

- For the comprehensive evaluation of muscle fibres (i.e. to allow access to the full range of staining and enzymatic techniques), biopsy samples should be rapidly frozen. Many laboratories recommend the rapid (overnight) submission of chilled fresh biopsy material and/or samples preserved in 10% buffered neutral formalin (BNF), which has implications for transportation. If rapid transportation to the laboratory is not available, snap-freezing the samples at the time of collection may be considered; although, this requires specialist techniques and material (e.g. isopentane, liquid nitrogen). Submitting frozen samples also has implications for transportation.
- For the comprehensive evaluation of nerve tissue, frozen, preserved (including specialist preservation techniques such as the use of glutaraldehyde; see Nerve biopsy) and fresh (for teased fibre preparations) material should be submitted. Consequently, laboratories may recommend the submission of chilled fresh material and/or samples preserved in 10% BNF, which has implications for transportation.

It is therefore important that the clinician seeks advice from relevant specialists in this field to identify suitable laboratories, and plan the biopsy procedure carefully. It is also important that the veterinary surgeon understands the preferences and requirements of the laboratory that will be processing the samples; laboratory websites are an excellent source of such specific information.

Samples sent cooled on dry ice and in fixatives are considered hazardous and legal requirements for packaging and labelling must be fulfilled. In addition, it may be desirable to send samples internationally for expert examination and in this situation customs requirements must also be met. For these reasons the clinician must arrange a suitable carrier, who has experience in transporting potentially hazardous biological specimens, beforehand. The time delay between taking the sample and its arrival at the laboratory must also be considered when being sent internationally to avoid the sample arriving at its destination outside of normal working hours or during a weekend/holiday and therefore being subject to deterioration. In addition, it may be desirable to send samples internationally for expert examination and, in this situation, customs requirements must also be met.

Muscle biopsy

Indications

The decision to proceed to biopsy is clear where muscle involvement is easy to identify. Clinical signs of muscle disease include:

- Muscle hypertrophy
- Muscle atrophy
- Contractures.

Other indications for muscle biopsy include:

- Weakness, stiffness or pain localizing to the neuromuscular system
- Results of diagnostic tests that support muscle disease (e.g. electromyography, persistently elevated creatine kinase concentration and myoglobinuria).

Tissue selection

The selection of tissue to biopsy depends on whether the underlying problem is:

- Generalized
- Localized to a specific muscle
- Restricted to a particular muscle group (e.g. temporalis muscles in masticatory muscle myositis).

With generalized disease, muscles should be selected for biopsy so that the diagnostic yield is maximized but morbidity is minimized; most laboratories prefer biopsy samples from two different muscles. Histological and histochemical characteristics vary between individual muscles reflecting their physiology; ideally, the selected muscle should be well characterized to aid interpretation (i.e. normal structure should be known).

Standard biopsy sites from the pelvic limb include the proximal muscles such as the vastus lateralis or biceps femoris, and from the thoracic limb include the triceps muscle. If neuropathy is likely, biopsy of the distal limb muscles, such as the cranial tibial muscle from the pelvic limb and the extensor carpii radialis from the thoracic limb, is suggested. Alternatively, the selection of biopsy site may be guided by electromyography. If nerve pathology is also suspected, a combined nerve and muscle biopsy should be considered; this may determine which muscle to biopsy if both are to be undertaken through one incision.

Severely fibrotic (end-stage) tissue should be avoided as it is unlikely to be informative with regard to the nature of the process or aetiology of the disease. Areas that have been subject to invasive investigations, such as the insertion of electromyogram (EMG) needles or previous biopsy should also be avoided (EMG studies should be planned with potential for biopsy in mind). Specimens should be harvested away from tendinous insertions as the normal histology of these areas can be confusing.

Techniques

Open biopsy

An open approach (Figure 6.1) is the standard method for muscle biopsy as it provides good and safe access, leading to confident identification of the sample tissue. This approach also allows an adequate tissue volume to be collected. The use of special clamps has been advocated to maintain the orientation and prevent contraction of the muscle; however, the use of such clamps demands a relatively large biopsy site and diagnostic samples can be obtained without their use. The disadvantages of the open approach are the need for general anaesthesia and the relatively invasive nature of the technique, which mitigates against sampling multiple sites.

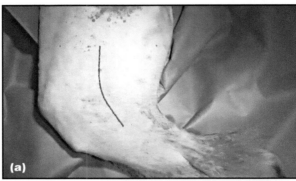
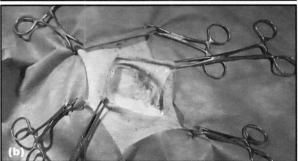

6.1 Open muscle biopsy procedure. **(a)** Position of the leg prior to draping. The incision site is indicated. **(b)** The leg following draping and skin incision. The vastus lateralis is exposed.

Once the skin and overlying fascia have been incised to expose the muscle, the orientation of the fibres should be established. Parallel incisions are then made in the direction of the fibres. A specimen should be approximately 0.5 x 0.5–1.0 cm in width and depth and 1–2 cm in length. Some authors recommend obtaining smaller samples (0.25 x 0.25 cm in cross-section and 1–2 cm in length); however, larger samples can be trimmed in the laboratory if necessary. The ends are sharply transected and the sample lifted clear, with care being taken to manipulate it by the ends only and thus minimize crush artefacts. The defect and overlying tissues are closed routinely.

Needle biopsy

Needle biopsy has been described in the dog for research purposes but has not become adopted as routine practice. Although there are the advantages of low morbidity and the possibility of performing the technique under sedation, disadvantages include the requirement for specialized equipment, potential problems with confidence in the tissue sampled, difficulties with sample orientation, and potentially poor tissue yields.

Complications

Complications following muscle biopsy are rare; if performed correctly, this is a minor procedure. Haemorrhage, swelling and haematoma formation are potential complications but are uncommon. Such events are usually related to either insufficient haemostasis during the procedure or patient interference with the surgery site and are managed in a routine fashion. Although open muscle biopsy may result in an appreciable defect at a single site in a large muscle, this is not a significant problem for the majority of patients. An appropriate biopsy is unlikely to result in long-term muscle dysfunction.

Tissue handling and processing

A complete histopathological examination of muscle involves many techniques that cannot be performed on traditional formalin-fixed material alone and require fresh-frozen tissue. The sample is usually placed in saline-moistened gauze and shipped overnight under refrigeration. Freezing is only undertaken if liquid nitrogen and isopentane are available. Specimens fixed in formalin (10% buffered formal saline) are not without value, although they cannot be characterized as extensively as frozen tissue. Samples for examination by electron microscopy should be collected into special fixatives containing 2.5% glutaraldehyde. Samples that are immersion-fixed should be attached to a splint, such as a tongue depressor, using a 25-gauge needle, to prevent contraction during fixation and reduce artefacts.

Examination and interpretation

In most cases, examination of a muscle biopsy sample should confirm or deny the presence of a myopathy or neuropathy. The value of having biopsy material from a representative nerve and associated muscle is self-evident. Non-specific myofibre atrophy is occasionally found since atrophy may be the result of many different insults including disuse and cachexia, and interpreting this finding is dependent upon good clinical detail and thorough investigation.

Establishing whether a process is inflammatory represents a significant step in assessing the nature of the disease and may indicate a specific diagnosis or a rationale for therapy, even if the specific aetiology remains uncertain. The major decision to be made is whether evidence of inflammation suggests an infectious or immune-mediated aetiology. Being able to put the findings in context of the clinical scenario is important for the pathologist in advising the veterinary surgeon and, perhaps, suggesting further avenues of investigation.

Frozen tissue is required to take advantage of the full range of enzymatic and immunohistochemical techniques that have been developed for the characterization of muscle biopsy specimens. A general morphological examination can be undertaken on both frozen and fixed tissues. The major features of morphological interest are:

- Muscle fibre type and distribution
- Muscle fibre shape and size
- Presence of degeneration/regeneration ± necrosis
- Distribution of nuclei
- Presence of vacuoles or inclusions
- Cellular infiltrates.

Muscle fibre type and distribution

Myofibre typing is achieved by histochemical techniques that identify the presence of enzymes or substrate in the tissue. This technique is based on the myofibrillar adenosine triphosphatase (ATPase) reaction under different pH conditions, which identifies two major muscle fibre types and a number of subtypes (Figure 6.2). Most normal muscle fascicles contain a mixture of fibre types and hence

Muscle type	ATPase immunostaining	Physiological properties	Comments
I	pH 4.3 (reversal) dark pH 4.6 dark pH 9.8 light	Predominately aerobic with oxidative metabolism (slow contraction/fatigue-resistant/postural muscles)	
IIA	pH 4.3 (reversal) light pH 4.6 light pH 9.8 dark	Predominantly anaerobic with glycolytic metabolism (fast contraction/phasic movement/movement muscles)	
IIB	pH 4.3 (reversal) light pH 4.6 intermediate pH 9.8 dark		Not present in dogs
IIC	pH 4.3 (reversal) intermediate pH 4.6 intermediate pH 9.8 dark		Rare except in neonates or may be seen with myofibre regeneration
IIM	pH 4.3 intermediate pH 4.6 dark pH 9.8 dark	Specialized type II fibres that are primarily muscles of mastication	Specific to the dorsal muscles of first branchial arch origin

6.2 Classification of muscle fibre types. Optimum pH varies with species.

there is a mosaic appearance with ATPase staining (Figure 6.3). The proportion and distribution of myofibre types may be altered by disease and any changes must be put in context of the particular muscle sampled. There may be a general change in the proportion of myofibre types (e.g. type I fibre predominance in Labrador Retriever myopathy) or loss of the mosaic pattern, producing large groups of single fibre types (fibre type grouping) as a result of reinnervation. Determining whether there is a selective increase or loss of a particular myofibre type requires quantitative analysis, which is time-consuming.

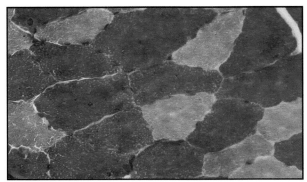

6.3 Mosaic appearance of normal muscle stained with ATPase (pH 9.8). The darker fibres are the 'fast' type II myofibrils. (Original magnification X80)

Muscle fibre shape and size

Healthy muscle fibres have a polygonal shape and smooth outline (Figure 6.4). Myofibre diameter is variable and reflects the specific muscle sampled, the region within the specific muscle, patient age and size. Changes in the shape and cross-sectional area of myofibres within fascicles suggest disease. The major patterns and their significance are described in Figure 6.5.

Angular atrophy of type I and type II muscle fibres is a hallmark of denervation. Atrophic fibres have a reduced cross-sectional area and sharp, pointed projections (see Figure 6.4b). In early denervation, single atrophic fibres are scattered throughout an affected muscle. As denervation progresses, small and large groups of atrophic fibres develop. Occasionally unaffected myofibres may develop compensatory hypertrophy, resulting in an excessive variation in muscle fibre size. If atrophy of all myofibres occurs at a similar time a round or polygonal shape is observed. Myofibres may undergo splitting as a non-specific event, usually associated with myopathic disease; although, this can be a normal finding at the musculotendinous junction. Depending on the plane of the section the nuclei may appear internalized.

Degeneration/regeneration ± necrosis

Regenerating muscle fibres are smaller in diameter than normal fibres, with a basophilic appearance on sections stained with haematoxylin and eosin (H&E) (Figure 6.6a). These immature fibres have an increased number of normally situated nuclei. In

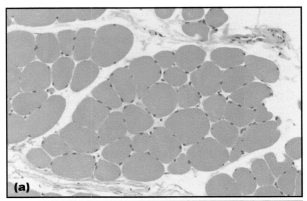

6.4 Normal muscle in transverse section is composed of groups of myofibrils with similar diameters, a smooth polygonal outline and peripherally located nuclei. Atrophy of specific myofibrils produces a characteristic angular cross-sectional outline. **(a)** Normal muscle. (H&E stain; original magnification X60) **(b)** Myopathy in a cat. Note the atrophied fibres scattered through the muscle. (H&E stain; original magnification X25)

Finding	Process

Atrophy:
    Angular
    Small group
    Large group
	Neuropathy but can be observed as a non-specific finding with myopathy

Necrosis	Myopathy
Infiltrate	Myopathy
Myofibril regeneration	Myopathy or neuropathy
Cellular infiltrates: accumulation of substrates (e.g. glycogen) or cellular organelles (e.g. mitochondria)	Myopathy

6.5 Pathological findings observed in myopathic and neuropathic muscle disease.

contrast, necrotic muscle fibres show a decreased intensity of staining with enzymatic and traditional histochemical techniques, giving rise to 'ghost fibres'. They tend to have an increased density of central nuclei (Figure 6.6b) and there may be a monocytic infiltrate. It should be noted that degeneration of muscle fibres does not necessarily lead to necrosis. End-stage degenerate muscle fibres are replaced with connective and adipose tissue in varying proportions.

Distribution of nuclei

Muscle fibre nuclei are normally distributed peripherally around the sarcolemma. A central location may be observed with both myopathies and neuropathies, but is not a finding specific to either (see Figure 6.6b). In general, if >1% of the nuclei are central, this is interpreted as abnormal.

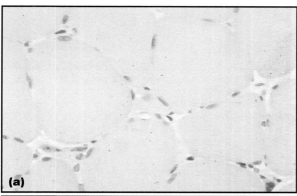

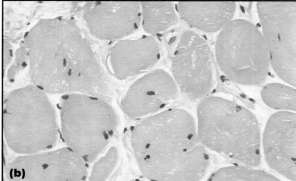

6.6 **(a)** Regenerating myofibrils are reduced in diameter and have a basophilic appearance on H&E staining. (Original magnification X100) **(b)** With some myopathies there is central migration of the nuclei. (H&E stain; original magnification X100)

Presence of vacuoles and inclusions

Abnormal deposits of substances, structures and organelles may be observed microscopically or ultrastructurally. Accumulations may represent excess substrate, product or abnormal cellular components, depending on the underlying disorder. Metabolic disorders result in the accumulation of substrate or product, depending on the point at which the pathways are disrupted, within the muscle fibres. These accumulations may be seen as vacuoles of material (e.g. glycogen or lipid) or accumulations of cytoskeletal elements (e.g. mitochondria in inherited myopathy of the Great Dane) (see Chapter 18).

Cellular infiltrates

Accumulations of lymphocytes, neutrophils, eosinophils and macrophages may occur with myositis. These may cluster around blood vessels or abnormal tissue components within either muscle or nerve fibres. Occasionally, neoplastic lymphocytes may be present with multicentric lymphoma. Primary muscle tumours are occasionally observed (Neravanda *et al.*, 2009), but muscle is not a common site for metastatic disease.

The presence of parasites is usually marked by inflammatory infiltrates and myofibre necrosis, but organisms are only occasionally observed on sections stained routinely (Figure 6.7). Immunostains are available for specific parasites (e.g. *Neospora*; Lindsay *et al.*, 1999). Parasitic and protozoal cysts can be found with no evidence of associated inflammation.

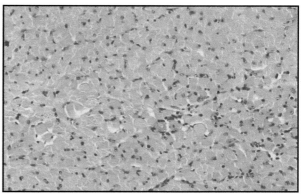

6.7 Inflammatory infiltrate in canine muscle affected by neosporosis. Note the increased density of nuclei (stained blue). (H&E stain; original magnification X25)

Staining

For a list of histological and enzymatic stains and their applications see Figure 6.8. The use of immunostains is of value in specific circumstances (e.g. confirmation of Duchenne's type muscular dystrophy by demonstration of loss of dystrophin). Panels of immunostains may be of value in describing unusual myopathies by further characterizing the nature of the abnormality.

Stain/enzyme	Applications
Haematoxylin and eosin (H&E)	General stain for morphological assessment of cells and nuclei of all tissue; necrotic fibres have reduced stain uptake; degenerating/regenerating fibres are basophilic
Modified Gomori trichrome	General stain for morphological assessment of cells and nuclei of all tissues; useful for demonstrating nemaline rods
Myofibre adenosine triphosphatase (ATPase)	Identifies functional fibre type (see Figure 6.2)
Periodic acid–Schiff (PAS)	Glycogen storage disorders
Acid phosphatase	Lysosomes in myofibrils and macrophages
Oil Red O	Triglyceride fats; identification of lipid storage disorders
Alkaline phosphatase	Identification of regenerating fibres and proliferating connective tissue (cats)

6.8 The application of histological and enzymatic staining to muscle samples. (continues) ▶

Stain/enzyme	Applications
Nicotinamide adenine dinucleotide–tetrazolium reductase (NAD–TR)	Identifies mitochondrial oxidative enzyme; stains mitochondria and sacroplasmic reticulum; highlights mitochondrial-rich fatigue-resistant fibres and angular atrophied fibres; useful for identifying mitochondrial aggregates, tubular aggregates and pyknotic nuclear clumps
Succinate dehydrogenase (SDH)	Identifies mitochondrial oxidative enzyme; specific to mitochondria
Cytochrome-c oxidase (CcO)	Identifies mitochondrial oxidative enzyme; specific to mitochondria
Staphylococcal protein A – horseradish peroxidase	Non-specific binding to deposits of immunoglobulin; may detect antibodies at the neuromuscular junction in myasthenia gravis
Esterase	Identifies neuromuscular junctions; also stains lysosomes of myofibrils and macrophages

6.8 (continued) The application of histological and enzymatic staining to muscle samples.

Peripheral nerve biopsy

Indications
Clinical evidence of peripheral nerve disease (see Chapters 2 and 15) supported by electrophysiological evidence of nerve dysfunction (see Chapter 4) are prerequisites for electing to perform a nerve biopsy.

Tissue selection
Theoretically, a biopsy can be performed on any nerve. However, the practicalities of surgical access and the potential for dysfunction following biopsy are major considerations. For example, a biopsy is rarely performed on the cranial nerves because of their surgical inaccessibility and the likelihood and consequences of subsequent dysfunction.

The tissue for biopsy may be indicated by localized dysfunction. Alternatively, for more generalized conditions the nerve selected should be based upon the following factors:

- Ease of surgical access
- Likely subsequent dysfunction
- Specific clinical deficit (motor *versus* sensory)
- The normal characteristics of the nerve under consideration as a basis for interpretation
- The normal characteristics of the associated muscle if a combined nerve/muscle biopsy is planned.

The common peroneal nerve is an example of a peripheral nerve with established morphological and electrophysiological data associated with a well characterized muscle (i.e. cranial tibial muscle). The common peroneal nerve has the advantage of being easily accessed and identified (Figure 6.9). However, as with the majority of peripheral nerves,

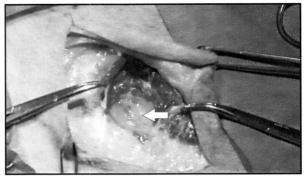

6.9 Common peroneal nerve biopsy. The use of self-retaining retractors is of great value. The nerve (arrowed) lies beneath the fascia of the biceps femoris muscle, which is incised to reveal the nerve. The nerve is divided longitudinally using fine sutures to support the extremities and reduce artefact.

the common peroneal nerve is a mixed nerve, i.e. contains both motor and sensory fibres. The availability of predominantly sensory nerves is limited; the caudal cutaneous antebrachial nerve (thoracic limb) and the caudal cutaneous sural nerve (pelvic limb) (Figure 6.10) are examples.

Biopsy of nervous structures where there is a high likelihood of subsequent dysfunction (e.g. cranial nerves) is usually avoided; although, it may be necessary on occasion during cytoreductive procedures. Biopsy of proximal peripheral nervous tissue and nerve roots, as indicated by electrophysiological studies, is possible but requires significant surgical dissection and experience in identifying the relevant tissue for sampling. If a nerve root biopsy is performed, ideally a dorsal root should be selected to minimize motor dysfunction, although single ventral nerve roots can be removed with little or no resulting dysfunction. Nerve tissue may also be found within

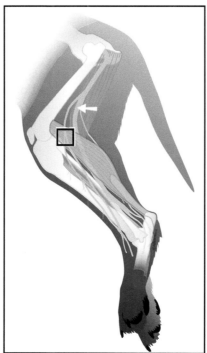

6.10 Nerves of the pelvic limb showing incision site for biopsy (black box) and the common peroneal nerve (arrowed). The vastus lateralis which lies over the peroneal nerve has been removed for clarity.

muscle biopsy material and is of potential value in assessing the distal nerve branches as well as the secondary consequences on muscle morphology.

Techniques

Peripheral nerves must be visualized using an open approach. The majority of nerves are biopsied by transecting approximately a third of the width of the nerve and removing fascicles about 1 cm in length, taking care not to transect the entire width of the nerve (see **Muscle and nerve biopsy** clip on DVD). Care in handling the specimen is important and the sample should only be handled at the ends to preserve a region free of potential artefact; this may be achieved by placing fine sutures in each extremity. Terminal branches of sensory nerves may be removed entirely. Prerequisites of this procedure are:

- Competent soft tissue handling skills
- Good condition of instruments.

Complete descriptions of this procedure have been published elsewhere (Dickinson and Le-Couteur, 2002).

Complications

Neurological dysfunction may be observed and reflects the nerve sampled. Biopsy of the common peroneal nerve (at the level of the stifle) rarely produces deleterious persistent dysfunction, although the biopsy site may be painful postoperatively. Wound problems similar to those found following muscle biopsy, primarily due to patient interference and excessive postoperative movement, may be observed and are managed in a routine fashion.

Tissue handling and processing

Nerve specimens should be fixed with a longitudinal orientation (e.g. by pinning to a piece of cork and floating tissue immersed in the fixative) to minimize artefacts; however, samples should not be placed under tension as this may itself create artefacts. The choice of fixative is significant. Traditional processing using 10% BNF and paraffin embedding removes lipids, which represent approximately 50% of the myelin sheath, impairing visualization of the myelin sheath structure. An alternative fixative and embedding technique, using glutaraldehyde and resin, is required for best preservation of anatomical detail (Figure 6.11). However, paraffin-embedded sections are of value in assessing infiltrates and may provide some information about the myelin structure.

Frozen sections can be prepared if chilled fresh tissue is submitted. Frozen sections may be required for special techniques (e.g. immunolabelling/enzymatic techniques) and might be recommended by the pathology laboratory, depending on the circumstances (see above). A teased nerve fibre preparation is a specialist technique, which is of value in assessing demyelination and/or the distribution of pathology along axons. However, this specialized technique is only available from selected laboratories.

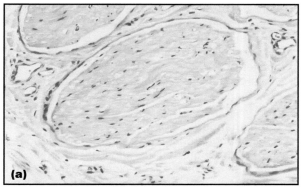

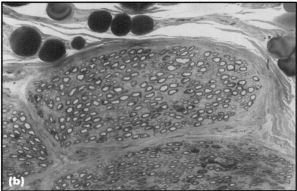

6.11 Transverse sections of a normal peripheral nerve showing the effects of fixation techniques on the appearance of the myelin sheath. **(a)** BNF fixation, paraffin embedding and H&E staining. (Original magnification x100) **(b)** 2.5% glutaraldehyde fixation, resin embedding and azure blue staining. Note the distinct appearance of the myelin sheath as a dark staining outline to each axon in the resin-embedded section. (Original magnification X100)

Examination and interpretation

The information gained from examination of the biopsy tissue may lead to a specific diagnosis. However, changes are often non-specific and may support the presence and nature of a disease, without revealing a specific cause, as well as suggesting a prognosis (e.g. if there is endoneurial fibrosis, marked nerve fibre loss and no regeneration, there is often a poor prognosis for recovery).

Paraffin-embedded samples are examined using routine stains for tissue structure and cellular components. Routine histopathological examination might establish axon density and myelin status. Resin embedding is more appropriate for examining myelin structure, at both the light microscope and ultrastructural (electron microscopy) level. Teased preparations are of value in ascertaining the distribution of pathology along an individual axon. Electron microscopy is of value for examining unmyelinated fibres in addition to cellular and myelin sheath ultrastructure (e.g. mitochondria). Neither electron microscopy nor teased preparations are undertaken routinely.

The major features of interest when evaluating a peripheral nerve are:

- Axon structure and density
- Myelin sheath thickness and integrity

- Schwann cell population (health and numbers)
- Support tissues (blood vessels and fibrous sheaths)
- Evidence of an infiltrate (distribution and nature of cells)
- Neuronal cell population (only relevant to dorsal root ganglion biopsy).

Axonal changes

Axonal changes observed range from evidence of dystrophy through degeneration to complete loss. These changes may affect axons of either large or small diameter, or may be generalized, and may be relevant to the underlying aetiology. Loss of axons may be secondary to traumatic, toxic or metabolic insults in addition to loss of motor neurons or axonopathies of undetermined cause. When an axon is transected, the distal axon undergoes a stereotypical sequence of degenerative cellular events with disappearance of the axon and myelin. This process is called Wallerian degeneration.

Axonal dystrophy may be seen as axonal swelling, referred to as spheroid formation, with secondary loss of myelin in the area of the swelling. Spheroids contain accumulated cell components, the nature of which can be confirmed by ultrastructural examination. Axonal dysfunction may also be accompanied by the formation of large myelin ovoids and myelin balls, with evidence of remyelination if the axon survives. Lipid accumulations in local macrophages may be noted (Figure 6.12).

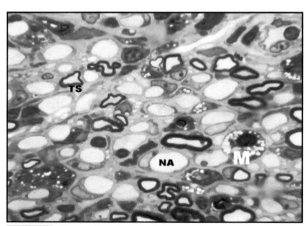

6.12 Demyelinating peripheral neuropathy in a dog. Myelin loss (naked axons, NA) and possible remyelination (thin myelin sheaths, TS) are evident. Note the macrophage with foamy cytoplasm (M); these inclusions contain lipid from the breakdown of myelin. (Resin-embedding and azure blue staining; original magnification approximately X250) (Courtesy of I Griffiths)

Myelin changes

Care must be taken when interpreting myelin changes because artefacts are common if the tissue is handled, fixed or processed suboptimally. Myelin changes may affect specific populations (sizes) of axons or may be a general event. Primary demyelination leaves the axons intact. The myelin sheath may be thinner or thicker than normal, show evidence of degeneration, or be absent.

- Hypomyelination (disproportionately thin myelin sheaths) may be due to:
  - Dysmyelination (failure of the proper development of myelin in developing animals)
  - Myelin loss (demyelination)
  - Remyelination (see Figure 6.12).
- Hypermyelination may be observed in the peripheral nervous system (PNS). Excessively thick myelin sheaths are usually related to repeated attempts at remyelination. Hypermyelination is a rare observation in animals (e.g. hypertrophic neuropathy in Tibetan Mastiffs; Cooper et al., 1984).

Disorders of myelination can be primary, but are often secondary to other processes, including endocrine (e.g. diabetes mellitus), compressive and inflammatory diseases.

Schwann cell changes

Specific pathological alteration of Schwann cells may be due to developmental abnormalities, storage diseases, toxins, immune dysfunction or neoplasia (malignant nerve sheath tumours).

Support tissues

The supporting tissues of nerves (meninges of proximal nerve roots, perineurium/endoneurium and blood vessels) may also reflect disease. Hypertrophy of these structures is the most common abnormality. Hypertrophy may reflect the duration of the process or may be secondary to an infiltrate.

Infiltration

The presence, distribution and nature of an infiltrate are important observations for understanding the disease process. Infiltrates generally reflect inflammation (Figure 6.13) or invasion by tumour cells. Special techniques may be required for detailed characterization of specific features (e.g. subtyping of lymphoma).

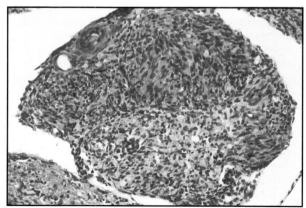

6.13 Nerve root affected by *Neospora canis*. The nerve has become thickened and there is an increased density of nuclei, suggesting a cellular infiltrate. (H&E stain; original magnification X60)

Brain biopsy

The veterinary neurologist relies heavily on computed tomography (CT) and magnetic resonance imaging (MRI) when diagnosing intracranial diseases. However, whilst imaging provides some information about the nature of a lesion (such as size, location and relationship to other intracranial structures), it can only provide, at best, circumstantial evidence as to the underlying pathology. Frequently the differential diagnoses list for a lesion found on imaging the brain includes sterile inflammation, infection, vascular conditions and neoplasia. Furthermore, ancillary tests such as cerebrospinal fluid (CSF) taps and electroencephalography are often unhelpful in distinguishing between these diagnoses. Given that different pathological processes require different therapeutic approaches and carry different prognoses, a definitive diagnosis should be sought, and this may require pathological examination of the tissue involved.

Indications

Generally, tissue may be biopsied for one of three reasons:

- To provide a diagnosis to determine optimal treatment
- To provide a diagnosis to give a more accurate prognosis for the patient
- As part of therapy (either excisional biopsy in an attempt to cure the disease or debulking to alleviate the clinical signs).

The lesions most suitable for biopsy are those that are easily visible on imaging studies, particularly with contrast medium. This includes the majority of brain tumours, as well as lesions of an inflammatory and/or infectious nature, especially if the inflammation is focal, superficial and well defined. Examples include the focal form of granulomatous meningoencephalitis (GME), abscesses and localized encephalitis/meningitis (Figure 6.14). Diffuse lesions are less suitable for biopsy as the

Lesions well suited for intracranial biopsy
• Most tumours situated in superficial locations: meningioma, astrocytoma, oligodendroglioma, ependymoma, metastatic adenocarcinoma, some lymphoid tumours • Lesions caused by inflammatory diseases that are focal in nature: focal granulomatous meningoencephalitis (GME), abscesses, some forms of encephalitis

Lesions poorly suited for intracranial biopsy
• Tumours in deep-seated areas: medulloblastoma within the cerebellum/medulla, other tumours in the thalamus, hypothalamus or brainstem • Vascular tumours: choroid plexus papilloma, metastatic haemangiosarcoma • Vascular lesions: cerebral haematoma, cerebrovascular malformation • Diffuse lesions: diffuse GME, some lymphomas, gliomatosis cerebri

6.14 Suitability of various lesions for intracranial biopsy.

selection of representative sample areas is more difficult and the tissue taken may not yield a definitive diagnosis. Examples include some tumours (e.g. gliomatosis cerebri and some forms of lymphoma), diffuse GME and viral encephalitides (Figure 6.15). It should also be remembered that biopsy is more risky with lesions which are likely to bleed significantly. This includes some tumours (e.g. choroid plexus papilloma) and lesions involving the cerebral vasculature (e.g. vascular hamartoma).

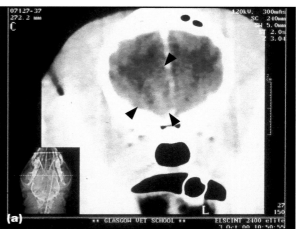
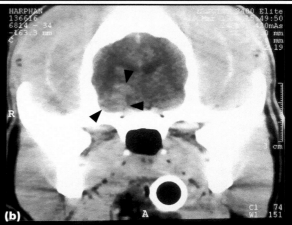

6.15 Lesions unsuitable for biopsy.
(a) Granulomatous meningoencephalitis. Post-contrast CT image showing patchy, mild contrast medium uptake diffusely (arrowheads) with white matter oedema but no obvious focus to target.
(b) Intraparenchymal haemorrhage. Following contrast medium administration, this CT image appeared similar to pre-contrast images with minimal uptake of contrast medium but a poorly defined area of hyperintensity (arrowheads).

Tissue selection

When biopsying intracranial lesions, it is important to select areas that are likely to contain the most active (and therefore representative) pathological processes. The presence of hypodense or hypointense areas within a lesion following contrast medium administration is suggestive of necrosis, fluid accumulation or possibly oedema. Consequently, samples taken from these areas may be non-diagnostic and yield little more than fragments of necrotic brain tissue. However, samples taken from regions that are enhanced by contrast medium are more likely to yield tissue with a good vascular supply, and consequently represent those areas that are involved in the active pathological process. These principles are particularly important when performing stereotactic needle biopsy, where the volume of tissue yielded is limited and the chance of sampling non-representative tissue is relatively high. When sampling deep lesions, even needle biopsy may prove a risk. It has been recommended in humans that only one needle biopsy sample be taken from the brainstem or other high-risk areas. This is to decrease the risk of haemorrhage and compromise of adjacent vital structures such as the cardiovascular and respiratory centres (Kondziolka *et al.*, 1998). Consequently, selecting the site from which the sample is to be taken in order to maximize the diagnostic yield becomes critical.

Techniques

Open craniectomy
Open craniectomy is a relatively common procedure, usually performed in order to carry out excision or debulking of a lesion, although it may also be undertaken for other reasons, such as decompression following cranial trauma. Many parts of the brain are accessible via open craniectomy, including the olfactory bulb, frontal, temporal, parietal and occipital lobes (via a frontal sinus, lateral or extended lateral approach) and the cerebellum (via a suboccipital or caudotentorial approach). Lesions located deep to the surface of the brain, which are not visible at surgery, can be localized accurately using ultrasonography. However, in general, these approaches do not allow access to the deeper parts of the brain, such as the thalamus, or the brainstem.

Needle biopsy
Needle biopsy may be performed either 'freehand', usually to access very superficial lesions through a burr hole created following imaging and localization (with or without the assistance of ultrasonography), or using a stereotactic frame to guide the needle, again following imaging and localization (Figure 6.16). Freehand fine-needle aspiration may also be performed on superficial lesions.

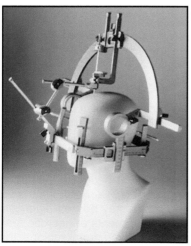

6.16

Leksell stereotactic frame. This is one of the most commonly used frames for image-guided needle biopsy in human patients. (Courtesy of Elekta UK)

Stereotactic biopsy is generally performed using a side-cutting brain cannula. The cannula is a blunt-ended needle with an inner and outer sheath, both of which contain a lateral window. Once the cannula is introduced into the region to be sampled, tissue is drawn into the inner sheath using gentle suction applied via a syringe attached to the end of the cannula. The inner sheath is then rotated through 180 degrees in relation to the outer sheath; the sharp edges of the lateral window of the inner sheath excise the brain fragment within the inner sheath using a guillotine action. The sample is then collected by withdrawing the inner sheath from the outer sheath. Stereotactic needle biopsy has been used in human neurosurgical institutions extensively over the past two decades, and stereotactic frames and biopsy systems have now been developed for use with dogs and cats, although they are not yet widely available (Koblik *et al.*, 1999a; Moissonnier *et al.*, 2002; Chen *et al.*, 2011).

Frameless stereotactic systems have also been developed which utilize cameras and fiducial markers placed on the skin to triangulate the position of the tip of the biopsy needle in three-dimensional (3D) space and reference this to pre-acquired CT or MRI images in real-time. The Brainsight™ system is an example of a frameless stereotactic device developed for use in animals, and has the advantage of allowing both needle biopsy and intraoperative navigation to be performed during open craniectomy (Figure 6.17; see also **Stereotactic needle biopsy** clip on DVD). Stereotactic biopsy allows access to lesions in parts of the brain that are inaccessible via open craniectomy, and is generally regarded as being a safe and reliable technique, with figures for morbidity and mortality in humans ranging from 2–6% and 0–2.3%, respectively (Burger and Nelson, 1997; Kondziolka *et al.*, 1998). The mean needle placement error distance is 1.8 mm based on a recent study using the Brainsight™ system (Chen *et al.*, 2011). Stereotactic biopsy may also allow aspiration of fluid from fluid-filled lesions and can be used to introduce treatment agents into lesions, bypassing the blood–brain barrier.

Choice of technique
The decision regarding which method to use is dictated primarily by the facilities available to the neurosurgeon. Other factors that need to be considered include the appearance of the lesion on CT and/or MRI, the location of the lesion (intra-axial *versus* extra-axial) and the neurological status of the patient (Figure 6.18). If the neurological status of the patient is poor and raised intracranial pressure (ICP) is suspected, a craniectomy and biopsy may be performed to allow decompression and alleviation of the clinical signs, in addition to providing tissue for diagnosis. However, lesions in deep structures may be difficult to biopsy via an open craniectomy. This particularly applies to lesions in the deep grey matter of the forebrain (e.g. thalamus and hypothalamus) or brainstem (e.g. medulla oblongata). In this situation, stereotactic needle biopsy may be preferable, if available, as it causes less damage to vital

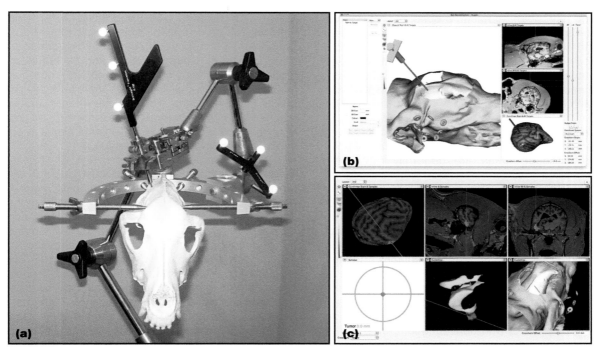

6.17 An MRI stereotactic biopsy system. **(a)** During surgery, the head of the animal is held rigidly in place using a c-clamp and skull screws, which press against the animal's skull. The c-clamp is attached to a standard operating table using a large adjustable arm. An articulated surgical arm is attached the c-clamp to guide tools to the target. In conjunction with the neuronavigation software and the position sensor, a path is set to target the brain of the animal. **(b)** Brainsight™ software enables the 3D reconstruction of imaging data, which is then used to target a tumour with a biopsy needle. Reconstructions of the skin, skull and brain are generated from MR images. **(c)** A lesion or tumour is identified as a target (red) in the right temporal region using MR images of the dog and the Brainsight™ software. The centre of the target is visualized in 3D and the most appropriate trajectory to the tumour (avoiding key structures such as the ventricular system (yellow)) is saved by the software. Co-registration of the animal to the MR images is performed by identifying homologous points between the images and the subject with the help of fiducial markers that are rigidly fixed to the animal's head. Once registered, neuronavigation is performed in real-time with the aid of a position sensor in the operating suite to precisely target the tumour. (Courtesy of S Frey, Rogue Research Inc.)

Technique	Advantages	Disadvantages
Open craniectomy	Allows decompression for patients with deteriorating neurological status Requires less specialized equipment and facilities Allows control of haemorrhage intraoperatively Provides large tissue samples	Only able to access superficial lesions More invasive with higher morbidity
Needle biopsy	Minimally invasive with low morbidity and mortality Allows sampling of lesions in deep areas of the brain	Requires specialized equipment Does not allow decompression for patients with deteriorating neurological status Provides smaller tissue samples Does not allow control of haemorrhage intraoperatively

6.18 Advantages and disadvantages of brain biopsy.

structures. With lesions that are thought to be very vascular, based on their imaging characteristics, conventional biopsy obtained via a craniectomy may be more desirable than a needle biopsy as haemorrhage can be controlled intraoperatively.

Complications

Craniectomy
Complications associated with conventional craniectomy have been well described. The majority of these are the result of damage to important structures during surgery, either through direct trauma or following secondary haemorrhage and/or infarction. Primary damage that occurs during surgery may be followed by more significant and progressive secondary damage. Secondary damage is mediated by biochemical, vascular and inflammatory events, all of which contribute to the end results of neuronal and glial necrosis, ischaemia or infarction, cerebral oedema and raised ICP. Ultimately, if this process is not interrupted or reversed, cerebral or cerebellar herniation may result, leading to death of the patient. Less severe damage may result in postoperative seizures, which may necessitate long-term anticonvulsant therapy (Kostolich and Dulish, 1987).

As with any open surgical procedure, iatrogenic infection may occur following surgery, which is serious and commonly fatal. A significant complication reported with intracranial surgery is aspiration pneumonia associated with prolonged periods of recumbency and possible megaoesophagus; this may be seen with brainstem lesions (Fransson *et al.*, 2001).

Needle biopsy

Stereotactic biopsy is also associated with complications, although these are generally rare. The most common problem is haemorrhage caused by the biopsy procedure; this may lead to significant neurological deficits and can be life-threatening. To prevent this the trajectory of the biopsy needle must be planned carefully in order to avoid major blood vessels and care should be taken if imaging findings suggest the lesion is highly vascular (e.g. choroid plexus papilloma; Figure 6.19). In addition, it is important to maintain normal systemic blood pressure during surgery, as hypertension in humans has been reported to increase the risk of haemorrhage following biopsy. As with conventional craniectomy, postoperative imaging is recommended following needle biopsy to detect haemorrhage. Close monitoring of the patient's neurological status should also be performed for 48 hours following the procedure and scanning should be repeated if any deterioration in the level of consciousness occurs. In rare cases, a craniectomy may be required to alleviate raised ICP or to adequately control haemorrhage. Other complications reported in dogs include:

- Transient worsening of clinical signs
- Seizures
- Cardiac arrythmias
- Epistaxis
- Hypercapnia
- Apnoea.

A rare complication reported in humans is 'seeding' of a tumour along the needle tract. Morbidity and mortality rates in dogs and cats range from 12–26% and 7–8%, respectively, and are higher than in humans (morbidity: 3.5%; mortality: <1%) (Hall, 1998; Koblik *et al.*, 1999b; Moissonnier *et al.*, 2002). In addition, it should be remembered that due to the small volume of tissue yielded during needle biopsy procedures, it is fairly common to obtain a non-diagnostic sample, especially if a non-representative part of the tumour is targeted. It is therefore extremely helpful to perform cytology or to examine frozen sections during the procedure to ensure that a representative sample has been obtained.

Tissue handling and processing

Samples obtained by conventional biopsy or stereotactic needle biopsy may be submitted for either frozen sections or smear cytology, in addition to routine histopathological examination. Fine-needle aspirates are generally submitted for conventional cytological examination. Fixation of biopsy samples in 10% BNF is most common, allowing standard H&E and a range of immunohistochemical stains to be used. Samples submitted for snap-freezing in liquid nitrogen can be subjected to specific immunohistochemical stains if a particular disease is suspected and facilities for snap-freezing are available.

As standard formalin fixation and paraffin embedding is relatively time-consuming, a portion of the sample may be examined intraoperatively to provide a provisional diagnosis. The aims of intraoperative evaluation are two-fold:

- To confirm the diagnostic value of the sample in order to minimize the number of samples taken
- To provide a provisional diagnosis that facilitates patient management in the early postoperative period.

The most common form of intraoperative diagnosis utilizes frozen sections, which requires specialized equipment and the ability to snap-freeze samples in liquid nitrogen soon after their acquisition. Turnaround time from sample submission to staining and examination is approximately 20–30 minutes.

An alternative to frozen sections is the use of smear preparations. Smear preparations are created by placing the sample on one glass slide and, applying pressure, quickly and firmly 'smearing' the sample with the end of a second glass slide. Smear preparations can be performed rapidly, with a turnaround time of approximately 90 seconds depending on the stain used. Rapid stains such as Romanovsky-type (e.g. Diff-Quik®) or toluidine blue may be used, as well as standard H&E staining.

Smear preparations are also useful for confirming the presence of disease and differentiating inflammation from neoplasia (Long *et al.*, 2002). Viewing smear preparations at low power often provides valuable information as different lesions smear in characteristic ways (Figure 6.20). In the case of tumours, whilst they may suggest a particular type of neoplasm, smear preparations may be less useful in providing an accurate grading of malignancy due to the small tissue sample examined. The reader is

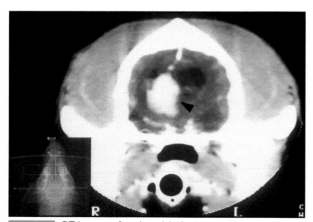

6.19 CT image of a choroid plexus papilloma following the injection of contrast medium. Note that there is marked contrast medium uptake, resulting in the extremely hyperdense appearance of the lesion (arrowhead). This is consistent with a highly vascular lesion.

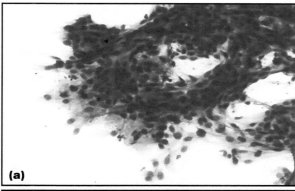

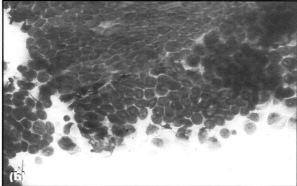

6.20 Smear cytology characteristics of intracranial tumours at low power. **(a)** Meningioma. Note the cohesive nature of this tumour and the tumour cells adhering to branching capillaries. (Diff-Quik® stain; original magnification X50) **(b)** Metastatic carcinoma. Note the appearance of sheets of tumour cells and 'moulding' of cell nuclei to each other. (Diff-Quik® stain; original magnification X50)

referred to the comprehensive report by Vernau *et al.* (2001) for a description of the cytological appearance of those lesions characterized in the dog.

Interpretation

In some circumstances, interpretation may not give a definitive diagnosis or could be misleading. This occurs particularly when an area of a lesion is sampled that is not representative of the underlying pathology. For example, the periphery of certain lesions (including tumours) may show non-specific reactive inflammation with hypercellularity due to an increase in the number of astrocytes that are reactive in nature. If this area is sampled, it may be difficult to determine whether the lesion is inflammatory or neoplastic in nature, as benign astrocytic tumours may appear to be very similar to non-specific reactive inflammation.

The histological characteristics of most intracranial lesions in dogs and cats have been well described (Summers *et al.*, 1995). Important features of brain biopsy samples, which may help to achieve a diagnosis, include:

- Number of cells
- Presence of abnormal cells (neoplastic cells)
- Presence of inflammation (either diffusely within the brain parenchyma or clustered around blood vessels)

- Appearance of brain cells (e.g. chromatolytic neurons, hypertrophic astrocytes)
- Appearance of background tissue (e.g. oedema, necrosis)
- Presence of special features (e.g. inclusion bodies).

Number of cells

The number of cells in a given part of the brain may provide an important clue to the underlying pathology. Hypercellularity may occur with an increase in the population of cells normally resident in the brain (usually astrocytes, oligodendrocytes or microglia), an increase in inflammatory cells migrating into the brain from elsewhere, and an increase due to proliferation of neoplastic cells. It may be difficult to distinguish between inflammation and neoplasia on the basis of cell number alone.

Abnormal cells

Abnormal cells are most commonly neoplastic. They may be of a single morphological type or may vary widely in shape and size. More uniform cells are suggestive of a well differentiated tumour, whilst variation in size and shape suggests a more malignant, poorly differentiated tumour. Other hallmarks of neoplasia may also be seen, including mitotic figures, vascular changes (predominantly endothelial hyperplasia) and necrosis.

Inflammation

Inflammatory cells may arise from normal brain tissue or may migrate into the brain from the blood vessels. Cells within the normal brain that have inflammatory functions include astrocytes and microglia. An increase in the number of either of these cells is often seen with certain types of intraparenchymal inflammation. Inflammation may also be characterized by the presence of large numbers of inflammatory cells surrounding the blood vessels (Figure 6.21); these cells most commonly consist of a mixture of lymphocytes, macrophages and plasma cells, and the majority enter the brain via the bloodstream.

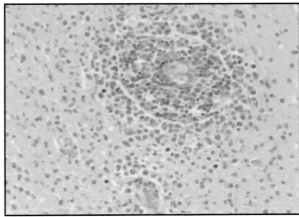

6.21 Biopsy sample taken at craniectomy showing marked perivascular cuffing with mononuclear inflammatory cells, predominately lymphocytes and plasma cells, in GME. (H&E stain; original magnification X50)

Brain cell appearance

The population of cells normally resident in the brain may also exhibit changes. Neurons undergoing degeneration may show pale areas within the cell body with loss of the normal granular Nissl substance and eccentric nuclei; this change is termed chromatolysis. Neurons undergoing hypoxic or ischaemic damage may appear shrunken and brightly eosinophilic. Astrocytes may also display a variety of appearances in certain lesions. Large, swollen astrocytes containing eosinophilic material within their cytoplasm are termed gemistocytes and these may be a feature of chronic inflammation or neoplasia (gemistocytic astrocytoma).

Background tissue appearance

The neuropil may show areas of vacuolation and pallor comprising oedema, or may show areas of necrosis, becoming degenerate and fragmented. Necrosis occurs as a result of inadequate perfusion of the tissue and can be a component of many different disease processes including neoplasia.

Other features

Specific features may also be identified within sections that suggest a particular diagnosis. These include the inclusion bodies seen with viral encephalitis and the presence of intracellular vacuoles containing storage products in certain storage diseases.

References and further reading

Available on accompanying DVD

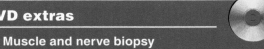

DVD extras

- Muscle and nerve biopsy
- Stereotactic needle biopsy

7

Genetic diseases

Dennis O'Brien

Genetic diseases are being recognized with increasing frequency in veterinary medicine (Patterson, 2000; O'Brien, 2011). This is due, in part, to heightened awareness and control of environmental diseases such as infections and nutritional deficiencies. It may also be the result of the influence that a popular sire can have on a breed (similar to the 'founder effect' that a patriarch might have on an isolated human population). An animal will win a show or field trial circuit because they have the characteristics that the fanciers of the breed value. It is only natural that other breeders will want to capture those traits within their line as well. If the winning animal is a male dog, the ease of artificial insemination and shipping of frozen semen allows breeders throughout the world to utilize the services of the stud.

Unfortunately, most of the genetic diseases identified in animals are recessive traits, and it is estimated that any individual is likely to carry five or more disease-causing mutations in one of the alleles (one form of a particular gene) (Patterson, 2000; Meyers-Wallen, 2003). Unless the mutant allele is already prevalent in the population, it is unlikely that the disease will be recognized in the first generation from the sire, but 50% of the offspring will be carriers of the disease-causing allele. When the carriers begin to breed with one another, affected offspring will be produced; however, it may not be immediately apparent that the disease is hereditary, especially if the age of onset is delayed. Thus, a disease can become widespread within the population by the time is it recognized as hereditary.

Advances in animal genomics have allowed the identification of disease-causing mutations and the development of a DNA test to detect the mutant allele. This in turn has simplified the diagnosis of hereditary conditions. These advances have also provided breeders with the tools to develop wise breeding strategies aimed at decreasing the incidence of these diseases whilst maintaining desirable genetic diversity within the breed. Breeders can request DNA tests be performed on cheek swab samples, but often lack the background to understand the full meaning of the results.

Recognizing genetic diseases

Genetic diseases can present with a wide array of clinical signs at any age; although, there are certain disease characteristics which should raise suspicion of a hereditary disease. Some mutant alleles, such as the *SOD1* mutation which causes degenerative myelopathy (Awano *et al.*, 2009), appear to have originated early in canine evolution and are widespread throughout many breeds. However, more commonly, hereditary diseases originated after breeds were formed or were concentrated within a breed due to a popular sire effect. For further information on breed-associated diseases, the reader is referred to Appendix 1. Inbreeding *per se* does not cause inherited disease, but the more inbred a line is, the more likely it is that a recessive trait will be expressed. This can either be the desirable trait that the breeder is trying to establish in the line or a disease-causing mutation.

Families share more than their genetics; infectious diseases, nutritional deficiencies and toxicities may affect multiple puppies in a litter (Figure 7.1a). Conversely, random breeding does not insure against hereditary disease as demonstrated by

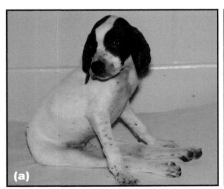
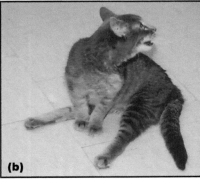

7.1 Patients presented with young-onset spastic paraplegia. It is critical to consider all the differential diagnoses and investigate the extended family history before concluding that a disease is hereditary. **(a)** Pure-bred English Pointer with a history of littermates similarly affected. Although the history makes a hereditary disease more likely, this patient had an infectious disease (*Neospora caninum*). **(b)** Stray cat from the streets of St. Louis with hereditary muscular dystrophy.

laminin-deficient muscular dystrophy, which was recognized in a breeding population of cats from the streets of St. Louis (O'Brien *et al.*, 2001; Figure 7.1b). Thus, an extended family history must be considered when deciding whether a disease is likely to be hereditary, and other differential diagnoses need to be excluded. The age of onset, progression and nature of the clinical signs in hereditary diseases tend to be highly stereotyped and have certain characteristics which raise suspicion that the condition is genetic. It is beyond the scope of this chapter to provide details on all known hereditary diseases, but selected examples are discussed below.

Congenital diseases

Many hereditary diseases are congenital, with clinical signs apparent from the neonatal period. Developing a functional nervous system is an extraordinarily complex process and many genes are expressed only during brief periods of development to direct this process. Mutations that disrupt this process can cause alterations in the structure or function of the central nervous system (CNS), which become apparent before weaning. Neonatal neurological diseases have not received a great deal of attention in the past due to the difficulty in making a definitive diagnosis in a neonate and the perception on the part of many breeders and veterinary surgeons that a certain amount of neonatal mortality is unavoidable in some breeds. Improvements in our understanding of these diseases and in brain imaging have led to a greater appreciation of the importance of neonatal diseases and the development of DNA tests (O'Brien, 2009; Gross *et al.*, 2010).

Congenital structural malformations are best diagnosed using advanced imaging or on necropsy. Care must be taken in interpreting images since

magnetic resonance imaging (MRI) characteristics of the developing nervous system can be very different from those of the adult (Gross *et al.*, 2010). The simplest forms of congenital malformation are hypoplasia (e.g. agenesis of the vermis in Dandy–Walker syndrome; Summers *et al.*, 1995) and dysplasia (e.g. polymicrogyria in Standard Poodles; Van Winkle *et al.*, 1994). In some conditions, such as congenital tremors in Chow Chows (Vandevelde *et al.*, 1981) or a form of congenital myasthenia gravis in Dachshunds (Dickinson *et al.*, 2005), development is delayed but the affected dogs eventually function normally. An animal can 'grow out of' such a hereditary disease when an impaired embryonic/neonatal form of a protein (e.g. an ion channel or myelin protein) is replaced by the adult form as part of normal development. Other congenital diseases such as vertebral anomalies or hydrocephalus may be present from birth, but can show deteriorating clinical signs later in life as a result of chronic instability or progressive loss of brain tissue, respectively.

Inborn errors of metabolism

A hereditary deficiency in a key enzyme involved in brain metabolism can disrupt normal function without necessarily affecting structure. Whilst a myriad of syndromes are possible, inborn errors of metabolism are generally divided into organic acidurias and lysosomal storage diseases, depending on what aspect of metabolism is affected and the fate of the abnormal byproducts.

Organic acidurias

With organic acidurias, the pathways for intermediate metabolism of nutrients are affected (O'Brien, 2005; Figure 7.2). The enzyme deficiency disrupts the pathway, leading to a lack of downstream substrates and/or energy production from the Krebs

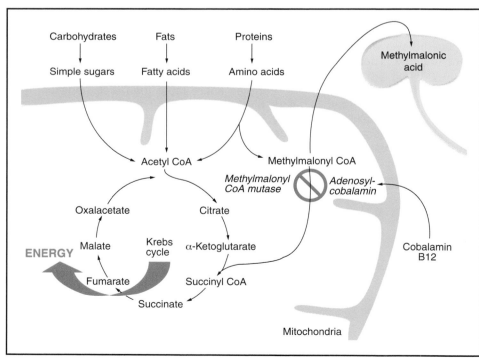

7.2 Organic acids are intermediary steps in the metabolism of nutrients to produce energy and substrates for synthesis. Methylmalonic acid is a step in the metabolism of branched chain amino acids. A hereditary deficiency in the enzyme methylmalonyl CoA mutase or a dietary deficiency of cobalamin (a key cofactor), results in the accumulation of methylmalonic acid which can be detected in the urine (O'Brien, 2011).

cycle. The organic acid immediately upstream of the metabolic 'roadblock' accumulates. One or more of these disturbances results in clinical signs and in some cases may produce changes in routine clinical pathology tests (Figure 7.3). Inborn errors may be evident in neonates but are often written off as 'fading puppies or kittens' without adequate diagnostic tests to identify the underlying cause (O'Brien, 2009). Although a deficiency may have been present from birth, some organic acidurias may have a progressive course, a delayed onset of signs, or a waxing and waning course, which can be influenced by diet. The latter can resemble more common conditions such as portosystemic shunts.

Clinical signs
• Waxing/waning encephalopathy • Muscle weakness • Strong dietary influences • Young-onset seizures
Unexplained clinical pathology findings
• Decreased total CO_2 or bicarbonate • Increased anion gap • Metabolic acidosis • Ketonuria • Hypoglycaemia • Hyperammonaemia

7.3 Findings suggestive of organic aciduria.

Clinical signs vary depending on the specific disease, but often include altered consciousness, dementia, weakness and seizures. MR images may show signal changes: when present, such changes are generally symmetrical and may affect specific areas, for example grey matter lesions in L-2 hydroxyglutaric aciduria (Abramson *et al.*, 2003). Organic acids are small molecules that are readily excreted in the urine, where they can be detected with appropriate screening tests for abnormal metabolites (see **Useful websites** on DVD). The organic acid identified may point towards the underlying deficiency, which can sometimes be confirmed with appropriate biochemical assays of tissue, leucocyte and fibroblast samples. However, care must be taken to rule out potential acquired causes of such conditions.

• Many B vitamins are cofactors in the Krebs cycle and deficiencies can result in neurological signs and abnormal organic acids in the urine (O'Brien, 2005).
• Methylmalonic aciduria (see Figure 7.2) can arise from impaired absorption of cobalamin secondary to gastrointestinal disease (Simpson *et al.*, 2001) or from a hereditary deficiency in cobalamin transport proteins (Fyfe *et al.*, 1991).

Identifying the deficiency may suggest an alternative pathway that could be exploited through dietary manipulation. For example, Maltese dogs with malonic aciduria cannot utilize fats as an energy source, thus, clinical signs can be ameliorated by ensuring a constant source of carbohydrate in the diet (O'Brien *et al.*, 1999).

Lysosomal storage diseases

Lysosomal storage diseases are caused by a disruption in the degradation of normally formed macromolecules within the lysosomes (O'Brien, 2010). Since large macromolecules are involved, the substrates upstream of the disruption are not excreted, but accumulate within the lysosome. Since the macromolecules are formed normally, the affected animal typically develops normally. Clinical signs develop as the accumulated material or the lack of recycled substrates interferes with cell function. The delay in the onset of clinical signs is typically months to 1–2 years, but in some cases can be ≥5 years (e.g. neuronal ceroid lipofuscinosis in Tibetan Terriers; Katz *et al.*, 2005). Signs vary with the specific disease, but can include ataxia, dementia, blindness and seizures. The signs are inexorably progressive and seizures may be poorly responsive to therapy. Brain imaging may show non-specific atrophy.

Whilst many storage diseases only affect the nervous system, other organs may be affected, leading to organomegaly or musculoskeletal abnormalities. In these cases, storage material may be detected in the leucocytes or in a liver/muscle biopsy sample, and in a few cases abnormal metabolites can be detected in the urine (Skelly and Franklin, 2002). However, most commonly, brain biopsy or necropsy is necessary for a definitive diagnosis. Treatment is still largely symptomatic, although various enzyme replacement, stem cell and gene therapies are being investigated.

Channelopathies

Excitable membranes rely on ion channels to set their resting potential and transmit excitation along the membranes. Neurotransmitter receptors linked to ion channels and second messenger systems permit communication between neurons or peripheral nerves and muscles. The diseases that result from mutations in the genes for these proteins are sometimes referred to as channelopathies. By altering the electrical properties of the muscle or nerve membranes, such mutations can produce excessive or deficient excitability and clinical signs. For example, the mutation in the chloride channel in Miniature Schnauzers with myotonia congenita reduces chloride conductance across muscle membranes (Bhalerao *et al.*, 2002). This delays relaxation following a contraction and results in the muscle stiffness and hypertrophy characteristic of the disease. Such mutations do not typically cause structural changes that can be detected on histopathology; thus, the condition must be diagnosed based on the clinical signs and/or electrophysiological studies. Drugs that alter membrane excitability are used for symptomatic treatment.

Channelopathies are thought to underlie other disorders of neuronal excitability, such as idiopathic epilepsy and episodic ataxias, although no mutations have been identified in domestic animals to date; however, reports are starting to appear in the human literature (Noh *et al.*, 2012). Although the mutant ion channel would not change, other factors influence the overall excitability of the nervous system and explain the episodic nature of these conditions. Bandera's neonatal ataxia in Coton de Tulear dogs is caused by a mutation in a metabotropic glutamate receptor: a receptor linked to a G-protein second messenger system (Zeng *et al.*, 2011). Rather than affecting short-term ion conductances, this mutation is thought to influence long-term changes underlying motor learning in the cerebellum. Thus, although the cerebellum appears normal on histology, affected pups never learn to coordinate movements normally and never develop the ability to walk.

Hereditary neurodegenerative diseases

In addition to lysosomal storage diseases, other hereditary diseases may have a delayed onset of clinical signs accompanied by degenerative changes on histopathology. The mutation affects cell function, leading to premature cell death and signs of disease. Terms such as dystrophy, amyotrophy or abiotrophy are sometimes used to describe these conditions. The Greek root –*trophia* means nourishment and reflects the prevailing view when the terms were coined that the degeneration was due to a lack of nutrients. As the hereditary nature of these conditions was recognized, the nomenclature shifted towards one based on the clinical signs or identified genetic locus (see below).

The clinical signs of hereditary neurodegenerative diseases depend upon the specific cell type or types affected.

- Some diseases are very selective, such as hereditary ataxia in Old English Sheepdogs where only Purkinje cells in the cerebellum degenerate (Steinberg *et al.*, 2000).
- Others can affect a specific subset of neurons, such as multiple system degeneration in Kerry Blue Terriers and Chinese Crested dogs, which affects not only the Purkinje cells but also the basal nuclei resulting in cerebellar ataxia, followed by difficulty initiating movements (O'Brien *et al.*, 2005).
- Whereas diseases such as chromatolytic degeneration in Cairn Terriers have widespread effects (Cummings *et al.,* 1991).

The age of onset can vary widely, from weaning in some of the hereditary ataxias and muscular dystrophies to old age in diseases such as degenerative myelopathy. The latter may reflect an increased susceptibility to environmental insults or age-related changes. The older the animal is at the onset of clinical signs, the more difficult it may be to recognize a disease as having a hereditary basis; however, a strong breed predisposition to a disease suggests that the genetic makeup of the breed may be playing an important role.

Whilst the nature of the clinical signs may be pathognomonic for some diseases, histopathology is often necessary for a definitive diagnosis. In some neurodegenerative diseases, abnormal material may accumulate in the cell. However, in contrast to lysosomal storage diseases, any inclusions are free within the cytoplasm rather than enclosed within a lysosomal membrane. When axonal transport is impaired, spheroids may be present within the axons. Spongiform changes are seen when empty vacuoles are present within neurons or myelin layers. In other diseases, such as the hereditary cerebellar ataxias, the cells appear simply to undergo apoptosis, without any clear preceding degenerative changes. The changes in some of these diseases can be subtle, so it is best to consult a pathologist who has an interest in neuropathology when submitting tissue samples for examination.

Basic genetics: segregation analysis

If a hereditary disease is suspected based on the nature of the condition, the family history should be investigated. Breeders can become defensive at the suggestion that there may be a hereditary problem in their line, thus, it is important for the clinician to be open to other aetiologies and to approach the breeder with the idea of helping them solve the problem if one is identified. As breeders see the value of DNA testing to improve their breed, they are becoming more amenable to assisting in investigating hereditary diseases. Information on the number and phenotype (physical manifestation of an individual's genetic makeup) of animals from previous or subsequent litters, the sex ratios, the phenotype of the parents and the degree of inbreeding allows segregation analysis.

Segregation analysis compares the pattern of disease seen in a family to what would be predicted with different modes of inheritance. Punnett squares are used to depict the possible combinations of alleles from a breeding pair of animals (where the genotypes are known) and to predict the probable percentages of each genotype. The genotypes of the parents are shown on the top and side of the square, and the possible combinations of the offspring within the square (see Figures 7.4 to 7.6). However, it should be remembered that these are only probabilities and that in any given litter, any combination is possible.

Autosomal recessive traits

Most hereditary diseases seen in animals are autosomal recessive traits because carriers of a single copy of the mutant allele do not show clinical signs of disease. Both parents must be carriers of the mutant allele to produce affected offspring, and on average 25% are affected (Figure 7.4). Typically, 25% of the litter are homozygous for the normal allele and 50% are carriers (heterozygous). If the affected animals are readily recognized, this means that 66% of the clinically normal offspring are carriers of the mutant allele. Males and females are equally affected.

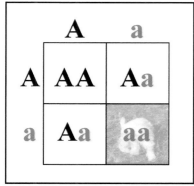

7.4 Neonatal ataxia in Coton de Tulear dogs is an autosomal recessive trait. The parents are carriers with one normal allele (A) and one mutant allele (a). On average 25% of the offspring receive two normal alleles and are normal; 50% of the offspring receive one normal and one mutant allele and are carriers; and 25% of the offspring receive two mutant alleles and are affected. Since the affected puppies are readily identified, 66% of clinically normal puppies are carriers (O'Brien, 2011).

Autosomal dominant traits

If the disease is an autosomal dominant trait, one mutant allele is sufficient to produce the disease (Figure 7.5). Thus, affected offspring have at least one affected parent. When one affected and one normal animal are mated, on average 50% of the offspring are affected. There is no difference in the sex ratio. If both parents are heterozygous for the mutant allele, 75% of the offspring are expected to have at least one mutant allele and be affected. Dominant diseases are uncommon in domestic animals since animals carrying the mutant allele can be recognized by their phenotype and removed from the breeding programme, unless the onset of disease occurs after breeding age.

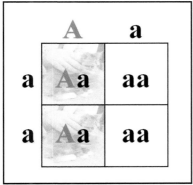

7.5 The tailless trait in Manx cats is an autosomal dominant trait. One parent is affected with one mutant allele (A) and one parent is homozygous for the normal allele (a). On average 50% of the offspring receive the mutant allele from the affected parent and are affected. The other 50% are homozygous for the normal allele and are clinically normal (O'Brien, 2011).

Sex-linked traits

If the mutant allele is located on the X chromosome, there is a sex bias amongst affected animals. Since males only have one X chromosome, and the Y chromosome carries little genetic information, they will always express the mutant allele. If a female carrier of a recessive X-linked allele is mated with a normal male, she will pass on the mutant allele to 50% of the male offspring, who then become affected with the disease. A clinically normal male only has the normal allele and cannot pass the trait on to the offspring. The female offspring are, on average, 50% homozygous for the normal allele and 50% heterozygous (i.e. have one normal and one mutant allele) and thus are carriers of the mutant allele (Figure 7.6). If a female carrier is mated with an affected male, 50% of the female offspring also inherit the mutant allele and are affected.

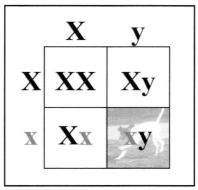

7.6 Hereditary cerebellar ataxia in English Pointers is an X-linked trait. The female parent is heterozygous for the recessive trait (x). The male parent is normal. On average 50% of the female offspring receive the mutant allele and are carriers. In addition, 50% of the male offspring receive the mutant allele, but since the Y chromosome does not contain a normal allele, these animals are affected (O'Brien, 2011).

Females that are heterozygous for the mutant allele may show a milder form of the disease due to the process of X-inactivation (lyonization). In females, for any given cell, the alleles of only one X chromosome are expressed; the other X chromosome is inactivated. A familiar example of this process is the coat colour in tortoiseshell cats. The orange coat colour allele is on the X chromosome, so a female that is heterozygous for orange shows a mosaic of expression of this colour, depending on which X chromosome is inactivated in the melanocytes. Female carriers of a mutant X-linked gene for a myelin protein (proteolipid protein) show a similar mosaic of myelination in the peripheral nerves and mild clinical signs (Cuddon *et al.*, 1998).

Mitochondrial traits

The mitochondria contain their own complement of DNA, which codes for some of the mitochondrial enzymes. Within a given cell, there is a mix of mitochondria with different genomes. Since sperm do not transmit mitochondria, the mitochondrial DNA is inherited exclusively from the egg. Thus, if the female is a carrier of a mitochondrial DNA mutation, she can pass mitochondria with that mutation on to her offspring (maternal pattern of inheritance). The percentage of affected offspring varies depending upon what 'dose' of mutant mitochondria are present in the egg. Disruption of the respiratory chain function within the mitochondria can produce clinical signs of encephalopathy, neuropathy and/or myopathy. A mutation in the mitochondrial gene cytochrome b has been associated with spongiform leukodystrophy in Australian Cattle Dogs and Shetland Sheepdogs (Li *et al.*, 2006); other encephalopathies are also suspected to be caused by mitochondrial mutations.

Factors affecting segregation analysis

A number of factors such as ascertainment bias and variable penetrance can influence the actual percentage of affected offspring identified when performing segregation analysis.

Ascertainment bias

Ascertainment bias is the failure to take into account all the potential outcomes from a mating. For example, mating two carriers of a particular trait could result in affected offspring, but by chance did not. As a result, these offspring may not have been included in the calculations for segregation analysis because they were not ascertained to be from a family where the mutant allele was segregating. Formulas such as the Davie correction can be used to account for such bias (Davie, 1979). This correction is based on the number of probands identified. A proband is the first affected individual that brings the family to the attention of the geneticist. Thus, it is important when collecting data to note whether an affected individual comes from a family where the mutant allele is known to be segregating, or whether the individual is from a new family and therefore another proband.

Penetrance

Not all genetic diseases are fully penetrant: i.e. an individual could have the genotype that should cause the disease, but they are clinically normal. Presumably there are other genetic or environmental factors that protect the individual from the disease.

Expressivity

Expressivity refers to the degree of expression of a mutant disease. For example, in the Manx cat variable expression of the mutant allele leads to cats with varying degrees of caudal vertebral/spinal cord agenesis. This ranges from cats with a slightly shortened tail (stubbies, which cannot be entered into shows) to desirable cats with no tail (rumpies), through to cats with sacral cord agenesis and neurological signs. Animals with low expression of the disease could easily be overlooked when performing the segregation analysis. Some dominant traits (such as Manx cat taillessness and Chinese Crested Dog hairlessness) are lethal when homozygous. If two animals that are heterozygous for the mutant allele are mated, the percentage of surviving offspring with the trait will be different to that anticipated if the homozygous animals die *in utero* and are not counted.

Gene discovery strategies

Once a genetic disease has been identified, the next step is to identify the mutation responsible. Knowing which gene is affected can lead to a better understanding of the disease process and may suggest therapeutic interventions. DNA tests can be developed to diagnose the disease and detect carriers of the trait.

Candidate gene approach

Currently, the candidate gene approach and gene mapping strategies (see below) are used to identify the mutation. The candidate gene approach involves selecting specific genes to investigate based on the similarities between the newly recognized disease and a disease in another breed or species where a mutation has been identified. The more accurate and molecular the diagnosis is, the more easily the field of candidates can be narrowed, and the more likely the mutant allele is to be indentified. For example, identification of autofluorescent lysosomal storage material in the neurons of a Dachshund with progressive neurodegenerative disease suggests that the condition is likely to be neuronal ceroid lipofuscinosis. On electron microscopy, the curvilinear bodies within the lysosome appear very similar to those seen in humans with one form of the disease caused by a deficiency of the lysosomal enzyme tripeptidyl-peptidase 1 (TPP1). This finding makes the gene which codes for TPP1 a prime candidate gene. Sequencing the gene revealed a premature stop codon (the signal for the end of a gene), which abolished all activity of the enzyme (Awano *et al.*, 2006). In this case, the mutation was identified with the information and samples collected from a single affected individual. A DNA test is now available to Dachshund breeders.

Gene mapping

However, often the candidate gene approach is not successful. There may be too many genes associated with the syndrome in question (e.g. epilepsy, where hundreds of genes have been associated with seizures in both mice and humans). Alternatively, the gene responsible may not be known in any species or those that are known may have been ruled out as candidates for the family being studied. The approach then turns to searching for an unknown gene using mapping strategies such as linkage mapping or genome wide association studies (GWAS).

Linkage mapping

Microsatellites are repeated DNA elements that vary in the number of repetitions. Since they typically occur in regions of the genome that are not translated into RNA, this variability does not affect function, but it does result in highly variable (polymorphic) markers spread throughout the chromosomes, which can be tracked through a pedigree. When the mutant allele resides close to one of these markers, they tend to stay together (linkage) during meiosis since the probability of a recombination occurring between the two is low (Figure 7.7). A linked marker identifies a locus (an area where the mutation is likely to reside) which is then named for the disease caused by the mutant allele. For example, the first locus to be identified as causing neuronal ceroid lipofuscinosis in humans was named *CLN1* (ceroid lipofuscinosis, neuronal 1). Subsequently, if a new family for a particular disease is investigated and the mutation is found to be linked to markers in a different region of the genome, then a new locus is reported and numbered sequentially (i.e. *CLN2, CLN3*).

Although microsatellites are highly polymorphic, and thus likely to be informative within a family, they occur relatively infrequently within the genome. This can result in large gaps between the microsatellite markers. If the disease causing allele is not close to a marker, recombinations may be frequent and a large family may be necessary to show an association. In addition, the chemistry involved does not lend itself as well to automation as the single nucleotide polymorphisms (SNPs) used in next generation gene mapping techniques (e.g. GWAS).

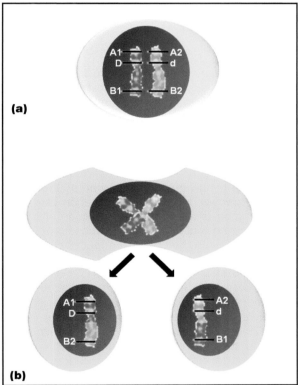

(a)

(b)

7.7 Markers are DNA sequences that can vary between individual chromosomes. **(a)** In this pair of chromosomes, markers A and B are polymorphic and the different alleles (1 and 2) have been labeled. Markers A1 and B1 are on the chromosome with the normal allele (D). Markers A2 and B2 are on the chromosome with the disease causing recessive allele (d). A2 and B2 tend to segregate with the disease and thus are markers for the mutant allele. **(b)** When the chromosomes undergo meiosis, they separate and recombine, producing a different combination of markers. In this case, the marker A2 is closer to the disease causing allele (d) and thus more tightly linked. Recombination is more likely to occur between the disease causing allele (d) and the marker B2, which is further away. Such recombinations are helpful in narrowing the locus in linkage studies, but can lead to error when using linked markers to identify carriers of a trait (O'Brien, 2011).

Genome wide association studies

SNPs are variations in a single base pair in a gene and can occur anywhere in the genome. If they occur in a coding region (the region that is translated into RNA and then protein), and if that change significantly alters the protein structure, an SNP could be a disease causing mutation. However, typically the change is of no consequence. Either it is in a region of the genome which is not translated into a protein, or if it does change an amino acid in a protein, that change does not affect the function of the protein.

As with microsatellites, SNPs can be used to detect differences in the genome between individuals. Although SNPs are not as polymorphic, they are much more prevalent than microsatellites and amenable to automation in microarrays ('SNP chips'). With this technology, thousands of SNP markers can be screened in a cost-effective manner. In GWAS, the pedigree is not as critical; instead, the constellation of markers across the entire genome (hence the term genome wide) in affected individuals is compared with normal controls, and the markers that are more likely to be found in affected dogs identified. If a group of SNP markers is significantly more common in the diseased animals than in the control animals, then there may be an association between those markers and the disease (Figure 7.8). This area then becomes the locus to be investigated. The unique characteristics associated with evolution of the canine genome, with particular reference to the establishment of pure breeds, make it ideally suited for the identification of disease causing mutations using this approach (Karlsson *et al.*, 2007).

Additional markers

Once a locus has been identified with linkage mapping or GWAS, additional markers within that area are investigated in the individual dogs to look for recombinations that define the borders of the region where the gene is likely to reside. The genes within this area then become candidates for disease based on their location on the chromosome. These genes are prioritized for sequencing based on criteria such as whether they are expressed in the nervous system or whether they are involved in a pathway likely to result in disease. Typically, the coding regions are sequenced and the results examined for changes that are likely to be consequential. A deletion or insertion that results in a premature stop codon is liable to produce a truncated and non-functional protein. A single nucleotide change in the sequence could be significant, depending on whether it results in a change in an amino acid that is important to the normal function of the protein.

Screening

When a suspected disease causing mutation is identified, all dogs in the family should be examined to determine whether the mutation segregates as expected, and a large number of randomly selected dogs should be screened to ensure that the mutation is not found in healthy animals. Ideally, biochemical studies should be undertaken to demonstrate that

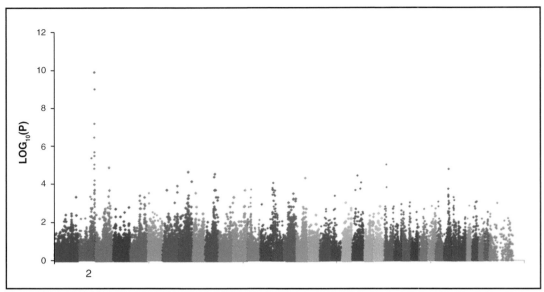

7.8 In GWAS the probability that an SNP marker is more common in an affected animal than in a control animal is represented graphically in a 'Manhattan plot', where each individual chromosome is expressed in a different colour along the Y axis. The peak of significant association seen in chromosome two (red dots, second from the left) indicates that the disease causing mutation resides within this area of the chromosome.

the function of the protein is altered by the mutation. Once a mutation has been proven to be associated with a disease, a DNA test can be devised to identify whether dogs are:

- Homozygous for the mutant allele and at risk for the disease
- Carriers of the mutant allele (if the mutant allele is dominant, the dog will be at risk for the disease; if the mutant allele is recessive, the dog will be clinically normal)
- Homozygous for the normal allele.

How this information is used depends on the reason why the test was performed.

DNA tests

A variety of DNA tests are now available for specific neurological diseases, and the number is likely to increase dramatically in the future. A list of **Useful websites** and the DNA tests available can be found on the DVD. When advising a client on the results of a DNA test, the clinician must understand the strengths and limitations of DNA testing.

Types of test

Linked marker tests
Initially, the only DNA test available may be a linked marker for the locus. For such a test to be reliable, the marker must be in close proximity on the chromosome to the gene which contains the mutation, so that the probability of a recombination between the two is very low. This probability is expressed as a recombination fraction and needs to be <5% for the test to be of value. However,

even then recombinations can occur resulting in false-positive and false-negative results. In addition, the marker may be present in some families without the associated disease causing mutation, leading to false-positive results. Thus, linked markers are of most value when evaluating an entire family where the mutant allele is known to segregate, and not very accurate in determining whether an isolated individual is a carrier of the mutant allele. However, typically, identification of a linked marker soon leads to the identification of the disease causing mutation within a specific gene, and the mutation can then be tested for directly.

Direct mutation tests
Direct DNA tests for a specific mutation are highly specific and sensitive in determining the genotype of an animal. However, there are several caveats when interpreting test results. False-positive results could be the consequence of variable penetrance of the mutant allele. Over time, the degree of penetrance for a given disease can be ascertained and true sensitivity calculated.

False-negative results can occur when attempting to use a DNA test developed for one breed in another, since a different mutation in the same gene could result in an identical disease phenotype. As the DNA test only detects the specific mutation it was designed for, it does not detect a different mutation in the second breed. For example, a mutation in the superoxide dismutase gene (*SOD1*) that changes the negatively charged amino acid glutamic acid to the positively charged amino acid lysine at position 40 leads to degenerative myelopathy in numerous breeds, suggesting that the mutation probably originated in ancestral dogs before the separate breeds were formed (Awano *et al.*, 2009). A new mutation could occur in the gene; however, this would not be detected by the currently available test but it could still affect function and lead to disease. In a recent study, Bernese Mountain Dogs with confirmed degenerative myelopathy were consistently negative for the known mutation. Sequencing the *SOD1* gene in affected individuals demonstrated a different mutation in the same gene, and a DNA test for this mutation is now also available (Wininger *et al.*, 2011).

Alternatively, a mutation in a different gene could produce the same disease phenotype (phenocopy) and thus a false-negative result on testing, even in the same breed. In Dachshunds, mutations in two different genes, *CLN1* and *CLN2*, have been identified as causing the lysosomal storage disease neuronal ceroid lipofuscinosis. These genes code for different enzymes (palmitoyl protein thioesterase 1 and tripeptidyl-peptidase 1, respectively) that affect different steps in the degradation of protein within the lysosome (Awano *et al.*, 2006; Sanders *et al.*, 2010). However, since they affect different steps in the same pathway, the clinical signs are virtually identical. The DNA test for *CLN1* is highly specific and sensitive for that mutation, and thus would not detect the mutation in *CLN2*, and *vice versa*. A brain biopsy would be very sensitive for detecting the characteristic storage material, but it is less invasive and expensive to perform DNA tests for both mutations.

Acquired conditions

Phenocopy can also refer to acquired diseases which resemble the genetic disease being tested for and may need to be ruled out as part of the diagnostic approach. For example, neonatal encephalopathy with seizures is a syndrome in Standard Poodles caused by a mutation in the transcription factor gene *ATF2* (Chen *et al.*, 2008), but neonatal seizures can also be caused by other conditions such as hypoglycaemia. A readily treatable condition like hypoglycaemia should be excluded before a DNA test, which may take weeks to return results, is considered.

False-positive results can also occur with an acquired phenocopy. A dog that is homozygous for the mutation in *SOD1* that causes degenerative myelopathy is at high risk of developing the disease, but the trait does not appear to be completely penetrant and the age of onset can vary. Other diseases, such as neoplasia or type II intervertebral disc disease, can present with identical clinical signs in old age. Thus, a dog may be homozygous for the mutant allele and at high risk of developing degenerative myelopathy, but still have ataxia and paraparesis as a result of a different disease process. Therefore, it is always important to consider all the differential diagnoses for a clinical problem and ensure that potentially treatable conditions are excluded and/or treated. However, the caveat is that before surgery is performed for intervertebral disc disease in an 11-year-old Corgi that is homozygous for the *SOD1* mutation, the owner must be aware that the dog is at high risk of developing degenerative myelopathy as well.

Genetic counselling

When providing genetic counselling to breeders, the aim should be never to produce an animal affected with the disease, whilst continuing to select for the best characteristics of the breed and maintaining desirable genetic diversity. Decreasing the incidence of the mutant allele in the population is also desirable but secondary to the other objectives.

- If a disease is suspected to have a hereditary basis, but the mode of inheritance is unknown, it is difficult to give sound advice to a breeder. Affected dogs should not be bred from, but the odds of family members being carriers cannot be accurately predicted.
- When the mode of inheritance is known, but a DNA test is not available, a breeder can be counselled on the probability of affected and/or carrier offspring if the genotype of the parents is known.
- With dominant traits, the genotype is readily apparent, unless the onset of disease is delayed, and simply not breeding from affected dogs quickly eliminates the mutant allele from the population.
- With recessive traits, an affected animal should not be bred from since all the offspring will be carriers, or they could be affected if the affected animal is mated with a carrier animal.

For a normal animal that has not been bred from before, breeding trials with a known carrier of the mutant allele are needed to establish whether the new breeding animal is a carrier. When such trials are performed, the offspring have a 50% chance of being carriers of the trait and if the animal being tested is a carrier, then 25% of the offspring will be homozygous for the mutant allele. Thus, breeding trials result in numerous carriers of the mutant allele and may produce affected animals.

When a specific DNA test is available, carriers of a recessive trait can be easily identified, but this information should be used with the health of the population as a whole in mind. If the mutant allele is rare in the breed, and the breeding population large enough, it may be acceptable to exclude carriers of the trait from the breeding programme. However, more commonly, either the mutant allele is widespread in the population or the breeding pool is small (as with the more uncommon breeds). In this case it is best to continue to use carriers in the breeding programme to maintain the desirable genetic diversity in the population. The best strategy is to mate carriers with animals that are free from the mutation, test the offspring to determine whether they are carriers of the mutant allele, and use carrier status as one of the factors when considering who will be used for future breeding stock. Other factors, such as the desirable breed characteristics in an individual animal or the genotype for other hereditary diseases, should also be considered. By gradually selecting future breeding stock clear of the mutant allele, the frequency of occurrence of the allele within the population decreases, whilst the genetic diversity and desirable characteristics of a particular line are maintained. If the frequency of a mutant allele is very high in a breed, it may be difficult to find animals that are clear of the mutation but have the other traits desirable in the breed. In these unusual situations, mating two carriers with a recessive trait, or a normal animal with an animal that has a dominant trait could be considered. DNA testing of all offspring is essential to identify those affected with the disease.

Polygenic traits and the risk of disease

With fully penetrant, simple Mendelian traits, a single gene controls whether an animal develops a disease. However, in some conditions such as degenerative myelopathy the onset of disease is delayed until old age; in addition, the *SOD1* mutation is not fully penetrant, since a small number of animals that are homozygous for the mutation never develop the disease. Environmental factors such as accumulated oxidative stresses or the declining ability of a cell to deal with such stresses due to ageing may influence the expression of the mutation. Alternatively, other genes may affect which individuals show clinical signs of disease.

Quantitative traits or polygenic inheritance refers to a disease attributable to the interaction between multiple genes and the environment. As advances in technology and our understanding of genomics progress, genes that influence the risk of disease in such a quantitative sense will be increasingly identified. In some diseases (e.g. autoimmune diseases) a complex interplay between genes regulating immune function, cell surface antigens and environmental triggers is involved.

In multiple sclerosis (an immune-mediated disease of the nervous system) in humans, only approximately 30% of the risk of developing the disease can be explained by genetics (Milo and Kahana, 2010); thus, environmental factors play a significant role.

In systemic lupus erythematosus, dozens of loci have been associated with the risk of developing the disease (Flesher *et al.*, 2010).

Thus, the discovery that necrotizing meningoencephalitis in Pugs is associated with the dog leucocyte antigen class II locus (Greer *et al.*, 2010) may not be of much value in diagnosing the disease, since it is likely one of many factors involved. Nonetheless, by using a DNA test for that locus when considering which animals to breed from, Pug breeders may be able to decrease the susceptibility of the breed to this fatal condition. Meanwhile, further mapping studies may identify other loci which could also be used to select breeding animals and decrease the risk of disease further. By knowing which animals are at risk for developing such a disease, the environmental factors that also contribute can be more easily identified. As our knowledge of canine genomics expands, hopefully the contribution of genetics to other diseases such as epilepsy will be elucidated and then used to produce healthier animals.

References and further reading

Available on accompanying DVD

8

Seizures

Michael Podell

The approach to and treatment of seizure disorders in small animals is similar in many respects to the treatment of various other ailments in veterinary medicine: an antecedent historical problem arises, a proper diagnosis is made to confirm the condition, and therapy is initiated to treat the underlying disease or signs of the disease. However, important differences arise specific to the diagnosis and treatment of seizure disorders. Firstly, a specific underlying aetiology is often not identified. Secondly, the clinician must often make a therapeutic decision based on historical accounts alone. Thirdly, treatment is often initiated when the animal is otherwise normal, with little ability to predict frequency of seizure recurrence. Finally, the quality of life of both the pet and the owner during the interictal period must be balanced with the ability to limit the severity, frequency and duration of future seizure events.

Clinical signs

Classification of seizures and epilepsy into a universally accepted, coherent and relevant scheme for clinicians has been an ongoing dynamic process in human epilepsy since the early 1980s. The standardized classification scheme for seizures and epilepsy established by the International League Against Epilepsy (ILAE) in the 1980s (Commission for ILAE, 1981, 1989) provided the first basis for a taxonomic foundation for an analytical approach in the diagnosis and treatment of epilepsy. This classification scheme is restricted by the following limitations:

- The reliance on the clinician's ability to classify seizure types based on the presence of 'impaired consciousness'
- The reliance on electroencephalographic features to classify seizure type
- The difficulty in distinguishing an 'idiopathic' disorder of confirmed undetermined aetiology from a 'cryptogenic' cause of highly suspect morphological disease of the brain (Engel, 2001).

The goal is to attempt to piece together a rational categorization for use in small animal epileptic patients adapted from the recommendations of the ILAE Task Force on Classification and Terminology (Engel, 2001). The purpose is to establish a common-ground mode of communication to allow diagnostic and therapeutic data to be tabulated for clinical outcome measures. The proposed scheme for seizure investigation consists of five considerations or 'axes' (Figure 8.1) as proposed by Engel (2001) and recently revised by Berg et al. (2010).

Axis 1: Seizure (ictal) phenomenology

• Seizure:
  – Epileptic seizure
  – Non-epileptic episodes
• Epilepsy
• Status epilepticus

Axis 2: Seizure type

• Self-limiting (isolated)
  – Focal:
    o Sensory
    o Motor:
      • Elementary
      • Automatisms
    o Reflex
  – Generalized:
    o Tonic–clonic
    o Clonic
    o Myoclonic
    o Atonic
    o Absence
    o Reflex
• Clustered or continuous (status epilepticus):
  – Focal:
    o Sensory: aura continua
    o Motor: epilepsia pars continua
  – Generalized

Axis 3: Seizure syndrome

• Familial (genetic) epilepsies
• Idiopathic epilepsies:
  – Focal
  – Generalized
• Reflex epilepsies
• Epileptic encephalopathies (progressive neurological dysfunction)
• Myoclonic epilepsies

Axis 4: Aetiology
• Genetic • Structural or metabolic • Unknown

8.1 Proposed diagnostic scheme (five axes) for dogs and cats with epileptic seizures (adapted from Engel, 2001). (continues) ▶

Axis 5: Impairment from epilepsy

• Temporary:
  – Motor
  – Sensory
  – Other
• Permanent:
  – Motor
  – Sensory
  – Other

8.1 (continued) Proposed diagnostic scheme (five axes) for dogs and cats with epileptic seizures (adapted from Engel, 2001).

Axis 1: Seizure (ictal) phenomenology (is it a seizure?)

A seizure can be defined as a non-specific, paroxysmal, abnormal event of the body. An epileptic seizure is defined by the ILAE as 'a transient occurrence of signs and/or symptoms due to abnormal excessive or synchronous neuronal activity in the brain' (Fischer et al., 2005). Thus, an epileptic seizure has a specific neural origin. Absolute confirmation that a seizure is epileptic may be difficult as it requires simultaneous observation of behavioural and electroencephalographic changes. As a result, historical information is often used to diagnose an epileptic seizure. The clinical features of epileptic seizures can be separated into four components (Engel, 1989; Podell, 1996).

1. The prodrome is the time period prior to the onset of seizure activity. Owners report that they can 'predict' the onset of their pet's seizures based on behaviour exhibited during this time, such as increased anxiety-related behaviour (i.e. attention-seeking, whining), reluctance to perform normal activity patterns and increased hiding (especially in cats).
2. The aura is the initial manifestation of a seizure. During this period, which can last from minutes to hours, animals can exhibit stereotypical sensory or motor behaviour (e.g. pacing, licking), autonomic patterns (e.g. salivating, urinating, vomiting) and even unusual psychiatric events (e.g. excessive barking, increased/decreased attention-seeking).
3. The ictal period is the actual seizure event, manifested by involuntary muscle tone or movement and/or abnormal sensations or behaviour, lasting usually from seconds to minutes.
4. The postictal period follows the actual seizure and can last from minutes to days. During this time an animal can exhibit unusual behaviour, disorientation, inappropriate bowel and/or bladder activity, excessive or depressed thirst and appetite, or actual neurological deficits including weakness, blindness and sensory or motor disturbances. The latter problems are known as Todd's paralysis and are often an indicator of a focal, contralateral cortical epileptic focus. Often owners observe only the postictal period as evidence that their pet has had a seizure.

Regardless of the cause, a patient's epileptic seizures may be recurrent over time or may occur as a single event. If the patient has a chronic brain disorder characterized by recurrent epileptic seizures, then that patient has epilepsy. It should be noted that neither the term seizure nor epilepsy connotes the underlying aetiology of the disorder.

Status epilepticus can be defined as a state of continuous seizure activity lasting for 5 minutes or longer, or repeated seizures with failure to return to normality within 30 minutes (Huff and Fountain, 2011) (see Chapter 20). Epilepsia partialis continua is a continuous focal seizure involving the motor cortex (Engel, 2001). Although not well documented by an electroencephalogram (EEG) in animals, typical manifestations include facial muscle movements with 'chewing gum' activity, repetitive eye and/or lip twitching and myoclonic jerking of limb muscles.

Several other paroxysmal 'episodes' of altered behaviour, body movement or neurological status may mimic epileptic seizures (see Chapter 18). Distinguishing these 'episodes' from epileptic seizures is just as important because an incorrect diagnosis could lead to failure to identify another serious medical condition, the administration of unnecessary medication to the patient, or undue emotional and financial strain on the owner. Some common causes of paroxysms include syncope of cardiac origin, metabolic-related weakness (e.g. transient hypoglycaemia, endocrine diseases) and acute toxicities. One helpful distinguishing feature is the lack of a postictal period following these 'episodes'. With syncope, a rapid return to consciousness or ability to walk within seconds to a minute is typical, although some animals will urinate during or immediately after the event. Neurological episodes that are not epileptic seizures may be acute vestibular attacks (with ataxia, falling, rolling, etc.), cataplectic/narcoleptic events (sudden loss of consciousness with excitement), hypertonic syndromes in Cavalier King Charles Spaniels and Soft-coated Wheaton Terriers, muscle cramping syndromes in Scottish and Border Terriers or fulminant myasthenia gravis (rapid loss of the ability to walk; see Chapter 9).

Axis 2: Seizure type

Seizures are classified as:

- Self-limiting (isolated) – one seizure within 24 hours
- Clustered – two or more seizures, lasting <5 minutes each, within 24 hours but separated by a normal interictal period
- Continuous – seizures lasting 5 minutes or longer, or without return to a normal interictal period between seizures (see **Status multiple seizure types** clip on DVD).

Within each category, seizures are divided into either focal or generalized. Focal seizures are the manifestation of a discrete, epileptogenic event in the cerebral cortex (Cascino, 1992). The focal nature of this seizure type is associated with a higher incidence of focal intracranial pathology

(Podell *et al.*, 1995). Focal seizures can be elementary motor seizures, commonly seen as facial muscle twitching, or manifested by more abnormal behavioural disorders (see **Focal motor seizure** clip on DVD). Progressive involvement of the facial, neck and/or shoulder or limb muscles is known as a 'Jacksonian' march seizure event. More complex behaviour patterns with focal seizures include impaired consciousness, often with bizarre behavioural activity. Previously termed complex partial or psychomotor seizures, these events are now classified as automatisms or automotor seizures (Engel, 2001) (see **Complex partial seizure (automatism)** clip on DVD). Animals may show 'fly-biting' behaviour patterns, become aggressive without provocation, howl incessantly, become restless or exhibit a variety of motor disturbances. Cats may show a variety of abnormal behaviours or motor signs, including drooling, hippus, excessive vocalization or random, rapid running behaviours indoors. Whenever a focal seizure is suspected, the clinician should be suspicious of a focal cerebral disturbance and plan the diagnostic work-up accordingly.

Generalized seizures are subdivided into tonic–clonic, clonic, myoclonic, atonic or absence types (Berg *et al.*, 2010; Poma *et al.*, 2010) (see **Generalized tonic–clonic seizure** and **Myoclonic and atonic seizures** clips on DVD). The terms convulsive (*grand mal*) and non-convulsive (*petit mal*) seizures are no longer in use. Generalized seizures originate from both cerebral hemispheres from the start, or more commonly progress secondarily from focal seizures (Engel, 1989; Berendt and Gram, 1999) (Figure 8.2). Unlike focal seizures, generalized seizures are not necessarily associated with focal cerebrocortical disease.

Reflex seizures can be focal or generalized and occur in response to a trigger (e.g. photostimulation). Whilst this type of seizure is well described in human medicine, with numerous different triggers reported (Engel, 2001), recognized triggers have not been reported commonly in veterinary medicine. A notable exception is myoclonic epilepsy in Wirehaired Dachshunds with Lafora disease in which seizures are triggered by auditory and visual stimuli (Lohi *et al.*, 2005; Webb *et al.*, 2009). Another phenomenon reported in human medicine is epileptic spasms. Epileptic spasms are currently classified as a discrete seizure type, as it has yet to be determined whether these events have a focal or generalized onset based on electroclinical data from humans (Berg *et al.*, 2010).

Axis 3: Seizure syndrome

By definition, a syndrome is a group of signs or characteristics that defines a particular abnormality. Epilepsy syndromes are not well defined in veterinary medicine, although familial (genetic) epilepsies are now being identified with segregation analysis (see Chapter 7). A number of dog breeds have been identified with either proven or highly suspect familial epilepsy, including Belgian Tervuerens (Famula and Oberbauer, 2000), Vizslas (Patterson *et al.*, 2003), Keeshonds (Hall and

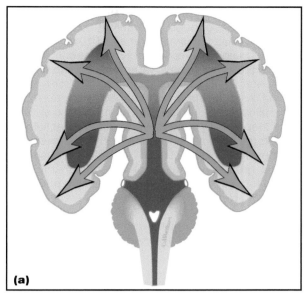

(a)

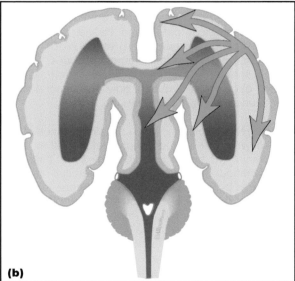

(b)

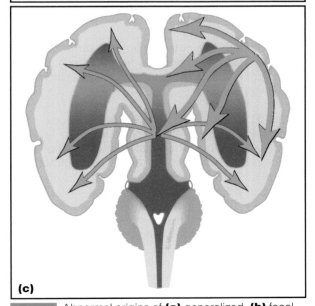

(c)

8.2 Abnormal origins of **(a)** generalized, **(b)** focal and **(c)** focal progressing to generalized seizure discharges.

Wallace, 1996), Retrievers (Jaggy *et al.*, 1998), Shetland Sheepdogs (Morita *et al.*, 2002) and Border Collies (Hulsmeyer *et al.*, 2010).

The majority of epileptic syndromes in dogs are suspected to be genetic in nature and are currently classified as idiopathic; although, this term is now falling out of favour in human medicine (see Axis 4). An epileptic syndrome (such as myoclonic epilepsy) can theoretically have several different aetiologies. The term epileptic encephalopathy has been used to describe electroclinical syndromes associated with a greater probability of encephalopathic signs attributable to the onset and progression of epileptic seizures (Hermann *et al.*, 2006). Inherent with this term is the ability to reverse the clinical signs with improvement of cognition and behaviour, especially with early and effective seizure control with drug therapy (see Axis 5).

Axis 4: Aetiology

The differential diagnosis of epileptic seizures due to underlying brain disease can be divided into three main aetiological categories based on the ILAE reclassification scheme (Berg *et al.*, 2010): genetic, structural/metabolic, and unknown causes. The goal of this scheme is to create a classification system in which each cause contains only one dimension and is not used to imply other causes.

- Genetic – epilepsy that is the direct result of a known or presumed genetic defect. Either precise molecular genetic studies that have identified a genetic mutation or familial studies that appropriately demonstrate a genetic component are acceptable criteria for inclusion.
- Structural or metabolic (formerly symptomatic/ secondary or reactive) – epileptic seizures that are directly related to either an underlying brain or metabolic disease.
- Unknown (formerly probable symptomatic/ cryptogenic) – the cause of the epileptic seizures has yet to be determined.

It should be noted that the term idiopathic epilepsy has been removed from this scheme as it only connotes our inability to determine the underlying cause.

Axis 5: Impairment from epilepsy

Inclusion of signs that are related to epilepsy allows evaluation for persistence of functional and structural neurological changes associated with seizures. The majority of signs in cats and dogs are transient, such as disorientation, visual impairment, salivation, incontinence and altered behaviour. Dogs have been found to demonstrate transient structural changes such as cerebral oedema of the temporal lobe on magnetic resonance imaging (MRI) of the brain (Mellema *et al.*, 1999), and altered cerebral metabolism on proton MR spectroscopy after seizures (Neppl *et al.*, 2001). Symptomatic temporal lobe epilepsy with associated hippocampal neuronal loss appears not to be present in idiopathic epileptic dogs

(Buckmaster *et al.*, 2002). More permanent neuro-pathological deficits can occur, especially in dogs or cats with very prolonged seizure activity (Koestner, 1989).

Lesion localization

Seizures are the manifestation of a change in forebrain activity. Thus, by default, all animals with epileptic seizures are classified as having a forebrain neurolocalization (Figure 8.3). For this discussion, the forebrain is defined as the diencephalon and telencephalon as one functional unit. Neurological deficits associated with forebrain lesions include changes in behaviour, wide circling patterns, head turns to the side of the lesion, contralateral hemiparesis and conscious proprioceptive deficits, as well as contralateral vision loss (cranial nerve (CN) II), facial muscle weakness (CN VII) and facial hypoalgesia (CN V) (see Chapters 2 and 9). Any combination of these signs should alert the clinician to the possibility of a forebrain lesion.

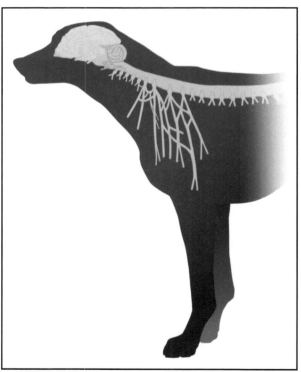

8.3 Lesion localization for seizure disorders. The forebrain comprising the cerebrum and diencephalon is highlighted.

Pathophysiology

Epilepsy represents a heterogeneous disease consisting of diverse aetiologies, electrophysiological and behavioural seizure patterns, and responses to pharmacological intervention. As such, the pathogenesis of epilepsy is multifactorial. Genetically determined seizure susceptibility factors play a crucial role in the response of the brain to triggering or precipitating factors, also known as the seizure threshold. The seizure threshold in humans has been shown to decrease during sleep (in particular stage 2 sleep), where the hypersynchrony of sleep facilitates both the initiation and propagation of focal seizures in the parietal and occipital lobes (Herman *et al.*, 2001). Seizures in these individuals may be activated by unrecognized changes in neuronal activity, or intrinsic neurochemical transmission, or by environmental stimuli or stresses that do not cause seizures in the normal brain.

A basic tenet in the mechanism of epilepsy is the presence of an imbalance in excitatory and inhibitory neurotransmission. A seizure develops when the balance shifts towards excessive excitation. Much research has been focused on the role of glutamate and its receptor complex, the *N*-methyl-D-aspartate receptor (Lipton and Rosenburg, 1994). Glutamate is the principal excitatory neurotransmitter in the brain and plays an important role in the modulation of cognitive, motor, memory and sensory functions of the central nervous system (CNS) (Figure 8.4). The overabundance of excitatory influences in the immature brain is also important in developmental neuronal plasticity of the mammalian nervous system (Lipton and Rosenburg, 1994; Veliskova *et al.*, 1994).

As the brain matures, the balance of excitation and inhibition becomes a finely tuned process. Conditions leading to excessive excitation or loss of inhibition result in depolarization of neurons without normal regulatory feedback mechanisms. The result is a paroxysmal depolarization shift of a neuronal aggregate. In response to this sudden change in brain activity, local surrounding inhibitory zones are established to try to prevent the spread of this epileptogenic activity (Figure 8.5). Gamma-aminobutyric acid (GABA) is the main inhibitory neurotransmitter in the brain involved in this process. If inhibition is unsuccessful, other neuronal aggregates are excited through thalamocortical recruitment, intrahemispheric association pathways or interhemispheric commissural pathways. Successful recruitment of a critical number of areas with synchronized depolarization then leads to a seizure (Figure 8.6).

Ion channel mutations have been linked to a variety of epilepsies considered idiopathic in humans (Escayg and Goldin, 2010; Meisler *et al.*, 2010). The majority of genes identified to date for human idiopathic epilepsy are inherited disorders of ion channels, known as channelopathies (Noebels, 2003). Each ion channel is a protein complex comprising several subunits. Excessive influx of sodium, blockade of efflux of potassium or altered calcium flux can lead to repetitive neuronal firing. Specific functional genetic mutations have been identified for each of these ion channels in humans (Noebels, 2003). Although similar mutations have yet to be identified in animals, the presence of familial epilepsy in the dog makes this possibility a high likelihood in the near future.

In the initial stages of epilepsy, an animal may possess only a single or limited number of epileptic foci. With recurrent seizure activity, the number of cells with an intrinsic pattern of high spontaneous firing activity (pacemaker cells) increase in the epileptic focus (known as kindling). An increase in the number of pacemaker cells is highly correlated with an increase in seizure frequency in experimental

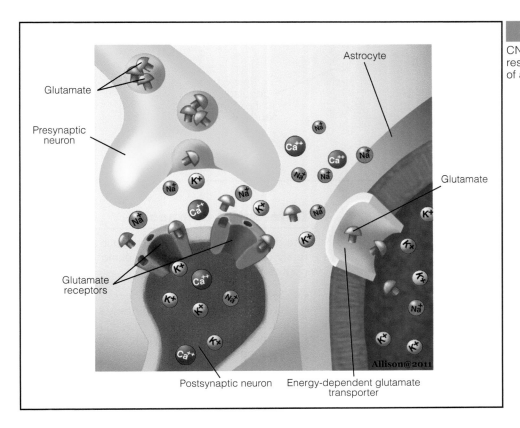

8.4 Glutamate receptors in the CNS generally responsible for excitation of associated neurons.

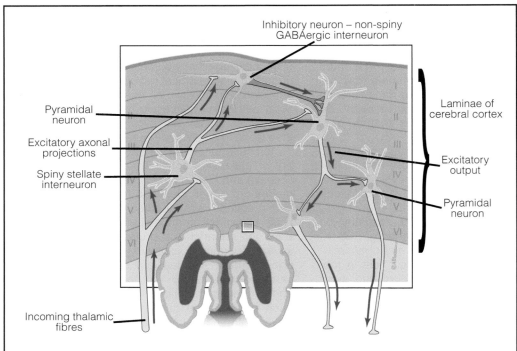

8.5 The neuronal circuitry in the cerebrum responsible for feed-forward inhibition. An imbalance in the levels of excitation and inhibition can lead to seizure discharges. (Modified from March 1998)

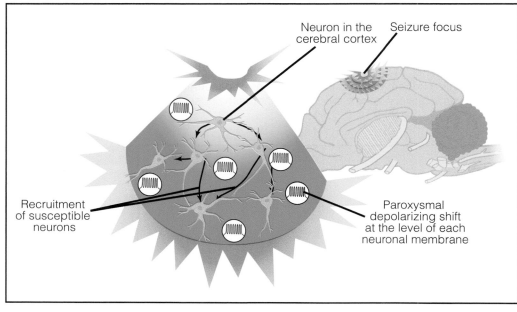

8.6 Recruitment of groups of neurons undergoing a paroxysmal depolarizing shift can be responsible for extension of the seizure focus.

models of epilepsy (Wyler *et al.*, 1978). Furthermore, a mirror focus of actively firing epileptogenic neurons may develop in a homologous region on the opposite hemisphere. If this happens, the number of epileptic foci can multiply rapidly. The significance of these changes is that, as a patient continues to seizure, there is an increased number of areas of the brain that are randomly and spontaneously able to initiate a seizure. Thus, the successful medical management of this patient will be challenged. Prevention of this sequence relies primarily on the early identification of the underlying aetiology of the seizure disorder, followed by the initiation of appropriate medical therapy.

Differential diagnosis

The differential diagnosis of epileptic seizures is currently divided into three main aetiological categories (Figure 8.7):

- Genetic (formerly idiopathic)
- Structural or metabolic (formerly symptomatic/secondary and reactive)
- Unknown (formerly probable symptomatic/cryptogenic).

Genetic epilepsy

A diagnosis of genetic epilepsy is most common in purebred dogs with the first onset of seizures

Genetic

- Channelopathies [8]
- Unknown genetic causes [8]

Structural or metabolic

- Developmental anomaly [9]:
  - Hydrocephalus
  - Cortical dysplasia
  - Lissencephaly
- Neoplasia [9]:
  - Extra-axial: meningioma, bone tumours
  - Intra-axial: glial tumours, metastasis
  - Intraventricular: ependymoma, choroid plexus tumours
- Infectious [11]:
  - Viral
  - Bacterial
  - Rickettsial
  - Fungal
  - Protozoal
  - Parasitic
- Inflammatory diseases [11]:
  - Granulomatous meningoencephalitis
  - Necrotizing meningoencephalitis
  - Eosinophilic meningoencephalitis
  - Meningoencephalitis of unknown origin
- Toxicity:
  - Lead [9]
  - Organophosphates
  - Ethylene glycol
- Traumatic [20]
- Vascular [9]
  - Ischaemic:
    o Thromboembolic
    o Idiopathic:
      • Feline ischaemic encephalopathy
  - Haemorrhagic:
    o Hypertension related
    o Coagulopathy
- Organ failure:
  - Hepatic [9]
  - Renal [9]
- Electrolyte imbalance:
  - Hyponatraemia or hypernatraemia [9]
  - Hypocalcaemia [13]
- Energy deprivation:
  - Hypoglycaemia [9]
  - Thiamine deficiency [11]

Unknown

- Prior head trauma in patients with normal imaging
- Post-encephalitic seizures developing months to years later
- Undetected hypoxic or vascular events of the brain post-anaesthesia
- *In utero* or birth trauma

8.7 Differential diagnosis of seizures in the dog and cat. The numbers in square brackets denote chapters where these conditions are discussed in detail.

between 1 and 5 years old, a normal interictal neurological examination, and if there is a lengthy initial interictal period (>4 weeks) (Podell *et al.*, 1995). A genetic basis has been reported in numerous dog breeds, including: Belgian Shepherd Dogs, Poodles, Beagles, Springer Spaniels, Vizslas, Irish Wolfhounds, Lagotto Romagnolos and Retrievers (Patterson *et al.*, 2003, 2005; Casal *et al.*, 2006; Jokinen *et al.*, 2007; Licht *et al.*, 2007; Berendt *et al.*, 2008, 2009; Oberbauer *et al.*, 2010). The mutation

causing myoclonic epilepsy in Miniature Wirehaired Dachshunds has been determined. These dogs suffer from Lafora disease and have a mutation in the *EPM2* gene (Lohi *et al.*, 2005). True genetic epilepsy is much less common in cats due to their more diverse genetic background (Quesnel *et al.*, 1997; Schriefl *et al.*, 2008; Kuwabara *et al.*, 2010). As such, all cats should be evaluated for underlying structural or metabolic seizures before a diagnosis of genetic epilepsy is made (Pákozdy *et al.*, 2010).

Structural or metabolic epileptic seizures

These types of epileptic seizures are the direct result of either structural brain pathology or metabolic disease. Dogs of any age can develop structural epileptic seizures. Younger animals are more prone to developmental and encephalitic diseases, whilst older dogs (>7 years of age) are more likely to develop intracranial neoplasia. As expected with underlying cerebral pathology, these animals are more likely to exhibit focal or multifocal neurological deficits. However, focal lesions in 'silent' cortical areas of the brain (e.g. olfactory, pyriform and occipital lobes) may have seizures as the only neurological problem. This type of seizure is common in cats and can be caused by feline infectious peritonitis (FIP) and meningioma (Barnes *et al.*, 2004; Tomek *et al.*, 2006; Timmann *et al.*, 2008).

Metabolic (formerly reactive) epileptic seizures are a reaction of the normal brain to transient systemic insult, toxic reaction or physiological stresses. Animals of any age may be affected. Small-breed dogs are more predisposed to develop seizures secondary to portosystemic shunts at a younger age. Typically, a higher seizure frequency occurs initially until the underlying metabolic or toxic insult is corrected, but evidence of systemic illness is often present concurrently (Brauer *et al.*, 2011).

Unknown cause of epileptic seizures

A variety of epileptic seizures arise without a cause but are thought to have a more specific aetiology. Previously termed probable symptomatic (or cryptogenic) epileptic seizures, these events are believed to be due to an underlying unidentified brain disease. Whilst this sounds like a somewhat nebulous disease category, it has particular implications when understanding why certain animals may be refractory to therapy. Examples of cases that may fit into this category are prior head trauma in patients with normal imaging studies, post-encephalitic seizures developing at a later date, undetected hypoxic or vascular events in the brain following anaesthesia or birth-related trauma.

Neurodiagnostic investigation

Historical data

The most important component in approaching a seizure case is acquiring a thorough and accurate history. Enquiries regarding the seizure event should address a description of the event, time of day, duration and post-ictal effects. The purpose is to establish overall frequency, seizure type, patterns of occurrence, relationship to daily activity (e.g. exercise, sleep) and severity of post-ictal effects. It is recommended that a charting technique measuring seizure frequency and severity should be developed to aid objective evaluation of future therapeutic success. Owners should be provided with a calendar to record the frequency and description of all observed and suspected seizures.

The interictal status of cerebrocortical function (between seizures and after the post-ictal period) can be evaluated by asking questions concerning the animal's behaviour, vision, gait and sleep/wake patterns. For example, if the dog is more withdrawn or attention seeking, showing any unusual episodes of aggression or irritability, or fails to follow simple commands, then a structural cerebral problem should be suspected. Likewise, subtle gait disturbances (stumbling up or down the stairs), visual disturbances (occasionally bumping into objects on one side) and restless sleep patterns may indicate structural forebrain problems.

Diagnostic evaluation
The sequence of diagnostic testing for any animal with seizures should proceed from the least to the most invasive (and expensive) modality.

- A complete blood count (CBC), biochemistry panel (including blood glucose), urinalysis and blood pressure measurement should be performed for all animals being evaluated for an epileptic seizure. For dogs, additional testing is based upon the age, breed, seizure type, seizure frequency and neurological examination findings.
- Dogs <1 year of age and those being initiated on hepatic metabolized antiepileptic drug (AED) therapy should also be evaluated for hepatic disease using a serum bile acid study or resting serum NH_4 concentration.
- Other individual tests for toxin exposure (e.g. plasma lead, serum cholinesterase assay), parasitic or rickettsial infection, or systemic illness are based on the clinical picture at the time of presentation.
- For cats, basic screening should include a retroviral screen for feline leukaemia and feline immunodeficiency virus and testing for serum antibodies to *Toxoplasma gondii*. Testing for the virus that causes feline infectious peritonitis is not recommended, as the correlation between a positive titre and active CNS infection is low.
- All dogs ≥7 years old with an initial onset of seizures, regardless of the seizure pattern or frequency or neurological examination, should undergo advanced imaging of the brain with MRI or computed tomography (CT). Due to the high incidence of symptomatic epilepsy in cats, the author recommends that advanced imaging of the brain be performed in all epileptic cats.
- Cerebrospinal fluid (CSF) analysis is recommended in any animal with multifocal neurological deficits or lesions observed on MRI or CT. The presence of an abnormal CSF

analysis has been found to be highly associated with the presence of underlying brain parenchymal lesions as detected on MR images (Bush *et al.*, 2002). In addition, CSF can also be abnormal due to the seizures themselves (Goncalves *et al.*, 2010).
- Although EEG analysis is beneficial for identifying underlying epileptic foci in the dog (Berendt *et al.*, 1999), the overall usefulness of this test for determining diagnosis and treatment has yet to be proven. For further information on EEG, see Chapter 4.

In addition, video segments of events can be extremely helpful for clinicians to determine whether an epileptic event has occurred. Owners should be encouraged to video an event if possible and to try and distract the animal to determine whether the event can be terminated with external stimuli. Distractability often implies a non-epileptic event.

Treatment

Management of epilepsy in cats and dogs often requires a lifetime commitment by the owners. The owner must be willing to medicate their pet several times per day, travel to emergency clinics at unpredictable times, follow up with periodic re-evaluations and diagnostic testing, and watch their pet carefully for adverse effects of therapy. The balance between quality of life and therapeutic success is often a key issue for an owner to continue treating their pet (Chang *et al.*, 2006). Despite all of the time, financial and emotional commitment, a significant portion of dogs may still continue to have seizures. Thus, proper client education is critical in preparing owners for understanding their pet's condition and the potential associated lifestyle changes. In particular, owners need to know that a diagnosis of epilepsy implies an increased risk of premature death with the prognosis dependent on a combination of veterinary expertise, therapeutic success and the motivation of the owner (Berendt *et al.*, 2007).

Decision-making strategies for AED therapy
The decision regarding when to start AED treatment is based on a number of factors, including aetiology, risk of recurrence, seizure type and its effect on the patient, as well as the risk of treatment. Risk factors for seizure recurrence are not well established for cats and dogs. A number of relative risk factors have been identified in epileptic people, including current or previously defined cerebral lesions or trauma, the presence of interictal EEG epileptic discharges (up to 90% recurrence rate) and a history of marked post-ictal adverse effects (Todd's paralysis) (Scottish Intercollegiate Guidelines Network – Guideline 70). Evidence-based guidelines from several international groups are well established for humans based on the risk:benefit ratio and predictability factors of drug effect (American Academy of Neurology (AAN),

2004). From these guidelines, several commonalities exist for guiding clinical practice including confirmation of an epileptic seizure event and seizure type, obtaining a definitive diagnosis, knowledge that recurrent seizure activity is correlated with poorer long-term treatment success, and the influence of treatment on the patient's quality of life (Stephen and Brodie, 2009). Thus, the decision to treat is a reflection of the treatment goals to reduce or eliminate epileptic events, reduce seizure severity, avoid adverse effects, and reduce seizure-related mortality and morbidity.

Initiating treatment

Whilst similar information is not as readily available for the veterinary patient population, extrapolation is possible to provide rationale treatment guidelines. Overwhelming evidence exists in humans that there is no benefit in starting treatment after a single unprovoked event (Glauser et al., 2006). However, the earlier AED therapy is initiated, the better the potential outcome may be for seizure control (Freitag and Tuxhorn, 2005; Chadwick, 2008).

Reasons to initiate AED therapy include:

- Structural epilepsy is diagnosed
- Status epilepticus has occurred
- Two or more isolated seizures occur within a 6-month period
- Two or more cluster seizure events occur within a 12-month period
- The first seizure is within 1 month of a traumatic event
- Severe or unusual post-ictal effects are present (e.g. prolonged blindness, aggression).

Drug selection

AED selection is based on a number of factors, including seizure type, efficacy and tolerability.

Evidence-based guidelines established by the ILAE, AAN and Standard and New AED Trials (SANAD) provide probability-based recommendations. Despite these guidelines, no evidence exists that any single AED provides a better outcome for adults with unprovoked epilepsy when early treatment is initiated. Monotherapy is still the recommendation for new onset epilepsy. The use of a single AED has the advantages of no drug interactions, more predictable pharmacokinetic and pharmacodynamic properties, less potential for adverse effects, and less expense to the client.

AEDs are classified into three broad mechanistic categories which decrease either the seizure onset or spread of seizures (Figure 8.8):

- Enhancement of inhibitory processes via facilitation of the action of GABA (Figure 8.9)
- Reduction of excitatory transmission
- Modulation of membrane cation conductance.

Unfortunately, several limitations exist in the selection of AEDs for use in veterinary medicine, including toxicity, tolerance, inappropriate pharmacokinetics and expense (Podell, 1998). In the past, many of the AEDs useful for humans could not be prescribed for small animals, due either to inappropriate pharmacokinetics (too rapid an elimination) or potential hepatotoxicity. The result was that the most commonly used AEDs in veterinary medicine were from the same mechanistic category, that of enhancing inhibition of the brain. However, newer AEDs with alternative mechanisms of action are now available, allowing a broader selection of treatment options.

The efficacy and safety profiles of AEDs are determined in large part by their pharmacokinetic properties. Drugs that are the easiest to use by the general population are ones that have the most

Drug	Decreased seizure onset		Decreased seizure spread	
	Enhanced Na+ channel inactivation	*Enhanced GABA activated Cl- conductance*	*Reduced current through Ca2+ channels*	*Reduced glutamate-mediated excitation*
Benzodiazepines		++		
Bromide		++ [a]		
Felbamate	+	+		++
Gabapentin	+	++ [b]	+	+
Lacosamide	++			
Levetiracetam		++ [b]		++
Phenobarbital		++	+	+
Rufinamide			++	
Topiramate	+	+		+
Zonisamide	+		++	

8.8 Summary of the mechanism of action of several currently available antiepileptic drugs. [a] Competitive displacement of chloride through activated GABA receptors. [b] Indirect GABA receptor activation via increased GABA activity. + = secondary mechanism; ++ = postulated primary mechanism.

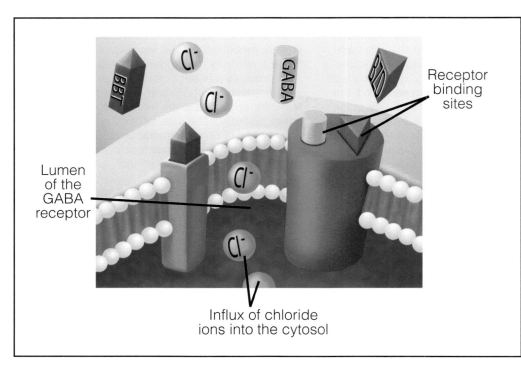

8.9 GABA$_A$ receptor in the CNS generally responsible for increasing local chloride levels and causing a surrounding inhibition. The receptor can be bound by barbiturates (BBT) and benzodiazepines (BZD).

favourable pharmacokinetic properties (Bourgeois, 2000). Ultimately, an AED with the most desirable pharmacokinetic profile has complete bioavailability, is available as a parenteral formulation, and has an elimination half-life suitable for daily or twice-daily dosing, linear elimination kinetics, no autoinduction of enzymatic biotransformation, no pharmacokinetic interactions with other drugs, rapid brain penetration, a volume of distribution with a single compartment, low and non-saturable protein binding, and no active metabolites. The ideal AED has not yet been formulated for any species.

Tolerability is a major consideration for drug selection. Adverse effects can be divided into transient, persistent and life-threatening (idiosyncratic or predictable). Most transient adverse effects are avoidable with titration dosing and dissipate within several weeks. Persistent effects are either CNS dose-dependent associated with sedation, ataxia, vertigo or cognitive impairment, or metabolic-related with hormonal imbalances, metabolic syndromes and degenerative effects (e.g. osteoporosis). Severe life-threatening effects are mainly associated with either idiosyncratic bone marrow disease (e.g. aplastic anaemia) or predictable organ damage over time (e.g. hepatotoxicity).

AED generations
From the introduction of bromide in 1857 by Charles Locock to treat 'hysterical' epileptic fits in women, to the development of phenobarbital in the early 1900s, and the introduction of phenytoin, valproate and carbamazepine in the early 1970s, the use of first-generation AEDs was limited by mechanism, benefit and adverse effects. Not until the early 1990s did a revolution in drug development occur with the introduction of felbamate. The succession of second-generation drugs over the

following two decades resulted in greater treatment success with a significant improvement in tolerability. Third-generation AEDs aimed at improving seizure control and patient quality of life are now available (Figure 8.10).

First-generation AEDs
• Benzodiazepines
• Bromide
• Carbamazepine
• Phenobarbital
• Phenytoin
• Valproate

Second-generation AEDs
• Felbamate
• Gabapentin
• Lamotrigine
• Levetiracetam
• Oxcarbazepine
• Pregabalin
• Topiramate
• Zonisamide

Third-generation AEDs
• Lacosamide
• Rufinamide

Next generation AEDs
• Brivacetam
• Carisbamate
• Flurofelbamate
• Losigamone
• Remacemide
• Retigabine
• Seletracetam
• Tiagabine

8.10 Categorization of AEDs by generation of drug development.

Success parameters

The treatment of epilepsy should be goal-oriented and approached in an objective fashion. Eliminating or significantly reducing the number and severity of seizures and maintaining a normal lifestyle for both the patient and owner are all important considerations. Whilst many drugs may provide initial improvement in seizure control, long-term efficacy is dependent on many factors. With only approximately 60–80% of human and canine epileptic patients responding to treatment, evaluating the reasons for recurrent seizure activity (refractory epilepsy) is important (Brodie *et al.*, 2007).

These factors can be separated into three main variables:

- Disease-related
- Drug-related
- Patient-related.

Disease-related factors

Disease-related factors include the presence of an undiagnosed underlying brain disease, such as cortical malformation, prior trauma or an active disease process. Occult conditions can lead to localization-related epilepsy, where epileptic foci develop drug resistance due to architectural brain changes.

Drug-related factors

Drug-related factors include an ineffective mechanism of action, development of tolerance and alteration of the drug target or uptake over time (Loscher and Schmidt, 2006). Seizure-specific therapy targets a drug for a specific seizure type, and inappropriate drug selection may result in poor control.

The reasons for drug tolerance or loss of effectiveness can be categorized as either metabolic (pharmacokinetic) or functional (pharmacodynamic). Metabolic tolerance is due to altered drug metabolism, which occurs in an unpredictable fashion. As such, a change in drug dosage does not result in a parallel change in serum drug level; for example, the autoinduction phase seen with phenobarbital in dogs occurs typically during the first 60 days of treatment. During this time, autoinduction of the cytochrome p450 enzyme system increases drug clearance and is not dose-dependent. Serum drug levels decline over time with the same dose until steady state clearance is achieved. Concomitant drug usage that either inhibits or stimulates the p450 system also alters hepatic metabolized AED levels.

Functional drug tolerance, also known as drug-resistant epilepsy, is due to reduced drug transport through the blood–brain barrier, long term downregulation of the target receptor or genetic factors that alter cellular metabolism of the drug.

Patient-related factors

Patient-related factors are now being discovered in relation to gene polymorphisms that affect AED pharmacokinetic or pharmacodynamic properties. As a result, altered drug metabolism or action is no longer predictable when compared with the general patient population. In addition, a placebo effect has been demonstrated in epileptic dogs, indicating that non-pharmacological therapeutic effects may play a role in canine epilepsy treatment (Munana *et al.*, 2010). Not all epileptic patients can be controlled with a single AED and some animals require multiple medications for successful treatment.

Specific AED treatment for dogs

Figure 8.11 summarizes the AEDs available for the treatment of dogs; Figure 8.12 details those drugs not recommended.

First-generation AEDs

Phenobarbital: This drug, a phenyl barbiturate, has the longest history of chronic use of all AEDs in veterinary medicine. It is a relatively inexpensive, well tolerated drug that can be administered two or three times per day and has well documented success in preventing seizures (Farnbach, 1984; Schwartz-Porsche *et al.*, 1985; Parent and Quesnel, 1996; Boothe *et al.*, 2012).

Pharmacology: Phenobarbital has a high bioavailability, being rapidly absorbed within 2 hours and with a maximal plasma concentration obtained within 4–8 hours following oral administration (Ravis *et al.*, 1989). Almost one-half of the drug is protein bound. The majority of phenobarbital is metabolized by the liver, with approximately one-third excreted unchanged in the urine. Phenobarbital is an autoinducer of hepatic microsomal enzymes (p450 system), which can progressively reduce the elimination half-life with chronic dosing.

Side-effects: Overall, phenobarbital is well tolerated at therapeutic serum concentrations in the dog. Idiosyncratic drug reactions to phenobarbital can be either behavioural or biochemically mediated. Behavioural changes, such as hyperexcitability, restlessness or sedation, may occur after starting treatment with the drug, but they appear not to be dose-related and resolve typically within 1 week. A more serious idiosyncratic reaction is development of an immune-mediated neutropenia or thrombocytopenia in dogs (Jacobs *et al.*, 1998), as well as anaemia. Typically, this reversible blood dyscrasia occurs within the first 6 months of dosing. Rare acute, idiosyncratic hepatotoxic reactions may also be present, as evidenced by a rapid elevation of alanine aminotransferase (ALT) and abnormal dynamic bile acid levels. The drug should be stopped immediately if either neutropenia or dramatic elevations in ALT are noted, and the animal should be loaded with an additional AED, such as potassium bromide (see below). Phenobarbital may also be a risk factor for the development of superficial necrolytic dermatitis in dogs (March *et al.*, 2004).

Chronic adverse historical effects usually revolve around polydipsic and polyphagic behaviour. As a result, dogs may develop psychogenic polydipsia with associated polyuria. The most common serum biochemical change with chronic phenobarbital therapy is elevation of the serum alkaline phosphatase

Drug	Clinical pharmacology				Therapeutic range	Dosage	Efficacy	Major possible adverse effects
	$T_{1/2}$ (hr)	Tss (d)	Vd (l/kg)	Protein binding (%)				
Bromide	20–46 days	100–200	0.45	0	Monotherapy: 1000–3000 mg/l with phenobarbital at 1500–2500 mg/l	40–60 mg/ kg orally q24h	Generalized seizures	Sedation; weakness; polydipsia; possible pancreatitis; possible behavioural disorders
Clorazepate	5–6	1–2	1.6	85	20–75 µg/ml (nordiazepam)	2–4 mg/kg orally q12h	Add on; generalized and partial seizures	Sedation; withdrawal seizures
Felbamate	5–6	1–2	1.0	25	25–100 mg/l	20 mg/kg orally q8h	Partial seizures	Blood dyscrasia; liver toxicity; induces p450 system
Gabapentin	2–4	1	0.2	0	4–16 mg/l	10–20 mg/ kg orally q8–12h	Generalized and partial seizures	Sedation; ataxia
Levetiracetam	2–4	2–3	0.5	<10	Variable	20 mg/kg orally q8–12h	Add on or first line; generalized and partial seizures	Not greater than placebo; sedation; ataxia
Phenobarbital	24–40	10–14	0.8	40	20–40 mg/dl	2.5 mg/kg orally q12h	Generalized seizures	Sedation; polydipsia; liver toxicity; induces p450 system; blood dyscrasias
Zonisamide	15–20	3–4	1.5	50	10–40 µg/ml	5–10 mg/ kg orally q12h	Add on or first line; generalized and partial seizures	Sedation; ataxia; loss of appetite; keraconjunctivitis sicca; vomiting

8.11 AEDs available for treating epilepsy in dogs. $T_{1/2}$ = elimination half-life; Tss = approximate time to steady state; Vd = volume of distribution.

Inappropriate

- Toxicity:
  - Phenytoin (hepatic)
  - Primidone (hepatic)
  - Lamotrigine (cardiac)
  - Vigabatrin (blood dyscrasia)
- Inappropriate pharmacokinetics:
  - Carbamazepine (short elimination half-life)
  - Phenytoin (short elimination half-life)
  - Oral diazepam (inability to achieve therapeutic serum concentration)

Use with caution

- Synergistic hepatic toxicity:
  - Phenobarbital and:
    o Felbamate
    o Zonisamide
- Withdrawal seizures:
  - Phenobarbital
  - Clorazepate
  - Felbamate

8.12 AEDs inappropriate for use in the dog.

level (Bunch *et al.*, 1985). These changes can occur as soon as 2 weeks after initiating therapy. Neither endogenous adrenocorticotropic hormone (ACTH) nor the exogenous response to ACTH is altered by phenobarbital dosing (Dyer *et al.*, 1994). Moreover,

phenobarbital does not interfere with the low-dose dexamethasone suppression test, regardless of dose or treatment time (Foster *et al.*, 2000). Serum total and free thyroxine (T4) concentrations may be low in dogs treated with phenobarbital (and in a few dogs the serum thyroid-stimulating hormone concentration may be elevated), resulting in a mistaken diagnosis of hypothyroidism (Kantrowitz *et al.*, 1999).

Three serious and potentially life-threatening complications can occur with long-term phenobarbital therapy:

- With time, physical dependence on the drug develops. Withdrawal seizures can occur as serum phenobarbital concentrations decline to between 15 and 20 µg/ml
- There may be the development of functional tolerance to the drug. Functional tolerance is the loss of drug effectiveness due to changes in drug–receptor interaction, change in drug distribution into the brain, or progression of an underlying disease state
- Potentially, the most life-threatening complication is drug-induced hepatotoxicity. Hepatotoxicity to primidone (which is metabolized predominantly to phenobarbital), either alone or in combination with other AEDs, has been shown to occur in experimental and

clinical conditions in dogs (Bunch *et al.*, 1985; Poffenbarger, 1985; Gaskill *et al.*, 2005). Documentation of a serum phenobarbital concentration >35 µg/ml had the highest correlation with the development of hepatotoxicity (Dayrell-Hart *et al.*, 1991). All animals on chronic phenobarbital therapy should have a routine biochemistry panel performed every 6–12 months to monitor for the development of chronic hepatotoxicity. Bile acid and/or ammonia concentrations should be analysed to evaluate liver function if ALT levels suddenly increase or if the serum albumin level starts to decrease.

Administration and monitoring: The appropriate starting dose of phenobarbital for dogs is 2.5 mg/kg orally q12h (see Figures 8.11 and 8.13). An intravenous loading dose can be used to produce a rapid rise in serum blood concentration. This starting dose is the only time a weight-based dosage is used. All future adjustments should be based on serum drug concentrations in conjunction with clinical assessment. The objectives of monitoring trough serum concentrations of any AED are:

- To determine whether a therapeutic value is present at the time when the lowest serum concentration is present, as dogs are most likely to seizure at this time
- To record that serum concentration fluctuates within the established therapeutic range for that drug when chronically administered (steady-state concentration)
- To prevent toxic effects from occurring
- To individualize therapy.

Serial serum trough phenobarbital concentrations should be evaluated at: 14, 45, 90, 180 and 360 days after the initiation of treatment, at 6-month intervals thereafter, if the pet has more than two seizure events between these times, and at 2 weeks after a dosage change. Although blood level fluctuations may not be dramatic throughout the day in dogs with steady-state concentrations (Levitski and Trepanier, 2000), blood samples are best taken in the early morning, prior to dosing, in a fasted dog, to increase consistency in comparison with published information, maintain consistency in interpretation and remove diurnal or dietary-induced fluctuations of absorption (Maguire *et al.*, 2000).

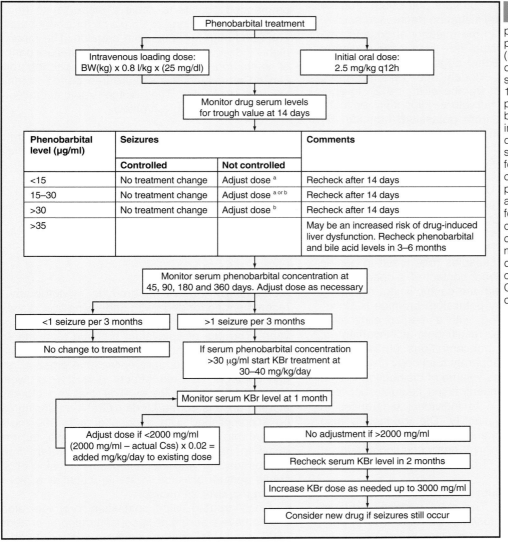

8.13 Algorithm for use of phenobarbital and potassium bromide (KBr) in the dog. [a] The dose of phenobarbital should be increased by 10–25%. [b] The dose of phenobarbital should be cautiously increased or a second drug, such as KBr, should be given. The formula used to calculate the phenobarbital dose adjustments is as follows: (Desired concentration/Actual concentration) x total mg phenobarbital per day = Oral daily dose of phenobarbital (mg). Css = steady-state concentration.

Adjustments in AED dosages are undertaken either to enhance the effect or to reduce the adverse effects. The most efficacious and safe trough therapeutic phenobarbital range for the dog is 15–30 µg/ml. An optimal starting level is between 20 and 25 µg/ml. Increments of 5 µg/ml are beneficial if seizures are occurring at an equal frequency or worsening after 30 days of therapy. Adjustments of the trough phenobarbital levels can be calculated with the following formula:

(Desired concentration/Actual concentration) x
total mg phenobarbital per day =
Oral daily dose of phenobarbital (mg)

A ≥20% drop in the trough serum concentration is often an indicator of poor administration compliance. Overall, phenobarbital is an AED that can provide excellent seizure control in idiopathic epileptic dogs (in approximately 85% of dogs seizures are eradicated) with careful serial monitoring of trough serum drug concentrations (Boothe et al., 2012).

Potassium bromide: Potassium bromide can be used as either monotherapy or as an add-on AED of choice in the dog. Concomitant potassium bromide and phenobarbital administration decreased seizure number and severity in the majority of dogs in several studies, with seizure-free status ranging from 21% to 72% of all treated dogs (Schwartz-Porsche and Jurgens, 1991; Podell and Fenner, 1993; Trepanier et al., 1998; Boothe et al., 2012). In general, many canine refractory idiopathic epileptic patients may benefit from potassium bromide. By allowing a reduction in the use of drugs metabolized by the liver, potassium bromide therapy may also reduce the incidence of hepatotoxicity.

Pharmacology: In the USA, bromide is typically given as the inorganic salt potassium bromide, usually as a solution of 200–250 mg/ml dissolved in double distilled water. In the UK several commercial formulations are available. Potassium bromide is a known mucosal irritant and capsules may result in gastric irritation due to the direct contact of a concentrated amount of the drug with the gastric lining. A starting dose of 40 mg/kg/day potassium bromide is slowly metabolized in the dog, with a median elimination half-life of 15.2 days, resulting in achievement of median steady-state concentrations of 2450 mg/l (March et al., 2002); apparent total body clearance is 16.4 ml/kg/day and the volume of distribution is 0.40 l/kg. Steady-state concentrations fluctuate between dogs, most likely due to individual differences in clearance and bioavailability. Dietary factors also alter serum drug concentrations, with high chloride diets resulting in excessive renal secretion and lower serum concentrations (Trepanier and Babish, 1995).

Side-effects: Potassium bromide is generally well tolerated in the dog. The most common adverse effects seen with potassium bromide and phenobarbital combination therapy are polydipsia, poly-phagia, increased lethargy and mild ataxia with increasing serum concentration. Pancreatitis and gastrointestinal intolerance have also been reported (Gaskill and Cribb, 2000; Baird-Heinz et al., 2012). Potassium bromide may cause skin problems (bromoderma), although no substantiated reports exist currently. Intoxication to the point of stupor is rare, but pelvic limb ataxia, weakness and altered behaviour are more likely with serum concentrations >3000 mg/l (Rossmeisl and Inzana, 2009). Caution should be used when treating dogs with underlying renal insufficiency, due to reduced renal elimination (Nichols et al., 1996). Therapy for potassium bromide intoxication consists of intravenous normal saline administration to enhance renal excretion. Careful monitoring is advised as dogs may become more susceptible to seizure activity with lowering of the serum concentration.

Administration and monitoring: Potassium bromide can be administered at a starting dose of 40 mg/kg/day when used as sole therapy or 30 mg/kg/day when used as an add-on drug to phenobarbital. Potassium bromide serum concentration should be measured at 1 month and at the first steady-state concentration (approximately 8–12 weeks). The recommended goal is to achieve steady-state trough serum concentrations of 25 µg/ml for phenobarbital and 2000 mg/l for potassium bromide. The range is highly individualized according to the seizure pattern of each dog. Further reductions in phenobarbital can be attempted if a seizure-free period is maintained for 6 months. The dosage is adjusted according to the formulae given below.

Combined therapy: For concomitant phenobarbital and potassium bromide treatment, the new maintenance dose can be calculated as follows:

(Target Css – Actual Css) x (Clearance/Bioavailability) =
(2000 mg/l – Actual Css) x 0.02 = mg/kg/day added to
existing dose
Where Css = steady-state concentration.

Monotherapy: Potassium bromide monotherapy is recommended for dogs with underlying liver disease and those with less frequent seizure activity (<3 per year). The use of potassium bromide monotherapy is not recommended for high initial frequency seizure activity, if secondary epilepsy is present, or if unacceptable adverse effects persist (e.g. weakness, extreme polydipsia). The oral monotherapy starting dose is 40 mg/kg/day. Oral load dosing can be accomplished with a dose of 400–800 mg/kg divided into equal doses q4h over 4 days, but may result in gastric upset. The author prefers intravenous loading with a constant rate infusion of 3% sterile sodium bromide in sterile water at a rate of 900 mg/kg over 24 hours.

Dogs treated with potassium bromide alone should have a serum drug concentration at or above 2500 mg/l for optimal seizure control. Gradual increases in dose allow for better adaptation to the drug. For monotherapy, the new maintenance dose can be calculated as follows:

(Target Css – Actual Css) x (Clearance/Bioavailability) =
(2500 mg/l – Actual Css) x 0.02 = mg/kg/day added to
existing dose
Where Css = steady-state concentration.

Benzodiazepines: These are a class of AEDs that interact with specific CNS benzodiazepine receptors which activate the GABA$_A$ chloride channel to hyperpolarize neuronal membranes (see Figure 8.9). Diazepam is the most widely used benzodiazepine in veterinary medicine and is best suited for the emergency treatment of seizures by intravenous and/or per rectum administration (see also Chapter 20). Chronic oral administration of diazepam is not recommended in the dog due to its lack of effectiveness in stopping seizures, its very short half-life, the potential for increased hepatic enzyme inhibition, physical dependence, and cross-tolerance preventing effective use of intravenous diazepam in stopping seizures in an emergency (see Figure 8.12). Clorazepate, a long-acting benzodiazepine, is a diazepam pro-drug with more suitable pharmacokinetic properties for chronic use in the dog, but similar problems may arise as with chronic oral diazepam, especially the potential for severe withdrawal seizure activity (Scherkl et al., 1989). Pulse dosing of clorazepate in dogs has the potential to stop cluster seizure events that are separated by several hours with a normal interictal period. A dose of 1 mg/kg q8h is recommended at the onset of the first seizure. Treatment is maintained for 24 hours, followed by tapering to every 12 hours for 24 hours and then every 24 hours for one dose to prevent withdrawal seizure reaction (Scherkel et al., 1989). Unfortunately, this drug is no longer available in some countries.

Second-generation AEDs

Felbamate: This is a dicarbamate with proven ability to block seizures induced by a variety of methods. Felbamate is believed to increase the seizure threshold and prevent seizures from spreading by reducing excitatory neurotransmission in the brain. Neuroprotective effects have also been demonstrated through this ability to alter excitatory neurotransmission. In human clinical trials, felbamate has been shown to be most useful as monotherapy for the treatment of uncontrolled focal epilepsy.

Felbamate is metabolized by the hepatic microsomal p450 enzymes, with increased metabolism in younger animals (Adusumalli et al., 1992). In dogs, the drug has a high bioavailability and protein-binding capability (see Figure 8.11 for dose). Effective control of complex focal seizure activity (automatisms) with documented therapeutic serum concentrations has been shown with felbamate therapy in dogs (Ruehlmann et al., 2001). Felbamate is a non-sedating drug.

A higher incidence of aplastic anaemia and liver toxicity has been reported in humans, but these adverse effects have not been documented in dogs. Serial monitoring of the CBC and biochemistry panel is recommended at 1 month and every 3 months during treatment. The trough serum drug concentration is typically measured 1–2 weeks after initiation of treatment, with a therapeutic range between 25 and 100 mg/l. This drug is not currently available in the UK and needs to be imported on a special licence.

Gabapentin: This AED is most commonly used for neuropathic pain relief in small animals. Initially designed to mimic GABA in the brain, gabapentin can readily pass through the blood–brain barrier. However, once in the brain, gabapentin does not mimic the pharmacological properties of GABA nor does it bind to the GABA receptors. In preclinical studies, gabapentin effectively blocked seizures induced by a variety of proconvulsant methods. Evidence also suggests that gabapentin may facilitate the extracellular transport of GABA out of cells to act on the GABA$_A$ receptor (Honmou et al., 1995). The dog is the only known species to partially biotransform the drug to N-methyl-gabapentin in the liver (Radulovic et al., 1995). A major benefit of the drug is that both the parent and metabolites are excreted renally; thus, it does not induce drug–drug interactions with other AEDs with hepatic metabolism (e.g. phenobarbital).

Gabapentin may also be beneficial as an add-on therapy for epileptic seizures secondary to hepatic disease (e.g. portosystemic shunting) and post-traumatic or post-hypoxic delirium. Dosing every 8 hours is necessary due to the rapid elimination half-life (Kukanich and Cohen, 2011). Lower starting doses with gradual adaptation over time (e.g. once daily dosing for 3 days, then twice daily dosing for 3 days and then thrice daily dosing thereafter) is recommended to avoid excessive sedation, which is seen as a side effect in many dogs (see Figure 8.11). Reduced doses may be needed in patients with renal insufficiency. Serum monitoring is not recommended as the drug has a very high therapeutic index and little drug–drug interaction. Preliminary clinical evaluation of this drug as an add-on therapy for refractory idiopathic epileptic dogs recorded an improvement in seizure frequency in approximately 50% of cases (Govendir et al., 2005; Platt et al., 2006). Pharmaceutical suspension formulations of gabapentin contain the artificial sweetener xylitol, which can induce hypoglycaemia and should be avoided in the dog and cat.

Topiramate: This is a sulphamate-substituted monosaccharide which blocks the spread of seizures via rapidly potentiated GABA activity in the brain (Petroff et al., 2001). In humans, topiramate is well absorbed and primarily excreted renally as an unchanged drug. With a relatively long half-life of 20–30 hours, twice-daily dosing is recommended. With a relatively broad-spectrum activity against many seizure types and minimal adverse effects, topiramate is approved for use in both adult and paediatric human patients. Dosing ranges are between 25 and 50 mg/day per patient (Holland, 2001) but gradual dose titration is better tolerated (see Figure 8.14). No clinical studies have been published on the use of this drug in small animals to date; although, pharmacokinetics in Beagles have demonstrated a terminal half-life of 2–3.8 hours, no accumulation and no autoinduction or inhibition of enzymes (Streeter *et al.*, 1995).

Zonisamide: This is a substituted 1,2-benzisoxazole derivative that works by both blocking the propagation of epileptic discharges and suppressing focal epileptogenic activity (Ito *et al.*, 1980). Broad-spectrum antiepileptic activity has been reported against a variety of seizure types, with particular improvement in the treatment of adult myoclonus epilepsy (Henry *et al.*, 1988). Zonisamide can be an efficacious and well tolerated drug in dogs with recurrent generalized seizures refractory to phenobarbital or potassium bromide therapy. Over 70% of dogs with refractory idiopathic epilepsy responded well to zonisamide addon therapy in one study, with 58% responding favourably in another (Dewey *et al.*, 2003; von Klopmann *et al.*, 2007).

Pharmacology: Zonisamide is well absorbed, has a relatively long half-life (18–28 hours) and high protein-binding affinity (70%) (Booth and Perkins, 2008). The drug is highly concentrated in red blood cells due to high binding to carbonic anhydrase and other red cell protein components (Patsalos and Sander, 1994). Zonisamide is metabolized hepatically and thus influenced by concurrent administration of other similarly metabolized drugs (Walker *et al.*, 1988).

Side-effects: The major adverse effects include sedation, dry eye, ataxia, inappetence and vomiting. A higher incidence of renal calculi formation and gastrointestinal disorders is found in humans, but has not been documented in dogs. Metabolic acidosis and liver dysfunction has been documented in dogs receiving this medication (Cook *et al.*, 2011; Miller *et al.*, 2011; Schwartz *et al.*, 2011). Patients with a history of sulfa drug hypersensitivity should not be prescribed zonisamide.

Administration and monitoring: Zonisamide is available as a generic medication in dosages of 25 mg, 50 mg and 100 mg. Parental and suspension formulations are not commercially available. A preliminary study demonstrated that dogs responded to treatment with a blood level close to 20 µg/ml (Dewey *et al.*, 2003); a recent experimental study revealed that stable plasma concentrations were achieved in 3–4 days in dogs following oral administration (Fukunaga *et al.*, 2010).

Combination therapy: Phenobarbital dosages should be reduced by 25% at the time of starting zonisamide due to the enhanced hepatic enzyme induction and clearance of zonisamide (Orito *et al.*, 2008).

Levetiracetam: This is the *S*-enantiomer of the ethyl analogue of piracetam and has a unique mechanism of action mediated by binding to the presynaptic vesicular protein, SV2A, which decreases glutamate neurotransmitter release (Lynch *et al.*, 2004). In dogs, the drug is well absorbed, is rapidly metabolized with an estimated elimination half-life of 4–8 hours, and is predominantly excreted renally (>80%) (Volk *et al.*, 2008). However, wide fluctuations of drug metabolism occur in the dog. The initial dose of 10–20 mg/kg orally q12h is gradually incremented to ≥20 mg/kg orally q8h. The therapeutic range is not well defined and drug monitoring is recommended only to establish the pharmacokinetic pattern of the individual patient.

The drug is well tolerated, with sedation noted as the most common adverse effect (Patterson *et al.*, 2008). The oral dose should be increased when dogs are receiving phenobarbital concurrently as lower serum levels can potentially be related to the induction of serum hydrolases (Moore *et al.*, 2010, 2011). A parenteral formulation is available for intramuscular dosing or intravenous loading at 40–60 mg/kg over 15–30 minutes in a 1:1 diluted saline solution (Patterson *et al.*, 2008). An oral syrup formulation is also available. Recent work suggests that levetiracetam may need to be given at higher doses in dogs refractory to phenobarbital therapy as it may not offer any advantage compared with a placebo at routine doses (Muñana *et al.*, 2012). A new extended release formulation of levetiracetam has been shown to have a half-life in excess of 7 hours in dogs following oral administration, giving rise to the potential for once or twice daily administration (Platt *et al.*, 2011).

Lamotrigine: This novel drug is chemically unrelated to any current AEDs. Although efficacious in human epileptic patients, the drug is converted to a cardiotoxic 2-*N*-methyl metabolite in dogs (Wong and Lhatoo, 2000), which is not found in humans. This drug is not recommended for use in dogs (see Figure 8.12).

Pregabalin: This is a structural analogue of GABA with a mechanism of action of voltage-gated calcium channel modulation, which decreases depolarization-induced calcium influx at the nerve terminals and ultimately reduces excitatory neurotransmitter release. The mean elimination half-life is estimated at 7 hours in dogs (Salazar *et al.*, 2009). Metabolism appears to be predominantly via renal excretion with minimal protein binding and drug interaction. Efficacy as an add-on therapy for refractory partial seizures was found in several studies in humans and in a recent study in dogs (Dewey *et al.*, 2009). A definitive therapeutic range has yet to be determined for humans and dogs. The initial dose recommendation is 4 mg/kg orally q8–12 hours. Adverse effects appear to be limited to sedation and ataxia.

Third-generation AEDs

Lacosamide: This is a functionalized amino acid proven to decrease neuronal discharge frequency and synaptic excitability (Halford and Lapointe, 2009). The postulated mechanisms of action include selective slow inactivation of sodium channels and novel binding to collapsin response mediator protein-2. In humans, the drug is well absorbed, has minimal first-pass effect with predominant renal excretion, low protein binding, favourable drug–drug interactions with other AEDs, and is well tolerated. Clinical trials in humans have demonstrated a comparable decrease in seizure frequency with that of levetiracetam and zonisamide at a dose of 100–200 mg orally q12h. A parenteral formulation is available for intravenous loading. The author has used lacosamide successfully to treat refractory idiopathic epilepsy in dogs at a dose range of 5–10 mg/kg orally q12h.

Rufinamide: This novel drug is structurally unrelated to any other AED. Its main mechanism of action is related to prolongation of the inactive state of the sodium channel, thus preventing neuronal depolarization. In humans, the drug is absorbed slowly and has low bioavailability. Renal excretion is high and no induction of the hepatic p450 system has been found, although other hepatically metabolized drugs decrease the serum concentration. Of a total of 9 double-blinded studies in humans, 5 revealed a positive effect of rufinamide to treat refractory partial seizures but not generalized seizures (Biton, 2009). Initial dosing ranged from 10–40 mg/kg orally q24h, with dose-dependent adverse effects of sedation, fatigue and dizziness noted. A parenteral formulation is not available. No data were found regarding clinical use in dogs or cats.

Specific AED treatment for cats

Figure 8.14 summarizes the AEDs available for the treatment of cats.

First-generation AEDs

Phenobarbital: As with dogs, phenobarbital is the recommended first-line AED in the epileptic cat (Parent and Quesnel, 1996). The pharmacokinetic properties are similar to those in the dog, but with a more prolonged elimination half-life range. In addition, cats are more sensitive to the sedative effects and eliminate the drug more slowly. Thus, the therapeutic range is lower, typically between 10 and 20 µg/ml, and dosing can be highly individualized. Most cats can be treated with 1–2 mg/kg/day orally, with once-daily dosing, initially at night. A subsequent increase to twice-daily dosing can be instituted as needed. Idiosyncratic reactions include blood dyscrasias, dermatitis, lymphadenopathy and persistent unusual behaviours. Predictable dose-dependent adverse effects include polydipsia, polyuria and polyphagia. More severe problems may include hepatotoxicity, although this has not been reported to date. Overall, phenobarbital can be used successfully in the cat with proper monitoring.

Benzodiazepines: Diazepam is recommended for cats refractory to phenobarbital as an alternative but not concomitant AED. The dose range is 0.5–2.0 mg/kg orally q8–12h. Gradual adaptation is necessary to prevent excess sedation. Diazepam is metabolized to the active metabolites nordiazepam and oxazepam. Trough serum nordiazepam concentrations should be in the therapeutic range of 200–500 ng/ml. Potential complications include similar behavioural problems to those described for phenobarbital therapy, physical dependence and possible withdrawal seizure activity, and acute fulminant hepatic necrosis. The latter problem is an idiosyncratic reaction that can be fatal (Center *et al.*, 1995). Therefore, all cats treated with diazepam should have liver enzymes monitored within the first week of therapy and again within 1 month. The drug should be discontinued if any liver enzyme elevation is observed.

Drug	$T_{1/2}$ (hr)	Therapeutic range	Initial dose	Potential adverse effects
Clonazepam	Unknown	500–700 ng/ml (nordiazepam)	0.5–1 mg orally q12–24h	Acute hepatic necrosis; sedation
Diazepam	15–20	500–700 ng/ml (nordiazepam)	2.5–10 mg orally q8–12h	Acute hepatic necrosis; sedation
Gabapentin	3	Unknown	5–10 mg/kg orally q8–12h	Sedation; ataxia
Levetiracetam	2–5	10–50 µg/ml	10–20 mg/kg orally q8–12h	Sedation
Phenobarbital	34–43	10–30 mg/dl	1–2 mg orally q12–24h	Sedation; hepatotoxicity; blood dyscrasia
Topiramate	Unknown	Unknown	12.5–25 mg orally q8–12h	Sedation; inappetence
Zonisamide	35	Unknown	5–10 mg/kg orally q24h	Sedation; anorexia; vomiting; somnolence; ataxia; diarrhoea (Hasegawa *et al.*, 2008)

8.14 AEDs available for treating epilepsy in cats. $T_{1/2}$ = elimination half-life.

Clonazepam can be used as an alternative to diazepam in the cat, as it does not undergo hepatic microsomal metabolism, has a more prolonged elimination half-life and, therefore, may not produce an idiosyncratic hepatic reaction. The recommended starting dose is 0.5 mg/cat orally q12–24h. Clorazepate is another long-acting benzodiazepine that the author has successfully used, although the precise pharmacokinetic properties of this drug are not well understood in the cat. The recommended dose range is 3.75–7.5 mg/cat orally q12–24h. Similar precautions as described for diazepam are necessary.

Potassium bromide: This is not recommended as a standard therapy in cats due to the relatively high prevalence of adverse respiratory problems (Boothe and George, 2002). Cats can develop a cough and more severe respiratory signs suggestive of an allergic asthmatic disease, which can be fatal in some cases (Wagner, 2001). The author no longer recommends the use of potassium bromide in cats.

Second-generation AEDs

Gabapentin: This is a useful AED in the cat due to its exclusive renal excretion. However, cats may exhibit increased sedation and benefit from a gradual increment in dosing over 1–2 weeks. The author recommends starting at 5–10 mg/kg orally q24h for 3–5 days, then increasing to twice daily dosing. Gabapentin has an approximate half-life of 3 hours in cats (Siao et al., 2010). Further increases are dependent upon the response to therapy. Both solution and capsular formulations of the drug are available, but the oral solution is not recommended. The drug can be used both as monotherapy and an add-on medication.

Levetiracetam: This is an effective add-on AED and is well tolerated in cats (Bailey et al., 2008). Levetiracetam appears to be rapidly metabolized and has an elimination half-life of under 4 hours. Up-titration dosing starting at 10 mg/kg orally q24h to eventually achieve a dose of 20 mg/kg orally q8h over a 10-day period is recommended. Monitoring drug levels is typically not necessary due to the high degree of safety and non-hepatic metabolism. However, caution should be used in cats with renal disease.

Treatments in development

The future of epilepsy treatment is undergoing multifaceted, exponential growth. Many new AEDs are currently in clinical trials throughout the world. A common denominator for drug development is the ability to define pharmacoresistant therapy by both drug action and patient pharmacogenomics. Brivaracetam and selacetam are analogue drugs of levetiracetam formulated with significantly greater SV2A protein binding for higher potency. Preliminary studies in humans have demonstrated efficacy against refractory complex partial and myoclonic seizures (French et al., 2007). However, brivaracetam has been found to have a low margin of safety for hepatotoxicity in a small number of normal dogs (von Rosenstiel, 2007). Carisbamate blocks voltage-gated neuronal calcium channels and, in humans, is predominantly excreted renally with minimal adverse effects. It is effective against a wide range of seizure types (Luszckzi, 2009). Retiagabine directly activates voltage-gated potassium channels (Kv7 subunit), preventing paroxysmal burst discharges. It is also useful against a variety of seizures (Luszckzi, 2009).

With the advent of more advanced diagnostic capabilities to map localization-related epilepsy, conventional surgical and radiosurgical intervention can now provide curative outcomes previously never imagined. Vagal and brain stimulators have introduced a physiological method of changing the baseline seizure threshold of the brain, by altering cholinergic synaptic release to produce an inhibitory influence on the ascending thalamocortical pathways (Muñana et al., 2002). Whilst veterinary surgeons may not incorporate all of these modalities into clinical practice as yet, the future potential to help our patients grows every day as well.

Emergency treatment

Hospital emergency treatment for seizures

A rapid, reliable protocol for the emergency management of seizures in dogs and cats is provided in Chapter 20. The physiological sequelae of frequent or continuous seizure activity (status epilepticus) leading to increased intracranial pressure and neuronal necrosis include systemic arterial hypertension, loss of cerebrovascular regulation, disruption of the blood–brain barrier and cerebral oedema.

At-home emergency treatment for seizures

The financial and emotional constraints of providing recurrent emergency therapy can be overwhelming for the owner and result in euthanasia of the animal. It is important to discuss methods by which the owner can provide emergency treatment for their pet at home if the animal is prone to cluster seizures. Diazepam per rectum (DZPR) therapy by owners of dogs with primary epilepsy and generalized cluster seizures has been associated with a significant decrease in the number of cluster seizure events in a 24-hour period, and a decrease in the total number of seizure events when compared with an identical time period without such therapy (Podell, 1995). As a consequence of this there was a significant decrease in the total cost for emergency care per dog, when compared with a similar period prior to the onset of use of DZPR therapy.

Pharmacokinetic studies of DZPR therapy in normal dogs have demonstrated that chronic phenobarbital therapy in the dog reduces the total benzodiazepine concentration after intravenous and per rectum administration, presumably due to the increased hepatic clearance of diazepam and/or its metabolites, oxazepam and nordiazepam (Wagner et al., 1998). Administration of diazepam at a dosage of 2 mg/kg per rectum for dogs on chronic phenobarbital therapy achieved effective plasma benzodiazepine concentrations >300 µg/l with minimal adverse effects. A dose of 1 mg/kg is recommended without concurrent phenobarbital therapy. This dose can be given up to three times in a 24-hour period but should not be given within 10 minutes of a prior dose. No information is reported for rectal AED therapy in the cat.

References and further reading

Available on accompanying DVD

DVD extras

- Complex partial seizure (automatism)
- Focal motor seizure
- Generalized tonic–clonic seizure
- Myoclonic and atonic seizures
- Status multiple seizure types

9

Coma, stupor and mentation change

Rodney S. Bagley and Simon Platt

'Consciousness' and 'awareness' are terms with numerous connotations. In a medical setting, these terms are used to describe the mental state generated through the normal functions of the intracranial nervous system. Consciousness and awareness refer to a state of being able to recognize and respond to a variety of internal and external nervous system stimuli.

Terminology

In veterinary medicine the terminology used to describe abnormal mentation and consciousness is not standardized and can be confusing.

The following terms are commonly used to describe stages or levels of consciousness, mentation and the behaviours associated with neurological function:

- Alert – a patient that pays attention to its surroundings and is quick to respond in a predictable fashion to external stimuli
- Consciousness – the state of being conscious (fully alert, aware, oriented and responsive to the environment)
- Awareness – the ability to 'take account' of an object, but does not imply assessment of the nature of the object
- Behaviour – the observable response of an animal to a given situation or stimulus
- Cognition – the mental process of 'knowing', which includes perception, recognition, judgement and sensation
- Delirium – mental disturbance denoted by illusions, hallucinations, cerebral excitement, physical restlessness and incoherence
- Dementia – impaired intellectual function involving memory and judgement (confusion) as well as changes in personality. This term should not be used in veterinary medicine as memory and judgement are difficult qualities to assess in veterinary patients. A more useful and accurate term is 'inappropriate'

Aetiology

Abnormalities in consciousness and cognition can result from a variety of intracranial disease processes. In addition, normal intracranial nervous system function responsible for consciousness is influenced by multiple extracranial body systems and organs. Disease or dysfunction of these non-neurological body systems can indirectly alter the willingness or ability of the animal to respond appropriately to a variety of endogenous and environmental stimuli.

Thus, disorders of consciousness and/or behaviour may result from many primary intracranial diseases or may reflect a variety of disease states. In an animal with altered consciousness, it is important to determine whether the inciting abnormality resides primarily within the intracranial nervous system or is the result of non-nervous system disease. As disorders that tend to cause severe alterations in consciousness are often life-threatening, coma and stupor are considered emergency situations.

Clinical signs

Altered consciousness

Clinical signs of altered consciousness range from subtle (e.g. an animal that is just less active than normal) to severe (e.g. comatose and unable to respond to any external stimuli) (Thomas, 2010). The 'normal' state of consciousness is dynamic and dependent on a complex interaction between stimuli and response, which varies from individual to individual and, in some cases, from moment to moment. Therefore, clinical assessments of consciousness are often crudely categorized into general groups of responses (Figure 9.1).

Normal

An animal is assessed as alert if they respond in a predictable fashion to a given stimulus. Normal

Mental status	Interpretation
Quantity	
Alert	Normal
Depressed	Reduced level of consciousness but appropriate responses to stimuli
Stuporous	Remains unresponsive to environmental stimulation but responsive to painful stimulation
Comatose	Non-responsive to both environmental and painful stimulation
Quality	
Appropriate	Responses to environmental stimuli are considered normal for the individual
Inappropriate	Responses are not normal to some environmental stimuli. The responses can be reduced to absent, bizarre or exaggerated

9.1 Mental status categories of animals.

animals that are alert are acutely aware of changes in their environment. They orient themselves to alterations in activity, sound and light. Unless the clinician is very familiar with the normal personality and response of the animal to a range of environmental stimuli, subtle abnormalities of consciousness are more difficult to determine. It is often only through owner questioning to establish the 'normal' personality of the animal that subtle alterations of consciousness are elucidated.

Abnormal

Animals with depressed consciousness tend to stay in one location (see **Severe depression (1)** and **(2)** clips on DVD), may sleep more than normal, and are less responsive to external stimuli such as light, touch and sound. These animals may not eat or drink appropriately (Nelson *et al.*, 1981; Bagley, 1994). Stuporous animals remain in sternal or lateral recumbency and are relatively unresponsive to environmental stimuli. However, these animals still react to painful stimuli. Comatose animals are similarly unresponsive to environmental stimuli, but in addition do not react to painful stimuli. Abnormalities of cranial nerve (CN) reflexes and pupil reactivity, posture and proprioception may also be present with intracranial derangements (see Lesion localization). Decerebrate rigidity (associated with opisthotonus, extensor rigidity of all limbs and either stupor or coma) is present with severe midbrain or bilateral cerebral hemisphere lesions.

In addition to an altered level of consciousness, patients may have concurrent respiratory, cardiovascular and pupillary changes, which can be helpful in assessing the location and severity of the lesion.

Altered respiration: There are a number of abnormal respiratory patterns which may be associated with alterations in consciousness; although, these have not been consistently recognized in animals.

- Cheyne–Stokes respiration is characterized by a waxing and waning depth of respiration with regularly occurring periods of hyperpnoea and apnoea (Ropper and Samuels, 2009; Hall, 2010).
- Biot's breathing manifests as irregular periods of apnoea alternating with periods of 4–5 breaths of identical depth. This is seen with increased intracranial pressure (ICP).
- Central neurogenic hyperventilation is due to mesencephalic lesions. Tachypnoea to the point of panting can be seen.
- Apneustic breathing occurs with pontine lesions and is characterized by periods of breathing and apnoea that are very short, with cycles of respiration consisting of only 1–2 breaths interposed with periods of apnoea.
- Ataxic breathing with an irregular rate and rhythm can be caused by caudal brainstem (medulla oblongata) lesions involving the respiratory centres.

Altered cardiovascular function: Alterations in heart rate and rhythm (such as bradycardia and

tachyarrhythmias) may be evident in animals with increased ICP and brain–heart syndrome, respectively (Shapiro, 1975; King *et al.*, 1982; Kornegay, 1993; van Loon *et al.*, 1993; Bagley, 1996abc). Animals with a significant increase in ICP may also have systemic hypertension in an attempt to increase cerebral blood flow. For further information of the regulation of ICP, the reader is referred to Chapter 21.

Altered pupil function: Pupillary changes may be present in animals with alterations in consciousness (Neer and Carter, 1987; Collins and O'Brien, 1990; Scagliotti, 1990). With bilateral, usually severe, cerebrocortical disease, the pupils are often smaller than normal (miotic). At least two theories exist to explain this clinical finding:

1. There is a bilateral central sympathetic system abnormality, possibly at the hypothalamus or brainstem level.
2. It is the result of the supratentorial structures, which normally exert a negative influence on pupillary constriction. With supratentorial disease, upper motor neuron (UMN) influence over CN III function is lost and, therefore, the pupillary constrictor muscle becomes hyperresponsive (excessive parasympathetic tone).

If unilateral transtentorial brain herniation occurs, the ipsilateral pupil dilates and becomes non-responsive to light because of the pressure exerted on CN III from the herniated parahippocampal gyrus (Kornegay *et al.*, 1983) or because CN III is stretched by the lateral (falcine) herniation of the cerebral hemisphere. As the midbrain is further compressed or damaged, fixed mid-range or dilated (in some instances) pupils result (deLahunta and Glass, 2008).

Transient alterations in consciousness

Episodic or short-term loss of consciousness with periods of normal consciousness in between may be found with narcolepsy, syncope and seizures.

- Narcolepsy (excessive daytime sleepiness) is an episodic disorder that results in rapid progression to deep sleep, usually following a triggering (exciting) stimulus such as eating (see Chapter 13).
- Syncope is a short, episodic loss of consciousness that results from transient cerebral hypoxia or anoxia. Syncope may mimic a seizure (see Chapter 8) or a narcoleptic/cataplectic event. If the hypoxia is prolonged, actual seizures may result and confound the clinical interpretation. Syncope is most often the result of a cardiopulmonary disorder (usually a bradyarrhythmia) and, therefore, attention should be paid to the cardiopulmonary system during the routine physical examination (Ropper and Samuels, 2009).

Behaviour

Normal behaviour is a generalization determined for a population of animals, but is also individual (Thomas, 2010). Alterations in behaviour may include aggression, vocalization, excessive or abnormal sexual activity, changes in eating, chewing, drinking, urinating and defecating, as well as changes in personality. Frenzied activity and repeated unusual behaviour, such as tail chasing or 'fly-biting' (see 'Fly-biting' clip on DVD), may also occur. Changes in behaviour related to stimulating events, such as following eating in animals with hepatic encephalopathy, may be important clues to the underlying metabolic disease process.

Changes in behaviour may be due to structural or functional cerebral disease. A subgroup of functional disorders, well described in human medicine, used to be termed psychoneuroses and later just neuroses. However, more recently, even in veterinary medicine, the terms neuroses and neuropsychiatric disorders have been replaced by terms such as anxiety disorders, phobic states and obsessive–compulsive disorders. The genesis of these disorders is often unknown, but it is generally accepted that they do not arise *de novo* in otherwise normal animals.

Animals can show behavioural abnormalities as a result of 'stress' (stereotypical behaviours). This type of abnormality can be difficult to differentiate from those alterations in behaviour associated with abnormalities of cognition; however, they usually have a repeated pattern of activity that can be terminated through interaction with the owner or clinician.

In general, clues to an underlying behavioural problem may be suggested by whether the abnormality occurs when the owner (audience) is not present, the movements of the animal can be interrupted, and whether the abnormality occurs at a consistent time or in response to a consistent stimulus or context (i.e. the owners leaving or coming home). Animals with episodic abnormalities which only occur in the presence of the owner/audience, who can be interrupted from the activity, or where the abnormality only arises in response to a specific stimulus are likely to have a behavioural problem.

Lesion localization

For an animal to be alert and oriented to its environment (i.e. normal level of consciousness and behaviour), neurons in the cerebral hemispheres, thalamus and brainstem need to function appropriately (King, 1987; Oliver *et al.*, 1997; deLahunta and Glass, 2008; Thomas, 2010) (Figure 9.2). Thus, disease affecting the structure or function of the brain can result in alterations in consciousness and behaviour.

Consciousness

Brainstem disease involving the ascending reticular activating system (ARAS) can significantly alter consciousness (deLahunta and Glass, 2008). The ARAS within the brainstem provides stimulatory input to the cerebral cortex via the thalamus to maintain consciousness or wakefulness (Figure 9.3). The

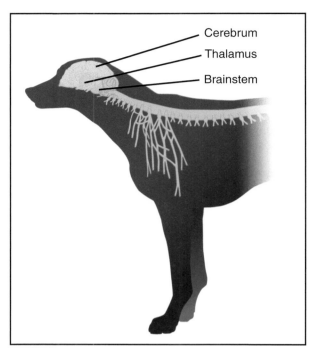

Cerebrum
Thalamus
Brainstem

9.2 Lesion localization for coma and stupor: the cerebrum, thalamus (diencephalon) and brainstem are indicated.

ARAS lies in the central portion of the brainstem from the medulla to the diencephalon. Many of these areas are ill defined and lie within the reticular formation. Afferent neurons to this area come from all pathways that project ascending sensory information. The ARAS projects to either the thalamic reticular or hyposubthalamic reticular system. The diencephalic portion stimulates the entire cerebral cortex diffusely. The ARAS awakens the cortex to prepare it to receive sensory information. This system may allow the discrimination of stimuli, sorting out which stimuli to recognize and/or reject.

Behaviour

Perception and cognition

Perception and cognition occur primarily through the activity of cortical neurons, with input from additional neurons in regions such as the thalamus and brainstem. With specific intracranial lesions, animals may only perceive portions of their environment (i.e. hemi-inattention/hemi-neglect) (Holliday, 1991; O'Brien, 1993) and may show abnormal behaviours as a result. For example, animals with unilateral supratentorial or forebrain disease turn their head toward the side of lesion and tend to turn or circle in that direction when walking (aversion syndrome). This is believed to result from a loss of cortical integration of sensory information from the contralateral side of the body. Other clinical signs include seizures, behavioural abnormalities, lack of conscious recognition of touch and pain on one side of the face (usually contralateral to the unilateral lesion; Figure 9.4), contralateral menace deficits and deficits of conscious proprioception (usually contralateral to the unilateral lesion). In addition, the animal may pace compulsively but its gait is usually normal.

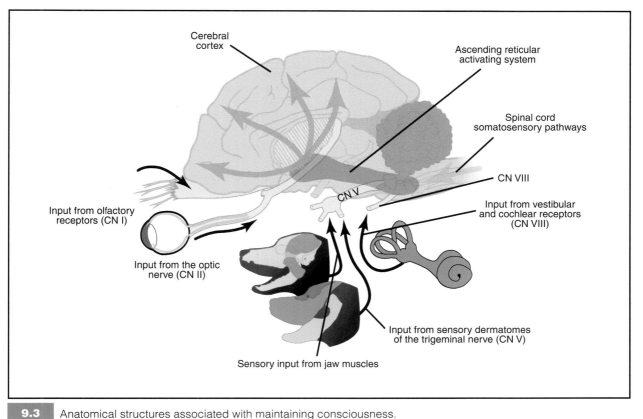

9.3 Anatomical structures associated with maintaining consciousness.

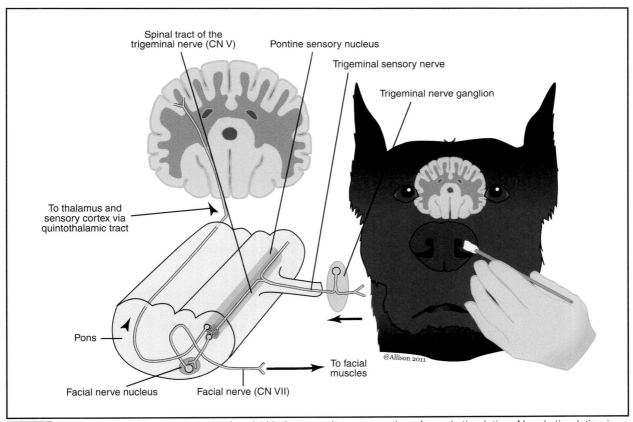

9.4 Neuroanatomical pathways associated with the conscious perception of nasal stimulation. Nasal stimulation is used to both test the sensory innervation to the nares and observe the behavioural response to the stimulation. If the observer knows that the animal has sensation to its head and face based on brainstem reflexes, then lack of a behavioural response can indicate a failure to integrate sensory information at the cortical level due to a lesion in the contralateral hemisphere.

Emotional and visceral behaviour

The limbic system is associated with emotional and behavioural patterns in animals. It functions in the non-olfactory part of the rhinencephalon (the part of the brain once thought to be concerned entirely with olfactory functions). The name limbic (edge or border) is used because the nuclei that primarily comprise the non-olfactory rhinencephalon lie in two incomplete rings on the medial aspect of the telencephalon at its border with the diencephalon. The term now includes other anatomically distant nuclei such as those in the brainstem. The major structures of the limbic system include the amygdaloid, hippocampus and cingulate gyrus in the telencephalon, the thalamus and hypothalamus in the diencephalon, and the reticular formation of the mesencephalon.

The function of the limbic system is to influence visceral motor activity, primarily through its influence on the hypothalamus. Neurons in this system receive projections from the olfactory, optic, auditory, exteroceptive and interoceptive sensory systems. It is the portion of the brain in humans that is involved in basic drives, sexual activity, emotional experiences, memories, fears and pleasures. Normal behaviour also requires the complex interaction of numerous components of the thalamus and cerebral cortex.

Intracranial pathophysiology

Intracranial dysfunction may result from a single primary lesion, from secondary intracranial pathophysiological sequelae to a focal lesion (e.g. increased ICP) or from global central nervous system (CNS) dysfunction as a consequence of extracranial systemic disease (Bagley, 1996ab). Secondary pathophysiological alterations include, but are not limited to:

- Physical invasion and/or destruction of neurons
- Metabolic alterations in neuronal or glial cells
- Impairment of vascular supply to normal tissue (ischaemia or hypoxia)
- Impairment of autoregulation
- Haemorrhage
- Irritation (seizure generation)
- Obstruction of the ventricular system
- Oedema formation
- Production of physiologically active substances.

Many of these processes increase the relative volume within the intracranial cavity, ultimately affecting ICP. An increase in ICP can result in a decrease in cerebral blood flow, perpetuating cerebral ischaemia and hypoxia. As a terminal consequence, increases in ICP lead to brain herniation causing brain dysfunction and death.

There are several types of brain herniation (Kornegay *et al.*, 1983) (Figure 9.5).

1. Transtentorial herniation occurs when the parahippocampal gyrus herniates caudally underneath the tentorium cerebelli. This causes compression of the midbrain and CN III, resulting in loss of consciousness and dilated pupils unresponsive to light.
2. The most devastating type of herniation occurs when the caudal cerebellum herniates caudally into the foramen magnum. The associated compression of the brainstem affects the respiratory centres in the medulla oblongata and the animal usually ceases voluntary respiration.
3. Falcine herniaton occurs when one cerebral hemisphere herniates laterally ventral to the falx cerebri as a result of a unilateral hemispheric lesion.
4. Herniation from a craniotomy site can also occur perioperatively.

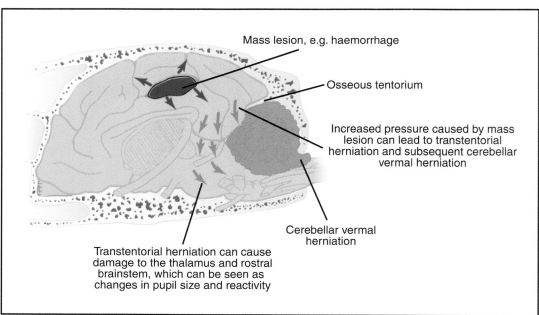

9.5
Various types of brain herniation.

Mass lesion, e.g. haemorrhage

Osseous tentorium

Increased pressure caused by mass lesion can lead to transtentorial herniation and subsequent cerebellar vermal herniation

Cerebellar vermal herniation

Transtentorial herniation can cause damage to the thalamus and rostral brainstem, which can be seen as changes in pupil size and reactivity

Differential diagnosis

Once dysfunction of consciousness and/or behaviour has been established, it is important to determine whether the primary problem lies within the intracranial nervous system or is the result of dysfunction within a non-neural body system (Figure 9.6). Further discussion is limited to important diseases within the nervous system that result in abnormalities of consciousness and/or behaviour. It is accepted that any disease process which results in life-threatening changes in systemic metabolic or cardiovascular function ultimately affects consciousness in the terminal stages of the disease.

Mechanism of disease	Specific diseases
Degenerative	Inherited neurodegenerative diseases (e.g. lysosomal storage diseases) [9, 15, Appendix 1]
Anomalous	Hydrocephalus [9] Intracranial intra-arachnoid cyst [11]
Metabolic/endocrine	Hepatic encephalopathy [8] Hypoglycaemia [9, 20] Electrolyte disturbances [9, 19] CNS perfusion abnormalities (hypoxia, polycythemia vera, carbon monoxide toxicity) [9] Hypothyroid myxoedema coma [9]
Neoplastic	Primary – meningiomas, gliomas, choroid plexus tumours, ependymomas, pituitary gland tumours, lymphomas [9] Metastatic – haemangiosarcomas, lymphomas, carcinomas [9] Local extension – multilobular osteochondromas (MLOs), ceruminous gland adenocarcinomas
Nutritional	Thiamine deficiency [11]
Idiopathic	Narcolepsy/cataplexy [17]
Infectious/ inflammatory	Infectious – viral, rickettsial, bacterial, protozoal, fungal, parasitic [11, 15] Inflammatory – granulomatous meningoencephalitis, necrotizing encephalitides (e.g. Pug dog encephalitis) [11]
Toxic	Lead [9] Avermectins [9] Metronidazole [11] Organophosphates/carbamates
Trauma	Head trauma [20] Intracranial haemorrhage [20] Subdural haematoma [20]
Vascular	Arteriovenous malformation Infarction [9] Feline ischaemic encephalopathy [9] Haemorrhage [9] Hypertensive encephalopathy [9]

9.6 Causes of coma, stupor and behavioural change. The numbers in square brackets denote chapters where these conditions are discussed in detail.

Neurodiagnostic investigation

Depending on the localization of the disease, appropriate diagnostic tests should be performed to rule in or out each disease on the differential diagnosis list (Figure 9.7). Sometimes the underlying disorder is evident such as with cranial trauma; however, all too often animals with stupor or coma can present a diagnostic challenge. If the animal presents in a coma, emergency evaluation of airway patency and vital signs including cardiac function and respiration should be undertaken, as for animals with head trauma. Although limited in many ways, the neurological examination of the stuporous or comatose patient is of crucial importance. The important aspects of the evaluation include:

- Response to noxious stimulation
- The presence of voluntary motor movement
- Posture (i.e. decerebrate rigidity)
- Pupil reactivity to light
- Eye movements (physiological nystagmus)
- Segmental spinal reflexes.

This evaluation is very similar to that of the patient with severe head trauma and in some respects the Modified Glasgow Coma Score System may be useful; although, it has not been universally utilized or validated. Unless the diagnosis is established from the history (e.g. toxin ingestion), further testing is usually necessary.

- Routine laboratory analysis is essential – the minimal acceptable information should include packed cell volume (PCV), total protein concentration, blood urea nitrogen (BUN), electrolytes and glucose concentrations.
- Urinalysis and urine production rate should be assessed, which may necessitate urethral catheterization.
- Liver function tests.
- Thoracic and abdominal radiographs may be useful to supplement physical examination findings.
- Cerebrospinal fluid (CSF) analysis is indicated primarily to confirm an inflammatory lesion. Although such analysis is rarely specific, when it is assessed in conjunction with the patient's signalment, history, neurological signs and the results of other diagnostic tests (such as serological assays) it can help to better define the underlying aetiology. If there is evidence or even a suspicion of increased ICP (anisocoria, lack of pupil response to light, reduced or absent physiological nystagmus, decreased or absent response to noxious stimulation), diagnostic imaging should be performed prior to cisterna magna or lumbar puncture, which risks promoting further herniation. In these cases, reducing the ICP using mannitol (0.25–1 g/kg i.v.) should be considered.
- Advanced imaging studies such as computed tomography (CT) and magnetic resonance imaging (MRI) are strongly indicated to assess the integrity of the intracranial structures.

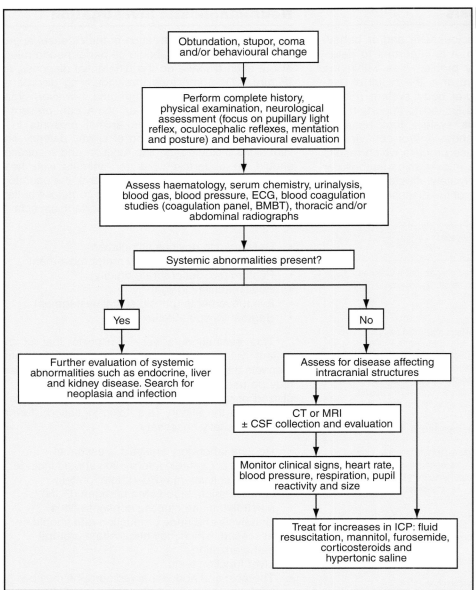

9.7 Clinical approach to patients with altered consciousness and/or behaviour. BMBT = buccal mucosal bleeding time; CSF = cerebrospinal fluid; CT = computed tomography; ECG = electrocardiogram; ICP = intracranial pressure; MRI = magnetic resonance imaging.

- An electroencephalogram (EEG) records the electrical activity associated with forebrain structures. An EEG is rarely specific and with certain cerebral conditions it also lacks sensitivity. Although rarely used as a diagnostic tool, electroencephalography can provide confirmation of brain death (flat or isoelectric EEG). However, other factors such as patient body temperature, concurrent drug administration and cardiac function must be considered before brain death is diagnosed. Further information on electroencephalography can be found in Chapter 4.

Comatose animals

Monitoring

Monitoring the animal that is comatose requires recognition, understanding and treatment of the secondary pathophysiological sequelae of intracranial disease. Life-threatening systemic complications should be recognized and treated. Neurological assessments should be frequently recorded to ensure recognition of trends in intracranial function. A coma scale is used as a guide to determine treatment and prognosis in humans with brain injury. A similar scale has been adapted for use in dogs; however, its role in determining treatment and prognosis is less clear (see Chapter 20). A common sense approach based upon diligent and repeated assessment of major neurological functions, such as the level of consciousness and voluntary movement, is usually most important.

Animals are usually monitored in a critical care or intensive care area for signs of neurological deterioration. Parameters commonly monitored include heart rate and rhythm, respiratory rate and pattern, blood pressure, urine production and pain. Neurological parameters monitored include pupil size and responsiveness to light, level of consciousness, behaviour and the ability to move and walk.

Intravenous fluid therapy is given to maintain normal hydration and cerebral perfusion. Both dehydration and over-hydration should be avoided. Monitoring of systemic blood pressure and central venous pressure may aid in re-establishment of normovolaemia. Insertion of a central venous catheter should be performed cautiously in animals with increased ICP, as manipulation or occlusion of the jugular vein for catheter placement may elevate ICP. Quick, efficient, and atraumatic jugular catheterization is imperative in this situation.

Routine evaluations such as complete blood count (CBC), serum chemistry panel, urinalysis, blood pressure, electrocardiography and bile acid testing are performed initially to determine overall systemic health. Thoracic and abdominal radiography is often helpful to quickly assess these body cavities. If no obvious abnormality is detected on routine screening tests, an advanced imaging study (CT or MRI) is indicated to determine whether there are any structural intracranial causes for the coma. If these studies are unavailable or not feasible, or if the clinical signs are mild, the animal should be periodically monitored (hourly, if necessary) for deteriorating neurological function. If the clinical signs are severe from the outset or worsen progressively, treatment for elevated ICP (e.g. fluid therapy to maintain normal blood pressure, mannitol and oxygen) should be initiated (see Chapter 20 for further information).

Management
Smaller animals are often better candidates for prolonged nursing care compared with larger animals due to the ease of manipulation. Good nursing care includes the prevention of decubital ulcers in the recumbent animal and monitoring for secondary infections, particularly of the pulmonary and urogenital systems. Recumbent animals should be placed on clean, soft bedding and turned frequently (ideally every hour). Physical therapy should begin as soon as possible if there are no unstable vertebral injuries. Physical therapy is tailored to the individual needs of the animal and may include supported or non-supported walking, passive flexion and extension of the limbs, massage and swimming. A daily record of physical therapy should be kept to ensure that it is not overlooked and to allow multiple individuals (including the owner) to become involved in the healing process.

Prognosis
The prognosis for a comatose animal ultimately depends upon the underlying cause of the coma. If the coma is the result of a process which is no longer progressing (i.e. head trauma), and if the secondary effects of intracranial disease can be recognized and controlled, the animal has a reasonable chance of recovery. In general, lesions of forebrain structures or the cerebellum have a better overall prognosis for recovery than lesions involving the brainstem (deLahunta and Glass, 2008). After the acute effects of brain disease are controlled (usually within 7 days), the goal is to allow time for brain healing and recovery of function to occur; this is a continual process which takes place over the following 1–3 months.

In general, clinical signs of unilateral forebrain injury improve within the first 2 weeks following trauma. Usually the animal is ambulatory within 4 weeks post-injury; although, residual gait deficits and blindness may continue. A tendency to circle may also persist, being especially prominent when the animal is distressed or excited. Recovery from brainstem injury may be less complete and residual signs commonly remain, including vestibular dysfunction, facial paresis, laryngeal paresis and megaoesophagus. Recovery from cerebellar injury often occurs in a similar timeframe as for supratentorial injury. If the secondary effects of brain injury are controlled, many animals can recover from the primary brain insult associated with trauma.

Degenerative diseases

Inherited neurodegenerative diseases

Clinical signs
The majority of degenerative diseases involving the nervous system result in clinical signs early in life, usually with an onset at <1 year of age. Many are breed-related and presumed inherited (see Appendix 1 for a complete list). Clinical signs are slowly progressive with severe alterations in consciousness occurring relatively late in the disease course. Most diseases cause multifocal neurological signs and many affect the cerebellum (see **Neuronal ceroid lipofuscinosis** clip on DVD).

Pathogenesis
Neurodegenerative diseases can affect any part of the nervous system and commonly result in dysfunction of the brain (Braund, 2003). Examples include multisystem neuronal degeneration of Cocker Spaniels, spongiform degenerations in Labrador Retrievers, Samoyeds, Silky Terriers, Dalmatians (cavitating leucodystrophy), mixed-breed dogs and Egyptian Mau kittens, and multisystemic chromatolytic neuronal degeneration in Cairn Terriers. The pathogenic mechanisms of many of these diseases have not been fully elucidated.

Storage diseases are due to an inborn error of metabolism and the absence of a vital enzyme necessary to breakdown endogenous body substances (Braund, 1987, 1994, 2003; March, 1996; Skelly and Franklin, 2002) (see Chapter 19 and Appendix 1). These substances then accumulate within the neuron or other cells associated with the nervous system and eventually cause cellular dysfunction (Figure 9.8). The numerous storage diseases of small animals have been reviewed in detail previously (March, 1996; Skelly and Franklin, 2002).

Diagnosis
Antemortem diagnosis requires biopsy of the affected tissue. Determination of the lysosomal enzyme activity within the brain and other cells may

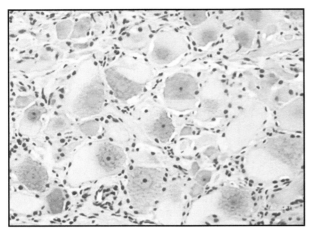

9.8 Swollen neurons in the cerebellum of a dog with the lysosomal storage disease GM2 gangliosidosis. (H&E stain; original magnification X40)

be helpful, but is not universally clinically available (see Appendix 1).

Blood and urine screening: Screening blood and urine for accumulation of products indicative of inborn errors of metabolism may suggest the presence of a lysosomal storage disease, and in some cases can be diagnostic. Depending on the disease, abnormal accumulations may be evident within cells (particularly macrophages), on Buffy coat blood smears and in biopsy samples from the liver, spleen, lymph nodes, bone marrow or nerves. Screening tests performed on fresh urine samples should include evaluation for the following analytes:

- Urinary organic acids – the accumulation of organic acids within the body fluids (particularly urine) is indicative of inborn errors of metabolism such as L-2-hydroxyglutaric aciduria in Staffordshire Bull Terriers (Abramson *et al.*, 2003)
- Urinary oligosaccharides – the accumulation of mannose-containing oligosaccharides in cats is indicative of mannosidosis. The accumulation of high molecular weight oligosaccharides in dogs and cats is indicative of GM1 and GM2 gangliosidosis, and of fucosidosis in English Springer Spaniels
- Urinary glycosaminoglycans – the accumulation of dermatan sulphate is indicative of mucopolysaccharidosis (MPS) I, II, VI and VII. The accumulation of heparin sulphate is indicative of MPS IIIA and IIIB.

Enzyme analysis: Where the signalment and neurological signs are suggestive of one or more lysosomal storage disease, and where the underlying enzyme defect is known for those diseases, then an enzyme analysis can be performed against known normal control animals. A reduction in the level of enzyme activity is indicative of that particular lysosomal storage disease. Washed white blood cells or cultured skin fibroblasts are usually the most appropriate cell source and can be assayed either fresh or fresh-frozen.

Magnetic resonance imaging: Characteristic MRI changes may be apparent with some canine and feline genetic diseases, although the changes are rarely specific for a single disease. The lesions usually appear bilaterally symmetrical (as seen with L-2-hydroxyglutaric aciduria in Staffordshire Bull Terriers; Figure 9.9) and often result in a decrease in the apparent size of the cerebellum. Fucosidosis in English Springer Spaniels and some of the gangliosidoses can also result in notable MRI abnormalities.

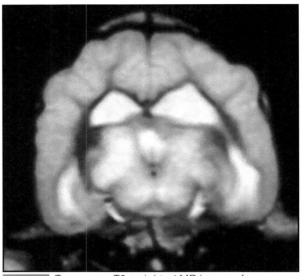

9.9 Transverse T2-weighted MR image of a Staffordshire Bull Terrier with L-2-hydroxyglutaric aciduria. Note the diffuse symmetrical hyperintense areas within the grey matter structures. The white matter seems relatively reduced in size and has a more hypointense signal.

Treatment and prognosis

Currently there is no effective treatment for degenerative diseases of the CNS. Symptomatic therapy, such as anticonvulsants and anti-anxiety drugs, can help alleviate clinical signs but these diseases are inevitably progressive. Often helping the owner decide when to elect euthanasia for a dog affected by a slowly progressive brain disease is the most challenging aspect of these diseases.

Gene therapy: In the future, gene therapy may play a role in the treatment of these diseases. Gene therapy would not necessarily need to transfect every neuron to result in improvement because some of the enzymes involved are soluble and can be taken up from the interstitial fluids. Thus, enzyme replacement in the CSF could potentially deliver the enzyme to the neurons. Trials are under way at several institutions to develop such therapies for dogs.

Cognitive disorder

Clinical signs

This syndrome affects older dogs and cats (Nielson *et al.*, 2001; Gunn-Moore *et al.*, 2007; Osella *et al.*, 2007; Landsberg *et al.*, 2010; Salvin *et al.*, 2010;

Gunn-Moore, 2011). Affected animals show chronic progressive behavioural abnormalities such as loss of learned behaviour, failure to recognize their owners and disturbed sleep cycles (Ruehl *et al.*, 1997; Landsberg *et al.*, 2011) (Figure 9.10).

Clinical sign	Behavioural abnormality
Disorientation	Reduced spatial orientation
Interaction	Altered social interactions with people and/or other pets, including aggression and irritability
Sleep–wake cycle	Increased night time waking
House soiling	Loss of toilet training; may be related to confusion or disorientation
Activity	Increased repetitive activity, restlessness or decreased activity levels
Miscellaneous	Excessive vocalization; decreased self-hygiene; alterations in appetite

Note:
Based on an owner survey, 75 dogs from a random geriatric population of 124 dogs exhibited at least one of the above categories of clinical signs; thus, it has been suggested that cognitive disorder is an under-diagnosed phenomenon in older pets (Osella *et al.*, 2007). However, many such prevalence studies are not supported by pathological confirmation of a senile-related degeneration of the brain

9.10 Clinical signs compatible with cognitive dysfunction in dogs and cats. These signs are not specific for a diagnosis, which must be made by the exclusion of other brain diseases.

Pathogenesis
The normal ageing brain progressively accumulates oxidative damage and other types of neuropathology that ultimately result in neuronal dysfunction and cognitive decline. This syndrome has been likened to the early stages of Alzheimer's disease in humans. In fact, diffuse beta-amyloid plaques may develop in the temporoparietal and entorhinal cortex in dogs (Cotman *et al.*, 2002), but the neurofibrillary tangles seen in humans have not been reported in dogs. In dogs, the frontal lobe volume decreases, ventricular size increases and there is evidence of meningeal calcification, demyelination, increased lipofuscin and apoptotic bodies, neuroaxonal degeneration and a reduction in the number of neurons (Borras *et al.*, 1999). The aetiology and clinical consequences of these pathological changes is unclear in dogs. There is also evidence of age-associated brain pathology in cats. Imaging studies have identified an increased ventricular size and widened sulci (Landsberg *et al.*, 2010). A loss of neurons and a decrease in the number of dendrites in the Purkinje cells have also been shown to occur in the feline cerebellum associated with age. The pathological significance of these findings is again up for debate.

Diagnosis
Cognitive disorder is diagnosed by excluding other causes of the behavioural abnormalities. However, due to the non-specific clinical signs associated with this clinical syndrome, it is difficult to make a definitive diagnosis. An extensive evaluation for other causes of intracranial signs in older dogs, such as brain tumours, metabolic disorders, vascular-based diseases and hypertension-associated intracranial disease, should be undertaken. Measurement of the interthalamic adhesion thickness using MRI has been suggested as a criterion for the confirmation of brain atrophy in dogs as it is significantly smaller in older dogs with cognitive dysfunction (Hasegawa *et al.*, 2005).

Treatment and prognosis
Diets rich in antioxidants have been useful in slowing age-related behavioural changes in experimental colonies of dogs (Cotman *et al.*, 2002; Landsberg, 2005). The use of L-deprenyl has also been advocated (Ruehl *et al.*, 1997). Antidepressant and anti-anxiety medications may be beneficial in the symptomatic management of some animals (Landsberg *et al.*, 2011). Coupled with the difficulty in definitive antemortem diagnosis, and the fact that the natural course of this syndrome has yet to be described in the pet dog population, it is often difficult to objectively determine whether any treatment for this disorder is beneficial.

Anomalous diseases

Anomalous conditions such as exencephaly (mass of skin-covered meninges and cerebral hemispheres that project through an opening in the cranial cavity), hydranencephaly (each cerebral hemisphere is reduced to a fluid-filled sac with the wall of the sac containing the leptomeninges, glial membrane and ependyma), anencephaly (lack of cerebral hemispheres) and other severe malformations of the intracranial structures often result in early fetal or neonatal death (deLahunta and Glass, 2008). If animals survive birth, they may have significant alterations in consciousness and behavioural development.

Hydrocephalus
Hydrocephalus is the term used to describe a condition of abnormal dilatation of the ventricular system within the cranium (Rekate, 2009). It can be further subdivided into obstructive and non-obstructive types. Ventricular dilatation occurs with some frequency in dogs and cats due to a variety of intracranial disease processes (Harrington *et al.*, 1996; Thomas, 2010). Some breeds are predisposed to congenital hydrocephalus, including Chihuahuas, Pomeranians, Yorkshire Terriers, English Bulldogs, Lhasa Apsos, Toy Poodles, Cairn Terriers, Boston Terriers, Pugs, Pekingese and Maltese dogs (Thomas, 2010).

Clinical signs
Hydrocephalus can result in clinical signs due to loss of neurons or neuronal function and/or alterations in ICP and all of its consequences. Clinical signs of hydrocephalus can reflect the anatomical

level of disease involvement or can represent a diffuse disease process. The severity of the clinical signs is not necessarily dependent upon the degree of ventricular dilatation, but rather on a host of concurrent abnormalities including the underlying disease process, associated ICP changes, intraventricular haemorrhage and the acuity of ventricular obstruction. In animals with severe hydrocephalus, the compressed layer of cortex is prone to tearing either spontaneously or with minor trauma, causing a sudden onset of focal signs of forebrain disease.

- In young dogs prior to ossification of the cranial sutures, hydrocephalus may contribute to abnormalities of skull development such as a thinning of the bone structure, a dome-shaped or bossed appearance to the head, or a persistent fontanelle.
- A ventral and/or lateral strabismus has been noted in humans and animals with hydrocephalus (Figure 9.11). This is sometimes referred to as the 'setting sun sign' (Ropper and Samuels, 2009). Confusion remains as to the underlying reason for this clinical finding. It has been suggested that this appearance is associated with skull deformity and distortion of the orbits. Others suggest that because this abnormality can be improved with shunting of the lateral and third ventricles, the strabismus is associated with pressure on the mesencephalic tegmentum (deLahunta and Glass, 2008).
- As a result of the involvement of the forebrain and brainstem structures in hydrocephalus, alterations in awareness and cognition are common. Many congenitally affected animals may appear less intelligent than normal and be difficult to house train. In addition to alterations in consciousness, aggression, circling, paresis and seizures may also be seen. Central visual dysfunction can occur with compression of the optic radiations and occipital cortex.
- Occasionally, when hydrocephalus is associated with fourth ventricle enlargement, there may be pronounced vestibular dysfunction.

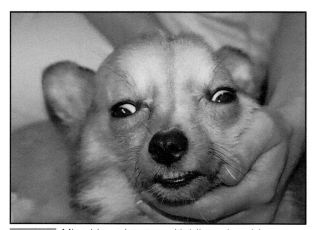

9.11 Mixed-breed puppy with bilateral strabismus ('setting sun sign') associated with hydrocephalus.

Pathogenesis

Hydrocephalus can result from:

- Obstruction (intraventricular or extraventricular) of the ventricular system (e.g. brain tumour)
- Increased size of the ventricles due to loss of brain parenchyma (hydrocephalus *ex vacuo*)
- No obvious cause (congenital)
- The overproduction of CSF associated with a choroid plexus tumour (rare)
- Obstruction of CSF flow as a result of ependymitis and vasculitis (e.g. associated with CNS infection with feline coronavirus, which causes feline infectious peritonitis).

Diffuse ventricular enlargement suggests congenital ventricular dilatation or obstruction at the level of the lateral apertures or foramen magnum. Focal ventricular enlargement suggests focal obstruction or loss of parenchymal cells. It is not uncommon to have asymmetrical bilateral lateral ventricle enlargement. Animals with an asymmetrical appearance of the ventricles should be critically evaluated for focal obstruction of, or impingement on, the ventricular system due to mass effect. Elevation of ICP associated with hydrocephalus can occur in cases of acute severe obstruction to CSF flow or chronically enlarged ventricles with little cortical mantle remaining to absorb pressure (Thomas, 2010).

Initial pathological changes are found in the ependyma at the angles of the lateral ventricles. Loss of integrity of the ependymal surface allows fluid to leak into the periventricular white matter, causing oedema. Further enlargement of the ventricles causes direct damage to the white matter due to compression. Treatment needs to be considered prior to damage affecting the cerebral cortex.

Diagnosis

The diagnosis of hydrocephalus is aided by information obtained from a variety of imaging and electrophysiological studies. Historical, invasive techniques (such as pneumoventriculography and contrast ventriculography) have been replaced by non-invasive evaluations (deLahunta and Glass, 2008; Thomas, 2010).

Ultrasonography: This can be used to diagnose hydrocephalus (Hudson *et al.*, 1990; Spaulding and Sharp, 1990) (see **Hydrocephalus** clip on DVD). This is most readily accomplished when a fontanelle is present, as it provides an acoustic window (ultrasound waves do not adequately penetrate the skull). Measurements of lateral ventricle size have been recorded in normal neonatal dogs and those with hydrocephalus. In general, correlation of the degree of ventricular enlargement and clinical signs is poor (Hudson *et al.*, 1990). However, in one study, ventricular enlargement (ventricle to brain (VB) ratio) was correlated to the severity of clinical signs using transcranial Doppler ultrasonography in small-breed dogs (Saito *et al.*, 2003). Perhaps, more importantly, asymptomatic dogs with a VB ratio >60% all went on to develop neurological signs related to the hydrocephalus, and surgical shunting (see below) could be considered in these cases. The resistance index of the basilar artery, which directly correlates with ICP, can also be measured with transcranial Doppler ultrasonography. This index also correlates with the neurological status of dogs with congenital hydrocephalus (Saito *et al.*, 2003).

Computed tomography: This non-invasive intracranial imaging modality is often useful for defining ventricular size (Figure 9.12). As CSF has a lower CT number (i.e. is less attenuating) than brain parenchyma, the ventricular system is usually readily identifiable due to its relatively dark signal in comparison with the parenchyma. CT evaluation also affords the ability to examine the majority of the ventricular system as well as additional intracranial structures. However, as stated above, ventricular size alone does not always correlate with clinical signs and the significance of ventricular enlargement is difficult to predict.

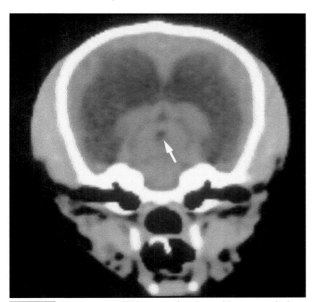

9.12 Transverse CT image of a dog with congenital hydrocephalus at the level of the midbrain. There is obvious dilatation of the lateral ventricles. The mesencephalic aqueduct is visible (arrowed) and is not dilated.

Magnetic resonance imaging: This also affords evaluation of the ventricular system (Figure 9.13). MRI provides superior neural parenchymal resolution and is especially useful for the evaluation of infratentorial structures. It is now recognized that many toy breeds that are predisposed to hydrocephalus also have infratentorial anomalies such as Chiari-like malformations, which can potentially complicate their management and are only detected on MRI.

Treatment and prognosis

Although the prognosis for resolution of hydrocephalus is uncertain, there are several medical and surgical options which may be beneficial. The choice of treatment is generally dictated by physical status, age of the animal and cause of the hydrocephalus.

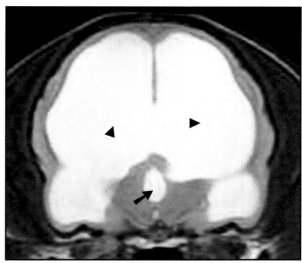

9.13 Transverse T2-weighted MR image of a dog with congenital hydrocephalus. The CSF appears white, highlighting marked dilatation of the lateral (arrowheads) and third ventricles (arrowed).

Medical treatment may include general supportive care and drugs to limit CSF production and reduce ICP. Surgical treatment is designed to provide drainage of CSF from the brain to another site for absorption (Thomas, 2010).

Medical management: Glucocorticoids are often used for medical treatment (Harrington *et al.*, 1996). Prednisone may be given at a dose of 0.25–0.5 mg/kg orally q12h. The dose is gradually reduced at weekly intervals to 0.1 mg/kg orally q48h. This dose is continued for at least 1 month, after which time it is discontinued if possible. Alternatively, dexamethasone may be given at a dose of 0.05 mg/kg orally q6–8h. The dose can be gradually reduced over 2–4 weeks. Some animals can be adequately managed with long-term glucocorticoid administration at low doses. If no clinical benefits are observed within 2 weeks, or if side effects develop, other forms of therapy should be tried.

Acetazolamide (a carbonic anhydrase inhibitor) is thought to reduce CSF pressure by decreasing CSF production. Its effectiveness in treating hydrocephalus is inconsistent. Omeprazole has also been administered for the treatment of clinical signs related to hydrocephalus; however, positive outcomes are also inconsistent (Javaheri *et al.*, 1997). Mannitol, hypertonic saline and furosemide may be administered to provide a temporary decrease in ICP and thus are reserved for emergency cases.

Surgical management: Surgery is generally required by those animals that do not improve within 2 weeks, if deterioration occurs during corticosteroid therapy or if there is an obstructive cause such as a tumour that cannot be resected. As a successful outcome may be more likely in animals that have minimal clinical signs, surgery may be appropriate in animals with a VB ratio >60%; although, few owners are willing to undergo the expense and risk of shunt placement if their dog appears healthy.

The surgical procedures are designed to provide controlled CSF flow from the ventricles of the brain to either the peritoneal cavity or right atrium of the heart. Shunt systems which have been designed for use in humans seem to work well in animals. The shunts have not been proven to be more effective than medical management, but only surgical treatment offers the possibility of long-term control of the clinical signs. Ventriculoperitoneal (VP) shunts (Figure 9.14) are most commonly used in small animals. Complications of shunt placement occur in

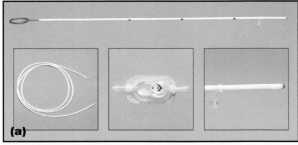
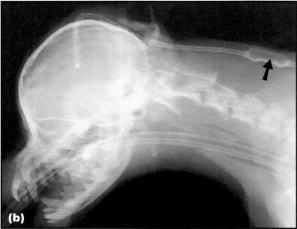
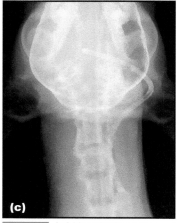

9.14 **(a)** Ventriculoperitoneal (VP) shunt with stylet in place. There are fenestrated ventricular (right inset) and abdominal (left inset) segments, which both connect to a unidirectional valve (centre inset). Some shunts come as one piece and some valves are programmable so that the pressure at which they open can be altered based on the status of the patient. **(b)** Lateral and **(c)** ventrodorsal radiographs of a dog following VP shunt placement to treat congenital hydrocephalus. The shunt reservoir (valve) is visible in the cervical region (arrowed). (b, c courtesy of N Olby)

approximately 20% of cases and include excessive trauma to the cerebral parenchyma, over-shunting, migration of the shunt, infection (Figure 9.15) and shunt blockage. Migration of the shunt is the most common of these complications and care should be taken when anchoring it to the skull (de Stefani et al., 2011). In one study, 9 out of 12 dogs with hydrocephalus had sustained clinical improvement and only 17% (two dogs) had neurological postoperative complications (Shihab et al., 2011). These dogs had no identifiable cause of the hydrocephalus.

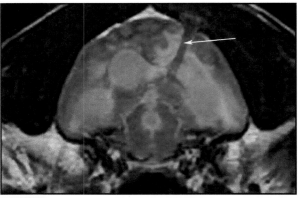

9.15 Transverse T2-weighted FLAIR MR image of a dog with hydrocephalus and an intraventricular shunt (arrowed). The dog acquired an infection as a result of the procedure, which can be seen to have caused hyperintense ventricular signals, periventricular hyperintensities and peri-shunt oedema.

Metabolic diseases

Numerous metabolic abnormalities may alter cerebrocortical and brainstem function (Cuddon, 1996; Lorenz et al., 2011). Liver disease (hepatic encephalopathy), renal disease (renal encephalopathy), pancreatic disease (pancreatic encephalopathy), glucose abnormalities (hyperglycaemia or hypoglycaemia), electrolyte abnormalities (sodium, potassium, chloride, calcium, magnesium), cardiovascular diseases (resulting in ischaemia and hypoxia) and acid–base abnormalities are examples of metabolic diseases. Endocrine abnormalities (thyroid hormones and cortisol) may also affect consciousness (Joseph and Peterson, 1992; Jaggy et al., 1994; Feldman and Nelson, 1996). The following discussion of metabolic encephalopathies addresses the basic diagnostic and treatment regimens for the underlying diseases, but an in-depth description of these subjects is beyond the scope of this text; further details can be found in standard internal medicine texts.

Hepatic encephalopathy
When liver function is compromised due to organ failure, hepatic microvascular dysplasia or portosystemic shunting, CNS signs quickly ensue (Windsor and Olby, 2007; Mertens et al., 2010).

Clinical signs
Animals with hepatic encephalopathy are most often admitted for seizures, ptyalism (especially in cats) and

mentation changes, which range from behavioural abnormalities to coma (see **Portosystemic shunt** clip on DVD). Signs of hepatic dysfunction such as weight loss, polydipsia, anorexia and vomiting may be present. These animals are often sensitive to the administration of benzodiazepines and barbiturates as both these types of drug are metabolized by the liver. Overzealous administration of these drugs may result in stupor and coma due to CNS depression.

Pathogenesis
Hepatic encephalopathy occurs when numerous putative neurotoxins reach the brain without being metabolized as a result of passing through an abnormally functioning liver (Cuddon, 1996). Suspected toxins include neurotransmitters (such as gamma-aminobutyric acid (GABA) and glutamate), aromatic amino acids, mercaptans, ammonia, manganese and skatoles (Gow et al., 2010).

Diagnosis
The diagnosis of hepatic encephalopathy is supported by abnormal liver function studies such as bile acid testing and resting ammonia levels (Torisu et al., 2008; Ruland et al., 2010). Other associated abnormalities may include microcytic red blood cells, low albumin, cholesterol, glucose and urea concentrations, and elevated liver enzymes if there is parenchymal damage. The preferred imaging studies to confirm a diagnosis of portosystemic shunt include mesenteric portography, abdominal ultrasonography and per rectal scintigraphy (Lee et al., 2006). Transcranial colour-coded duplex ultrasonography and MRI have also been used to characterize the brain tissue of animals with hepatic encephalopathy (Torisu et al., 2005; Lee et al., 2006; Duque et al., 2011).

Treatment and prognosis
Treatment of hepatic encephalopathy aims to:

- Treat the underlying liver disease
- Treat any associated seizures
- Reduce the level of haematogenous neurotoxins (e.g. ammonia).

A diet of high quality, low quantity protein can help to minimize ammonia production in the gut (Proot et al., 2009). Lactulose (0.5–1.0 ml/kg orally q8h) is frequently used to assist with this aim as it reduces the amount of colonic ammonia produced and 'traps' ammonia by creating an acidic environment within the gut. Lactulose can also be administered as an enema to comatose patients (1–2 ml/kg q4–6h until loose stool is seen). In addition, neomycin (20 mg/kg orally q8h), ampicillin (22 mg/kg orally q8h) or metronidazole (7.5 mg/kg orally q8h) can be given to reduce the number of urea splitting bacteria in the colon. Potassium bromide can be used in these cases, but requires load-dosing to rapidly attain steady-state levels. Levetiracetam is also a safe choice of antiepileptic drug (see Chapters 8 and 20).

Seizures following surgical ligation of portosystemic shunts can be especially severe and difficult to effectively treat. Cautious use of a constant rate infusion of diazepam or midazolam may be used for status epilepticus in this situation; however, it can be difficult to dose due to the underlying alterations in liver function. Reduced dosages titrated to effect can be helpful but require vigilant patient monitoring and assessment. Mannitol is usually administered concurrently and seems to provide an added benefit in these animals. In addition, newer anticonvulsants such as levetiracetam have been used as they are not metabolized through the liver (see Chapter 8).

The prognosis depends on the underlying hepatic disease and the initial response to medical therapy.

Hypoglycaemia
The neurons in the brain require glucose for energy metabolism. A decrease in the availability of glucose to the brain neurons can cause a constellation of clinical abnormalities as a result of abnormal neuronal function (neuroglycopenic signs) and activation of the sympathetic nervous system.

Clinical signs
Hypoglycaemia can cause a variety of neurological signs, including anxiety, a ravenous appetite, lethargy or depression, tremors, seizures and coma. Exercise or fasting may precipitate signs. The speed with which the glucose concentration changes influences signs to a certain extent. A sudden drop in the blood glucose level causes a sympathetic discharge, hence anxiety and hunger; whereas, a chronically low glucose concentration causes lethargy. A peripheral neuropathy causing a stilted pelvic limb gait has been reported in dogs with insulinoma (Shahar et al., 1985; Braund et al., 1987; Bergman et al., 1994; Schrauwen et al., 1996; Madarame et al., 2009) (see Chapter 15). Central blindness is a frequent finding in animals that present with hypoglycaemic seizures. This can be a permanent residual deficit if severe damage has occurred.

Pathogenesis
Decreases in the blood glucose level alter intracranial neuronal function (Howerton and Shell, 1992). Hypoglycaemia can occur secondary to insulinoma, liver disease, hypoadrenocorticism, glycogen storage diseases, insulin overdose in diabetic animals, toxicity (e.g. xylitol), infectious diseases (e.g. babesiosis; Keller et al., 2004) and extrapancreatic neoplasia (Zini et al., 2007; Rossi et al., 2010). Toy breeds and neonates may become hypoglycaemic during times of stress. Some dogs that undertake significant exercise (e.g. hunting dogs) and young animals with metabolic stresses (such as caused by a parasitic infestation) are also at risk of developing hypoglycaemia.

Diagnosis
Serum glucose concentrations <3.3 mmol/l (<60 mg/dl) accompanied by consistent neurological signs are suggestive of significant hypoglycaemia. If the glucose level decreases slowly, some animals can tolerate a lower concentration (<2 mmol/l; <35 mg/dl) without serious clinical problems. Any single glucose concentration that is

abnormally low should be rechecked to eliminate sample handling or laboratory error. If the glucose concentration is consistently low, further investigation of the underlying cause is indicated.

Treatment and prognosis
Treatment and prognosis depend on the underlying cause. Feeding multiple small meals can help dogs with insulinomas. Direct correction of hypoglycaemia is indicated in emergency situations. Syrup can be applied to the gums when intravenous access is not available. (For further information on the intravenous administration of glucose, the reader is referred to Chapter 20.) It should be noted that if the suspected diagnosis is insulinoma, giving large amounts of glucose, either in the form of a large meal or intravenously, can cause a further increase in insulin release into the circulation and exacerbate the problem.

Electrolyte disturbances

Sodium abnormalities
Both hypernatraemia and hyponatraemia may affect the CNS and result in abnormalities of mentation.

Hypernatraemia:

Clinical signs: The clinical signs of hypernatraemia include lethargy and irritability progressing to ataxia, tremors, myoclonus, seizures, blindness, coma and death.

Pathogenesis: Hypernatraemia is most extreme in animals with abnormalities of thirst and drinking, which may also be associated with hypothalamic disease (Bagley, 1994). Hypernatraemia is synonymous with hyperosmolality and can lead to shrinkage of the brain parenchymal cells, which in turn can cause stretching of the small intracranial blood vessels and haemorrhage. After 2–3 days, the brain attempts to compensate for the altered extracellular sodium level by producing osmotically active intracellular substances (idiogenic osmoles). Thus, overly rapid correction of chronic hypernatraemia can cause sudden swelling of the brain parenchyma and ultimately be fatal.

Diagnosis: Demonstration of an abnormal electrolyte level in the presence of an encephalopathy which improves with appropriate correction confirms the diagnosis.

Treatment and prognosis: Guidelines for the treatment of sodium abnormalities have been suggested but are crude. Appropriate therapy is based upon replacement of the water deficit (calculated using the following equation) in conjunction with addressing the underlying cause.

$$\text{Water deficit (l)} = 0.6 \times \text{bodyweight (kg)} \times \left(\frac{\text{patient's sodium concentration}}{\text{normal sodium concentration}} - 1 \right)$$

However, calculations such as this are only used as a guide to begin therapy. With chronic serum sodium abnormalities, cautious fluid therapy with frequent patient monitoring for neurological deterioration is imperative. In an animal with established hypernatraemia, the water deficit should be corrected either orally or by fluid therapy administered conservatively over 2–3 days. An isotonic maintenance fluid should be used, initially at 1.5 times the normal maintenance rate. Serum sodium concentrations should be monitored every 4–6 hours and the rate of fluid therapy administration adjusted up or down accordingly. If the serum sodium concentration is lowered too rapidly, cerebral oedema may result with clinical deterioration in consciousness. Therapies such as mannitol (0.25–1.0 g/kg i.v. as needed q4–6h, but not more than 1.0 g/kg q24h) are often necessary for treatment of these animals.

Hyponatraemia:

Clinical signs: The clinical signs of hyponatraemia include lethargy, nausea and vomiting progressing to seizures, coma and death.

Pathogenesis: Hyponatraemia is synonymous with hypo-osmolality and can result in swelling of the brain parenchymal cells with subsequent oedema. After 2–3 days, the brain tries to compensate for this by actively extruding osmotically active intracellular components. As with hypernatraemia, rapid correction of hyponatraemia can be fatal.

Diagnosis: Demonstration of an abnormal electrolyte level in the presence of an encephalopathy which improves with appropriate correction confirms the diagnosis. T2-weighted and fluid-attenuated inversion recovery (FLAIR) MR images of the thalamic area of the brain reveal characteristic bilateral hyperintense abnormalities. These abnormalities are often focal and oval.

Treatment and prognosis: Appropriate therapy is based upon correction of the sodium deficit (calculated using the following equation) in conjunction with addressing the underlying cause.

$$\text{Sodium deficit (mEq/l)} = 0.6 \times \text{bodyweight (kg)} \times (\text{normal sodium concentration} - \text{patient's sodium concentration})$$

As for hypernatraemia, cautious fluid therapy and frequent patient monitoring are paramount. Too rapid correction of established hyponatraemia can result in thalamic lesions thought to be similar to central pontine myelinolysis (osmotic demyelination syndrome) in humans (O'Brien *et al.*, 1994).

Potassium abnormalities
Alterations in potassium concentration tend to affect muscle function more than CNS function. However, poor cerebral blood flow secondary to cardiac arrhythmias caused by alterations in the potassium

concentration may affect intracranial function. Clinical signs reflect lack of oxygen to the brain (see below).

Calcium abnormalities
Hypercalcaemia may result in nervous system depression. Hypocalcaemia can result in increased nervous system excitability manifest as seizures and tremors, as well as abnormal neurotransmission.

Central nervous system perfusion
Alterations in cerebral blood flow and perfusion, including ischaemia and hypoxia, can affect neuronal function. These alterations may occur as a result of systemic hypoperfusion due to cardiac or pulmonary disease and anaesthetic accidents. Hyperviscosity due to increased red blood cell numbers (polycythemia vera) may also result in intracranial disease, which affects the oxygen-carrying capacity of the red blood cells. Anaemia and haemoglobin-related toxicity (e.g. cyanide toxicosis) can also affect oxygen delivery to the brain. Smoke inhalation may also result in intracranial clinical signs, usually in associated with significant respiratory abnormalities (Drobatz et al., 1999ab; Kent et al., 2010). In addition, primary abnormalities of neuronal metabolic function and energy metabolism may result in abnormal cerebrocortical function.

Hypothyroid-associated central nervous system dysfunction

Clinical signs
Hypothyroid-associated CNS dysfunction (myxoedema coma) is an extremely rare presentation in dogs. Dobermanns seem to be over-represented. Affected animals can become stuporous to comatose, severely hypothermic (with an absence of shivering), bradycardic and exhibit CN dysfunction. More classic signs of hypothyroidism are also present.

Pathogenesis
Myxoedema coma occurs in severely hypothyroid animals as a result of a hypometabolic state. The aetiology of the coma is not understood, but clinical signs seem to be triggered by a stressful event (Finora and Greco, 2007).

Diagnosis
The diagnosis is confirmed by measurement of thyroxine levels, which should be extremely low. The response to parenteral thyroxine therapy can also help establish the diagnosis.

Treatment and prognosis
Thyroxine levels can be increased rapidly in an emergency situation by intravenous administration of levothyroxine (Henik and Dixon, 2000). Unfortunately, this disease carries a poor prognosis.

Neoplastic diseases

Brain tumours primarily affect older dogs and cats. While some estimates exist for the frequency of

brain tumours in dogs (Vandevelde, 1984), the actual incidence is not known. Brain tumours may arise primarily from the brain or surrounding tissues, extend into the brain from adjacent structures, or metastasize to the brain from another location in the body. Tumours result in clinical signs either through primary mechanical damage or as a consequence of secondary pathophysiological events such as oedema and haemorrhage (Dickinson et al., 2008b). The increased reporting of brain tumours is no doubt the result of increased diligence on the part of the owner to pursue the causes of clinical signs, coupled with the increased availability and use of advanced imaging modalities such as CT and MRI for antemortem diagnosis of intracranial disease.

In a retrospective review of 97 dogs diagnosed with brain tumours, 95% of the affected dogs were ≥5 years old at the time of diagnosis (Bagley et al., 1999). The median age of the dogs diagnosed with a brain tumour was 9 years (range: 4–13 years). The most commonly affected breeds included Golden Retrievers, Labrador Retrievers, Boxers, Collies, Dobermanns, Schnauzers, Airedale Terriers and mixed-breed dogs. A retrospective review of 160 cats with intracranial neoplasia found the median age at the time of diagnosis was 11.3 years (± 3.8 years) (Troxel et al., 2003).

Clinical signs
Most dogs with brain tumours (76%) have lesions of the supratentorial space. The most common presenting complaint in these cases is seizures. However, whilst seizures are often reported to be a clinical manifestation of brain tumours in dogs, the actual incidence of seizures associated with intracranial tumours is not well established. In one study, McGrath (1960) described the clinical features of 79 dogs with brain tumours, 36 (46%) of which had seizures. In another series of 43 dogs with rostral cerebral tumours, 22 (51%) had seizures (Foster et al., 1988). Seizures are sometimes the only sign of a structural intracranial abnormality, with the remainder of the neurological examination findings being normal. This is particularly true with more rostral and olfactory lobe lesions (Palmer et al., 1974; Foster et al., 1988). Thus, the onset of seizures in dogs >5 years old, regardless of the associated neurological examination abnormalities, should raise suspicion for the presence of a brain tumour.

Most feline intracranial neoplasia (87.3%) affects the supratentorial space (Troxel et al., 2003). The most common neurological signs observed in these animals include altered consciousness (depression, stupor or coma – 26%), circling (22.5%), seizures (22.5%), ataxia (16.9%) and behavioural changes (15.6%).

Pathogenesis
Tumours of the intracranial space may be primary (arise from tissues in the intracranial space) or secondary (arise from tissues adjacent to the intracranial

space or from metastasis) (Bagley *et al.*, 1992; Moore *et al.*, 1996). Primary intracranial tumours include:

- Meningiomas
- Gliomas (glioblastomas, astrocytomas, oligodendrogliomas)
- Ependymomas
- Choroid plexus tumours
- Pituitary gland tumours.

Secondary intracranial lesions arise as a result of metastasis or direct extension from extraneural sites. Primary tumours within the skull, nasal cavity or frontal sinuses can extend directly into the brain (Smith *et al.*, 1989; Moore *et al.*, 1991). With caudal nasal cavity tumours, often signs of intracranial extension such as seizures occur prior to, or without, other signs of nasal disease.

Numerous tumours in older animals metastasize to the brain, including haemangiosarcomas, lymphomas and mammary gland and other carcinomas (Moore and Taylor, 1988; Waters *et al.*, 1989; Fenner, 1990; Snyder *et al.*, 2008). The incidence of intracranial metastasis is often underestimated as the brain is not always examined during routine necropsy. One study of 160 cases of feline intracranial neoplasia found that 5.6% of all tumours were the result of metastatic disease (Troxel *et al.*, 2003). In this study, lymphoma comprised 16% of the lesions identified: of these 13% were focal masses with the remainder being diffuse diseases of the cerebrum or brainstem, and approximately 70% of cases represented multicentric lymphoma.

Tumours that readily metastasize to the lungs may be more likely to metastasize to the brain (Waters *et al.*, 1989). The cortical grey/white matter junction is a common area of metastasis due to the increased vascularity; metastasis to the brainstem and spinal cord occurs less frequently. Choroid plexus tumours may metastasize through the CSF to other areas of the brain or spinal cord ('drop-mets') (Ropper and Samuels, 2009). In some instances, spinal cord dysfunction may be the first sign of choroid plexus metastasis. Diffuse intracranial neoplasia (such as carcinomatosis) is also possible.

Other tumours involving the brain are uncommon but include germ cell tumours, dermoid and epidermoid cysts, and craniopharyngiomas. Many of these tumours are primarily seen in younger animals.

Meningiomas

Meningiomas are the most common brain tumours in dogs and cats (Bagley *et al.*, 2002; Troxel *et al.*, 2003; Montoliu *et al.*, 2006; Matiasek *et al.*, 2009; Sessums and Mariani, 2009). These tumours arise from the arachnoid layer of the meninges, originating at the periphery of the brain parenchyma and expanding inwards. In dogs, meningiomas tend to infiltrate the cortical parenchyma; in cats, meningiomas are often well encapsulated. Predominantly cystic meningiomas, often involving the olfactory area, have also been described (Bagley *et al.*, 1996) (Figure 9.16). Meningiomas are usually histologically benign.

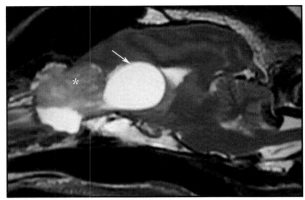

9.16 Sagittal T2-weighted MR image demonstrating a mass (✳) in the olfactory lobe associated with a more caudal cyst (arrowed). Histopathology of the mass confirmed a meningioma.

Gene expression: Gene expression patterns of meningiomas in dogs have been evaluated using a canine brain-specific cDNA microarray: up-regulation of ribosomal proteins was documented (Thomson *et al.*, 2005). Recent studies demonstrated that canine meningioma genome deletions spanned the chromosomal regions syntenic to those most often deleted in human meningiomas (Courtay-Cahan *et al.*, 2008; Thomas *et al.*, 2009). In the first of these studies, the quantitative loss of DNA was associated with the shortest progression-free survival time. The level of *NF-2* gene expression has been evaluated in canine meningiomas but no significant difference was noted relative to normal canine tissues, and no specific pattern of transcript expression was seen relative to tumour grade or subtype, even though several tumour samples had decreased expression of NF-2 protein on western blot analysis (Campbell *et al.*, 2006).

Gliomas

Gliomas arise from the supporting cells of the brain parenchyma. These include astrocytes and oligodendrocytes forming astrocytomas, oligodendrogliomas and the extremely malignant glioblastoma multiforme. Brachycephalic breeds such as Boxers and Boston Terriers may be more often affected with these tumours.

Ependymomas and choroid plexus tumours

Ependymomas and choroid plexus tumours originate in or around the ventricular system. Choroid plexus tumours arise from areas where the choroid plexus is concentrated (the lateral, third and fourth ventricles) (Ribas *et al.*, 1989; Westworth *et al.*, 2008). Due to their association with the ventricular system, obstructive hydrocephalus is commonly seen with choroid plexus tumours.

Pituitary gland tumours

Pituitary gland tumours may result in signs of endocrine disease (e.g. hyperadrenocorticism, acromegaly) or signs primarily related to CNS dysfunction (Sarfaty *et al.*, 1988; Davidson *et al.*, 1991). Macroadenomas may enlarge dorsally from the sella and compress the diencephalon. Neurological impairment can be surprisingly minimal. The relative size of the tumour cannot be predicted from the endocrine test results (Kipperman *et al.*, 1992).

Diagnosis

Imaging studies
Advanced imaging modalities, such as CT and MRI, are most commonly used to investigate cases of suspected neoplasia. Features of primary brain tumours have been reviewed elsewhere (Turrel *et al.*, 1986; Gavin *et al.*, 1995; Tucker and Gavin, 1996; McDonnell *et al.*, 2007; Rossmeisl *et al.*, 2007; Sturges *et al.*, 2008; Ródenas *et al.*, 2011; Sutherland-Smith *et al.*, 2011).

Meningiomas: These most commonly appear as broad-based, extra-axial (arising outside and pushing into the parenchyma) contrast-enhancing masses on CT and MRI (Figure 9.17). These tumours may contain haemorrhage or be calcified, in

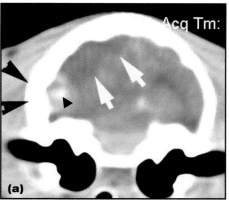
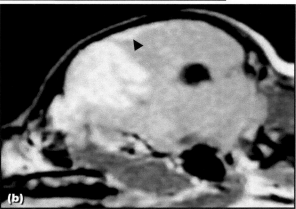

9.17 **(a)** Transverse contrast-enhanced CT image of the brain of a 14-year-old cat that presented with seizures. There is a small contrast-enhanced mass in the right temporal lobe with a mineralized centre (arrowhead). The overlying skull is thickened (hyperostosis; black arrows). As the meningioma is lying in the subarachnoid space, the brain has been pushed away from the skull (white arrows) and there is an accumulation of CSF in the resultant space. (Courtesy of N Olby)
(b) Sagittal contrast-enhanced T1-weighted MR image of an 8-year-old Bichon Frise with a meningioma. There is a large contrast-enhancing mass with a broad base in contact with the surface of the brain and extending along the meninges (arrowhead) (dural tail sign).

addition to having large cystic areas. On pre-contrast CT images, haemorrhage and calcification have a hyperattenuating (white) appearance. Haemorrhage may have a varied appearance on MRI, depending upon its duration (Figure 9.18).

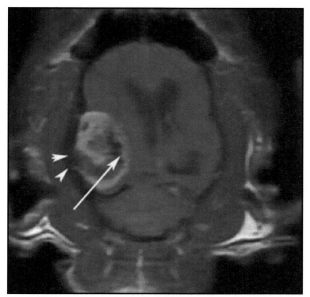

9.18 Dorsal post-contrast T1-weighted MR image of a cat with a large well delineated mass in the cerebral cortex. The areas with minimal to no signal (arrowed) are suggestive of haemorrhage and/or mineralization based on the histopathology. The lesion was confirmed to be a meningioma. Note the adjacent hyperostosis (arrowheads) of the skull, which is sometimes seen in response to intracranial meningiomas.

Gliomas: The CT and MRI appearance of gliomas is varied and enhancement after contrast medium administration is not consistently seen (Figure 9.19). A mass confined within the parenchyma of the brain is characteristic for this type of tumour. Gliomas are not always visible on CT, thus MRI is advised in older brachycephalic breeds with clinical signs of a focal forebrain lesion (Figure 9.20).

Choroid plexus tumours: Choroid plexus tumours (e.g. papillomas, carcinomas) often markedly enhance following intravenous contrast medium administration because of the concentration of blood vessels with the tumour (Figure 9.21).

Pituitary gland tumours: These tumours may be identified in the sella or in a suprasellar location. Smaller tumours are more readily seen with MRI than CT, especially with dynamic contrast studies (Figure 9.22).

Biopsy

CT-guided biopsy: CT-guided, free-hand needle biopsy of brain tumours has been reported in dogs with intracranial lesions to obtain a histological diagnosis prior to treatment. Although CT-guided, free-hand needle biopsy is a relatively safe procedure, the diagnostic yield is low and up to 62% of samples produce a false-negative result.

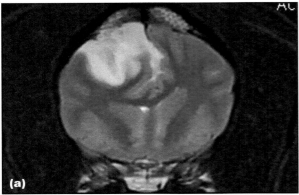

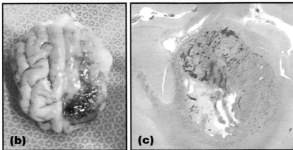

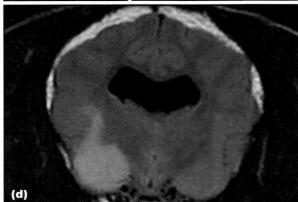

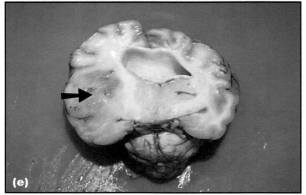

9.19 **(a)** Transverse T2-weighted FLAIR MR image of the brain of a Boston Terrier presented with seizures and inappropriate mentation. A large hyperintense lesion predominantly affecting the grey matter and causing a mass effect can be seen.
(b) Dorsal view of the gross brain of the dog in (a).
(c) Histopathology confirmed the lesion as an oligodendroglioma. (H&E stain; original magnification X10)
(d) Transverse T2-weighted FLAIR MR image of the brain of a dog with a large piriform lobe hyperintensity, which was confirmed as an astrocytoma on histopathology.
(e) Transverse section of a gross brain showing an astrocytoma in the piriform lobe (arrowed).

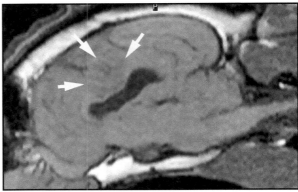

9.20 Sagittal contrast-enhanced T1-weighted MR image of a 9-year-old mixed-breed dog. The mass is an indistinct hypoattenuating area lying in the parietal lobe (arrowed) that has not been enhanced by contrast medium. Histopathology confirmed the mass as a high grade glioma.

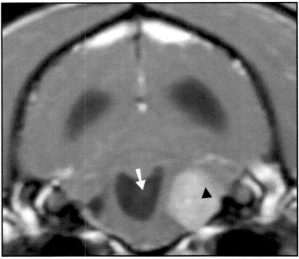

9.21 Transverse contrast-enhanced T1-weighted MR image at the level of the pons in a 7-year-old Border Collie. There is a large homogeneous contrast-enhanced mass in the left cerebellopontine angle (arrowhead) and the fourth ventricle is dilated (arrowed). Histopathology confirmed the mass as a choroid plexus papilloma.

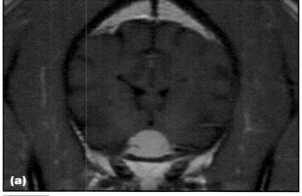

9.22 **(a)** Transverse post-contrast T1-weighted MR image of a dog with a pituitary gland-based mass. The uniform contrast medium enhancement with well defined borders suggests a lesion outside the parenchyma. (Courtesy of N Olby) (continues) ▶

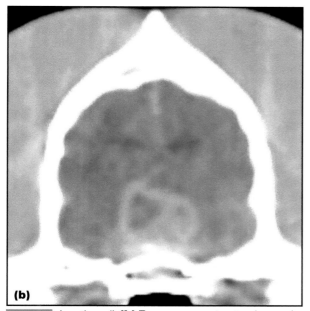

9.22 (continued) **(b)** Transverse contrast-enhanced CT image of a 6-year-old Labrador Retriever that presented with unexplained pain and compulsive pacing. A large contrast-enhancing mass is visible over the pituitary fossa. The mass has a cystic area and was confirmed at necropsy to be a pituitary adenocarcinoma. (Courtesy of N Olby)

Recent modifications to human CT-guided systems have allowed them to be used successfully to obtain brain biopsy samples from dogs and cats (Koblik *et al.*, 1999; Moissonnier *et al.*, 2000, 2002; Flegel *et al.*, 2002; Giroux *et al.*, 2002; Troxel and Vite, 2008). Modifications to human systems are required to accommodate the 90% shift in orientation of the canine head (compared with the human head) during CT imaging and to facilitate other components of the biopsy procedures that are affected by the uneven and variable size and shape of canine and feline skulls. The safe and accurate performance of CT-guided stereotactic brain biopsy has been reported in 50 dogs with intracranial lesions with an overall diagnostic yield of 91% (Koblik *et al.*, 1999). This is similar to the diagnostic yield reported in humans.

MRI-guided biopsy: An MRI-compatible stereotactic brain biopsy system has recently been validated for use in dogs. This modified frameless stereotactic system has been shown to have acceptable precision for obtaining biopsy samples and has been used successfully in a clinical setting (for further information, the reader is referred to Chapter 6).

Cytology
The rapid cytological evaluation of a brain biopsy sample can provide critical information with reference to treatment. In human medicine, the intraoperative cytological evaluation of smear preparations (supported by frozen and paraffin-embedded tissue samples) has become routine. Smear preparations are generally wet fixed in 95% alcohol and stained with haematoxylin and eosin (H&E) stain; although,

toluidine blue, Giemsa or Papanicolaou stains may also be used.

In one study, tissue samples were obtained from lesions either via CT-guided stereotactic brain biopsy (44 samples) or intraoperatively during craniotomy (49 samples) and the results from smear preparations were compared with those from sections of paraffin-embedded tissue (Vernau *et al.*, 2001). The overall diagnostic accuracy of the samples obtained by both stereotactic biopsy and craniotomy was 80%. This compares favourably with the 64–94% accuracy reported in some large series human studies.

The main advantages of intraoperative cytological evaluation of smear preparations are speed, ease of preparation, technical simplicity, need for minimal equipment, high degree of cytological resolution compared with frozen preparations, low cost and the small sample size required. The limitation of this diagnostic technique is that it is difficult to prepare adequate smear preparations of certain tough and coherent tumours (e.g. fibrillary astrocytomas and some meningiomas). In addition, although smear preparations provide excellent cytological detail, they differ from the conventional histological appearance of H&E-stained paraffin-embedded tissue samples. Thus, experience is required for the correct interpretation of smear preparations.

Immunohistochemistry
Immunohistochemical analysis has been performed on brain tumours in dogs and cats to assist with classification (Ribas *et al.*, 1989; Barnhart *et al.*, 2002; Cantile *et al.*, 2002; Mandrioli *et al.*, 2007; Dickinson *et al.*, 2009; Rossmeisl *et al.*, 2009; Thomas *et al.*, 2009; Higgins *et al.*, 2010; Ide *et al.*, 2010; Ramos-Vara *et al.*, 2010).

Cerebrospinal fluid analysis
CSF analysis is often not helpful for the definitive diagnosis of a brain tumour, and in some instances can even be misleading. Typically, CSF in dogs with a brain tumour contains an increased level of protein without a concurrent pleocytosis (albuminocytological dissociation). However, in a significant proportion of these cases cellular changes consistent with inflammation are present and, interpreted alone, may falsely suggest a primary inflammatory disease (e.g. encephalitis or meningitis) (Bailey and Higgins, 1986; Carrillo *et al.*, 1986). Occasionally, CSF in a dog with a brain tumour is normal. The presence of neoplastic cells in the CSF is specific; however, it is a very rare finding. This may occur more often with lymphomas, carcinomatosis and choroid plexus tumours. Median CSF total protein and nucleated cell count in 28 cats with variable types of intracranial neoplasia were 38.0 mg/dl (range: 16–427 mg/dl; reference interval: <25 mg/dl) and 5 cells/μl (range: 0–162 cells/μl; reference interval: <5 cells/μl) (Troxel *et al.*, 2003; Dickinson *et al.*, 2006a).

Treatment
Treatment for brain tumours in dogs depends upon tumour type, location, natural history of the tumour,

associated morbidity/mortality with the treatment modality, and cost. Whilst studies of brain tumour treatment in dogs and cats exist in the veterinary literature, many have incomplete diagnoses, non-standardized treatment protocols, lack of a control population and different tumour types being grouped together to increase overall case numbers. These problems make it difficult to make definitive statements regarding treatment efficacy.

Glucocorticoid administration

Glucocorticoid therapy has been deemed only to provide minimal supportive care for patients with brain tumours; although, its use can often be necessary and helpful. The aims of glucocorticoid treatment are to control the secondary conditions of acquired hydrocephalus and peritumoral oedema, and to reduce ICP. At anti-inflammatory doses, glucocorticoids can reduce CSF production as well as oedema and blood supply to the tumour within 24 hours. The use of high potency glucocorticoids has a beneficial effect upon oedema associated with both primary and metastatic tumours. Glucocorticoids are presumed to act directly on endothelial cells, reducing their permeability, as well as shrinking normal brain tissue, leading to an overall decrease in ICP. In humans with brain tumours, there is no rigid schedule for the administration of high potency steroids (e.g. methylprednisolone): drugs are administered at bedtime to suppress headaches and focal symptoms.

Clinical signs in many patients improve following the initiation of steroid treatment, which may give some indication of tumour invasion and what could be achieved with surgery. Data concerning the survival of dogs and cats with brain tumours that received only steroids as palliative therapy are scarce. The results of one study indicated a mean and median survival time of 81 days and 56 days, respectively, following CT diagnosis of a primary brain tumour (Turrel *et al.*, 1984). In this study, 6 of the 8 dogs died or were euthanased within 64 days of diagnosis. In another study that included 13 dogs with intracranial meningiomas, survival times from initial clinical signs to necropsy varied from 1 day to 405 days with a mean survival time of 75 days (Foster *et al.*, 1988).

In human patients, glucocorticoids are always administered at least 1 week prior to intracranial surgery, to reduce cerebral oedema and thereby facilitate cerebral retraction for improved exposure. If adequate surgical decompression is achieved, the steroid dosage can be tapered off rapidly and discontinued within the first week or two following the operation. However, some patients require a maintenance dosage of steroids because a large volume of the tumour remains, because the tumour occupies the brainstem or because of steroid-dependence as a result of long-term prior use. Patients who no longer require glucocorticoids following surgery may require them during or after radiation therapy, as reactive oedema may occur during irradiation, which can cause transient clinical deterioration. The lowest dosage of glucocorticoid that maintains patients at their maximum level of comfort and function is used in human patients. Typically, this is determined by decreasing the dosage until symptoms increase or become apparent and then increasing the dosage until they subside. If deterioration is secondary to tumour growth or treatment-induced effects, the dose of glucocorticoids may have to be increased to keep the patient comfortable.

Surgery

Surgery is ideal for superficially located, encapsulated, relatively small, benign tumours, of which meningiomas are the most common example. Unfortunately, in dogs, even when meningiomas are histologically benign, these tumours are often not well encapsulated and hence difficult to surgically remove; microscopic and even macroscopic disease can remain after surgery.

Median survival times reported in dogs following surgery for all types of brain tumour vary, but tend to cluster around 140–150 days (Heidner *et al.*, 1991; Niebauer *et al.*, 1991; Jeffery and Brearley, 1993; Axlund *et al.*, 2002; Greco *et al.*, 2006). For meningiomas, median survival times may be slightly longer (240 days) and there is evidence that improving surgical excision using ultrasonic aspiration or endoscopy results in prolonged median survival times of 1254 days (Greco *et al.*, 2006) and 2104 days (Klopp and Rao, 2009), respectively. There is significant mortality within the first 30 days following surgery of animals with infratentorial tumours compared with supratentorial tumours.

Surgical excision is more readily accomplished in cats as meningiomas in this species tend to be well encapsulated and easily delineated from normal brain tissue. Studies have determined the median survival time in cats following meningioma resection to be between 22 and 27 months (Gallagher *et al.*, 1993; Gordon *et al.*, 1994).

Conventional radiation therapy

Conventional radiation therapy has been shown to be effective for brain tumours in dogs (Evans *et al.*, 1993; LaRue and Gillette, 2001). Radiation therapy is more apt to control tumour progression; however, in some rare instances, it may eradicate the tumour completely. The main goal of treatment is to administer the highest possible dose to the tumour whilst minimizing the dose to the surrounding normal tissue. Treatment protocols and survival analysis for radiation therapy of brain tumours have been reviewed. From these limited studies, median survival times in dogs are around 150 to 350 days (for further information, see Chapter 24).

Radiosurgery using a stereotactic head frame system has been documented in a small number of dogs; survival data cannot be interpreted, but it was documented to be a feasible and safe technique (Lester *et al.*, 2001). Boron neutron capture therapy has also been evaluated in dogs in a phase I trial; initial clinical results similar to those achieved with conventional radiation have been documented (Gavin *et al.*, 1989; Kraft *et al.*, 1992).

Dogs have also been involved in radiation treatment trials evaluating hyperthermia and photodynamic therapy (Whelan *et al.*, 1993; Thrall *et al.*, 1999; Kangasniemi *et al.*, 2004). In one study, 25 dogs received radiation therapy and 20 dogs received a combination of radiation and whole body hyperthermia (Thrall *et al.*, 1999). The total radiation dose (44, 48, 52, 56 or 60 Gy) was randomly assigned. For whole body hyperthermia, the target rectal temperature was 42°C and three treatments were planned. Whole body hyperthermia toxicity was severe in 6 dogs and resulted in the interruption of treatment or death. There was no survival difference between the groups. The 1-year survival probability (95% confidence interval) for dogs receiving radiation therapy along was 0.44 (0.25–0.63) compared with 0.40 (0.19–0.63) for dogs receiving radiation and whole body hyperthermia. The results suggested that the use of whole body hyperthermia alone to increase the temperature of intracranial tumours as a means of improving radiation therapy outcome was not a successful strategy.

Chemotherapy

Chemotherapy is used as a primary therapy or as an adjunct to surgery in selected instances in animals with brain tumours (Dimiski and Cook, 1990; Fulton, 1991). Chemotherapeutic agents are primarily used for the treatment of gliomas in humans; although reports on the use of chemotherapy to treat gliomas and meningiomas in dogs exist in the veterinary literature. Carmustine (BCNU) and lomustine (CCNU) are alkylating agents that have some effectiveness against gliomas. They are administered either intravenously or orally (CCNU) at 3–6 week intervals (depending on the protocol). Side effects include bone marrow suppression, liver disease and pulmonary fibrosis. Temozolomide is an alkylating agent that is used to treat aggressive gliomas in humans. It has been used anecdotally in dogs, but there is no clinical information available on the appropriate dosing regimen and efficacy. However, temozolomide has been used in dogs with refractory lymphoma and has been documented to be safe (Dervisis *et al.*, 2007). Hydroxyurea at a dose of 30–45 mg/kg orally three times a week is gaining popularity for the treatment of meningiomas (Tamura *et al.*, 2007). The blood cell count should be monitored for evidence of myelosuppression. Other chemotherapeutic agents that have been used to treat primary CNS lymphoma include cytosine arabinoside (which readily crosses the blood–brain barrier) and methotrexate. There is little data available on the effectiveness of chemotherapy for canine and feline brain tumours.

Novel treatment options

Convection-enhanced delivery: Convection-enhanced delivery, also referred to as high flow microinfusion, is a promising local delivery technique which uses the bulk flow of molecules of various sizes to target specific areas within the CNS (Dickinson *et al.*, 2008a; Fiandaca *et al.*, 2008). This delivery technique aids the passage of significant volumes of drug through the blood–brain barrier, reaching the target tissues with minimal toxicity. This technique has been documented in normal dogs using real-time MR monitoring of drug delivery for optimization of the infusion (Dickinson *et al.*, 2008a) (Figure 9.23). A pilot clinical trial investigating the intratumoral convection-enhanced delivery of liposomal CPT-11 (irinotecan) in spontaneous canine gliomas has also been reported in the literature (Dickinson *et al.*, 2010). Irinotecan (a topoisomerase 1 inhibitor) delivered in this manner was well tolerated and resulted in improved clinical examinations and decreased tumour volumes on MRI assessment.

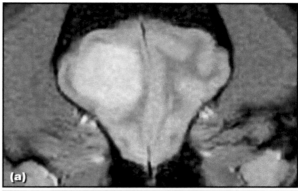
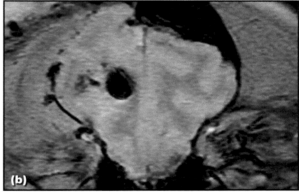

9.23 **(a)** Transverse gradient echo MR image of the frontal lobe of a dog with an oligodendroglioma. **(b)** Post-surgery the lesion has reduced in size. Note the focal signal void where iron oxide nanoparticle tracers have been used to help follow the administration of a novel treatment by convection-enhanced delivery into the tumour bed.

Non-thermal irreversible electroporation: Non-thermal irreversible electroporation has shown promise as an ablative therapy for a variety of soft tissue neoplasms. Minimally invasive CT-guided non-thermal irreversible electroporation has been reported as safe in normal canine brain tissue; the non-thermal aspect of the technique was confirmed with real-time temperature data measured at the electrode–tissue interface (Garcia *et al.*, 2010). Non-thermal irreversible electroporation has also been reported to have safely and effectively reduced the volume of a brain tumour and associated intracranial hypertension in a dog (Garcia *et al.*, 2011). The authors reported the potential benefits of non-thermal irreversible electroporation for *in vivo* ablation of brain tumours and suggested it as an option when traditional methods of cyto-reductive surgery are not possible or ideal. This process may also act as a radiosensitizing therapy.

Prognosis

The prognosis for an animal with a brain tumour depends upon the adequacy of local tumour control. Currently, radiation therapy and surgery have resulted in the longest survival times in dogs with brain tumours; however, rarely is the median survival time >1 year. In a minority of cases, the survival time is >1 year and this should be the goal for treatment in the future. Cats appear to have a better overall prognosis than dogs, primarily because feline brain tumours are often benign meningiomas that can be readily removed via surgery.

Surgical removal of brain tumours is associated with a higher rate of morbidity compared with radiation therapy. However, surgery also has the potential to be curative and the decompression afforded can be life-saving in animals with severe deficits. It is hoped that increased early recognition of lesions through more widespread use of advanced intracranial studies coupled with improvements in surgical and radiation therapies will increase both the quantity and quality of life of animals with brain tumours.

Molecular studies

Several molecules have been identified and investigated as markers of malignancy, including:

- Oestrogen, progesterone and androgen receptors (Speciale *et al.*, 1990; Mandara *et al.*, 2002; Adamo *et al.*, 2003)
- Vascular endothelial growth factor (VEGF) and its receptors (FLT-1 and KDR) (Platt *et al.*, 2006; Dickinson *et al.*, 2008b)
- Endothelial growth factor receptor-1 (EGDR-1)
- Platelet-derived growth factor α (PDGFRα) (Dickinson *et al.*, 2006b)
- H-telomerase reverse transcriptase (Long *et al.*, 2006)
- Ki-67.

The majority of canine meningiomas express progesterone receptors but not oestrogen receptors. The presence of an increased number of progesterone receptors has been associated with lower cell proliferation rates and longer survival times (Theon *et al.*, 2000; Mandara *et al.*, 2002). VEGF expression has been detected in all meningiomas examined, with >50% of cells staining positively; shorter survival times have been associated with increased expression (Platt *et al.*, 2006). VEGFR, EGFR-1, PDGFRα and h-telomerase reverse transcriptase expression have all been associated with cell proliferation and malignancy in canine meningiomas, but not with survival times (Dickinson *et al.*, 2006b; Mandrioli *et al.*, 2007; Rossmeisl *et al.*, 2007). In addition, matrix metallinoproteinase 2, cathepsin and STAT3-TYR705 markers have been identified, but as yet no attempt has been made to investigate the associated survival times.

Nutritional diseases

Thiamine deficiency

Thiamine deficiency occurs most commonly in anorexic cats or cats that are fed an all-fish diet containing thiaminase (Palus, 2010). More recently, it has been associated with the feeding of canned cat food (Marks *et al.*, 2011). Thiamine deficiency can also occur in dogs (Hazlett *et al.*, 2005; Singh *et al.*, 2005). This deficiency results in polioencephalomalacia of the oculomotor and vestibular nuclei, the caudal colliculus and the lateral geniculate body (deLahunta and Glass, 2008). Early, non-specific signs typically include lethargy and inappetence. The earliest neurological sign is bilateral vestibular ataxia, which manifests as an abnormal broad-based stance, a ventroflexed neck in cats and loss of balance. If untreated, signs progress to semi-coma, persistent vocalization, opisthotonus and death. The diagnosis and treatment of this disorder are discussed in Chapter 11.

Infectious diseases

Encephalitis and meningitis

Encephalitis and meningitis (see Chapters 10, 12 and 14) often exist concurrently in dogs and cats. Numerous agents have been implicated, including both infectious and non-infectious aetiologies (Meric, 1986; Muñana, 1996). The incidence of infectious agents causing meningitis varies with geographic location. Most meningitis syndromes (approximately 60%) in small animals do not have a definable infectious cause.

Infectious agents that can cause brain disease include (Kornegay, 1978; Greene *et al.*, 1985; Meric, 1986; Dow et al., 1988; Hass et al., 1989; Hoskins *et al.*, 1991; Baroni and Heinold, 1995; Muñana, 1996):

- Viral – distemper, parvovirus, parainfluenza, herpesvirus, feline coronavirus (which causes feline infectious peritonitis), West Nile virus, pseudorabies and rabies
- Bacterial
- Rickettsial – Rocky Mountain spotted fever and *Ehrlichia*
- Fungal – blastomycosis, histoplasmosis, cryptococcosis, coccidioidomycosis and aspergillosis
- Protozoal – toxoplasmosis and neosporosis
- Unclassified organisms – prototheocosis.

Non-infectious causes of disease of the supratentorial structures include granulomatous meningoencephalitis (GME), breed-specific encephalitis and meningitis, and many non-specific entities (Oliver *et al.*, 1997). For further information on the diagnosis, treatment and prognosis of these conditions, see Chapters 10, 12 and 14.

Rabies

Rabies is caused by an enveloped RNA neurotropic virus of the genus *Lyssavirus* in the family

Rhabdoviridae. All warm blooded animals are vulnerable to infection with rabies, but species susceptibility varies tremendously. Foxes, coyotes, jackals and wolves are amongst the most susceptible animals with skunks, raccoons, bats and cattle also having a high susceptibility. Dogs and cats have a moderate susceptibility; in 2009, 81 dogs and 300 cats were reported with rabies infection in the USA (Blanton *et al.*, 2010). In the northern hemisphere, rabies is predominantly a disease of wildlife, whereas in the southern hemisphere, the dog is the primary species involved in transmission of the disease. The highest incidence of canine and feline rabies cases generally occurs in areas where wildlife rabies is epidemic. Recent animal control programmes and pet vaccination have been responsible for a decline in the number of domestic animal infections; although, occasional vaccine breakthroughs have been reported in dogs and cats (McQuiston *et al.*, 2001; Murray *et al.*, 2009).

Clinical signs
There are several overlapping phases during the progression of the disease. In dogs there is usually a prodromal phase (lasts for 2–3 days) during which clinical signs such as apprehension, nervousness, anxiety and variable fever may be seen. Overall, a significant change in the normal behaviour of the animal is noted by the owner. Affected animals can be seen to constantly lick the site of viral inoculation. Cats may also exhibit this prodromal phase, but it more commonly consists of erratic behaviour for 1–2 days.

The furious or psychotic form of rabies usually lasts up to a week in dogs and is manifest by cerebral dysfunction with exaggerated responses to sound and touch. Affected animals can bite at imaginary objects or their cage and become extremely irritable. At this stage they frequently exhibit generalized tonic–clonic seizure activity, during which they can die. Occasionally, dogs can exhibit a predeath paralyzed state. Cats typically develop the furious stage, resulting in unprovoked attacks and appearing 'disconnected' from the environment.

The paralytic or dumb form of rabies is often seen within 2–4 days following the onset of clinical signs and is manifest by flaccid paralysis. In both dogs and cats, a bite to the neck or head may more commonly result in CN dysfunction. Dysphonia, dysphagia, excessive salivation and a dropped jaw may be seen, and these clinical signs are also classed as part of the paralytic form. Coma and death usually follow these signs within 2–4 days.

Pathogenesis
Infection most often occurs as a result of being bitten by an infected animal with rabies virus in its saliva. The incubation period is influenced by multiple factors, including patient age, bite site, the variant and the amount of virus inoculated. After intramuscular inoculation, the virus enters the neuromuscular junctions following a variable period (from days to 6 months) of replication in the local tissues. The virus rapidly spreads up the peripheral nerves and then spinal cord to the forebrain, causing damage to the nervous tissue *en route* and resulting in progressive nervous system signs.

Diagnosis
Rabies should always be suspected in any animal presenting with neurological dysfunction living in an area known to have a virus reservoir in the local wildlife. Particular concern should be raised for animals that are known to be unvaccinated and that have exhibited clinical signs for <5 days.

There are no antemortem tests sensitive enough to be consistently reliable for confirming a diagnosis of rabies, and there are no haematological or serum biochemical changes characteristic of the disease. CSF analysis may reveal elevated protein levels and white blood cell count with a lymphocytic predominance. Serological tests are rarely performed because of the low percentage of animals that have time to develop antibodies. However, a serological assay can be used to assess vaccine efficacy.

A direct fluorescent antibody assay test of the nervous tissue can be performed on thin touch impression smears and is rapid and sensitive for a definitive diagnosis (Lackay *et al.*, 2008). The most commonly affected areas on examination are the brainstem, hippocampus, cerebrum and cerebellum (Stein *et al.*, 2010). Reverse transcriptase polymerase chain reaction (RT-PCR) is a relatively new method for rabies diagnosis and is very useful when the sample size is small (e.g. CSF sample) (Lackay *et al.*, 2008).

No gross lesions are detectable in the CNS of animals with rabies infection. Acute polioencephalitis (grey matter or neuronal disease) characterized by lymphocytic inflammation, perivascular cuffing, minimal neuronophagia, neuronal degeneration and non-suppurative inflammation is seen early during the disease process followed by necrotizing encephalitis. Negri bodies (ovoid eosinophilic intracytoplasmic inclusion bodies) are definitive for rabies diagnosis, but are absent in up to 60% of cases (Lackay *et al.*, 2008; Stein *et al.*, 2010) (Figure 9.24).

Treatment and prognosis
There is no specific treatment for this fatal disease. A dog or cat suspected of contracting the disease should be quarantined as recommended by the local heath authorities or euthanased and the brain submitted for examination. Exposure of all healthcare providers to the animal and/or its tissues should be restricted.

Parasitic disease
Parasites (e.g. *Toxocara*, *Dirofilaria* and *Cuterebra* larva) most commonly affect the forebrain during aberrant migration (Meric, 1986). *Cuterebra* is speculated to be associated with intracranial disease in cats (Glass *et al.*, 1998). Treatment is directed at parasite removal and reducing the potential for an inflammatory reaction to parasite death. Anthelmintics are rarely effective when the CNS is involved.

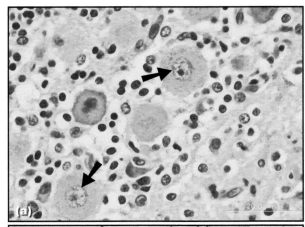
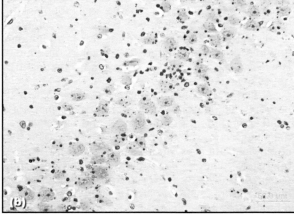

9.24 **(a)** Hippocampus of a dog with rabies showing several intracytoplasmic inclusion bodies (arrowed). (H&E stain; original magnification X20) **(b)** Hippocampus of a dog demonstrating distinct labelling for rabies virus antigen within the perikaryon of several neurons. (Immunohistochemistry labelled streptavidin biotin method with diaminobenzine substrate; Mayer's haematoxylin counterstain; original magnification X40) (Courtesy of R Rech)

Idiopathic diseases

Narcolepsy and cataplexy
Narcolepsy (excessive daytime sleepiness) and cataplexy (periods of acute muscular hypotonia) are episodic disorders that may mimic syncope and seizures (deLahunta and Glass, 2008) (see Chapter 13). An abnormal sleep/awake cycle is causative.

Traumatic injury

Traumatic injury remains a common cause of brain dysfunction in dogs and cats (Dewey et al., 1993). Trauma to the brain can occur from exogenous or endogenous conditions. Exogenous injuries most commonly result from automobile trauma; although injuries from gunshot wounds, kicks, animal bites and falls can also occur. All of these insults cause mechanical disruption of the intracranial tissues (primary injury). The primary injury may initiate a number of secondary pathophysiological sequelae such as metabolic alterations in the neuronal or glial cells, impairment of vascular supply to the normal tissues

(ischaemia), impairment of cerebrovascular autoregulation, haemorrhage (intraparenchymal, intraventricular, extradural or subdural), irritation (seizure generation), obstruction of the ventricular system, oedema formation, production of physiologically active products and increased ICP (Bagley, 1996b). For a full discussion on the management of head trauma, the reader is referred to Chapter 20.

Toxic diseases

Numerous toxins can affect the nervous system either primarily or secondarily (Dorman, 1993; Dorman and Fikes, 1993). Primary toxins include organophosphates, metaldehyde, lead, bromethalin and hexachlorophene. A thorough history is essential in the investigation of possible toxin exposure. For further information on toxicities that cause ataxia and tremors, see Chapter 18.

Lead toxicity
Lead toxicity usually results from the ingestion of lead-containing products (e.g. removal of paint containing lead via sanding may produce lead-laden dust. If this dust contaminates the fur of the animal, sufficient lead may be ingested during normal grooming to result in toxicity).

Clinical signs
Nervous system signs of lead toxicity include depression, seizures, ataxia and blindness. Gastrointestinal signs, weight loss and haematological abnormalities may accompany CNS signs.

Pathogenesis
Lead inhibits the sulphydryl group of enzymes, which are important for metabolism.

Diagnosis
The diagnosis is best supported by demonstrating an increased level of lead in the blood.

Treatment and prognosis
Chelation therapy with calcium EDTA or penicillamine may be necessary to improve the clinical signs. Treatment is usually successful.

Avermectin toxicity
Avermectin (particularly ivermectin) administration has been associated with intracranial signs and seizures in dogs (Yas-Natan et al., 2003; Sartor et al., 2004; Snowden et al., 2006; Geyer et al., 2007; Lehner et al., 2009).

Clinical signs
Clinical signs reported in mildly affected animals include salivation, vomiting, tremors, mydriasis, bradycardia, confusion and ataxia. More severely affected animals may have seizures and become comatose, requiring mechanical ventilation. Clinical signs can deteriorate for up to 6 days following subcutaneous administration of ivermectin and take 3 weeks to resolve (Hopper et al., 2002).

Collies and similar breeds are more susceptible to the toxic effects of ivermectin, most likely due to alterations in the cellular transport mechanisms (e.g. P-glycoprotein abnormalities as a result of mutations in the *ABCB1* gene (formerly the multiple drug resistance *(MDR1)* gene)) (Mealey *et al.*, 2001, 2003). Such breeds can therefore develop side effects when administered doses as low as 100 μg/kg (normal dose range: 50-300 μg/kg).

Pathogenesis
Ivermectin is believed to be a GABA agonist that binds to the postsynaptic GABA receptor. Penetration of the CNS is normally poor in mammals unless administered at high doses or given to an animal with a mutation in the *ABCB1* gene.

Diagnosis
The diagnosis is based upon a history of exposure or iatrogenic administration of these drugs. Testing for the *ABCB1* genotype can be performed to evaluate for dysfunctional P-glycoprotein. Some laboratories can assay blood levels of avermectins and, recently, a rapid, sensitive semi-quantitative ElectroSpray Ionization Mass Spectrometry (ESI/MS) method has been developed for ivermectin detection in canine tissue samples (Lehner *et al.*, 2009).

Treatment and prognosis
Treatment focuses on the provision of adequate supportive care, which can mean prolonged mechanical ventilation in severely affected dogs. Additional drug therapy is controversial: temporary (30–90 minutes) reversal of coma can sometimes be achieved by the administration of physostigmine. Picrotoxin (a GABA antagonist) has also been used in one dog to reverse coma: it can improve the level of consciousness but can also cause seizures. Some dogs develop severe tremors and both diazepam and phenobarbital have been used to treat this problem. However, as both of these drugs act at the GABA receptor, there are concerns that this worsens the level of consciousness. In general, if adequate supportive care can be provided, the prognosis is good; although, protected ventilation may be necessary in the most severely affected dogs.

Vascular diseases

Vascular-related conditions are increasingly recognized as a cause of intracranial disease (Garosi *et al.*, 2005, 2006; Garosi and McConnell, 2005; Wessmann *et al.*, 2009; Garosi, 2010; Altay *et al.*, 2011; Gonçalves *et al.*, 2011). A variety of pathological conditions can result in disruption of blood flow to the intracranial structures and cause clinical signs.

Anatomy
The major afferent blood supply to the brain arises from the two internal carotid arteries and the two vertebral arteries in the dog (Figure 9.25). The bilateral sources of blood supply are indirectly joined at the base of the brain by the cerebral arterial circle (circle of Willis). The carotid and vertebral arteries are situated so that the internal carotid arteries and their branches supply the middle and rostral areas of the brain, whilst the branches from the vertebral and basilar arteries supply the caudal cerebral cortex, the cerebellum and the more caudal divisions of the brainstem. The internal carotid and vertebral arteries are joined on each side by the caudal communicating arteries. At the termination of the internal carotid arteries with the circle of Willis, there is a trifurcation which represents the origin of the rostral and middle cerebral arteries as well as the caudal communicating artery (Jenkins, 1978). In addition to the two main sources of blood supply to the brain, in the dog and cat there are large anastomoses between the intracranial and extracranial blood vessels. These extensive anastomoses are the principal reason why catastrophic cerebral vascular accidents are seen less frequently in dogs and cats.

Vascularization in the feline brain is different to that in the canine brain, rendering differences in lesion distribution feasible. In the cat, the arterial circle is supplied by anastomoses with the maxillary and pharyngeal arteries, which arise from the external carotid artery. The proximal portion of the internal carotid artery, which is the main supply vessel in the dog, becomes obliterated in cats soon after birth. The maxillary artery supplies the arterial circle by an anastomosing ramus, which includes a rete mirabile (i.e. a network of fine arterioles). The arterial circle in the cat is not a closed ring because of the lack of a rostral communicating artery, which is normally present in other species (Jenkins, 1978). In addition, the direction of flow in the basilar artery is away from the arterial circle, so maxillary blood from the external carotid artery supplies the entire brain, except for the caudal portion of the brainstem which is supplied by the vertebral arteries (King, 1987).

Clinical signs
The clinical signs reflect an abnormality in the area of the CNS affected and are most commonly acute in onset. Cerebrovascular disease primarily results in ischaemia and haemorrhage. Focal ischaemia or haemorrhage may result in hemiparesis, vestibular signs or visual deficits. Other secondary consequences include oedema formation, mass effect and increased ICP. In addition, behavioural changes, alterations in consciousness, seizures, salivation and CN abnormalities are often present. Signs may be initially progressive as the vascular event results in secondary brain disease and oedema, but are often static after the first 24 hours. If the degree of ischaemia and the associated pathophysiological sequelae are more severe, clinical signs may be rapidly progressive and often fatal.

In a study of 40 dogs with suspected brain infarctions, MRI was used to identify the location of the lesions (Garosi *et al.*, 2006).

- Forebrain (11 of 40 lesions) – clinical signs included abnormal mental status, contralateral postural reaction deficits, contralateral nasal

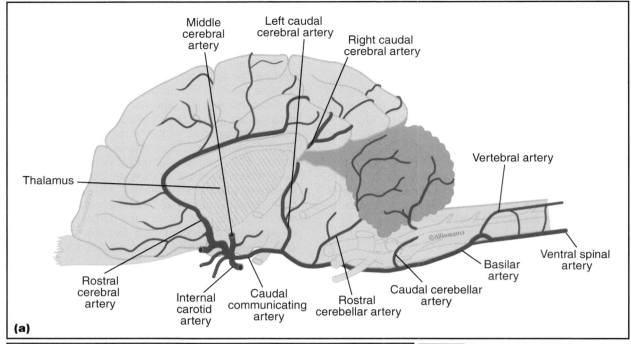

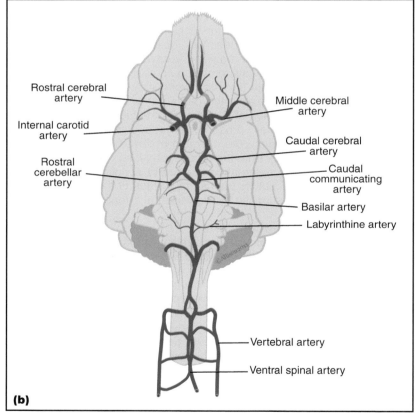

9.25 **(a)** Lateral and **(b)** ventral views of arterial blood supply to the canine brain.

hypoalgesia, contralateral menace deficit and ipsilateral circling.
- Thalamus/midbrain (8 of 40 lesions) – clinical signs included contralateral or ipsilateral postural reaction deficits, contralateral menace deficit, ipsilateral head tilt or turn, nystagmus, ventrolateral strabismus and anisocoria.
- Cerebellum (18 of 40 lesions) – clinical signs included ipsilateral asymmetrical cerebellar ataxia, head tilt, intermittent opisthotonus, nystagmus and ipsilateral menace deficit with apparent normal vision.
- Multifocal (3 of 40 lesions).

In a recent study, MRI was used to identify the location of thalamic infarctions in 16 dogs (Gonçalves *et al.*, 2011). The lesions were grouped into three thalamic regions: paramedian (8 of 16 lesions), extensive dorsal (5 of 16 lesions) and ventrolateral (3 of 16 lesions). Paramedian lesions resulted in clinical signs typical of vestibular dysfunction; whereas, extensive dorsal lesions were associated with vestibular ataxia, circling and contralateral menace response deficits.

Striatocapsular infarctions have been reported in 6 dogs, all of which exhibited acute onset non-progressive homonymous hemianopia (a type of partial blindness resulting in a loss of vision in the same visual field in both eyes), contralateral proprioceptive deficits or hemiparesis and facial hypoalgesia (Rossmeisl et al., 2007).

In a recent study of 16 cats, 7 had ischaemic infarctions, 5 had haemorrhagic infarctions and 4 were diagnosed with intracranial haemorrhage (Altay et al., 2011). The median age was 8 years and 9.5 years in cats with infarctions and intracranial haemorrhage, respectively. Clinical signs were severe, acute, consistent with the localization of the cerebrovascular lesion and influenced by the underlying pathology. Asymmetrical or lateralized clinical signs (including hemiparesis, anisocoria, unilateral menace response and head tilt) were noted in 4 of the 12 cats with infarction.

Pathogenesis

Diseases of the cerebral vasculature may result from excessive blood flow through the cerebral vessels (hypertension), transmural extravasation of blood, ischaemia, thrombosis and embolization (Bagley, 2000; Sager et al., 2009; Wessmann et al., 2009; Garosi, 2010; Hecht and Adams, 2010; Paul et al., 2010; Altay et al., 2011; Cervera et al., 2011; Martin-Vaquero et al., 2011). The common sites of infarction are the corona radiata, internal capsule, the periventricular white matter of the cerebrum and the white matter of the cerebellum. A breed predisposition in spaniels and Greyhounds has been suggested (McConnell et al., 2005; Garosi et al., 2006).

Hypertension (associated with a variety of conditions such as renal disease and hyperadrenocorticism) can result in an increase in cerebrovascular hydrostatic forces leading to intracranial haemorrhage and interstitial oedema. Disorders of coagulation (e.g. disseminated intravascular coagulation, DIC) and platelet (e.g. thrombocytopenia) function can also result in cerebral haemorrhage. Diseases that predispose to hypercoagulability (such as glomerulonephritis) may result in intramural emboli and subsequent thrombosis of cerebral vessels. Bacteraemia (e.g. endocarditis) may predispose to septic embolization of intracranial vessels. Vessel wall integrity can be disrupted by neoplastic infiltration or inflammatory diseases (including vasculitis syndromes) resulting in thrombosis and haemorrhage. Less commonly, arteriovenous malformations and aneurysms have been reported in dogs. All these intracranial vascular abnormalities may predispose to cerebral hypoxia and ischaemia, as well as intracranial haemorrhage. In a study of 33 dogs with brain infarction, a concurrent medical condition was detected in 55% (18 dogs), with chronic kidney disease (24%; 8 dogs) and hyperadrenocorticism (18%; 6 dogs) being most commonly encountered (Garosi et al., 2005). In a recent study, all cats with haemorrhagic infarcts had severe liver pathology, and nephritis was identified in 25% (4 of 16 cats) of cases (Altay et al., 2011).

Ischaemic damage (regardless of cause) results in endothelial cell damage, predisposing to thrombosis, necrosis and haemorrhage. One of the most devastating effects of severe intracranial vascular disease is intracranial haemorrhage. Haemorrhage into and around the brain can result in an associated inflammatory reaction, an overall increase in intracranial contents, and an increase in ICP. Systemic vascular disease (such as bleeding disorders) may also increase the risk of haemorrhagic injury to the brain and, in some instances, nervous system signs occur prior to any obvious systemic signs. Intraventricular bleeding and bleeding into the CSF irritates the local nervous tissue and may result in inflammation (meningitis, myelitis or encephalitis). Haemorrhage into the third ventricle is often associated with fever, most likely due to local alterations in the thermoregulatory centre. If the bleed is substantial, haematomas may be formed. This additional volume within the intracranial space can alter CNS volume/pressure relationships, resulting in increased ICP and decreased cerebral blood flow. Intracranial haemorrhage may also be the first sign of systemic infection with Angiostrongylus vasorum, a lungworm detected in much of Europe and Canada (Garosi et al., 2005; Wessmann et al., 2006; Lowrie et al., 2012). This parasite can cause thrombocytopenia and/or dysfunction of coagulation factors, resembling chronic DIC. Other causes which should be considered include chronic kidney disease and endocrine diseases.

Diagnosis

Cerebrovascular disease should be suspected in any animal with acute neurological signs.

Examination

A thorough physical examination for petechiae is important and should include the mucous membranes (particularly the penis, prepuce and vulva) and retina. Pallor, low grade heart murmurs, weakness and tachycardia are characteristic of large volume haemorrhage into the body cavities as a result of a coagulopathy. Thoracic auscultation for pleural fluid and abdominal palpation for haemoperitoneum are important. Radiography and ultrasonography may be useful when the physical examination is unrewarding but a large volume of internal bleeding is suspected. Large amounts of blood can be lost through the gastrointestinal tract, so examination of the stool for haematochezia and melaena should be performed. Blood pressure measurement (via either direct or indirect methods) should be undertaken to determine whether hypertension is present. A faecal examination should be performed to rule out Angiostrongylus infection.

Haematology and biochemistry

A complete blood count, with particular reference to red blood cell and platelet counts, is often helpful. Specific coagulation testing (e.g. bleeding time, prothrombin time, partial thromboplastin time and fibrin degradation products) is also commonly performed. A biochemical panel to evaluate for the presence of a hypercoagulability (such as proteinuria) should be undertaken.

Imaging studies

As cerebrovascular disease often alters the structural integrity of the brain, clarification of the cause of the clinical signs tends to require advanced imaging studies (such as CT and MRI) (Hecht and Adams, 2010; Paul *et al.*, 2010). The imaging characteristics of cerebrovascular disease may vary depending upon the degree of disease (e.g. ischaemia versus overt haemorrhage) and the time between the onset of clinical signs and the imaging studies being performed.

Small vessel damage without overt haemorrhage most commonly causes cerebral oedema, but can result in no acute imaging abnormalities. If overt infarction or haemorrhage occurs, oedema may be seen in association with a cerebral mass effect.

Ischaemia:

Computed tomography: CT images are frequently normal during the acute phase of ischaemia; therefore, the diagnosis of ischaemic stroke relies upon the exclusion of other diseases. Early CT signs of ischaemia include:

* Parenchymal hypoattenuation
* Loss of differentiation between the grey and white matter
* Subtle effacement of the cortical sulci
* Local mass effect.

Magnetic resonance imaging: On MR images, the appearance of cerebrovascular disease varies from a focal mass to diffuse or multifocal changes. Conventional MRI can be used to visualize ischaemic stroke within 12–24 hours of the onset of clinical signs and to distinguish haemorrhagic lesions from infarction (Figure 9.26). T2-weighted and FLAIR MR images are particularly useful as they allow evaluation of the anatomy of the brain and depict oedema, old infarcts, microangiopathic changes, tumours and other pathology. With these sequences, ischaemic infarction appears as a hyperintense lesion. Often there is evidence of oedema (which may be cytotoxic or vasogenic) in the area of the cerebrovascular damage. Typically, a wedge-shaped lesion is visible with the point of the wedge directed centrally. In addition, T2-weighted (gradient echo) images are used to rule in or out the presence of intracranial haemorrhage.

Contrast enhancement following gadolinium administration depends on the interval between the vascular damage and the MRI examination, the resulting inflammatory response, and the degree of vascular disruption (break in the blood–brain barrier). In most

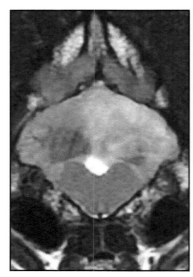

9.26 Transverse T2-weighted MR image of a dog following the sudden onset of cerebello-vestibular dysfunction. There is a well defined region of hyperintensity within the cerebellar parenchyma compatible with ischaemic infarction.

cases, imaging studies are performed within 48 hours following the insult due to the severity of the clinical signs and thus contrast enhancement is uncommon. When present, contrast enhancement of cerebrovascular lesions is minimal, heterogeneous and peripheral or ring-like. In addition, focal inflammatory brain disease and some neoplastic lesions (such as gliomas) may have a similar appearance on MR images (Cervera *et al.*, 2011).

Diffusion and perfusion MRI are new techniques that monitor water transport in the microenvironment at the cellular or capillary level and can be used to more definitively diagnose ischaemia. These techniques provide complementary information about the pathophysiological processes that occur following cerebral ischaemia. Diffusion-weighted imaging (DWI) has improved sensitivity and specificity for the diagnosis of acute stroke, making it the ideal sequence for positive identification of hyperacute stroke (Figure 9.27). The temporal evolution of the DWI signal also allows discrimination of acute and chronic lesions.

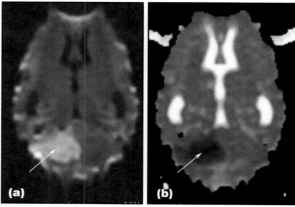

9.27 **(a)** Dorsal diffusion-weighted MR image of the same dog as in Figure 9.26. A focal hyperintense lesion (arrowed) is visible, compatible with oedema related to ischaemia. **(b)** The lesion (arrowed) appears hypointense on apparent diffusion coefficient (ADC) mapping, confirming the presence of an ischaemic infarction.

Haemorrhage:

Computed tomography: CT is very sensitive for the detection of acute haemorrhage, which appears as a hyperdensity due to the hyperattenuation of X-rays by the globin portion of blood. The attenuation decreases until the haematoma is isodense (approximately 1 month after onset). The periphery of the haematoma enhances following contrast medium administration from 6 days to 6 weeks after onset due to revascularization.

Magnetic resonance imaging: On MR images, haemorrhage <12–24 hours old cannot be differentiated from vasogenic oedema (Figure 9.28). In the blood circulation, haemoglobin is present in either an oxyhaemoglobin or deoxyhaemoglobin state. The heme iron in both oxyhaemoglobin and deoxyhaemoglobin is in the ferrous (Fe^{2+}) state. When haemoglobin is removed from the high oxygen environment of the blood circulation, the heme iron undergoes oxidation to the ferric (Fe^{3+}) state, forming methaemoglobin. Continued oxidative denaturation results in the formation of ferric hemichromes (haemosiderin).

As the red blood cells break down, the various forms of haemoglobin (which have different paramagnetic properties) influence the appearance of the clot on MRI. As different regions of the haemorrhage may contain haemoglobin at different stages

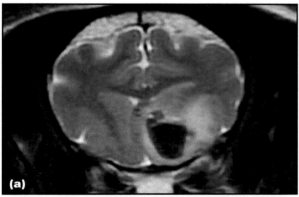
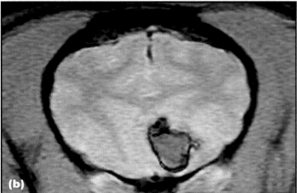

9.28 **(a)** Transverse T2-weighted MR image of the brain of a dog with a haemorrhagic lesion. The lesion appears as an area of hypointensity or signal void. Note also the peri-lesional hyperintensity compatible with oedema. **(b)** Gradient echo MR image showing the lesion as a hypointense structure, confirming the presence of haem.

of breakdown, a heterogeneous appearance to the lesion can be encountered. In addition to the form of haemoglobin present, the signal intensity of a blood clot may vary depending upon the operating field strength, the type of sequence and the technique used. The appearance of the haemorrhage may also vary depending on where the bleed originated (e.g. subdural, intraparenchymal or subarachnoid location). However, most infarcts in dogs are not associated with an appreciable haemorrhage.

Treatment

Therapy for cerebrovascular disease includes management of any predisposing factors as well as treatment of the secondary intracranial consequences such as haemorrhage and oedema. These secondary consequences often result in an increase in ICP and subsequent decrease in cerebral blood flow. Treatment to decrease elevated ICP often restores cerebral blood flow (see Chapter 20 for further information). However, if haemorrhage is a component of the disease process, then an increase in cerebral blood flow may perpetuate active haemorrhage and worsen the clinical course.

Treatment for a localized haematoma within the CNS involves surgical evacuation, usually via craniectomy. If the underlying bleeding disorder is still active, a dilemma exists between the need for surgical drainage of the haematoma and the risk of causing increased haemorrhage. Short-term haemostatic support with blood products or platelets may provide a window of patient stability for the surgical procedure to be performed. Ultimately, if the accumulation of blood within the CNS becomes life-threatening, surgical drainage is a necessity that is undertaken in view of the increased risk of haemorrhagic complications.

Whilst it is impossible to reverse all of the effects of the haemorrhage, decreasing the size of an expanding haematoma with the resultant decrease in nervous system pressure may improve clinical signs. However, the following should be considered:

- By decreasing the intraparenchymal pressure, blood flow to the area may be restored and a rebound haemorrhage may occur
- If the original cause of the bleeding was a ruptured vessel (aneurysm or arteriovenous malformation), removal of the haematoma may result in the bleed restarting.

However, in both of these situations, haemostasis can hopefully be employed intraoperatively to decrease this possibility.

Hypertensive encephalopathy

Systemic hypertension is increasingly recognized in small animals. The pathological effect of systemic hypertension on tissues is referred to as target organ damage. Target organ damage can result when the systolic blood pressure reaches 150–160 mmHg. A variety of tissues can be affected, including the kidneys, eyes, cardiovascular system and the CNS.

Hypertensive encephalopathy is well recognized in humans. In addition to the observation of systemic hypertension concurrently with CNS dysfunction, the best criterion for confirming the diagnosis is resolution of the clinical signs with appropriate anti-hypertensive therapy. The clinical signs of hypertensive encephalopathy are often reversible, with resolution of the neurological signs occurring within hours to the first few days following initiation of therapy. Given the reversibility of the clinical signs and the anatomical distribution of the pathology in the caudal portion of the cerebellum, hypertensive encephalopathy in humans is often referred to as posterior reversible encephalopathy. Although underlying hypertension is present in the majority of cases, 20–30% of affected individuals are normotensive at the time of diagnosis.

Hypertensive encephalopathy has been reported in dogs and cats (O'Neill *et al.*, 2012). It is associated with either an acute (>30 mmHg from resting level) or a sustained (>180 mmHg) elevation in systolic arterial blood pressure. The clinical signs reflect involvement of the prosencephalon and include seizures, altered mentation and blindness. In addition, signs may also relate to dysfunction of the CNS structures of the caudal fossa and include altered mentation, vestibular or cerebellar ataxia and abnormal nystagmus.

Although the pathogenesis of hypertensive encephalopathy is not completely understood, the most widely held explanation suggests that the lesions are probably the consequence of vasogenic and interstitial cerebral oedema, which occurs as a result of failed autoregulation of the cerebral vasculature. When the myogenic autoregulatory mechanisms for cerebral perfusion are compromised, hyperperfusion ensues. Hyperperfusion results in alteration of the blood–brain barrier, leading to development of vasogenic oedema. An alternative explanation has been proposed in humans – lesions may be the consequence of initial hypoperfusion secondary to a systemic inflammatory response and endothelial activation and injury. Consequently, systemic vasoconstriction ensues to increase perfusion and reverse brain hypoxaemia. Autoregulatory vasoconstriction in response to the initial hypoperfusion may further reduce brain perfusion and induce ischaemia, which leads to the development of oedema.

Vasogenic oedema typically results in an increased signal intensity within the white matter on T2-weighted MR images. In addition, lesions related to vasogenic oedema are hyperintense on both DWI and apparent diffusion coefficient (ADC) mapping, which suggests a T2 shine through phenomenon related to restricted diffusion of protons (stationary protons). In contrast, cytotoxic oedema results in a hyperintensity on DWI and a hypointensity on ADC mapping. Hyperintensity of the white matter of the cerebrum has been observed on both DWI and ADC mapping with hypertensive encephalopathy in humans and dogs (O'Neill *et al.*, 2012).

Feline ischaemic encephalopathy

Feline ischaemic encephalopathy has historically been classified as a vascular disorder and involves ischaemic necrosis of the cerebral hemisphere in cats (deLahunta and Glass, 2008). The infarction is usually located in the area of the brain supplied by the middle cerebral artery; however, vascular lesions are infrequently found at necropsy. The cause of this condition is unknown; although, there is speculation that in some cats it may be related to the migration of *Cuterebra* larvae (Glass *et al.*, 1998).

References and further reading

Available on accompanying DVD

DVD extras

- 'Fly-biting'
- Hydrocephalus
- Neuronal ceroid lipofuscinosis
- Portosystemic shunt
- Severe depression (1)
- Severe depression (2)

10

Disorders of eyes and vision

Jacques Penderis

The neuro-ophthalmological examination combines aspects of the neurological examination and ophthalmic assessment in order to identify ophthalmic disorders arising from diseases affecting the nervous system. From a neurological viewpoint, the visual system is both fascinating and unique, in that the retina and optic disc are the only components of the nervous system directly visible in the normal patient. Therefore, even in the absence of overt neuro-ophthalmological abnormalities, a thorough evaluation of the eyes, including a fundic examination, should always be performed in the neurological patient, as the underlying cause of the neurological disease may be evident. This is particularly important with inflammatory and infectious central nervous system (CNS) diseases (Figure 10.1). Conversely, a full neurological examination should be performed in any animal with ocular abnormalities that do not have an obvious ophthalmic cause.

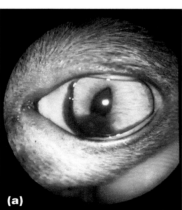

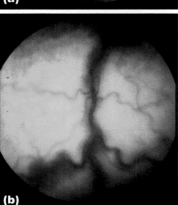

10.1 Evaluation of the eyes should be performed even when neuro-ophthalmological abnormalities are not suspected. The **(a)** anterior uveitis and **(b)** retinal vasculitis evident in this cat with episodes of opisthotonus are suggestive of infection, most probably with feline coronavirus (the causative agent of feline infectious peritonitis, FIP). FIP was confirmed at post-mortem examination. (Courtesy of J Mould, Eye Veterinary Practice)

Terminology

Terms that are commonly used in clinical neuro-ophthalmology include:

- Anisocoria – pupils of unequal or asymmetrical size
- Blepharospasm – spasm of the orbicularis oculi muscle
- Consensual (indirect) pupillary light reflex (PLR) – application of a light stimulus to one eye causing reflex constriction of the opposite pupil
- Direct PLR – application of a light stimulus to one eye causing reflex constriction of the ipsilateral pupil
- Enophthalmos – abnormal displacement or sinking of the eyeball into the orbit
- Esotropia – convergent strabismus: deviation of the visual axis of one or both eyes toward that of the opposite eye (also called cross-eye)
- Exophthalmos – abnormal displacement or protrusion of the eyeball out of the orbit
- Exotropia – divergent strabismus: deviation of the visual axis of one or both eyes away from that of the opposite eye (also called wall-eye)
- Miosis – abnormal or excessive constriction of the pupil
- Miotic – drug or agent that causes pupillary constriction
- Mydriasis – abnormal or excessive dilatation of the pupil
- Mydriatic – drug or agent that causes pupillary dilation
- Nystagmus – rhythmical, involuntary movements of the eyeball with either fast and slow phases (jerk nystagmus) or, less commonly, equal oscillations (pendular nystagmus)
- Ophthalmoplegia – paralysis of the eye muscles
- Ophthalmoplegia interna – paralysis of the iris and ciliary muscles
- Ophthalmoplegia externa – paralysis of the extraocular muscles
- Opsoclonus – rapid, uncontrolled and unpredictable eye movements in multiple directions
- Pan-ophthalmoplegia – paralysis of the iris, ciliary muscles and extraocular muscles (also called total ophthalmoplegia)
- Pupillary light reflex (PLR) – also called the photomotor reflex
- Ptosis – abnormal or paralytic drooping of the upper eyelid
- Saccade – rapid, simultaneous eye movements with both eyes moving in the same direction. Saccades allow rapid eye fixation on an object of interest during rapid eye movements and the fast phase of jerk nystagmus
- Strabismus – abnormal deviation of the visual axis of the eye that the animal cannot overcome
- Xeromycteria – abnormal dryness of the nasal mucous membrane and planum.

Neuro-ophthalmological assessment

Before performing a detailed neuro-ophthalmological examination, it is essential first to observe the animal from a distance. This allows assessment of the patient's interaction with its surroundings, giving an indication as to the level of consciousness, as well as evaluation of any localizing signs (e.g. circling, hypermetria or head tilt). Identifying animals with decreased levels of consciousness is important, as these animals may respond inappropriately to tests requiring conscious input without there actually being a lesion within the pathway being tested.

Vision

Vision is supplied by cranial nerve (CN) II (optic nerve). The structure of the retina is detailed in Figure 10.2. The optic nerve supplies conscious perception of vision as well as visual input into unconscious reflex pathways, including the PLR, visual startle reflex and dazzle reflex. The visual pathways are demonstrated in Figure 10.3. As part of the hands-off assessment, vision should be appraised by observing the animal interacting with and negotiating a strange environment (usually the consulting room) and navigating an obstacle course, and by performing the tracking response (evaluating whether the patient is able visually to follow moving but silent objects, such as a dropped piece of cotton wool).

The clinical assessment of vision includes the following:

- Visual placing response – the patient is held under its chest and brought up towards a table edge, but without letting the thoracic limbs touch the table. The normal patient should see the table and attempt to place its thoracic limbs on the surface of the table. This test assesses vision, appropriate mentation and the postural control of the forelimbs, and is particularly useful in smaller patients
- Menace response – this learned response may not be present in normal animals <12 weeks of age. The test is performed by making a threatening movement towards each eye in turn whilst closing the other eye, without touching the patient (Figure 10.4). The normal response is for the patient to blink, with or without aversion of the head. Motor innervation of the muscles responsible for the blink is via the facial nerve (CN VII) and this test therefore also assesses the integrity of the facial nerve and cortical awareness (Figure 10.5). The menace response is coordinated in the cerebellum, and lesions of the cerebellum may result in ipsilateral loss of the menace response without loss of vision (Figure 10.6). The menace response is a cortical response and therefore may be abnormal (without a lesion in the visual pathways) in animals with a reduced level of consciousness
- Pupillary light reflex (PLR)
- Chromatic PLR
- Swinging flashlight test
- Dazzle reflex

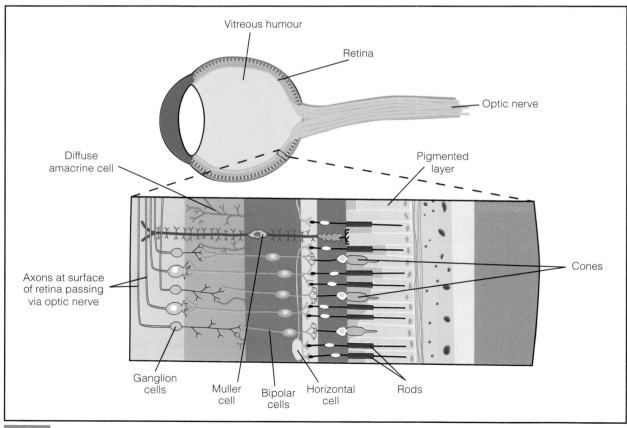

10.2   Structure of the retina.

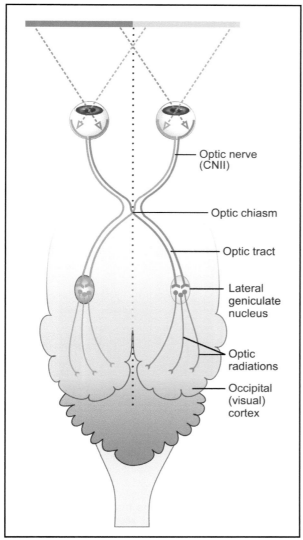

10.3 The visual pathways demonstrating how each side of the visual field is represented within the opposite occipital (visual) cortex. As the degree of binocular vision in different species decreases, so a greater proportion of optic nerve fibres decussate at the optic chiasm. (© Jacques Penderis)

Labels: Optic nerve (CNII); Optic chiasm; Optic tract; Lateral geniculate nucleus; Optic radiations; Occipital (visual) cortex

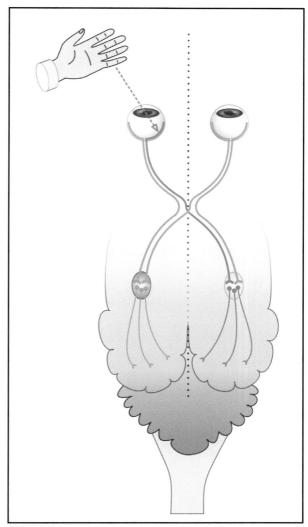

10.4 The menace response is assessed by making a threatening movement towards each eye in turn. Usually the visual stimulus is only directed at the nasal retina and not the temporal (lateral) retina and therefore only assesses the contralateral visual cortex. (© Jacques Penderis)

- Visual startle reflex – this subcortical reflex (also called the visual body reflex) represents reflex movements of the head and visual axis in the direction of a sudden visual stimulus
- Assessment of pupil size and symmetry – used to check for anisocoria and should include evaluation in both the light and the dark.

Pupillary light reflex

The size of the aperture of the iris (the pupil) is determined by a combination of the tone of the pupillary constrictors and the pupillary dilators. Constriction of the pupil is mediated by parasympathetic innervation via CN III (oculomotor nerve). Dilatation of the pupil is mediated by the sympathetic nervous system.

The PLR (the constriction of the pupil in response to light) tests the integrity of the parasympathetic pathway. It is supplied by CN II and the parasympathetic portion of CN III. The PLR evaluates the afferent visual pathways from the retina to just prior to the lateral geniculate nuclei in the thalamus (Figure 10.7), whilst the efferent outflow is mediated via the parasympathetic portion of CN III. The PLR is tested by shining a bright light into the pupil and assessing for constriction (direct reflex). The opposite pupil should constrict at the same time (consensual reflex), but it is not necessary to assess the consensual reflex if the direct reflex is intact in both eyes. However, excessive sympathetic tone (e.g. as seen in a very nervous animal) may antagonize the light stimulus and result in a PLR that appears reduced. A common cause of apparent failure of the PLR is using a light that is not bright enough in a nervous animal with high resting sympathetic tone.

The normal direct PLR response is initial pupillary constriction followed by slight dilatation. The

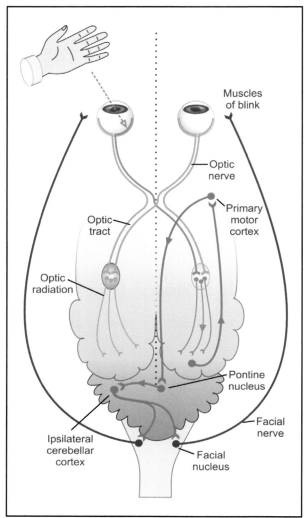

10.5 The menace response pathway – a lesion interrupting any part of the pathway may result in a menace deficit. (© Jacques Penderis)

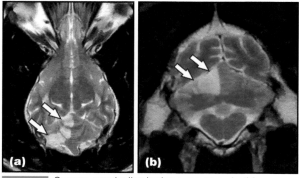

10.6 Severe cerebellar lesions, as seen in this example of a cerebrovascular incident within the right cerebellum, may result in ipsilateral loss of the menace response without causing visual or facial nerve deficits. (© Jacques Penderis)

degree of dilatation increases with decreasing brightness of light stimulation and with longer stimulation times: this is termed pupillary escape and is the consequence of light adaptation of the photoreceptors. It has been suggested that the PLR

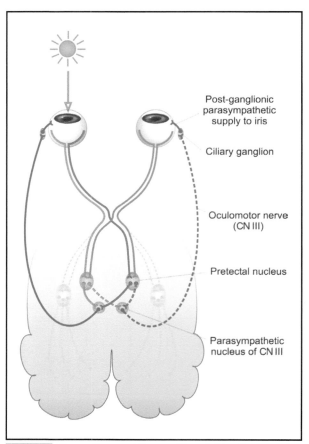

10.7 The pathway of the pupillary light reflex (divergence of the conscious visual pathway is detailed in light grey). (© Jacques Penderis)

requires fewer intact axons than conscious perception of vision and in partial lesions the situation may exist where there is loss of vision but the PLR is spared (Ferreira and Peterson-Jones, 2002).

Chromatic pupillary light reflex
In normal dogs, pupillary constriction occurs at low light intensities of both red and blue light, mediated via the rod and cone PLR. Following discrete loss of rod and cone cells (typically seen with sudden acquired retinal degeneration, SARD), there is loss of the PLR at low light intensities. However, the PLR is still evident in dogs with SARD at high blue light intensities. This occurs via the intrinsic, melanospin-mediated, retinal ganglion cell-mediated PLR. The chromatic PLR is therefore used to confirm that acute blindness is due to SARD when a PLR is still present at high light intensities. The PLR in dogs with SARD is elicited using light wavelengths within the melanopsin-sensitive light spectrum (blue light: ideal wavelength = 480 nm), but is absent when red light (ideal wavelength = 630 nm) is used. This implies the loss of the rod and cone-mediated PLR (Grozdanic *et al.*, 2007).

Swinging flashlight test
The swinging flashlight test, a variation of the PLR, allows evaluation of both the direct and consensual PLR. The test is performed by 'swinging' the light

stimulus from one eye to the other. If both the direct and consensual PLRs are intact, as the light stimulus is swung from one eye to the other each pupil can be seen to be already constricted as the light stimulus is directed at it (consensual response) and continue to remain constricted for the duration of the direct stimulus (direct response). As the pupil being directly stimulated tends to constrict to a slightly greater extent than the contralateral pupil, slight further constriction may be evident as the light stimulus is directed at each eye.

Dazzle reflex

The dazzle reflex (Figure 10.8), supplied by CNs II and VII, is similar to the PLR in that it does not evaluate the cortical aspects of the visual pathway. In contrast to the PLR, in which the efferent arm is mediated by the oculomotor nerve, the efferent pathway of the dazzle reflex is mediated via the facial nerve. The reflex is induced by flashing a very bright light into the eyes with the normal response being a blink response or blepharospasm. Loss of the dazzle reflex implies a subcortical lesion. Cortical lesions causing blindness may, in some cases, result in an exaggerated dazzle reflex through disinhibition due to loss of upper motor neuron (UMN) innervation.

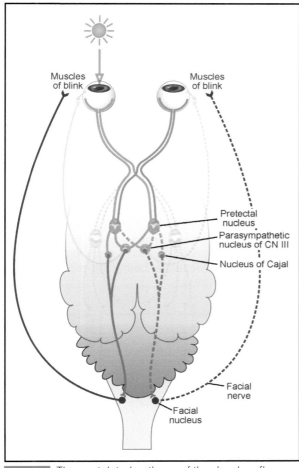

10.8 The postulated pathway of the dazzle reflex – a subcortical reflex blink associated with a bright light stimulus. (© Jacques Penderis)

Extraocular muscular control of eyeball position and movement

The parasympathetic portion of the oculomotor nerve supplies the iris muscle for the PLR as well as the ciliary muscle (see Figure 10.7). The oculomotor nerve also supplies motor innervation to the extraocular muscles (including the dorsal, medial and ventral rectus muscles and the ventral oblique muscle of the eyeball) and the levator palpebra muscle of the upper eyelid. The trochlear nerve (CN IV) innervates the dorsal oblique muscle. The abducent nerve (CN VI) innervates the lateral rectus and retractor bulbi muscles. The innervation to the extraocular muscles is detailed in Figure 10.9.

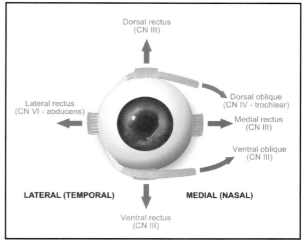

10.9 Innervation of the extraocular muscles (besides the retractor bulbi and levator palpebrae muscles). (© Jacques Penderis)

The innervation to the extraocular muscles can be assessed individually but it is more usual to assess them together, as in most cases CN III is affected in isolation or all three nerves are affected together (resulting in external ophthalmoplegia). Assessing eyeball movement is achieved by:

- Observing the eye movements as the patient looks around voluntarily and in response to induced movements (by holding the head fixed and creating a distraction on either side to see if the animal can appropriately fix its gaze on the visual stimulus in a bilaterally coordinated fashion)
- Assessing the eyes for any asymmetry of the visual axis between the left and right eyes (strabismus or squint)
- Evaluating the innervation to the retractor bulbi muscles (innervated by the abducent nerve) by observing for retraction of the globe during the corneal reflex (stimulated by touching the cornea – sensation is mediated via the ophthalmic branch of the trigeminal nerve (CN V))
- Retropulsion of eyeball to assess for the presence of a retrobulbar mass.

The normal eye movements can be further evaluated by inducing physiological nystagmus (vestibulo-ocular reflex, which also evaluates the vestibulocochlear nerve (CN VIII)). The evaluation of physiological nystagmus is detailed below under vestibular control of eyeball position and movement. The absence of normal physiological nystagmus indicates a vestibular lesion, a lesion affecting the extraocular muscles (or their innervation) or a lesion affecting the connection between the two.

Vestibular control of eyeball position and movement

Vestibular control of eyeball position and movement is supplied by the vestibulocochlear nerve. There is a close association between the vestibular system and the innervation of the extraocular muscles, which allows an animal to keep its gaze fixed on an object despite changes in head position. When the head is moved from side to side or up and down at a steady rate without the gaze being fixed on a single object, a nystagmus is induced with the fast phase movements of the eyeball being in the direction of head movement. This nystagmus is termed physiological nystagmus or the vestibulo-ocular reflex. These normal vestibular eye movements are independent of vision and are normally still present in animals with acquired visual loss. Physiological nystagmus allows the gaze to jump from object to object and to follow the object as the visual field moves past, instead of the visual input recording a constant blur of passing information. Physiological nystagmus should stop once the head movement stops. An exception to this is where the head movement continues for a prolonged period in the same direction and at a constant speed, such as being spun on a revolving chair. In this situation the vestibular system has time to adapt, with the physiological nystagmus stopping during the constant movement but briefly restarting when the speed or direction of movement changes or movement is stopped.

In contrast to normal physiological nystagmus, lesions affecting vestibular input to the extraocular muscles may result in a static alteration in gaze direction (strabismus or squint) or involuntary eye movements (nystagmus). The vestibular control of eyeball position and movement is therefore assessed by evaluating for strabismus, spontaneous nystagmus and the presence of normal physiological nystagmus. This should include elevating the animal's head (with the ears level) and holding it briefly elevated to see if a strabismus can be induced, as well as altering the animal's position (including turning it on its back) to assess for positional nystagmus. Other features of vestibular disease and associated CN deficits, including concurrent ipsilateral hearing deficits, facial nerve paresis and Horner's syndrome, may be present. With central (brainstem) lesions, other CNs and the ascending proprioceptive and descending motor tracts to the limbs or the cerebellum may be affected.

Somatosensory innervation of the eyeball and eyelid

The three branches of CN V (maxillary, mandibular and ophthalmic) are responsible for sensory information from the entire face (Figure 10.10a). The ophthalmic and maxillary branches also supply sensory information from the nasal mucosa, and the ophthalmic branch provides sensory information from the skin on the inner surface of the nostrils via the nasociliary nerve. In addition, the mandibular branch provides motor innervation to the masticatory muscles (masseter, temporal, pterygoids, rostral digastrics and mylohyoid) (Figure 10.10b).

The ophthalmic branch of the trigeminal nerve is evaluated by performing the palpebral and corneal reflexes and assessing the cutaneous sensation to the inner surface of the nostrils. The palpebral reflex is evaluated by touching the medial canthus of the eye and observing for the presence of a blink (mediated by CN VII); the response to touching the lateral canthus is variable and probably innervated by the maxillary branch. The corneal reflex is evaluated by holding the eyelids open and lightly touching the cornea with a finger or cotton swab. The normal response to the corneal reflex is to retract the globe (mediated by CN VI) and prolapse the third eyelid. A more objective assessment of corneal sensation can be obtained using a corneal aesthesiometer: both contact and non-contact corneal aesthesiometers are available (Golebiowski et al., 2011). However, it should be noted that differences exist between the different types of corneal aesthesiometer; thus, the readings are not comparable. Differences also exist between canine breeds (with dolichocephalic breeds being more sensitive than brachycephalic breeds) and regions of the cornea (with the centre being the most sensitive) (Barret et al., 1991).

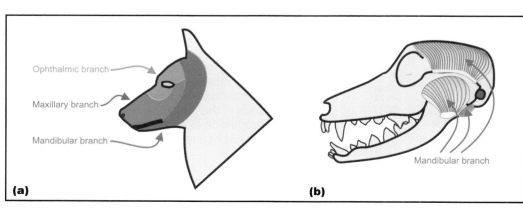

10.10 **(a)** Sensory innervation fields of the three branches of the trigeminal nerve. **(b)** Motor innervation of the mandibular branch of the trigeminal nerve to the muscles of mastication. (© Jacques Penderis)

Motor control of the eyelids

The motor innervation to the blink is supplied by CN VII, which also innervates the other muscles of facial expression, supplies parasympathetic innervation to (amongst other structures) the lacrimal gland and lateral nasal gland, and provides sensation to the rostral two-thirds of the tongue and inner surface of the pinna. The parasympathetic innervation to the lacrimal gland splits from the facial nerve in the facial canal just prior to the close approximation between the facial nerve and tympanic bulla.

Normal function of facial nerve innervation to the orbicularis oculi muscles controlling the blink is assessed by:

- Observing the animal for normal blinking
- The menace response
- The palpebral reflex.

Lacrimal gland function

The lacrimal gland is supplied by the sensory portion of CN V and the parasympathetic portion of CN VII. The parasympathetic portion of CN VII also innervates the lateral nasal gland (a serous secreting gland that functions to keep the nose moist). The normal function of facial nerve innervation to the lacrimal gland is assessed by performing a Schirmer tear test and examining the ipsilateral nostril for dryness.

There are two main types of tear production in veterinary species: basal tear production (keeps the cornea moist) and reflex tear production. Increased reflex tear production occurs in response to sensory stimuli (including direct corneal stimulation and exposure to cold and irritants) via the ophthalmic branch of the trigeminal nerve. Trigeminal lesions resulting in corneal anaesthesia do not usually affect basal tear production, but reflex tear production in response to corneal, conjunctival or nasal stimulation is lost. Blinking to spread the tear film in response to corneal drying is also reduced in animals with trigeminal lesions.

Sympathetic innervation to the eye and face

The sympathetic innervation to the head and eye is detailed in Figure 10.11. The pathway consists of first, second and third order neurons, with the first order neurons originating in the hypothalamus and rostral midbrain and travelling down the tectotegmental spinal tract. The first order neurons synapse with the second order neurons in the lateral horn of the spinal cord grey matter at the level of T1–T3. The second order axons then leave the spinal cord with the T1–T3 nerve roots. The brachial plexus, which innervates the thoracic limb, comprises contributions from nerve roots C6–T1 (and sometimes T2); part of the sympathetic supply leaving the spinal cord is therefore closely associated with innervation of the thoracic limb.

The sympathetic axons separate from the T1–T3 nerve roots as the ramus communicans and form the thoracic sympathetic trunk. The sympathetic trunk courses cranially in close apposition to the descending vagus nerve (CN X), together forming the vagosympathetic trunk within the carotid sheath. The sympathetic axons course rostrally through the caudal cervical ganglion and synapse in the cranial cervical ganglion, adjacent to the tympanic bulla. From here the third order sympathetic axons pass through the middle ear and enter the cranial cavity with the glossopharyngeal nerve (CN IX), then pass close to the cavernous sinus with the carotid artery, before leaving the cranial cavity via the orbital fissure in close approximation to the ophthalmic branch of the trigeminal nerve. The sympathetic supply to the eye and face innervates smooth muscle in the iris (dilator muscle), orbit, upper and lower eyelids (Müller's muscle), third eyelid and walls of blood vessels in the head. The effect is to contribute to the control of pupil and palpebral fissure size and maintain smooth muscle tone within the orbit (affecting eyeball position and third eyelid protrusion).

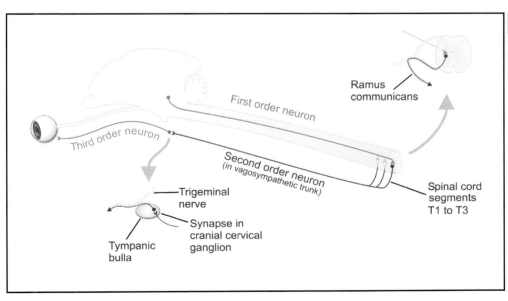

10.11 The pathway of the sympathetic innervation to the eye and adjacent structures of the head. (© Jacques Penderis)

Pharmacological evaluation of pupil function

Pharmacological testing of pupil function may be useful in two situations:

1. To confirm the neurological nature of a lesion, i.e. whether it is a sympathetic dysfunction (Horner's syndrome) or a parasympathetic dysfunction. However, in most cases the nature of the lesion can be ascertained based on the characteristic appearance and response of the pupils to light stimuli and the dark, and pharmacological testing is not required. Examination of pupil function must always be performed prior to pharmacological testing.
2. To ascertain the site of lesions affecting the efferent arm of the PLR and the sympathetic supply to the eye (Horner's syndrome). However, pharmacological testing is not an exact science and the time to a response should be used only as a guide to the site of the lesion. There are differences in opinion on the utility of this form of testing and, in particular, on the concentration of drugs used.

The basis of the tests lies in the development of denervation hypersensitivity (Rosenblueth and Cannon, 1936). There are a number of considerations when performing pharmacological testing:

- Testing should always be performed in both eyes, using the normal eye as a comparison
- The pharmacological agent should be instilled into the conjunctival sac at an equal volume and concentration in both eyes. A second dose should be instilled after a few minutes in case the first dose was washed away by induced tear production
- Contact with or manipulation of the eye should be avoided during pharmacological testing as this can affect drug absorption or induce tear production, which may dilute the pharmacological agent
- The light intensity and degree of stimulus should remain constant throughout the test.

Pharmacological testing of the sympathetic nervous system is discussed in more detail under Horner's syndrome. Lesions affecting the efferent arm of the PLR (parasympathetic lesions producing mydriasis) can be localized further by application of direct and indirect parasympathomimetics.

- The use of a direct parasympathomimetic (0.1% pilocarpine drops) may allow confirmation of a parasympathetic lesion and differentiation between pre- and post-ganglionic lesions. Iris constriction occurs rapidly in the affected eye with post-ganglionic lesions due to denervation hypersensitivity, but has little effect on the normal eye (Antonio-Santos *et al.*, 2005). The test depends on achieving a specific concentration of pilocarpine at the iris and therefore a formulation that includes a vehicle to enhance corneal penetration (e.g. benzalkonium chloride) should be used (Carter, 1979). In human patients false-positive responses are more common with pilocarpine concentrations >0.2%, and false-negative responses may occur at concentrations <0.05% (Younge and Bruski, 1976). In practice this test is often non-specific, with a response indicating only that the lesion is neurological, rather than specifying the site. For example, this test can be used to differentiate mydriasis due to iris disease or pharmacological blockade from atropine or atropine-like substances (both of which are unresponsive to pilocarpine) from neurological disease (Scagliotti, 2000). Topical pilocarpine can be irritant to the eye and may induce a blepharospasm that can last up to 12 hours; owners should be warned of this prior to performing the test.
- Differentiation between pre- and post-ganglionic lesions (ciliary ganglion) can be achieved by the topical administration of an indirect parasympathomimetic (0.5% physostigmine drops). Physostigmine inhibits cholinesterase, thereby increasing the concentration of acetylcholine at the neuromuscular junction. If the post-ganglionic neuron is preserved, it apparently releases low levels of acetylcholine continuously, the local concentration of which is increased by application of physostigmine. With pre-ganglionic lesions, iris constriction occurs before the control eye due to denervation hypersensitivity. However, with post-ganglionic lesions, physostigmine has no effect. Physostigmine causes peak pupil constriction at 30 minutes in human patients, with a return to normal at around 90 minutes. If neither pupil responds, the test is considered a false-negative and must be repeated.

Electrophysiological evaluation of the visual system

Electrophysiological evaluation of the visual system largely comprises electroretinography and visual evoked potentials (VEPs – also called visual evoked responses).

Electroretinography

Electroretinography tests retinal function and assesses both the rod and cone photoreceptors. It is useful for the identification of blindness due to retinal disease where the retina appears normal on ophthalmic examination (e.g. SARD). Electroretinography can be performed under general anaesthesia, or under sedation in a cooperative patient (see **Electroretinography** clip on DVD). A corneal contact lens electrode is used to record retinal voltage changes that occur in response to a defined flash of light or repeated flashes of light. The response is expressed as a waveform, with a and b waves most commonly recorded. The waveform and, in particular, the amplitude and latency of the a and b waves are measured when evaluating the electroretinogram (ERG) (Figure 10.12).

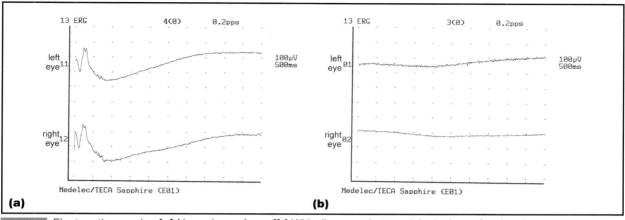

10.12 Electroretinography. **(a)** Normal waveform. **(b)** With diseases that result in the loss of rod and cone photoreceptors, the normal waveform is abolished. (© Jacques Penderis)

Visual evoked potentials

VEPs are recordings of occipital cortex potentials, which arise in response to brief flashes of light. VEPs are recorded using electrodes attached to the scalp and signal averaging techniques. The resulting waveform can be used to assess the function of the central retinal region and post-retinal structures, including the optic nerve, optic tracts and visual cortex. The VEP is largely a research procedure and its use in clinical neuro-ophthalmology is limited, but in generalized CNS disorders the VEP may be used to infer white matter conduction velocity within the CNS by determining conduction velocity within the optic nerve.

Magnetic resonance imaging and cerebrospinal fluid analysis

Magnetic resonance imaging (MRI) is important for evaluation of the visual pathways, including the optic nerve. In addition, MRI allows evaluation of the oculomotor nerve and can aid in the recognition of raised intracranial pressure (ICP), which may affect both vision and the oculomotor nerve. Cerebrospinal fluid (CSF) analysis is particularly important if infectious and/or inflammatory lesions are affecting the visual pathways.

Neuro-ophthalmic syndromes

Based on initial presentation, cases can be divided into the following (although some animals may have multiple deficits):

- Ophthalmic manifestations of neurological disease – there are a variety of neurological and systemic disorders in which ophthalmic changes are evident and the eye may provide evidence as to the underlying disease
- Blindness – these patients can be further subdivided:
  - Concurrent loss of subcortical visual reflexes (PLR and dazzle reflex) – indicates a lesion affecting the eye, optic nerve, optic chiasm or optic tract up to the synapse within the lateral geniculate nucleus. Consideration should be given to lesions of the subcortical pathways where there is still a weak PLR with bright light stimulation (e.g. SARD and partial lesions severe enough to interrupt the conscious visual pathways but not totally block the PLR pathway)
  - Intact subcortical visual reflexes – indicates a lesion of the lateral geniculate nucleus and associated optic tracts and/or optic radiations and the occipital cerebral cortex.
- Pupil abnormalities – the patient still has vision in both eyes but the pupils are an abnormal shape or size, or the pupils do not dilate in the dark or constrict in the light. Failure of constriction or dilatation usually implies either a parasympathetic CN III lesion or a sympathetic lesion, respectively, but may also relate to lesions affecting the iris itself
- Abnormal eyeball position or movement – common causes of abnormal eyeball position and movement include breed conformation, hydrocephalus, vestibular disease, extraocular muscle disease, space-occupying retrobulbar masses and diseases of CNs III, IV and VI
- Eyelid abnormalities – the inability of the eyelids to close normally or being in an abnormal position usually implies a facial nerve lesion, but may also imply a partial sympathetic or parasympathetic lesion
- Abnormal sensation of the medial canthus, the cornea or the inner nasal mucosa – abnormalities of sensation usually imply a trigeminal nerve lesion, but may also be seen with forebrain lesions. With trigeminal nerve lesions, neurogenic keratitis is common and can be very severe. With forebrain lesions, the subcortical reflexes are still intact (including the palpebral and corneal reflexes), but the voluntary cortical responses to sensory stimuli (including the response to nasal stimulation) are lost
- Third eyelid abnormalities – the most common abnormalities affecting the third eyelids include retrobulbar masses, Horner's syndrome and dysautonomia, which cause abnormalities of eyeball position, pupil size and pupil function, respectively

- Abnormal tear production – if tear production is reduced (most common), hydration of the nasal mucosa and mouth should be assessed. The main neurological causes of reduced tear production include damage to the parasympathetic portion of the facial nerve (with concurrent ipsilateral dry nose (xeromycteria)) and dysautonomia (bilaterally symmetrical with pupil abnormalities, dry mouth (xerostomia) and generalized clinical signs of dysautonomia).

Ophthalmic manifestations of neurological disease

The retina and optic nerve represent the only part of the CNS normally visible and disease processes that affect the CNS (and sometimes the peripheral nervous system, PNS) may result in concurrent ophthalmic changes. These changes may provide an important clue as to the nature of the neurological disease (Swanson, 1990).

Inborn errors of metabolism

Lysosomal storage diseases and other inborn errors of metabolism may present with a visible accumulation of storage products within the retinal cells, other cells of the eye or the cornea (Figure 10.13). These disorders should be suspected in any juvenile animal with progressive, symmetrical neurological disease and concurrent ocular changes. Pure-bred animals appear to be predisposed. GM1 and GM2 gangliosidosis and mucopolysaccharidosis are the most commonly reported lysosomal storage diseases in canine and feline patients with ocular changes (typically corneal clouding, but also lens and retinal changes).

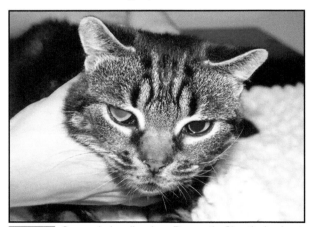

10.13 Corneal clouding in a Domestic Shorthaired cat with mucopolysaccharidosis type VI. (© Jacques Penderis)

Acquired metabolic diseases

A variety of acquired metabolic diseases may have concurrent neurological and ophthalmic changes, including peripheral neuropathies and cataracts associated with diabetes mellitus, peripheral neuropathies and lipaemia retinalis associated with hyperchylomicronaemia and hyperlipidaemia (Jones *et al.*, 1986), and copper-coloured irises and congenital portosystemic shunts in cats (Figure 10.14).

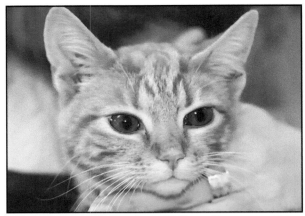

10.14 Domestic Shorthaired kitten with a congenital portosystemic shunt presented with copper-coloured irises. (© Jacques Penderis)

Ocular effects of neoplasia affecting the nervous system

Neoplasms arising from the nervous system or resulting in concurrent CNS or PNS signs may affect the eyes in a variety of manners, with the most obvious being direct and indirect tumour extension to the eyes. One of the more common tumours with ocular involvement in dogs and cats is lymphoma (Figure 10.15); however, lymphoma cells tend to infiltrate the ocular tissues and, less commonly, result in discrete masses or may present as uveitis (Massa *et al.*, 2002). The eye may also be affected as a paraneoplastic effect (e.g. papilloedema caused by intracranial mass lesions or retinal ischaemia as a result of serum hyperviscosity due to functional B-cell tumours) (Center and Smith, 1982).

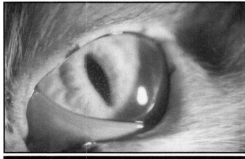
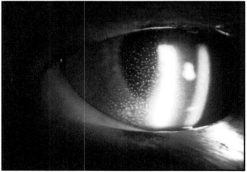

10.15 The iris thickening and corneal precipitates evident in this cat with central vestibular disease suggest that infectious agents or lymphoma may be the cause of the neurological deficits. CSF analysis confirmed the presence of lymphoma. (© Comparative Ophthalmology Unit, Animal Health Trust)

Infectious diseases

Infectious diseases most commonly present with concurrent ophthalmic and neurological signs, particularly in young dogs and cats (see Figure 10.1). The most important include:

- Viral infections – canine distemper virus, feline coronavirus (which causes feline infectious peritonitis, FIP), feline leukaemia virus (FeLV) and feline immunodeficiency virus (FIV)
- Coccidial infections – in particular toxoplasmosis and neosporosis. In one study of 100 cats with toxoplasmosis, histological examination revealed that 80% had CNS lesions and 82% had intraocular lesions (Dubey and Carpenter, 1993)
- Fungal diseases – in particular *Cryptococcus* in cats (most commonly in immunosuppressed individuals following systemic dissemination of the organisms).

Cardiovascular disease and hypertension

Cardiovascular disease may present with neurological signs, in particular as a risk factor for cerebrovascular insults and in association with partial seizure activity in cats. Long-standing hypertension may be evident as multifocal retinal ischaemia, whilst more severe hypertension may result in retinal haemorrhage, retinal detachment and even blindness. Coagulopathies may also result in conjunctival, scleral and retinal haemorrhage.

Decreased vision with concurrent loss of subcortical visual reflexes

Concurrent visual impairment and PLR deficits are suggestive of a lesion affecting the proximal portion of the visual pathway from the retina to just prior to the lateral geniculate nucleus.

Retinal, optic disc and optic nerve lesions

Unilateral lesions usually result in impaired vision and loss of the direct and consensual PLR in the affected eye. Both the direct and consensual PLR should still be present in the normal eye. Bilateral lesions usually result in impaired vision, mydriasis and loss of the direct and consensual PLR in both eyes.

Sudden acquired retinal degeneration: SARD occurs occasionally in dogs and is characterized by an acute loss of vision (although in some cases this may develop over a few days) (Mattson *et al.*, 1992). Affected dogs are typically middle-aged and present bilaterally blind with dilated unresponsive pupils (Montgomery *et al.*, 2008). Miniature Schnauzers and Dachshunds are commonly affected. In the acute stage, no abnormalities are evident on ophthalmoscopic examination, but over time (weeks) a bilaterally symmetrical retinal degeneration becomes evident with hyper-reflectivity of the tapetal fundus and attenuation of the retinal blood vessels. An ERG is required to demonstrate photoreceptor death in the acute stage, in order to differentiate SARD from other lesions responsible for acute-onset blindness (Miller *et al.*, 1998). The underlying cause is unknown; although, a substantial number of affected dogs have

concurrent hyperadrenocorticism or elevated sex hormones (Carter *et al.*, 2009). An elevated level of neuronal-specific enolase antibodies may be seen in 25% of affected dogs, and this may indicate either an autoimmune process or just reflect the degree of retinal damage (Braus *et al.*, 2008). There is no treatment for SARD and although the blindness is permanent, no further clinical signs develop.

Fluoroquinolone-induced acute retinal degeneration in cats: The antimicrobial enrofloxacin has been demonstrated to have a dose-dependent toxic effect on the retina (Gelatt *et al.*, 2001). In one experimental study, cats treated with 50 mg/kg enrofloxacin all developed retinal degeneration as early as 3 days following treatment (Ford *et al.*, 2007). High doses of the related fluoroquinolones orbifloxacin and marbofloxacin have also been reported to induce retinal degeneration in cats.

Clinically affected cats present with acute onset bilateral blindness, pupillary dilation and loss of the PLR. Fluoroquinolone toxicity induces necrosis of the retinal photoreceptors, outer nuclear layer and outer plexiform layer, but no retinal changes are initially evident on ophthalmic examination and only become apparent with time. An ERG is required to demonstrate photoreceptor death in the acute stage. Fluoroquinolones are normally actively transported by P-glycoprotein and *ABCG2* from the retinal capillary endothelial cells back into the blood vessel lumen, restricting their distribution to the retina. Four feline-specific amino acid changes have been demonstrated within conserved regions of *ABCG2* and are associated with impaired function (compared with human *ABCG2*). These changes may cause the toxic accumulation of fluoroquinolones within the retina in cats (Ramirez *et al.*, 2011).

Optic disc or nerve hypoplasia: Optic disc or nerve hypoplasia may be unilateral or bilateral. It occurs sporadically in many dog breeds and has been suggested to be inherited in the Miniature Poodle (Kern and Riis, 1981). Depending on the severity, optic disc hypoplasia may result in decreased to absent vision with a proportional decrease in the PLR. In unilateral cases, the owner may not notice the problem. In extreme cases, puppies can be bilaterally blind with bilaterally dilated and unresponsive pupils from the time their eyes first open. On ophthalmoscopic evaluation, affected optic discs appear small and grey (Peterson-Jones, 1995). There is no treatment, but in those cases with a possible hereditary cause, preventative measures should be taken against breeding. Optic nerve hypoplasia in human patients is usually identified in young children and almost invariably occurs concurrently with clinical signs of hypothalamic dysfunction and/or neurodevelopmental impairment (Borchert and Garcia-Filion, 2008).

Optic disc atrophy: Damage to the retinal ganglion cells, proximal axonal processes or optic nerve may occur due to a variety of causes, including generalized retinal degeneration, glaucoma, trauma and inflammatory lesions. The consequence of this is axonal loss or the development of Wallerian-like degeneration of axons, with loss of the surrounding myelin sheath. The amount of axonal loss determines the degree of optic disc atrophy, and the disc appears grey and shrunken-looking on ophthalmoscopic examination. This process is gradual and not immediately apparent at the time of insult.

Papilloedema: This is defined as oedema of the optic disc and usually results from raised ICP (due to cerebral tumours and inflammation) but may occur secondary to optic nerve tumours and inflammation and potentially in conditions that cause widespread myelin oedema (seen with certain metabolic and toxic disorders, such as hexachlorophene and triethyl tin acetate toxicity). Papilloedema is evident as an irregular and swollen optic disc margin (Figure 10.16), frequently with evidence of retinal congestion and haemorrhage (Palmer *et al.*, 1974).

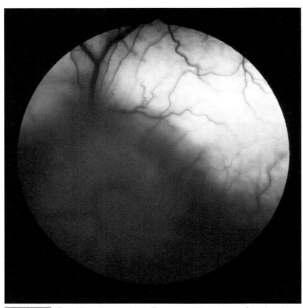

10.16 Papilloedema in a Boxer with a large forebrain tumour. Note the irregular and swollen optic disc margin. The identification of papilloedema should alert the clinician to the probability of raised intracranial pressure. (© Jacques Penderis)

Papilloedema needs to be differentiated from hypermyelination of the optic disc (pseudo-papilloedema), where myelination extends beyond the periphery of the optic disc, giving the disc margin an irregular and fluffy appearance. Hypermyelination is more evident in certain large-breed dogs, including Boxers, German Shepherd Dogs and Golden Retrievers. Papilloedema is frequently identified in humans and primates in association with raised ICP, but is less reliably present in dogs and does not appear to be useful in cats with increased ICP (Hedges and Zaren, 1969). Historically, it has been reported that papilloedema spares vision and this can be used to distinguish it from optic neuritis; however, in the majority of cases in clinical practice, any forebrain or optic

nerve lesion severe enough to cause papilloedema usually interrupts the visual pathways, resulting in concurrent visual deficits.

Optic neuritis: Optic neuritis or papillitis is defined as inflammation of the optic nerve and is characterized by visual loss in the presence of optic disc changes similar in appearance to those seen with papilloedema; thus, it can be difficult to distinguish optic neuritis from papilloedema on ophthalmoscopic examination (Fischer and Jones, 1972). Typically, the optic disc appears swollen with frequent haemorrhage. Swelling of the optic nerve may be evident on MRI (Seruca *et al.*, 2010) and consideration should be given to performing MRI and CSF analysis in any case with abnormalities of the optic disc evident on fundic examination. Potential causes include granulomatous meningoencephalitis (GME), canine distemper virus, cryptococcosis (Jergens *et al.*, 1986; Malik *et al.*, 1992) and histoplasmosis (Percy, 1981); although, often no underlying cause is identified and the disorder is presumed to be immune-mediated. Many cases respond to anti-inflammatory or immunosuppressive treatment, including the use of steroids in combination with other medications; however, the prognosis for recovery of vision remains guarded.

Miscellaneous causes:

- Retinal degeneration (also known as progressive retinal atrophy) and retinal dysplasia are hereditary in many different breeds of dogs and can result from taurine deficiency in cats. The reader is referred to standard ophthalmology textbooks for full details of retinal disease.
- Neoplasia (primary optic nerve neoplasia *versus* secondary compressive orbital neoplasms) may interrupt optic nerve function. Due to its meningeal covering, the optic nerve may be affected by meningiomas (Perez *et al.*, 2005; Montoliu *et al.*, 2006) as well as gliomas of the optic nerve itself (Naranjo *et al.*, 2008) (Figure 10.17).
- Trauma may cause optic nerve compression, traction or haemorrhage.

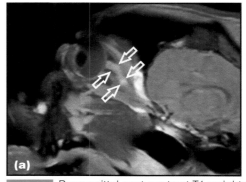

10.17 Parasagittal post-contrast T1-weighted fat saturation MR images of the optic nerves from a Golden Retriever with left blindness and a prominent optic nerve on fundic examination. **(a)** There is enlargement and increased contrast medium uptake in the left optic nerve (arrowed). The lesion is consistent with neoplasia or focal inflammation. (© Jacques Penderis) (continues) ▶

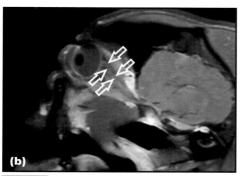

10.17 (continued) Parasagittal post-contrast T1-weighted fat saturation MR images of the optic nerves from a Golden Retriever with left blindness and a prominent optic nerve on fundic examination. **(b)** Compare the normal right optic nerve (arrowed) with the left optic nerve in (a). The lesion is consistent with neoplasia or focal inflammation. (© Jacques Penderis)

Optic chiasm lesions

Lesions affecting the optic chiasm usually result in decreased to absent vision and mydriasis with loss of both the direct and consensual PLR in both eyes.

Neoplasia and other space-occupying lesions: Space-occupying masses can occasionally occur at the level of the optic chiasm and, despite the slow development of the underlying disease process, some animals may present with acute onset of visual deficits (Davidson *et al.*, 1991). Lymphoma is a common cause in cats (Chang *et al.*, 2006) but consideration should be given to other tumours in both dogs and cats, including pituitary macroadenomas (Figure 10.18), meningiomas and tumours of the nasal cavity extending into the region of the optic chiasm. An unusual brain tumour called a suprasellar germ cell tumour has been reported in young adult dogs, in particular Dobermanns (Valentine *et al.*, 1988). This tumour expands in the region of the pituitary fossa and can become extremely large, causing compression of the optic chiasm, the adjacent cavernous sinus and associated CNs.

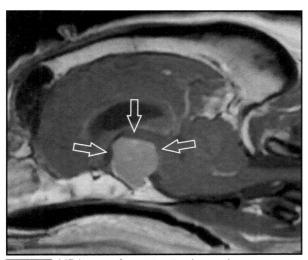

10.18 MR image of a contrast-enhanced mass (arrowed) at the level of the optic chiasm in a dog. The appearance and clinical findings were consistent with a pituitary macroadenoma. (© Jacques Penderis)

Miscellaneous causes:

- Inflammatory lesions.
- Vascular lesions.

Optic tract lesions

Optic tract lesions usually cause visual deficits in the lateral (temporal) visual field (corresponding to the medial retina) of the contralateral eye and the medial (nasal) visual field (corresponding to the lateral retina) of the ipsilateral eye. As the menace response tests the lateral visual field of the eye being assessed (see above), the response is usually reduced or absent in the eye contralateral to the optic tract lesion. The PLR is intact in both eyes but the degree of pupillary constriction may be slightly reduced in the contralateral eye (most evident on the swinging flashlight test).

Inflammatory lesions: The most common causes of CNS inflammation affecting the visual tracts in dogs include GME, necrotizing encephalitis and infectious agents such as *Toxoplasma*, *Neospora*, canine distemper virus, tick-borne agents and *Cryptococcus*. In cats, FIP is a significant cause but consideration should also be given to Borna virus, FeLV, FIV, toxoplasmosis, cryptococcosis and meningoencephalitis of unknown origin (see also Chapters 9 and 11).

Space-occupying masses: As for other CNS structures, the optic tracts are vulnerable to disruption or compression by mass lesions, including tumours and haemorrhage.

Decreased vision with intact subcortical visual reflexes

Lesions affecting the central projections of the visual pathway (from the lateral geniculate nucleus to the visual cortex) result in visual deficits but do not affect the PLR. The PLR requires fewer intact axons than conscious perception of vision; therefore, the situation may occasionally arise whereby with partial lesions of the proximal visual pathways there is loss of vision but the PLR is spared, creating the illusion of a more central lesion.

Unilateral lesions affecting the central projections of the visual pathways usually result in a diminished to absent lateral visual field in the contralateral eye and a (less obvious) diminished to absent medial visual field in the ipsilateral eye. Other clinical signs of forebrain disease, including decreased consciousness, seizures, circling, proprioceptive placing deficits and hemi-neglect/hemi-inattention syndrome, are usually evident with lesions severe enough to cause visual deficits.

Degenerative diseases

Central visual disturbances may also be a feature of some degenerative disorders, particularly lysosomal storage diseases (reported with gangliosidoses and sphingomyelinosis).

Anomalous diseases

Hydrocephalus: Congenital hydrocephalus, characterized by massive dilatation of the ventricular system of the brain (in particular the lateral ventricles), is typified by a dome-shaped forehead (Figure 10.19a). With congenital hydrocephalus, and to a lesser extent acquired hydrocephalus, the optic radiations (as they pass adjacent to the lateral ventricles) are particularly vulnerable to injury, and visual deficits are therefore one of the potential clinical signs (Figure 10.19b). Congenital hydrocephalus is further characterized by the presence of a bilateral ventrolateral strabismus ('setting sun sign'; see Chapter 9 for further details).

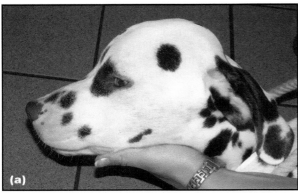
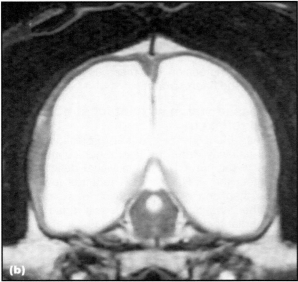

10.19 Central blindness may be seen in association with hydrocephalus. **(a)** Affected dogs have an enlarged, dome-shaped skull. **(b)** Blindness results from the vulnerability of the optic radiations adjacent to the enlarged lateral ventricles as evident in this MR image. (© Jacques Penderis)

Lissencephaly: This is a rare developmental disorder, described in the Lhasa Apso as a hereditary trait, where there is congenital absence of cerebrocortical convolutions. Neurological abnormalities become apparent within the first year of life and include seizures, behavioural abnormalities and cortical visual disturbances (Greene *et al.*, 1976). Treatment is limited to management of seizures, and the prognosis is grave for this progressive disorder. Lissencephaly has also been described sporadically in other breeds of dog and in cats (e.g. the Korat cat).

Metabolic diseases
Diffuse encephalopathies, most commonly secondary to metabolic disorders or hypoxic episodes, may present with visual deficits. Any animal with a metabolic encephalopathy severe enough to cause visual deficits usually demonstrates marked CNS depression. Potential metabolic encephalopathies that should be considered include: hepatic encephalopathy, hypoglycaemia, renal-associated encephalopathy, profound electrolyte derangements, endocrine-associated encephalopathies (hypothyroidism), profound acid–base disturbances and mitochondrial encephalopathies (see Chapter 9 for more details). Global cerebral ischaemia may occur as a consequence of anaesthetic accidents or following prolonged seizures. It is not unusual for such patients to have persistent cortical blindness. Post-ictal depression (functional forebrain suppression following seizure activity) may also present as central blindness.

Neoplastic diseases
Space-occupying lesions within the cerebral hemispheres are primarily tumours. The most common primary brain tumours include meningiomas (particularly in cats) and gliomas, but lymphoma, ependymomas, choroid plexus tumours and metastatic tumours should also be considered (see Chapter 9 for further information).

Inflammatory diseases
Immune-mediated (particularly GME in dogs) and infectious (including viral, bacterial, protozoal, rickettsial and fungal agents) causes of encephalitis should be considered (see Chapter 11 for more details).

Trauma
The forebrain is vulnerable to trauma, although it is relatively well protected (more so in dogs) by the skull and overlying masticatory muscles. Blindness, as one of the potential clinical signs of forebrain trauma, may be evident immediately following the injury or the onset may be delayed in the event of secondary processes, including CNS infection or abscessation.

Toxic diseases
Toxins are rare causes of cortical blindness, but in the presence of other suggestive clinical signs (particularly gastrointestinal disturbances), lead poisoning should be considered (Zook *et al.*, 1969).

Vascular diseases
Cerebrovascular disease is recognized with increasing frequency in dogs and typically presents as an acute onset of non-progressive neurological deficits (Garosi *et al.*, 2005). The site of the stroke lesion determines the clinical signs, but one of the predilection sites is the thalamus. Stroke lesions that involve the dorsal aspect of the thalamus in which the lateral geniculate nucleus is located (and in particular extensive lesions) usually result in a reduction or loss of the menace response (Goncalves *et al.*, 2011). Vascular lesions (haemorrhagic or ischaemic)

may occur secondary to underlying diseases, including hyperadrenocorticism, hypertension, renal disease, bleeding disorders (Figure 10.20) and trauma (Figure 10.21). However, in a substantial proportion of cases, no underlying cause is identified.

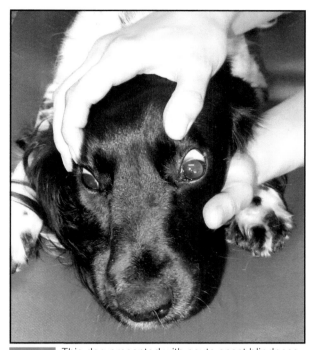

10.20 This dog presented with acute onset blindness and loss of the PLR, suggestive of a retinal, optic nerve or optic chiasm lesion. The evidence of scleral haemorrhage indicates the possibility of an underlying bleeding disorder and this was later confirmed as the cause of the blindness. (© Jacques Penderis)

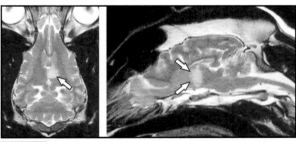

10.21 Cerebrovascular accidents are occasional findings in dogs and may result in blindness if the visual pathways are affected. One site of predilection is the thalamus (arrowed) and contralateral visual deficits, conscious proprioceptive deficits and vestibular dysfunction may be evident. (© Jacques Penderis)

Pupil abnormalities

Pupil abnormalities, usually evident as alterations in pupil size, in the absence of visual loss may affect one or both pupils (Figure 10.22). Pupil size is determined by a combination of the tone of the pupillary constrictors and dilators (see above). Anisocoria results when only one pupil is affected. In these cases, evaluation of the PLR is necessary in order to determine which pupil is abnormal. Before a neuro-ophthalmology assessment is performed, it is essential first to ascertain whether the pupil

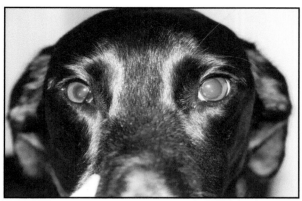

10.22 Right Horner's syndrome in a dog showing miosis, ptosis and protrusion of the third eyelid. Enophthalmos is the fourth feature associated with Horner's syndrome but cannot be appreciated on this image. (© Jacques Penderis)

abnormalities can be explained by non-neurological abnormalities of the iris (including iris atrophy, iris hypoplasia, uveitis and trauma) or globe (including lens luxation and glaucoma). Painful conditions of the cornea and conjunctiva may also cause miosis.

Hippus
Brief oscillations of pupillary size, referred to as hippus, may occur as a normal feature in response to light exposure. Very exaggerated hippus may be an indication of CNS disease, particularly if it occurs in conjunction with other neuro-ophthalmological abnormalities.

Pharmacological miosis and mydriasis
Pharmacological agents, accidentally or intentionally administered, may profoundly affect pupillary function. This includes pupillary dilation following administration of mydriatic (e.g. atropine) or cycloplegic (e.g. tropicamide) drugs and pupillary constriction following administration of miotic drugs (e.g. pilocarpine). Anaesthetic agents may also have a profound effect on pupillary size (e.g. miosis following the systemic administration of some opioids in dogs; Stephan *et al.*, 2003).

Resting anisocoria
Subtle resting anisocoria (idiopathic or benign anisocoria) is a common observation, particularly in cats, and is of no clinical significance. It is similar to the physiological anisocoria seen in up to 20% of the human population (Lepore, 2002) and is thought to be the consequence of an imbalance in basal sympathetic and parasympathetic tone between the two eyes. Resting anisocoria demonstrates no other neurological or ocular abnormalities and the pupils have a normal ability to dilate and constrict.

Horner's syndrome
Lesions affecting the sympathetic supply to the head result in Horner's syndrome (Figure 10.23) and loss of cutaneous vascular tone on the affected side with peripheral vasodilatation. The loss of cutaneous vascular tone in some dogs and cats is evident

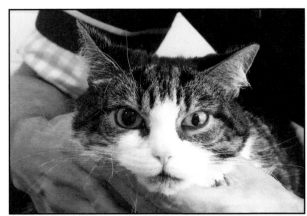

10.23 Left Horner's syndrome in a cat showing miosis, ptosis and protrusion of the third eyelid. Enophthalmos is the fourth feature associated with Horner's syndrome. (© Jacques Penderis)

as increased cutaneous temperature (the pinna on the affected side being warmer than the unaffected side) and hyperaemia. The effects of loss of cutaneous vascular tone on the eye include mild congestion of the scleral blood vessels and a decrease in intraocular pressure. Horner's syndrome describes the specific ophthalmic changes associated with loss of sympathetic innervation:

* Miosis (constriction of the affected pupil) – avulsion of the brachial plexus nerve roots usually causes only a partial Horner's syndrome, often with miosis as the only feature. This is typically because only the T1 nerve root of the T1–T3 sympathetic outflow is affected by brachial plexus avulsions. Partial Horner's syndrome (with miosis as the only feature) may also occur in dogs with acute and severe lateralized cervical spinal cord disease, but the expectation would still be for the majority of cases to have complete Horner's syndrome (Griffiths, 1970)
* Enophthalmos – loss of sympathetic innervation leads to the loss of orbital smooth muscle tone and sinking of the globe into the orbit
* Protrusion of the third eyelid (nictitating membrane) – whilst in the dog this occurs passively secondary to enophthalmos, in the cat, the protrusion is due to a combination of enophthalmos and loss of third eyelid retraction
* Ptosis (drooping) of the upper eyelid and decreased tone of the lower eyelid – this occurs as a result of loss of smooth muscle tone affecting the Müller's muscle.

Horner's syndrome is usually classified according to the level of the lesion along the sympathetic pathway (see Figure 10.11) as first order, second order (pre-ganglionic) or third order (post-ganglionic). Pharmacological testing or evidence of other neurological abnormalities can be used to localize the site of the lesion, but the times to a response should only be treated as a guide to the site of the lesion and other neurological signs should be taken into

consideration. In the majority of cases with apparent third order Horner's syndrome (based on pharmacological testing), no underlying cause has been identified. These cases have historically been termed idiopathic Horner's syndrome (Kern *et al.*, 1989; Morgan and Zanotti, 1989). The prognosis depends to a large degree on the underlying neurological disease, but is excellent in idiopathic Horner's syndrome (which is largely cosmetic and in many cases may resolve spontaneously). Treatment is rarely required but in cases with bilateral Horner's syndrome (Figure 10.24) and where vision is obscured by third eyelid protrusion, topical 1% or 10% phenylephrine can be used to provide occasional, short-term alleviation of the clinical signs. Maximal effect occurs for up to 2 hours and in some cases the effect may be maintained for up to 18 hours.

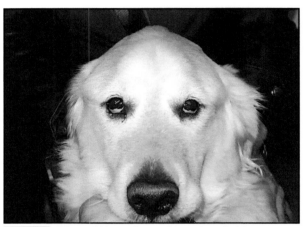

10.24 Bilateral Horner's syndrome in a Golden Retriever. Third eyelid protrusion may interfere with vision in cases of bilateral Horner's syndrome, whereas in unilateral cases it can be considered mainly cosmetic. (© Jacques Penderis)

Pharmacological testing: The guidelines for pharmacological testing (see Pharmacological evaluation of pupil function) should be followed. Confirmation of Horner's syndrome in cases where this is not immediately apparent can be achieved using topical cocaine; however, this is only rarely required as failure of the affected pupil to dilate in the dark and other features of Horner's syndrome are usually conclusive. Topical administration of 4% or 10% cocaine eye drops results in dilation of the pupil in normal patients, but no pupil dilation is seen with sympathetic dysfunction. Cocaine blocks noradrenaline (norepinephrine) reuptake, resulting in prolonged activity of noradrenaline in the synaptic cleft and consequently pupil dilation. However, in Horner's syndrome there is a lack of noradrenaline in the synaptic cleft and therefore the pupil fails to dilate. Pupil size should be determined prior to the administration of cocaine eye drops and again after 30–60 minutes.

In cases where Horner's syndrome has been present for some time (usually at least 7–14 days), denervation hypersensitivity resulting from sympathetic denervation enables pharmacological testing to be performed to predict the site of the lesion

based on increased sensitivity to topical phenylephrine. The time to pupillary dilation following topical
administration of 1% phenylephrine to both eyes
should be determined. Essentially, the shorter the
time to pupillary dilation, the closer the lesion is to
the iris:

- Less than 20 minutes suggests third order
  Horner's syndrome
- 20–45 minutes suggests second order Horner's
  syndrome
- 60–90 minutes suggests first order Horner's
  syndrome or no sympathetic denervation of the
  eye
- If 10% phenylephrine is used, mydriasis occurs
  in 5–8 minutes with post-ganglionic (third order
  neuron) lesions (Figure 10.25).

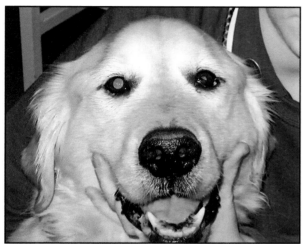

10.25 Following topical administration of
phenylephrine into the right eye of the bilateral
Horner's syndrome case from Figure 10.24, the miosis
resolved rapidly (<20 minutes) indicating a third order
neuron lesion. (© Jacques Penderis)

Pourfour du Petit syndrome

Mild pathological insult to the sympathetic supply to
the head (most likely adjacent to the middle ear)
may lead to irritation of the sympathetic fibres,
resulting in sympathetic hyperactivity rather than
sympathetic denervation. Pourfour du Petit syndrome (excessive sympathetic tone to the eye; the
opposite of Horner's syndrome) was first described
in human patients and has subsequently been
reported as a rare finding in cats (Boydell, 2000).
The excessive sympathetic tone to the eye results in
pupil dilatation, an enlarged palpebral fissure and
subtle exophthalmos of the affected side (Figure
10.26). The prognosis is good for a full recovery,
depending on the nature of the underlying cause.

Idiopathic internal ophthalmoplegia

Idiopathic lesions affecting the internal portion of
CN III (parasympathetic portion) are occasionally
identified in dogs, particularly Flat-coated Retrievers (Figure 10.27). These cases are characterized by pupil dilatation in the affected eye, with
intact vision, in the absence of other ophthalmic

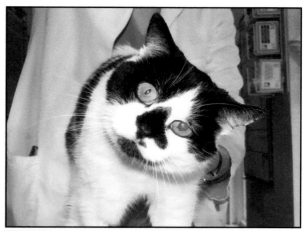

10.26 Pourfour du Petit syndrome in the left eye of a
cat. The cat has left peripheral vestibular
syndrome with irritation to the sympathetic supply at the
same level. The excessive sympathetic tone results in
pupil dilatation and (not apparent on this image) an
enlarged palpebral fissure and subtle exophthalmos on
the affected side. (© Jacques Penderis)

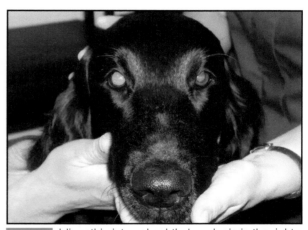

10.27 Idiopathic internal ophthalmoplegia in the right
eye of a Flat-coated Retriever. Pharmacological
testing confirmed a CN III parasympathetic lesion. No
other clinical signs were evident on examination, MRI and
other investigations were normal and the lesion resolved
spontaneously over the course of a month. (© Jacques
Penderis)

and neurological abnormalities. Pharmacological
testing with 0.1% pilocarpine drops results in rapid
constriction of the pupil due to denervation hypersensitivity. Spontaneous remission occurs in the
majority of cases.

Neoplasia of the oculomotor nerve

Neoplasms of the oculomotor nerve, in particular
malignant nerve sheath tumours, may have an
identical presentation to idiopathic internal ophthalmoplegia; however, these cases usually present
with additional signs of oculomotor nerve dysfunction, including lateral or ventrolateral strabismus
(either at presentation or developing over time)
(Figure 10.28). Neoplastic lesions affecting the
oculomotor nerve may be identified on advanced
imaging (Figure 10.29).

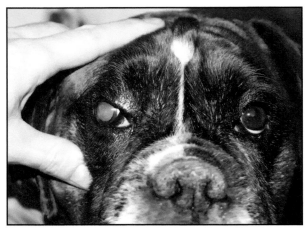

10.28 This dog presented with pupillary dilatation (which did not constrict on light stimulation), lateral strabismus and ptosis of the right eye. Vision was intact. These clinical signs are suggestive of a lesion affecting CN III. (© Jacques Penderis)

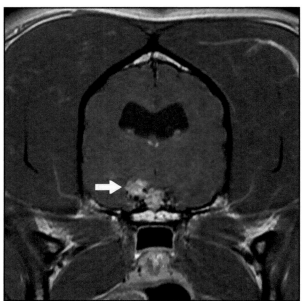

10.29 Transverse, post-gadolinium T1-weighted MR image at the level of the thalamus of the dog in Figure 10.28 demonstrating contrast enhancement and enlargement of the oculomotor nerve, which is suggestive of neoplasia. (© Jacques Penderis)

Static anisocoria

Static anisocoria (spastic pupil syndrome) occurs in cats and is associated with FeLV infection; although, it has also been suggested to occur in association with other viruses, including FIV. However, few documented cases of static anisocoria or hemidilated pupils (see below) appear in the literature (Brightman *et al.*, 1977, 1991) and the majority of textbooks which refer to the disorder provide largely anecdotal evidence. Cats with static anisocoria demonstrate moderate miosis (occasionally cats may show mydriasis) and anisocoria. The miosis typically only changes minimally, if at all, during dark adaptation. The clinical signs may be intermittent or change during the course of the disease and are thought to be the

result of either viral infection or lymphosarcoma infiltration of the short ciliary nerves or ganglion.

Hemidilated pupils

A hemidilated (D-shaped) pupil is the consequence of vulnerability to paralysis of the ciliary nerves supplying the iris constrictor muscles in cats. It is particularly seen with FeLV-associated lymphoma infiltration (Collins and O'Brien, 1990; Roberts, 1992). Either of the two ciliary nerves, the lateral (malar) ciliary nerve or medial (nasal) short ciliary nerve, may be affected and, depending on which nerve is affected, this results in either a D-shaped or a reverse D-shaped pupil (Figure 10.30). Hemidilated pupils have also been described with apparent lymphoma invasion of the medial iris stroma in both eyes of a cat (Nell and Suchy, 1998).

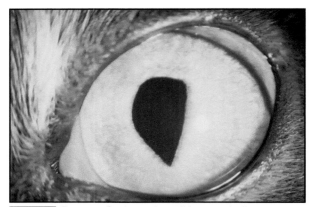

10.30 Reverse D-shaped pupil in a cat indicating damage to the nasal ciliary nerve of the left eye. Cats presenting with ciliary nerve damage should be investigated for FeLV as well as for other viral agents and lymphoma. (© Comparative Ophthalmology Unit, Animal Health Trust)

Organophosphate and carbamate toxicity

Alteration in pupil size is a feature of a variety of toxins, with the most common being the marked miosis associated with organophosphate and carbamate toxicity. Both substances inhibit cholinesterase and induce a variety of clinical signs, including salivation, gastrointestinal disturbances, muscle twitching, weakness and possibly seizures.

Cavernous sinus syndrome

The paired cavernous sinuses are situated on the floor of the calvarium and adjacent to the pituitary fossa. This area offers a convenient site for expansion of mass lesions (particularly tumours but also inflammatory lesions and vascular malformations) and, as it is the venous drainage from the frontal sinus and nose, there may be an increased likelihood of infectious and neoplastic diseases of these structures spreading to the cavernous sinus area. Neurological deficits develop when these lesions expand to incorporate the adjacent CNs III, IV and VI (innervating the extraocular muscles, iris and ciliary muscle), the first two branches of the trigeminal nerve and the post-ganglionic (third order) sympathetic supply to the eye. It is reported that cavernous sinus syndrome affects the ophthalmic and maxillary branches of the trigeminal nerve (Theisen *et al.*, 1996) but, in practice, lesions may expand and also involve the mandibular branch of the trigeminal nerve. Cavernous sinus syndrome is an anatomical diagnosis, not an aetiological diagnosis; the most common aetiology is neoplasia. The diagnostic criteria for cavernous sinus syndrome differ, but in veterinary species the diagnosis depends upon the demonstration of paralysis of CNs III, IV and VI and at least one branch of CN V.

Lesions in this area may therefore result in:

- Paralysis of the extraocular muscles (external ophthalmoplegia)
- Loss of iris and ciliary muscle function (internal ophthalmoplegia)
- Ipsilateral sensory deficits in the ophthalmic and maxillary branches of the trigeminal nerve
- Atrophy of the ipsilateral masticatory muscles (innervated by the mandibular branch of the trigeminal nerve) with associated deficits (seen with particularly large lesions).

The potential for involvement of both the parasympathetic (CN III) and sympathetic innervation of the pupil can produce either a fixed mydriatic or a mid-range pupil. Paralysis of the extraocular muscles, the ciliary muscle and the parasympathetic and sympathetic supply to the iris is termed total ophthalmoplegia or pan-ophthalmoplegia. As the optic nerve is distant from the cavernous sinus, vision is usually not lost, but the loss of lens accommodation and eyeball movement impairs vision and extensive mass lesions may involve the optic nerves, optic chiasm or optic tracts. Computed tomography (CT) or MRI of the brain should be performed in any animal with cavernous sinus syndrome, after retropulsion of the eyeball to determine whether the lesion is retrobulbar.

Pupillotonia
Pupillotonia (defined as a pupil that is slow to react to light on both direct and consensual stimulation) has been reported in the dog due to a suspected immune-mediated cause (Gerding *et al.*, 1986). This condition has not been reported since and may simply have represented a poor light source, fear or iris atrophy.

Cerebellar disease
Mydriasis of the contralateral pupil is an uncommon clinical sign associated with asymmetrical cerebellar disease (DeLahunta, 1983). This may also explain the intermittent mydriasis seen in cats with feline spongiform encephalopathy, in addition to diffuse cerebellar signs and altered behaviour.

Raised intracranial pressure
The oculomotor nerve, as it passes ventral to the brain and over the petroclinoid ligament, is vulnerable to compression as a result of increased ICP and following transtentorial brain herniation (most commonly caudal or descending transtentorial herniation). Direct compression of the oculomotor nucleus in the midbrain may also occur. Initial irritation or loss of inhibition of the oculomotor nerve as a result of raised ICP may be evident as a miotic pupil, but this rapidly progresses to complete paralysis with a fixed dilated pupil with continued elevation of ICP and herniation of the cortex under the tentorium. Such animals usually have other signs of increased ICP, most notably a reduced level of consciousness. The parasympathetic fibres surrounding the oculomotor nerve are compressed first. As compression progresses, there may be complete paralysis of the oculomotor nerve with reduced to absent eye movements. Extensive lesions which affect the origin of the sympathetic tectotegmental spinal tract as well as the oculomotor nerve result in mid-position fixed pupils.

Dysautonomia
Bilateral pupillary dilatation that is not responsive to light, protrusion of the third eyelids and decreased tear production, in the presence of normal vision, are features of canine and feline dysautonomia (also called Key–Gaskell syndrome in cats) (Wise and Lappin, 1990; Longshire *et al.*, 1996) (Figure 10.31). The ocular changes are also associated with profound systemic signs of autonomic dysfunction, in particular depression, anorexia, decreased saliva production, megaoesophagus, bradycardia and occasionally faecal and urinary incontinence. The canine and feline syndromes are both rare and occur sporadically. The treatment is purely supportive and the prognosis is guarded. Pharmacological testing may be useful to confirm sympathetic and parasympathetic dysfunction (see Chapter 19 for further details).

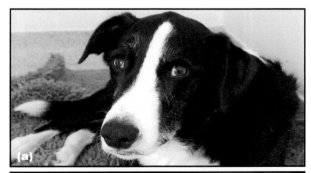

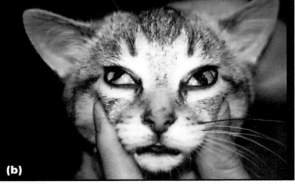

10.31 Dysautonomia in **(a)** a dog and **(b)** a cat with protrusion of the third eyelids, pupillary dilatation and bilateral xeromycteria (dry nose) (a = © Jacques Penderis; b = Courtesy of the Royal (Dick) Veterinary School)

Thiamine deficiency

Bilateral pupillary dilatation with the occasional presence of non-specific fundus changes, including peripapillary oedema and papillary neovascularization, are evident with thiamine (vitamin B1) deficiency in cats. Thiamine deficiency in dogs and cats is associated with evidence of central vestibular syndrome (nystagmus and strabismus) and systemic changes including anorexia, ataxia and cervical ventroflexion (in cats). The prognosis is good with early thiamine supplementation (see Chapter 11 for more information).

Abnormal eyeball position or movement

There is an intimate functional association between the innervation to the extraocular muscles and the vestibular system. The extraocular muscles are innervated by CNs III, IV and VI. Any strabismus due to a lesion in one or more of these CNs must be differentiated from lesions affecting the extraocular muscles (including traumatic rupture and extraocular myositis) (Figure 10.32).

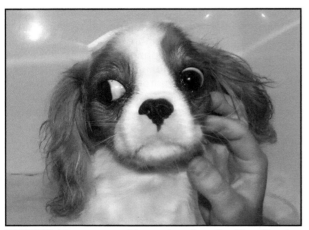

10.32 Divergent strabismus in a Cavalier King Charles Spaniel suggestive of a pathological cause. However, subsequent examination revealed normal eyeball movement and function. The strabismus was ascribed to an extreme form of divergent strabismus (exotropia) due to brachycephalia. (© Jacques Penderis)

- Lesions simultaneously affecting CNs III, IV and VI result in external ophthalmoplegia and internal ophthalmoplegia if the pupillary constrictor (CN III) is affected.
- Lesions with only CN III involvement may present with a lateral or ventrolateral strabismus (see Figure 10.28); more rarely, lesions may only affect single muscle groups, resulting in a strabismus opposite to the normal function of the denervated muscle.
- Lesions affecting the trochlear nerve in isolation are extremely rare but, where they do occur, result in loss of function of the ipsilateral dorsal oblique muscle (brainstem lesions may result in ipsilateral or contralateral loss of function). The dorsal oblique muscle functions to rotate the dorsal portion of the globe nasally (intorsion); therefore, lesions of the dorsal oblique muscle are evident upon rotation of the eyeball where the dorsal portion of the eyeball is deviated temporally (laterally). In cats, this is seen as rotation of the normally vertical pupils, but in dogs (which have round pupils) this is only apparent upon demonstrating lateral deviation of the dorsal retinal arteriole and vein on ophthalmoscopic examination (Figure 10.33).
- Abducent lesions are extremely rare in isolation but, where they do occur, result in medial strabismus of the affected eye (the abducent nerve innervates the lateral rectus and retractor bulbi muscles of the eyeball). Lesions of the abducent nerve can be distinguished from congenital medial strabismus by the absence of eyeball retraction in the affected eye upon performing the corneal reflex (Figure 10.34).

Eyeball movement is further controlled by the vestibular and saccadic systems. The function of the vestibular system with regard to vision is to maintain the visual image in a steady position on the retina in response to movements of the head. This is achieved by inducing eye movements, via the vestibulo-ocular reflex, that are equal to but in the opposite direction to the head movements. In contrast to the

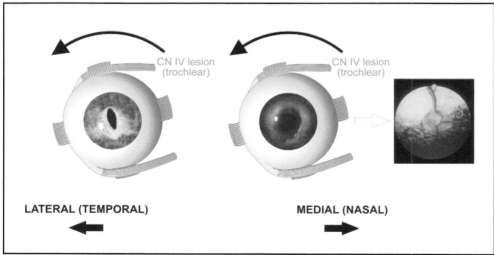

10.33 Trochlear nerve lesions in isolation are extremely rare. Lesions manifest as rotation of the contralateral eyeball with the dorsal portion (12 o'clock position) being temporally (laterally) deviated. This is apparent in cats as rotation of the vertical pupil (left) but in dogs is only apparent on fundic evaluation of the dorsal retinal arteriole and vein (right). (© Jacques Penderis)

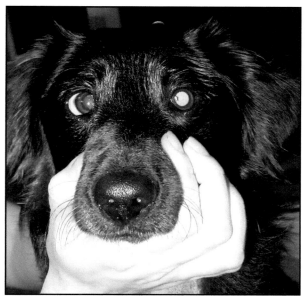

10.34 Lesions of the abducent nerve cause medial strabismus, but can be easily differentiated from the congenital medial strabismus in this cross-breed dog by assessing the corneal reflex. With abducent nerve lesions, eyeball retraction is absent when the reflex is performed. (© Jacques Penderis)

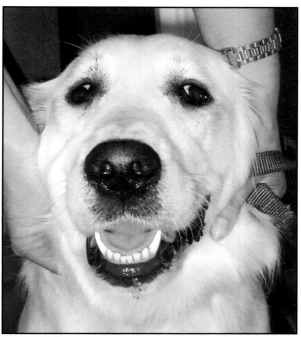

10.35 Congenital divergent strabismus (exotropia) in a Golden Retriever puppy. (© Jacques Penderis)

vestibular system, the saccadic system functions to change the line of sight to focus a new visual stimulus on the retinal region with the highest visual acuity (usually the area centralis). Saccadic eye movements occur in response to startle reflexes (sudden visual and auditory stimuli) and during the fast phase eye movements of the vestibulo-ocular reflex.

Congenital nystagmus
Congenital nystagmus may be recognized in association with ocular abnormalities and congenital visual deficits, particularly if complete blindness is present from birth. Idiopathic pendular or jerk nystagmus may occasionally be present in the absence of other ocular abnormalities. The nystagmus associated with congenital visual deficits is characterized as either a continuous fine oscillation of both globes (often rotary) or random eye movements (amaurotic nystagmus or 'searching nystagmus'). Rotary nystagmus has been described in association with microphthalmos and congenital cataracts in puppies, even though vision is not totally lost. Animals that lose their vision at a young age may also develop nystagmus (Ferreira and Peterson-Jones, 2002). Pendular nystagmus may occur secondary to congenital abnormalities of the visual pathway in Belgian Shepherd Dogs. In these dogs decussation is lost at the optic chiasm and all the retinal projections are into the ipsilateral optic tract (Hogan and Williams, 1995). Congenital nystagmus in Siamese and related cat breeds is discussed below.

Congenital strabismus
Congenital strabismus is seen occasionally in the absence of identifiable underlying causes (Figure 10.35) or may be associated with albinism or congenital vestibular syndrome of brachycephalic breeds.

Congenital visual pathway abnormalities in cats
Albino and imperfect albino animals (including Siamese, Birman and Himalayan cats) demonstrate congenital disorganization of the retina and visual pathways (Cucchiaro, 1985; Bacon *et al.*, 1999) (Figure 10.36). The consequent clinical anomalies seen in Siamese and related breeds include convergent strabismus (esotropia) (Figure 10.37) and occasionally spontaneous pendular nystagmus (see **Pendular nystagmus** clip on DVD). The majority of the axonal projections from the temporal retina usually do not cross at the level of the optic chiasm, but in melanin-deficient animals there is increased cross-over of these normally uncrossed pathways at the optic chiasm. During development there is disorganization of the retina, aberrant crossing of optic nerve axons at the optic chiasm, alterations in speed of axonal migration and misrouting of axonal processes within the rostral colliculus, lateral geniculate nucleus and visual cortex. Affected animals are able to make some sense of the conflicting visual inputs by blocking the projections of the inappropriately crossed afferents into the visual cortex and thus restore some vision. However, the consequence is that the consciously perceived visual field and binocularity are reduced.

Although the visual cortex projections of the misrouted visual afferents are blocked, this information is still available for the reflex control of eyeball position and may explain both the convergent strabismus and occasional spontaneous nystagmus present in these cases. Alternatively, the convergent strabismus may be the result of a compensatory attempt to obtain increased overlap of the left and right visual fields. The spontaneous nystagmus is the consequence of the misrouted information being mapped in reverse at the level of the lateral geniculate nucleus. If an animal

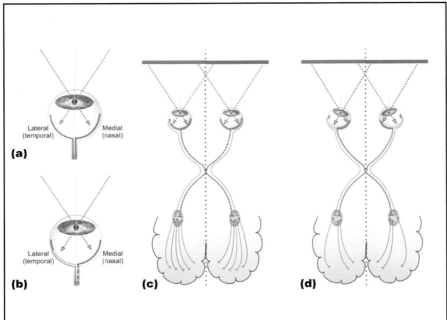

10.36 Visual pathway abnormalities in Siamese and related cat breeds. **(a)** In normal animals the temporal retinal afferents (blue) do not cross at the optic chiasm. **(b)** In Siamese and related cat breeds information from the temporal retina is abnormally crossed at the optic chiasm. **(c)** This misrouted information is then mapped to the wrong lateral geniculate nucleus and visual cortex. **(d)** Affected cats compensate by blocking the cortical projections of the incorrect afferent at the level of the lateral geniculate nucleus, but the result is that the perceived visual field and consequently binocularity are dramatically reduced. However, this inappropriately crossed visual information is still used for eyeball position and visual tracking and this may explain the medial strabismus and abnormal nystagmus. (© Jacques Penderis)

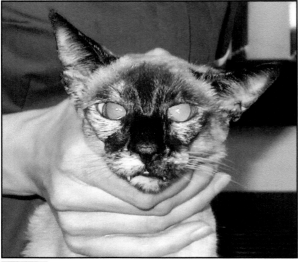

10.37 Convergent strabismus (esotropia) in a Siamese cat with congenital abnormalities of the visual pathways. (© Jacques Penderis)

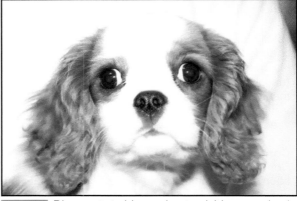

10.38 Divergent strabismus (exotropia) is recognized in brachycephalic dogs, but the underlying cause has yet to be fully elucidated. (© Jacques Penderis)

uses this misrouted and reversed information during attempts to fix the gaze on a visual target, the consequent eyeball movements are inverted and the eye moves in the opposite direction to the target. Repeated eyeball movements in the wrong direction are then made, resulting in nystagmus.

Divergent strabismus in brachycephalic breeds

Congenital divergent strabismus (exotropia), which may be unilateral or bilateral, occurs in brachycephalic breeds, including the Boston Terrier, English Bulldog and Pekingese (Figure 10.38). Vision and eye movements are normal and the condition appears non-progressive. Although no cause has been identified, paresis and abnormal caudal insertion of the medial rectus muscle have been suggested as possible explanations.

Vestibular disease

Disorders affecting the vestibular system may result in alterations in eyeball position and movement, typically the presence of nystagmus and/or strabismus (see **Central vestibular disease** clip on DVD). Nystagmus is categorized as vertical, horizontal or rotary (Figure 10.39). In vestibular disease the strabismus is characteristically ventrolateral in direction and can be induced or exacerbated by holding the head of the animal with the nose elevated (Figure 10.40). Bilateral vestibular disease may cause bilateral ventrolateral strabismus upon elevating the head (Figure 10.41).

Congenital hydrocephalus

In addition to the visual deficits (see above), congenital hydrocephalus is further characterized by the presence of a variable strabismus and abnormal gaze fixation. Strabismus is recognized in a high proportion of human neonates with hydrocephalus and most likely reflects the underlying brain damage

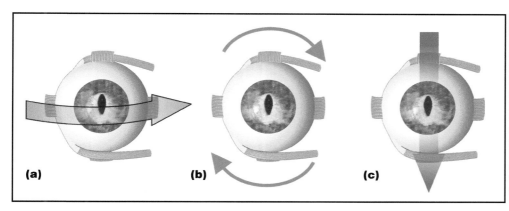

10.39 Spontaneous nystagmus associated with vestibular disease may indicate the site of the lesion. **(a)** Horizontal and **(b)** rotary nystagmus are seen with both peripheral and central vestibular disease, but **(c)** vertical nystagmus is only associated with central vestibular disease. (© Jacques Penderis)

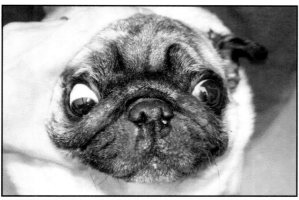

10.40 Ipsilateral ventrolateral strabismus in the right eye of a Pug induced by raising the head. This is a frequent feature of vestibular disease. (© Jacques Penderis)

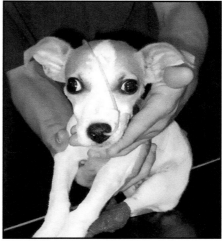

10.42 Congenital hydrocephalus in a Jack Russell Terrier puppy associated with bilateral ventrolateral strabismus ('setting-sun sign'). (© Jacques Penderis)

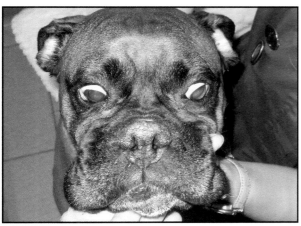

10.41 Bilateral ventrolateral strabismus in a Boxer, which occurred upon raising the head. This is an indication of bilateral vestibular disease. (© Jacques Penderis)

and conformational changes that occur during development (Aring *et al.*, 2007). The strabismus affects both eyes and is typically ventrolateral or ventromedial (the 'setting sun sign') (Harrington *et al.*, 1996) (Figure 10.42). In dogs, ventrolateral strabismus appears to be more common.

Ocular tremor secondary to cerebellar disease
A fine ocular tremor, usually only evident on ophthalmoscopic assessment, may be a feature of severe cerebellar disease. This is thought to be a form of cerebellar intention tremor affecting the extraocular muscles.

Cavernous sinus syndrome
Cavernous sinus syndrome is the most common cause of either external or total ophthalmoplegia (see above for further details).

Extraocular myositis
Inflammation of the extraocular muscles, with a presumed underlying immune-mediated aetiology similar to that of masticatory myositis, occurs occasionally in dogs. During the acute inflammatory phase, affected dogs present with exophthalmos, strabismus and a decreased range of eyeball movement due to the swelling of the extraocular muscles (Figure 10.43). During the chronic stage of the inflammatory disease, muscle tissue is largely replaced by fibrosis and subsequently marked strabismus often develops (despite the resolution of the exophthalmos). Golden Retrievers appear to be over-represented (Williams, 2008). The diagnosis is established by demonstrating enlargement and sometimes oedema of the extraocular muscles on MRI (Figure 10.44) and ultrasonography, demonstrating elevated muscle enzyme levels and confirming inflammatory changes on muscle biopsy

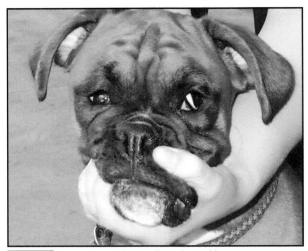

10.43 Lateral strabismus in a dog with acute extraocular myositis. The subsequent fibrosis of the extraocular muscles (following resolution of the acute inflammation) may also result in strabismus. (© Jacques Penderis)

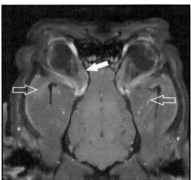

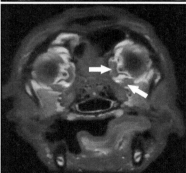

10.44 MR images showing the acute stage of extraocular myositis. Note the enlargement of the extraocular muscles (solid arrows) and more widespread inflammation in the masticatory muscles (open arrows). The masticatory muscles are more accessible, allowing a confirmatory muscle biopsy sample to be obtained. (© Jacques Penderis)

(Ramsey *et al.*, 1995). Although biopsy of the extraocular muscles is difficult, extraocular myositis may occur as part of a wider polymyositis; therefore, biopsy of the readily accessible masticatory muscles may be useful in some cases. Due to the presumed underlying immune-mediated aetiology, this disorder often responds to corticosteroid therapy (Carpenter *et al.*, 1989).

Fibrosing esotropia

Myositis and subsequent fibrosis of the extraocular muscles (with the medial rectus muscle most commonly affected) occurs in young Shar Peis and has also been described in the Irish Wolfhound, Dalmatian, Golden Retriever and Akita. The disease

may occur unilaterally or bilaterally and has a presumed immune-mediated basis. Due to the preferential involvement of the medial rectus muscle, affected dogs present with convergent strabismus (esotropia) and enophthalmos. The esotropia is often so severe that the cornea is obscured by the conjunctiva and vision is consequently impaired (Figure 10.45). Cases may respond to immunosuppressive levels of corticosteroids, but surgical resection of the medial rectus muscle may be required in the presence of severe fibrosis (Gelatt, 2000).

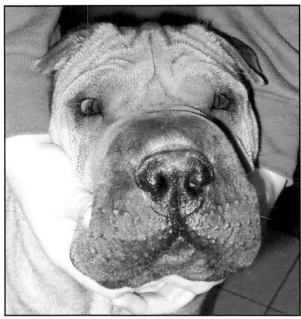

10.45 Fibrosing esotropia in a Shar Pei. The severe convergent strabismus in this case means that the pupils are occluded behind the medial canthus. The sclera is mainly visible. (© Jacques Penderis)

Retrobulbar swelling or trauma

Retrobulbar swelling or mass effect may interfere with normal eyeball movement with affected cases usually presenting with exophthalmos, protrusion of the third eyelid (Figure 10.46) and occasionally mechanical strabismus (Figure 10.47) (Gilger *et al.*, 1992).

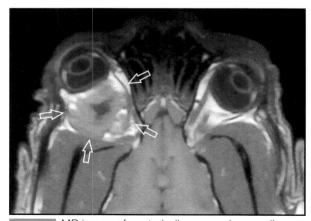

10.46 MR image of a retrobulbar mass (arrowed) causing exophthalmos and interfering with normal eyeball movement. (© Jacques Penderis)

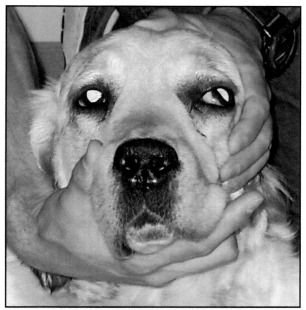

10.47   Left retrobulbar mass. Exophthalmos, protrusion of the third eyelid and mild lateral strabismus are evident in this case. (© Jacques Penderis)

Tetanus
Although the clinical signs of tetanus are usually characteristic, strabismus (Figure 10.48) and brief, intermittent protrusion of the third eyelid may occur (Timoney *et al.*, 1988).

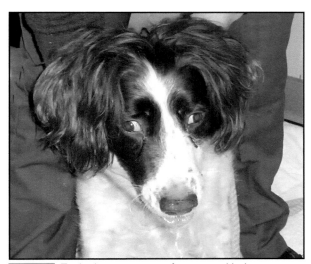

10.48   Typical appearance of tetanus with the ears held close together and the forehead wrinkled. Dogs with tetanus may demonstrate lateral strabismus (as in this case), intermittent protrusion of the third eyelids and photophobia. (© Jacques Penderis)

Intracranial lesions causing strabismus
Intracranial lesions may selectively affect the innervation to certain extraocular muscles, resulting in strabismus. Forebrain lesions causing circling and a head turn may be associated with a lateral strabismus in the direction of the head turn (Figure 10.49). The mechanism for this is uncertain; the neurological deficits responsible for the head turn and circling may induce the lateral strabismus.

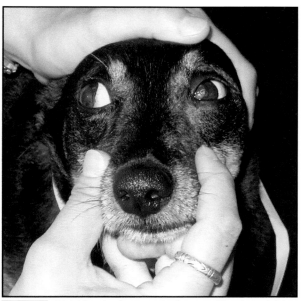

10.49   Right forebrain mass lesion resulting in a right lateral strabismus when the head is held facing forward. The underlying basis for the lateral strabismus ipsilateral to the side of the lesion is unclear, but may be related to a similar mechanism that causes ipsilateral circling and head turn with some asymmetrical forebrain lesions. (© Jacques Penderis)

Eyelid abnormalities
Abnormalities of the eyelids (including blink) are usually the result of lesions affecting CNs V or VII. The integrity of the blink pathway is evaluated by performing the palpebral reflex (afferent touch sensation via the trigeminal nerve and efferent motor function via the facial nerve) and the menace response (afferent visual stimulus via the optic nerve and efferent motor function via the facial nerve).

Sensory lesions
Lesions of the ophthalmic branch of the trigeminal nerve result in loss of sensation to the cornea and medial canthus of the eye (as well as the inner surface of the nostrils and nasal cavity). The consequence of this is loss of the corneal and palpebral reflexes. The menace response should still be intact if vision and the facial nerve are not involved. Exposure keratopathy, with rapid progression from neuroparalytic keratitis to ulcerative keratitis (Figure 10.50), is a frequent complication of ophthalmic branch lesions but is infrequently seen following facial nerve (motor) lesions (except in dog breeds with marked exophthalmos, e.g. Pugs). Although basal tear secretion should be normal, reflex tear production in response to stimulation of the cornea or nasal mucosa is lost as this is mediated via the ophthalmic branch of the trigeminal nerve. Blinking to spread the tear film is also reduced as the perception of corneal drying is reduced or lost. If the mandibular branch of the trigeminal nerve is affected, the resulting masticatory muscle atrophy causes an increase in the retrobulbar space and consequently a pronounced enophthalmos (Figure 10.51).

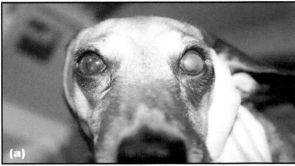

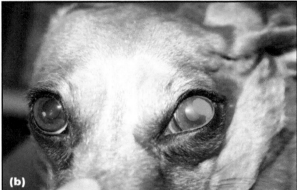

10.50 Neurogenic corneal ulcer (neuroparalytic keratitis) in the left eye of a Dachshund secondary to loss of corneal sensation due to a lesion affecting the ophthalmic branch of the trigeminal nerve. **(a)** Before and **(b)** after fluorescein staining. Neurogenic ulcers tend to be central, situated over the exposed region of the cornea. (© Jacques Penderis)

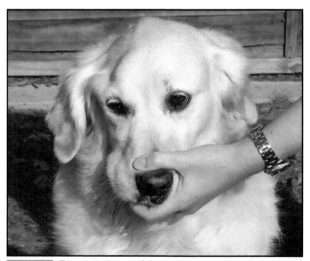

10.51 Enophthalmos of the right eye secondary to masticatory muscle atrophy as a result of a lesion affecting the mandibular branch of the trigeminal nerve. (© Jacques Penderis)

Neoplasia (in particular of the trigeminal nerve roots) is the most common cause of trigeminal nerve sensory lesions (Figure 10.52) but other possibilities should be considered, including trauma, fractures of the petrous temporal bone, inflammatory lesions and cranial polyneuropathies. The sensory portion of the trigeminal nerve is usually not affected in idiopathic trigeminal neuritis (dropped jaw; see Chapter 12 for more details).

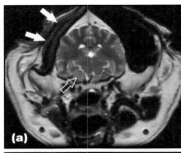

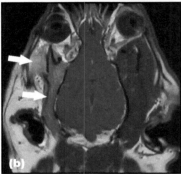

10.52 MR images showing **(a)** a tumour of the trigeminal nerve root (open arrow) and **(b)** consequent atrophy of the masticatory muscles on the affected side (closed arrows). (© Jacques Penderis)

Motor lesions
One of the functions of the facial nerve is innervation of the orbicularis oculi muscle, which is responsible for closing the eyelids. Decreased or absent function of the orbicularis oculi muscle results in a decrease in, or loss of, the menace response and palpebral reflex. The normal retraction of the globe during the corneal reflex is maintained if the trigeminal nerve is preserved. Blinking is responsible for spreading the tear film over the cornea; therefore, loss of blinking may predispose to exposure keratitis (although this is more common when there is concurrent reduced tear production or trigeminal nerve damage).

Hemifacial spasm
Hemifacial spasm (an unusual syndrome in dogs) is characterized by spasm of the muscles innervated by the facial nerve on one side, resulting in blepharospasm, contraction of the upper lip, elevation of the ear and deviation of the nasal philtrum to the affected side (Figure 10.53). The condition is usually intermittent and can often be induced by stimulation of the face on the affected side (Roberts and Vainisi, 1967; Parker *et al.*, 1973). It is thought to represent irritation of the facial nerve, potentially preceding facial nerve paralysis, but has also been described secondary to intracranial mass lesions (Van Meervenne *et al.*, 2008).

Disorders of eyelid opening
Ptosis may be evident with lesions affecting CN III and the sympathetic supply to the head (Horner's syndrome). The ptosis seen with CN III lesions is due to loss of innervation to the levator palpebrae superioris muscle and is easily differentiated from the ptosis seen with Horner's syndrome, primarily through the difference in pupil size (miosis with Horner's syndrome and mydriasis with oculomotor nerve lesions).

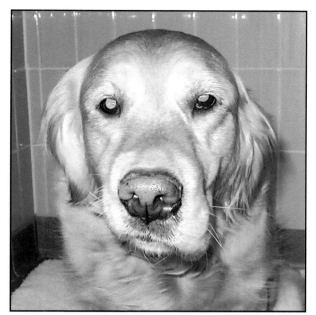

10.53 Right-sided hemifacial spasm in a Golden Retriever. Note the increased tone on the affected side of the face with the lip and ear pulled up in contrast with the normal left side. Although not apparent in this case, hemifacial spasm often causes a narrowed palpebral fissure on the affected side. (© Jacques Penderis)

Third eyelid abnormalities

Protrusion of the third eyelid may occur passively following loss of sympathetic tone to the orbit (Horner's syndrome, dysautonomia and systemic illness), in conditions causing enophthalmos and secondary to retrobulbar masses. Intermittent, brief protrusion of the third eyelid may occur in tetanus (Timoney *et al.*, 1988).

Haw's syndrome in young cats

Haw's syndrome is bilateral protrusion of the third eyelid of unknown cause and occurs in young cats in the absence of other systemic and ophthalmic abnormalities. It has been suggested to occur in dogs, in particular the Golden Retriever (Gelatt, 2000). The condition may develop following a history of diarrhoea and generally persists for some time before gradually resolving. Confirmation of the diagnosis is possible by demonstrating that topical administration of 1–2% adrenaline or 10% phenylephrine can temporarily abolish the third eyelid protrusion (by stimulating smooth muscle contraction). The disorder can be easily differentiated from bilateral Horner's syndrome by the absence of concurrent miosis and from dysautonomia by demonstrating normal pupil dilatation in the dark and constriction in the light.

Abnormal tear production

The normal production of tears can be subdivided into:

- Basal tear production – evaluated by a Schirmer II test, where tear production following anaesthesia of the cornea is measured

- Induced tear production – evaluated by a Schirmer I test, where the cornea is not anaesthetized and as a consequence the stimulation from placing a test strip in the eye induces reflex tear production.

Induced tear production occurs following stimulation of the ophthalmic branch of the trigeminal nerve (which innervates the surface of the cornea and the nasal mucosa) and in response to high light intensities. Loss of induced tear production most commonly occurs due to lesions of the ophthalmic branch of the trigeminal nerve (DeHaas, 1962), but the decreased tear production is less important than the loss of corneal sensation with consequent decreased blink frequency and development of neuroparalytic keratitis.

Decreased tear production

The lacrimal gland is innervated by the parasympathetic portion of the facial nerve, a branch of which also innervates the lateral nasal gland (a serous-secreting gland that functions to keep the nose moist). Lesions affecting the parasympathetic portion of the facial nerve therefore result in neurogenic keratoconjunctivitis sicca (as both basal and reflex tear production are lost) and an ipsilateral xeromycteria (dry nose) (Figure 10.54). The presence of an ipsilateral dry nostril allows differentiation from immune-mediated keratoconjunctivitis sicca, as nasal mucosa hydration is dependent upon the function of the lateral nasal gland and not tear production.

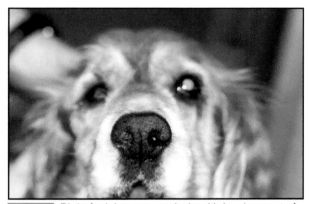

10.54 Right facial nerve paralysis with involvement of the parasympathetic innervation to the lacrimal gland and lateral nasal gland, resulting in neurogenic keratoconjunctivitis sicca and ipsilateral xeromycteria (dry nose). (© Jacques Penderis)

The majority of cases are idiopathic and resolve spontaneously. Those arising from an underlying cause usually improve if this is addressed, but supportive management with supplemental eye lubrication is essential. As there is no underlying immune-mediated process, ciclosporin A is unlikely to have any affect on the neurogenic keratoconjunctivitis sicca. The presence of denervation hypersensitivity following parasympathetic denervation of the lacrimal glands allows the opportunity to re-establish lacrimation in cases that do not spontaneously resolve with a direct parasympatho-mimetic. The drug most commonly used is 1% pilocarpine, given in food twice daily, but the dose should be carefully titrated to achieve an effect that stimulates tear production but avoids the development of deleterious side effects, such as vomiting and diarrhoea.

Increased tear production

Paradoxical tearing (gustatolacrimal reflex or 'crocodile tears') describes the syndrome of excessive tear production whilst eating or during anticipation of a meal. The syndrome has been recognized for a considerable time in humans (Lutman, 1947) and has subsequently been described in the cat (Hacker, 1990). The underlying cause in humans is thought to be aberrant regeneration of facial nerve fibres following trauma, with fibres that usually innervate the salivary glands being misrouted to the lacrimal gland. The name 'crocodile tears' was derived from the popular myth that crocodiles cry whilst eating their prey.

References and further reading

Available on accompanying DVD

DVD extras

- **Central vestibular disease**
- **Electroretinography**
- **Pendular nystagmus**

11

Head tilt and nystagmus

Karen R. Muñana

Head tilt and nystagmus are relatively common presentations in veterinary practice. These signs are typically associated with vestibular disease, although an intermittent head tilt alone may be due to otitis externa or other aural irritation. A thorough neurological evaluation is critical to successful management; by determining the location of the disturbance within the vestibular system, a list of differential diagnoses and a diagnostic plan can be formulated, in conjunction with recommendations for appropriate treatment and an accurate prognosis.

Clinical signs

Head tilt
Head tilt is described as a rotation of the head about the atlas (C1) vertebra, such that one of the ears is held lower than the other (Figure 11.1). Head tilt is indicative of vestibular disease and is the most consistent sign of a unilateral vestibular deficit.

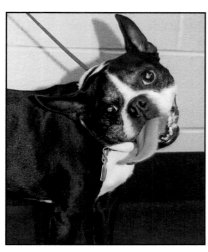

11.1 An 8-year-old Boston Terrier with a right-sided head tilt. (Courtesy of S Platt)

Nystagmus
Nystagmus is a term used to denote the involuntary rhythmic oscillation of the eyeballs.

- Jerk nystagmus – the eye movements have a slow phase in one direction and a rapid recovery in the opposite direction. This is commonly seen with vestibular disease and can be horizontal, rotary or vertical in character. The nystagmus is named according to the direction of the rapid recovery or fast phase of movement.
  - Spontaneous or resting nystagmus – observed when the head is in a normal static position (see **Spontaneous nystagmus (1)** and **(2)** clips on DVD).
  - Positional nystagmus – elicited by moving the head into an unusual position (see **Positional nystagmus** clip on DVD).
- Pendular nystagmus – characterized by small oscillations of the eyes with no fast or slow component and commonly observed as an incidental finding in Siamese, Birman and Himalayan cats. It is a manifestation of a congenital abnormality in the visual pathway, in which a larger percentage than normal of optic nerve axons cross in the chiasm. It can occasionally be seen with cerebellar disease and visual deficits.

Other signs
Other clinical signs of vestibular dysfunction include:

- Ataxia
- Wide-based stance
- Circling, leaning, falling or rolling toward the side of the head tilt (see **Vestibular disease** clip on DVD)
- Positional strabismus (i.e. the eye on the affected side deviates ventrally or ventrolaterally when the head is elevated; see **Positional strabismus** clip on DVD).

An animal with bilateral disease of the vestibular system has neither a head tilt nor a spontaneous or positional nystagmus. Wide excursions of the head from side to side are frequently seen, and the animal lacks a physiological nystagmus. Animals with acute vestibular disease can present with anorexia or vomiting associated with the disequilibrium. Meclozine (dogs: 25 mg/dog orally q24h; cats: 12.5 mg/cat orally q24h) or maropitant (dogs: 1 mg/kg s.c. q24h or 2 mg/kg orally q24h; cats: 1 mg/kg s.c., orally q24h) can be helpful in treatment of this clinical sign.

Lesion localization

The presence of a head tilt and jerk nystagmus is indicative of a disturbance of the vestibular system (Figure 11.2). Further evaluation is necessary to

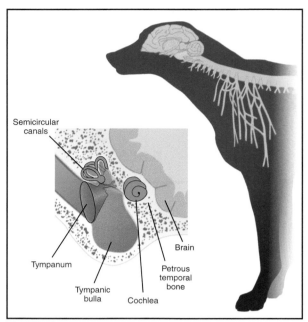

11.2 Lesion localization for head tilt and nystagmus; the brainstem is highlighted. The peripheral section of the vestibular system originates in the petrous temporal bone and the central section resides in the brainstem and flocculonodular lobe of the cerebellum. Inset: middle and inner ear structures (magnified). The membranous labyrinth (blue) contains the sensory receptors for vestibular function and hearing.

central and peripheral diseases, the head tilt, circling and any limb deficits typically occur ipsilateral to the lesion. The differentiation of central and peripheral vestibular disease based on clinical findings is summarized in Figure 11.3.

Clinical sign	Central vestibular disease	Peripheral vestibular disease
Paresis	Possible	No
Proprioceptive deficits	Possible	No
Consciousness	May be depressed, stuporous, comatose	Alert; may be disoriented
Cranial nerve (CN) deficits	CNs V–XII may be affected	CN VII only
Horner's syndrome	Rare	Possible
Nystagmus	Horizontal, rotary or vertical with fast phase in any direction; may change direction with changes in head position	Horizontal or rotary with fast phase away from side of the lesion; direction not altered with head position

11.3 Clinical findings associated with central and peripheral vestibular disease.

determine whether the central or peripheral components of the vestibular system are affected. The peripheral components include the sensory receptors for vestibular input located in the membranous labyrinth of the inner ear and the vestibular portion of cranial nerve (CN) VIII (vestibulocochlear nerve). These peripheral structures are encased within the petrous temporal bone. The central vestibular components include the nuclei and pathways located within the brainstem and cerebellum.

Animals with central vestibular disease typically have additional clinical signs reflective of brainstem involvement, including:

- Deficits of CNs V to XII
- Evidence of ipsilateral paresis or postural reaction deficits due to involvement of the upper motor neuron (UMN) pathways to the limbs
- Depression of consciousness due to disturbance of the ascending reticular activating system.

Nystagmus seen with central diseases can be horizontal, rotary or vertical and can change direction with different positions of the head. In contrast, animals with peripheral disease have a normal level of consciousness (although they can exhibit profound disorientation) and no evidence of weakness or postural reaction deficits. Facial nerve deficits and/or Horner's syndrome can be seen with peripheral disease, due to the proximity of CN VII (facial nerve) and the sympathetic nerve to CN VIII in the area of the petrous temporal bone. Either a horizontal or rotary nystagmus is seen. With both

Paradoxical vestibular disease

Vestibular signs can also be seen with cerebellar lesions that involve the flocculonodular lobe or the caudal cerebellar peduncle. This syndrome is called paradoxical vestibular disease because the head tilt and circling occur contralateral to the lesion. There is usually some evidence of cerebellar disease on neurological examination, such as ipsilateral dysmetria, a head tremor or a truncal sway. These lesions also often affect the proprioceptive and motor pathways in the region, resulting in postural reaction deficits ipsilateral to the lesion but contralateral to the head tilt. Chapter 13 contains further details on cerebellar disease.

Other causes of vestibular disease

Head tilt and nystagmus have also been described in dogs with ischaemic infarcts in the paramedian region of the thalamus. These clinical signs are believed to be due to damage to adjacent midbrain regions involved in vestibular function (Goncalves *et al.*, 2011). In addition, a head tilt can occasionally be seen with focal cervical lesions that affect the spinal muscles asymmetrically, although affected animals do not have other evidence of vestibular dysfunction.

Pathophysiology

The vestibular system functions to maintain an animal's balance and orientation with respect to gravity. The system detects linear acceleration and rotational movement of the head, and is responsible for maintaining the position of the eyes, trunk and limbs in reference to the position of the head.

The sensory receptors for vestibular input are located in the membranous labyrinth of the inner ear (Figure 11.4). The saccule and utricle are primarily responsible for detecting gravity and linear acceleration, and the semicircular canals detect rotation. Input from the receptors enters the brain

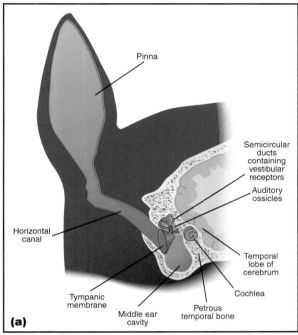

(a)

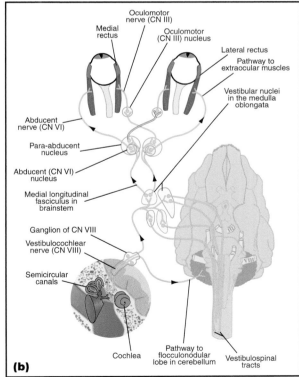

(b)

11.4 **(a)** Overview of the anatomy of the middle and inner ear. **(b)** Overview of the neuronal connections that form the peripheral and central vestibular systems. Stimulation of the peripheral vestibular system in the inner ear ultimately produces a conjugate deviation of the eyes to the ipsilateral side.

via the vestibular portion of CN VIII, where the majority of fibres terminate in one of four vestibular nuclei. The remaining axons terminate in the cerebellum. Pathways from the vestibular nuclei project to the nuclei of CNs III (oculomotor), IV (trochlear) and VI (abducent) to control eye movements, as well as to other brainstem centres and the cerebellum, cerebral cortex and spinal cord (Figure 11.4).

A head tilt results from the loss of anti-gravity muscle tone on one side of the neck. Jerk nystagmus develops from the dysfunction of the pathways responsible for integrating vestibular input with the extraocular eye muscles. The slow phase of the jerk nystagmus is the pathological phase, with the fast phase being corrective or compensatory. Dysfunction of these pathways can also result in a loss of normal physiological nystagmus and/or coordinated eye movements with movement of the head.

Animals use sight and proprioception to compensate for stable or slowly progressing vestibular disease. This might explain the improvement that can be seen in many animals after the onset of vestibular signs, regardless of the underlying cause of the disease (Kent *et al.*, 2010; Rossmeisl, 2010).

Differential diagnosis

The differential diagnoses for an animal with vestibular disease vary considerably depending on whether the vestibular deficits are determined to be central or peripheral in origin. The two most common disease processes that cause central vestibular signs are neoplasia and infection/inflammation, whilst the two most common diagnoses in animals with peripheral vestibular signs are otitis media/interna (OM/OI) and idiopathic vestibular disease. A complete list of differential diagnoses for central and peripheral vestibular localizations is given in Figure 11.5.

Mechanism of disease	Central vestibular disease	Peripheral vestibular disease
Degenerative	Lysosomal storage disorders Neurodegenerative diseases [13]	
Anomalous	Intra-arachnoid cysts [11] Chiari-like malformation [14, 15]	Congenital vestibular disease [11]
Metabolic		Hypothyroidism [11]
Nutritional	Thiamine deficiency [11]	
Neoplasia	Brain tumours [9]	Tumours of the middle or inner ear [11]

11.5 Differential diagnoses associated with central and peripheral vestibular system disease. Numbers in square brackets refer to chapters where details can be found. (continues) ▶

Mechanism of disease	Central vestibular disease	Peripheral vestibular disease
Inflammatory	Meningoencephalitis [11]	Otitis media/interna Nasopharyngeal polyps [11]
Idiopathic		Idiopathic vestibular disease [11]
Toxic	Metronidazole [11]	Aminoglycosides, topical iodophors, chlorhexidine, others [11]
Trauma	Head trauma [20]	Trauma to the middle or inner ear [11]
Vascular	Cerebrovascular disease	

11.5 (continued) Differential diagnoses associated with central and peripheral vestibular system disease. Numbers in square brackets refer to chapters where details can be found.

Neurodiagnostic investigation

A thorough history should be obtained to gain information with respect to the onset and progression of the disease, any history of trauma, vaccination history, presence of other clinical signs, history of ear disease and whether potentially ototoxic drugs have been administered.

A complete neurological examination is necessary to determine whether the vestibular deficits are due to a central or a peripheral disease, which then dictates the emphasis of further diagnostic testing. A complete blood count, blood chemistry, thyroid panel and urinalysis should be performed in all animals presenting with vestibular signs. This can be useful for identifying potential inflammatory or metabolic disturbances that might be responsible for the clinical signs, in addition to serving as a general health screen, because further diagnostic testing usually requires anaesthesia. Blood pressure measurements should also be obtained, as hypertension can manifest as vestibular dysfunction (Brown *et al.*, 2007; Bentley and March, 2011).

Peripheral vestibular disease

An animal determined to have peripheral vestibular disease should undergo a thorough otoscopic examination, performed under anaesthesia, along with radiographs of the tympanic bullae to assess for OM/OI. It should be noted that normal radiographs do not rule out OM/OI. If there is evidence of OM/OI, a sample of fluid should be obtained via myringotomy and submitted for cytology and bacterial culture (see **Myringotomy** clip on DVD).

Computed tomography (CT) and magnetic resonance imaging (MRI) of the tympanic bullae are the most sensitive means of identifying fluid within the middle ear, and can be considered in cases posing a diagnostic challenge. If the equipment is available, hearing can be assessed using a brainstem auditory evoked potential (BAEP) to evaluate for involvement of the cochlear branch of CN VIII. Cats should undergo a thorough pharyngeal examination to check for possible inflammatory polyps.

The diagnostic approach to an animal with peripheral vestibular disease is summarized in Figure 11.6.

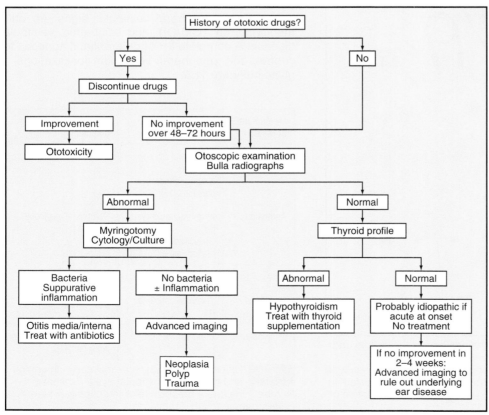

11.6 Diagnostic algorithm for the work-up of an animal presenting with signs of peripheral vestibular disease.

Central vestibular disease

Diagnostic testing in an animal determined to have central vestibular disease should include advanced imaging of the brain (preferably MRI) to identify any structural abnormalities. Analysis of cerebrospinal fluid (CSF) collected from the cerebellomedullary cistern can also be helpful. However, if any abnormality is identified on imaging that suggests increased intracranial pressure (ICP), such as a mass effect (shifting of structures across the midline), CSF should not be collected because of the risk of fatal brain herniation. When collected, CSF is tested for evidence of inflammation and increased protein concentrations (see Chapter 3). Serological ± CSF testing for potential infectious agents is indicated where CSF testing shows inflammation.

It should be noted that an animal with central vestibular disease can initially present with signs referable to the peripheral components. This is most commonly seen with extra-axial masses that compress CN VIII as it exits the brainstem. For this reason, it is recommended that an animal with apparent peripheral disease undergo brain imaging and possible CSF analysis if signs do not improve with treatment over the course of 2–4 weeks.

Peripheral vestibular diseases

Anomalous diseases

Congenital vestibular disease

Congenital vestibular diseases are seen infrequently in dogs and cats but have been reported in Siamese, Burmese and Tonkanese cats, and in Dobermanns (Figure 11.7), Cocker Spaniels, German Shepherd Dogs, Akitas, Smooth Fox Terriers and Beagles (see Appendix 1).

Clinical signs: The onset is usually first noticed between 3 and 12 weeks of age. Head tilt, ataxia and circling can be seen. Nystagmus is not a characteristic feature. In some animals, deafness accompanies the vestibular signs.

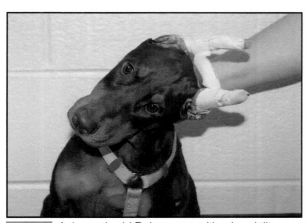

11.7 A 4-month-old Dobermann with a head tilt which the owner had identified when the dog was 2 months old. The diagnostic investigation suggested it was compatible with a congenital lesion seen in this breed. (Courtesy of S Platt)

Pathogenesis: The pathogenesis is not known. One study of Dobermanns demonstrated non-inflammatory cochlear degeneration in affected animals, with progressive loss of the auditory sensory hair cells (Wilkes and Palmer, 1992), whilst a separate study revealed the presence of lymphocytic labyrinthitis in affected Dobermann puppies (Forbes and Cooke, 1991).

Diagnosis: The diagnosis is confirmed by exclusion of other disorders and consideration of the signalment and history.

Treatment and prognosis: No treatment is available. Vestibular signs can improve over time; this is most likely due to compensation for a static vestibular deficit rather than disease resolution. Deafness, if present, tends to be permanent. Affected animals should not be bred from as the condition is presumed to be inherited.

Metabolic diseases

Hypothyroidism

Peripheral vestibular disease has occasionally been reported in association with hypothyroidism (Jaggy et al., 1994; Vitale et al., 2007).

Clinical signs: Clinical signs include head tilt, ataxia, circling and positional strabismus, unless the disease is bilateral, in which case wide excursions of the head and neck result. Facial nerve paresis has been reported in conjunction with vestibular signs in some dogs. Signs commonly attributed to hypothyroidism, such as lethargy, weight gain and poor hair coat, are frequently absent in affected dogs. The onset of signs can be either acute or chronic, and the disease course can be either progressive or non-progressive.

Pathogenesis: The pathogenesis of peripheral nerve disease associated with the hypothyroid state is not completely understood; however, it is believed to reflect a deficit in energy metabolism and the resultant disturbance in axonal transport.

Diagnosis: The diagnosis is based on laboratory evaluation of thyroid function and the response to treatment.

Treatment and prognosis: Supplementation with levothyroxine is the standard therapy. Resolution of most neurological deficits is expected within 2 months, although a residual head tilt and positional strabismus can persist.

Neoplastic diseases

Tumours of the middle or inner ear

Clinical signs: Neoplastic conditions of the inner or middle ear can cause peripheral vestibular signs in dogs and cats. Tumours that have been reported to cause vestibular disease include (Kirpensteijn, 1993; Garosi *et al.*, 2001):

- Fibrosarcoma, chondrosarcoma and osteosarcoma of the osseous bulla
- Squamous cell carcinoma
- Ceruminous gland adenocarcinoma
- Lymphoma.

Pathogenesis: Vestibular signs are caused by the destruction or compression of CN VIII by the tumour.

Diagnosis: Radiography of the skull often reveals destruction of the tympanic bulla; associated soft tissue swelling or periosteal reaction can also be evident. Advanced imaging via CT or MRI provides additional detail with respect to the origin and extent of the neoplastic process and determines whether the tumour has invaded the cranial vault (Figure 11.8).

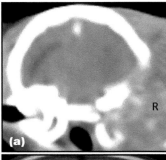
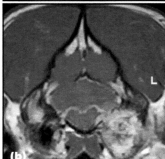

11.8 **(a)** CT image of a cat with an aggressive tumour involving the right tympanic bulla. There is bony destruction of the bulla, extensive soft tissue involvement and evidence of extension into the cranial cavity. **(b)** Contrast-enhanced transverse T1-weighted image of a dog with an aggressive tumour involving the left tympanic bulla. There is extensive soft tissue involvement and erosion of the adjacent calvarium with extension into the cranial vault.

Treatment and prognosis: Complete surgical resection of tumours involving the middle or inner ear is difficult. Adjunctive radiation therapy is recommended when complete surgical resection is not possible. Prognosis depends upon the tumour type and extent of the disease, but overall tends to be poor.

Inflammatory diseases

Otitis media/interna
OM/OI is one of the more commonly recognized causes of peripheral vestibular disease in both dogs and cats (Schlicksup *et al.*, 2009).

Clinical signs: Evidence of otitis externa (OE) can be apparent on general physical examination. Facial nerve paralysis, neurogenic keratoconjunctivitis sicca and/or Horner's syndrome can be seen in

association with the vestibular signs, due to the close association of CN VII and the sympathetic supply with the petrous temporal bone. Disease is most frequently unilateral, but bilateral disease can also occur.

Pathogenesis: OM/OI typically develops as an extension of OE, with common bacterial isolates including *Staphylococcus intermedius* and *Pseudomonas* spp. (Cole *et al.*, 1998). OM/OI can occur in the absence of OE, in which case it is believed to be due to the ascent of bacteria from the oral cavity through the auditory tube or by haematogenous spread.

Diagnosis: The diagnosis is based on thorough otoscopic examination and imaging of the tympanic bullae. Radiography of the tympanic bullae can reveal evidence of fluid density within, and sclerosis of, the bulla (Figure 11.9). However, radiographs can be normal in some cases, particularly early in the course of disease, and thus additional imaging techniques such as CT or MRI might be required to provide more sensitive imaging of the bone and soft tissue in the affected area (Figure 11.10).

Any exudate noted in the external ear canal should be removed by gentle saline irrigation to visualize the tympanic membrane. The tympanic membrane is frequently ruptured; if it is intact, it can appear to be bulging into the external ear canal. If fluid is visualized within the middle ear, an attempt should be made to obtain a sample via

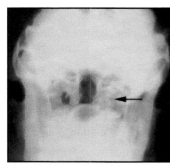

11.9 Open-mouth bulla view of a dog with unilateral OM/OI. The left tympanic bulla is obscured by bone and soft tissue density (arrowed) compared with the normal air-filled right bulla.

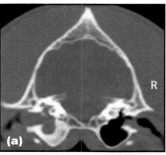

11.10 **(a)** CT image of a dog with chronic left-sided OM/OI. Note the bony sclerosis and soft tissue density within the tympanic bulla. **(b)** Transverse T2-weighted MR image of a cat with OM/OI. Note that the hyperintensity seen within the bulla is present within the ventromedial and dorsolateral cavities of the middle ear.

myringotomy. This can be performed under general anaesthesia by inserting a 22-gauge spinal needle or tomcat catheter through the ventral aspect of the tympanic membrane, using an otoscope for guidance. The fluid present can then be gently aspirated into a syringe and submitted for cytology and bacterial culture.

Treatment and prognosis: The treatment for bacterial OM/OI consists of a 4–6 week course of systemic antibacterial drugs. The choice of drugs should be based on the results of culture and sensitivity testing (if samples are successfully obtained via myringotomy). Otherwise, a drug that is effective against the most common causative organisms and that penetrates the tympanic bullae (e.g. amoxicillin/clavulanate, a cephalosporin or a fluoroquinolone) should be chosen. Otic cleansing products should not be used, particularly if the tympanic membrane initially cannot be visualized. If cleansing products escape into the middle ear, they can worsen the vestibular signs and cause deafness.

Prognosis is good for resolution of the infection, although neurological deficits can persist after effective medical therapy due to irreversible damage to the neural structures. Cases that are unresponsive to medical therapy might require surgical drainage and debridement via bulla osteotomy. Occasionally, an infection can extend into the cranial vault causing central rather than peripheral vestibular signs to predominate (Figure 11.11). Aggressive management, including surgical drainage of the tympanic bulla and cranial vault via a bulla osteotomy and appropriate drug therapy, can result in a favourable outcome in such cases (Sturges *et al.*, 2006).

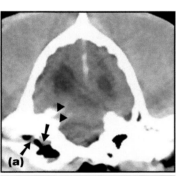
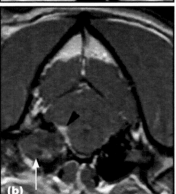

11.11 **(a)** Contrast-enhanced CT image of a dog with OM/OI with extension into the brain. Note the soft tissue density within the tympanic bulla (arrowed). The contrast medium has enhanced areas at the cerebellopontine medullary angle on the same side (arrowheads). **(b)** Contrast-enhanced transverse T1-weighted MR image of a dog with OM/OI with extension into the brain. Note the soft tissue density within the tympanic bulla (arrowed). There is evidence of linear peripheral enhancement in the caudal fossa on the same side (arrowhead).

Nasopharyngeal polyps

Nasopharyngeal (inflammatory) polyps comprise well vascularized fibrous tissue lined by epithelium.

Clinical signs: Disease is identified most frequently in cats from 1 to 5 years of age but has been reported in dogs. Polyps can cause signs of upper respiratory disease and dysphagia in addition to peripheral vestibular dysfunction. Evidence of OE is often present.

Pathogenesis: Nasopharyngeal polyps originate in the auditory tube or the lining of the tympanic cavity and grow passively into the nasopharynx or middle ear of cats and, very rarely, dogs. OM/OI can be a complication of auditory tube obstruction by the polyp.

Diagnosis: The diagnosis is based on visualizing the polyp in the nasopharynx or external ear canal during a thorough pharyngeal and otoscopic examination performed under anaesthesia. Radiography can reveal occlusion of the nasopharynx or sclerosis and soft tissue opacity within the tympanic bulla. Advanced imaging can provide additional information on the extent of soft tissue involvement associated with the polyp (Figure 11.12).

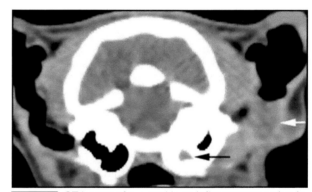

11.12 CT image of a cat with an inflammatory polyp in the right ear canal and secondary OM/OI. Note the soft tissue density within the tympanic bulla (black arrow) characteristic of OM/OI as well as the soft tissue density polyp obscuring the horizontal ear canal (white arrow).

Treatment and prognosis: Treatment involves removal of the polyp. Many polyps are attached to the auditory tube by a narrow stalk of tissue and this can be successfully removed with simple traction. More extensive polyps may require surgical removal via ventral bulla osteotomy (Anders *et al.*, 2008). Horner's syndrome is a common postoperative complication following ventral bulla osteotomy, but tends to be transient.

Overall prognosis is good. However, recurrence is possible, especially for polyps removed non-surgically.

Idiopathic diseases

Idiopathic vestibular disease

Idiopathic vestibular disease is a common cause of vestibular disturbance in both dogs and cats.

Clinical signs: These most commonly reflect unilateral involvement of the peripheral vestibular system and can be quite severe and acute at onset. Occasionally, bilateral disease is seen, especially in cats (Negrin *et al.*, 2010). In contrast with many of the other diseases that affect the peripheral vestibular system, facial paresis and Horner's syndrome are not features of idiopathic vestibular disease (Schunk and Averill, 1983; Burke *et al.*, 1985).

Pathogenesis: Idiopathic vestibular disease is characterized by the acute or even peracute onset of non-progressive peripheral vestibular signs.

- The canine form typically, but not exclusively, affects older dogs and is also known as canine geriatric vestibular disease.
- The feline form is seen in cats of all ages and is documented to be most common in the spring to autumn months, especially in the north-eastern USA (no such temporal association has been made in Europe).

The aetiology of these disorders has not been determined. However, it has been hypothesized that the feline disease in the USA may be caused by *Cuterebra* larval migration (Glass *et al.*, 1998). It should be emphasized, however, that idiopathic vestibular disease is a disorder of the peripheral vestibular system and that *Cuterebra* migration is often the cause of central nervous system (CNS) disease; although this may affect the vestibular system, it also causes progressive multifocal signs.

Diagnosis: The diagnosis is based on the presence of a compatible history and physical examination findings, and the exclusion of other causes of peripheral vestibular disease. Typically, improvement in clinical signs is seen within 2–3 days.

Treatment and prognosis: No treatment is recommended aside from supportive care, which consists of administering intravenous fluids to animals that are vomiting, and confining the animal to a well padded area in order to minimize self-trauma secondary to disorientation. Meclozine or maropitant can be given to treat nausea.

Prognosis is good as the condition resolves on its own within 2–4 weeks in dogs and 4–6 weeks in cats. A mild residual head tilt or ataxia can persist in some animals.

Toxic diseases

Ototoxicity

Clinical signs: Ototoxic agents can affect vestibular function, hearing or both.

Pathogenesis: The systemic administration of aminoglycosides is most commonly associated with ototoxicity. Prolonged therapy for >2 weeks with high doses of the drug is necessary to induce changes in normal animals; however, animals with renal impairment are more susceptible to developing toxicity.

Of the aminoglycosides, streptomycin is most often associated with damage to the vestibular system. Other agents can induce ototoxicity when used topically, the most notable of which are the iodophors and chlorhexidine. Due to the potential for ototoxicity, topical otic preparations should never be introduced into the ear when the tympanic membrane cannot be visualized or is determined to be ruptured.

Diagnosis: The diagnosis is based on the acute onset of compatible clinical signs in an animal that has recently been administered an ototoxic agent, in addition to the exclusion of other causes. Deafness can be confirmed with BAEP testing.

Treatment and prognosis: No definitive treatment is possible. Vestibular signs usually improve over time, due to resolution of the damage or compensatory mechanisms, but deafness tends to be permanent.

Traumatic diseases

Trauma to the middle and inner ear

Clinical signs: Traumatic injuries to the middle and inner ear can result in peripheral vestibular signs. Horner's syndrome and facial nerve involvement can also be seen due to the close association of these nerves to CN VIII in the area of the petrous temporal bone. Facial abrasions and swelling can be apparent in some animals, and haemorrhage can be present in the external ear canal on the affected side.

Pathogenesis: Vestibular signs are caused by direct damage to CN VIII or compression by bone fragments or haemorrhage.

Diagnosis: In addition to a suggested or confirmed history of trauma, radiography can reveal fractures of the tympanic bulla. CT and MRI (Figure 11.13) can be helpful in showing fractures not identified on skull radiography, as well as determining the extent of soft tissue involvement, respectively.

Treatment and prognosis: No specific treatment is typically recommended other than that required for the head trauma itself (see Chapter 20).

Prognosis depends upon the severity of the injury. In general, vestibular signs tend to improve over time but residual deficits can persist.

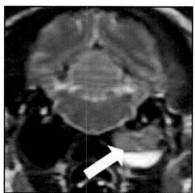

11.13

Transverse T2-weighted MR image of a cat following a traumatic head injury causing acute clinical vestibular signs and middle ear haemorrhage (arrowed).

Central vestibular diseases

Degenerative diseases

Lysosomal storage disorders and neurodegenerative diseases
Lysosomal storage disorders are inborn errors of metabolism in which specific deficiencies of degradative enzymes cause substrate accumulation and result in cellular and clinical dysfunction.

Neurodegenerative disorders are diseases associated with an abnormality in the metabolic pathway that leads to early death of the neuron. Several of these conditions can present with ataxia and incoordination suggestive of vestibular disease. (See Chapter 13 for a more detailed discussion of this class of disorders and Appendix 1 for a list of reported breed associations.)

Anomalous diseases

Chiari-like malformations
Chiari-like malformations are congenital defects characterized by caudal displacement of part of the cerebellum through the foramen magnum. This occurs as a result of occipital bone hypoplasia causing the caudal fossa to become abnormal in size or shape. This malformation can cause compression of the brainstem and cerebellum, and result in signs of central vestibular disease; although, this is clinically not commonly seen. A more thorough discussion of Chiari-like malformations can be found in Chapters 14 and 15.

Intracranial intra-arachnoid cysts
Intracranial intra-arachnoid (supracollicular or quadrigeminal) cysts are uncommon but have been described most frequently in small brachycephalic breeds of dog (Matiasek *et al.*, 2007). These cysts can also occur in cats. Intra-arachnoid cysts are accumulations of CSF that arise between two layers of the arachnoid membrane and cover the neural parenchyma. These cysts can occur anywhere along the CSF pathway, but in dogs are most commonly reported in the quadrigeminal cistern, a triangular space between the caudal cerebral hemispheres, dorsal to the midbrain and rostral to the cerebellum (Vernau *et al.*, 1997). Cysts in the quadrigeminal cistern can cause compression of the adjacent cerebellum and occipital lobe.

Clinical signs: Neurological findings in animals with quadrigeminal intra-arachnoid cysts often include cerebellar and/or vestibular signs attributable to compression of the cerebellum by the cyst. Hemiparesis and depression may be apparent with brainstem involvement. Dogs can also present with seizures, which are presumed to be associated with compression of the occipital cortex by the cyst. Seizures can occur alone or in combination with cerebellar or vestibular signs. Intracranial arachnoid cysts are often incidental findings and other causes of neurological disease should be excluded before attributing the clinical signs to compression from the cyst.

Pathogenesis: The cause of these cysts is not known, but in most cases it is believed to be congenital and reflects splitting of the arachnoid mater.

Diagnosis: The diagnosis is based on brain imaging. Both MRI and CT characteristics have been described in dogs (Vernau *et al.*, 1997; Matiasek *et al.*, 2007). Typically, cysts are located in an extra-axial position, have sharply delineated margins and contain a fluid that is either isodense or isointense compared with the CSF (Figure 11.14). The cyst wall and contents are not enhanced by intravenous administration of contrast medium.

Intra-arachnoid cysts within the quadrigeminal cistern can also be identified using ultrasonography, with images obtained through a persistent bregmatic fontanelle, the temporal window in the area of thin bone at the junction of the temporal and parietal bones, or the foramen magnum (Saito *et al.*, 2001). The majority of affected animals have enlarged lateral ventricles in addition to the fluid-filled cyst at the level of the quadrigeminal cistern (Figure 11.14). CSF should be analysed to rule out the possibility of underlying infectious or inflammatory diseases.

Treatment and prognosis: Reports on treatment for intracranial arachnoid cysts in dogs are limited. Medical management consists of administering antiepileptic drugs to animals with seizures and prednisolone to decrease CSF production. Surgical management has been described in dogs and consists of either fenestrating or shunting the cyst (Vernau *et al.*, 1997; Dewey *et al.*, 2007). Little information exists on long-term follow-up of dogs treated either medically or surgically and consequently the overall prognosis is unknown.

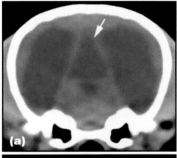
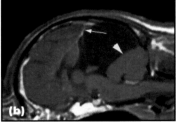

11.14 **(a)** CT image of a dog with an intracranial intra-arachnoid cyst in the region of the quadrigeminal cistern. The cistern is represented by the sharply delineated, triangular fluid-filled space (arrowed). Note the dilated lateral ventricles on either side. **(b)** Sagittal T1-weighted MR image of a dog with an intracranial intra-arachnoid cyst in the region of the quadrigeminal cistern. Note the compression of the occipital lobe of the cerebrum (arrowed) and the cerebellum (arrowhead).

Metabolic diseases

Hypothyroidism
Central vestibular signs have been reported as an uncommon manifestation of hypothyroidism in dogs.

Clinical signs: Affected dogs manifest with an acute onset of persistent or episodic vestibular disease. Signs tend to progress over time. Other physical abnormalities characteristic of hypothyroidism are typically not evident.

Pathogenesis: Some dogs with hypothyroid-associated central vestibular disease have evidence of brain infarction on MRI, which is believed to be secondary to atherosclerotic vascular disease. The pathogenesis in dogs without infarcts is poorly understood, but is believed to be multifactorial and may involve functional ischaemic lesions and metabolic derangements of neurons or glial cells within the brain secondary to thyroid hormone deficiency (Higgins *et al.*, 2006).

Diagnosis: MRI of the brain can reveal changes consistent with an infarct. A chemistry profile typically reveals hypercholesterolaemia. Analysis of CSF collected from the cerebellomedullary cistern can demonstrate albuminocytological dissociation. Thyroid function testing typically demonstrates a decrease in serum free and total T4, and an increase in thyroid-stimulating hormone (TSH) levels.

Treatment and prognosis: Treatment with levothyroxine results in improvement of vestibular signs, with resolution typically occurring within 4 weeks.

Neoplastic diseases

Brain tumours
Of the primary brain tumours seen in dogs, meningiomas and choroid plexus papillomas have a site predilection for the caudal fossa. As such, vestibular signs are commonly encountered in affected animals. The reader is referred to Chapter 9 for a more thorough discussion of brain tumours.

Brain cysts
Dermoid and epidermoid cysts are occasionally classified as neoplastic abnormalities. Many of the canine epidermoid cysts reported have been located in the cerebellomedullary pontine angle and can extend into the fourth ventricle (Platt *et al.*, 1999). Although these cysts can be incidental findings on post-mortem examination, dogs with clinical signs consistently have vestibular dysfunction. These cysts have a stratified squamous epithelium lining and expand by progressive exfoliation into the lumen. Definitive treatment is achieved by total surgical removal of the cyst; however, the success of surgical resection depends upon the location of the lesion.

Intracranial dermoid cysts are less common than epidermoid cysts in dogs. Dermoid cysts are neoplastic lesions with a complex cyst wall, containing both epidermoid tissue and adnexa. Due to the caudal fossa location of these lesions, they can be associated with vestibulocerebellar signs and obstructive hydrocephalus. Both types of cyst have characteristic MRI signs (Platt *et al.*, 1999; Targett *et al.*, 1999).

Nutritional diseases

Thiamine deficiency
Although now not commonly encountered, a deficiency of thiamine (vitamin B1) can cause a rapidly progressive encephalopathy in both dogs and cats.

Clinical signs: Initial clinical signs include anorexia and lethargy. Neurological deficits develop a few days later and commonly manifest as vestibular signs, along with pupillary dilatation and seizures. As this is a bilaterally symmetrical disease, the vestibular signs often present as wide excursions of the head and neck with poor to absent physiological nystagmus. Cats can develop marked ventroflexion of the head and neck (Figure 11.15) and curl up in a tight semicircular position. Paraparesis can also be seen in dogs.

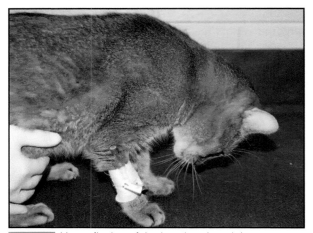

11.15 Ventroflexion of the head and neck in a cat presented with central vestibular disease due to thiamine deficiency. (Courtesy of S Platt)

Pathogenesis: Thiamine plays an essential role as a coenzyme in the metabolism of carbohydrates. Inhibition of carbohydrate metabolism in a thiamine-deficient state leads to energy depletion and results in neuronal necrosis.

Thiamine deficiency in cats most frequently results from feeding a raw fish diet that is rich in thiaminase. An excessive amount of cereal in the diet has also been shown to predispose cats to thiamine deficiency. Thiamine deficiency in dogs and cats can be caused by feeding cooked meat or canned food heated to excessive temperatures (>100°C) (Marks *et al.*, 2011). In addition, the use of sulphur dioxide as a preservative can destroy thiamine in food and cause signs of deficiency in both dogs and cats. Gastrointestinal or pancreatic disease with impaired absorption of dietary thiamine should also be considered as a potential underlying cause. More recently, there have been reports associated with feeding of canned cat food (Marks *et al.*, 2011).

Diagnosis: The diagnosis is based on historical findings suggesting a thiamine-deficient diet (although this might not always be evident), along with compatible examination findings and measurement of blood thiamine levels. MRI can demonstrate the presence of bilaterally symmetrical areas of haemorrhage and malacia within susceptible nuclei of the brain (Garosi *et al.*, 2003) (Figure 11.16).

Gross pathological findings include bilaterally symmetrical petechial haemorrhage in brainstem nuclei (including the vestibular, oculomotor and red nuclei) with the caudal colliculi most frequently affected. Microscopic lesions are confined to the grey matter and are characterized by focal, symmetrical areas of oedema and neuronal necrosis.

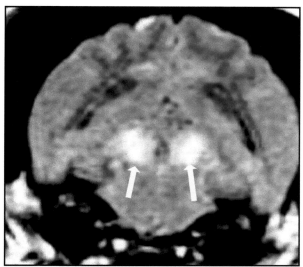

11.16 Transverse T2-weighted FLAIR MR cerebral image of a dog with confirmed thiamine deficiency. The caudal colliculi on both sides are hyperintense, compatible with cytotoxic oedema of these nuclei (arrowed). (Courtesy of L Garosi)

Treatment and prognosis: The disease is rapidly progressive and typically fatal if left untreated. However, treatment with thiamine (12.5–50 mg/dog or 12.5–25 mg/cat i.m. or s.c. q24h until oral supplementation is possible) in the early stages of disease can lead to rapid reversal of clinical signs; although, some signs, such as blindness and wide excursions of the head and neck, can be residual.

Inflammatory diseases

Meningoencephalitis
Meningoencephalitis refers to inflammation of the brain and surrounding meninges.

Clinical signs: As a general rule, inflammatory diseases tend to be acute in onset and progressive, with a multifocal or diffuse, often asymmetrical, distribution within the CNS. Neurological manifestations are quite variable and reflect the location of the inflammatory foci within the nervous system.

Central vestibular signs are commonly encountered and can be seen alone or in combination with other neurological signs. Neck pain can also be present as a manifestation of meningeal inflammation. Animals with CNS infections frequently do not have evidence of systemic involvement. Therefore, the absence of fever, anorexia and depression, and the presence of a normal haemogram cannot be used to exclude the possibility of an infectious aetiology in an animal with neurological signs.

Pathogenesis: Infectious causes of CNS inflammation in small animals include viral, protozoal, fungal, parasitic and bacterial organisms (Figure 11.17). The most commonly recognized CNS infections in dogs include:

- Canine distemper virus (uncommon if vaccinated)
- Rickettsial disease (e.g. ehrlichiosis and Rocky Mountain spotted fever; very rare in Europe)
- Protozoal infections (e.g. toxoplasmosis and neosporosis)
- Fungal diseases (e.g. cryptococcosis; rare in the UK).

Inflammatory, non-infectious causes of CNS dysfunction in dogs include such diseases as granulomatous meningoencephalomyelitis (GME) and necrotizing encephalitis. These diseases are often grouped together antemortem within the term meningoencephalitis of unknown origin (MUO). CNS infections in cats most commonly involve feline coronavirus (which causes feline infectious peritonitis, FIP), toxoplasmosis and cryptococcosis.

Diagnosis: A thorough ophthalmological examination should be performed in every neurological case to look for evidence of fundic changes or uveitis compatible with inflammatory disease. Definitive diagnosis of CNS inflammatory disease is typically based on finding an increased total nucleated cell count (TNCC) or an abnormal cell type distribution, with a concomitant increase in protein concentrations, on CSF analysis (see Chapter 3). In rare instances, normal CSF can be obtained from an animal with confirmed CNS inflammatory disease. This can occur if the inflammation does not involve the meninges or the ependymal lining of the ventricular system, or if the animal has been treated with corticosteroids prior to CSF collection. Elevations in protein concentration can result from breakdown of the blood–brain barrier or intrathecal antibody production. It is likely that both of these mechanisms contribute toward the elevated protein levels recognized with most CNS inflammatory disease.

Cytological evaluation of the fluid provides additional information as to possible causes:

- Viral diseases typically result in mild lymphocytic inflammation, with the exception of FIP, which can cause neutrophilic pleocytosis
- Bacterial infections usually cause a marked increase in neutrophils in the CSF, with cell counts often >500 cells/µl. There is also evidence of toxic changes in cell morphology. However, mixed neutrophilic and mononuclear

inflammation can be observed in animals with bacterial diseases that have been previously treated with antibacterial drugs
- Rickettsial infections frequently cause mild mononuclear inflammation, although neutrophilic inflammation can be seen with Rocky Mountain

Viral
• Canine distemper • Rabies • Pseudorabies • Canine herpesvirus • Canine parainfluenza • Canine parvovirus • Infectious canine hepatitis • Central European tick-borne encephalitis • Borna disease virus • Feline coronavirus (which causes FIP) • Feline immunodeficiency virus • Feline leukaemia virus

Protozoal
• Toxoplasmosis • Neosporosis • Encephalitozoonosis • Acanthamoebiasis • *Sarcocystis*-like organism • Trypanosomiasis • Babesiosis

Rickettsial
• Ehrlichiosis • Rocky Mountain spotted fever • Salmon poisoning disease

Bacterial
• Aerobes • Anaerobes • Leptospirosis

Fungal
• Cryptococcosis • Blastomycosis • Histoplasmosis • Coccidioidomycosis • Aspergillosis • Phaeohyphomycosis • Hyalohyphomycosis

Parasitic
• *Cuterebra* • *Dirofilaria immitis* • *Toxocara canis* • *Ancylostoma caninum* • *Angiostrongylus vasorum* (Europe) or *cantonensis* (Australia)

Algal
• Protothecosis

Idiopathic
• Granulomatous meningoencephalomyelitis • Necrotizing meningoencephalomyelitis • Polioencephalomyelitis • Pyogranulomatous meningoencephalomyelitis • Eosinophilic meningoencephalitis • Periventricular encephalitis

11.17 Causes of clinical meningoencephalitis in dogs and cats.

spotted fever, secondary to an associated vasculitis
- Protozoal diseases most often result in mild to moderate inflammation with a mixed population of neutrophils and mononuclear cells, with occasional eosinophils
- Fungal infections usually cause a mixed or primary neutrophilic inflammation. Eosinophils can also be seen, especially with cryptococcosis (Windsor *et al.*, 2009).

Additional testing, based on the cytological evaluation, is performed in an attempt to identify the infectious cause of the inflammation. These tests can include:

- CSF culture for bacterial or fungal organisms
- Serum and CSF antibody or antigen titres
- CSF polymerase chain reaction (PCR) analysis.

However, despite extensive testing, an underlying cause for the inflammation is not determined in most cases.

Treatment and prognosis: Treatment is aimed at the primary disease process. Treatment with clindamycin (10–15 mg/kg orally q12h) and/or trimethoprim/sulphonamide (15 mg/kg orally q12h) for potential protozoal infections can be initiated once a diagnosis of encephalomyelitis has been made based on CSF results, whilst additional test results are pending. If no infectious cause is discovered upon additional testing, or the animal does not respond to initial antimicrobial therapy, treatment with corticosteroids should be initiated. Anti-inflammatory doses are often effective at alleviating the clinical signs but higher immunosuppressive doses may be required in some instances to appropriately manage the immune-mediated disease.

Prognosis is variable and depends upon both the cause of the inflammation and the extent and severity of associated neurological deficits. Some infections, especially those caused by protozoal and fungal agents, are difficult to eradicate and relapses are common. In addition, residual neurological deficits can persist despite successful treatment of an infection due to irreversible damage caused by the inciting agent.

Bacterial encephalitis
Bacterial infection is a relatively rare cause of encephalitis in dogs and cats when compared with other species.

Clinical signs: Animals can exhibit a variety of signs including vestibular dysfunction, seizures, cerebellar signs, paresis, cervical hyperaesthesia and coma (Radaelli and Platt, 2002). Fever is present in approximately 50% of cases at presentation. The signs are usually rapidly progressive and frequently fatal.

Pathogenesis: Bacterial infection of the brain is usually a consequence of direct extension of infection from the middle ear or sinuses (Spangler and

Dewey, 2000; Sturges *et al.*, 2006) or a penetrating injury to the skull (surgical or traumatic). Haematogenous spread can occur less commonly. Both aerobic and anaerobic infections have been reported. It is possible for the infection to be limited to the extradural or subarachnoid space, especially following bite wounds, in which case the infection can remain localized (intracranial empyema or abscess) and signs might not be so rapidly progressive. Clinical signs are largely the result of the inflammatory reaction that bacteria incite.

Diagnosis: Routine blood work usually reflects an inflammatory process, but can be normal. A urine sample should be cultured if bacterial encephalitis is suspected and blood cultures are indicated in animals in which there is no obvious source of infection. Imaging of the brain (CT or MRI) is helpful to identify defects in the skull and OM/OI and can be suggestive of an inflammatory process. CSF analysis is the most useful test. Typically, there is a marked elevation in the protein level and TNCC and the majority of cells are degenerate neutrophils. Bacteria may be visible in the spinal fluid. However, CSF analysis can be unremarkable or show more non-specific inflammatory changes. CSF should be cultured if it contains degenerate neutrophils, although it is common for the cultures to be negative (Radaelli and Platt, 2002). Samples for culture should be obtained from the middle ear by myringotomy if OM/OI is present. PCR testing targeted at the genetic sequence common to the bacterial species has been recently utilized to obtain a diagnosis of bacterial meningoencephalitis in a case where cultures were negative (Messer *et al.*, 2008). Molecular diagnostic techniques are likely to assume a more significant role in the future.

Treatment and prognosis: Whilst culture results are pending, treatment with an antibacterial drug that penetrates the CNS should be initiated (see Chapter 22). The most common bacterial isolates are *Escherichia coli*, *Streptococcus* and *Klebsiella*, but anaerobic infections can also occur. Appropriate drugs include fluoroquinolones and third-generation cephalosporins. Many patients are in a critical condition and need intravenous fluids and anti-inflammatory drugs. Mechanical ventilation might be necessary in comatose patients.

Prognosis is poor in animals with rapidly progressing severe signs. Early appropriate treatment is vital to obtain a good outcome.

Canine distemper virus infection
Canine distemper virus (CDV) is a paramyxovirus that commonly infects the CNS of dogs.

Clinical signs:

- Neurological signs – seizures, visual deficits, vestibular dysfunction, cerebellar signs, paresis, and myoclonus. The presence of myoclonus is most commonly associated with CDV infection but is not pathognomonic as it has been described with other inflammatory CNS disorders. Neurological disease associated with CDV infection tends to have a progressive course. Disease can develop in well vaccinated animals, so previous vaccination history does not exclude the possibility of CDV-associated disease (Lan *et al.*, 2006).
- Systemic signs, such as respiratory and gastrointestinal involvement, are reported to precede the neurological signs by 2–3 weeks. However, many dogs have no previous history of disease prior to the onset of neurological signs.
- Extraneural signs – conjunctivitis, rhinitis, fever, respiratory signs, gastrointestinal signs, tonsillitis, cachexia, enamel hypoplasia and hyperkeratosis of the footpads or nose. These signs are frequently mild (Tipold *et al.*, 1992; Koutinas *et al.*, 2002).
- Fundic examination is recommended in all suspected cases, as many dogs have evidence of chorioretinitis.

Pathogenesis: The presence and severity of the neurological signs depend on factors such as the age and immunocompetence of the host and the neurovirulence of the virus strain. Many dogs probably develop transient CNS infections without concurrent clinical signs. In the CNS, CDV initially replicates in the neurons and glial cells, and can cause both grey and white matter lesions, with one usually predominating. These early degenerative lesions are not characteristically inflammatory. A chronic course of CNS infection results from a late or insufficient immune response to CDV, with characteristic inflammatory demyelinating lesions (Tipold *et al.*, 1992). Polioencephalomyelopathy (PEM) has been reported most frequently in immature dogs, whilst leucoencephalomyelopathy (LEM) or a combination of PEM and LEM is more common in mature animals (Thomas *et al.*, 1993).

Diagnosis: An indirect fluorescent antibody test for viral antigen in conjunctival smears can be positive in many dogs with CNS distemper, regardless of whether the disease is acute or chronic (Thomas *et al.*, 1993). Viral antigen can also be demonstrated in tracheal washings and urine sediment.

Results of CSF analysis are variable. During the acute stage of the disease, an inflammatory response is lacking and thus the cell count and protein levels can be normal. In the chronic stage of the disease, lymphocytic pleocytosis is more frequently identified. An elevated CSF titre of antibody against CDV relative to the serum titre is supportive of a diagnosis.

Biopsy samples of haired skin from the dorsal neck can be used antemortem for immunohistochemical testing for acute CDV infection (Haines *et al.*, 1999). PCR analysis of urine and CSF samples for CDV has proven most useful in the antemortem diagnosis of distemper-associated neurological disease (Amude *et al.*, 2006; Saito *et al.*, 2006). In addition, PCR analysis of infected nervous tissue often confirms the presence of viral RNA. MRI can demonstrate multifocal contrast-enhancing white or grey matter lesions (Figure 11.18). Histopathology can confirm the presence of acidophilic intracytoplasmic or intranuclear inclusion bodies within the neurons and occasionally the astroglia (Figure 11.19).

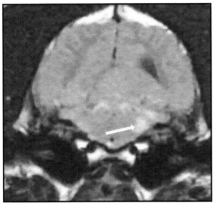

11.18 Contrast-enhanced transverse T1-weighted MR image of a dog showing hyperintense lesions (arrowed) in the region of the vestibular nuclei in the medulla oblongata due to CDV infection. (Courtesy of L Garosi)

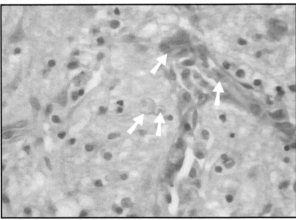

11.19 A histopathological section of the area of the medulla affected in Figure 11.18. The arrows indicate acidophilic intracytoplasmic CDV inclusion bodies. (H&E stain; original magnification X100) (Courtesy of M Bestbier and L Garosi)

Treatment and prognosis: There is no specific treatment for CDV-associated neurological disease. Overall, prognosis is poor, especially in cases with rapidly progressive signs. However, some dogs can survive with residual neurological deficits. Seizures are reported to be an unfavourable prognostic sign as they are often difficult to control with antiepileptic drugs (Tipold *et al.*, 1992). However, the disease is not fatal in all instances and some animals recover. Consequently, in cases where the neurological signs are not severe, it is recommended that the animal is provided with supportive care and the disease progression monitored over 1–2 weeks before considering euthanasia (Tipold *et al.*, 1992).

Feline coronavirus
Feline coronavirus is the causative agent of FIP, which is a common cause of meningoencephalitis in cats.

Clinical signs:

- Neurological signs – seizures, cerebellar signs, vestibular dysfunction and paresis. The disease often has an insidious onset and can lack distinct clinical signs.
- Affected cats may have concurrent systemic signs, including anorexia and weight loss.
- Ocular lesions have also been identified, including anterior uveitis, iritis, keratic precipitates, retinitis and anisocoria.

Pathogenesis: The disease occurs most commonly in cats <3 years old and from multiple cat households (Foley *et al.*, 1998); however, cats as old as 15 years have been diagnosed with the disease (Kline *et al.*, 1994). Neurological involvement is most common with the non-effusive or 'dry' form of the disease. Up to one-third of cats with the non-effusive form of the disease have been reported to have either primary neurological FIP or neurological signs as part of the overall disease presentation (Foley *et al.*, 1998). FIP induces a pyogranulomatous and immune complex-mediated vasculitis involving the meninges, ependymal lining, periventricular brain tissue and choroid plexus of the CNS. Secondary hydrocephalus can be seen due to obstruction of the ventricular system by the inflammation (Figure 11.20).

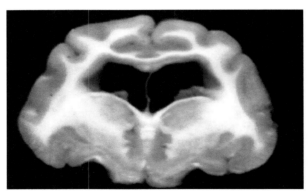

11.20 Pathological specimen from a cat with CNS FIP showing the marked dilatation of the lateral ventricles that is often seen with the disease secondary to obstruction of the ventricular system.

Diagnosis: Haematological findings can include anaemia, leucocytosis and hyperglobulinaemia; however, in some affected cats no abnormalities are present. Serum tests for anti-coronavirus antibodies are often positive but have low specificity. In addition, a negative serum titre (i.e. a complete absence of antibody) does not exclude the possibility of FIP-associated neurological disease because soluble antibodies can form immune complexes and escape detection by standard tests. Advanced imaging of the brain often reveals the presence of ventricular dilatation and periventricular contrast enhancement can be visible with MRI (Figure 11.21).

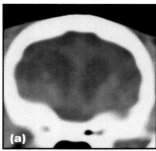
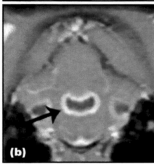

11.21 **(a)** CT image of a cat with CNS FIP showing evidence of dilated lateral ventricles. **(b)** Contrast-enhanced transverse T1-weighted MR image of a cat with CNS FIP showing evidence of dilatation of the fourth ventricle and periventricular contrast enhancement (arrowed).

Results of CSF analysis are variable. The characteristic finding is a marked neutrophilic to pyogranulomatous pleocytosis, with cell counts often in the hundreds, and an associated increase in protein concentration to >200 mg/dl (Rand *et al.*, 1994). However, the CSF can be normal, show a mild mononuclear pleocytosis or have a normal cell count with an elevated protein concentration. Positive CSF titres can be a useful antemortem indicator of neurological disease (Foley *et al.*, 1998). However, positive antibody titres must be interpreted with respect to the integrity of the blood–brain barrier (Boettcher *et al.*, 2007). PCR assays performed on CSF samples have not been shown to be reliable for confirming disease (Foley *et al.*, 1998).

Treatment and prognosis: Prognosis for cats with CNS FIP is poor. Definitive treatment is not available. The use of immunosuppressive drugs can slow the progression of disease. Affected animals should be isolated from other cats to prevent the spread of infection.

Toxoplasmosis and neosporosis
Toxoplasma gondii is an intracellular protozoan parasite of humans and animals that can cause encephalitis in infected dogs and cats. *Neospora caninum* is a protozoan parasite that is known to cause neurological disease in dogs but not cats.

Clinical signs: Signs of disease are seen most frequently in young or immunocompromised animals, and can occur with concurrent CDV infection or FIP (Kent, 2009).

- Neurological signs – seizures, behavioural changes, CN deficits, cerebellar signs and diffuse neuromuscular disease. A progressive cerebellar ataxia has been described in adult dogs with neosporosis (Garosi *et al.*, 2010).

- A characteristic early sign of disease is progressive rigidity of one or more limbs as a result of myositis and neuritis.
- Concurrent ocular abnormalities can be identified on fundoscopic examination.

Pathogenesis: Ingestion of tissue from infected intermediate hosts is the most common cause of *Toxoplasma gondii* infection in dogs and cats. In the case of *Neospora*, dogs are commonly infected *in utero*, although they can also be infected by ingestion of intermediate host tissue.

Diagnosis: Imaging can reveal the presence of either solitary or multiple mass lesions in the brains of affected animals (Figure 11.22). CSF analysis typically demonstrates pleocytosis with a mixed population of neutrophils and the presence of small and large mononuclear cells. Eosinophils can also be seen. With toxoplasmosis, a presumptive diagnosis is based on positive antibody titres in the CSF. However, a positive titre can be seen in animals previously exposed to the organism following nonspecific immune stimulation and therefore is not definitive evidence of active disease (Lappin *et al.*, 1996). Serum and CSF anti-*Neospora* antibody titres are more reliable than serum titres alone. However, for both infections, evidence of a rising titre should be obtained. PCR assays performed on CSF samples can aid in the antemortem diagnosis of these protozoal infections (Schatzberg *et al.*, 2003).

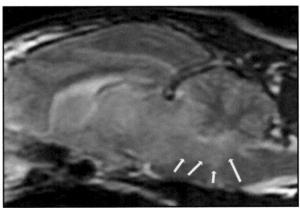

11.22 Sagittal T2-weighted cerebral MR image of a cat that presented with vestibular disease due to CNS toxoplasmosis. Arrows indicate a diffuse area of hyperintensity associated with infection within the brainstem, extending caudally to the area of the vestibular nuclei. (Courtesy of S Platt)

Treatment and prognosis: Clindamycin and/or trimethoprim/sulphonamide therapy is recommended in animals with CNS protozoal infections for a duration of 3–4 weeks. Trimethoprim/sulphonamide can be combined with pyrimethamine (0.5–1 mg/kg orally q24h for 2 days, then 0.25 mg/kg orally q24h for 2 weeks) and a folic acid supplement (5 mg/day orally) once the diagnosis has been confirmed. Neurological signs typically improve with treatment but might not resolve because of permanent damage caused by the organism. In addition, relapses are possible.

Cryptococcosis

Cryptococcus is a saprophytic yeast with a worldwide distribution. The organism can be isolated from several sources, although its main reservoir is pigeon droppings.

Clinical signs:

- Non-specific signs – anorexia, weight loss, lethargy, lymphadenopathy and pyrexia.
- Respiratory signs – nasal discharge, sneezing and coughing.
- Skin lesions.
- Ocular disease (including anterior uveitis, chorioretinitis and retinal detachment) can be seen in association with neurological signs.
- Neurological signs often reflect a diffuse or multifocal localization and frequently include altered mentation, CN deficits and gait abnormalities (Berthelin *et al.*, 1994a; Gerds-Grogan and Dayrell-Hart, 1997; Sykes *et al.*, 2010).

Pathogenesis: Dogs and cats most frequently become infected following inhalation of the organism. Neurological involvement results from haematogenous spread or local extension of an infection through the cribriform plate.

Diagnosis: MRI findings are variable and include multifocal or solitary lesions with uniform or peripheral contrast enhancement. Meningeal enhancement can also be observed (Sykes *et al.*, 2010). A haemogram can reveal the presence of monocytosis. In animals with extraneural disease, a definitive diagnosis can often be made based on cytology (Figure 11.23) and/or culture of urine, nasal discharge, lymph node aspirates or cutaneous masses. In addition, these animals often have positive CSF or serum titres for cryptococcal capsular antigen.

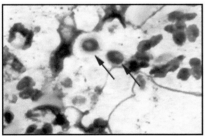

11.23 Impression smear from a cat with cryptococcosis showing the presence of several encapsulated cryptococcal organisms (arrowed). (Diff-Quik; original magnification X500)

Diagnosis of CNS cryptococcosis can often be made by cytological evaluation of the CSF. Neutrophilic, mononuclear or mixed pleocytosis can be seen, with neutrophilic pleocytosis most common in cats. Eosinophils are frequently present. The encapsulated organism can be seen in cytological preparations in the majority of cases (Berthelin *et al.*, 1994b; Sykes *et al.*, 2010). The use of India ink, new methylene blue or Gram stains allows the organisms to be identified more readily. In cases in which the organism is not observed on cytology, diagnosis can be made either by detecting cryptococcal capsular antigen in the CSF or by culturing CSF samples.

Treatment and prognosis: Treatment with amphotericin, fluconazole or itraconazole is recommended, although overall prognosis is fair to poor. Non-steroidal anti-inflammatory drugs (NSAIDs) should be administered when antifungal therapy is initiated, to counteract the intense inflammatory reaction that accompanies the killing of *Cryptococcus*. Long-term treatment is required, ranging from several months to years. It is difficult to completely rid the body of the organism and relapses are common. Treatment should be continued until serum cryptococcal titres are negative or for 2 months beyond the resolution of clinical signs.

Granulomatous meningoencephalomyelitis

GME is an inflammatory disease of unknown aetiology, which affects the CNS of dogs and, rarely, cats.

Clinical signs and pathogenesis: The disease is most common in middle-aged toy and small-breed dogs, with a possible breed predisposition in poodles and terriers. Three clinicopathological forms of the disease exist:

- The ocular form of the disease manifests with acute onset of dilated, unresponsive pupils due to optic neuritis
- The focal form of the disease presents with clinical signs suggestive of a single space-occupying mass, with areas of predilection in the pontomedullary region and forebrain
- The diffuse form of the disease presents with clinical signs suggestive of a multifocal CNS disorder, with the cerebrum, brainstem, cerebellum and cervical spinal cord most commonly involved. Clinical signs are usually acute in onset and progressive.

Although the cause of GME is unknown, characteristics of the lesion suggest a possible immunological basis for the disease (Vandevelde *et al.*, 1981). Infectious, autoimmune and neoplastic causes have also been proposed (Talarico and Schatzberg, 2010).

Diagnosis: CSF analysis typically reveals a mononuclear pleocytosis with an associated increase in protein concentration. However, both neutrophilic pleocytosis and normal CSF analysis have been reported (Bailey and Higgins, 1986). A mass lesion may be evident on imaging with the focal form of the disease, whilst the brain parenchyma can have a patchy, heterogeneous appearance with the diffuse form (Cherubini *et al.*, 2006). A definitive diagnosis can only be made histologically on postmortem examination or by biopsy. A definitive antemortem diagnosis cannot be made and so, when infectious aetiologies have been excluded, a diagnosis of meningoencephalitis of unknown origin (MUO) is made, of which GME is a leading cause (Figure 11.24).

Drug	Dosing regimen	Median survival (days)	Comments	Reference
Azathioprine Prednisone	2 mg/kg orally q24h for 2 wks then q48h 1 mg/kg q12h for 4wks then taper	1834 (range: 50–2469)	Excluded dogs that died in the first week; N = 40	Wong et al., 2010
Ciclosporin ± prednisone ± ketoconazole	3–15 mg/kg orally q12h; dose of prednisone not reported	930 (range: 60–1290)	Dosed to blood ciclosporin level of 200–400 ng/ml; N = 10	Adamo et al., 2007
Cytarabine Prednisone	50 mg/m² s.c. q12h for 48h, then q3wks 1–2 mg/kg q12h then taper	531 (range: 46–1025)	N = 10	Zarfoss et al., 2006
Lomustine + Prednisolone	60 mg/m² (range: 44–88) orally q6wks 2 mg/kg/day then taper	457 (range: 107–709)	GME only; N = 14	Flegel et al., 2011
Prednisolone	2 mg/kg/day orally then taper	323 (range: 39–542)	GME only; N = 11	Flegel et al., 2011
Prednisone	Range to 2 mg/kg orally q12h then taper	36 (range: 2–1200)	Pooled data; N = 26	Granger et al., 2010
Procarbazine Prednisone	25–50 mg/m² orally q24h 0.25–2 mg/kg q12h then taper	425 (range: 8–464)	N = 21	Coates et al., 2007

11.24 Summary of published data on treatment of MUO. Case series involving only ≥10 dogs have been included. Treatment regimes for prednisone vary widely and are frequently modulated according to the clinical progression of the disease. (Courtesy of N Olby)

Treatment and prognosis: The most commonly prescribed treatment for GME (or MUO) consists of immunosuppressive doses of corticosteroids. Other immunomodulatory drugs are frequently used in combination with corticosteroids, including cytosine arabinoside (Zarfoss et al., 2006; Smith et al., 2009), ciclosporin (Adamo and O'Brien, 2004), procarbazine (Coates et al., 2007), lomustine (Flegel et al., 2011) and azathioprine (Wong et al., 2010).

- Cytarabine (cytosine arabinoside) is administered at 50 mg/m² s.c. q12h for 2 consecutive days every 3 weeks. Recent studies suggest that more consistent serum levels are achieved using a constant rate infusion of 200 mg/m² over 8–12 hours.
- The recommended dose of ciclosporin is 6 mg/kg orally q12h.
- Procarbazine has been used at a dose of 25–50 mg/m² orally q24h, with an attempt to reduce the dose to every other day after 1 month of treatment.
- Both cytosine arabinoside and procarbazine are myelosuppressive and haemograms should be monitored regularly during the course of therapy.

Radiation therapy has also been recommended as a treatment for dogs with the focal form of the disease (Muñana and Luttgen, 1998). Overall, prognosis is poor, but survival times range from weeks to years. The diffuse form of the disease carries the worst prognosis with a survival time of weeks to months (Muñana and Luttgen, 1998).

Necrotizing meningoencephalitis
Necrotizing meningoencephalitis is a chronic progressive neurological disorder reported in Pugs (Pug encephalitis), Yorkshire Terriers, Chihuahuas and Maltese dogs. There are also sporadic reports of similar findings in other small-breed dogs, such as the Pekingese and Shih Tzu.

Clinical signs:

- Pug encephalitis is most commonly seen in juveniles to young adults, and causes seizures and other signs of forebrain dysfunction (Cordy and Holliday, 1989).
- The disease described in Maltese dogs also has a predilection for the forebrain (Stalis et al., 1995).
- The disease in Yorkshire Terriers causes signs of forebrain and brainstem involvement (Tipold et al., 1993).
- Chihuahuas present with neurological signs, including seizures, blindness, mentation changes and postural deficits (Higgins et al., 2008).
- Multifocal loss or collapse of cortical grey/white matter demarcation is identified on MRI.
- Multifocal asymmetrical areas of necrosis or collapse in both the grey and white matter of the cerebral hemispheres is seen on post-mortem examination.

Pathogenesis: The aetiology of the disease is unknown. Infection with an alpha-type herpesvirus has been suggested based on histological similarities with this type of infection in humans. However, attempts at viral isolation have been unsuccessful. The disease is associated with necrosis and a non-suppurative meningoencephalitis predominantly in the cortex. The subcortical white matter is frequently involved. Areas of necrosis can also be seen in the brainstem. Recent research suggests that genetics may play a role in disease susceptibility in Pugs (Greer et al., 2010; Barber et al., 2011).

Diagnosis: CT may reveal a focal hypodense area within the brain parenchyma relating to the area of necrosis (Figure 11.25). Multifocal, asymmetrical areas of high signal intensity in the brain can be seen on T2-weighted MR images, with variable contrast enhancement of the parenchyma and

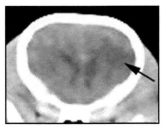

11.25 CT image of a Yorkshire Terrier diagnosed with necrotizing encephalomyelitis showing a focal area of hypoattenuation in the right forebrain (arrowed).

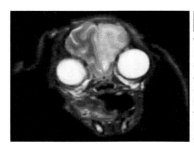

11.26 Transverse T2-weighted cerebral MR image of a Maltese dog with necrotizing encephalitis showing diffuse asymmetrical hyperintensity throughout the frontal lobe parenchyma. (Courtesy of S Platt)

meninges visible on T1-weighted images (Young *et al.*, 2009) (Figure 11.26). A lymphocytic pleocytosis is most frequently recognized on CSF analysis. A definitive diagnosis is based on histopathology.

Treatment and prognosis: Prognosis is poor and the disease is typically fatal. Combined immunosuppressive protocols similar to those utilized for the treatment of GME are recommended. As with GME, there is limited information on the efficacy of such treatments in cases of histologically confirmed disease (Jung *et al.*, 2007; Flegel *et al.*, 2011).

Toxic diseases

Metronidazole toxicity

Clinical signs: Central vestibular signs have been reported in dogs following administration of metronidazole (Dow *et al.*, 1989; Evans *et al.*, 2003). Initial clinical signs include anorexia and vomiting, and can progress rapidly to include bilateral central vestibular signs with either a symmetrical or asymmetrical generalized ataxia and a positional vertical nystagmus. Head tilt and seizures are observed less frequently.

The onset of clinical signs can occur as soon as 3 days after initiating treatment but can also be seen following chronic therapy. Dogs reported to have developed toxicity were typically treated with an oral dose of metronidazole >60 mg/kg/day (Dow *et al.*, 1989), although doses as low as 30 mg/kg/day have been incriminated (Evans *et al.*, 2003).

Metronidazole toxicity has also been reported in cats, but affected animals display signs of forebrain and cerebellar involvement rather than vestibular

signs (Saxon and Magne, 1993). Toxicity can be seen with lower doses than those reported for dogs.

Pathogenesis: The pathogenesis is poorly understood, but it is hypothesized to be related to the interaction of metronidazole with gamma-amino-butyric acid (GABA) receptors in the cerebellum and vestibular nuclei (Evans *et al.*, 2003).

Diagnosis: A history of metronidazole administration and compatible clinical signs should lead to a high suspicion for this disorder.

Treatment and prognosis: Treatment consists of discontinuation of the drug and provision of nursing care. In addition, administration of diazepam has been shown to shorten recovery times in dogs (Evans *et al.*, 2003). An intravenous injection of diazepam (0.43 mg/kg), followed by 0.43 mg/kg orally q8h for 3 days has been recommended. Recovery is typically seen within 1–3 days in dogs treated with diazepam, and within 2–3 weeks in dogs for which treatment only consists of drug discontinuation and supportive care. As with dogs, clinical signs in cats are reversible with discontinuation of the drug.

Trauma

Head trauma

Head trauma in dogs and cats is most often caused by automobile accidents. Injury to the brainstem can result in vestibular signs along with other signs of brainstem dysfunction. For details on the management of brain trauma, the reader is referred to Chapter 20.

Vascular diseases

Cerebrovascular disease

Cerebrovascular disease is being reported more frequently in dogs and cats as a result of the greater availability of MRI as a diagnostic tool. A review of cerebellar infarcts in dogs and cats found that the majority of animals had a vestibular component to the neurological signs, either in the form of paradoxical vestibular disease or cerebellovestibular signs (Berg, 2003). Vestibular signs have also been reported with thalamic infarcts in dogs (Goncalves *et al.*, 2011). The reader is referred to Chapter 9 for a more thorough review of cerebrovascular disease.

References and further reading

Available on accompanying DVD

DVD extras

- Myringotomy
- Positional nystagmus
- Positional strabismus
- Spontaneous nystagmus (1)
- Spontaneous nystagmus (2)
- Vestibular disease

12

Neurological abnormalities of the head and face

Nick Jeffery and Nicolas Granger

Recognition of neurological abnormalities of the head and face plays a key role in identifying the distribution of a neurological disease and thereby suggesting possible aetiologies. Due to the large number of neural structures involved in causing such deficits (Figure 12.1) many of the conditions affecting the head and face are described in greater detail in separate chapters. Vestibular dysfunction is covered in detail in Chapter 11 and ocular disorders are considered in Chapter 10. A key component of the diagnosis of neurological abnormalities of the head and face is to determine whether the lesion is located within the peripheral nervous system (PNS) or central nervous system (CNS). Signs of cranial nerve (CN) dysfunction may result from lesions within either system and therefore the aetiology and prognosis may differ greatly. Generalized disorders of the PNS may just be expressed in the CNs or in combination with peripheral nerve deficits elsewhere in the body; these conditions are considered in further detail in Chapter 15.

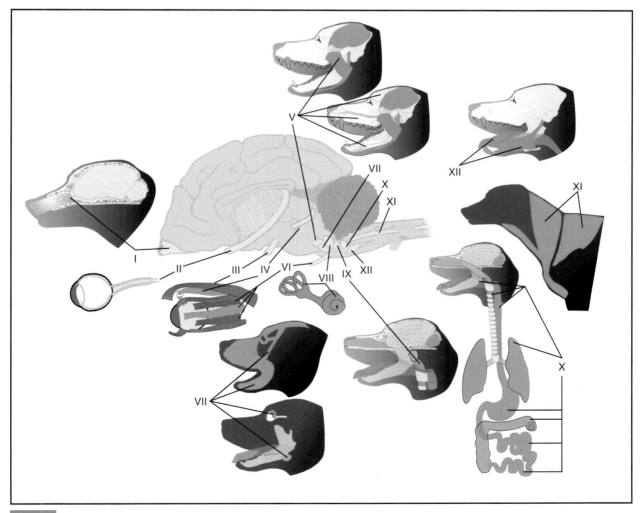

12.1 Overview of cranial nerve origins and distribution in the dog.

Anatomy and clinical signs

Anosmia

The olfactory portion of the rhinencephalon is the special visceral afferent (sensory) system designed for the conscious perception of smell. The chemoreceptor is located in the olfactory epithelium of the caudal nasal mucosa. The axon leaving the cell body joins with other axons to form CN I (olfactory nerve). These nerves pass through the cribriform plate into the olfactory bulbs. Axons from the olfactory bulbs project through the olfactory tract to the ipsilateral olfactory cortex over the pyriform lobe.

Loss of sense of smell is difficult to ascertain clinically because of the lack of widely available objective testing methods, and is often due to abnormalities of the nasal cavity rather than specific neurological abnormalities. Depressed appetite and, perhaps, changed patterns of behaviour might be predicted consequences of anosmia. However, even in animals in which a reduced sense of smell would be expected (i.e. those with large nasal tumours or nasal aspergillosis) such signs are often not apparent.

External ophthalmoplegia

External ophthalmoplegia (paralysis of the extraocular muscles) causes strabismus and deficiencies in eye movements in specific directions due to dysfunction of CNs III (oculomotor nerve), IV (trochlear nerve) and VI (abducent nerve) – these clinical signs are discussed in more detail in Chapter 10. It is important to differentiate disorders of specific extraocular eye muscles from vestibular lesions (see Chapter 11) as both can cause strabismus.

Reduced facial and head sensation

Sensation to the head and face is provided by the three branches of CN V (trigeminal nerve): mandibular (cheek, lower teeth, tongue); maxillary (most of the face, cheek, side of nose and lateral eyelids); and ophthalmic (orbit, medial part of upper eyelid, dorsum of nose) (Figure 12.2). Therefore, a lesion affecting the trigeminal nerve may, depending on its site, decrease sensation in any or all of these regions of the head. Decreased, or loss of, facial sensation may also cause dysphagia because of poor prehension of food and water, but this is not common. The pinna of the dog is innervated by CN VII (facial nerve) on the concave surface and by dorsal branches of the second cervical spinal nerve on the convex surface, and not by the trigeminal nerve.

The cell bodies of the trigeminal sensory neurons are located in the trigeminal ganglia. The trigeminal sensory axons enter the pons just rostral to the origin of the facial and vestibulocochlear (CN VIII) nerves and course caudally through the medulla in the spinal tract of the trigeminal nerve (see Figures 12.6 and 9.4). This tract continues caudally into the first cervical segment. Lesions in the medulla involving the spinal tract of the trigeminal nerve result in ipsilateral loss of facial sensation but no impairment of masticatory muscle function, which is controlled by the motor branches of this nerve. Lesions of the sensory cerebral cortex frequently cause subtle reductions in contralateral facial sensation, which can be most easily detected by touching the nasal mucosa using a small pair of forceps (see Figure 9.4). Such subtle loss of function should be differentiated from the more gross loss of function caused by lesions of the trigeminal nerve. This can be achieved by evaluating both the brainstem reflex and conscious response to facial stimulation. With trigeminal lesions, neither the typical reflex palpebral response, nor the conscious aversive response is seen with stimulation of the nasal mucosa. In contrast, cerebral lesions result in loss of the conscious aversive response but the palpebral response is unaffected.

The mandibular branch of CN V also provides motor innervation to the muscles of mastication. Sensory deficits, including diminished corneal and palpebral reflexes (Figure 12.3) may, therefore, occur in isolation or in conjunction with motor deficits, such as decreased jaw tone and/or loss of masticatory muscle bulk. Loss of sensory input from the cornea can result in neurogenic keratopathy (see Chapter 10 for further information).

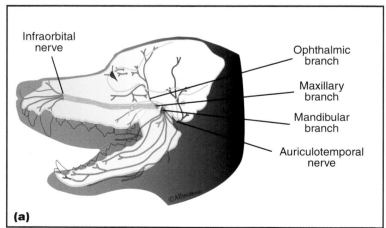

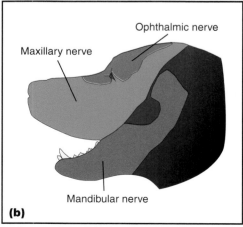

12.2 **(a)** CN V (trigemial nerve) and its branches. **(b)** Areas of cutaneous innervation of the head supplied by the branches of CN V.

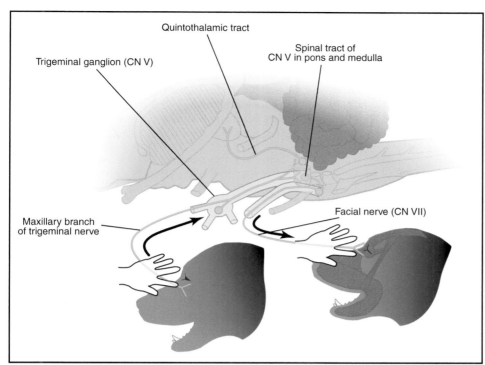

Trigeminal ganglion (CN V)

Quintothalamic tract

Spinal tract of
CN V in pons and medulla

Facial nerve (CN VII)

Maxillary branch
of trigeminal nerve

12.3 The palpebral reflex is elicited by touching and stimulating the skin of the medial and lateral canthus of the palpebrae. The sensory (afferent) portion of the pathway enters the brainstem via the trigeminal nerve and synapses in the sensory nucleus within the pons. The motor (efferent) portion of the pathway (facial nerve) is then stimulated, which causes a palpebral blink response. This is an interneuron facilitated reflex. There is also contralateral central recognition of the sensory stimulus from the trigeminal sensory nucleus.

Dropped jaw

Weakness of the jaw muscles may manifest as a reduction in voluntary movement of the jaw causing dysphagia or a complete loss of jaw muscle tone and inability to close the mouth (Figure 12.4; see also **Dropped jaw** clip on DVD). The inability to close the mouth implies a bilateral lesion affecting the motor component of CN V, since a unilateral lesion does not cause sufficient weakness to prevent mouth closure. The bilateral nature of the trigeminal lesion strongly implies that it involves the peripheral nerves rather than the brainstem (since a lesion in the brainstem large enough to affect both trigeminal nuclei would likely be fatal). The motor neurons of CN V are located in the pons near the rostral cerebellar peduncles and their axons are distributed to the muscles of mastication by the mandibular branch of CN V.

It is important to differentiate a lesion affecting only the trigeminal nerve from one affecting multiple CNs since both may cause an animal to drool. This can be achieved by examining the animal's ability to use its tongue and swallow food when its mouth is held partially closed; these functions are mediated by CN XII (hypoglossal nerve) and CN IX (glossopharyngeal nerve), respectively, which are not affected by an isolated motor trigeminal neuropathy. Apparent inability to close the mouth must also be distinguished from an unwillingness to close the mouth, which can be caused by painful conditions of the head, such as masticatory muscle myositis, retrobulbar lesions, temporomandibular joint disease or craniomandibular osteopathy.

Atrophy of the masticatory muscles

Masticatory muscle atrophy can occur bilaterally or unilaterally (Figure 12.5). In spite of dramatic muscle atrophy, the ability to close the mouth usually appears unimpaired. However, opening the mouth

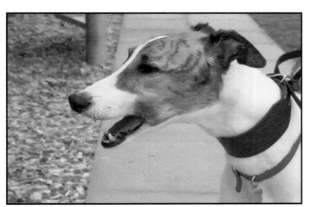

12.4 A 3-year-old male Greyhound presented with an acute onset of dropped jaw due to an underlying inflammatory disease of the central nervous system.

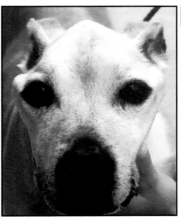

12.5 Severe atrophy of the masticatory muscles affects the profile of the dorsal aspect of the head. Enophthalmos may also occur and can cause periodic protrusion of the third eyelids.

may be very limited in cases in which there has been muscle inflammation and subsequent fibrosis. Masticatory muscle atrophy can result from impaired muscle innervation due to lesions of the motor branch of CN V, diseases of the muscles themselves or systemic disorders, such as cachexia or hyperadrenocorticism (or exogenous corticosteroid administration). Unilateral loss of temporal muscle mass can occur in the absence of any sensory signs.

Abnormal facial expression

Muscles that control facial expression and maintain the normal appearance of the palpebral fissures and mouth are innervated by the facial nerve. The neurons are located in the facial nuclei of the rostral medulla and axons leave the ventrolateral surface of the medulla ventral to CN VIII. CN VII enters the petrosal bone through the internal acoustic meatus on the dorsal aspect of CN VIII and emerges from the skull through the stylomastoid foramen (Figures 12.6 and 12.7).

Acute damage to the facial nerve in small animals causes widening of the palpebral fissure and laxity of the facial muscles of expression, often termed facial paresis. The lip may droop on the affected side and food or saliva may fall from that side of the mouth (Figure 12.8). The nasal philtrum can be deviated to the normal side in the early stages and drooping of the ears may be apparent in some breeds. Loss of the palpebral and corneal reflexes predisposes the animal to exposure keratitis (see **Palpebral reflex** clip on DVD). With chronicity, muscle contracture can lead to narrowing of the palpebral fissure, widening of the mouth and, in unilateral cases, deviation of the nostrils towards the affected side. The striking appearance of hemifacial spasm can be differentiated from chronic contracture by observing intact blink reflexes. In contrast to disease of CN VII itself, release of upper motor neuron (UMN) inhibition on this nerve (e.g. tetanus intoxication) increases muscle tone, producing a wide 'grimacing' mouth and narrowing of the palpebral fissures (through lateral distraction of the lateral margin of the eyelids).

There are some signs of CN VII dysfunction for which pet owners may seek veterinary attention that do not immediately suggest a facial nerve lesion:

- Owners may observe the third eyelid flicking over the eye. In these cases, the animal substitutes globe retraction (with concomitant third eyelid protrusion) for blinking with the paralysed lids
- Accumulation of food in cheeks that have poor muscle tone may lead to halitosis.

Keratoconjunctivitis sicca

Keratoconjunctivitis sicca ('dry eye') is discussed in more detail in Chapter 10.

Head tilt and spontaneous nystagmus

Head tilt and spontaneous nystagmus are caused by CN VIII disease and are discussed in detail in Chapter 11.

Deafness

Auditory sensation is provided by the cochlear portion of CN VIII; the cell bodies of the cochlear nerve form the spiral ganglion in the petrosal bone (Figure 12.9). Axons extend proximally to join the vestibular neurons in the internal acoustic meatus and enter the brainstem at the junction of the medulla and pons, terminating on the cochlear nuclei. The central pathway is bilateral and multisynaptic projecting to the medial geniculate nucleus of the thalamus. Other axons project to several brainstem nuclei and

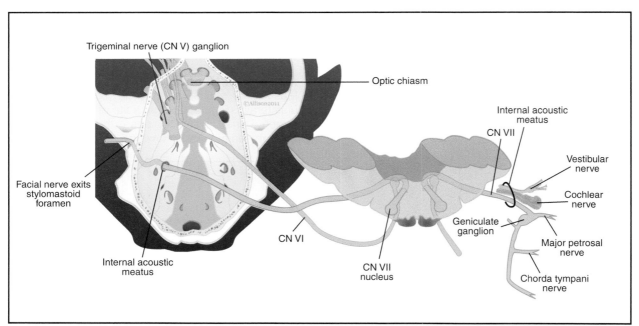

12.6 The facial nerve (CN VII) exits the brainstem at the level of the medulla and exits the intracranial cavity via the internal acoustic meatus, where it becomes three branches: the major petrosal nerve before the geniculate ganglion, the chorda tympani nerve and the main branch of the facial nerve (as shown). It then leaves the calvaria via the stylomastoid foramen.

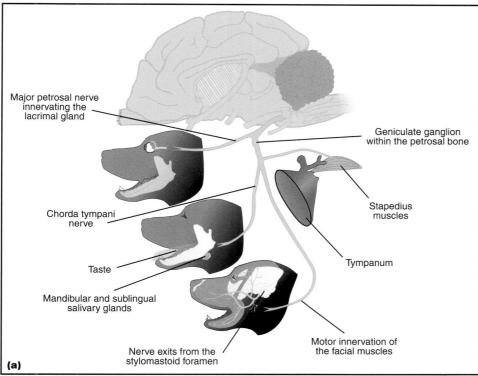

Major petrosal nerve innervating the lacrimal gland

Chorda tympani nerve

Taste

Mandibular and sublingual salivary glands

Nerve exits from the stylomastoid foramen

Geniculate ganglion within the petrosal bone

Stapedius muscles

Tympanum

Motor innervation of the facial muscles

(a)

12.7 **(a)** CN VII is shown to exit from the medulla oblongata of the brainstem and its branches are depicted innervating the lacrimal glands, the stapedius muscle and the mandibular and sublingual salivary glands. The main component of CN VII exits the stylomastoid foramen to innervate the muscles of facial expression. **(b)** The superficial branches of CN VII.

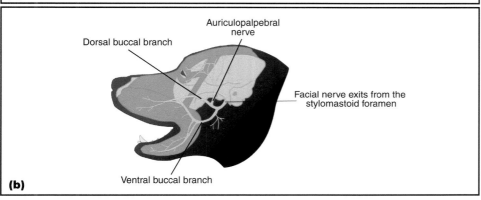

Auriculopalpebral nerve

Dorsal buccal branch

Facial nerve exits from the stylomastoid foramen

Ventral buccal branch

(b)

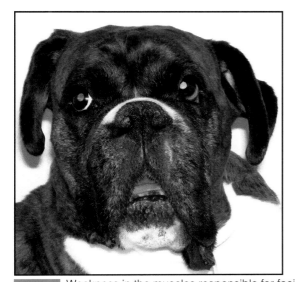

12.8 Weakness in the muscles responsible for facial expression causes drooping of the lip, widening of the palpebral fissure and poor movement of the pinna. This can be observed even in loose-skinned breeds such as the Boxer.

the caudal colliculus in the midbrain (see Figure 4.17). The conscious perception of sound is served by the projection from the geniculate nucleus to the temporal lobe of the cerebral cortex, largely from the contralateral ear.

Owners usually only recognize deafness if it affects both ears. Typically, owners report that the animal fails to respond to commands and sleeps very heavily, only waking when touched. Astute owners sometimes suspect unilateral deafness: unilaterally affected animals may be unable to localize the origin of noise or voice commands, even though they can be seen to react to sounds in general. Deafness is discussed in more detail below.

Dysphagia and regurgitation

Many types of lesion around the head and neck can cause dysphagia; probably the most common is a physical obstruction caused, for instance, by foreign bodies or neoplastic masses. Nevertheless, primary neurological dysfunction of one or multiple CNs should not be overlooked. The functions of CNs IX and X (vagus nerve) are integral to the function of

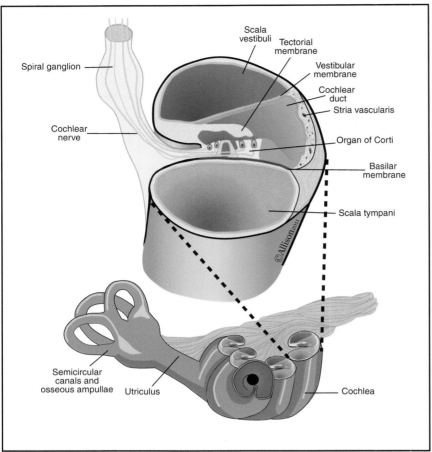

Cross-section of a cochlear coil. The scala vestibuli and tympani are filled with perilymph and the cochlear duct is filled with endolymph.

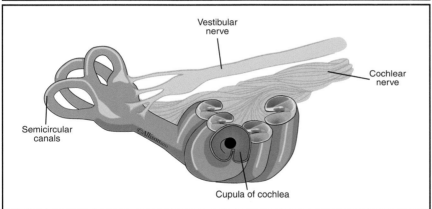

the pharynx, larynx and oesophagus (Figure 12.10). These nerves together with CN XI (spinal accessory nerve) originate from the same medullary nucleus (nucleus ambiguus). The rostral two-thirds of this nucleus is involved in swallowing by means of motor impulses through the glossopharyngeal and vagus nerves. The caudal nucleus ambiguus controls the laryngeal and oesophageal muscles through the vagus nerve and its branches (recurrent laryngeal nerves) with a minor contribution from the spinal accessory nerve.

Careful questioning of the owner may help to distinguish disorders of prehension (suggesting trigeminal or hypoglossal lesions) from those of swallowing (more likely glossopharyngeal or vagus lesions). For instance, swallowing disorders result in coughing

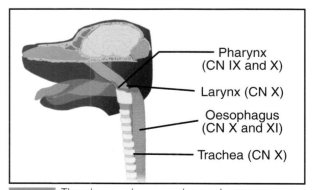

12.10 The pharynx, larynx and oesophagus are innervated by the glossopharyngeal nerve (CN IX) and vagus nerve (CN X). The spinal accessory nerve (CN XI) sends a few fibres to join the vagus nerve.

after eating or drinking (more common), and there may be excessive saliva in the pharynx. Whereas, animals that have difficulty with prehension have often been observed spending an inordinate amount of time drinking (although often without success); this sign may be so prominent as to be interpreted by the owner as polydipsia. Inspiratory dyspnoea can occur in conjunction with dysphagia if CNs IX and X are also involved.

Regurgitation must be distinguished from true vomiting. This can usually be achieved by eliciting details from the owner about the event but also by measuring the pH of the ejected material.

Dysphonia and inspiratory stridor
The laryngeal muscles are innervated by branches of the vagus nerve and the abductor muscles are innervated by the recurrent laryngeal nerve. Lesions affecting the recurrent laryngeal nerve frequently lead to dysphonia or signs of overt respiratory distress. However, other conditions (such as myopathies or masses in the airway) can also result in this sign. Dysphonia and laryngeal paralysis are commonly encountered as a feature of both acute and chronic generalized neuropathies (see Chapter 15).

Dysphonia may be a primary complaint of the owner but is more likely to require careful questioning (i.e. avoidance of leading questions) to confirm. Upper respiratory tract signs may be sufficiently severe to be noted by the owners but may be subtle in dogs presented primarily for exercise intolerance or collapse during activity. The function of the larynx is most compromised in the inspiratory phase during forced exercise. Upper respiratory tract noise associated with inspiration is called stridor and can occur in combination with dyspnoea and cyanosis. Animals in which laryngeal function is severely compromised may require prompt intervention, ranging from provision of supplementary oxygen through to emergency tracheotomy. In addition, affected animals are at risk of inhaling food or water, with the consequent development of aspiration pneumonia. Concurrent deficits in the function of CNs IX and X greatly increase the risk of aspiration.

Tongue abnormalities
The tongue muscles are innervated by CN XII. This nerve originates from cell bodies located in the medulla and exits the brainstem at a site just caudal to the accessory nerve traversing through the hypoglossal canal to the exterior. Bilateral weakness of the tongue is manifest by the inability to retain the tongue in the mouth (Figure 12.11). Unilateral abnormalities cause marked asymmetry of movement or muscle fasciculations on the affected side; this is best seen when a dog is panting. Animals cannot prehend food or water so may be presented for dysphagia prior to the presence of physical abnormalities. In chronic unilateral disease there may be marked atrophy and contracture of the tongue muscles causing permanent deviation towards the affected side.

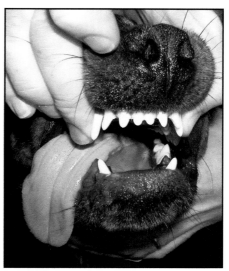

12.11 This dog has such profound tongue weakness that it cannot be withdrawn into the mouth voluntarily. Attempting to grasp the tongue may provide more information in less severe cases.

Horner's syndrome
The characteristic combination of a miotic pupil, prolapsed third eyelid (resulting from globe retraction; i.e. enophthalmos) and an imperfectly elevated upper eyelid comprises complete Horner's syndrome. It is not necessary for all components to be present. The most persistent sign is miosis, and the consequent anisocoria can be exaggerated by placing the animal in dim lighting conditions. This syndrome is discussed in detail in Chapter 10.

Autonomic anatomy of the head
Sympathetic nerve supply to the head, face and eye originates in nuclei in the caudal part of the hypothalamus. Axons descend through the lateral funiculus of the spinal cord to synapse with preganglionic neurons in the intermediate grey matter of the T1–T3 region of the spinal cord (Figure 12.12). The axons of these neurons ascend in the sympathetic trunk (alongside the vagus nerve) to synapse in the cranial cervical ganglion, from where they pass through the middle ear and are distributed with the ophthalmic nerve (a branch of the trigeminal nerve) to the smooth muscles of the head. Normal tone in this smooth muscle maintains a protruded globe, wide palpebral fissure, third eyelid retraction and a degree of pupil dilatation.

Parasympathetic nerve supply to the head is provided by CNs III, VII, IX and XI and originates from neurons located in separate, but poorly defined, nuclei adjacent to the somatic efferent nuclei of each nerve. The parasympathetic fibres synapse in the ganglia lying close to the structures that they innervate (Figure 12.13). Thus, parasympathetic fibres in the:

- Oculomotor nerve synapse in the ciliary ganglion. The postganglionic fibres run along the optic nerve (CN II) to innervate the ciliary muscle and pupillary constrictors

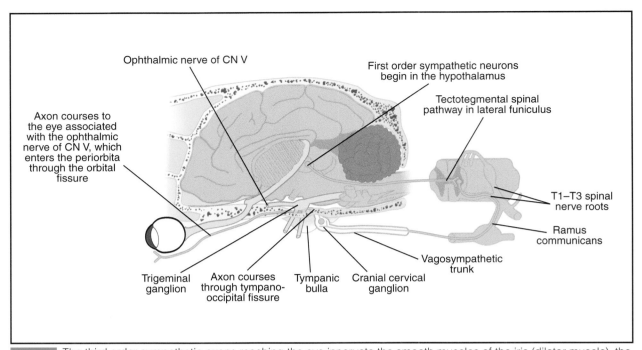

12.12 The third order sympathetic axons reaching the eye innervate the smooth muscles of the iris (dilator muscle), the periorbita, the upper and lower eyelids (tarsal muscles) and the third eyelid.

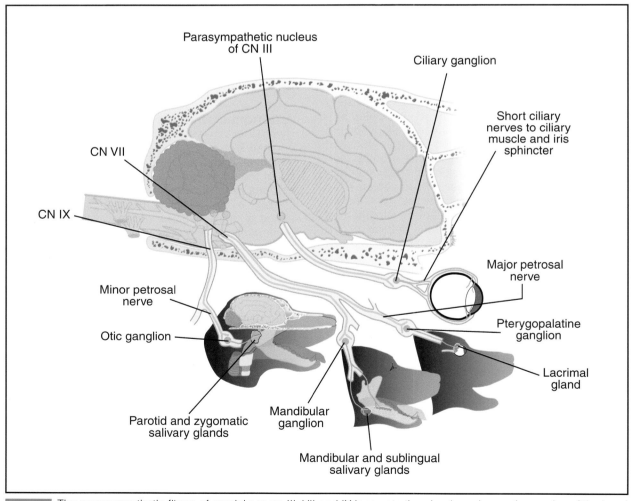

12.13 The parasympathetic fibres of cranial nerves III, VII and IX innervate the glands and smooth muscles of the head and eye.

- Facial nerve synapse in the pterygopalatine, mandibular and sublingual ganglia. The postganglionic fibres innervate the lacrimal, palatine and nasal glands and the mandibular and sublingual salivary glands (distributed via branches of the trigeminal nerve)
- Glossopharyngeal nerve synapse in the otic ganglion. Postganglionic fibres innervate the zygomatic and parotid salivary glands (distributed via branches of the trigeminal nerve)
- Vagus nerve run in the main vagal part of the vagosympathetic trunk to reach ganglia in the walls of the abdominal viscera and oesophagus. A few postganglionic fibres course in the internal branch of CN XI and join those of CN X.

Lesion localization

The CNs are numbered from rostral to caudal according to the location of their nuclei (motor and/or sensory) within the brain; the majority of these (from the trigeminal nerve to hypoglossal nerve) lie within the most caudal parts of the brainstem (the pons and medulla). The exceptions are: the oculomotor and trochlear nuclei, which lie within the mesencephalon (midbrain); the optic nerve, which enters the diencephalon; and the olfactory nerves, whose axons enter the telencephalon (forebrain) directly (Figure 12.14).

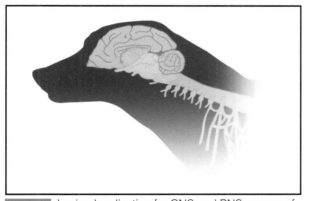

12.14 Lesion localization for CNS and PNS causes of disorders of the face and head. The brainstem and CNs are highlighted.

Thus, lesions located within the brainstem (especially those within the medulla) or along the course of the peripheral nerves can cause signs of neurological dysfunction of the head and face. It is crucial to differentiate peripheral nerve lesions from those within the brainstem (i.e. CNS lesion) (Figure 12.15). The types of disease that affect the CNS and PNS differ considerably in aetiology and therefore in prognosis. It should also be noted that, histologically, the optic nerve is part of the CNS and therefore is susceptible to diseases of the CNS such as granulomatous meningoencephalitis.

During clinical examination the most useful test to differentiate central from peripheral lesions is the evaluation of postural reactions. Animals that have a lesion located within the brainstem are likely,

Parameter	Peripheral CN disease	Brainstem (central) CN disease [a]
Consciousness	Normal	Depression; stupor; coma
Postural reactions	Normal	Frequently abnormal on ipsilateral side
Segmental spinal reflexes	May be abnormal if the underlying aetiology also causes a generalized peripheral neuropathy	Intact
Neck pain	May be a feature if the aetiology involves the nerve roots or meninges	May be a feature if the aetiology involves the nerve roots or meninges, or causes an elevation of intracranial pressure
Gait	Commonly normal unless there is a concurrent generalized peripheral neuropathy	Ipsilateral paresis
Cranial nerves	Frequently just one CN involved	Multiple ipsilateral CNs can be involved

12.15 Neurological examination results indicative of peripheral *versus* brainstem (central) CN disease. [a] Central CN disease implies disease of the CN nuclei or the nerve roots as they leave the brainstem. Intracranial extra-axial disease affecting the cavernous sinus or retro-orbital areas can also cause signs that may be central in origin.

because of the close proximity of the relevant tracts, to have deficits in postural reactions in addition to signs of CN dysfunction. For instance, a lesion located in the medulla that causes facial paralysis usually also results in postural reaction deficits (i.e. hopping, proprioceptive placing) in the ipsilateral limbs.

Unfortunately, the absence of postural reaction deficits cannot be used to definitely rule out a central lesion, since occasionally lesions within the brain (especially within the fourth ventricle) and intracranial extra-axial masses may not initially cause a concomitant postural reaction deficit. Furthermore, animals may have postural reaction deficits due to unrelated lesions elsewhere in the nervous system (e.g. chronic disc disease).

Additional features of the neurological examination may provide further evidence to differentiate brainstem from peripheral nerve disease. For instance, finding deficits in several CNs located close to one another in the brainstem (e.g. CN III–VII), or perhaps finding unusual patterns of nystagmus (e.g. vertical), would suggest a CNS lesion. More general examination may suggest a specific localization, most notably the combination of Horner's syndrome, facial nerve paralysis and head tilt strongly suggests middle ear disease since that is the only site at which the three relevant neural pathways are co-located.

Pathophysiology

Diseases that cause neurological abnormalities of the head and face can affect any component of the innervation, from the cell body (contained within CN ganglia or the CNS) to the tips of the axons, which may lie within either the CNS or the PNS. Thus, there is a wide range of possible pathological insults that may be responsible for the observed deficits (similar to those described for tetraparesis in Chapter 15). In general, it is useful to subdivide the diseases into those affecting the CNS and those affecting the PNS.

Central nervous system diseases

Many different types of CNS disease may be responsible for inducing neurological abnormalities of the head and face, particularly trauma (although brainstem signs are less common than those of the forebrain), neoplasia and various forms of encephalitis; these conditions are reviewed in Chapters 20, 9 and 11, respectively.

Peripheral nervous system diseases

PNS diseases that cause neurological abnormalities of the head and face include those that can also cause deficits in limb function (see Chapter 15). However, there are specific features of cranial innervation that render specific disease processes more likely:

- The peripheral components of the CNs are generally more superficial than those elsewhere in the body and are therefore more susceptible to trauma. Nerve swelling due to any aetiology is particularly deleterious since it can cause secondary compromise of blood flow as nerves pass through the foramina in the skull. The foramina are susceptible to fractures
- Certain CNs appear to be more susceptible to myasthenia gravis, in particular those innervating the oesophagus and muscles of facial expression
- Idiopathic mononeuropathies occur more commonly amongst the CNs (specifically the trigeminal, facial and vestibulocochlear nerves) than other peripheral nerves.

Differential diagnosis

Generally, the underlying causes of neurological abnormalities of the head and face are similar whichever nerve (or nucleus) is affected, but there are a few conditions which are specific to, or more commonly affect, certain nerves. Figure 12.16 details the differential diagnoses for different presenting problems.

Neurodiagnostic investigation

A complete neurological examination is a prerequisite for investigating suspected neurological disease of the head and face (see Chapters 1 and 2). However, several features may require particular

Presenting problem	Differential diagnosis
Deafness	Congenital deafness [12] Senility (presbycusis) [12] Neoplasia of the middle ear [12] Otitis media/externa [11, 12] Nasopharyngeal polyp [12] Toxicity (aminoglycoside, others) [12]
Laryngeal paralysis	Congenital laryngeal paralysis [12] Laryngeal paralysis polyneuropathy complex [15] Encephalitis: brainstem [11] Idiopathic laryngeal paralysis [12] Neoplasia: thyroid [12]; brainstem [9] Surgical trauma to vagus nerve [12] Toxicity (lead, organophosphate) [12]
Regurgitation/ megaoesophagus	Dysautonomia [19] Congenital megaoesophagus [12] Persistent right aortic arch [12] Hypoadrenocorticism [12] Polymyopathy [12, 18] Oesophagitis [12] Myasthenia gravis [18] Encephalitis: brainstem [11] Neoplasia: brainstem [9] Botulism [12, 15]
Masticatory muscle atrophy	Idiopathic age-related atrophy [12] Neoplasia: cachexia (bilateral); CN V nerve root tumour [12]; cerebellomedullary pontine angle meningioma (unilateral) [9] Hyperadrenocorticism/exogenous administration of corticosteroids [12] Masticatory myositis [12] Generalized myopathies [18]
Dropped jaw	Idiopathic trigeminal nerve palsy [12] Encephalitis: brainstem [11]
Dysphagia (difficulty swallowing)	Polymyositis [18] Myasthenia gravis [18] Encephalitis: brainstem [11] Neoplasia: brainstem [9] Botulism [15]
Facial paralysis	Neoplasia: brainstem [9]; middle ear [12] Idiopathic facial paralysis [12] Encephalitis: brainstem [11] Otitis media/interna [11, 12] Trauma: surgical or external [12]
Multiple cranial nerve deficits	Ipsilateral CNs VII and VIII and Horner's syndrome: middle ear; otitis media/interna; neoplasia of the middle ear [12] Ipsilateral CNs III, IV, V and VI: cavernous sinus syndrome; neoplasia and infection [10] Multiple ipsilateral CN deficits: neoplasia (brainstem, nerve root tumour, round cell tumour) [9]; encephalitis [11] Multiple CN deficits plus generalized lower motor neuron signs: polyneuropathy [15]

12.16 Neurological differential diagnoses for different presenting problems. The numbers in square brackets denote the chapters in the Manual where these conditions are discussed in detail.

attention (see below). The diagnostic approach to abnormalities of the head and face is summarized in Figure 12.17.

History

A thorough history is essential because certain neurological disorders of the head and face may result in signs that cannot be observed by the veterinary surgeon during a consultation. For instance, if an animal is reported to be vomiting it is crucial to determine whether it is 'true' vomiting or regurgitation. The owner of any animal in which generalized weakness or exercise intolerance is reported should be questioned about the animal's vocalization since dysphonia resulting from laryngeal dysfunction occurs commonly in association with peripheral neuropathy.

Observations

Before conducting a 'hands on' examination, several observations may aid in recognizing or classifying disorders of the head and face.

- As the animal walks around the consulting room, the position of the head and neck can be observed. The presence of a head tilt or generalized tremors (as these may also affect the head) should be noted.
- Examination for symmetry provides important clues with regard to the function of the nerves innervating the musculature of the head and face. This examination should focus on the relative size of the masticatory muscle mass, symmetry of facial expression and the size of the palpebral fissure and pupils.
- The ability of the animal to close their jaw (dependent on the motor component of the trigeminal nerve) and maintain a normal tongue position (mediated by the hypoglossal nerve) may also be apparent from simple observation.

Neurological examination

Innervation of the head and face can be assessed using the menace response, blink (palpebral) reflex, oculovestibular reflexes and gag reflex (see

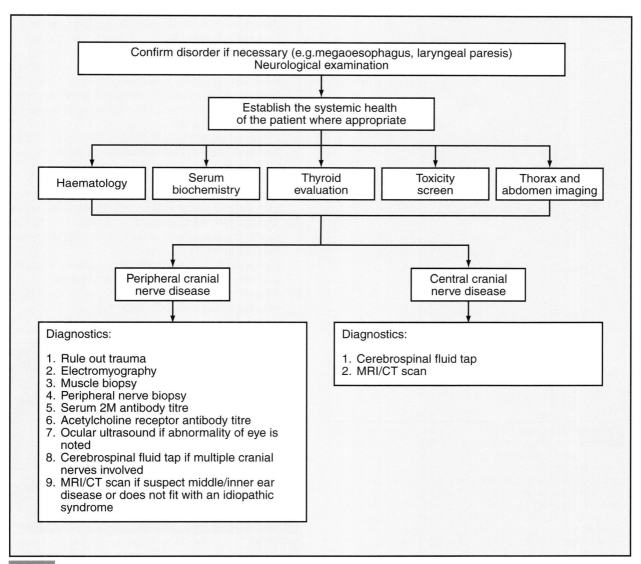

12.17 Diagnostic approach to cases with abnormalities of the head and face.

Confirm disorder if necessary (e.g.megaoesophagus, laryngeal paresis)
Neurological examination

↓

Establish the systemic health of the patient where appropriate

Haematology | Serum biochemistry | Thyroid evaluation | Toxicity screen | Thorax and abdomen imaging

Peripheral cranial nerve disease

Diagnostics:

1. Rule out trauma
2. Electromyography
3. Muscle biopsy
4. Peripheral nerve biopsy
5. Serum 2M antibody titre
6. Acetylcholine receptor antibody titre
7. Ocular ultrasound if abnormality of eye is noted
8. Cerebrospinal fluid tap if multiple cranial nerves involved
9. MRI/CT scan if suspect middle/inner ear disease or does not fit with an idiopathic syndrome

Central cranial nerve disease

Diagnostics:

1. Cerebrospinal fluid tap
2. MRI/CT scan

Chapters 1 and 10 for further information). Several other tests may be of value in detecting neurological abnormalities of the head and face.

- Olfaction can be tested in a crude manner by observing the response to concealed food (e.g. by blindfolding the animal). Substances such as surgical spirit should not be used since they are irritant and may stimulate the nociceptive pathways in the trigeminal nerve rather than the olfactory receptors.
- Masticatory muscle tone can be evaluated by opening the jaws.
- Tongue strength can be evaluated by attempting to hold the tongue: normal animals can easily withdraw the tongue as it is wet and slippery.

Ancillary diagnostic tests
- Hearing can be tested in a crude manner by observing how an animal responds to noise. However, a more sophisticated and objective test is the brainstem auditory evoked potential (BAEP) (Figure 12.18; see also Chapter 4).
- Schirmer tear tests can be used to detect deficits in tear production (see Chapter 10).

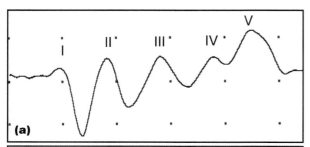

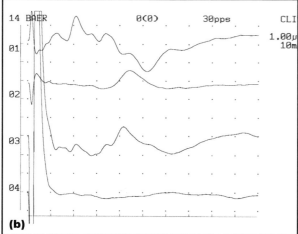

12.18 **(a)** Normal BAEP tracing showing the five peaks that are typically detected. **(b)** BAEPs obtained from a 6-week-old Dalmatian puppy with unilateral deafness in the left ear. Trace 01 = normal trace from the right ear stimulated at 80 dB. Trace 02 = recorded after stimulating the left ear at 80 dB. Trace 03 = recorded after stimulating the left ear at 100 dB. Traces 02 and 03 show only wave V. This wave originates from the contralateral (normal) ear due to decussation of the auditory pathways in the rostral brainstem. The absence of waves I to IV in traces 02 and 03 indicates deafness in the left ear. Trace 04 = an abnormal response in the left ear after stimulation at 100 dB with the right ear masked at 30 dB. (continues) ▶

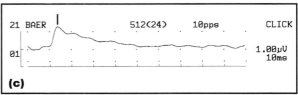

12.18 (continued) **(c)** Abnormal BAEP obtained from an 8-year-old cross-breed dog with severe brainstem compression. Only wave I is clearly discernible.

- Pharmacological testing with adrenergic agonists is occasionally helpful in the investigation of Horner's syndrome (see Chapter 10).
- Measurement of the number of antibodies to the acetylcholine receptor can be used to substantiate the diagnosis of immune-mediated myasthenia gravis. Currently, the test for dogs and cats can only be reliably performed by a few laboratories in the world (see Chapter 18).
- Measurement of serum antibodies to type 2M muscle fibres can be used to aid diagnosis of masticatory muscle myositis.
- Magnetic resonance imaging (MRI) and computed tomography (CT) can be used to detect lesions, particularly within the CNS (e.g. tumours) (Figure 12.19), as well as abnormal structures in the PNS. MRI can be used to evaluate the CNs and special sequences have been described for examining the inner ear. CT is particularly useful for detecting bone lesions (such as destruction or proliferation adjacent to the skull foramina).
- Cisternal cerebrospinal fluid (CSF) analysis can be used to detect inflammatory disease of the CNS or nerve roots (see Chapter 3).
- Electrodiagnostics (electromyography, nerve conduction velocity) can be used to diagnose generalized peripheral neuropathies or to assess specific CN function (such as that related to the facial, trigeminal and recurrent laryngeal nerves) (see Chapter 4).
- Serum and CSF antibody titres against various infectious agents, including *Toxoplasma*, *Neospora* and canine distemper virus, can be measured (see also Chapter 11).

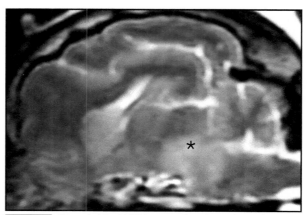

12.19 T2-weighted MR image showing a hyperintense lesion (✶) in the brainstem of a dog that had reduced facial sensation. The lesion was later confirmed to be granulomatous meningoencephalitis.

Specific neurological syndromes of the head and face

Specific diseases of the eyes and the vestibular system are described in Chapters 10 and 11, respectively, and are not considered here.

Deafness

A list of differential diagnoses and their diagnostic features can be found in Figure 12.20.

Cause of deafness	Distinguishing diagnostic features
Congenital	Usually deaf from birth; no waveforms on BAEP
Neoplasia of the middle or inner ear	Lysis on bulla radiography; bulla mass on CT/MRI; cytology on myringotomy
Otitis media/interna	Abnormal otic examination; soft tissue in bulla on CT/MRI; cytology on myringotomy
Nasopharyngeal polyp	Young cats; mass visible on otic/pharyngeal examination
Toxicity (aminoglycosides, furosemide, cisplatin)	History of exposure; rule out other causes

12.20 Specific diagnostic features of different causes of deafness.

Clinical signs

Owners usually only detect hearing loss if it is bilateral, although perceptive owners may notice a change in their pet's behaviour with unilateral loss. If hearing loss is associated with otitis media/interna (OM/OI), the animal may show signs of pain and develop signs of vestibular disease and Horner's syndrome. Occasionally, unilateral deafness is associated with signs of brainstem disease.

Pathogenesis

Deafness can be classified as conductive (failure of conduction of sound) or sensorineural (dysfunction of the sensory organ), depending on the underlying pathogenesis.

Congenital disease: Congenital lesions of the peripheral vestibular system or auditory apparatus are well recognized in certain breeds. Congenital deafness occurs in blue-eyed white cats, Dalmatians, Border Collies, white Boxers, Dobermanns, English Setters and many other breeds of dog. There appears to be an association between blue eyes and localized patches of white coat in many affected individuals (Strain, 1996, 2004; Famula *et al.*, 2000, 2007; Saunders and Bagley, 2003; Cargill *et al.*, 2004; Platt *et al.*, 2006; Cvejic *et al.*, 2009; Strain *et al.*, 2009; De Risio *et al.*, 2010).

The genetic basis for congenital deafness is not known (Rak, 2005). In Dalmatians, deafness develops during the first 3–4 weeks postpartum, during which time there is degeneration of the stria vascularis causing secondary destruction of hair cells with the organ of Corti (Strain, 1996). Congenital vestibular dysfunction is discussed in Chapter 11.

Acquired disease: Deafness in adult animals is most commonly caused by otitis externa (OE) or OM, which impairs conduction of sound to the tympanum (i.e. conductive deafness) or by OI, which causes direct damage to the organ of Corti (i.e. sensorineural deafness). Such cases often have long-standing evidence of ear disease and frequently exhibit pain or irritation in the region of the ears. However, otitis cannot be ruled out simply because of an absence of otoscopically detectable disease. Older animals occasionally develop tumours in the middle ear cavity (ceruminous gland adenocarcinoma, squamous cell carcinoma) and nasopharyngeal polyps (inflammatory lesions) are sometimes found in cats (see Chapter 11).

It is well recognized that geriatric animals can become deaf because of senile degeneration of the middle ear ossicles (Strain, 1996) or age-associated degeneration of the organ of Corti (also called presbycusis) (Knowles *et al.*, 1989). Sensorineural deafness in young adults is most likely to be caused by exposure to systemic toxins (in particular aminoglycosides and cisplatin) or local toxins administered topically or used as cleansing agents (such as chlorhexidine).

Diseases affecting the ascending pathways through the brainstem (such as trauma, neoplasia or encephalitis) rarely cause complete deafness, and other signs of brainstem disease tend to overshadow any loss of hearing that does occur. On rare occasions, middle ear infections can extend through the temporal bone to invade the intracranial cavity (Sturges *et al.*, 2006).

Diagnosis

Deafness as a result of disease of the brainstem or middle and inner ear can be readily confirmed by BAEP recordings (see Figure 12.18 and Chapter 4). During this procedure, which can be carried out when the animal is conscious, sedated or anaesthetized, clicking noises are played through headphones into the ear canals (or vibration applied to the temporal bone). The responses of the brainstem are recorded via fine subcutaneous needle electrodes. This test can be used to determine the site and severity of any hearing loss.

OM and neoplasia of the middle ear can be diagnosed by careful otoscopic examination and radiography. MRI and CT are more sensitive imaging modalities and can also be used to confirm the diagnosis where available. Myringotomy can be performed to obtain a sample from the middle ear for cytology and culture (see Chapter 11) but requires anaesthesia.

Treatment and prognosis

Many causes of deafness are not amendable to treatment, such as genetic or toxin-mediated degeneration of the hair cells. Infection in the middle ear can be treated with antimicrobials or, more commonly, requires surgical treatment (bulla osteotomy). Following severe OM there may never be restoration of full hearing acuity.

Laryngeal paresis and paralysis

A list of differential diagnoses and their diagnostic features can be found in Figure 12.21.

Causes of laryngeal paresis and paralysis	Distinguishing diagnostic features
Congenital	Specific breed; early onset; rule out other causes
Laryngeal paralysis polyneuropathy complex	Specific breed; progressive lower motor neuron tetraparesis; rule out other causes
Neoplasia (thyroid)	Presence of thyroid mass
Idiopathic laryngeal paralysis	Rule out other causes
Surgical trauma to vagus nerve	Recent history of neck surgery
Toxicity (lead, organophosphate)	History of exposure; blood lead levels; blood cholinesterase activity
Brainstem disease (neoplasia, encephalitis)	Presence of other signs of brainstem disease; CT/MRI of brain; CSF analysis

12.21 Specific diagnostic features of different causes of laryngeal paresis and paralysis.

Clinical signs

Inspiratory stridor and dysphonia are the classic clinical signs associated with laryngeal paresis and paralysis; although, severe inspiratory dyspnoea, cyanosis and collapse occur on occasion. These signs may be sufficiently mild that animals only present for treatment following particular periods of respiratory stress, such as prolonged exercise or extreme hot weather, at which time they may present in a hyperthermic crisis. Affected animals may also cough (especially when drinking water) and can develop clinical signs related to the secondary development of aspiration pneumonia.

Pathogenesis

Suspected hereditary disease: Laryngeal paralysis in dogs <1 year of age has been reported in several breeds, including Bouviers des Flandres, Siberian Huskies (and Husky cross-breeds), Dalmatians, Alaskan Malamutes, Rottweilers, Pyrenean Mountain Dogs, Russian Black Terriers, Miniature Schnauzers, Tibetan Mastiffs and Bull Terriers (see Appendix 1). In Bouviers des Flandres and Huskies there is evidence of degeneration of neuronal cell bodies within the nucleus ambiguus in the medulla oblongata (Venker-van Haagan et al., 1978; O'Brien and Hendriks, 1986) with subsequent Wallerian-like degeneration of the laryngeal nerves; whereas, in other breeds it occurs as part of a generalized axonal or demyelinating neuropathy (Braund et al., 1989; Granger, 2010). In Leonbergers and Italian Spinones, the onset of clinical signs can occur later in life (up to 8 years old).

Acquired disease: Laryngeal paralysis occurs most commonly as an acquired disease in middle-aged and older large-breed dogs, notably Labrador Retrievers. Although laryngeal paralysis in mature animals was often previously considered to be idiopathic, there is now strong evidence that it occurs as one, particularly prominent, component of a generalized neuropathy (Jeffery et al., 2006; Shelton, 2010; Thieman et al., 2010). One study has also demonstrated an association between laryngeal paralysis, polyneuropathy and oesophageal dysfunction (Stanley et al., 2010). Since the recurrent laryngeal nerve is particularly long, it has been proposed that it is more susceptible that other peripheral nerves to axonal 'dying back' diseases, in which transport of vital substances to the tip of the axon is compromised. Therefore, it is important to consider an investigation for systemic diseases that can cause polyneuropathies in dogs with laryngeal paralysis (see Chapter 15).

Acquired laryngeal paralysis occasionally occurs as a consequence of trauma to the vagus nerve during cervical surgery, lead and organophosphate toxicity, retropharyngeal infection or neoplasia in the vicinity of the recurrent laryngeal nerve; thyroid carcinoma is the most common tumour type. Laryngeal paresis and/or paralysis can occasionally result from brainstem disease. In these cases other CNs are usually involved and there is often a profound alteration in the consciousness of the dog.

Diagnosis

Laryngeal paralysis is usually diagnosed by examination of the movement of the vocal cords, either directly through the mouth when the animal is lightly anaesthetized (see **Laryngeal hemiparesis** clip on DVD) or using ultrasonography when the patient is conscious (Figure 12.22). In equivocal cases, electromyography is helpful, not only in

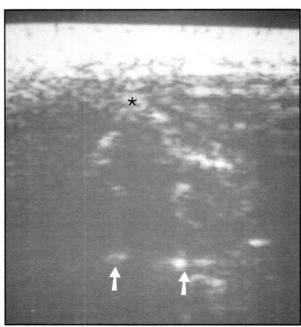

12.22 Poor abduction of the arytenoid cartilages during inspiration can often be detected by real-time ultrasound examination. Note the position of the cuneiform processes (arrowed). ★ = thyroid cartilage.

identifying denervation of the larynx but also in detecting more generalized disease both of the cranial structures (especially the pharynx) and throughout the body. Palpation, ultrasonography and biopsy can readily diagnose thyroid tumours.

Treatment and prognosis

Treatment of laryngeal paralysis requires surgical lateralization of the arytenoid cartilage (Monnet, 2003), regardless of the underlying cause, as it is usually a permanent defect. Nevertheless, surgical lateralization of the arytenoids should not be undertaken lightly in cases in which deglutition is compromised since it dramatically increases the risk of food aspiration. Surgery is only a short-term measure in those breeds with concurrent progressive tetraparesis, and owners should be made aware that exercise intolerance frequently persists after arytenoid lateralization in dogs with generalized neuropathies. Some thyroid tumours can be excised surgically but others are extremely locally invasive, implying that other anti-cancer treatment modalities should be considered.

Megaoesophagus

A list of differential diagnoses and their diagnostic features can be found in Figure 12.23.

Causes of megaoesphagus	Distinguishing diagnostic features
Dysautonomia	Other signs of autonomic dysfunction
Congenital	No other neurological deficits; certain breeds predisposed
Persistent right aortic arch	Radiographic appearance
Hypoadrenocorticism	Generalized weakness; electrolyte abnormalities; negative adrenocorticotropic hormone stimulation test
Myasthenia gravis	± Exercise intolerance; response to tensilon test; positive acetylcholine receptor antibody titre
Polymyositis	Generalized weakness; increased creatine kinase; generalized electromyogram abnormalities; myositis on muscle biopsy
Oesophagitis	History of vomiting; endoscopic evidence
Botulism	Generalized lower motor neuron signs
Brainstem disease (neoplasia, encephalitis)	Other signs of brainstem disease; CT/MRI of brain; CSF analysis

12.23 Specific diagnostic features of different causes of megaoesophagus.

Clinical signs

The characteristic sign of megaoesophagus is regurgitation, usually involving both food and fluid. During the initial investigation it is critical to differentiate regurgitation from true vomiting. There may be several other clinical signs associated with regurgitation including weight loss (or failure to gain weight) and coughing due to aspiration pneumonia.

Pathogenesis

Congenital disease: The underlying cause of congenital megaoesophagus is unknown, but some studies have suggested that afferent function may be aberrant (Holland *et al.*, 1996, 2002). Congenital megaoesophagus can arise as a secondary consequence of a persistent right aortic arch or as one aspect of congenital myasthenia gravis (although not all affected breeds develop megaoesophagus). Congenital megaoesophagus may also form part of a suspected hereditary generalized neuropathy in a number of breeds (Granger, 2010).

Acquired disease: Acquired megaoesophagus can result from a wide range of lesions, including brainstem and systemic disease. The most common cause is myasthenia gravis, in which there is immune-mediated destruction of the acetylcholine receptor. Deficient oesophageal motility is also being increasingly recognized in ageing dogs with laryngeal paralysis (Stanley *et al.*, 2010).

Diagnosis

Megaoesophagus is readily diagnosed on radiography, especially with contrast studies (Figure 12.24). Nevertheless, careful examination is required because abnormal oesophageal motility can occur without obvious signs of megaoesophagus, especially in young terriers (Bexfield *et al.*, 2006). Determining the cause of megaoesophagus relies on detecting and investigating other signs of systemic or brainstem disease. For instance, routine blood analysis and blood chemistry may reveal hypoadrenocorticism, myositis or systemic lupus erythematosus. Hypothyroidism and myasthenia gravis can be detected by specific blood tests. If the neurological examination identifies generalized peripheral nerve disease, then botulism or generalized peripheral neuropathies (see Chapter 15) should be considered; if nearby CNs show deficits, then brainstem disease may be suspected and can be diagnosed using advanced imaging techniques and CSF analysis. The possibility of

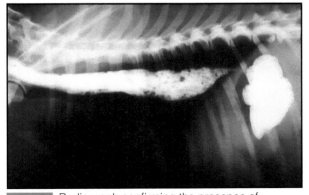

12.24 Radiograph confirming the presence of megaoesophagus. Contrast medium (barium mixed with food) was administered prior to exposure.

dysautonomia should be considered, particularly if other signs of autonomic dysfunction are evident. If all of these conditions can be ruled out, then idiopathic disease must be assumed.

Treatment and prognosis

For many acquired cases of megaoesophagus, treatment of the underlying disease may be possible (i.e. immunosuppressive corticosteroids or other immuno-modulating drugs for systemic lupus erythematosus or polymyositis). With congenital myasthenia gravis, although the disease can be treated using anticho-linesterases, it can be difficult to achieve the correct dose to restore satisfactory swallowing function (Miller *et al.*, 1983). Similarly, unless persistent aortic arches are surgically treated early, the associated megaoesophagus will not resolve adequately. No matter what the cause of megaoesophagus, postural feeding (i.e. feeding the animal with its head directly above its stomach) and feeding a diet that is of a gelatine-like consistency are highly recommended to aid passage of food from the mouth to the stomach and to avoid inhalation.

The prognosis for animals with mega-oesophagus is guarded because of the very high incidence of aspiration pneumonia, which is life-threatening. Many animals succumb within a few weeks to months of starting therapy. It has been suggested that since spontaneous remission can occur in myasthenia gravis it may be preferable to avoid immunosuppressive therapy because it may promote respiratory tract infection (Shelton, 2002) (see Chapter 18).

Abnormalities in the muscles of mastication

A list of differential diagnoses and their diagnostic features can be found in Figure 12.25.

Causes of abnormalities in the muscles of mastication	Distinguishing diagnostic features
Age-related atrophy	Rule out other causes
Hyperadrenocorticism or exogenous administration of corticosteroids	Other signs of hyperadrenocorticism: elevated alkaline phosphatase; positive adrenocorticotropic hormone stimulation test; recent history of corticosteroid administration
Neoplasia: cachexia (bilateral); CN V nerve root tumour or cerebellomedullary pontine angle meningioma (unilateral)	Development of ipsilateral facial sensory deficits and neurogenic keratitis; spontaneous activity on electromyogram; presence of mass on imaging of the brain (CT/MRI)
Masticatory myositis	May have muscle pain and swelling at onset of signs; antibodies against type 2M myofibres; inflammatory infiltrate on muscle biopsy; elevated creatine kinase; difficulty opening jaw
Generalized myopathy	Signs of a generalized myopathy (see Chapter 18)

12.25 Specific diagnostic features of different causes of abnormalities in the muscles of mastication.

Clinical signs

Atrophy of the masticatory muscles can occur unilaterally or bilaterally. Bilateral atrophy is not associated with failure to close the mouth but some individuals exhibit limited mouth opening (trismus). Third eyelid protrusion may follow severe temporal and masseter muscle atrophy, resulting in enophthalmos (due to loss of muscle support to the orbit) which may be sufficiently severe to impair vision. Swelling of the muscles of mastication can occur in the acute phase of masticatory myositis with trismus and exophthalmos. Palpation of the muscles or attempting to open the jaws may cause pain and occasionally a 'locked jaw' syndrome can result, in which animals are unable to either open or close their mouth (Gatineau *et al.*, 2008). Exophthalmos in the absence of masticatory muscle swelling can result from myositis of the extraocular muscles. Young Golden Retrievers may be predisposed to this unusual disease (see Chapter 10).

Pathogenesis

The differential diagnoses for masticatory muscle atrophy include all causes of generalized and localized myopathies (see Chapter 18) as well as diseases of the trigeminal nerve and its nucleus. The absence of other detectable neurological deficits confirms that brainstem involvement is improbable in most cases.

Bilateral atrophy: Bilateral atrophy can be caused by many systemic diseases, most notably cachexia (associated with cancer) and hyperadrenocorticism (associated with prolonged use of exogenous, or high levels of endogenous, corticosteroids). However, bilateral atrophy most commonly occurs as a consequence of masticatory myositis due to the destruction of muscle fibres and scarring, which can occur rapidly. This is an immune-mediated disorder in which antibody-directed inflammation is targeted at the muscles of mastication, including the masseter, temporalis and pterygoid muscles. The specific antigen is part of the unique myofibre (type 2M) contained within these muscles. There is no gender predisposition documented for masticatory myositis and breeds noted to have a predisposition include the German Shepherd Dog, Hungarian Vizsla (Haley *et al.*, 2011) and Cavalier King Charles Spaniel (Pitcher and Hahn, 2007). Most affected dogs are of large breeds and are often young adults; cats are infrequently affected.

Unilateral atrophy: Unilateral atrophy is occasionally encountered and, although many animals live for years without developing other signs, it is recognized that nerve sheath tumours may be responsible (Bagley *et al.*, 1998).

Diagnosis

Detection of a significant concentration of anti-type 2M muscle fibre antibodies confirms masticatory myositis; although, by the time the chronic phase is reached, the antibody response may well have subsided. Serum creatine kinase levels may also be elevated. Muscle biopsy may reveal an inflammatory infiltrate, myofibre necrosis and phagocytosis. It may also specifically identify antibody localization to the type 2M myofibres. Electromyography often identifies spontaneous abnormalities and should always be performed to evaluate the rest of the musculature in cases where a more generalized myopathy is suspected. CT or MRI is required to diagnose nerve sheath tumours in cases with unilateral masticatory muscle atrophy.

Treatment and prognosis

Masticatory muscle atrophy as a result of systemic disease does not appear to be reversible but does not often cause significant deficits. Masticatory myositis is treated with immunosuppressive doses of corticosteroids, but some cases of atrophy are too far advanced for this therapy to be effective. The recommended dose of prednisolone is 1–2 mg/kg orally q12h for 3–4 weeks, after which the dosage is tapered slowly to achieve the lowest dosage q48h that eliminates the clinical signs. Most dogs treated aggressively in the early stages show a good response to therapy but relapses are possible. Some cases require the addition of a further immunosuppressive medication, such as azathioprine (see Chapter 18).

Whilst cases that respond rapidly often have a favourable prognosis, chronic loss of muscle may lead to trismus and permanent dysphagia. Feeding regimens should be discussed with the owner as even in the early stages of a responsive condition feeding tubes may be necessary, if only to reduce the potential for aspiration pneumonia. Additional therapy such as vigorous physiotherapy of the jaw muscles (by encouraging the dog to chew rawhides or play with tennis balls) is advisable.

Idiopathic trigeminal nerve palsy

Clinical signs

Motor deficits caused by trigeminal nerve palsy are recognized in the syndrome of 'dropped jaw', in which the patient (almost always a dog) cannot close its mouth or prehend food properly (see **Dropped jaw** clip on DVD). Other CNs are rarely affected but there can be a variable degree of sensory loss (sensory trigeminal distribution) and some animals display Horner's syndrome. Golden Retrievers are over-represented (Mayhew *et al.*, 2002).

Pathogenesis

The cause of idiopathic trigeminal nerve palsy is thought to be an idiopathic neuritis, although lymphoma and *Neospora caninum* infection have been reported (Mayhew *et al.*, 2002) and older texts suggest an unsubstantiated link with dogs carrying heavy loads in their mouths.

Diagnosis

The diagnosis is made largely through recognition of the typical pattern of clinical signs, absence of any other neurological disease and allowing a period of time to elapse in which recovery can occur. MRI and CSF analysis can be helpful to rule out other causes.

Treatment and prognosis

Treatment is supportive: helping the animal to eat by offering boluses of soft food and assisting with drinking, or the placement of a temporary feeding tube. It has been suggested that holding the mouth partially closed with a muzzle facilitates eating and drinking during recovery. Most animals recover rapidly and are able to eat unassisted within 3 weeks.

Facial paralysis

Facial nerve dysfunction may be due to disease of the peripheral facial nerve caused by OM/OI (see Chapter 11), trauma, neoplasia of the middle/inner ear or polyneuropathies (see Chapter 15). Disease of the facial nerve nucleus in the medulla of the brainstem can result from any disease affecting the CNS. The most common cause of peripheral facial nerve paralysis has been reported to be idiopathic (75% of dogs and 25% of cats with facial paralysis). A list of differential diagnoses and their diagnostic features can be found in Figure 12.26.

Causes of facial paresis	Distinguishing diagnostic features
Myasthenia gravis	Regurgitation; megaoesophagus; exercise intolerance; response to tensilon test; positive acetylcholine receptor antibody titre
Neoplasia of middle or inner ear	Lysis on bulla radiographs; bulla mass on CT/MRI; cytology on myringotomy
Idiopathic	Normal tear production; rule out other causes
Otitis media/interna	May have decreased tear production; abnormal otic examination; soft tissue on bulla CT/MRI; cytology on myringotomy
Trauma (surgical or external)	Recent history of trauma or surgery
Brainstem disease (neoplasia, encephalitis)	Other signs of brainstem disease; CT/MRI of brain; CSF analysis
Other generalized lower motor neuron (LMN) diseases	Generalized signs of LMN dysfunction

12.26 Specific diagnostic features of different causes of facial paresis.

Idiopathic facial paralysis

Clinical signs: Idiopathic facial nerve paralysis or palsy may be unilateral or bilateral, but usually occurs in the absence of other neurological deficits (sometimes affected animals also develop idiopathic vestibular syndrome). Exposure keratitis can occur subsequent to improper lubrication of the cornea, despite normal tear production. Clinical signs are usually maximal within 7 days and recovery can take 3–6 weeks if it occurs at all (Varejão *et al.*, 2006). Since unilateral facial nerve palsy can also develop in association with CNS diseases, it is essential to consider the possibility of CNS lesions; typically, these are associated with postural reaction abnormalities (see Lesion localization). In addition, facial nerve palsy is sometimes observed in animals with more generalized peripheral neuropathies (e.g. those affecting multiple limbs).

Pathogenesis: In early reports on idiopathic facial nerve palsy, biopsy revealed marked depletion of large diameter myelinated axons (Braund *et al.*, 1979).

Diagnosis: All possible causes of facial paresis and/or paralysis should be excluded before this specific diagnosis can be made. A thorough investigation for ear disease should be undertaken in addition to electromyography to rule out polyneuropathies. MRI may reveal contrast enhancement of the intratemporal facial nerve, which has been proposed to suggest a poorer prognosis (Varejão *et al.*, 2006).

Treatment and prognosis: There is no effective treatment for the underlying disease but it is important to ensure that the cornea is adequately lubricated (either by endogenous production or eye drops). The prognosis for idiopathic facial palsy varies, many animals make a gradual recovery (weeks to months) but some are left with permanent deficits. These deficits may progress to muscle contracture and deform the facial ex-pression permanently. This can be mistakenly interpreted as hemifacial spasm, an uncommon syndrome in dogs and cats.

Hemifacial spasm
Clinical signs of this syndrome include blepharospasm, elevation of the ear, deviation of the nose to the affected side and wrinkling or displacement of the upper lip. The signs may precede facial paralysis but the spasm must be differentiated from contracture secondary to denervation atrophy and fibrosis. Hemifacial spasm may be due to lesions of the middle/inner ear or the brainstem and should be investigated thoroughly. Control of hemifacial spasm depends on identifying and treating the underlying cause.

Multiple cranial nerve deficits
Various combinations of unilateral or bilateral CN deficits are sometimes detected; almost any combination of signs is possible depending on the underlying cause (see **Facial hyperaesthesia** clip on DVD). In some instances there is concomitant reduction of ipsilateral postural reactions and some animals may exhibit stupor.

It is important to recognize the significance of bilateral CN disorders and postural reaction deficits. Bilateral CN deficits suggest that the lesion is not located within the CNS (a lesion within the brainstem large enough to cause bilateral deficits would probably be fatal), and postural reaction deficits in

combination with CN deficits suggest that the lesion is located within the CNS.

Generalized peripheral neuropathies (see Chapter 15) can cause any combination of CN deficits. Therefore, it is of the utmost importance to examine all peripheral nerve reflexes in any animal that has a CN disorder. Occasionally, the most prominent signs are confined to the CNs. For instance, there are uncommon idiopathic diseases that can affect multiple CNs, most notably:

- Feline dysautonomia – pupillary dilatation and megaoesophagus are characteristic signs (see Chapter 19)
- Polyganglioneuritis – reported as a cause of multiple somatic CN deficits (see Chapter 14).

Brain tumours may occasionally cause multiple CN signs, especially if they develop within the caudal part of the brainstem; in most instances these signs are accompanied by postural reaction deficits. A more confusing presentation is that associated with skull-base tumours (sometimes known by the misnomer 'cavernous sinus syndrome', see Chapter 10) in which there may be multiple, often bilateral, CN deficits (Figure 12.27) without evidence of brainstem involvement. Such animals are often also very depressed because of elevated intracranial pressure.

Iatrogenic cranial nerve lesions
Several CNs and associated structures are susceptible to injury during surgical procedures around the head and neck.

- The facial nerve is vulnerable because of its superficial location on the side of the face. Surgery around the deep portions of the external auditory canal and middle ear (see **Palpebral reflex** clip on DVD), or parotid duct transposition are common causes of facial nerve palsy. Clinical signs due to neurapraxia usually improve within 2 weeks.
- The sympathetic supply is vulnerable to injury during bulla osteotomy (especially in cats) and during any deep neck surgery that involves prolonged retraction of the soft tissues, including the sympathetic truck where it is contained within a common sheath alongside the vagus nerve. Occasionally, dogs appear to develop Horner's syndrome after vigorous restraint using choke chains.
- The recurrent laryngeal nerve may be injured during approaches to, or around, the trachea (especially during extraluminal stenting procedures for tracheal collapse).
- The hypoglossal nerve is susceptible to injury during mandibular surgery, particularly hemimandibulectomy. Bilateral injury can lead to dramatic drooping of the tongue from the mouth.
- The peripheral vestibular system can be damaged by over vigorous curettage during bulla osteotomy.

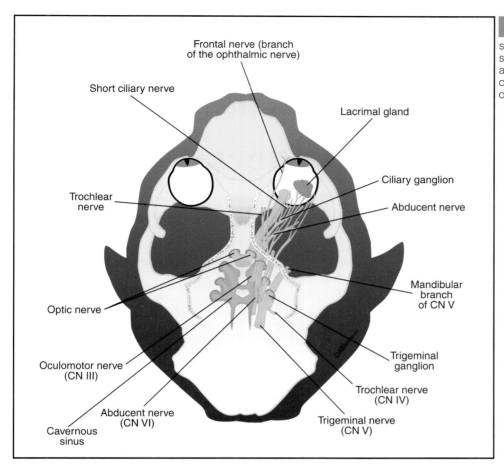

Nerve supply to the eye and surrounding muscles and structures. Note the close approximation of multiple cranial nerves at the base of the skull.

References and further reading

Available on accompanying DVD

DVD extras

- Dropped jaw
- Facial hyperaesthesia
- Laryngeal hemiparesis
- Palpebral reflex

13

Tremors, involuntary movements and paroxysmal disorders

Rodney S. Bagley and Simon Platt

Involuntary movement abnormalities result in some of the most dramatic clinical presentations in veterinary medicine. Classically, involuntary movement disorders are present during periods of inactivity rather than during normal movement. Some involuntary movements are persistent whilst others are episodic. Certain involuntary movements have characteristics that allow for identification of specific causes, whereas others are only a reflection of dysfunction of the nervous or musculoskeletal systems. Clinically, it is important to first identify the type of involuntary movement present. Subsequently, a more directed approach can be used to establish the cause of the movement disorder.

Paroxysmal events are characterized by the sudden and reversible onset of neurological dysfunction in an otherwise normal animal, which can be manifest as an involuntary movement. The animal does not lose consciousness and, rarely, has a structural lesion identifiable within the central nervous system (CNS). The underlying cause of many of these events may be a functional abnormality related to neurotransmitter imbalances or receptor abnormalities and dysfunction. Several stereotypical events have been described in specific breeds (see below). Confirmation of the specific syndrome is difficult or impossible in the clinical setting and depends heavily on the exclusion of structural CNS abnormalities such as neoplasia, inflammation and cerebrovascular disease.

Types of involuntary movement

Terms such as tic, twitch, shivering, shuddering and fasciculation are often used to describe episodic, irregular muscle movements associated with 'local' muscle contractions. Involuntary movements, however, are usually manifest through abnormal motion of the limbs, trunk or head.

Terminology

The clinical signs commonly associated with involuntary movement disorders include:

- Cramp – muscle cramps are involuntary and forcibly contracted muscles that do not relax

▶

- Dyskinesia – difficulty or distortion in performing voluntary movements
- Dystonia – sustained muscle contractions causing twisting and repetitive movements or abnormal postures
- Fasciculation – involuntary contractions or twisting of groups of muscle fibres
- Myoclonus – rhythmic movement of a portion of the body resulting from sudden involuntary contraction and relaxation of muscle groups
- Myokymia – continuous involuntary muscle twitching that gives the appearance of worm-like rippling of the muscles
- Myotonia – sustained muscular contraction following an initiating stimulus
- Rigidity – increased resistance to change in position or angle of joint(s)
- Spasm – a brief, automatic jerking movement
- Spasticity – a state of increased tone of a muscle
- Tetanus – sustained muscle contraction without a period of relaxation
- Tetany – intermittent tonic muscular contractions
- Tremor – any abnormal repetitive shaking movement of the body.

Myoclonus

Myoclonus is a shock-like contraction of a muscle or muscles that tends to occur repeatedly in a rhythmic pattern (see **Myoclonus (1)** clip on DVD) and may persist during sleep. It is akin to the rhythmic depolarization and contraction that occurs in the heart with each beat. Myoclonus can be focal, multifocal or generalized. It often presents in the thoracic limbs; however, the pelvic limbs or facial muscles including the tongue may also be involved (deLahunta and Glass, 2008). Myoclonus may be physiological (such as that seen when falling asleep or during sleep), epileptic (see **Myoclonus (2)** clip on DVD) or symptomatic, associated with CNS disease. An idiopathic (essential) myoclonus has been recognized in humans but has not yet been described in veterinary medicine. Myoclonus in dogs is usually the result of distemper virus infection, which establishes a pacemaker-like depolarization of local motor neurons; however, it has also been associated with lead toxicity and other causes of CNS inflammation.

Seizures

Seizure activity also results in spontaneous involuntary movements (see Chapter 8). With generalized seizures, the clinical pattern is fairly characteristic, including falling to a lateral recumbent position, rigidity and eventually paddling or gaiting movements of the limbs. However, with focal seizures, localized involuntary movements such as twitching of a single limb or part of the face may be present. Electroencephalography (see Chapter 4) must be performed at the time of the movement to confirm the cerebral aetiology of the disorder, but this is rarely practical in veterinary medicine.

Tremors

Tremor is one of the most common involuntary movement disorders in humans, and is also a surprisingly common clinical abnormality in dogs. A tremor is an involuntary rhythmic, oscillating movement of fixed frequency, resulting from alternate or synchronous contraction of reciprocally innervated antagonistic muscles (Jankovic and Fahnn, 1980; deLahunta *et al.*, 2006; Ropper and Samuels, 2009). It can be focal (e.g. affecting just one limb or the head) or generalized. Electromyographically, a tremor is characterized by rhythmic bursts of motor neuron activity occurring in opposing muscle groups. This biphasic character differentiates tremors from other movement abnormalities. Whilst seen during the awake state, true tremors should cease with sleep. As for myoclonus, tremors may be physiological, idiopathic (essential; such as that seen in senile dogs) or pathological (due to nervous system disease).

Intention tremors

Intention tremors occur or become worse when an animal intends to perform a function in a goal-oriented manner. This type of tremor is usually most evident when the animal attempts to eat or drink (see **Intention tremor** clip on DVD). Intention tremors usually occur at a frequency of between 2 and 6 times per second and are typically associated with diseases of the cerebellum. Other signs of cerebellar disease that may accompany tremors include:

- Ataxia (incoordination, swaying from side to side)
- Dysmetria ('goose-stepping', overflexing of the limbs when walking)
- Menace deficits (with normal vision and pupillary light reflexes)
- Head tilt (can be paradoxical; see Chapter 8)
- Nystagmus (fast followed by slow movement of the eyes) (Holliday, 1979/1980; deLahunta and Glass, 2008)
- Truncal sway
- Anisocoria (infrequent).

Myokymia and neuromyotonia

Myokymia (involuntary rippling of muscles) and neuromyotonia (abnormal muscle tone) can persist even during sleep and under anaesthesia (Vanhaesebrouck *et al.*, 2010) (see **Myokymia and neuromyotonia** clip on DVD). These disorders represent a continuum of signs that result from motor axon or terminal hyperexcitability. This hyperexcitability can be caused by a wide variety of CNS and peripheral nervous system (PNS) disorders, but is particularly related to ion channel dysfunction. On electromyography, myokymia is characterized by short bursts of ectopically generated motor unit potentials, firing at a rate of 5–62 Hz, which appear as doublets, triplets or multiplets. These bursts fire rhythmically or semi-rhythmically and sound like soldiers marching. Neuromyotonia is characterized by muscle stiffness and persistent contraction related to underlying spontaneous repetitive firing of motor unit potentials. On electromyography, there are prolonged bursts of motor unit potentials, firing at a rapid rate of 150–300 Hz, which begin and end abruptly, do not occur repetitively in a rhythmic fashion and have a characteristic waning amplitude. There are few descriptions in companion animals (Van Ham *et al.*, 2006; Walmsley *et al.*, 2006) but it appears to be an emerging problem in Jack Russell Terriers (Vanhaesebrouck *et al.*, 2010; Bhatti *et al.*, 2011).

Dyskinesia

Dyskinesia is defined as impairment of the power of voluntary movements, resulting in fragmented or incomplete movements (Ramsey *et al.*, 1999; Penderis and Franklin, 2001). Dyskinesia occurs spontaneously during activity or when the animal is at rest, and can be triggered by excitement or exercise. The most common clinical sign is dystonia (increased muscle tone in one or several limbs) and it can lead to collapse. Dogs with these abnormalities may exhibit an abnormal posture such as holding up a limb in an attempt to move or kyphosis of the spine without being able to initiate movement (see **Dyskinesia** clip on DVD). The impaired movement can appear as and has been termed muscle 'cramp', which is defined as paroxysmal, prolonged and severe contraction of muscles that may be painful and can be either focal or generalized (Shelton, 2004). Examples of diseases associated with 'cramp' that may be dyskinesias include:

- Scotty cramp
- Episodic hypertonicity of Cavalier King Charles Spaniels
- Canine epileptoid cramping syndrome in Border Terriers (see **Useful websites** on DVD)
- Extreme generalized muscular stiffness in male Labrador Retrievers (Vanhaesebrouck *et al.*, 2011).

Muscle cramp has also been described secondary to systemic diseases such as hypoadrenocorticism.

Lesion localization

Myoclonus

Myoclonus is often considered as originating from spinal cord disease causing a localized persistent movement abnormality due to abnormal lower motor neuron (LMN) discharges (Podell, 2004). It can also arise from apparent cerebral disease as a type of seizure.

Tremors

Tremor is ultimately a disorder of movement (Jankovic and Fahnn, 1980; Podell, 2004; Ropper and Samuels, 2009; Lorenz *et al.*, 2011). Therefore, lesions in any region of the CNS, PNS or the musculoskeletal system primarily responsible for normal movement may generate a tremor. This makes localization challenging when considering the clinical signs alone. In humans, important motor areas include the basal nuclei and other components of the extrapyramidal system, the cerebellum, diffuse neuronal cell bodies involved in segmental and supraspinal reflex mechanisms, components of the LMN and the interconnecting pathways. In addition, abnormalities of the mechanical apparatus of the limbs (e.g. bones, joints and tendons) may also lead to tremors as a result of pain and weakness. However, species differences do exist and it is important to note that lesions involving the basal nuclei and substantia nigra commonly result in tremor in humans but apparently not in dogs (Ropper and Samuels, 2009).

Intention tremors are most often associated with cerebellar disease and can involve the head or entire body (deLahunta and Glass, 2008) (Figure 13.1). Fine tremors (decreased amplitude and increased frequency) are more often associated with diffuse neuronal disease or muscle weakness (Garosi *et al.*, 2005). The causative lesion may also give rise to other signs of neurological dysfunction that can help further define the localization.

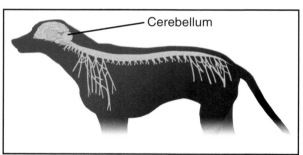

Cerebellum

13.1 Lesion localization for tremors. The CNS (including the cerebrum, cerebellum and meninges) and the diffuse peripheral nervous tissue are highlighted.

Myokymia and fasciculations

Myokymia is the result of spontaneous discharges from large motor units (see above) and indicates neuronal disease followed by sprouting of the motor unit territory in response to denervation. The term neuromyokymia has been used to implicate the role of the neuronal axon in this disorder (deLahunta *et al.*, 2006). Fasciculations arise from ectopic electrical activity in the distal axon and are typically the manifestation of irritability of the neuronal cell body and its associated axons (Podell, 2004).

Dyskinesia

Dyskinesias are episodes of abnormal involuntary hyperkinetic movement or muscle tone. These events are distinguished from seizures by the presence of normal consciousness, although an electroencephalogram (EEG) is necessary for confirmation. The functional lesions responsible for these diseases are not well documented, but are suspected to be located in the thalamocortex and/or the spinal cord. The pathophysiological mechanisms underlying these movements are poorly understood, but may represent a central neurotransmitter or pathway abnormality, or possibly a local muscular abnormality. The localization of the purported functional neurotransmitter-based abnormalities responsible for these disorders may be within the CNS or PNS. In addition, several drugs (including phenobarbital and propofol) have been reported to cause similar dyskinesias in dogs (Smedile *et al.*, 1996; Kube *et al.*, 2006). These disorders are usually reversible with drug tapering or withdrawal.

A movement disorder has been described in young Bichon Frises, which has a variable frequency and random occurrence (Penderis and Franklin, 2001) (see **Dyskinesia** clip on DVD). Rapid muscle contractions cause hyperflexion and/or extension of an individual limb. In addition, the thoracolumbar spinal column can be affected by altered muscle tone during the event, resulting in the animal adopting a kyphotic posture. A similar condition has also been described in young Boxer puppies, which is triggered by excitement and results in abnormal facial, truncal and limb movements with sustained hyperflexion (Ramsey *et al.*, 1999). No successful treatment regimens have been described.

Paroxysmal disorders

Paroxysmal disorders may result from abnormalities in various locations within the nervous system. In some instances, the particular movement abnormality may be associated with a more specific localization (e.g. intention tremors result from a disorder of the cerebellum).

Pathophysiology

Physiological tremors

Several hypotheses have been proposed to explain physiological (essential) tremors. Traditionally, they were thought to represent the passive vibration of the body tissues produced by mechanical activity of cardiac origin. However, of greater significance is probably the contribution of spontaneous firing of groups of motor neurons and the natural resonating frequencies of the muscle fibres. Certain abnormal tremors (e.g. metabolic action tremors due to hypoglycaemia and phaeochromocytoma) are believed to be exaggerations of the physiological tremor. These tremors are also seen in older dogs and so could be considered a progressive disorder.

Cerebellar dysfunction

The cerebellum functions to control movement once it has been initiated (King, 1987; deLahunta and Glass, 2008). The cerebellum also assists with regulation of posture, unconscious proprioception and muscle tone. Structurally, the cerebellum contains two lateral hemispheres (primarily responsible for limb movements), a median portion or vermis (primarily responsible for regulating posture and muscle tone) and a ventral portion (the flocculonodular lobe, primarily responsible for the maintenance of equilibrium and coordination of head and eye movements; Figure 13.2). The cerebellar cortex consists of an outer molecular layer, a middle Purkinje cell layer and an inner granule cell layer (Figure 13.3). The cerebellar cortex has a predominantly inhibitory influence on the three paired cerebellar nuclei of the subcortical white matter (fastigial, interposital and

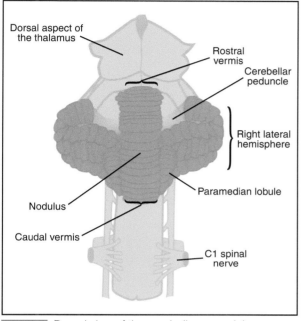

13.2 Dorsal view of the cerebellum, caudal brainstem and cranial cervical spinal cord.

dentate), which are responsible for the control of head and limb movements, but not the initiation of motor movements. Afferent and efferent information to the cerebellum is transmitted via three paired cerebellar peduncles, which attach the cerebellum to the brainstem.

Lesions are most commonly located within the cerebellar hemispheres. Signs of dysfunction of any area of the cerebellum usually include abnormalities of the rate, range, direction and force of motor movements. There are no signs of weakness or paresis seen with 'pure' cerebellar dysfunction. Other signs of cerebellar dysfunction (e.g. ataxia and hypermetria) may also be seen.

Cerebral, spinal cord and peripheral nerve dysfunction
A common underlying theme to the generation of tremors or other involuntary movements is spontaneous neuronal or axonal discharges in the CNS and/or PNS. This increased excitability can be caused by disorders that interfere with normal myelination, ion channel function, electrolyte concentrations (especially potassium, calcium and sodium) and neurotransmission. Inherited (e.g. dysmyelination in Chow Chows and Weimaraners), inflammatory and compressive disorders can all affect any one or more of these parameters, resulting in tremors or other involuntary movements.

The underlying cause of the clinical signs associated with myokymia is thought to involve biochemical alterations in the microenvironment of the axon membrane at the level of the motor unit, which is suggested to affect the local voltage gated potassium channels (Bhatti *et al.*, 2011). Potassium channel damage may be due to autoantibodies in inherited or congenital conditions. Paroxysmal dyskinesias in humans appear to result from mutations

13.3 Magnification of the neuronal circuitry present in the cerebellum. The arrows indicate the direction of impulse transmission.

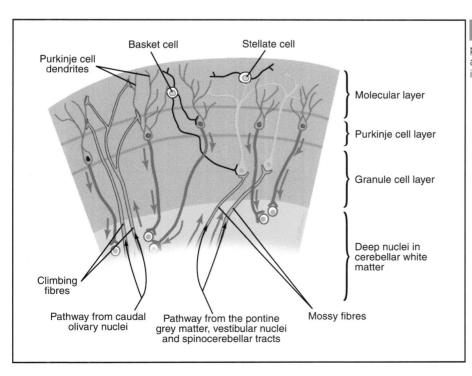

235

in various ion channels, although other mutations have been identified including those affecting glutamate transporter function. As some dyskinesias coexist with seizure disorders, an underlying channelopathy is a plausible pathophysiological mechanism (Packer *et al.*, 2010).

Differential diagnosis

The differential diagnosis is based upon the type of tremor or involuntary movement present (Figure 13.4). Tremors tend to be localized or generalized and categorizing movement disorders in this way

Clinical sign	Frequency	Differential diagnoses
Tremor	See Figure 13.4b	
Rigidity	Constant	Spinal cord disease; tetanus; decerebrate and decerebellate postures
	Intermittent	Tetany; neuromyotonia; vestibulocerebellar events; dyskinesia; endocrine muscle disease (e.g. hypoadrenocorticism)
Myoclonus	Constant	Spinal cord disease (e.g. distemper, pseudorabies); toxicity/drugs
	Intermittent	Cerebral disease (e.g. seizure events caused by Lafora disease in Miniature Wirehaired Dachshunds)
Myotonia	Constant	Myotonia; congenital muscle disease; endocrine muscle disease
	Intermittent	Seizure events; electrolyte aberrations
Myokymia/ fasciculation		Motor neuron disease (e.g. spinal muscular atrophy); peripheral nerve diseases; congenital/ inherited (Jack Russell Terriers); toxicity; inflammation; neoplasia
Dyskinesia		Toxicity; metabolic disorders **Breed-related diseases:** Bichon Frises/Chinooks –dyskinesia Cavalier King Charles Spaniels – episodic falling Dobermanns – dancing Irish Wolfhounds – startle disease Labrador Retrievers – general muscle stiffness Miniature Wirehaired Dachshunds – Lafora disease Norwich Terriers – epileptoid cramping Scottish Terriers – cramping

(a)

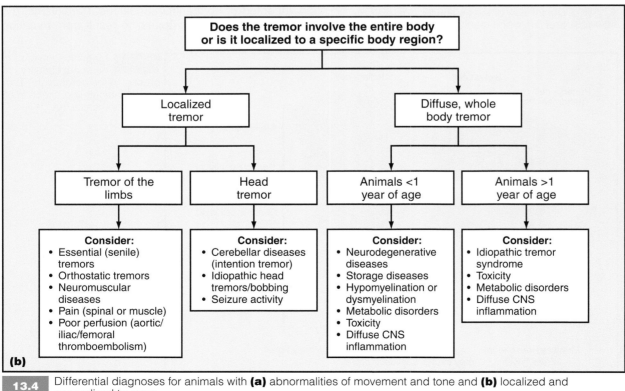

(b)

13.4 Differential diagnoses for animals with **(a)** abnormalities of movement and tone and **(b)** localized and generalized tremors.

helps to determine the list of differential diagnoses (Bagley, 1992; Podell, 2004). Consideration of whether tremors or other movement disorders are continuous or paroxysmal can also assist in determining the possible differential diagnoses.

Neurodiagnostic investigation

Obtaining an accurate history is important to define the onset and progression of the condition, in addition to elucidating any underlying systemic health problems that could be causing the disorder (Figure 13.5).

Tremors and involuntary movements

- Was the onset of the condition acute?
- Has the condition been progressive?
- Has the condition been constant or intermittent?
- Do the tremors disappear during sleep?
- If the animal is young, is there any information available about the littermates?
- Is there are possibility of exposure to toxins?
- What medications is the patient on?
- Is the patient on a standard diet?
- Have there been any recent changes in personality or behaviour?
- Are there any recent changes in the patient's appetite or thirst?

Paroxysmal disorders

- What did the event look like?
- Has this happened before?
- How often has this happened?
- Has it always had the same characteristics?
- Is the animal 'normal' immediately after these events?
- Is there any type of trigger factor that can be identified?
- Is the animal 'normal' in between the events?
- Are any other littermates known to be affected?
- Is the animal stiff or floppy at the time of the event?
- Are the gums pale at the time of the event?
- What are the heart and pulse rates at the time of the event?

13.5 Important questions to ask when establishing a diagnosis. Often dogs and cats are normal at the time of veterinary examination, thus history taking is imperative.

Physical examination is essential as some tremor/movement disorders can be associated with systemic disease. Many syndromes may also be seen in conjunction with neurological deficits; therefore, a neurological examination can help localize the causative lesion or associated deficits and determine the next stages necessary in the diagnostic work-up.

- Haematology, serum chemistry and urinalysis can help rule out systemic diseases, including hypoglycaemia, hypocalcaemia and electrolyte abnormalities.
- Testing for possible toxin exposure can be difficult without knowing which toxin to look for:
  - With organophosphate toxicity, serum cholinesterase activity can be dramatically lowered
  - With a possible history of exposure, blood lead concentrations should be evaluated

  - Home-testing drug kits are available over-the-counter in many USA pharmacies and online in Europe. These kits can rapidly determine the presence of prescription drugs (e.g. tricyclic antidepressants, barbiturates, benzodiazepines, methadone and oxycodone) as well as illicit drugs (e.g. marijuana, cocaine, opioids, methamphetamine, ecstasy, amphetamines and phencyclidine). These drug testing kits for humans have not been validated in animals.
- Thoracic and abdominal radiography and ultrasonography should be performed to rule out systemic neoplasia.
- Cerebrospinal fluid (CSF) analysis is necessary to rule out CNS inflammatory diseases.
- Serum and CSF immunoassays can confirm the infectious nature of a CNS inflammatory disease.
- Advanced imaging techniques such as computed tomography (CT) and magnetic resonance imaging (MRI) can help rule out destructive inflammatory lesions in the CNS as well as focal mass lesions such as neoplasia.

Localized tremor syndromes

Limb tremors and myoclonus

Recent classification schemes have suggested calling tremors a form of myoclonus (often action-related, indicating that they are more pronounced with activity). In this chapter, tremors and myoclonus are kept as separate entities with myoclonus referring to the rhythmic activity of large groups of muscles causing flexion and extension of the limbs, as opposed to diseases causing more 'fine' movement abnormalities of small muscle groups (tremor). There are many different causes of limb tremors. In addition, it should be remembered that focal seizures can cause involuntary movements of a single limb.

Spinal disease

Tremors restricted to only the pelvic limbs may be seen in dogs with lumbar and sacral spinal segment disease. The tremor may result in part from muscle weakness secondary to spinal cord or peripheral nerve impingement, or may possibly occur in response to pain. Pelvic limb tremors may also result from compressive diseases such as lumbosacral vertebral canal stenosis, neoplasia and discospondylitis (Bagley, 1992).

Senile tremors

Older dogs may exhibit tremors of the pelvic limbs (senile tremor); however, the aetiology and the pathogenesis of this syndrome remain unknown (Kornegay, 1986a; Podell, 2004).

Vascular diseases

Limb tremors may be seen with poor perfusion to the limb, resulting from anaemia, or cardiac, pulmonary or vascular disease. Localized cyanosis secondary to a right-to-left shunting patent ductus arteriosus can also result in pelvic limb tremors, most commonly seen during or following exercise. Partial vascular thrombosis and occlusion of the femoral arteries may result in a similar tremor.

Neuromuscular diseases

Diseases associated with muscle weakness such as neuropathy and myopathy may be seen in conjunction with muscle tremors (see Chapter 18). However, tremors associated with these diseases are often of short duration, episodic and present during attempts at muscle activity.

Myokymia and neuromyotonia: Neuromyotonia is clinically characterized by a combination of myokymia, persistent muscle contraction, muscle stiffness or cramp, and impaired muscle relaxation (Bhatti *et al.*, 2011) (see **Myokymia and neuromyotonia** clip on DVD). Axonal voltage gated potassium channel abnormalities may be responsible for this condition, secondary to autoantibody damage, toxicity or genetic mutation. Focal myokymia is generally caused by a structural lesion of the corresponding LMN.

Myokymia and neuromyotonia has been sporadically reported in dogs and cats but is most well documented in Jack Russell Terriers (Van Ham *et al.*, 2004; Galano *et al.*, 2005; Walmsley *et al.*, 2006; Vanhaesebrouck *et al.*, 2010ab). The clinical and clinicopathological findings, treatment and outcome of myokymia and neuromyotonia in 37 Jack Russell Terriers have recently been reported (Bhatti *et al.*, 2011). The most characteristic clinical signs were episodes of rhythmic, undulating muscle contractions which induced vermicular movements of the overlying skin. Collapse and recumbency were also seen in dogs that exhibited rigidity. The majority of episodes were triggered by excitement, exercise or hot weather.

Drugs that have a stabilizing effect on cell membranes, including those of the peripheral nerves, have been used to treat this condition. Sodium channel blockers (e.g. procainamide and mexilitine) as well as slow-release phenytoin have been used in dogs with variable effects (Bhatti *et al.*, 2011). Cold water baths have been more uniformly successful, especially when combined with general anaesthesia.

Orthostatic tremors

This disorder has been recognized in young Great Danes and Scottish Deerhounds (Garosi *et al.*, 2005; Platt *et al.*, 2006). This is a postural tremor seen only in the limbs when the dog is weight-bearing (see **Orthostatic tremor** clip on DVD). The tremors are absent when walking, leaning or lying down. The neurological examination of affected dogs is normal. Characteristic electromyogram (EMG) readings have been reported with motor unit action potentials of 13–16 Hz (Figure 13.6).

Head tremors

Dogs occasionally have tremors involving only the head (Bagley, 1992; Lorenz *et al.*, 2011). This type of tremor most likely results from tremor of the neck

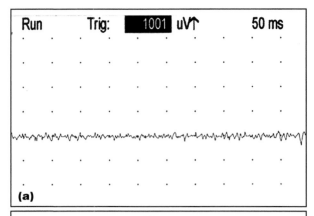

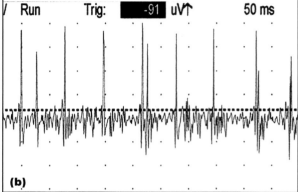

13.6 **(a)** Surface electromyogram (EMG) tracing of a normal dog, recorded when the patient was awake. **(b)** Surface EMG tracing from the pelvic limbs of a dog with orthostatic tremors, recorded whilst the animal was standing.

muscles, but its pathophysiology is poorly understood. Head tremors which are exacerbated by an intentional movement such as eating or drinking are termed intention or ataxic tremors. This abnormality indicates cerebellar dysfunction. Paroxysmal or continuous non-ataxic tremors of the head are often considered to result from cerebral or thalamic diseases. Focal facial movement abnormalities or intermittent head movements/jerks should also be considered as potential seizure disorders and investigated appropriately.

Non-ataxic head tremors

Metabolic, systemic and toxic diseases: Head tremors or bobbing have been reported in a dog undergoing peritoneal dialysis for renal failure and in a dog with iatrogenic hypoparathyroidism. The author [RB] has seen dogs with a variety of systemic illnesses receiving multiple drug therapies that have similar tremors. Metaclopromide treatment and doxorubicin administration are notable examples. In addition, a dog evaluated at the author's [RB] hospital with syncope due to third degree heart block had an intermittent affirmation head tremor.

Idiopathic head tremors/bobbing: This type of head tremor appears to occur without a definable cause in some breeds such as the Dobermann (especially in dogs <1 year of age), Boxers and

Bulldogs; however, a variety of breeds can be affected (Kornegay, 1986a; Bagley, 1992) (see **Idiopathic head tremor** clip on DVD). These dogs have no other clinical abnormalities and are usually young. Head tremors may be either in a vertical or lateral plane and are sometimes referred to as a head bob. Head tremors are usually more prominent when the dog is less active. In addition, dogs seem to be able to stop this movement if they desire, are conscious, can walk and can respond to verbal commands. This is almost the opposite of an intention tremor, as the tremor can be stopped when the dog is focused on a goal-oriented task such as eating.

The pathogenesis of the disease is not known. In humans, a nodding of the head can occur with lesions of the thalamus, and one author [SP] has seen this in a dog with a thalamic lesion. A 'yes' tremor may also accompany midline cerebellar lesions. A full diagnostic work-up (blood work, CSF analysis and imaging of the brain) is normal with the idiopathic condition. There is little information on the most appropriate treatment and although there may be a partial response to antiepileptic drugs, they are usually ineffective (Lorenz *et al.*, 2011). Fortunately, these tremors rarely impact on the quality of life of the animal.

Infectious and inflammatory causes: Although unusual, animals with a head tremor or bob as the only clinical sign can have an inflammatory or infectious disease (see Chapter 11 for further information on encephalitis). In addition, myoclonus of the head or face can be seen with inflammatory diseases of the CNS. This may be more common with distemper virus infections and has been called 'chewing gum fits' due to the rhythmic jaw movements seen. However, it may be difficult to distinguish this form of localized myoclonus from continuous focal seizure activity. Focal facial movement abnormalities or intermittent head movements/jerks should always be considered as potential seizure disorders and investigated appropriately (see **Focal motor seizure** clip on DVD).

Ataxic head tremors

Intention tremors are most often the result of cerebellar disease (deLahunta and Glass, 2008). The tremor may involve the whole body but is most obvious in the head. The head usually moves in a vertical plane at a frequency of 2–4 Hz. This is most likely a dysmetria of head movement.

Diseases of the cerebellum

Degenerative diseases

Primary cerebellar cortical degeneration: Cerebellar cortical degeneration (also called cerebellar abiotrophy) is usually an inherited disease in dogs (deLahunta, 1980) with few reports in cats.

Clinical signs: These diseases are recognized syndromes in the Kerry Blue Terrier, Gordon Setter, Rough-coated Collie, Border Collie, Old English Sheepdog, Brittany Spaniel, Scottish Terrier and Bull Mastiff, and occur rarely in the Samoyed, Airedale Terrier, Finnish Harrier, Labrador Retriever, Golden Retriever, Beagle, Cocker Spaniel, Great Dane and Pomeranian (deLahunta, 1980; Gandini *et al.*, 2005; Urkasemsin *et al.*, 2010). Clinical signs usually appear between 3 and 12 months of age. However, a subset of adult-onset diseases occur in the Brittany Spaniel (Higgins *et al.*, 1998), Gordon Setter (deLahunta *et al.*, 1980), Old English Sheepdog (Steinberg *et al.*, 2000) and Scottish Terrier (van der Merwe and Lane, 2001; Urkasemsin *et al.*, 2010, 2011) with clinical signs arising from 2–8 years of age. Beagles, Samoyeds, Jack Russell Terriers and Chow Chows are initially able to ambulate but are grossly ataxic. Coton de Tulears, Rhodesian Ridgebacks, Miniature Poodles and Irish Setters are non-ambulatory and exhibit severe motor deficits. Other signs of cerebellar disease that accompany tremor include ataxia, dysmetria, menace deficits, head tilt, nystagmus (deLahunta and Glass, 2008; Lorenz *et al.*, 2011), truncal sway and anisocoria (infrequent). Clinical signs associated with degenerative cerebellar diseases progressively worsen.

Pathogenesis: Primary cerebellar cortical degeneration refers to degeneration and loss of the Purkinje cells, molecular cells and/or granule cells. Scottish Terriers have also been found to have increased polyglucosan bodies in the cerebellum (Urkasemsin *et al.*, 2011). Abiotrophy is a process by which cells develop normally but later degenerate because of an intrinsic cellular defect necessary for continued life of the neuron (deLahunta and Glass, 2008). Many of these diseases may result from underlying abnormalities of cellular metabolism or function and are known to be inherited in the Old English Sheepdog, Gordon Setter and Brittany Spaniel. Recently, a homozygous 8 base pair deletion in a candidate gene previously associated with spinocerebellar ataxia in humans has been identified in Beagles with neonatal cerebellar ataxia. The encoded protein is critical for Purkinje cell development, and its absence can lead to cell damage through excitotoxicity. This explains the observed Purkinje cell neuron loss, degeneration of dendritic processes and associated neurological dysfunction (Beltran *et al.*, 2012). A mutation in a gene important for endoplasmic reticulum-associated protein degradation has been linked to early onset cerebellar degeneration in Finnish Hounds (Kyöstilä *et al.*, 2012). A similar mutation in a gene important for autophagy has been associated with cerebellar degeneration in Gordon Setters and Old English Sheepdogs (Olby, personal communication).

Diagnosis: Antemortem testing for these diseases often results in negative or normal findings. A definitive diagnosis is only possible at necropsy with histopathological examination of the nervous tissue. In some instances of cerebellar atrophy, a smaller than normal cerebellum may be seen on MRI of the intracranial nervous system (Thames *et al.*, 2010) (Figure 13.7). This is most readily seen on a sagittal view. CSF analysis is normal with degenerative cerebellar

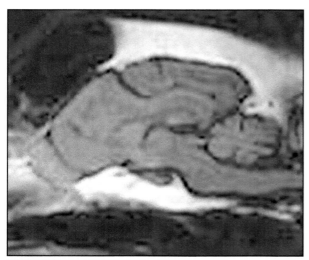

13.7 Sagittal T1-weighted MR image of the brain of a 6-year-old male castrated American Staffordshire Terrier with cortical degeneration. The cerebellar folia are clearly visible as a result of the CSF lying between them, reflecting the cerebellar atrophy. (Courtesy of N Olby)

conditions, but can help rule out inflammatory conditions. Genetic tests are now available for the Finnish Hound, Italian Spinone, Beagle, Old English Sheepdog and Gordon Setter.

Treatment and prognosis: There are no effective treatments for this group of disorders and the prognosis is guarded to grave.

Storage diseases: Storage diseases (Figure 13.8) can result in cerebellar degeneration (March, 1996; Vite and Braund, 2003). Cellular products accumulate and affect neuronal cells either physiologically or mechanically, resulting in cellular dysfunction and the appearance of clinical signs. The clinical signs are of a progressive cerebellar disease, and are most commonly seen in young pure breed dogs. Diagnosis is based upon the examination of biopsy or necropsy samples and/or genetic tests where available (see Chapter 9 for details on diagnosis). No treatment is effective. Breed specificities can be found in Appendix 1.

Storage disease	Subgroup	Enzyme deficiency	Clinical signs
Fucosidosis	Glycoproteinoses	Alpha-L-fucosidase	Progressive motor and mental deterioration from 6–12 months old. Ataxia, hypermetria and proprioceptive deficits at 12–18 months leading to dysphonia, dysphagia, nystagmus and seizures
Galactosialidosis		Beta-galactosidase	Ataxia, dysmetria and intention tremors
Mannosidosis		Alpha-D-mannosidase	Ataxia, dysmetria, intention tremors, skeletal anomalies, neuropathies, corneal opacity and progressive dementia
Mucopolysaccharidosis (MPS) I	Mucopolysaccharidoses	Alpha-L-iduronidase	Stunted, corneal clouding, degenerative disc disease, collapse of disc spaces, vertebral osteoporosis and spondylosis
MPS II		Iduronate-2-sulphate sulphatase	Cerebellar ataxia, exercise intolerance, corneal opacity and facial dysmorphism
MPS III		Sulphamidase	Cerebellar ataxia, tremors, retinal degeneration and corneal opacity
MPS VI		Arylsulphatase B	Growth retardation, facial deformity, corneal opacity and spinal fusion
MPS VII		Beta-D-glucuronidase	Growth retardation, facial deformity, corneal opacity, spinal fusion and paraparesis
Ceroid lipofuscinosis (CLN, Batten disease)	Proteinoses	CLN 1: palitoyl protein thioesterase I CLN 2: tripeptidyl-peptidase CLN 4: arylsulphatase G CLN 5: soluble lysosomal membrane protein CLN 6: endoplasmic reticulum membrane protein CLN 10: cathepsin D	Visual deficits, cerebellar ataxia, myoclonus, seizures and dementia of varying degree

13.8 Lysosomal storage diseases documented in dogs and cats. (continues) ▶

Storage disease	Subgroup	Enzyme deficiency	Clinical signs
Glucocerebrosidosis (Gaucher disease)	Sphingolipidoses	Beta-D-glucocerebrosidase	Cerebellar ataxia
Globoid cell leucodystrophy (Krabbe disease)		Beta-D-glucocerebrosidase galatosylceramidase	Multifocal signs, progressive paraparesis to tetraparesis, cerebellar dysfunction, hyporeflexia and muscle atrophy
GM1 gangliosidosis		Beta-D-galactosidase	Cerebellar ataxia, corneal clouding, tremors, seizures, paralysis, skeletal and facial dysmorphism
GM2 gangliosidosis (B, O, AB, B^{-1})		Beta-N-acetyl-hexosaminidase GM2-AB: GM activator protein deficiency	Cerebellar ataxia
Niemann–Pick disease		Beta-D-galactocerebrosidase; sphingomyelinase	Hyporeflexia to areflexia, fine tremors, hypotonia and plantigrade stance

13.8 (continued) Lysosomal storage diseases documented in dogs and cats.

Neuroaxonal dystrophy:

Clinical signs: This is a disease of Rottweilers (Chrisman, 1986), collies, Chihuahuas, Jack Russell Terriers, Papillons and domestic cats (Diaz *et al.*, 2007; Nibe *et al.*, 2007, 2009, 2010; Fyfe *et al.*, 2010). In Rottweilers, this disease is characterized by cerebellar signs (ataxia, hypermetria, loss of menace reflex and head tremor) with an onset at 1–2 years of age (ataxia) and progressing over the next 2–4 years (menace deficits and intention tremors). Conscious proprioception frequently remains intact.

Pathogenesis: The underlying pathogenesis is unknown. The cell bodies in the grey matter are affected throughout the nervous system (becoming axonal spheroids), except in the cerebral cortex. The most severe lesions are located within the spinocerebellar tracts and the Purkinje cells.

Diagnosis: A definitive diagnosis is usually only achieved post-mortem. Recognition of the characteristic clinical signs in young Rottweilers is suggestive of this disease, but a full diagnostic work-up (imaging and CSF analysis) is needed to rule out treatable diseases (e.g. encephalitis). It is important to note that Rottweilers also suffer from leucoencephalopathy (a neurodegenerative disease), which causes progressive tetraparesis at a young (1–4 years old) age (Chrisman, 1986; Slocombe *et al.*, 1989; Davies and Irwin, 2003). MRI characteristics of this disease have recently been described (Eagleson *et al.*, 2012). Younger Rottweilers (3–8 months old) can develop a disease called neuronal vacuolation, which causes a combination of laryngeal paralysis, progressive tetraparesis and microphthalmia (Kortz *et al.*, 1997). A non-specific diffuse cerebellar atrophy has been documented on MRI in cases with chronic clinical signs (Tamura *et al.*, 2007).

Treatment and prognosis: No treatment is known and the long-term prognosis is poor.

Anomalous diseases

Congenital malformations of the cerebellum are occasionally seen. These include aplasia (absence of cerebellar tissue) and partial agenesis or hypoplasia (partial or uniform lack of cerebellar tissue). Cerebellar hypoplasia has been associated with infection or toxin exposure during a critical stage of cerebellum development *in utero*. Caudal vermian hypoplasia is described in some dogs with associated ventricular dilatation (Dandy–Walker malformation; Figure 13.9) (Kornegay, 1986b). Cerebellar hypoplasia has been recognized in Chow Chows, Irish Setters and Wirehaired Fox Terriers. The latter two breeds may have concurrent lissencephaly.

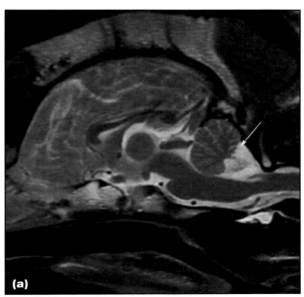

(a)

13.9 **(a)** Sagittal T2-weighted MR image of a Bull Terrier with cerebellar vermal hypoplasia (arrowed). (continues) ▶

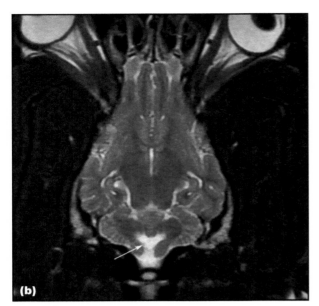

13.9 (continued) **(b)** Dorsal T2-weighted MR image demonstrating replacement of the cerebellum with CSF (arrowed).

Cerebellar aplasia has been reported in Siberian Huskies. Herniation of the cerebellar vermis is a component of Chiari malformations that has been reported in various small-breed dogs, particularly Cavalier King Charles Spaniels (see Chapter 14). However, rarely do cerebellar signs accompany the disease.

Feline cerebellar hypoplasia:

Clinical signs: The clinical signs are most apparent when the cat begins purposeful movement and attempts to walk. Tremors accompanying the disease usually have a slow frequency (2–6 times per second) and a large amplitude. The tremors worsen (increase in frequency or amplitude) when the cat moves in a goal-oriented manner (see **Intention tremor** clip on DVD). Other signs include ataxia, hypermetria, menace deficits, head tilt and nystagmus. Clinical signs usually remain static or improve with growth as the cat compensates, causing the tremor to become less apparent.

Pathogenesis: Feline cerebellar hypoplasia is caused by an *in utero* infection with the panleucopenia virus (parvovirus), which destroys the external germinal layer of the cerebellum and prevents formation of the granular layer (deLahunta and Glass, 2008). Some affected cats have concurrent hydrocephalus and hydranencephaly. Infection of the fetus may occur when a pregnant queen is vaccinated with a modified-live panleucopenia virus vaccination.

Diagnosis: Antemortem testing for this disease often results in negative or normal findings. Occasionally, inflammatory cells may be present in the CSF in cats with active panleucopenia infection. CSF analysis with other degenerative cerebellar conditions and with inactive panleucopenia infection is usually normal. MRI can confirm the presence of a small cerebellum, but this is not specific for this disease.

Treatment and prognosis: There is no treatment for this disorder. Some cases are mild but others can be quite severe (walking and eating may be difficult). As the signs do not progress with time, the prognosis may be fair if the animal is only mildly affected. To help prevent this condition, queens should not be vaccinated with a modified-live panleucopenia virus vaccine.

Neonatal ataxia (Bandera's ataxia) in Coton de Tulear dogs:

Clinical signs: Clinical signs become evident at 2 weeks of age once the puppies start to move around (Coates *et al.*, 2002). Signs include head and intention tremors, severe ataxia and vertical nystagmus. These signs are not progressive but are so severe that most dogs cannot walk and are euthanased.

Pathogenesis: The disease has been mapped to a gene for metabotropic glutamate receptor 1 (*GRM1*) (Zeng *et al.*, 2011), but the mechanism via which dysfunction of this gene causes clinical signs is yet to be elucidated.

Diagnosis: The diagnosis is confirmed by recognition of the clinical signs and ruling out other possible causes. Histopathological findings may be minimal using light microscopy, but electron microscopy reveals synaptic abnormalities.

Treatment and prognosis: There is no effective treatment. Although the disease is not progressive, the clinical signs are so severe that the prognosis is grave.

Neoplastic diseases

Primary or secondary neoplasia involving the cerebellum is uncommon. More common is primary neoplasia of the infratentorial region that may subsequently affect the cerebellum, including meningiomas and choroid plexus tumours. These tumours arise from the meninges and choroid plexus of the fourth ventricle, respectively. Gliomas and medulloblastomas rarely involve the cerebellum in dogs. Other mass lesions such as dermoid and epidermoid cysts may arise within or around the fourth ventricle and compress the cerebellum. Diagnosis is suggested using CT (Figure 13.10) or MRI and confirmed with histopathology.

Inflammatory diseases

The cerebellum can be involved with the same infectious and immune-mediated processes that result in encephalitis (Meric, 1986; Muñana, 1996; Garosi *et al.*, 2010) (see Chapter 11 for a full description of these diseases). The cerebellum may also be affected by inflammation causing generalized tremor syndromes (see below) that have been called idiopathic cerebellitis by some authors. No definitive cause for this inflammation has been elucidated in many cases.

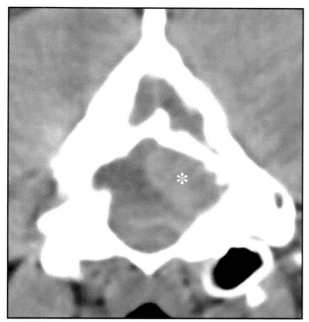

13.10 Transverse contrast-enhanced CT image of the caudal fossa in a neutered 10-year-old Boxer bitch. There is a contrast-enhancing mass (✱) compressing the dorsal cerebellum. The mass was removed surgically and confirmed to be a meningioma.

Presumed immune-mediated cerebellar granulo-prival degeneration in the Coton de Tulear breed:

Clinical signs: In this unusual disease of male Coton de Tulear dogs, the onset of progressive cerebellar signs was noted at 8 weeks of age (Tipold *et al.*, 2000).

Pathogenesis: Clusters of T lymphocytes are identified in the cerebellar cortex leading to the suggestion that this disease results from a genetically determined immune reaction against the granule cells.

Diagnosis: The diagnosis is obtained by the histopathological examination of the brain post-mortem.

Treatment and prognosis: No treatment has been reported.

Toxic diseases
With the exception of metronidazole, toxicity rarely specifically affects the cerebellum, but cerebellar dysfunction may be part of the clinical syndrome of many toxin exposures.

Metronidazole toxicity: Metronidazole toxicity may result in central vestibular and cerebellar signs in both dogs and cats (see Chapter 11). Generally, this is associated with relatively high doses of the drug. However, as metronidazole is metabolized by the liver, toxic serum concentrations can occur with appropriate doses in animals with liver dysfunction. Ataxia is usually the initial clinical sign, progressing to nystagmus and more severe vestibular and cerebellar dysfunction. Clinical signs

often reflect central vestibular dysfunction and morphological lesions have been found in the brainstem of affected animals.

Vascular diseases
Thromboembolic and vascular disease can involve the cerebellum (Bagley *et al.*, 1988; Berg and Joseph, 2003; McConnell *et al.*, 2005) (Figure 13.11). Clinical signs often occur acutely and rarely cause tremors alone. See Chapter 9 for more details of vascular disease.

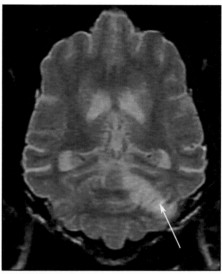

13.11 Dorsal T2-weighted MR image of a Springer Spaniel with acute onset of cerebellar dysfunction. A well delineated hyperintensity (arrowed) is visible in the lateral hemisphere, which is compatible with ischaemic infarction.

Generalized tremor syndromes

Generalized tremors are surprisingly common in dogs (Farrow, 1986; Bagley, 1992; Bagley *et al.*, 1993; Wagner *et al.*, 1997). These types of tremors can result secondary to intoxication, drug therapy, congenital myelin abnormalities, storage diseases and encephalitis, or may arise without a definable cause.

Degenerative diseases

Lysosomal storage diseases
Lysosomal storage diseases of the nervous system may have tremor as a presenting abnormality (Braund, 1987; March, 1996) (see Figure 13.8). These include:

- Globoid cell leucodystrophy
- Neuronal ceroid leucodystrophy in cats
- Mannosidosis
- Gangliosidosis.

Clinical signs: These diseases are often breed-related (see Appendix 1) with clinical signs occurring in animals <1 year old, but they can occur at any age. Many of these diseases involve the cerebellum, and the resulting tremor is more characteristic of cerebellar disease.

Pathogenesis: The accumulation of metabolic by-products within neurons or the surrounding neuropil usually results from an inherited deficiency of a specific catabolic enzyme. The accumulation causes dysfunction of the cells and regions of the nervous system affected.

Diagnosis: Antemortem testing for many of these diseases often results in negative or normal findings. CSF analysis is normal. Advanced imaging may reveal signs of symmetrical, anatomically defined, pathology but the characteristics are non-specific. A definitive diagnosis is often only achieved at necropsy with histopathological examination of the nervous tissue. However, there are specific blood and urine tests for many of these diseases, which can be performed at specialist laboratories. For information on these tests, the reader is referred to Appendix 1.

Treatment and prognosis: Typically, there is no effective treatment for affected animals and clinical signs associated with degenerative diseases progressively worsen. Animals are commonly euthanased due to the progressive incapacitation.

Motor neuronopathies

Motor neuronopathies are degenerative diseases that affect the cell bodies of the LMN, leading to degeneration of the cell in the ventral horn of the spinal cord and occasionally the CN nuclei (Olby, 2004). This is an inherited condition in the Brittany Spaniel and Swedish Lapland Dog but also occurs in the pointers, Cairn Terrier, Rottweiler, German Shepherd Dog, Briquet Griffon Vendeen and giant cross-breeds. Several cats have been reported with a motor neuronopathy that can appear in adulthood (Shelton *et al.*, 1998). Histopathological examination reveals that lesions are most severe in the ventral spinal grey matter and consist of neuronal cell loss and gliosis. Signs of motor neuronopathies include tremor, progressive weakness, cervical ventroflexion, dysphagia and muscle atrophy (Shelton *et al.*, 1998). In some cases, mild to moderate fibrillation potentials may be found in the appendicular and paraspinal muscles on electromyography. CSF analysis is normal, as are imaging studies. There is no known treatment.

Feline encephalomyelopathy

Encephalomyelopathy of young cats has been reported in the UK (Palmer and Cavanagh, 1995). Wallerian degeneration, primarily involving the spinocerebellar pathways and ventral funiculus of the spinal cord, was noted. A viral aetiology was suggested but not proven. Cats aged from 3 to 12 months were affected; however, the disease was seen in cats up to 3 years old. The clinical signs were usually progressive over weeks to months and included ataxia, paresis and head shaking. Ataxia of the pelvic limbs was the initial clinical sign noted. Currently, the commonality of this condition is unknown.

Anomalous diseases

Dysmyelination and hypomyelination

In this group of diseases, the axons within the CNS may be thinly myelinated (hypomyelination), myelinated with abnormal myelin (dysmyelination) or unmyelinated.

Clinical signs: Many breeds of dog are affected by this group of congenital disorders of myelination including the Chow Chow, Springer Spaniel, Samoyed, Bernese Mountain Dog and Weimaraner (Millán *et al.*, 2010). Signs are usually evident as soon as the animal starts to walk. Tremors in these animals affect the whole body and are classed as action tremors as they are usually worse with excitement or movement and stop during sleep. Some affected animals appear as though they are 'bouncing'. In some breeds with dysmyelination, such as Chow Chows, signs slowly dissipate over the first year of life and dogs are normal by 12–18 months of age.

Pathogenesis: Abnormal myelination of the CNS can affect nerve impulse conduction and cause tremors (Duncan, 1987; deLahunta and Glass, 2008). It is possible that altered impulse conduction or spontaneous discharge of non-myelinated axons (e.g. as a result of increased extracellular potassium concentrations) may generate the tremor. The degree of tremor correlates with the severity of the myelin abnormality. The underlying cause of most of these syndromes is unknown but as these diseases are believed to be inherited, a genetic defect of myelination is suspected (Duncan, 1987). In Springer Spaniels it has been confirmed as a recessive X-linked condition due to a point mutation in the proteolipid (*PLP*) gene (Nadon *et al.*, 1990).

Diagnosis: A definitive diagnosis is only reached by histopathological evaluation of the CNS. The classic presentation in young dogs of the correct breeds is very suggestive. However, infectious, inflammatory, systemic and toxic diseases should be ruled out.

Treatment and prognosis: There is no known treatment for this group of diseases. In breeds with dysmyelination, improvement occurs with age and the tremor may resolve when the animal becomes an adult and the myelin sheaths reach normal thickness.

Metabolic diseases

Changes in the metabolic environment may result in alterations of the muscle and nerve membrane resting potentials with subsequent spontaneous depolarization. Electrolyte (hypocalcaemia, hypercalcaemia, hyponatraemia and hypernatraemia), glucose and acid–base imbalances are the most common metabolic abnormalities resulting in tremor. Tremors and fasciculation with metabolic conditions tend to be episodic and irregular in frequency. In addition, they are also more common with hypocalcaemia than hypercalcaemia.

Hypocalcaemia

Clinical signs: The clinical signs include weakness, tetany and tremors. Spontaneous muscle depolarization can manifest as muscle fasciculation, cramping, rigidity and twitching. Signs can progress to include focal (e.g. ears or facial muscles) or generalized muscle tremors, seizures, weakness or ataxia.

Pathogenesis: Hypocalcaemia often results from iatrogenic injury to the parathyroid gland during the surgical removal of thyroid tumours (especially in cats) but can also be associated with lactation (eclampsia; most commonly seen in dogs). Primary hypoparathyroidism is rare (Forbes *et al.*, 1990; Peterson *et al.*, 1991; Russell *et al.*, 2006). Hypocalcaemia decreases the threshold for neuronal and muscle depolarization due to alterations in sodium flux and membrane potentials (Peterson *et al.*, 1991; Feldman and Nelson, 1996; Schaer, 2008).

Diagnosis: The diagnosis is supported by finding a decreased (usually <1.5 mmol/l (6 mg/dl)) serum ionized calcium concentration on biochemical analysis, in conjunction with the presence of calcium and phosphate in the urine (Schenck and Chew, 2008).

Treatment and prognosis: Treatment involves calcium supplementation and vitamin D therapy. If clinical signs are present, rapid institution of treatment is indicated with 0.5–1.5 ml/kg i.v. of 10% calcium gluconate. Intravenous calcium should be administered slowly over 10 minutes while monitoring heart rate. The infusion should be stopped if bradycardia occurs. Longer term maintenance requires oral calcium (25 mg/kg q8–12h) and vitamin D supplementation. The active form of endogenous vitamin D3 (calcitrol or 1,25 dihydroxycolecalciferol) can be given at a dose of 2.5–10 ng/kg orally q24h or alternatively, synthetic vitamin D3 (dihydrotachysterol) can be given at a dose of 0.02–0.03 mg/kg orally q24h for 3 days and then 0.01–0.02 mg/kg orally q6–24h.

Serum calcium concentrations should be monitored carefully as hypercalcaemia is nephrotoxic. Adjustments to the dose should be made every 1–3 days based on calcium concentrations. If hypocalcaemia is the result of thyroidectomy, calcium and vitamin D therapy can be reduced gradually over 2–3 weeks, and stopped if calcium levels remain within the reference range. Acute hypocalcaemia following bilateral thyroidectomy can be fatal if it is not recognized early and appropriate treatment initiated.

Hyponatraemia and hypernatraemia

Sodium salts represent the major osmotically active solutes in the body. Clinical hyponatraemia is synonymous with hypo-osmolality and hypernatraemia is commonly associated with hyperosmolality. Neurological signs usually include changes in the animal's level of awareness and seizure activity but can also include tremors.

Hepatic encephalopathy

Liver dysfunction affecting the nervous system more often results in changes in mentation and seizures than tremors, but these may occur in association with cerebral signs of disease.

Hypoglycaemia

Hypoglycaemia is more likely to cause changes in mentation, stupor, coma or seizures than tremors, but should always be considered as part of the differential diagnosis. This is particularly relevant in dogs with insulinomas associated with a paraneoplastic peripheral neuropathy (Madarame *et al.*, 2009).

Neoplasia

Neoplastic disease of any area of the nervous system has the potential to cause tremors usually, but not always, in the presence of more specific signs referable to the location of the tumour.

Inflammatory diseases

Generalized tremors without other definable systemic causes are most often secondary to inflammatory CNS disease (Farrow, 1986; Bagley, 1992; Bagley *et al.*, 1993; Wagner *et al.*, 1997).

Generalized tremor syndrome of dogs

Clinical signs: This idiopathic condition was historically identified in small-breed (<15 kg) dogs with white hair coats (e.g. Maltese dogs), hence these dogs were described as 'white shakers'. However, dogs with various other hair coat colours may be similarly affected and thus the term 'generalized tremor syndrome' is often used to describe the disease. Miniature Pinschers appear to be predisposed to this condition. Affected dogs are usually <2 years old when the generalized tremors begin. Early in the course of the disease, owners may interpret the tremor as the animal being 'scared' or 'cold'. When the tremors become more persistent, owners may elect veterinary evaluation.

The tremors in these dogs usually occur multiple times per second and are not associated with large to-and-fro movements (see **Generalized tremor** clip on DVD). This low amplitude, relatively rapid tremor is sometimes described as 'fine'. Tremors tend to worsen with excitement and improve with sleep. However, the author [RB] has evaluated two dogs with generalized tremors when awake that had a persistent thoracic limb myoclonus whilst under general anaesthesia. Other clinical signs may suggest a diffuse CNS problem. These include menace deficits, hypermetria, ataxia, nystagmus, conscious proprioception deficits and seizures.

Pathogenesis: Generalized tremor syndrome is often associated with a mild degree of CNS inflammation. Histological examination may reveal a mild, non-suppurative meningoencephalomyelitis, but in some cases no pathological changes in the CNS are evident.

Diagnosis: CSF analysis usually reveals a mild increase in nucleated cell counts and a mild to normal protein content. No obvious infectious or immune aetiology for the encephalitis has been identified.

Treatment and prognosis: Clinical signs usually respond to corticosteroids (prednisolone at a dose of 1–2 mg/kg orally q12h). This dose is administered for 1–2 weeks or until the clinical signs have resolved. Following resolution of the clinical signs, the corticosteroid dosage can be slowly decreased (over weeks to months) to prevent recurrence. Too rapid a reduction in the corticosteroid dose can result in the recurrence of clinical signs. The disease in some dogs only remains in remission with continual corticosteroid administration (as with other autoimmune diseases). Some dogs never show 100% improvement and some relapse at the end of steroid treatment or with dose reduction; relapse has been reported to be associated with vaccination in some dogs, but repeat treatment has been documented as effective. Other drugs prescribed in humans such as propranolol (0.5–1.0 mg/kg orally q8h), diazepam (0.5–1 mg/kg orally q8h) and phenobarbital (2–4 mg/kg orally q12h) have been used too infrequently to assess the therapeutic response or are not effective at controlling generalized tremors in dogs.

Feline encephalomyelitis
Encephalomyelitis is a more infrequent cause of tremors in cats compared with dogs.

Clinical signs: Cats of any age can be affected. Diffuse, whole body, low amplitude (fine), high frequency tremors are present. Cats may also twitch periodically. Other neurological signs that may be present in cats with encephalomyelitis include seizures, blindness, conscious proprioceptive deficits and CN deficits. Neurological signs may not be localized to a single area within the nervous system.

Pathogenesis: As for dogs, there may be an unknown or poorly defined cause of CNS inflammation which results in tremors. The underlying pathogenesis of these generalized tremors is poorly understood.

Diagnosis: CSF analysis may reveal increased numbers of nucleated cells (reference range = <2–5 cells/µl; mild inflammation = 5–20 cells/µl; severe inflammation = >50 cells/µl) and/or elevated protein concentrations. The nucleated cell type is variable, but most often it is a mononuclear cell population. Neutrophils may also be seen. This syndrome is associated with histological evidence of inflammation of the CNS. However, a consistent infectious aetiology has not been identified.

Treatment and prognosis: Treatment with corticosteroids (prednisolone at a dose of 2 mg/kg orally q12h initially) may improve clinical signs. If clinical signs improve, corticosteroid therapy should be slowly tapered (over months) to prevent recurrence. Poor response or relapse may be frequent.

Polioencephalomyelitis
Young to middle-aged cats have been diagnosed with tremors due to polioencephalomyelitis (Vandevelde and Braund, 1979). Currently, the commonality and geographical spread of this disease is unknown.

Clinical signs: Affected cats have slow onset, chronically progressive clinical signs including pelvic limb ataxia, seizures, paresis, hypermetria, intention tremors, decreased pupillary light reflexes and hyperaesthesia over the thoracolumbar area. Seizures are characterized by staring, clawing, biting and hissing, and may be noted during sleep.

Pathogenesis: Lesions primarily occur within the spinal cord and include severe degeneration and loss of neurons, perivascular mononuclear cuffing, lymphocytic meningitis, neuronophagia and glial nodules. A viral aetiology has been suggested but not proven.

Diagnosis: CSF analysis may reveal an elevated protein content but any changes in cell count or protein levels are non-specific. MRI may reveal a non-specific pattern of multifocal inflammatory change. Definitive diagnosis is often only made at necropsy. Histological examination can determine the type and severity of the lesion.

Treatment and prognosis: No treatment is known or has been attempted. Animals are usually euthanased due to the progressive nature of the clinical signs.

Feline spongiform encephalopathy
A spongiform encephalopathy has been reported in older cats in Europe and it is thought that a prion may be the cause (Leggett *et al.*, 1990; Kelly *et al.*, 2005; Lulini *et al.*, 2008; Hilbe *et al.*, 2009). Clinical signs include muscle tremors, ataxia, dilated unresponsive pupils, jaw champing, salivation and behavioural abnormalities. This condition is now considered rare.

Idiopathic diseases

Essential and geriatric tremors
Physiological and essential tremors are most common in humans. Essential tremors are considered exaggerated forms of physiological tremors, and when they occur in later life they are termed senile tremors. Some older dogs exhibit a fine tremor of the pelvic limbs as they age and the condition can be slowly progressive. It is a posture-related tremor and as such is only present when the dog is standing. There is no effect on strength or gait in these dogs and no pain is detected. No treatment is necessary unless symptomatic therapy is required to improve the perceived quality of life (see above).

Toxic disorders
Some acute toxicities may result in generalized tremors (Dorman, 1993; Dorman and Fikes, 1993).

Pathogenesis

Tremor is possible with multiple intoxications, including organophosphates, permethrins, hexachlorophene and bromethalin (Segev *et al.*, 2006; Boland and Angles, 2010). Metaldehyde and strychnine usually cause tetany and seizures, but tremors may also be seen. Mycotoxins such as penitrem-A have been associated with tremors in dogs (Wagner *et al.*, 1997; Boysen *et al.*, 2002; Eriksen *et al.*, 2010). Avermectin toxicosis has resulted in generalized ataxia, tremor, weakness, incoordination and miosis in dogs and cats (Snowden *et al.*, 2006). Other toxicities that result in nervous system stimulation (such as chocolate, amphetamines and caffeine) may have tremors as an associated clinical sign.

The mechanism responsible for generating the tremor with many of these toxic substances is not known. Toxins may lower the threshold for stimulation or directly stimulate muscles and nerves, resulting in tremor. Organophosphate intoxication potentiates the effect of acetylcholine at the neuromuscular junction and other synapses by binding with and inactivating acetylcholinesterase. This leads to increased acetylcholine concentrations at the neuromuscular junction, increased receptor stimulation and fatigue. Hexachlorophene causes vacuolation of the white matter. Pathological alterations in the nervous system (such as intramyelinic oedema caused by hexachlorophene and bromethalin) could potentially alter nerve impulse conduction, leading to tremors. Other substances most likely result in imbalances in neurotransmitter concentrations. Avermectins increase the concentration and effect of gamma-aminobutyric acid (GABA, inhibitory neurotransmitter) in the CNS. Numerous drug therapies (e.g. fentanyl/droperidol, adrenaline (epinephrine), isoproterenol and 5-fluorouracil) may cause tremors as a side-effect, possibly through alterations in the normal function of the extrapyramidal system or in the balance of normal neurotransmitter levels (Bagley, 1992).

Diagnosis

History of exposure to a toxic product is most helpful in establishing a diagnosis. Specific blood testing may be possible in these cases. With organophosphate toxicity, a decreased concentration of serum cholinesterase (<50% of normal) may lend support to the diagnosis. Depending on the laboratory, a concentration <500 IU/l (reference range = 900–1200 IU/l) is considered consistent with organophosphate toxicity.

Treatment and prognosis

For organophosphate toxicity causing neuromuscular signs (nicotinic overstimulation), treatment includes protopam or pralidoxime chloride at a dose of 10–20 mg/kg i.m. q12h, which reactivates cholinesterase, and diphenhydramine at a dose of 1–2 mg/kg orally q8–12h, which reduces muscle fasciculation. This treatment should be continued until clinical signs are abolished or additional benefit is no longer observed. However, it should be noted that enzyme reactivators may not be effective beyond 24 hours following exposure as they are only helpful if covalent binding of the insecticide and acetylcholinesterase has not yet occurred.

For cases of acute toxicity, atropine sulphate (0.2–0.4 mg/kg i.v., i.m. q4–6h) can be administered to decrease muscarinic autonomic signs, but this will not abolish the muscle tremors due to the excessive nicotinic stimulation. Current recommendations are that atropine should only be used if marked bradycardia is present because it may precipitate respiratory arrest. Salivation and defecation are not life-threatening and generally do not require atropine. Diazepam should be avoided in cats with organophosphate toxicity as it may result in generalized muscle tremors, hypersalivation, miotic pupils and vomiting, similar to the acute muscarinic signs of organophosphate toxicosis (Jaggy and Oliver, 1990). It is important to avoid further exposure to organophosphate toxicity until the animal has clinically recovered. No specific antidote exists for the other toxicities described here, but general supportive measures for toxin exposure should be provided. Prognosis is variable depending on the specific toxin (Hovda and Hooser, 2002).

Specific paroxysmal disorders

Head bobbing

Vertical (up and down nodding) and lateral (side to side shaking) plane head tremors have been noted in dogs (see **Idiopathic head tremor** clip on DVD). It has been suggested that thalamic lesions could be the cause of this movement disorder (see above). However, frequently no underlying cause can be determined and this condition is currently considered idiopathic in Boxers, Bulldogs and Dobermanns.

Neuromyotonia

This condition can result in paroxysmal collapse associated with rigidity and myokymia. Neuromyotonia is well described in Jack Russell Terriers (see above).

Feline hyperaesthesia syndrome

Clinical signs

Feline hyperaesthesia syndrome is a unique disease that may result in episodic behavioural twitching and fasciculation (deLahunta and Glass, 2008). Cats may become agitated and aggressive, and exhibit skin rippling and muscle spasms, usually over the lumbar area, in response to stimulation (e.g. stroking) of the thoracolumbar region. Cats may appear as though they have been startled and demonstrate frenzied behaviour such as licking or biting of the flanks, back and tail, or running (see **Feline hyperaesthesia syndrome** clip on DVD). Cats may appear as if they are hallucinating and have dilated pupils. Sudden startling, running, frantic meowing, growling, hissing and swishing of the tail may also occur. Episodes may occur multiple times a day and last between 1 and 5 minutes.

Pathogenesis

The cause of this syndrome is unknown. One theory suggests that it is a manifestation of a focal seizure; another suggests that it is similar to the obsessive–compulsive behaviour associated with Tourette's syndrome in humans, which is the result of dopaminergic hyperinnervation. Similar clinical signs have been associated with toxoplasmosis and vacuolar myopathy in cats. Some have suggested that this may be a primary behavioural disorder; whilst others believe that it begins with an inflammatory stimulus such as flea or food allergy dermatitis.

Diagnosis

The diagnosis is usually made based on the clinical signs and by ruling out underlying diseases such as dermatitis, lumbosacral spinal or nerve root compression, and intracranial disease. It is also important to determine whether the cat is exhibiting normal behaviour during oestrus.

Treatment and prognosis

Initial treatment should be with anti-inflammatory drugs. Corticosteroid therapy (prednisolone) may help if a flea allergy or other inflammatory stimulus is suspected. Non-steroidal anti-inflammatory drugs (NSAIDs) such as meloxicam and piroxicam, or megoestrol acetate can also be tried. Strict flea control may improve clinical signs. Behaviour-modifying drugs, such as the tricyclic antidepressants amitriptyline (2 mg/kg or 5–10 mg/cat orally q24h) and clomipramine (1–5 mg/cat orally q12–24h) or the selective serotonin uptake inhibitors fluoxetine (0.5–4 mg/cat orally q24h) and paroxetine (0.5 mg/kg orally q24h), may be helpful in some cats.

Anticonvulsants, such as phenobarbital (initially 3 mg/kg orally q12h followed by dose adjustments to maintain trough serum levels at 20–40 µg/ml), gabapentin, pregabalin and levetiracetam, may be helpful if anti-inflammatory and behaviour-modifying drugs are unsuccessful, but may sedate the cat. Feeding foods without preservatives has also been suggested. Carnitine/co-enzyme Q10 can help cats with vacuolar myopathy, and antioxidants and omega-3 fatty acids may also be useful (see Chapter 18). In addition, decreasing environmental stress may be important. The prognosis depends on the identification of the underlying disease and the initial response to medication, as well as the frequency and severity of the events.

Reflex myoclonus

Clinical signs

This rare disease is characterized by episodic, stimulation-evoked, extensor rigidity of the body. It has been suggested that rather than myoclonus, this condition should be considered a form of myotonia, although no muscle dimpling can be elicited. However, it is probable that this disorder is actually a type of dyskinesia. Reflex myoclonus has been reported in Labrador Retrievers (Fox *et al.*, 1984; March *et al.*, 1993) with onset of progressive signs at approximately 12 weeks. Affected animals become stiff, usually when excited or stimulated, and the signs become so severe that the animal is unable to walk or even stand. Other breeds (e.g. Dalmatians) are occasionally affected.

Pathogenesis

This condition appears to be a familial disorder in Labrador Retrievers. The pathogenesis is unknown, but it has been suggested that there is a loss of inhibitory neurotransmission at the level of the spinal cord.

Diagnosis

The diagnosis is confirmed by recognition of the typical clinical signs and electromyography. The EMG reveals bursts of giant polyphasic motor units.

Treatment and prognosis

Although the extensor rigidity is partially responsive to diazepam and phenobarbital, resolution of signs is unlikely and the prognosis is poor. As this may be a form of myotonia, the use of drugs such as procainamide should be considered.

Breed-related disorders

Scotty cramp

Clinical signs: Clinical episodes of dystonia are most commonly seen in Scottish Terriers from 6 weeks to 3 years of age and may be elicited by stress, excitement or exercise. The thoracic limbs are initially affected, becoming abducted shortly after the initiation of exercise (see **Scotty cramp** clip on DVD). This is followed by arching of the lumbar spine and pelvic limb stiffness, which can progress to somersaults, falling and tightly flexed pelvic limbs. Loss of consciousness is not a feature and clinical signs resolve within 10 minutes, but can recur multiple times in a 24-hour period. Similar conditions have been described in Dalmatians, Cocker Spaniels, Wirehaired Terriers, Wheaton Terriers, Norwich Terriers and Border Terriers. In Border Terriers, the disease has been termed 'spikes' disease or canine epileptoid cramping syndrome (CECS) (see **Canine epileptoid cramping syndrome** clip on DVD).

Pathophysiology: This recessive, inherited, non-progressive disorder is thought to be associated with relative deficiencies of the inhibitory neurotransmitter 5-hydroxytryptamine (serotonin) (Meyers *et al.*, 1973).

Diagnosis: A presumptive diagnosis is based on clinical signs and breed. All laboratory tests are within normal limits. Signs can be induced with exercise 2 hours after the administration of methylsergide at a dose of 0.3 mg/kg orally (a serotonin antagonist).

Treatment and prognosis: Treatment consists of daily oral dosing with acepromazine maleate (0.1–0.75 mg/kg q12h) or diazepam (0.5 mg/kg q8h).

Vitamin E (125 IU/kg q24h) has also been advised for these dogs. Serotonin reuptake inhibitors such as fluoxetine may be useful in affected dogs. NSAIDs are contraindicated. Prognosis is fair as the disease is non-progressive and appropriate lifestyle changes can result in a good quality of life. With CECS, dietary modification to provide hypoallergenic foods has been suggested, but no evidence exists for this at the current time.

Episodic hypertonicity in Cavalier King Charles Spaniels

This condition, also known as episodic falling syndrome in Cavalier King Charles Spaniels, has been described in the UK, USA and Australia, and is suspected to have an inherited component. The genetic locus for this condition has recently been mapped to canine chromosome 7 with approximately 13% of the breed suggested to be carriers for the disease (Gill *et al.*, 2011).

Clinical signs: This syndrome is often seen in animals between 3 and 7 months of age but can affect animals up to 4 years old. Variable periods of exercise induce a bounding pelvic limb gait in which the limbs may be abducted and appear stiff. The may progress to 'bunny-hopping', arching of the spine and collapse (see **Episodic hypertonicity** clip on DVD). As with Scotty cramp, the animals are normal between events, there is no loss of consciousness and the events may be triggered by exercise, stress and excitement.

Pathophysiology: Recent work has identified a genetic deletion in the *BCAN* gene, which codes for the protein brevican, in affected dogs and confirmed the disease as autosomal recessive (Forman *et al.*, 2012; Gill *et al.*, 2012). Brevican belongs to a family of aggregating extracellular matrix proteoglycans where it has a role in governing synapse stability. It is highly expressed in the CNS.

Diagnosis: Laboratory tests and electrodiagnostic examinations are normal. Thus, diagnosis is by exclusion of other conditions and correlation with an appropriate history and clinical signs.

Treatment and prognosis: Treatment with the benzodiazepine clonazepam (0.5 mg/kg orally q8h) can result in almost complete remission of the signs but tolerance to this drug does develop. The carbonic anhydrase inhibitor acetazolamide may also have a therapeutic benefit in these dogs.

Startle disease in Irish Wolfhounds

Hyperekplexia or startle disease is characterized by noise- or touch-induced non-epileptic seizures that result in muscle stiffness and apnoea in humans. Defective inhibitory glycinergic transmission due to genetic mutations affecting the glycine receptor is usually the cause. It has been suggested that the familial reflex myoclonus in Labrador Retrievers could be a glycinergic transmission disorder and represent a startle disorder. A

startle disease has recently been documented in Irish Wolfhounds in the USA with a microdeletion in the gene encoding a presynaptic glycine transporter (Gill *et al.*, 2011). The condition was seen to develop in 5–7-day-old puppies, evoked by handling and abating when relaxed or sleeping. The affected puppies could not stand and had a rigid posture in all four limbs with generalized tremor. Progressive feeding difficulty was noted and euthanasia was performed by 3 months of age. Carriers of this disease can now be identified.

Generalized muscle stiffness in male Labrador Retrievers

Young male Labrador Retrievers have been described with a paroxysmal generalized rigidity of CNS origin.

Clinical signs: Clinical signs have been seen to arise between 2 and 41 months of age, with a mean age of onset of 17 months (Vanhaesebrouck *et al.*, 2011). The clinical signs stabilize in adulthood. The disease appears to initially affect the pelvic limbs and then progresses to the thoracic limbs, causing the dog to be presented for exercise intolerance (see **Paroxysmal generalized rigidity** clip on DVD). Affected dogs seem to exhibit generalized muscle stiffness, persisting at rest and resulting in restricted joint movements. These animals have a flexed posture and bradykinesia (extremely slow movements and reflexes).

Pathophysiology: Currently, it is thought that this condition arises from basal nuclei and reticular formation abnormalities together with motor neuron dysinhibition caused by a decrease in the number of spinal cord interneurons. Initial pedigree analysis suggests an X-linked hereditary disease.

Diagnosis: The EMG shows continuous motor unit activity in the proximal limb and epaxial muscles, whilst the dogs are standing or in lateral recumbency (Vanhaesebrouck et al., 2011). Serum creatine kinase levels are normal as is the complete blood count, serum chemistry and CSF analysis. Thus, diagnosis is by exclusion of other conditions and correlation with an appropriate history and clinical signs.

Treatment and prognosis: A poor quality of life can lead to requests for euthanasia. Clinical signs can progress but have been seen to stabilize. Treatment with NSAIDs has been shown to provide partial and temporary improvement in some dogs. No specific and uniformly successful treatment is known.

Paroxysmal dyskinesia in Chinooks

A paroxysmal dyskinesia has been described in related Chinooks and is characterized by an inability to stand or ambulate, head tremors and involuntary flexion of one or multiple limbs, without autonomic signs or loss of consciousness (Packer *et al.*, 2010) (see **Paroxysmal dyskinesia** clip on DVD). Episode duration varies from minutes to an hour. Based on pedigree analysis, the disorder is considered to be consistent with a partially penetrant autosomal recessive or polygenic trait. There has been some consideration given as to whether this disorder is an atypical seizure episode but the same can be said for any of the aforementioned dyskinesias.

Lafora disease (myoclonic epilepsy) in Miniature Wirehaired Dachshunds

Familial myoclonic epilepsy with similarities to Lafora disease in humans has been reported in several Miniature Wirehaired Dachshunds (Webb *et al.*, 2009).

Clinical signs: Presenting clinical signs include repetitive muscle contractions (twitching), seizures and jerks in response to visual, auditory or sensory stimuli. Age of onset ranges from 6 to 13 years, and both males and females are affected.

Pathophysiology: An expanded repeat genetic mutation of the *EPM2B* genes that code for the protein malin has been reported in Miniature Wirehaired Dachshunds and Bassett Hounds with Lafora disease (Lohi *et al.*, 2005). Malin is an important enzyme in ubiquitination (ubiquitin ligase), the system by which proteins are recycled.

Diagnosis: Neurological examination and routine laboratory and CSF evaluations are within the normal range. MRI may reveal generalized ventricular dilatation and cortical atrophy, but these are not specific findings. EEG activity in dogs with Lafora disease is characterized by bilateral synchronous polyspike wave paroxysms. The presence of intense periodic acid–Schiff positive, diastase-resistant inclusions (polyglycosan bodies, Lafora bodies) in fresh-frozen muscle biopsy specimens may aid in establishing the diagnosis in cases with a consistent clinical phenotype. Some laboratories and human hospitals test for the *EPM2B* mutation (Webb *et al.*, 2009).

Treatment and prognosis: Phenobarbital therapy at standard anticonvulsant doses may result in some clinical improvement of the seizure activity, but has not been completely successful in the author's [SP] experience. Equivocal efficacy has also been reported with the use of gabapentin and potassium bromide. A diet high in antioxidants has been shown to slow the progression of the clinical signs. The prognosis depends on the frequency and severity of the events and how these affect the quality of life of the dog. Similar pathology has been described in older Beagles and Bassett Hounds.

Dancing Dobermann disease

A condition causing intermittent flexion of one or both pelvic limbs has been reported in Dobermanns (Chrisman, 1990) (see **Dancing Dobermann** clip on DVD). Muscle atrophy, weakness and postural reaction deficits may be seen in chronic cases. The gastrocnemius muscle appears to be the primary focus of the disease with EMG detectable changes including positive sharps, fibrillation potentials and complex repetitive discharges. The underlying cause is not known, but sciatic–tibial nerve biopsy samples may reveal axonal disease, which can be primary or secondary in origin.

Sleep disorders

Narcolepsy–cataplexy

Narcolepsy is a disorder of sleep/wake control characterized by a tendency to fall asleep during the day, disturbed night-time sleep patterns and cataplexy (Dauvilliers *et al.*, 2007; Nishino, 2007; Tonokura *et al.*, 2007). Cataplexy refers to sudden loss of motor tone, ranging in severity from a dropped jaw to complete collapse without loss of consciousness, and represents a disorder of rapid eye movement (REM) sleep. Narcolepsy has been reported in many canine breeds, including Dobermanns, Labrador Retrievers, Miniature Poodles, Beagles and Dachshunds.

Clinical signs: The predominant sign in dogs and cats is cataplexy, but excessive daytime sleepiness and fragmented sleep patterns have also been reported. Cataplexy is characterized by paroxysmal attacks of flaccid paralysis without loss of consciousness and may last up to 20 minutes, with a sudden return to normality (see **Narcolepsy–cataplexy** clip on DVD). The event is not accompanied by faecal or urinary incontinence, salivation or rigidity of muscle groups. These episodes, which may occur multiple times per day, are frequently induced by excitement such as eating or playing and can be reversed by verbal or tactile stimuli. Cataplexy has been recorded in puppies and adult dogs, but usually begins within the first 6 months following birth with the establishment of REM sleep.

Pathophysiology: The pathogenesis of this disorder remains uncertain; however, an imbalance between the cholinergic and catecholaminergic neurotransmitter systems within the CNS appears to be involved. Studies point to hypocretins (orexins) as important sleep-modulating neurotransmitters (Lin *et al.*, 1999; Wu *et al.*, 2002, 2011; Mishima *et al.*, 2008; Kroeger and de Lecea, 2009). The hypocretins are two novel hypothalamic neuropeptides (Hcrt-1 and Hcrt-2), derived from the same precursor gene, which are synthesized by hypothalamic neurons. Hypocretin secretion increases during wakeful states and decreases during sleep. Defects in hypocretin neurotransmission and hypocretin deficiency appear to play an important role in narcolepsy (Lindberg *et al.*, 2007).

Inherited forms of canine narcolepsy have a hypocretin receptor abnormality and sporadic forms have decreased hypocretin concentrations in the CSF (Tonakura *et al.*, 2003; John *et al.*, 2004). In addition, autoimmunity is considered by some researchers to play a role in the development of narcolepsy, in view of the rarity of hypocretin receptor mutations in humans and a genetic link to a human leucocyte antigen (HLA) locus. However, such an association has not been found in dogs and immunosuppressive treatment is not effective. Autosomal recessive inheritance with full penetrance has been established in both Dobermanns and Labrador Retrievers and is linked to a region of chromosome 12 termed the *canarc-1* gene. Subsequent studies have shown that there are mutations in the hypocretin receptor-2 (*Hcrt-2*) gene in this region (Lin *et al.*, 1999). Dogs with the inherited form have normal hypocretin concentrations within the CSF. A familial form exists in the Dachshund.

Diagnosis: The diagnosis is based on typical clinical signs, although routine CSF analysis to determine hypocretin levels may become available in the future. Episodes can be induced in most affected animals by exercise or eating. Signs can be alleviated for up to 45 minutes with imipramine (0.5 mg/kg i.v.). Atropine sulphate (0.1 mg/kg i.v.) is also reported to be a useful diagnostic test, providing immediate temporary remission of signs for up to 3 hours.

Treatment and prognosis: The disease may not be progressive with respect to frequency or severity of the events, but it can obviously affect the quality of life of the animal. Long-term treatment with tricyclic antidepressants such as imipramine hydrochloride (0.5–1.5 mg/kg orally q8–12h) and desipramine (3 mg/kg orally q12h) has been recommended based on their ability to inhibit noradrenaline (norepinephrine) reuptake in the brain. Methylphenidate hydrochloride has also been described as effective at a dose of 0.25 mg/kg orally q12–24h (Mignot, 2004). Venlafaxine has recently been reported as a potential treatment for narcolepsy in dogs (Delucchi *et al.*, 2010). Hypocretin replacement therapy has been attempted but without much success at this time (Fujiki *et al.*, 2003; Schatzberg *et al.*, 2004; Brisbare-Roch *et al.*, 2007).

REM sleep disorders
Normal sleep is divided into two stages: non-REM and REM (Schubert *et al.*, 2011). Non-REM sleep is the first stage of sleep and lasts about 20 minutes. During non-REM sleep there is a decrease in body temperature, heart rate and respiratory rate, and

animals are immobile but retain muscle tone. REM sleep lasts approximately 15 minutes during which time there is an increase in body temperature, heart rate and respiratory rate coincident with eye movements and atonia of the postural muscles (Lorenz *et al.*, 2011). Normal movements seen during this phase can include twitching of the eyelids, face, larynx and paws with occasional rhythmic paddling of all four limbs and yelping.

Clinical signs: REM sleep behavioural disorders have been documented in dogs (Bush *et al.*, 2004; Schubert *et al.*, 2011). Almost 30% of dogs in one study were Golden Retrievers. The episodes were predominately seen in young dogs (64% were <1 year old) but affected animals may be aged between 2 months and 7.5 years. Violent limb movements, howling, barking, growling, chewing or biting during sleep is seen in most affected dogs (see **REM sleep disorder** clip on DVD). Most dogs can be easily aroused and when awake are completely alert.

Pathophysiology: The cerebral cortex is highly active during REM sleep and if the cells of the ventral horn of the LMN in the brainstem and spinal cord are not inhibited (as normally occurs), uncontrolled limb movements are seen (Boeve *et al.*, 2007). Normally, the pons and medulla control this inhibition and disease of any of these structures could result in REM sleep abnormalities.

Diagnosis: The diagnosis can be made based on the clinical signs, but confirmation depends on EMG and EEG studies during the event, which is logistically difficult in veterinary medicine.

Treatment and prognosis: Treatment with oral potassium bromide at a dose of 40 mg/kg q24h reduced the severity and frequency of events in nearly 80% of dogs. Phenobarbital appears to have a minimal effect on this disorder in dogs, but tricyclic antidepressants such as amitriptyline may be helpful. Spontaneous recovery has not been reported.

References and further reading

Available on accompanying DVD

DVD extras
- Canine epileptoid cramping syndrome
- Dancing Dobermann
- Dyskinesia
- Episodic hypertonicity
- Feline hyperaesthesia syndrome
- Focal motor seizure
- Generalized tremor
- Idiopathic head tremor
- Intention tremor
- Myoclonus (1)
- Myoclonus (2)
- Myokymia and neuromyotonia
- Narcolepsy–cataplexy
- Orthostatic tremor
- Paroxysmal dyskinesia
- Paroxysmal generalized rigidity
- REM sleep disorder
- Scotty cramp

14

Neck and back pain

Simon Platt and A. Courtenay Freeman

Many diseases encountered in veterinary medicine cause spinal pain, including multiple neurological diseases and non-neurological conditions such as polyarthritis. Lesion localization is very important in cases of spinal pain, in order to ensure that the correct diagnostic tests are performed. The results of these tests should be interpreted in conjunction with the neurological examination findings. Treatment of spinal pain must address both the underlying disease and the alleviation of discomfort (see Chapter 21).

Terminology

- Allodynia – a condition in which pain arises from a stimulus that would not normally be experienced as painful or that is not noxious (e.g. light touch of the skin).
- Anaesthesia – complete loss of all forms of sensation.
- Dysthesia – impairment of sensation, especially of the sense of touch. It also describes an unpleasant sensation produced by ordinary stimuli.
- Hyperaesthesia – increased sensitivity to a normal level of stimulation, which is seen in the behavioural reaction of the animal (e.g. palpation of the spine during a physical examination).
- Hyperpathia – behavioural response to an injurious or noxious stimulation.
- Hypoaesthesia – diminution of sensation.
- Neuropathic pain – this results from central nervous system (CNS) or peripheral nervous system (PNS) disease or injury. It occurs from direct stimulation of (somatosensory) nervous tissue and is generally felt as burning or tingling in humans. It is often present in an area of sensory loss.
- Pain – this is a perception, rather than a quantifiable entity, which results from a noxious stimulus.
- Paraesthesia – altered sensation often described in humans as burning, tingling or pin pricks. It is often suggested to be a sensory pathway disease.

These conditions are difficult to objectively define in animals and thus are subjectively assumed to be present or inferred based on behavioural responses to touch and palpation as well as the presence of self-mutilation.

Clinical signs

Recognition of the signs of spinal pain in animals can be made difficult by the variable reaction to pain seen between individuals. Some animals may give no outward indication that they are in pain, but there are several clinical signs that may be present which are useful for determining the presence of neck and back pain (Figure 14.1). Neck pain can be intermittent because of the dynamic nature of the cervical spine. In these cases, an accurate history in addition to video recordings of the episodes (see **Behavioural response** clip on DVD) can be very helpful.

- Decreased general activity levels
- Depressed mentation
- Change in normal attitude (e.g. aggression or withdrawal) and unexplained vocalization
- Ventroflexion of the neck
- Stiff neck posture
- Increased cervical muscle tone
- Intermittent jerks/spasms of the neck related to movement
- Pain on palpation of cervical vertebrae and musculature
- Pain on dorsal and lateral flexion of the cervical vertebrae
- Gait abnormality – thoracic limb lameness (nerve root signature); stilted; stiff limbs; paresis if concurrent spinal cord disease
- Historical reluctance to go up and down stairs, climb into a vehicle or on to the furniture, or jump up
- Historical observation of difficulty to get into resting position; may seem restless
- Autonomic signs such as salivation, increased respiratory and heart rates, and pupillary dilatation
- Unwilling or unable to drink/eat from bowls on the floor

14.1 Clinical signs associated with neck or back pain.

Lesion localization

Possible structural origins of pain are shown in Figure 14.2. Spinal pain may result from disease of any of the numerous structures in the vertebral column, including:

- The meninges over the spinal cord and nerve roots
- The nerve roots themselves
- The annulus of the intervertebral discs
- Vertebral periosteum
- Joint capsules (especially those of the diarthrodial joints of the articular process)
- The epaxial musculature
- The ligamentous structures surrounding the vertebrae.

It should also be noted that intracranial disease may cause a 'referred' type of neck pain in circumstances or diseases which result in elevated intracranial pressure (ICP) as a result of compression

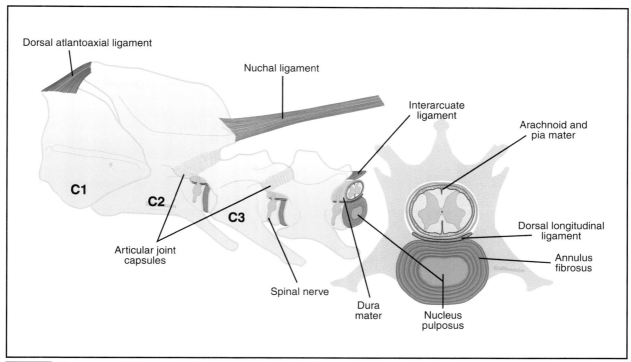

14.2 There are multiple origins of spinal pain, including ligaments, bone, nerve roots and spinal nerves, meninges, disc material and articular joints.

or stretching of the cerebral vasculature and meninges, which are densely innervated with nociceptors. In addition, neck pain can occur due to Chiari-like malformations of the skull, leading to the formation of a syrinx in the cervical spinal cord.

Localization of painful areas is accomplished by a combination of historical evidence, observation (Figure 14.3; see also **Behavioural response** clip on DVD), palpation and manipulation. After determining whether any clinical signs (see Figure 14.1) are present, the clinician must systematically palpate the animal, paying special attention to the appendicular muscle bellies and appendicular joints. It is usually best to start caudally and work cranially to

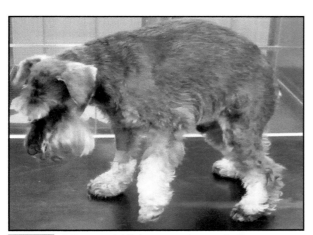

14.3 A 9-year-old Schnauzer demonstrating severe neck pain with a stiff and flexed neck posture accompanied by poor weight bearing on the left thoracic limb, sometimes referred to as 'nerve root signature'.

localize the pain. The vertebral column is palpated by pressing on the spinous processes or squeezing the articular or transverse processes, depending on the size and temperament of the animal (Figure 14.4a). Evaluation of the neck should also include cautious flexion, extension and lateral turning of the head and neck with the palm of the hand placed on the side of the neck to evaluate any resistance to movement (see **Flexion and extension of neck** clip on DVD). This can also be assessed by tempting the animal with a piece of food held in the hand and moved from side to side to monitor voluntary movement. If possible, the pain should be localized to the cranial, middle or caudal cervical segments.

When palpating the thoracolumbar spine to rule out diffuse spinal pain, a hand should be placed on the abdomen to detect increased tension in the muscles as painful areas are approached (Figure 14.4b). Pressing on the ribs may also be helpful in detecting thoracic vertebral pain. A few animals will be in so much pain that localization is impossible. Palpation of the head, temporal muscles and mandible, and opening the mouth are important in assessing the cranial structures (see Chapter 1), and manipulation of the tail and the hips are important in assessing the lumbar and lumbosacral structures (see Chapter 19). Some clinicians prefer to evaluate the lumbosacral spine when the animal is in lateral recumbency, so the transference of pressure to the hips is reduced. Dorsiflexion of the tail may exacerbate lumbosacral joint pain by 'tipping' the craniodorsal aspect of the sacrum forwards and forcing any associated soft tissue proliferation to compress the nervous structures.

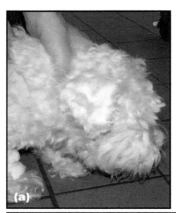

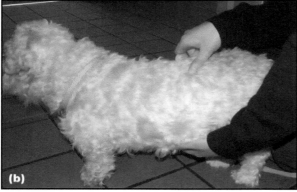

14.4 Vertebral palpation. **(a)** Palpation of the cervical vertebrae can be accomplished with one hand in small dogs. Pain may be exhibited by an increase in muscle tone associated with palpation, vocalization or a caudal 'flicking' of the ears. **(b)** Palpation of the thoracolumbar vertebrae should be performed with one hand underneath the abdomen of the patient, so as to detect any increase in muscle tone in this region. Pain may also be noted as vocalization or the animal turning toward the examiner.

Pathophysiology

Pain receptors (nociceptors) are free nerve endings that are especially numerous in the superficial layers of the skin, periosteum, arterial walls, joint capsules, muscles, tendons and meninges. Five types of nociceptors exist in the tissues:

- Mechanical – those responding to excessive mechanical stress
- Thermal – those responding to heat or cold
- Chemical – those responding to stimulatory chemicals, including bradykinin, serotonin, histamine, potassium ions and acids, as well as prostaglandins, leucotrienes and proteolytic enzymes released in various quantities during inflammation
- Polymodal – those responding to more than one class of stimulus
- Sleeping – those responding only in conditions of tissue injury or inflammation.

Nociceptors do not 'adapt' to the initial stimulus. They discharge continuously in the face of a persistent stimulus and are capable of responding to

repeated stimuli. The sensation of pain is transmitted centrally by small type A-delta myelinated fibres at a rate of 6–30 m/s (perceived as a sharp or pricking sensation) and by type C unmyelinated fibres at a rate of 0.5–2.0 m/s (perceived as a slow burning sensation). Both types of pain can be felt simultaneously. The conscious recognition of these sensations is due to their transmission up the multisynaptic and bilateral spinothalamic and spinoreticular tracts. These tracts pass to the brainstem reticular system with ongoing pathways to the thalamus, hypothalamus and several cortical areas of the brain, which reinforce the 'emotional' aspects of pain based on studies performed in humans.

Our current understanding of the various neurotransmitters released at different sites in the neuronal pathways mediating pain sensation (Figure 14.5), can be summarized as follows:

- The neurotransmitters released in the dorsal horn of the spinal cord, at the terminals of the central processes of the first order nociceptive neurons (located in the dorsal root ganglia), are believed to be glutamate and substance P. These neurotransmitters primarily excite second order spinothalamic dorsal horn neurons, the axons of which travel cranially in the spinothalamic tracts projecting cranially to the nuclei in the thalamus
- There are systems in place to modulate nociception. Opiate receptors are present on the terminals of the central processes of the first order nociceptive dorsal root ganglion neurons (presynaptic opiate receptors) and on the dendrites of the second order spinothalamic neurons (postsynaptic opiate receptors). The encephalinergic interneurons in the dorsal horn of the spinal cord (Figure 14.5) are activated by serotonergic projections from the medullary nucleus raphe magnus and by pontine locus ceruleus noradrenergic neurons. Encephalin released from the terminals of the encephalinergic dorsal horn interneurons acts on the opiate receptors located on the central processes of the nociceptive neurons within the dorsal root ganglia, to reduce calcium entry into the terminal and decrease the concentration of neurotransmitters (glutamate and/or substance P) released. Encephalin released from the terminals of these dorsal horn interneurons also activates the postsynaptic opiate receptors on the dendrites of the second order spinothalamic neurons, resulting in hyperpolarization by increasing potassium conductance, and inhibition. These actions of encephalin attenuate the effects of nociceptive stimuli. Thus, stimulation of descending serotonergic and noradrenergic projections to the dorsal horn causes the release of encephalin, which inhibits second order spinothalamic neurons by presynaptic and postsynaptic mechanisms.

Tissue damage or inflammation produces pain through stimulation of mechanosensitive, thermo-

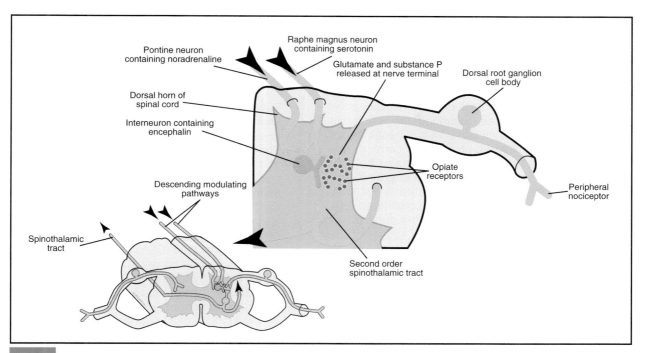

14.5 Neuroanatomy of the spinal cord dorsal horn associated with pain transmission and modulation.

sensitive and chemosensitive nociceptors. The presence and intensity of pain are dependent on two variables:

- The presence of nociceptors (it should be noted that the CNS does not have nociceptors, so damage to grey and white matter is not painful if other structures are not involved)
- The density of nociceptors (e.g. the meninges have a high density of nociceptors and are a source of spinal pain).

Occasionally, damage to the CNS can produce pain indirectly as a result of muscle spasm, which stimulates mechanosensitive nociceptors, and so pain relief must be directed toward muscle relaxation. Unlike back pain, neck pain can commonly be present in the absence of any neurological signs. It has been suggested that this may be due to a lower spinal cord-to-vertebral canal diameter ratio, which allows for space-occupying lesions to irritate the meninges and nerve roots without compressing them (Drost *et al.*, 2002). However, magnetic resonance imaging (MRI) reveals that there are minimal differences in the spinal cord-to-vertebral canal diameter ratio along the length of the spine (Figure 14.6). In the lumbosacral spine there is a relatively large epidural space, allowing the nerves or cauda equina in this region to avoid compressive lesions (Figure 14.6). The nerve roots, however, do not have a lot of space as they pass through the intervertebral foramen, meaning that small lesions causing foraminal stenosis can cause marked discomfort. There is a difference between dog breeds, with small breeds having a higher cervical cord-to-canal ratio than large breeds, meaning that smaller breeds are more likely to have concurrent neurological signs and neck pain (Fourie and Kirberger, 1999).

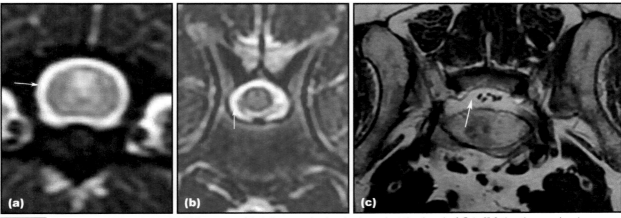

14.6 Transverse T2-weighted MR images of **(a)** the cervical spinal cord at the level of C4, **(b)** the thoracolumbar spine at the level of L3 and **(c)** the cauda equina. The size of the respective epidural spaces can be estimated based upon the presence of hyperintense fat (arrowed).

Differential diagnosis

The diseases that frequently cause spinal pain are listed in Figure 14.7. Many of these conditions are discussed in other chapters, as they often cause neurological signs in addition to pain. There are several notable exceptions, including meningitis, polyarthritis and polymyositis, although the latter two disorders may be associated with a weak flexor withdrawal reflex due to physical discomfort and weakness. These two conditions may also be difficult to evaluate for the 'true' absence of proprioceptive deficits due to the associated weakness. Intracranial disease should also be considered as a cause of cervical pain, especially in the presence of a compatible history and clinical signs.

Disease process	Specific diseases
Degenerative	Calcinosis circumscripta [15] Disc disease (Hansen types I and II) [15, 16] Wobbler syndrome [15] Spondylosis deformans [14] Synovial cysts [15]
Anomalous	Atlantoaxial instability [15] Intra-arachnoid cysts [15] Chiari-like malformations Dermoid sinus [16] Osteochondromatosis [16] Perineurial (Tarlov) cysts [14] Scoliosis/vertebral anomalies [16] Syringo(hydro)myelia [14]
Neoplastic	Extradural [16]: metastasis; vertebral tumours (sarcomas, plasma cell tumours); lymphoma Intradural/extramedullary: meningiomas [16]; nerve sheath tumours [17]; metastasis [16] Intramedullary [16]: ependymomas; gliomas; metastasis; round cell tumours Brain tumours: primary or secondary with increased ICP [9]
Nutritional	Hypervitaminosis A [14]
Inflammatory	Infectious meningitis/meningomyelitis [11] Steroid-responsive meningitis–arteritis [14] Granulomatous meningoencephalomyelitis [11] Discospondylitis/osteomyelitis [14]; physitis [16] Empyema [16] Polyarthritis Polymyositis [18]
Trauma	Fractures/luxations [15, 16, 20] Spinal cord contusions [14, 20] Traumatic disc herniations [15]
Vascular	Spinal haemorrhage [14]

14.7 Causes of neck and back pain. Numbers in brackets refer to the chapters in which diseases are discussed further.

Neurodiagnostic investigation

The approach and subsequent tests required to 'work-up' the patient with spinal pain depend on the history, clinical signs, physical and neurological examinations and the lesion or system localization. A general algorithm is shown in Figure 14.8. Polymyopathies, polyarthritides and soft tissue abnormalities, in addition to neurological disease, all need to be considered as causes of spinal pain. Certain diagnostic tests are appropriate in cases with spinal pain:

- For all cases, initial clinicopathological tests should include haematology, serum biochemistry (including creatine kinase) and urinalysis
- Thoracic radiographs should be obtained as part of the minimum database in dogs and cats with spinal pain. This is particularly useful in older animals and in those with suspected cardiorespiratory disease
- Survey spinal radiography is essential if a neurological disease is suspected
- Cerebrospinal fluid (CSF) collection and analysis is essential when survey radiographs are normal to rule out meningitis (see Chapter 3)
- Myelography, plain and contrast-enhanced computed tomography (CT) or MRI are often necessary to evaluate patients with spinal pain if the above tests do not establish a diagnosis, especially if surgery is a consideration
- Muscle disease requires systemic investigation: electrophysiological testing and muscle biopsy may be needed to determine the underlying aetiology (see Chapters 4, 6 and 18). MRI can be useful to target pathological areas for muscle biopsy
- Joint disease should be investigated with the aid of survey radiographs and arthrocentesis, in conjunction with an evaluation for systemic and infectious diseases. A joint capsule biopsy can be of assistance in some cases.

Degenerative diseases

Intervertebral disc disease
Spinal cord compression secondary to intervertebral disc protrusion or extrusion is one of the most common clinical neurological disorders. Protrusion describes a disc that is 'bulging' into the vertebral canal, whereas extrusion describes a situation where the central nuclear material of the disc has ruptured through the dorsal fibrous structures into the vertebral canal. Acute (type I) cervical disc herniations commonly cause pain, which may manifest as a 'nerve root signature', without obvious neurological deficits; the severity of the pain may be such that surgery is required. Although acute non-compressive nucleus pulposus extrusions (high velocity, low volume disc extrusion) can result in hyperpathia, affected dogs exhibit neurological dysfunction secondary to the spinal cord concussion. The pathophysiology, diagnosis and treatment of disc disease are discussed in Chapters 15 and 16.

Cervical spondylomyelopathy (Wobbler syndrome)
Cervical spondylomyelopathy, also termed cervical stenotic myelopathy, cervical spondylopathy, cervical spondylolisthesis, cervical malformation/malarticulation

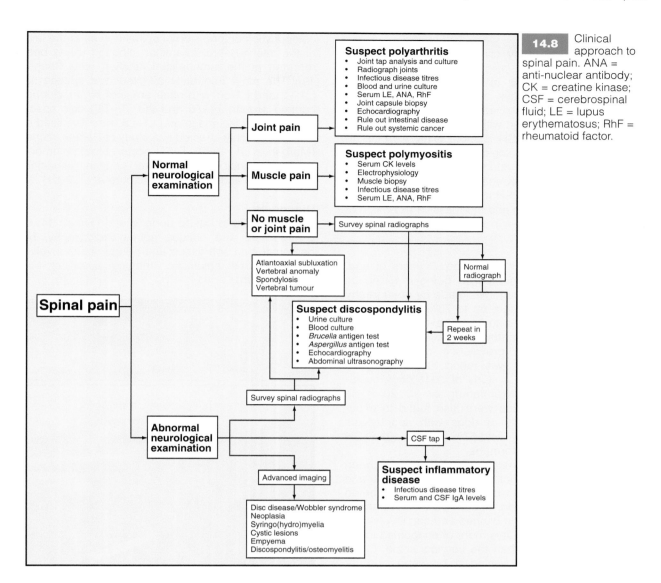

14.8 Clinical approach to spinal pain. ANA = anti-nuclear antibody; CK = creatine kinase; CSF = cerebrospinal fluid; LE = lupus erythematosus; RhF = rheumatoid factor.

and disc-associated Wobbler disease, most commonly affects Dobermanns and Great Danes, but many other breeds have been recognized with similar abnormalities such as the Bernese Mountain Dog, Weimaraner and Dalmatian. The age of onset of the disease is variable, ranging from 3 months to 9 years; the mean age for Dobermanns is 6.8 years and for all large breeds is 7.9 years. Neck pain may be the only clinical sign; however, pelvic limb ataxia, pelvic limb paresis and ambulatory tetraparesis are commonly associated with the discomfort. For a complete discussion of the pathophysiology, diagnosis and treatment of this disease, the reader is directed to Chapter 15.

Spinal synovial cysts

Extradural spinal (juxtafacet) synovial cysts, originating from articular facet joint capsules, that cause compression of the spinal cord have been described in dogs. They are most commonly found in the cervical vertebrae, especially in giant-breed dogs with cervical spondylomyelopathy (Levitski *et al.*, 1999; Dickinson *et al.*, 2001; Sale and Smith, 2007), but can occur in the lumbosacral spinal canal (Forterre *et al.*, 2006). Ganglion cysts are also classified as extradural synovial cysts, but histologically do not have a synovium-like lining of epithelial cells. These cysts are thought to result from mucinous degeneration of articular cartilage. All reported dogs with cervical extradural synovial cysts had cervical pain, but pain does not appear to be common with thoracolumbar cysts. Further information can be found in Chapters 15 and 16.

Spondylosis deformans

Spondylosis deformans is a degenerative, non-inflammatory, proliferative disease associated with the cartilaginous joints of the vertebral column. It is characterized by the presence of vertebral osteophytes at the intervertebral disc spaces, resulting in the formation of spurs or complete bony ridges. A similar but more severe condition called ankylosing hyperostosis or diffuse idiopathic skeletal hyperostosis (DISH) can also occur in dogs. DISH affects both the axial and appendicular skeleton, resulting in ossification of the soft tissues including the ventral longitudinal ligament and other attachments to bone. The new bone formation (enthesiophyte) that affects the ventral longitudinal ligament continues ventrally for at least four vertebral bodies.

Clinical signs

The condition is rarely clinical, although stiffness, restricted motion and pain might be attributed to spondylosis deformans in a small percentage of patients. It is imperative that all other causes of spinal pain should be ruled out before spondylosis is definitively associated with the signs. Unlike spondylosis deformans, DISH is more likely to result in stiffness, pain, neurological and/or orthopaedic abnormalities, with one study reporting clinical signs in a third of patients (Kranenburg *et al.*, 2011). The pain associated with DISH may be due to the involvement of the periosteum and the massive extension of the ossification into the surrounding soft tissues.

Pathogenesis

This disease occurs in dogs from 2 years of age, with 18–33% of the population being reported as affected based on a diagnosis made by radiography alone. By 9 years of age, up to 75% of dogs have spondylosis deformans to some extent based on necropsy studies (Romatowsky, 1986; Levine *et al.*, 2006). Recently, the prevalence of spondylosis deformans and DISH was found to be 18% and 3.8%, respectively, in a study of 2041 dogs evaluated retrospectively (Kranenburg *et al.*, 2011). In addition, these diseases were also found to occur concurrently, with 14% of dogs with spondylosis deformans having DISH and 67% of dogs with DISH having spondylosis deformans.

Spondylosis deformans and DISH have been reported with a high incidence in Boxers (55% and 40%, respectively), in which they may be inherited conditions. In this breed, spondylosis deformans is more commonly seen in bitches and can involve the whole spine; although, it is more often located in the thoracolumbar spine than the cervical spine. Other breeds suspected of having a predisposition for developing spondylosis deformans include the German Shepherd Dog, Cocker Spaniel, Flat-Coated Retriever and Airedale Terrier.

Trauma, degenerative disc disease and intervertebral disc fenestration have all been associated with the formation of spondylosis deformans; however, it may also occur in the absence of these conditions. Dogs with type II disc disease have a greater number of affected sites and more severe changes compared with dogs that have type I disc herniation, which is not thought to be associated with spondylosis deformans (Levine *et al.*, 2006). In general, the spatial relationship between sites of spondylosis and those of disc disease is currently thought to be coincidental or associated with vertebral column biomechanics.

Osteophyte formation is thought to be initiated by abnormalities at the site of attachment of peripheral annular fibres to the vertebral endplate. Weakened disc to endplate attachments lead to annular tears and result in small ventral or ventrolateral disc herniations (Levine *et al.*, 2006). The combination of annular tearing and small volume disc herniation is probably the cause of spondylosis. Osteophytic projections into the spinal canal causing compression of the spinal cord are rare, as is

osteophytic compression of spinal nerves at the level of the intervertebral foramina, although it has been reported at the lumbosacral junction (see Chapter 19). The most frequently affected disc spaces are L2–L3 and L7–S1 with other areas of high incidence centred around T4–T6 and the T9–T10 disc space. The C6–C7 disc space and L1–L6 were identified as being commonly affected in a study of Beagle bitches (Morgan *et al.*, 1989). DISH occurs most commonly in the thoracolumbar vertebral column, especially from T6–T10 and L2–L6 (Kranenburg *et al.*, 2011).

Diagnosis

The diagnosis is based upon lateral (Figure 14.9a) ventrodorsal and oblique spinal radiography, but demonstrating soft tissue and neural tissue involvement requires advanced imaging such as MRI (Figure 14.9b).

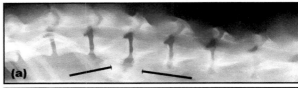

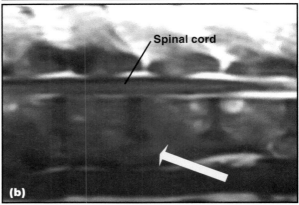

14.9 Spondylosis in a 7-year-old Golden Retriever. **(a)** Lateral radiograph showing marked ventral vertebral body spondylosis (arrowed). Other causes of back pain should be investigated as this osseous proliferation rarely causes neural tissue compression. **(b)** Sagittal T2-weighted MR image showing spondylosis (arrowed) but there is no evidence of cord compression.

Treatment and prognosis

Treatment relies on analgesia (if needed) and surgical decompression (but this is rarely required). Non-steroidal anti-inflammatory drugs (NSAIDs) and weight reduction are used for conservative management of DISH in humans; however, this has not been evaluated in dogs. Surgical decompression of DISH may be required in cases refractory to conservative management or with neurological deficits as compression of the spinal cord and nerves may be more likely.

Dural ossification

Dural ossification is a degenerative condition of dogs of unknown aetiology, characterized by deposition of bone plaques on the inner surface of the dura mater (Figure 14.10). These plaques occur

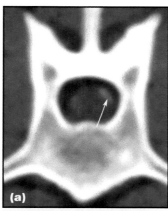

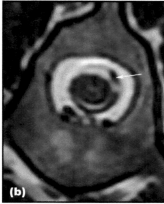

14.10
(a) Transverse CT image of the lumbar spine of a dog with dural ossification (arrowed). **(b)** T2-weighted MR image of the same spinal region. The dural ossification is represented as a signal void (arrowed).

most commonly in the cervical and lumbar regions of the spine and are common incidental findings on radiographic and CT studies of the spine (Jones and Inzana, 2000). Although clinical disease has been documented due to associated spinal cord compression (Wilson *et al.*, 1975), this should primarily be regarded as an incidental finding.

Calcinosis circumscripta
Calcinosis circumscripta is an uncommon syndrome of ectopic idiopathic, dystrophic, metastatic or iatrogenic mineralization characterized by deposition of calcium salts in the soft tissues. Sometimes called tumoral calcinosis, calcinosis circumscripta has been reported to cause spinal cord compression in several breeds of dog (Bernese Mountain Dogs, German Shepherd Dogs, English Springer Spaniels, Rottweilers and Great Danes) with many animals <1 year old and most <4 years old at the onset of clinical signs (Tafti *et al.*, 2005). Compressive disease is usually localized dorsally at the atlantoaxial articulation (Lewis and Kelly, 1990). Further information is available in Chapter 15.

Anomalous diseases

Atlantoaxial instability
Atlantoaxial instability can lead to subluxation of the first and second cervical vertebrae; the cranial aspect of the axis often rotates dorsally with respect to the atlas, into the vertebral canal. Subsequent spinal cord compression results in a variety of neurological

signs, but may just cause cervical pain. The pathogenesis, diagnosis and treatment of this disease are discussed in Chapter 15.

Atlanto-occipital overlapping
A decreased distance between the dorsal arch of the atlas and the supraoccipital bone is seen in some toy and small-breed dogs with congenital atlanto-occipital overlapping. The rostral aspect of the atlas can be located ventral to the foramen magnum or within the caudal fossa, resulting in compression of the cerebellum and obliteration of the cisterna magna. There is no evident vertebral malformation and the atlanto-occipital bones are not fused. However, atlanto-occipital overlapping can be accompanied by other abnormalities such as Chiari-like malformation and occipital dysplasia (Cerda-Gonzalez and Dewey, 2010). A study of 274 dogs with Chiari-like malformations confirmed the presence of atlanto-occipital overlapping in 28% of cases (Marino *et al.*, 2012).

Clinical signs consist of head and neck pain, and cervical myelopathy. Advanced imaging is necessary to diagnose the abnormality. MRI can be used to identify overlapping of the dorsal arch of the atlas with the supraoccipital bone, along with any accompanying nervous tissue compression and/or abnormality (Cerda-Gonzalez *et al.*, 2009b) (Figure 14.11). Medical management, similar to that for Chiari-like malformations, can help to control the neck and head pain. However, surgical stabilization may be necessary in some cases.

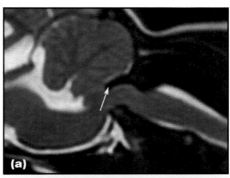

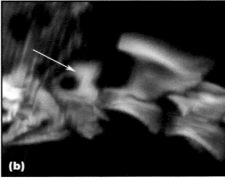

14.11 **(a)** Sagittal T2-weighted MR image of a dog with atlanto-occipital overlapping. The dorsal arch of C1 can be seen extending into the foramen (arrowed). **(b)** 3D reconstructed CT image demonstrating the relationship between the dorsal arch of C1 (arrowed) and the foramen magnum. (Courtesy of Drs S Cerda-Gonzalez and C Dewey)

Intra-arachnoid cysts

Intra-arachnoid cysts (also called subarachnoid cysts, meningeal cysts, leptomeningeal cysts and arachnoid diverticula) are developmental abnormalities that have been documented in dogs (Rylander *et al.*, 2002; Skeen *et al.*, 2003) and, less commonly, cats. Spinal pain is a rare feature of this disease. Further information on this disease is provided in Chapter 15.

Chiari-like malformation and syringomyelia

Chiari-like malformation (also known as caudal occipital malformation syndrome) and syringomyelia often occur together, although both conditions may also occur independently. Chiari-like malformation is defined as a decreased caudal fossa volume, due to congenital hypoplasia of the supraoccipital bone, with herniation of the cerebellum into or through the foramen magnum (Cappello and Rusbridge, 2007). The cerebellum can also be 'indented' by the osseous malformation, a feature which can exist without cerebellar herniation. Other concurrent structural abnormalities include obliteration of the dorsal subarachnoid space, 'kinking' of the medulla and compression of the craniocervical dural/fibrous band (Figure 14.12). A recent study identified medullary kinking in 68% and dorsal compression in 38% of dogs with Chiari-like malformations (Marino *et al.*, 2012). In humans, a similar condition is referred to as Chiari malformation and has several documented types. Human Chiari type I malformations are most similar to those seen in dogs and are characterized by the elongation and caudal displacement of the cerebellar tonsils (vermis and paravermal lobes) through the foramen magnum into the cranial cervical vertebral canal.

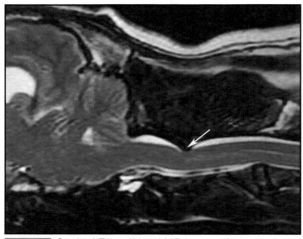

14.12 Sagittal T2-weighted MR image of the caudal skull and cranial cervical spine of a dog with a Chiari-like malformation. Note the dorsal compressive soft tissue lesion (arrowed) at the level of C1–C2.

Syringomyelia is a condition characterized by the presence of a fluid-filled cavity (syrinx) or cavities within the parenchyma of the spinal cord. Syringomyelia occurs secondary to abnormal CSF movement and is usually associated with Chiari-like malformation, although may also be seen with trauma, inflammation and neoplasia. The CSF, which normally flows through the foramen magnum during systole, becomes turbulent as laminar flow is interrupted by the obstruction at the craniocervical junction due to the Chiari-like malformation. The altered fluid flow in the subarachnoid space leads to fluid accumulation within the spinal cord.

Clinical signs

Chiari-like malformation and syringomyelia are most common in toy and small-breed dogs, particularly Cavalier King Charles Spaniels and Brussels Griffons (Rusbridge *et al.*, 2005, 2009). The onset of clinical signs may be acute or chronic in dogs aged between 6 months and 10 years old, but no sex predisposition has been identified. Clinical signs in dogs with Chiari-like malformations alone are usually related to neuropathic pain syndromes. In the presence of syringomyelia, neuropathic pain syndromes and neurological deficits related to spinal cord destruction can present variably. The most common sign of Chiari-like malformation and syringomyelia is pain, predominantly isolated to the cervical region, and this has been reported to occur in 35% of affected dogs and 80% of humans with a similar condition (Todor *et al.*, 2000; Rusbridge *et al.*, 2007).

Dogs may vocalize spontaneously without apparent stimulation or when the neck or shoulders are touched. Sensory abnormalities, including rubbing the face, chewing the feet and intolerance to neck collars or touch, have been described in some dogs and are particularly evident during times of stress or excitement. 'Phantom scratching', where dogs attempt to scratch often without making contact with their skin, is the most notable manifestation of these neuropathic pain abnormalities and has been described in affected dogs ranging from an infrequent to a near constant problem (see '**Phantom scratching**' clip on DVD). Other clinical signs include scoliosis and neurological deficits relating to cervical spinal cord dysfunction. Tetraparesis, sensory ataxia and abnormal proprioceptive positioning in all limbs have been noted in dogs with Chiari-like malformation and syringomyelia, but are uncommon. Intracranial signs, such as facial paresis and vestibular dysfunction, have also been reported.

However, some dogs may be completely asymptomatic with Chiari-like malformation and syringomyelia. Syringomyelia can be present in up to 44% of clinically normal Cavalier King Charles Spaniels (Couturier *et al.*, 2008; Cerda-Gonzalez *et al.*, 2009a) and in 24% of clinically normal Brussels Griffons (Freeman *et al.*, 2011).

Pathogenesis

In Cavalier King Charles Spaniels, Chiari-like malformations and syringomyelia are hereditary conditions, suggested to be autosomal recessive with incomplete penetrance (Rusbridge and Knowler, 2003; Rusbridge *et al.*, 2005; Lewis *et al.*, 2009). Chiari-like malformations are caused by congenital hypoplasia of the supraoccipital bone, resulting in overcrowding of the structures within the caudal fossa. From the results of one study, it appears that Cavalier King Charles Spaniels may actually have a caudal fossa suitable for the size of dog but have too much parenchyma compared with other similar sized breeds (Cerda-Gonzalez *et al.*, 2009a). As a result, the cerebellum herniates into or through the foramen magnum, the medulla becomes kinked and the dorsal subarachnoid space at the craniocervical junction is obstructed. This leads to the disruption of CSF flow through the foramen magnum. The pathogenesis of syringomyelia appears to be multifactorial as its dorsoventral size and sagittal extent do not correlate well with a single morphological abnormality (Shaw *et al.*, 2012).

Pain associated with Chiari-like malformations alone may be secondary to compression of the brainstem or first cervical nerve (Todor *et al.*, 2000; Taylor and Larkins, 2002). With syringomyelia, syrinx width (as measured on MRI) has been reported to be the strongest predictor of pain, with a wide syrinx being significantly associated with discomfort (Rusbridge *et al.*, 2007). In this study, >95% of dogs with a syrinx >6.4 mm demonstrated clinical signs. The location of the syrinx within the dorsal aspect of the spinal cord affecting the dorsal horn is thought to be one mechanism behind the development of pain (Rusbridge *et al.*, 2007; Rusbridge and Jeffrey, 2008). Neuropathic pain is secondary to disordered processing of sensory information within the nervous system and results in spontaneous pain, paraesthesia, dysthesia, allodynia or hyperpathia.

Dogs with Chiari-like malformations and syringomyelia may also develop scoliosis (Cerda-Gonzales and Dewey, 2010) (see below). Scoliosis occurs most commonly in the cervical spine; however, in a recent study, 76% of Cavalier King Charles Spaniels with a cranial cervical syrinx also had a syrinx affecting the more caudal regions of the spinal cord, resulting in clinical signs related to multifocal or diffuse CNS damage (Loderstedt *et al.*, 2011). Thus, restricting MRI studies to the cervical region of the spinal cord may underestimate the extent of the syringomyelia and the severity of the disease process.

Diagnosis

Chiari-like malformations are best diagnosed with MRI (Figure 14.13). Imaging findings include cerebellar herniation through the foramen magnum, cerebellar indentation by the supraoccipital bone, and obstruction of the foramen with obliteration of the subarachnoid space at the level of the craniocervical junction (Cerda-Gonzalez and Dewey, 2010). Kinking of the brainstem may also be evident. However, these findings seem to correlate poorly with clinical status (Cerda-Gonzalez *et al.*, 2009a), and in some cases these structural abnormalities may be clinically silent; therefore, their significance must be carefully considered (Lu *et al.*, 2003). Quadrigeminal intra-arachnoid cysts (Figure 14.14) and ventriculomegaly are suggested to be incidental findings.

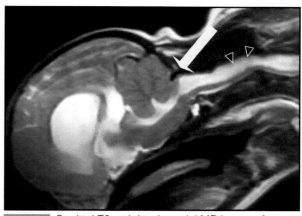

14.13 Sagittal T2-weighted cranial MR image of a 6-year-old Cavalier King Charles Spaniel. There is evident hydrocephalus and marked replacement of the spinal cord parenchyma with fluid-filled cavities (arrowheads). Note the caudal displacement of the vermis of the cerebellum (arrowed) associated with occipital dysplasia of the calvarium. This is compatible with a Chiari-like malformation.

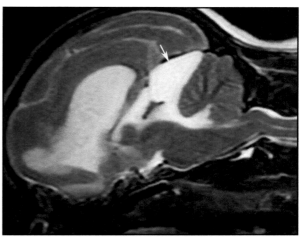

14.14 Sagittal T2-weighted MR image of the brain of a dog with a Chiari-like malformation and a large quadrigeminal intra-arachnoid cyst (arrowed).

Syringomyelia is seen as a hyperintensity on T2-weighted MR images and as a hypointensity on T1-weighted images. A prominent or dilated canal may be seen in some dogs. The extent of the syringomyelia can vary from a focal cyst-like structure, most commonly located in the grey matter of the dorsal cervical cord, to multifocal, multilobulated lesions located throughout the spinal cord (holocord syringomyelia). A localized area of hyperintensity associated with the central canal on T2-weighted FLAIR images is suggestive of a 'pre-syrinx'.

Evaluating the clinical significance of the MRI findings is difficult. However, two dimensional (2D) measurements of the skull and cerebellum, along with volumetric ratios relating to the size of the caudal fossa, can be useful to determine whether there is an association between the lesions and the clinical signs. In one study, a ratio of caudal fossa size to total cranial cavity volume of 13.3 had a sensitivity of 70% and a specificity of 92% when used to differentiate between clinically affected and unaffected Cavalier King Charles Spaniels with Chiari-like malformations (Cerda-Gonzalez et al., 2009a). In the Brussels Griffon, radiographically determined caudal fossa height to length ratios have been reported to predict Chiari-like malformations with a sensitivity of 87% and a specificity of 78% (Rusbridge et al., 2009). MRI based volume analysis is contentious in the human literature, but several studies have demonstrated a significant difference in the volume of the posterior fossa in patients with Chiari malformations compared with those without (Vega et al., 1990). A recent veterinary study investigating three dimensional (3D) skull volumes suggests that volumes alone cannot be used to assess the clinical significance of lesions in a particular patient as yet, but this work does lay the foundation for this to be possible in the future (Cross et al., 2009). This study determined that the percentage of herniated cerebellum was not related to the caudal fossa parenchymal volume in dogs.

It is important to rule out other concurrent diseases as the cause of the clinical signs. In toy and small-breed dogs, CSF analysis should be performed to investigate the possibility of an inflammatory disease, along with imaging to rule out disc disease. Recent studies suggest that there may be mild elevations in the CSF cell count and protein concentration in both Cavalier King Charles Spaniels (Whittaker et al., 2011) and Brussels Griffons (Freeman et al., 2011) with Chiari-like malformations and syringomyelia.

Ongoing studies in both the human and veterinary fields are investigating the role of CSF dynamics in the development of syringomyelia and its associated clinical signs. It is hoped that these studies will not only lead to a greater understanding of this complicated triad, but also provide appropriate long-term monitoring parameters to aid the treatment decision-making process and assess the success of therapeutic interventions. Phase-contrast MRI may be used to evaluate the velocity and pattern of CSF flow in dogs with Chiari-like malformations and to determine whether flow is obstructed (Cerda-Gonzalez et al., 2009c) (see **CSF flow study** clip on DVD). In the future, genetic tests for these conditions may become available.

Treatment and prognosis

Treatment may not be necessary in asymptomatic dogs or those with mild, non-progressive signs. Dogs exhibiting pain, severe neurological deficits or progressive signs can be treated either medically or surgically. Typically, initial medical therapy involves the use of analgesics and drugs to reduce the production of CSF. Furosemide (1–2 mg/kg orally q12h) and prednisone (0.5–1 mg/kg orally q24h) are frequently used. Other drugs used to decrease CSF production include acetazolamide and omeprazole. Treatment of the neuropathic pain with drugs such as gabapentin (10–20 mg/kg orally q8h) is also an important aspect of therapy. Pregabalin may be a useful alternative to gabapentin. Further options for controlling neuropathic pain include other anticonvulsants, tricyclic antidepressants, cyclooxygenase (COX)-2 inhibitors (e.g. meloxicam), amantadine and acupuncture (Cerda-Gonzalez and Dewey, 2010). Approximately 70% of patients show some improvement, but it is rarely complete and does not prevent disease progression.

If medical therapy does not alleviate the clinical signs, surgical decompression of the foramen magnum has been suggested (suboccipital craniectomy) and is the treatment of choice in humans. Foramen magnum decompression (Figure 14.15) has been performed in dogs with success rates reported to be approximately 80%; however, recurrence is common in the long term and neuropathic pain (along with the associated scratching) may persist requiring continued medical therapy (Dewey et al., 2005, 2007; Rusbridge et al., 2007). In addition,

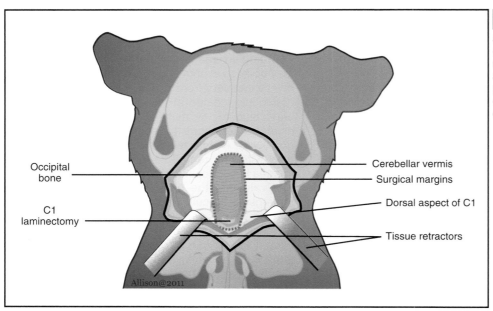

14.15 Dorsal view of the caudal skull and cervical vertebrae demonstrating the margins for craniectomy and laminectomy performed for decompression of the caudal fossa.

Occipital bone

C1 laminectomy

Cerebellar vermis

Surgical margins

Dorsal aspect of C1

Tissue retractors

Allison@2011

multiple surgical procedures may be necessary if scar tissue develops at the surgical site and obstructs CSF flow; although, cranioplasty may reduce the likelihood of this complication. Clinical improvement may not result in reduction of the size of the syrinx, which usually persists.

Perineurial cysts

Perineurial (Tarlov) cysts are rare lesions of the nerve roots that have been reported in two dogs (Platt *et al.*, 2003). Tarlov cysts are distinguished from other extradural meningeal lesions on the basis that:

- They arise at the junction of the dorsal root ganglion and the nerve root
- They develop between the endoneurium and perineurium
- Their lining contains nerve fibres and/or ganglion cells.

In humans, excision or fenestration of these cysts is recommended, although recurrence is possible. In the author's [SP] study, a 4-year-old neutered Scottish Deerhound bitch and an 8-month-old St Bernard bitch presented with chronic neck pain. MRI revealed fluid-filled structures at the level of vertebrae C6 and C7 (Figure 14.16). The cysts, which were attached to the nerve roots, were fenestrated. Histopathology of the capsules was compatible with perineurial cysts. On follow-up examination 1 year after surgery, neither dog had evidence of cervical pain.

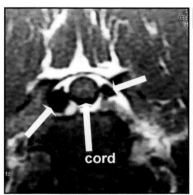

14.16 Transverse T1-weighted MR image of the spinal cord of a young Deerhound showing fluid-filled structures (arrowed) either side of the spinal cord at the level of the nerve roots.

Spinal cord anomalies

Spinal cord anomalies include spinal dysraphism, myelodysplasia, spina bifida and syringo(hydro) myelia. The first three conditions usually present with neurological deficits and are described in Chapter 16.

Syringomyelia

Syringomyelia (cavitation of the spinal cord) and hydromyelia (dilatation of the central canal) can result in similar signs of spinal cord dysfunction. Syringomyelia may exist as a distinct entity or in communication with the central canal (syringohydromyelia) (Figure 14.17). However, because it is often difficult to differentiate between these two

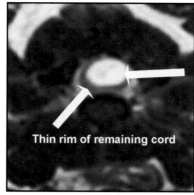

14.17 Transverse T2-weighted MR image of the dog in Figure 14.13 at the level of the second cervical vertebra. Note the large fluid-filled cavity within the parenchyma of the spinal cord (right arrow).

conditions, the term syringomyelia is preferred (Cappello and Rusbridge, 2007). The causes of this condition include Chiari-like malformations (see above), other congenital malformations, trauma, inflammation and neoplasia, but it can also be idiopathic. Clinical signs depend on the location of the lesion and can include pain, persistent scratching of the neck and flank, and neurological deficits. Spinal pain is present in approximately 40% of cases (Dewey, 2003).

Scoliosis

Scoliosis may be subclinical but can cause spinal discomfort (Figure 14.18). Neurological deficits may be present and depend on the underlying cause. Scoliosis may occur in animals with a hemivertebra. There are also numerous reports of scoliosis occurring in animals with congenital or acquired cystic lesions involving the spinal cord (e.g. syringomyelia) (Child *et al.*, 1986). This association has been suggested to be due to progressive destruction of grey matter by cavitation, resulting in denervation and unilateral atrophy of the epaxial muscles, followed by asymmetrical contralateral muscle spasticity and subsequent vertebral deviation. Diagnosis of the structural cause of the scoliosis necessitates imaging studies. Treatment, if any is possible, should be directed at the underlying cause. The prognosis is guarded.

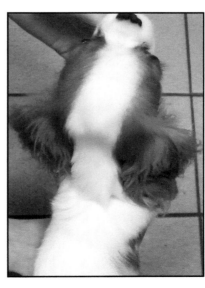

14.18 Lateral deviation of the cervical vertebrae in relation to the skill and thoracic vertebrae, compatible with scoliosis, in a 6-month-old Cavalier King Charles Spaniel.

Vertebral anomalies

Many spinal anomalies do not result in clinical signs and are detected as incidental findings. However, if a vertebral malformation is discovered in the presence of spinal pain, with or without neurological deficits, it should be thoroughly investigated. The presence of a vertebral anomaly may be a sporadic occurrence, but the potential for heritability must be considered. With the exception of atlantoaxial instability, many of the documented anomalies in veterinary patients occur in the thoracolumbosacral vertebrae, but have the potential to occur anywhere in the vertebral column. These anomalies often result in clinical signs due to associated spinal canal stenosis, progressive spinal deformity with growth or ageing, or instability exacerbated by degenerative disc disease. Important vertebral anomalies include hemivertebrae, block vertebrae, occipitoatlantoaxial malformation, hypoplasia or aplasia of the dens, transitional vertebrae and congenital spinal stenosis. These anomalies are described in Chapters 5, 15 and 16.

Neoplastic diseases

Spinal cord tumours are relatively common in cats and dogs and are usually classified according to their position in relation to the spinal cord and meninges as either extradural, intradural–extramedullary or intramedullary (Figure 14.19). Intramedullary neoplasia is rarely painful. Further details on the classification, diagnosis, treatment and prognosis of spinal tumours can be found in Chapter 16. Peripheral nerve sheath tumours are discussed in Chapter 17.

Nutritional diseases

Hypervitaminosis A

Abnormally high levels of vitamin A have been reported in cats fed on predominantly liver diets. This may cause hypertrophic bone formation on the vertebrae, leading to ankylosing spondylosis, primarily of the cervical vertebrae but in some cases this may extend to the lumbar region. Clinical signs relate to the rigidity of the spinal column and the associated pain. Treatment involves dietary modification, but this does not dramatically reverse the bone formation. Pain relief is recommended.

Inflammatory diseases

Infectious meningitis/meningomyelitis

Meningitis (inflammation of the meninges) and meningomyelitis (inflammation of the spinal cord and the meninges) can cause severe spinal pain. Meningomyelitis also causes neurological deficits. CSF analysis is the most reliable ante-mortem diagnostic test available for identifying CNS inflammation. It often reveals an increase in the white blood cell numbers as well as an elevation in

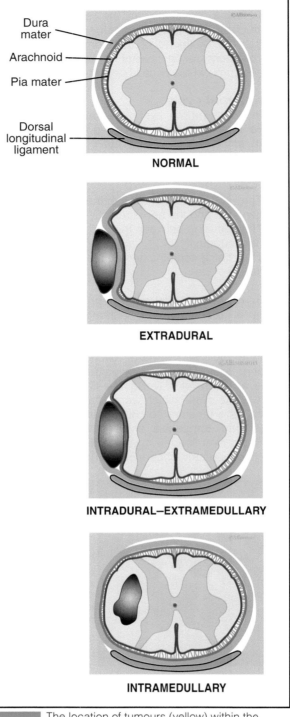

14.19 The location of tumours (yellow) within the spinal canal is classified according to their location relative to the spinal cord and the dura mater.

protein levels. A complete discussion of the diagnosis, treatment and prognosis of infectious CNS disease can be found in Chapters 11 and 16.

Steroid-responsive meningitis–arteritis

Clinical signs

Steroid-responsive meningitis–arteritis (SRMA), also known as necrotizing vasculitis, juvenile polyarteritis syndrome, corticosteroid-responsive meningitis/meningomyelitis, aseptic suppurative meningitis, panarteritis and pain syndrome, is a non-infectious inflammatory condition reported in Beagles, Bernese Mountain Dogs, Boxers, German Shorthaired Pointers and Nova Scotia Duck Tolling Retrievers (Tipold and Jaggy, 1994; Anfinsen *et al.*, 2008; Tipold and Stein, 2010) but has been noted in other medium to large dog breeds.

Affected dogs are often young adults (8–18 months old) but may be of any age, and are usually febrile and hyperaesthetic with cervical rigidity and anorexia (Figure 14.20). Neurological deficits can be seen with the chronic form of this disease and, rarely, severe motor dysfunction may result from spontaneous bleeding into the subarachnoid space (Tipold and Stein, 2010). Some dogs (up to 46%) with immune-mediated polyarthritis, especially Bernese Mountain Dogs, Boxers and Akitas, may show similar clinical signs to dogs with SRMA and have concurrent meningitis (Webb *et al.*, 2002). Some dogs may have concurrent glomerulonephritis.

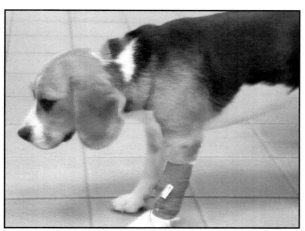

14.20 A 7-month-old Beagle exhibiting a stiff neck posture due to the inflammatory condition SRMA (sometimes called Beagle pain syndrome in this breed).

Pathogenesis
An immunological cause of this disease is suspected, resulting in vasculitis. The aetiopathogenesis is unknown, but an as yet unidentified infectious cause has been suggested. Notably increased levels of CSF and serum immunoglobulin (Ig) A, increased CSF and blood B cell:T cell ratios, and increased CSF levels of interleukin (IL)-8 are all thought to be compatible with immune system stimulation (Schwartz *et al.*, 2008a, 2011). High CD11a expression on polymorphonuclear cells appears to be an important factor in the pathogenesis of SRMA and may be involved in the enhanced passage of neutrophils into the subarachnoid space, leading to meningitis and clinical signs (Schwartz *et al.*, 2008b). Matrix metalloproteinase (MMP)-2 seems to also be involved in the neutrophilic invasion into the subarachnoid space (Schwartz *et al.*, 2010). Involvement of such molecular markers provides a potential therapeutic target. Subsequent to neutrophilic invasion of the subarachnoid space, there is development of fibrinoid arteritis and leptomeningeal

inflammation in the spinal cord and to a lesser degree the brain. With chronic progression of the lesions, rupture and haemorrhage of the weakened vasculature may occur accompanied by thickened leptomeninges with less severe inflammation.

Diagnosis
A marked peripheral neutrophilia with a left shift may be seen at the time of the clinical signs. CSF analysis often reveals a marked neutrophilic pleo-cytosis and protein elevations. Cell counts >100 cells/µl are common. Neutrophils are non-degenerative, unlike those seen with bacterial meningitis. In the majority of dogs with either acute or chronic disease, there are elevated IgA levels in both the CSF and serum; however, this is not specific for this disease. IgA concentrations in the CSF are significantly higher in dogs with SRMA compared with other disease processes, with the exception of inflammatory CNS disease, and must therefore be considered non-specific. The sensitivity for IgA concentrations in the CSF and serum was 91% with a specificity of only 78% in a study that evaluated 311 dogs with SRMA (Maiolini *et al.*, 2012).

C-reactive protein (CRP) is the primary major canine acute phase protein (APP) and has been shown to respond immediately to both the onset and resolution of inflammation. Other APPs include serum amyloid-A (SAA), haptoglobin and alpha-1-acid glycoprotein (AGP). Serum CRP levels have been reported to be significantly higher in dogs with SRMA compared with dogs with other neurological diseases (Bathen-Noethen *et al.*, 2008). Results of a recent study of 9 dogs with SRMA demonstrated a significant increase in all serum APPs above normal concentrations, which all decreased (with the exception of haptoglobin) in response to corticosteroid treatment (Lowrie *et al.*, 2009a). Serum CRP and SAA were also found to be consistently elevated in all patients exhibiting signs consistent with a relapse during treatment in the presence of normal CSF and leucograms. However, as with IgA, elevations in CRP are considered to be non-specific as this can also occur in sepsis, and so can only be used as a supportive diagnostic test (Eckersall and Bell, 2010).

Treatment and prognosis
The prognosis can be good if dogs are treated early and aggressively with immunosuppressive doses of corticosteroids (Figure 14.21), with up to 80% of cases going into long-term remission (Cizinauskas *et al.*, 2000; Lowrie *et al.*, 2009b). Infectious diseases should be ruled out before this treatment is initiated. The treatment is long-term and has been reported to be required for >2 years in some dogs; however, after this time, serum and CSF levels of IgA were still elevated in some cases and thus are not considered valuable for disease monitoring (Cizinauskas *et al.*, 2000). Monitoring the CSF cell count in dogs with this condition is a sensitive indicator of the success of treatment. In refractory cases or in patients with steroid-related side effects, alternative immunomodulation therapy such as azathioprine should be considered.

Drug	Dosing regimen
Prednisolone	4 mg/kg orally or i.v. q24h for 2 days
	2 mg/kg orally q24h for 14 days. If clinical signs have improved, a further reduction can be considered
	1 mg/kg orally q24h for 28 days. If clinical signs are normal, a further reduction can be considered
	0.5 mg/kg orally q24h for 28 days. If clinical signs are normal, a further reduction can be considered
	0.5 mg/kg orally q48h for 2 months. If clinical signs are normal, the medication can be stopped
Azathioprine	1.5 mg/kg orally q48h if clinical signs are refractory to the steroid medication

14.21 Treatment recommendations for SRMA.

Granulomatous meningoencephalomyelitis

Granulomatous meningoencephalomyelitis (GME) is a non-suppurative CNS inflammatory disease of undetermined aetiology in dogs. It is suggested to be the result of a T cell-mediated delayed-type hypersensitivity (Kipar *et al.*, 1998). It is most commonly seen in small-breed dogs (often terriers, toy breeds and Poodles), although any breed may be affected (Muñana and Luttgen, 1998; Adamo *et al.*, 2007). GME may involve the spinal cord at any level; however, lesions appear to be most severe in the cervical spinal cord (Figure 14.22). Findings include apparent cervical pain, rigidity, reluctance to move, hyperaesthesia, cervical paraspinal muscle spasms and neurological deficits. Further information on the pathophysiology, diagnosis and prognosis of this disease can be found in Chapter 11.

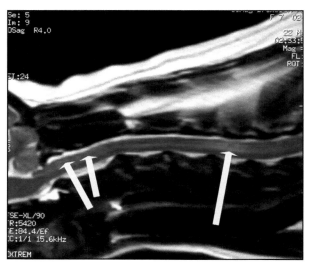

14.22 Sagittal T2-weighted MR image of the cervical spinal cord of an 8-year-old West Highland White Terrier with severe neck pain due to GME. Note the multifocal hyperintense inflammatory lesions within the cord (arrowed). This is not specific for this disease. CSF analysis is always necessary to document the inflammatory nature of the condition.

Discospondylitis/osteomyelitis

Clinical signs
Spinal pain is the most common initial clinical sign with this disease, which frequently occurs in large, intact male, young to middle-aged dogs (Burkert *et al.*, 2005). With proliferation of inflammatory tissue, compression of neural tissue can lead to ataxia, paresis and occasionally paralysis, depending on where the lesion is located (see **Discospondylitis** clip on DVD). Although it can occur in any animal, the condition is less common in toy and chondrodystrophic breeds of dog and rare in cats. Purebred dogs seem more commonly affected than mixed-breeds. Approximately 30% of dogs have signs of systemic illness such as fever and weight loss.

Pathogenesis
Discospondylitis is due to infection of the intervertebral disc and adjacent vertebral endplates. If the infection is confined to the vertebral body, it is called osteomyelitis or spondylitis (Thomas, 2000). Coagulase positive *Staphylococcus* spp. (*S. intermedius* or *S. aureus*) are the most common aetiological agents associated with canine discospondylitis (Tipold and Stein, 2010). Other less commonly identified organisms include *Streptococcus* spp., *Escherichia coli*, *Actinomyces* spp., *Brucella canis* and *Aspergillus* spp. Young German Shepherd bitches seem to be predisposed to aspergillosis (Berry and Leisewitz, 1996), whereas young Basset Hounds contract discospondylitis due to systemic tuberculosis (Carpenter *et al.*, 1988). Haematogenous spread from distant foci of infection (urogenital tract, skin, oral cavity), penetrating wounds, surgery or plant material migration can cause direct infection of the disc spaces or vertebrae, the latter of which is usually seen at the level of L2–L4 at the insertion of the diaphragmatic crus. Immunosuppression due to factors such as hyperadrenocorticism is considered a predisposing cause.

The sites most commonly affected are L7–S1, and the caudal cervical, mid-thoracic and thoracolumbar spine (Tipold and Stein, 2010). The infection is usually slowly progressive but can result in acute signs due to secondary pathological vertebral factures and intervertebral disc disease. An association with empyema has been documented in several dogs, which may represent an extension of the disease and should be taken into consideration when deciding which diagnostic tests to perform and/or when dealing with a refractory case (Lavely *et al.*, 2006; De Stefani *et al.*, 2007).

Diagnosis
- Haematological changes are usually not present unless there are concurrent conditions (such as endocarditis).
- Urine cytology may reveal bacterial or fungal agents.
- Blood and urine cultures should be performed in all suspected cases and are positive in up to 75% and 50% of cases, respectively (Thomas, 2000; Tipold and Stein, 2010). Ideally, these

tests should be performed prior to initiating antibiotic therapy.
- Serology for brucellosis should also be performed, especially in view of its zoonotic potential. It has been reported to be positive in up to 10% of cases.

In all cases, diagnostic investigation of potential systemic infectious foci should be considered. This should include abdominal ultrasonography for prostatic or renal disease, thoracic radiography for pulmonary disease, and cardiac ultrasonography for endocarditis.

Radiography: A definitive diagnosis is usually made with spinal radiographs, although radiographic changes may not be evident in the first 2–4 weeks of infection. As this can be a multifocal disease, the entire spine should be imaged. Radiographic evidence of disease includes narrowing of the disc space, accompanied by subtle irregularity of both endplates through to gross lysis and osseous proliferation of the adjacent vertebral bone (Figure 14.23) and even fractures (see Chapter 5). Radiography can also be used to monitor the response to treatment or the progression of the disease (Shamir *et al.*, 2001), although clinical progression is equally important as radiographic changes can lag behind clinical improvement.

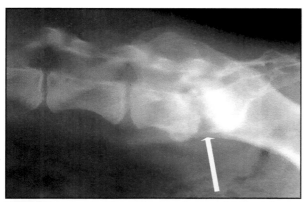

14.23 Lateral radiograph of an 8-year-old Airedale Terrier with lumbar pain. Gross irregular lysis and osseous proliferation of the vertebral endplates of L7 and S1 (arrowed) can be seen, which are compatible with discospondylitis.

Myelography used to be recommended in patients with substantial neurological deficits to rule out concurrent disc disease and subluxation affecting the neural tissues; however, this should now be reserved for when CT and MRI are unavailable. A study of 27 dogs with discospondylitis found that contrast-enhanced radiographs revealed only a 5% median cord compression, which was not related to the clinical signs or outcome (Davis *et al.*, 2000).

Advanced imaging: CT can identify subtle endplate erosion and paravertebral soft tissue swelling more readily than radiography. In addition, both contrast-enhanced CT and MRI (Figure 14.24) clearly define compression of the neural tissues by

infectious tissues. MRI can also highlight inflammation in the surrounding muscles. Discospondylitis appears to have an increased signal intensity on T2-weighted MR images and a decreased signal intensity on T1-weighted images. Contrast enhancement was seen in the endplates of affected vertebrae in 15 of 17 (88%) sites in one study (Carrera *et al.*, 2011), as was endplate erosion and hypointense bone marrow on T2-weighted images (Figure 14.24). Changes in the paravertebral tissues were also noted in all cases.

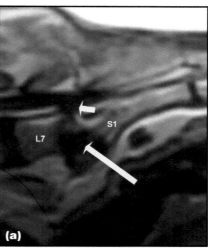
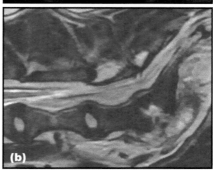
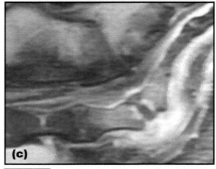

14.24 **(a)** Sagittal T2-weighted MR image of the same region of the dog shown in Figure 14.23. The bony detail is not as good as with radiography. A loss of signal is seen in the region of the osseous proliferation (long arrow) which is not specific for vertebral infection. However, in cases unresponsive to antibiotic therapy, MRI may help identify associated neural compression (short arrow). **(b)** Sagittal T2-weighted and **(c)** T1-weighted post-contrast lumbosacral MR images revealing pathology at the endplates compatible with discospondylitis. Note the hyperintensity within the disc and endplates (b) and contrast enhancement of the endplates and the soft tissues ventral to the lumbosacral junction (c).

Another diagnostic imaging option in dogs with discospondylitis is technetium-99m bone scanning (scintigraphy), which shows an increased uptake of the radiopharmaceutical at the affected disc space and endplates (Figure 14.25). However, care must be taken when interpreting this finding as spondylosis can also cause an increase in radioisotope uptake.

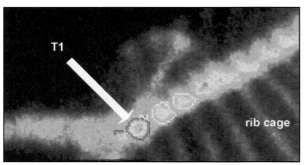

14.25 Scintigraphy can be performed to investigate for vertebral lesions, as demonstrated in this lateral view of the cervicothoracic spine of a 10-year-old Ibizan hound. The accumulation of the radioisotope within the body of the first thoracic vertebra (arrowed) is not specific for discospondylitis, and vertebral tumours can have a similar appearance.

Culture and cytology: If urine and blood culture, and brucellosis serology, have not identified an aetiological agent in cases of discospondylitis, percutaneous needle aspiration of the disc space can be performed to obtain tissue for bacterial and fungal culture and cytology. However, this procedure requires general anaesthesia, sterile surgical preparation and fluoroscopic (Figure 14.26) or CT guidance of the needle, and is usually only performed in patients who are unresponsive to initial broad-spectrum antibiotics. The procedure has

been documented to be up to 75% sensitive (Fischer *et al.*, 1997). Open biopsy of the vertebrae may be considered if needle aspiration is unrewarding. This procedure has yielded positive cultures in approximately 80% of patients (Kornegay and Barber, 1980).

Treatment and prognosis

If there is radiographic evidence of discospondylitis, treatment for the common pathogen *Staphylococcus intermedius* should be initiated. The treatment consists of antibiotics (potentiated amoxicillin or cefalexin), cage rest and analgesics (Figure 14.27). The choice of antibiotics may need to be altered in light of the results of culture and sensitivity testing.

Infectious agent	Antibiotic	Dosage
Staphylococcus intermedius	Cefalexin	20–30 mg/kg orally q8h
	Cefazolin	20 mg/kg i.v., i.m. or s.c. q6h
	Amoxicillin	20 mg/kg orally q12h
Beta-haemolytic *Streptococcus* spp.	Amoxicillin	20 mg/kg orally q12h
Escherichia coli	Enrofloxacin	5–11 mg/kg orally q12h
Brucella canis	Enrofloxacin	10–20 mg/kg orally q24h
	Doxycycline	25 mg/kg orally q24h
Aspergillus spp.	Fluconazole	2.5–5 mg/kg orally q24h
	Itraconazole	5 mg/kg orally q24h

14.27   Drug therapy for discospondylitis/osteomyelitis.

Intravenous antibiotics should be considered if severe neurological compromise or signs of sepsis are present; otherwise, oral antibiotics are acceptable. However quickly the patient improves, continuation of the antibiotics for 8–16 weeks is recommended (Thomas, 2000; Tipold and Stein, 2010); one study evaluating 513 cases noted a mean duration of treatment of 54 weeks (Burkert *et al.*, 2005). Resolution of clinical signs, such as pain and fever, should be expected within 5 days of initiating therapy; however, complete neurological resolution may take 2–3 months. Residual deficits may remain, but persistent pain indicates an active disease, and these patients should be treated with an additional antibiotic and considered for further diagnostics as they may have a potential fungal infection or a lesion that requires surgical decompression. Discospondylitis associated with *Aspergillus* spp. has been treated with itraconazole, although long-term reports of success are lacking and it has been suggested that chronic recurrence and progression are likely.

Surgical decompression is rarely needed and should only be considered in refractory cases or those with severe neurological deficits that show no signs of improvement within 3–5 days. Although internal fixation may be acceptable even at the

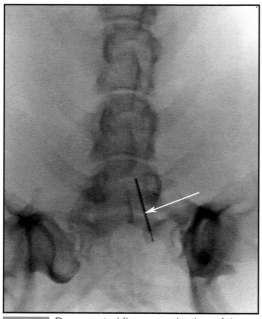

14.26   Dorsoventral fluoroscopic view of the lumbosacral vertebrae of a dog with discospondylitis. A needle (arrowed) is being directed to the disc space to obtain a sample for an aspiration study.

site of infection (Figure 14.28), it may be more appropriate to consider external skeletal fixation. External fixation has been reported to be successful in dogs with lumbosacral discospondylitis (Auger *et al.*, 2000). A fluoroscopy-guided percutaneous discectomy technique has been described and evaluated for 10 dogs with discospondylitis (Kinzel *et al.*, 2005). A 5 mm Mitchel trephine was used to obtain tissue and make a lesion into which parenteral antibiotics were administered. No side effects were noted after the procedure and a marked improvement was evident within 9 days in all dogs. The placement of an antibiotic impregnated gelatine sponge into the disc space has been described as a successful adjunct to decompressive and/or stabilization surgery (Renwick *et al.*, 2010).

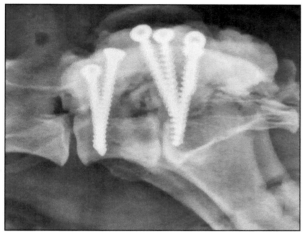

14.28 Lateral radiograph of the lumbosacral spinal vertebrae of a dog which had discospondylitis at L7–S1 that required surgical stabilization. Note that the discospondylitis has nearly completely resolved.

NSAIDs should be considered in dogs for the treatment of pain whilst awaiting the effect of the antibiotics, but should not be necessary after 5 days and should be discontinued to allow clinical assessment of the patient. Corticosteroids are not appropriate anti-inflammatory drugs for the treatment of this disease.

The prognosis for this disease is generally very good unless the aetiology is fungal, there are multiple lesions, vertebral fractures or subluxations are present, or there is endocarditis. The potential for recurrence should be considered, especially if brucellosis has been diagnosed or an underlying immunosuppressive condition is present. In those cases with severe residual neurological deficits associated with the infection, the prognosis should initially be guarded.

Empyema
Infection of the CNS may result in an abscess or empyema in subdural or epidural locations. Epidural infections can follow skin disease, vertebral osteomyelitis, discospondylitis or a paraspinal abscess. Clinical signs may include fever, anorexia, lethargy and apparent spinal pain, as well as neurological compromise; however, there may not be a systemic reaction. Further information on this condition can be found in Chapter 16.

Polymyositis/polymyopathy
The main clinical sign of disease affecting the skeletal muscles is weakness; however, muscle pain (myalgia), which can present as spinal pain, may also be a feature. The weakness that accompanies muscle disease may be discrete, causing an abnormal posture such as neck ventroflexion (particularly in cats), leading the clinician to focus on a cervical disease. For a complete discussion of muscle disease, the reader is directed to Chapter 18.

Polyarthritis
Arthritis is generally classified as either non-inflammatory or inflammatory (Johnson and Mackin, 2012ab) (Figure 14.29). Inflammatory joint diseases can affect multiple joints (polyarthritis) and are either infectious or immune-mediated. Immune-mediated polyarthritides can be further classified as erosive or non-erosive, based on the presence or absence of joint cartilage destruction and typical bone erosion visible on radiographs. Polyarthritis can often present as a spinal pain syndrome, but there is commonly concurrent appendicular joint pain. Typically, animals appear to be 'walking on eggshells', and are reluctant to lie down or rise once down. All appendicular joints should be carefully palpated but the absence of joint effusion does not rule out polyarthritis. The prevalence of spinal pain in dogs with non-infectious, non-erosive, idiopathic immune-mediated polyarthritis is approximately 30% (Webb *et al.*, 2002). The reader is directed to internal medicine and orthopaedic texts for a more complete discussion on the diagnosis and management of these conditions.

Type of arthritis	Condition
Non-inflammatory	Degenerative joint disease
Inflammatory	Infectious (septic)

	Immune-mediated (non-septic)
	
	Erosive:
	• Canine rheumatoid arthritis
	• Feline progressive polyarthritis
	• Periosteal proliferative polyarthritis
	• Polyarthritis of Greyhounds
	
	Non-erosive:
	• Systemic lupus erythematosus
	• Polyarthritis nodosa
	• Polyarthritis/meningitis
	• Lymphocytic–plasmacytic synovitis
	• Amyloidosis of Shar Peis
	• Idiopathic:
	  – Type I (uncomplicated)
	  – Type II (reactive)
	  – Type III (enteropathic)
	  – Type IV (malignant)

	Vaccine reactions Drug-induced

14.29 Classification of arthritis.

Traumatic diseases

Spinal facture or luxation

Vehicle-related injury is the most common exogenous cause of trauma to the spine in small animals; however, falls, trauma from falling objects, attacks by dogs and kicks from farm animals and horses are also possible. Depending on the type of force, the area of impact and the inherent strengths and weaknesses of the vertebral column, exogenous spinal injury often results in vertebral fracture, subluxation or luxation. Cervical and thoracolumbar vertebral injuries are discussed in detail in Chapters 15 and 16, respectively. The medical considerations for patients with spinal fractures and luxations are discussed in Chapter 20.

Vascular diseases

Spinal haemorrhage

Intramedullary, intrameningeal or epidural haemorrhage may be due to coagulopathies or associated with tumours, vascular malformations, acute intervertebral disc protrusion, trauma, parasitic migration or meningitis. Neurological deficits depend on the location of the haemorrhage and usually indicate an acute focal or multifocal myelopathy accompanied by severe pain. A more detailed description of these diseases is given in Chapter 15.

References and further reading

Available on accompanying DVD

DVD extras

- Behavioural response
- CSF flow study
- Discospondylitis
- Flexion and extension of neck
- 'Phantom scratching'

15

Tetraparesis

Natasha Olby

Terminology

- Tetraparesis is defined as reduced voluntary motor function in all four limbs and can be further subdivided into non-ambulatory and ambulatory categories.
- Tetraplegia indicates total absence of voluntary motor function in all four limbs.

Tetraparesis can result from focal or diffuse diseases of the brainstem and spinal cord, and generalized diseases of the peripheral nervous system (PNS) including diseases of the neuromuscular junction and muscle, but can also be caused by non-neurological diseases (Figure 15.1). A careful physical and neurological examination is therefore needed to localize the source of weakness. An additional concern in tetraplegic animals is the potential for the involvement of the respiratory muscles. Tetraplegic animals are at serious risk of respiratory failure due to:

- Paresis of the intercostal muscles and diaphragm
- Atelectasis as a result of recumbency
- Aspiration pneumonia
- Failure of respiratory drive if the brainstem is involved.

- Polymyositis (see Chapter 18)
- Polyarthritis
- Hypertrophic osteodystrophy
- Hypoglycaemia
- Hypoxaemia
- Hypotension

15.1 Non-neurological conditions that can cause tetraparesis.

This chapter discusses how to approach a tetraparetic animal and describes the features, treatment and prognosis of the more commonly encountered diseases. Management issues specific to the recumbent animal are discussed further in Chapter 25. Surgery is the recommended treatment for many spinal diseases; basic approaches to the spine, and the indications for and complications of spinal surgery are discussed in Chapter 22, but readers are referred to surgical texts for additional specific details (Sharp and Wheeler, 2005; Tobias and Johnston, 2011).

Clinical signs

In tetraparetic animals the pelvic limbs are often affected earlier and more severely than the thoracic limbs, and the severity of signs can range from mild weakness and ataxia to tetraplegia with respiratory failure. Animals with central nervous system (CNS) causes of tetraparesis have a general proprioceptive ataxia with proprioceptive placing and postural reaction deficits in all four limbs. Neck pain may be present depending on the aetiology of the signs and the individual (see Chapter 14). Myotatic and withdrawal reflexes and muscle tone in the pelvic limbs are normal to increased, and may be normal to increased, or decreased in the thoracic limbs depending on the neurolocalization (C1–C5 *versus* C6–T2, respectively). Caudal cervical lesions can cause lameness in one or both thoracic limbs, a short, stilted thoracic limb gait, atrophy of the supraspinatus, infraspinatus and biceps brachii muscles, and at rest animals may hold the affected limb(s) off the ground. These signs are a result of compression of the nerve roots causing pain and weakness (nerve root signature). Lateralized cervical spinal cord lesions can cause partial Horner's syndrome (miosis) on the affected side as a result of involvement of the sympathetic fibres running in the lateral funiculus of the spinal cord and emerging from the spinal cord at segments T1–T3. Lesions affecting spinal cord segments C8–T2 can affect the motor (effector) arm of the cutaneous trunci reflex, the lateral thoracic nerve, leading to a complete loss of the reflex on the affected side. In addition to tetraparesis, brainstem involvement can cause cranial nerve (CN) deficits, in particular vestibular dysfunction, and can cause changes in mentation. With both brainstem and spinal cord disease, lateralized lesions result in ipsilateral deficits (e.g. hemiparesis).

Generalized lower motor neuron (LMN) diseases cause weakness characterized by decreased muscle tone (flaccidity) and decreased or absent myotatic and withdrawal reflexes. With severe generalized neuropathies, ataxia and postural reaction and proprioceptive deficits may also be present. However, if adequate weight support is provided, typically the patient has normal postural reactions and proprioceptive placing, and ataxia is not a common feature. Involvement of the recurrent laryngeal nerve can cause a change in or loss of voice (dysphonia) and increased inspiratory noise (stridor). The development of megaoesophagus can cause regurgitation often with accompanying aspiration pneumonia, particularly if there is concurrent involvement of the pharyngeal and laryngeal muscles. Other CN deficits such as facial paresis may be present. As the disease progresses dramatic muscle atrophy develops, although in some myopathies and peripheral neuropathies, muscle hypertrophy occurs. Myopathies can generally be distinguished from neuropathies as with these disorders myotatic reflexes are usually normal whilst withdrawal reflexes are reduced in strength, and there are no proprioceptive placing deficits. Exercise intolerance may be the only presenting sign in some myopathies and disorders of neuromuscular transmission such as myasthenia gravis (see Chapter 18 for further details).

Any tetraplegic animal, whether the cause is spinal or peripheral in origin, is at risk from hypoventilation, and arterial blood gas analysis should be performed to measure the partial pressure of carbon dioxide (P_aCO_2). Ventilatory support by means of a mechanical ventilator may be necessary in animals with an elevated P_aCO_2. In small animals (<5 kg) a transtracheal catheter can be used in place of a ventilator. The catheter is advanced via the cricothyroid ligament to the level of the bronchial bifurcation and a humidified oxygen/air mixture is passed through the catheter at a rate sufficient to exchange CO_2 adequately. Any animal that is regurgitating is at risk of developing aspiration pneumonia: the lung fields should be auscultated carefully, and thoracic radiography, pulse oximetry and/or arterial blood gas analysis performed if there is any suspicion of aspiration.

Non-neurological causes of tetraparesis should be suspected whenever proprioceptive placing is normal. Careful palpation of the joints and long bones enables the clinician to identify orthopaedic diseases such as polyarthritis and hypertrophic osteodystrophy.

Lesion localization

Tetraparesis can result from focal lesions in the cervical spinal cord or brainstem, diffuse spinal cord diseases, and generalized diseases of the PNS, neuromuscular junction and muscle (Figure 15.2). Details of the neurological examination and lesion localization are covered in Chapters 1 and 2. Once the neurological examination has been completed, spinal cord disease should be differentiated from generalized LMN disease (Figure 15.3). Brainstem disease is considered in Chapter 11.

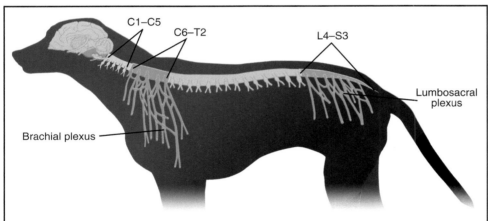

15.2 Lesion localization for tetraparesis. The brainstem, cervical spinal cord and PNS are highlighted.

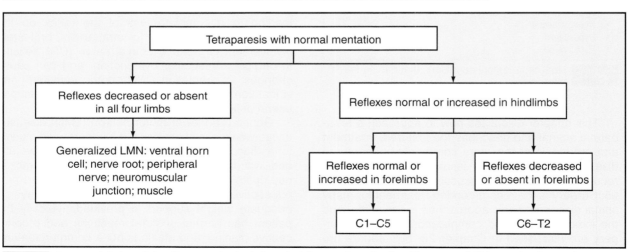

15.3 Approach to localizing the neurological signs in tetraparetic animals with a normal CN examination and mentation. Note: some animals with a generalized LMN disorder may also have CN dysfunction, especially facial and laryngeal paresis.

Pathophysiology

Conduction of nerve impulses is dependent on the integrity of the neuronal cell body, the axon, the myelin sheath and the junction between the neuron and its target. Neurons have excitable membranes due to selective ionic permeability. In the resting state, the membrane is polarized to a potential of approximately −70 mV as a result of partial permeability to potassium and active extrusion of sodium in exchange for potassium. Action potentials are generated by a rapid influx of sodium through voltage-dependent channels, which open in response to depolarization of the membrane. This membrane depolarization results from the activation of receptors by either excitatory (causing membrane depolarization) or inhibitory (causing membrane hyperpolarization) neurotransmitters (Figure 15.4). The membrane is repolarized by closure of the sodium channels (halting the influx of sodium) and opening of the voltage-dependent potassium channels (resulting in an efflux of potassium).

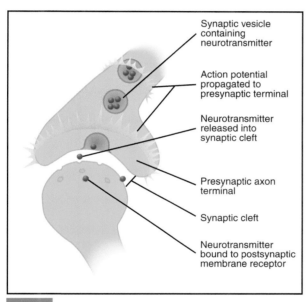

15.4 Propagation of a neuronal axon potential.

Action potentials that conduct down the axon are triggered at the axon hillock (the junction between the axon and neuronal cell body) (Figure 15.5). Speed of conduction is largely dependent on axon diameter (larger diameter conducts more quickly) and degree of myelination. Myelin (produced by oligodendrocytes in the CNS and Schwann cells in the PNS) insulates axons, increasing their membrane resistance (Figure 15.6). This causes action potentials to conduct along the axoplasm in a simple cable fashion to the next region of exposed axon membrane (node), where depolarization of the membrane produces a new action potential. The result is conduction of the impulse from node to node in a saltatory fashion, dramatically increasing the speed of conduction.

Spinal cord dysfunction most commonly results from compression, contusion, laceration, ischaemia

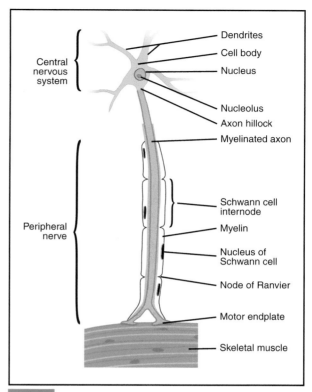

15.5 The structure of a somatic neuron.

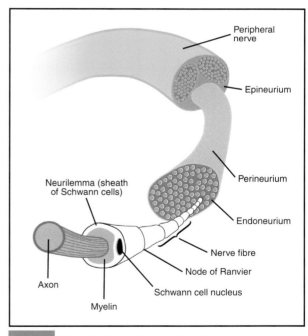

15.6 The structure of a peripheral nerve.

or inflammation with many diseases causing a combination of these problems. Neurodegenerative and toxic disorders can also affect the spinal cord (less common). Neurons within the CNS cannot effectively regenerate axons, and so recovery following axonal transection or neuronal death is dependent on developing alternative routes of conduction through the surviving tissue. As a result, prognosis in spinal cord disease, no matter what the aetiology, is greatly influenced by the severity of the damage at the time of evaluation. Treatment of spinal cord diseases focuses on surgical decompression of compressive lesions, appropriate treatment of infectious and inflammatory diseases and physical rehabilitation to facilitate and maximize recovery.

Neurons in the PNS are more resistant to injury than their CNS counterparts and are able to regenerate axons at a speed of 1–4 mm a day, if they are regenerating within an intact endoneural and Schwann cell tube. However, when an axon is completely severed and displaced (neurotmesis), successful regeneration to a target only occurs if the axon is able to locate the distal stump of the nerve.

Although the same basic injury types apply to peripheral nerves, metabolic, inherited and toxic disorders assume a greater clinical importance than in the spinal cord. In most peripheral neuropathies a mixture of demyelination and axonal degeneration is present. The distal ends of axons are particularly susceptible to degeneration as a result of their distance from the neuronal cell body, with longer nerves (e.g. recurrent laryngeal and sciatic nerves) often clinically affected first in toxic, degenerative and metabolic disorders.

Neurodiagnostic investigation

The history and findings of the physical and neurological examinations allow identification of a neurological problem and localization to the brainstem (see Chapter 11), spinal cord or PNS.

Spinal cord disease
The diagnostic evaluation of animals with evidence of spinal cord disease starts with routine blood work (complete blood count, serum biochemical analysis), urinalysis and survey spinal radiographs. Spinal radiographs can also be helpful to determine what further diagnostic tests are required (Figure 15.7).

Survey thoracic radiographs should be obtained for any animal in which neoplasia is a differential diagnosis to look for metastatic disease. As a general rule, if a diagnosis cannot be reached from survey radiographs, the animal should be referred to a specialist centre for further evaluation, including advanced imaging studies.

Lower motor neuron disease
The minimum diagnostic workup for dogs with generalized LMN signs includes a complete blood count, serum biochemical analysis (including

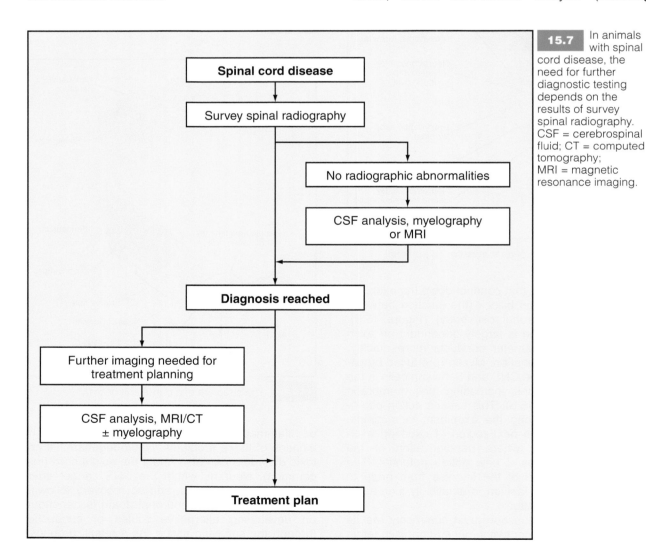

15.7 In animals with spinal cord disease, the need for further diagnostic testing depends on the results of survey spinal radiography. CSF = cerebrospinal fluid; CT = computed tomography; MRI = magnetic resonance imaging.

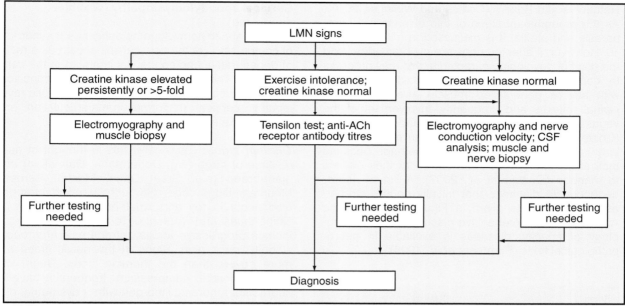

15.8 Animals with LMN signs often need an electrophysiological evaluation coupled with a nerve or muscle biopsy to determine the most appropriate treatment. ACh = acetylcholine; CSF = cerebrospinal fluid.

creatine kinase), urinalysis and thoracic radiographs to identify megaoesophagus, aspiration pneumonia and pulmonary metastases. Figure 15.8 illustrates the diagnostic approach to evaluate these cases further. Although nerve and muscle biopsies may provide a definitive diagnosis, further testing is often needed based on the results (see Chapter 6 for biopsy techniques).

Spinal cord diseases

Spinal cord diseases that can cause tetraparesis are listed in Figure 15.9.

Mechanism of disease	Specific diseases
Degenerative	Inherited neurodegenerative diseases [15] Degenerative myelopathy [16] Cervical spondylomyelopathy (Wobbler syndrome) [15] Intervertebral disc disease (Hansen types I and II) [15, 16] Discal cysts [15] Calcinosis circumscripta [15] Synovial cysts [15]
Anomalous	Atlantoaxial instability [15] Atlanto-occipital overlap [14] Intra-arachnoid cysts [15] Dermoid sinus [15, 16] Osteochondromatosis [16] Chiari-like malformation and syringo(hydro) myelia [14] Vertebral and spinal cord anomalies [5, 15, 16]

15.9 Spinal cord diseases that can cause tetraparesis. The numbers in square brackets denote the chapters in which the conditions are discussed in detail. (continues) ▶

Mechanism of disease	Specific diseases
Neoplastic	Extradural [16]: metastasis; vertebral tumours (sarcomas, plasma cell tumours); lymphoma Intradural–extramedullary [16]: meningiomas; nerve sheath tumours; metastasis Intramedullary [16]: ependymomas; gliomas; metastasis; round cell tumours
Inflammatory	Discospondylitis/osteomyelitis/physitis [14] Empyema [16] Granulomatous meningoencephalomyelitis [11] Infectious meningoencephalomyelitis [11, 16] Steroid-responsive meningitis–arteritis [14]
Toxic	Tetanus [15]
Trauma	Vertebral fractures/luxations [15, 16, 20] Epidural haemorrhage [15] Spinal cord contusion [15, 20] Traumatic disc herniation [15]
Vascular	Fibrocartilaginous embolism [15, 16] Spinal cord/epidural haemorrhage [15] Thromboembolic disease [16]

15.9 (continued) Spinal cord diseases that can cause tetraparesis. The numbers in square brackets denote the chapters in which the conditions are discussed in detail.

Degenerative diseases

Breed-specific spinal cord diseases
These are degenerative CNS diseases that are often inherited. They cause progressive signs and usually involve many areas of the CNS. The most common neurodegenerative disease specific to the spinal cord is degenerative myelopathy, which occurs in a wide range of breeds including German Shepherd Dogs, Pembroke Welsh Corgis, Chesapeake Bay

Retrievers and Boxers (Coates and Wininger, 2010). As the predominant signs of this disease are paraparesis and ataxia, it is discussed in full in Chapter 16. However, if affected dogs are maintained beyond the point of developing paraplegia, this may progress to generalized LMN signs of flaccid tetraparesis with severe generalized muscle atrophy, loss of jspinal reflexes and, frequently, involvement of the vagus nerve causing loss of bark and regurgitation (Coates *et al.*, 2007). This has been noted particularly in Pembroke Welsh Corgis, perhaps because their small size makes them easier for their owners to manage (Coates *et al.*, 2007). A list of neurodegenerative diseases that initially cause tetraparesis and ataxia is given in Figure 15.10 and the Appendix. A comprehensive discussion of the pathology of specific diseases is available in neuropathological texts (Summers *et al.*, 1995).

Breed	Disease
Boxer; Chesapeake Bay Retriever; German Shepherd Dog; Pembroke Welsh Corgi; Rhodesian Ridgeback; Siberian Husky; others	Degenerative myelopathy
Rottweiler	Leucoencephalomyelopathy
Dalmatian; Labrador Retriever	Leucodystrophy
Miniature Poodle	Demyelinating myelopathy
Afghan Hound; Kooiker Hound	Myelopathy
Labrador Retriever	Axonopathy
Beagle; Fox Hound; Harrier Hound	Hound ataxia
Cairn Terrier; West Highland White Terrier	Globoid cell leucodystrophy

15.10 Inherited diseases that can cause UMN signs. Many of these diseases also affect other areas of the CNS and therefore cause other (e.g. cerebellar) signs.

Cervical spondylomyelopathy (Wobbler syndrome)

Cervical spondylomyelopathy describes a syndrome of compression of the cervical spinal cord as a result of degenerative and congenital changes in the cervical spine. There are many names for this condition, including Wobbler syndrome, cervical stenotic myelopathy, cervical malformation/malarticulation and disc-associated Wobbler syndrome.

Clinical signs: Classically, this is thought of as a disease of large (e.g. Dobermann, Dalmatian) and giant-breed (e.g. Great Dane, Mastiff, Bernese Mountain Dog) dogs, although identical changes also occur in toy and small-breed dogs such as Chihuahuas and Yorkshire Terriers. Clinical signs include progressive ataxia, tetraparesis and, occasionally, neck pain. Signs in the pelvic limbs are more severe than the thoracic limbs. Dogs with caudal cervical compression frequently have a short stilted thoracic limb gait with a dysmetric, disconnected pelvic limb gait (see **Caudal cervical spondylomyelopathy** clip on DVD). Nerve root entrapment can cause thoracic limb lameness and muscle atrophy; in particular, compression of the suprascapular nerve can result in marked atrophy of the supraspinatus and infraspinatus muscles, making the scapular spine easily palpable. Although this is typically a chronic progressive disease, acute onset of severe signs can occur.

Pathogenesis: Progressive spinal cord compression results from both congenital stenosis and degenerative changes in the vertebral column (Trotter *et al.*, 1976; da Costa, 2010). The changes (Figure 15.11) can include:

- Hypertrophy and protrusion of the annulus fibrosus (Hansen type II disease), often associated with 'tipping' of the vertebrae. This change is classically seen with disc-associated Wobbler syndrome in Dobermanns

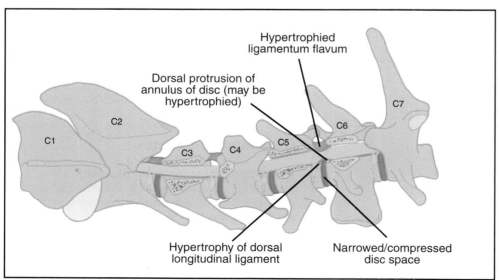

Hypertrophied ligamentum flavum

Dorsal protrusion of annulus of disc (may be hypertrophied)

C1 C2 C3 C4 C5 C6 C7

Hypertrophy of dorsal longitudinal ligament

Narrowed/compressed disc space

15.11 Soft tissue abnormalities that may contribute to cervical stenotic myelopathy in the caudal cervical spine are shown at C5–C6. The normal relationship of the soft tissues is shown at C2–C3 and C3–C4.

- Hypertrophy of the ligamentum flavum and dorsal longitudinal ligament. These changes are also common in disc-associated Wobbler syndrome
- Hypertrophy of synovial membrane and formation of synovial cysts at the articular facets. This is commonly seen with stenotic myelopathy in giant-breed dogs and is associated with remodelling of the facets (Dickinson *et al.*, 2001)
- Stenosis of the vertebral canal. Historically, this has been described in giant-breed dogs with stenotic myelopathy; however, there is evidence that Dobermanns also have a relative stenosis of the cervical vertebral canal (da Costa *et al.*, 2006a; De Decker *et al.*, 2011)
- Degenerative joint disease and remodelling of the articular facets. This is commonly seen with stenotic myelopathy in giant-breed dogs.

The aetiology of these changes is most likely multifactorial. Genetic factors probably play a role as the disease is seen in specific breeds of dog, although a pattern of inheritance has not been established in commonly affected breeds (Burbidge *et al.*, 1994). Over nutrition and excess calcium supplementation in the first year of life has been implicated in Great Danes (Hedhammer *et al.*, 1974), but correction of these feeding patterns has not prevented occurrence of the disease in this breed. It has been postulated that head and neck conformation influences the development of lesions. However, a study on Dobermanns failed to find a correlation between various body dimensions and radiographic or neurological signs (Burbidge *et al.*, 1994). It is believed by many that the degenerative changes seen with this syndrome ultimately result from relative 'instability' in the cervical spine.

In general, giant-breed dogs present within the first 3 years of life with degenerative changes of the articular facets and their associated synovium, synovial cysts and stenosis of the vertebral canal, affecting C3–T1 (da Costa *et al.*, 2011; Gutierrez-Quintana and Penderis, 2012). Large-breed dogs are more likely to present with disc-associated Wobbler syndrome or caudal cervical spondylomyelopathy. They develop signs in middle-age or older as a result of hypertrophy and protrusion of the annulus, and ligamentous hypertrophy affecting the caudal cervical vertebrae. The changes can be described as static (spinal cord compression not altered by flexion, extension or traction) or dynamic (compression altered by flexion, extension or traction). In approximately 50% of large-breed and 80% of giant-breed dogs, compressive lesions may be present at more than one site (da Costa *et al.*, 2011).

Diagnosis: Survey radiographs of the cervical spine may show degenerative changes typical of this syndrome (Figure 15.12), but cannot be used to identify sites of spinal cord compression (De Decker *et al.*, 2011; da Costa and Johnson, 2012). Stressed (dorsal and ventral flexion) views should not be taken as compression of the spinal cord can be exacerbated. Myelography combined with computed tomography (CT) used to be the gold standard for

diagnosis of cervical spondylomyelopathy (da Costa *et al.*, 2012) and for surgical planning (Figure 15.13). Linear traction views with myelography are used to determine whether compression can be addressed

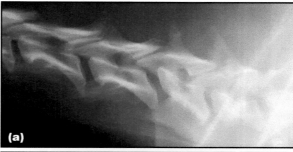
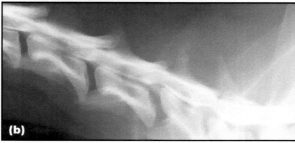

15.12 **(a)** Lateral cervical radiograph and **(b)** myelogram from an 8-year-old Dobermann with cervical stenotic myelopathy. Note the tipping of C6. The myelogram reveals severe compression of the spinal cord at C5–C6 and C6–C7.

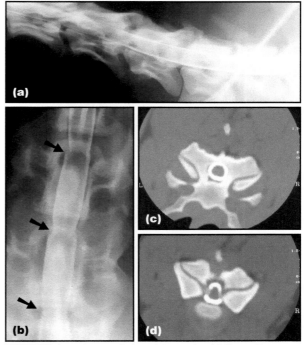

15.13 Imaging study in a 14-month-old Great Dane with ataxia and tetraparesis. **(a)** The lateral myelogram does not reveal any sites of compression but **(b)** the ventrodorsal view shows three sites of lateral compression of the caudal cervical spinal cord (arrowed). **(c)** Transverse CT myelogram at the centre of the vertebral body at C5 showing the normal appearance of the spinal cord. **(d)** Transverse CT myelogram at the level of the articular processes, highlighting the lateral compression of the spinal cord by the enlarged processes.

by distraction and fusion of the vertebrae (i.e. a dynamic lesion) (Sharp *et al.*, 1992). However, magnetic resonance imaging (MRI) (Figure 15.14) has largely replaced CT and myelography (Lipsitz *et al.*, 2001; Penderis and Dennis, 2004; da Costa *et al.*, 2006ab). The advantages of MRI include greater accuracy at detecting spinal cord compression and parenchymal disease. In addition, this imaging modality is associated with decreased morbidity (da Costa *et al.*, 2006b).

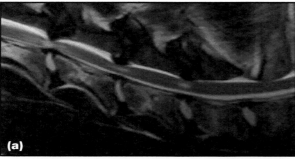
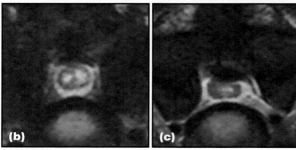

15.14 T2-weighted MR images of a 7-year-old male neutered Great Dane with dorsal compressive lesions at C4–C5, C5–C6 and C6–C7. **(a)** The dorsal compressive lesions (due to hypertrophied ligamentum flavum) are clearly visible on the sagittal view. **(b)** Focal parenchymal damage is also visible on the sagittal view and on the axial images at C6–C7 and **(c)** at C5–C6.

Treatment and prognosis: It is recommended that dogs with neurological deficits be treated surgically as this is a chronic progressive disease (da Costa *et al.*, 2008; De Decker *et al.*, 2009). However, many owners cannot afford or do not wish to have surgery performed, and medical therapy can be considered in such cases as well as in dogs with mild deficits.

Medical management: Medical management includes treatment of pain with anti-inflammatory drugs and muscle relaxants, along with restriction of unmonitored activity combined with controlled exercise and physical therapy (see Chapter 25). Anti-inflammatory doses of corticosteroids have been used to reduce vasogenic oedema (da Costa *et al.*, 2008; De Decker *et al.*, 2009) but do not appear to influence the outcome. Acupuncture can be useful to control chronic pain in some dogs. Dogs managed in this way should be monitored once or twice weekly to ensure early recognition of deterioration and allow recommendation for surgical intervention.

In a large study comparing surgical (n = 37) and medical management (n = 67) of cervical spondylomyelopathy, 54% of dogs treated medically improved compared with 81% of dogs treated surgically (da Costa *et al.*, 2008). However, the median survival time of the two groups was the same (36 months), suggesting that whilst surgery might provide early benefits, in the longer term the therapeutic advantages are lost. These findings are supported by another study of medical therapy in which 45% of 51 dogs with disc-associated Wobbler syndrome had a successful outcome without surgical intervention and the overall median survival time was 47 months (De Decker *et al.*, 2009), but in a third study only 8 of 21 dogs (38%) had a successful outcome with medical management (De Decker *et al.*, 2012).

Surgical management: The aims of surgery are to decompress and/or stabilize the cervical spine. Surgical strategies include the ventral slot (to remove disc material from the canal), distraction/stabilization techniques (to treat lesions responsive to traction) and dorsal laminectomy (to eliminate dorsal compression or address multiple disc protrusions). Cervical arthroplasty, using a titanium prosthesis to replace the disc, has been introduced more recently (Adamo, 2011). Surgical decisions are based on the type and number of lesions present, and surgeon preference; a full discussion of the different surgical procedures can be found elsewhere (McKee and Sharp, 2003; da Costa, 2010; Tobias and Johnson, 2011).

One significant problem of surgery is the development of new lesions adjacent to the previous surgical site (the domino effect) (Rusbridge *et al.*, 1998). Whilst there is controversy as to whether the development of domino lesions purely reflects the natural course of the disease (Jeffery and McKee, 2001), there is some evidence that surgical intervention does lead to the development of new lesions at adjacent sites (da Costa and Parent, 2007). Early surgical fusion of suspicious sites adjacent to the main lesion or procedures that preserve motion of the vertebral units (such as cervical arthroplasty) may help to reduce this problem in the future. Postoperative rehabilitation of patients is critical to their recovery and owners need to be fully informed about the implications of rehabilitating a non-ambulatory large or giant-breed dog (see Chapter 25). Rehabilitation includes passive range of motion exercises and massage in the recumbent dog, hydrotherapy and controlled exercise. Recovery of these dogs can be prolonged (6–12 weeks or more) due to the chronic nature of the disease.

Surgical success rates for dogs with disc-associated Wobbler syndrome (ventral slot, distraction/fusion techniques and dorsal laminectomy) are about 80% in the short-term (<1 year) (Jeffrey and McKee, 2001; da Costa *et al.*, 2008; da Costa, 2010). The presence of multiple lesions and severe neurological deficits (non-ambulatory) worsens the prognosis. The prognosis in the long term is not as good with a recurrence of signs developing in about 20% of dogs. There is less information available regarding the prognosis of giant-breed dogs with cervical stenotic myelopathy treated surgically, but outcomes appear to be comparable with those of dogs with disc-associated Wobbler syndrome (de Risio *et al.*, 2002; da Costa *et al.*, 2008).

Acute cervical disc disease

Acute cervical disc disease is a common problem in dogs, with few reports in cats. Hansen type II disc disease is addressed in the section on disc-associated Wobbler syndrome (see above). Hansen type I disc disease is described here.

Clinical signs: Cervical disc disease is a common problem in chondrodystrophoid breeds of dog such as Dachshunds, Shih Tzus and Pekingese. It is also frequently seen in Beagles and Cocker Spaniels, but can occur sporadically in almost any breed. Although thoracolumbar disc herniations have been reported in cats (see Chapter 16), cervical disc herniations have not been described in this species.

Onset of signs can occur from 18 months of age, with a peak incidence between 3 and 7 years old. It is unusual for a disc herniation to occur in dogs <2 years of age as the predisposing degenerative changes have not yet occurred. The most common presenting sign is severe neck pain (Cherrone *et al.*, 2004). The usual explanation for the lack of neurological deficits is that there is enough space within the cervical vertebral canal for herniation of disc material without compression of the spinal cord (see Chapter 14). The dog may adopt a stance with the head held down, neck rigid and back arched as the weight is shifted to the pelvic limbs (see **Cervical disc herniation** clip on DVD). Entrapment of nerve roots can cause a nerve root signature (holding up a thoracic limbs and lameness). The neck pain is so severe that dogs avoid moving their heads; spasm and rigidity of the cervical musculature are easily palpable. Neurological deficits are less common but can occur when the spinal cord is sufficiently compressed and include tetraparesis/hemiparesis, tetraplegia/hemiplegia, ataxia, and conscious proprioceptive and postural reaction deficits.

Pathogenesis: The intervertebral disc comprises an outer fibrous portion (the annulus fibrosus) and a gelatinous centre (the nucleus pulposus). With normal ageing the nucleus is slowly replaced by fibrocartilage, but in chondrodystrophoid breeds the nucleus ages prematurely and the nucleus matrix degenerates and mineralizes (Figure 15.15) (Bray and Burbidge, 1998ab; Brisson, 2010). There is also evidence of differences in the cellular characteristics and morphometry of the nucleus and annulus fibrosus in chondrodystrophoid breeds (Johnson *et al.*, 2010). For example, in the cervical spine, the nucleus pulposus occupies a smaller proportion of the intervertebral disc in chondrodystrophoid breeds compared with non-chondrodystrophoid breeds. As a result of these morphometric and degenerative changes, affected dogs are prone to extrusion of the mineralized nucleus pulposus into the spinal canal (Hansen type I disc herniations) causing spinal cord concussion and compression. The C2–C3 disc is

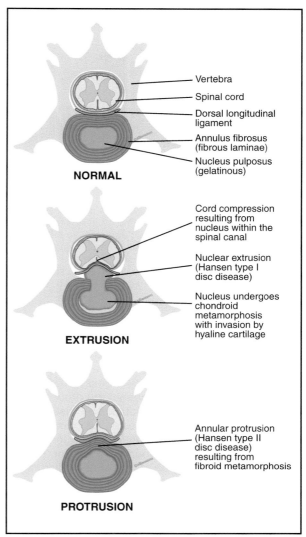

15.15 Normal structure and anatomical relationship of the intervertebral disc and the pathological changes seen with disc extrusion and protrusion.

most commonly affected in small breeds with the incidence decreasing further caudally in the cervical spine, whilst large breeds frequently suffer disc herniations at C6–C7 (Dallman *et al.*, 1992; Cherrone *et al.*, 2004).

Diagnosis: Survey radiographs should be taken to identify degenerative changes typical of disc herniation and to rule out other causes of the signs. Changes indicative of disc herniation include narrowing of the intervertebral disc space, narrowing of the intervertebral foramen and the presence of mineralized material within the vertebral canal and disc space (see Chapter 5). However, a definitive diagnosis cannot be reached with survey radiographs alone. Indeed, one study found that the correct site of disc extrusion was located only 35% of the time (Somerville *et al.*, 2001). Advanced imaging modalities such as myelography, CT and MRI (Ryan *et al.*, 2008) are necessary to identify the site of spinal cord compression (Figure 15.16).

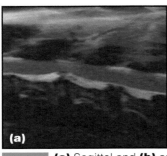 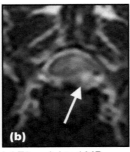

15.16 **(a)** Sagittal and **(b)** axial T2-weighted MR images of a 14-year-old neutered Dachshund bitch with an acute onset of tetraparesis and neck pain. The spinal cord is deviated dorsally by herniated disc material on the sagittal view and there is a hyperintensity within the spinal cord parenchyma overlying the herniated disc. The material is clearly visible in the ventrolateral aspect of the canal on the axial image (arrowed). The disc material is isointense and hypointense compared with the spinal cord, suggesting that it is not mineralized. This was confirmed at surgery.

Treatment and prognosis:

Medical management: Dogs can be managed medically with strict cage rest for 4 weeks combined with pain relief using anti-inflammatory drugs, opioids and/or muscle relaxants. Judicious use of anti-inflammatory doses of corticosteroids combined with appropriate cage confinement can be attempted if a definitive diagnosis has been reached and the pain is not responsive to non-steroidal anti-inflammatory drugs (NSAIDs). Muscle spasms can also be responsive to gentle massage and hot packing of the neck. Administration of an H2 receptor antagonist (such as famotidine) or a proton pump inhibitor (for example, omeprazole or pantoprazole) may help to prevent the development of gastric ulceration.

The aim of cage rest is to allow defects in the annulus fibrosus to heal, and resolution of pain does not mean that confinement should be discontinued. If this approach is successful, a gradual reintroduction to controlled exercise can be attempted and the owners should be cautioned to prevent their pet from taking part in activities that involve jumping in the long term.

Dogs should be monitored weekly and if the pain is unresponsive to medical therapy in the first week, recurs, or neurological deficits develop, surgery should be recommended. The prognosis for dogs treated medically is unknown, although one study of dogs presumptively diagnosed with cervical disc disease found that approximately 50% recovered with medical management alone (Levine *et al.*, 2007).

Surgical management: Indications for surgery include unremitting or severe pain, recurrent pain or neurological deficits. Once the site of disc extrusion has been confirmed, a ventral slot is performed to remove the herniated disc material (see Chapter 22 for a description of the surgical technique). Adjacent discs are fenestrated to prevent recurrence of the problem. Other surgical approaches have been advocated, including hemilaminectomy to address lateralized disc herniations (Rossmeisl *et al.*, 2005), ventral slot decompression combined with stabilization (Fitch *et al.*, 2000) and dorsal laminectomy (Gill *et al.*, 1996).

Postoperatively, dogs are provided with pain relief and confined for 4 weeks (2 weeks of strict confinement and then, if the animal is doing well, 2 weeks of increasing controlled exercise). Dogs are then gradually re-introduced to normal activity. If the dog has neurological deficits, postoperative care includes performing passive range of motion exercises, massage, hydrotherapy and controlled exercise (see Chapter 25 for further information). Whilst typically successful, disc surgery on the cervical spine is fraught with potentially severe complications, including the development of aspiration pneumonia (Java *et al.*, 2009), cardiac arrhythmias (Stauffer *et al.*, 1988) and luxation following ventral slot procedures (Lemarie *et al.*, 2000). Video-assisted techniques are being developed to allow a minimally invasive approach to the cervical spine, thus reducing the risk of luxation (Leperlier *et al.*, 2011).

The prognosis for dogs treated surgically is excellent with resolution of cervical hyperaesthesia and the return of normal ambulation in 99% of cases (Cherrone *et al.*, 2004). Predictors of outcome include severity of neurological deficits and size of the dog (small-breed dogs show a more complete recovery than large breeds) (Hillman *et al.*, 2009).

Discal cysts

This newly recognized condition (also called ventral intraspinal cysts) is characterized by the presence of a cyst directly overlying an intervertebral disc (Konar *et al.*, 2008). Whilst this is most commonly a cervical spinal disease, thoracolumbar discal cysts can also occur.

Clinical signs: Typically these cases have an acute or subacute (progression over 7–10 days) clinical course. Affected dogs present with cervical pain and paresis (Konar *et al.*, 2008).

Pathogenesis: The pathogenesis of this disease is poorly understood. Theories for the equivalent disease in humans include the proposal that the cyst develops secondary to an epidural haemorrhage as a result of sinus damage secondary to disc herniation, and that the cyst forms around a small disc herniation.

Diagnosis: Discal cysts have a characteristic appearance on MRI. The spinal cord is compressed by a cystic structure that lies directly over an intervertebral disc, which has a contrast-enhancing wall (Figure 15.17).

Treatment and prognosis: Dogs respond to surgical decompression via a ventral slot approach. The prognosis appears to be good (Konar *et al.*, 2008).

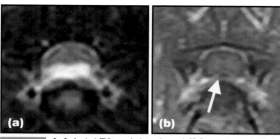

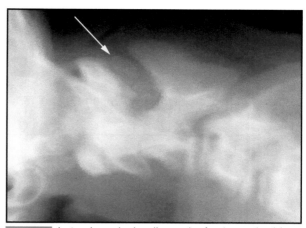

15.17 **(a)** Axial T2-weighted and **(b)** post-gadolinium T1-weighted MR images of a 10-year-old Miniature Pinscher with an acute onset of non-ambulatory tetraparesis and pain. (a) A cyst is visible as a hyperintense structure on the ventral floor of the canal causing compression of the overlying spinal cord. (b) The contrast-enhanced capsule (arrowed) surrounding the hypointense fluid centre is visible.

15.18 Lateral cervical radiograph of a 4-month-old Viszla with calcinosis circumscripta. Note the focus of mineralization dorsal to the atlas (arrowed).

Synovial cysts

Clinical signs: Affected animals are typically either young giant-breed dogs with multiple cysts present in the cervical spine, or older large-breed dogs with a single cyst in the thoracolumbar spine (Dickinson *et al.*, 2001) (see Chapter 16). Neurological deficits include spinal hyperaesthesia and signs of a chronic and progressive myelopathy, reflecting the site of the lesion.

Pathogenesis: Large cysts can develop from the synovial membranes around the articular processes, causing dorsolateral compression of the spinal cord. This can occur as a component of cervical spondylo-myelopathy (see above) or be an isolated disorder.

Diagnosis: Degenerative joint disease of the affected articular processes is usually visible on survey radiographs. Extradural lesions causing dorsolateral spinal cord compression are visible on myelography (± CT) and MRI. There are non-specific changes on cerebrospinal fluid (CSF) analysis. The precise nature of the lesion is confirmed at surgery.

Treatment and prognosis: The spinal cord can be decompressed by surgical removal of the cysts. This is usually achieved by dorsal laminectomy in the cervical spine and hemilaminectomy in the thoracolumbar spine. Prognosis is usually good in uncomplicated cases that are addressed before the neurological deficits become advanced.

Calcinosis circumscripta

Clinical signs: This is an unusual disease of young, large-breed dogs such as German Shepherd Dogs and Rottweilers. Affected dogs show progressive tetraparesis or paraparesis, depending on the location of the lesion.

Pathogenesis: Mineralization of the ligamentous structures of the vertebral column, usually either dorsal to the atlantoaxial junction or dorsal to the mid-thoracic spine (Figure 15.18), causes pain and compression of the spinal cord (Lewis and Kelly, 1990). Renal disease and trauma are both known to cause ectopic mineralization, but there is no evidence of either problem in these dogs. Postulated causes include a foreign body reaction to aberrant mesenchymal tissue and an as yet unidentified inherited defect of calcium and phosphate homeostasis (De Risio and Olby, 2000).

Diagnosis: The diagnosis can be made from a survey spinal radiograph. Routine blood work should be performed to rule out renal disease and to check calcium and phosphate levels. Parathyroid hormone concentrations can also be measured. Radiographs of the limbs should be obtained to identify other sites of soft tissue mineralization.

Treatment and prognosis: Surgical decompression is recommended and is successful in dogs with single lesions, mild to moderate neurological deficits and no evidence of an underlying cause.

Anomalous diseases

Atlantoaxial instability

Clinical signs: Onset of signs in dogs with the congenital form of the disease usually occurs in young animals (<2 years of age), although problems can develop at any age. Signs can develop acutely or gradually, and waxing and waning of signs is often reported (presumably a reflection of instability at the atlantoaxial junction causing repeated injury to the spinal cord). Signs include neck pain (variably present), ataxia, tetraparesis, and postural reaction and conscious proprioceptive deficits with normal to increased muscle tone and myotatic reflexes in all four legs. In severe cases, animals can present with tetraplegia and difficulty breathing, and may die as a result of respiratory failure. Some animals present with seizure-like episodes that involve sudden-onset opisthotonus and vocalization, presumably reflecting intermittent compression of the spinal cord and nerve roots, causing severe but transient pain and paresis.

Pathogenesis: The atlas and axis are bound together by ligaments that run from the dens of the axis to the atlas (apical ligament) and the skull, over the dens binding it to the floor of the atlas (the transverse ligament) and between the dorsal lamina of the atlas and the dorsal spinous process of the axis (dorsal atlantoaxial ligament) (Figure 15.19).

The dens is a bony projection from the cranial aspect of the body of the axis and develops from a separate growth plate. Subluxation of the atlanto-axial junction is a relatively common problem and can be caused by trauma or, more commonly, congenital malformations (Figure 15.20). It is not uncommon to see additional congenital malformations of

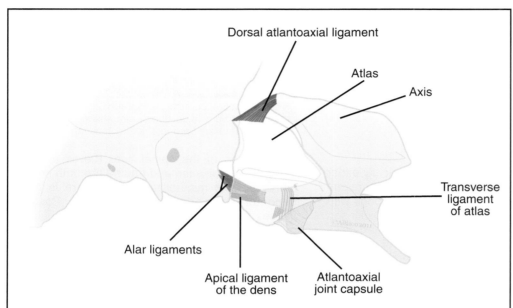

15.19 Ligaments of the atlas and axis vertebrae.

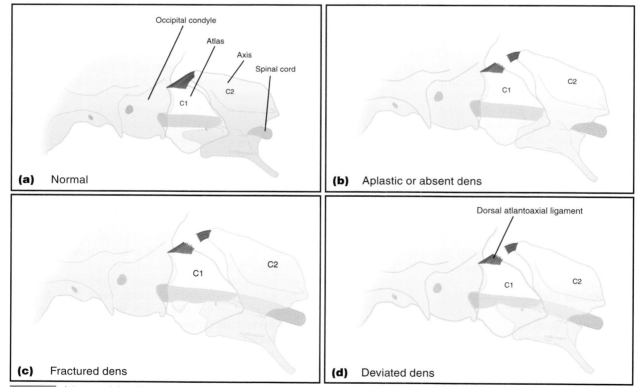

15.20 Atlantoaxial subluxation. **(a)** Normal relationship of the axis (C2) to the atlas (C1) and the spinal cord. **(b)** Subluxation associated with an aplastic or absent odontoid process (dens). Clinical signs may not be severe as there is minimal compression. However, concussion is always possible and can lead to severe motor and sensory dysfunction. **(c)** Subluxation due to traumatic fracture. Trauma may lead to fracture of the dens but is often associated with ligament rupture. **(d)** Subluxation associated with a dorsally deviated dens. Compression of the spinal cord can be exacerbated by such a subluxation. (Modified from Wheeler and Sharp, 1994)

the cervical spine, such as block vertebrae (see Chapter 5). The atlantoaxial and atlanto-occipital regions are prone to congenital defects, and atlanto-occipital overlapping can occur as a developmental disorder in this region (see Chapter 14 for full details). Aplasia, hypoplasia or dorsal angulation of the dens may be seen (particularly in toy and small breeds of dog). In addition, there may also be congenital absence of the transverse ligament and incomplete ossification of the atlas (Warren-Smith *et al.*, 2009; Parry *et al.*, 2010).

Diagnosis: Atlantoaxial subluxation can be diagnosed from survey radiographs of the cervical spine, although extreme care must be taken when restraining and moving dogs in which this condition is suspected. If the animal is sedated or anaesthetized, the head and neck should be supported in slight extension to avoid further spinal cord injury. On lateral radiographs an increased space can be seen between the dorsal lamina of the atlas and the dorsal spinous process of the axis. In severe cases, malalignment of the bodies of the atlas and axis is clearly visible (see Chapter 5). The presence and size of the dens can be evaluated most accurately on ventrodorsal (VD) views. If there is no evidence of subluxation on the lateral views, the neck can be carefully flexed to check for instability (the space between the dorsal lamina of the atlas and the dorsal spinous process of the axis should be evaluated). It is preferable to conduct this examination using fluoroscopy, so that movement can be monitored in order to prevent iatrogenic subluxation. Advanced imaging is commonly performed to aid decision-making for surgery. CT allows clear identification of the bony components of the atlantoaxial region, facilitating surgical planning for implant placement. MRI highlights the spinal cord and brainstem parenchyma, allowing diagnosis of concurrent abnormalities such as Chiari-like malformations and hydrocephalus, which might complicate recovery from surgery.

Treatment and prognosis:

Medical management: Dogs with mild signs can be treated conservatively by placing an external splint for at least 6 weeks. The splint must immobilize the atlantoaxial junction, so must come over the head cranial to the ears and go back to the level of the chest (Figure 15.21). The aim is to stabilize the junction whilst the ligamentous structures heal. The dog and splint should be checked daily for signs of decubital ulcers by the owner and weekly by the veterinary surgeon, with regular bandage changes if necessary. Splint placement addresses the instability and can produce an immediate improvement, although severe displacement of the atlantoaxial junction may not be adequately addressed. In one study, 6 of 16 dogs failed to improve following splint placement and were euthanased; the remaining 10 dogs responded well and maintained a good outcome 1 year following splint removal (Havig *et al.*, 2005).

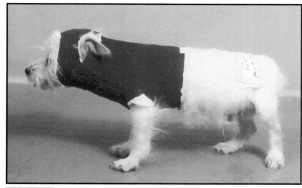

15.21 An 8-month-old West Highland White Terrier with a splint placed to prevent movement of the atlantoaxial junction. A thick layer of cast padding was placed first, then a splint was modelled to run ventral to the chin, neck and sternum. This was then held in place with another layer of bandage.

Surgical management: Surgery is recommended in dogs with neurological deficits, although it can be associated with high perioperative morbidity and mortality (Thomas *et al.*, 1991; Beaver *et al.*, 2000). Dorsal and ventral approaches to the atlantoaxial junction have both been described. However, dorsal approaches, although requiring less dissection and retraction of important soft tissue structures (e.g. oesophagus, pharynx and larynx), are associated with a greater risk of causing spinal cord injury during surgery and a higher incidence of implant failure. Newer implants designed for dorsal placement, such as the Kishigami Atlantoaxial Tension Band, have shown promise (Pujol *et al.*, 2010). With ventral approaches, subluxation is reduced and the atlantoaxial articular surfaces are curetted to promote bony fusion. The two bones are fused using transarticular screws or Kirschner wires and a cancellous bone graft is placed over the junction (Figure 15.22). In cases of traumatic injury or poor bone purchase, screws or Kirschner wires are placed in the bodies of the atlas and the axis, and the junction is stabilized with polymethylmethacrylate cement (Figure 15.23) (Platt *et al.*, 2004; Sanders *et al.*,

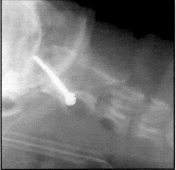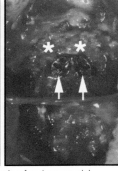

15.22 Lateral cervical radiograph of a 1-year-old Yorkshire Terrier showing surgical repair of an atlantoaxial subluxation. Two transarticular screws were placed once the subluxation was reduced. The heads of the screws are denoted with arrows in the surgical image. A cancellous bone graft was placed over the articulation between C1 and C2 (✱).

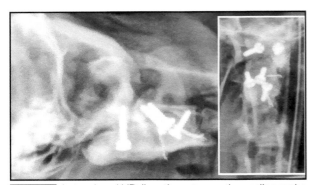

15.23 Lateral and VD (inset) postoperative radiographs of the atlantoaxial junction in a 1-year-old Toy Poodle. The atlantoaxial subluxation was initially reduced using wires around screws placed in the body of C2. Two screws were needed to correct both the dorsal and lateral deviation of C2 on C1. Two screws were placed in C1 and all five screws were covered in polymethylmethacrylate. The dog made an excellent recovery.

2004) or locking plates. A neck splint may be placed postoperatively whilst fusion occurs if transarticular screws alone are used. This is a problematic area to repair surgically; bone quality is often poor, the bones are small, movement of the vertebrae may cause additional injury to the spinal cord, and the pharynx and larynx can be damaged during retraction. There is a risk of respiratory arrest and death in the perioperative period as a result of additional spinal cord injury or inflammation of the upper airways secondary to retraction.

Whilst this is a serious condition, dogs treated surgically have an excellent prognosis if they survive the 48-hour perioperative period. Although reported surgical success rates range from 50% to 90%, the majority report a mortality rate in the region of 20% with a large number of deaths occurring either during or immediately following surgery (Thomas *et al.*, 1991; Beaver *et al.*, 2000; Platt *et al.*, 2004; Sanders *et al.*, 2004). As with all spinal cord diseases, prognosis is worse in animals with severe and chronic neurological deficits. It has also been shown that prognosis is better in young dogs (<24 months) (Beaver *et al.*, 2000).

Intra-arachnoid cysts
Intra-arachnoid cysts are focal accumulations of CSF within the subarachnoid space. The term cyst is somewhat misleading, as frequently cyst walls are not evident, and so the term arachnoid diverticulum is occasionally used. Accumulation of CSF over time causes progressive compression of the spinal cord and neurological deficits related to the site of compression.

Clinical signs: Intra-arachnoid cysts occur most commonly in young large-breed dogs, frequently dorsal to the cranial cervical spinal cord, and in older small-breed dogs, typically dorsal to the thoracolumbar spinal cord (see also Chapter 16). There is an apparent predisposition to the disease in Rottweilers (Rylander *et al.*, 2002; Gnirs *et al.*, 2003; Jurina and Grevel, 2004) and Pugs (Skeen *et*

al., 2003), although cysts can occur at any site, any age and in any breed of dog. Onset of signs (including tetraparesis, paraparesis and ataxia) is typically chronic and it is notable that dogs can present with faecal and/or urinary incontinence as an early sign (Skeen *et al.*, 2003). Neck pain may be present.

Pathogenesis: The aetiology of these cysts is most likely multifactorial with inherited predisposition, trauma, intervertebral disc disease and arachnoiditis all postulated to play a role (Dyce *et al.*, 1991; Skeen *et al.*, 2003).

Diagnosis: Survey radiographs are unremarkable. Cysts are visible as focal accumulations of contrast medium in the subarachnoid space or as intradural filling defects on myelography. On MRI, cysts appear as accumulations of fluid within the subarachnoid space (Figure 15.24).

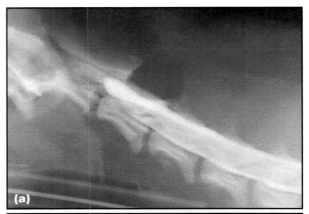
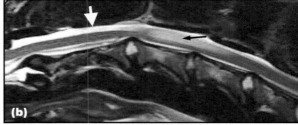

15.24 **(a)** Lateral cervical myelogram of a 1-year-old Labrador Retriever. The subarachnoid space is markedly dilated over C2–C3 as a result of an intra-arachnoid cyst. **(b)** Sagittal T2-weighted MR image of a similar subarachnoid cyst in a 9-month-old male Bloodhound. The parenchymal hyperintensity (black arrow) suggests a wider disturbance of CSF flow than simply obstruction of the subarachnoid space (white arrow).

Treatment and prognosis: The recommended treatment in dogs with progressive neurological deficits is surgical decompression by removal or fenestration and marsupialization of cysts. Medical management may improve a small proportion of dogs, but is only recommended in animals with mild neurological deficits. Medical management includes controlled exercise and anti-inflammatory doses of prednisone. Animals should be monitored regularly and surgery recommended if deterioration occurs.

The prognosis of dogs treated surgically depends on the severity and duration of the clinical signs and the age of the animal. Young dogs with mild signs have an excellent short-term prognosis when treated surgically (<1 year). Signs may recur in approximately one-third of dogs in the longer term (Skeen *et al.*, 2003). Outcome is not as good in older dogs with a long history of clinical signs and surgery should be approached with caution in these animals.

Dermoid sinus
Dermoid sinuses are inherited developmental defects in which there is a failure of separation of the skin and neural tube, leading to the formation of a sinus that extends to the supraspinous ligament or the subarachnoid space. This disease is described in full in Chapter 16.

Osteochondromatosis
Osteochondromatosis (also known as cartilaginous exostoses and multiple cartilaginous exostoses) is a disease of growing dogs in which bony protuberances, capped by cartilage, develop from the region near the growth plate of bones of endochondral origin. Vertebral lesions commonly arise, causing severe spinal cord compression. This disease is described in full in Chapter 16 and the associated radiographic changes are illustrated in Chapter 5.

Syringomyelia and Chiari-like malformations
Syringomyelia is characterized by the presence of a fluid-filled cavity within the parenchyma of the spinal cord. Hydromyelia refers to dilatation of the central canal. Syringomyelia may exist independently or in communication with the central canal (syringohydromyelia). As it can be difficult to differentiate the two conditions based on imaging studies alone, the term syringomyelia is preferred (Cappello and Rusbridge, 2007). This condition can be a secondary long-term complication of any spinal cord disease in which either a large volume of spinal cord tissue becomes necrotic or there is obstruction of normal CSF flow within the spinal cord. For example, syringomyelia may be seen with neoplasia (particularly intra-axial tumours) or feline coronavirus (the causative agent of feline infectious peritonitis) infection associated with ependymitis. The most common cause of syringomyelia in Cavalier King Charles Spaniels and other small breeds such as Pomeranians and Brussels Griffons is Chiari-like malformations. Neurological signs are caused by the progressive expansion of the fluid-filled cavities and relate to their location. The most common clinical signs are cervical pain and paraesthesia. For further information, see Chapter 14.

Vertebral and spinal cord anomalies
Atlantoaxial subluxation is the most common consequence of vertebral anomalies that cause tetraparesis (see above). Other vertebral anomalies include hemivertebrae, transitional, block and butterfly vertebrae, congenital spinal stenosis (often a component of cervical stenotic myelopathy) and vertebral facet dysplasia. These diseases are considered in full in Chapters 5 (radiographic appearance),

14 and 16. Syringomyelia is a common anomalous spinal cord disease that may cause tetraparesis and is described in Chapter 14. Other congenital spinal cord diseases (including spinal dysraphism) are described in full in Chapter 16. Anomalous diseases affecting the cauda equina (e.g. sacrocaudal dysgenesis) are considered in Chapter 19.

Neoplastic diseases
Spinal neoplasia can cause pain and tetraparesis or paraparesis depending on the location of the lesion. In dogs, extradural tumours (e.g. primary or metastatic sarcomas, metastatic carcinomas and phaeochromocytomas, and round cell tumours) account for approximately 50–60% of spinal tumours, intradural tumours (e.g. meningiomas and nerve sheath tumours) for approximately 30%, and intramedullary tumours (e.g. gliomas and ependymomas) account for approximately 10% (Prata, 1977). In cats, the most common spinal tumour is lymphoma. Spinal lymphoma is usually extradural and more likely to occur in the thoracolumbar spine, but can occur in the cervical spine and may infiltrate the brachial plexus (Spodnick *et al.*, 1992; Lane *et al.*, 1994). Neoplasia is more likely to affect older animals and can result in signs due to direct compression of the spinal cord, infiltration and destruction of the spinal cord parenchyma, intraparenchymal haemorrhage or by inducing pathological vertebral fractures. The diagnosis, treatment and prognosis of neoplasia affecting the vertebrae and spinal cord are addressed in detail in Chapter 16. Chapters 23 and 24 provide information on chemotherapy and radiotherapy, respectively.

Inflammatory diseases

Discospondylitis
Infection of the intervertebral disc and adjacent vertebral endplates by bacterial or fungal organisms is a common cause of spinal hyperaesthesia in dogs; cats are rarely affected. If left untreated, spinal cord dysfunction can occur as a result of local inflammation, compression from infected herniated disc material or local abscess formation, or pathological vertebral fractures. Discospondylitis can affect any site in the spine and caudal cervical lesions are common. Hyperaesthesia is the most common presenting sign. The diagnosis, treatment and prognosis of discospondylitis are covered in Chapter 14.

Spinal empyema
Epidural empyema is a rare but important cause of spinal cord disease and has been reported in both dogs and cats. Local bacterial infection of the epidural fat results in the accumulation of purulent material, which causes compression and inflammation of the adjacent spinal cord. This can be a result of local extension of infection from discospondylitis, grass awn migration, bites and other external trauma, or can result from haematogenous spread. In humans, it is also reported as a complication of spinal surgery and epidural catheter placement. Characteristic signs include a high fever, acute

progressive spinal hyperaesthesia and progressive myelopathy with the neurological deficits reflecting the site of infection. The diagnosis and treatment of spinal empyema are described in Chapter 16.

Meningoencephalomyelitis

Inflammatory conditions of the meninges and CNS can cause tetraparesis as a result of involvement of the brainstem and/or spinal cord. Typically signs are multifocal, but any inflammatory or infectious CNS disease can cause focal signs of spinal cord disease, including those caused by feline coronavirus, canine distemper virus, fungi (particularly *Cryptococcus neoformans*), protozoa (e.g. *Neospora caninum* and *Toxoplasma gondii*), Rickettsia and granulomatous meningoencephalomyelitis (GME). These diseases are diagnosed by CSF analysis in combination with appropriate titres and are considered in Chapters 11 and 16.

Steroid-responsive meningitis–arteritis

The predominant manifestation of steroid-responsive meningitis–arteritis (SRMA) is severe spinal hyperaesthesia. With chronic, severe disease, neurological deficits (ataxia, paraparesis or tetraparesis) can be present as a result of concurrent myelitis, but this is unusual (Cizinauskas *et al.*, 2000). For further information on this condition, see Chapter 14.

Toxic diseases

Tetanus

Clinical signs: Presenting signs include a generalized increase in extensor tone manifesting as a stiff, stilted gait, raised tail and a characteristic facial expression ('risus sardonicus') as a result of increased facial muscle tone (see **Tetanus** clip on DVD). The palpebral fissure is wider than usual, the pupils are miotic, the ears are rigid, the lips are drawn back and the forehead is wrinkled. The third eyelid may be protruded and there is often profuse salivation because the animal has difficulty swallowing. Owners most frequently report changes in the face and eyes as the first clinical signs that they notice (Burkitt *et al.*, 2007). Visual and tactile stimuli, and placing the animal on its side, often result in a further increase in muscle tone, resulting in muscle spasms (Coleman, 1998). As signs progress, the animal may become recumbent, have difficulty breathing and can develop a hiatal hernia and megaoesophagus as a result of increased diaphragmatic tone. Both bradycardia and tachycardia have been described in dogs with tetanus due to effects of the toxin on the autonomic nervous system. Cats are more likely to present with a focal form of the disease with signs limited to the area of the infection (e.g. monoparesis following distal limb injury, although this has also been reported in dogs) (Malik *et al.*, 1989).

Pathogenesis: Tetanus is caused by absorption of tetanus toxin (tetanospasmin) produced by the anaerobic bacterium *Clostridium tetani*. The source

of the bacterium is usually a penetrating wound or failure of sterile surgical technique providing both contamination with *Clostridium* and the conditions suitable for its growth (Bagley *et al.*, 1994). The toxin is absorbed into the bloodstream and from there is taken up by the nerves. In a similar fashion to botulinum toxin, tetanospasmin has zinc metalloproteinase activity and binds to and cleaves synaptobrevin (a SNARE protein that mediates fusion of synaptic vesicles with the presynaptic membrane), preventing the release of neurotransmitter and causing failure of synaptic transmission (Binz *et al.*, 2010). However, in tetanus the toxin is transported retrogradely up the motor neurons and from there to inhibitory interneurons (the Renshaw cells) where it blocks release of the inhibitory neurotransmitters glycine and gamma aminobutyric acid (GABA). As a result, there is loss of inhibition of the motor neurons, causing a state of rigidity, with superimposed muscle spasms with stimulation. Although both species develop clinical signs, dogs are more susceptible to tetanospasmin than cats (Coleman, 1998).

Diagnosis: The diagnosis is usually presumptive and based on the presence of classic clinical signs. The presence of a wound or history of recent surgery are supportive of the diagnosis. Attempts can be made to culture the organism, but are frequently unsuccessful due to low organism numbers and the need for anaerobic conditions. An infectious process may be suggested by the results of the complete blood count, and creatine kinase concentrations are often elevated due to the increased muscle tone. CSF analysis is unremarkable, nerve conduction studies are normal, but electromyography may reveal prolonged spontaneous motor unit potentials following needle insertion. This can be especially helpful in diagnosing mild or focal forms of the disease. Antibodies to the tetanus toxin can be measured by some laboratories.

Treatment and prognosis: If the source of infection can be identified it should be treated by surgical debridement (if necessary), flushing with hydrogen peroxide and intravenous administration of penicillin G (20,000–100,000 IU/kg q6–12h). Metronidazole, tetracycline and ampicillin are alternative choices of antibiotic if penicillin G is not available. Antitoxin should be administered intravenously (100–500 IU/kg, although a wide range of doses is cited by different authors) to inactivate any circulating toxin. A test dose of 0.1 ml should be given subcutaneously 20–30 minutes prior to the intravenous dose to check for adverse reactions. It is unclear whether antitoxin improves the outcome (Burkitt *et al.*, 2007).

Extensor tone can be reduced with a number of different drugs. Phenobarbital, pentobarbital, acepromazine, chlorpromazine, diazepam and methocarbamol have all been advocated. These drugs also help to reduce patient anxiety. If unable to prehend and swallow food, the animal may need to have a gastrostomy tube placed and in some instances a tracheostomy tube may also be necessary. The animal should be turned regularly and the environmental stimuli kept to a minimum by placing it in a quiet, dark room and putting cotton wool in its ears. Bladder expression or catheterization may be necessary.

Recovery is slow and signs may take up to 4 months to resolve completely, although most animals dramatically improve within a month of starting treatment. Reported outcomes of tetanus vary: in a review of 55 cases of tetanus in the dog, 58% recovered (Mason, 1964), whereas a more recent study of 38 cases reported a 77% survival rate 1 month after the onset of signs (Burkitt *et al.*, 2007). Younger dogs tend to develop more severe clinical signs, and the prognosis is worse in animals with more severe signs.

Traumatic diseases

Spinal cord contusion and traumatic disc herniation

Clinical signs: The signs reflect the site of injury and can be multifocal. A careful examination is therefore vital. A specific syndrome associated with dorsolateral explosion of cervical discs has been described (Griffiths, 1970). In this syndrome, there is acute onset of severe, dramatically lateralizing cervical myelopathy associated with differential hyperthermia (the affected side is 10°C warmer that the spared side due to the destruction of the ipsilateral sympathetic tracts) and positional dystonia (reflecting the destruction of the ipsilateral vestibulospinal tracts).

Pathogenesis: Traumatic injuries (e.g. road traffic accidents, falling from a height, horse kicks) often result in spinal cord injuries, usually with associated vertebral fractures and luxations. However, sometimes animals suffer an obvious traumatic event (either witnessed or other external evidence) associated with acute onset of focal signs of spinal cord dysfunction but there is no evidence of a vertebral fracture or luxation. It is possible for sudden flexion or extension or axial loading of the vertebral column to occur without causing fractures or permanent luxations, but causing contusions to the spinal cord, focal haemorrhage and/or traumatic disc herniations. In the case of cats and non-chondrodystrophic breeds of dog, the herniated nucleus pulposus is often not mineralized and therefore causes a primary contusive injury with little or no compression.

Diagnosis: This is a presumptive diagnosis in the face of a compatible history and clinical findings, with no evidence of vertebral fractures or luxations on survey radiography, CT or myelography. The patient should be handled with extreme care until survey radiographs rule out the presence of an unstable vertebral fracture or luxation. The atlantoaxial junction should be evaluated very carefully as this site is predisposed to injury. A collapsed disc space and focal extradural compression may indicate the presence of traumatic disc herniation and

focal swelling of the spinal cord. MRI can identify focal oedema within the spinal cord and surrounding musculature and may reveal changes in the nucleus pulposus indicating herniation (Figure 15.25).

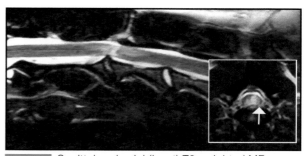

15.25 Sagittal and axial (inset) T2-weighted MR images of a 5-year-old mixed-breed dog that became acutely hemiplegic following a session of rough-housing with another dog. There is a hyperintensity within the spinal cord over the C2–C3 disc space and a small amount of hyperintense material (probably hydrated nucleus pulposus) visible in the canal ventrolateral to the cord (arrowed).

Treatment and prognosis: The protocols for medical management of acute spinal cord injuries are described in Chapter 20. If there is significant compression of the spinal cord by herniated disc material, decompressive surgery may be indicated. Management of the patient focuses on treatment of any other injuries and rehabilitation (see Chapter 25). Prognosis depends of the severity of the injury: it is guarded in the tetraplegic patient with associated hypoventilation, but good if there is any motor function present.

Cervical vertebral fractures and luxations

Clinical signs: Neurological deficits reflect the site of the injury, but as a result of the relatively spacious vertebral canal in the cervical region, quite dramatic luxations can be associated with only minimal neurological deficits and pain (Stone *et al.*, 1979; Hawthorne *et al.*, 1999).

Pathogenesis: Vertebral fractures and luxations can result from pathological processes such as vertebral neoplasia and discospondylitis, but most commonly result from external trauma. Cervical vertebral injuries are less common than thoracolumbar injuries (Selcer *et al.*, 1991), but the atlantoaxial junction relies on ligaments for stability (see above) and is therefore particularly at risk. The axis is the most commonly fractured cervical vertebra because it acts as a fulcrum between the caudal cervical spine and the so-called cervicocranium (the skull, atlas, dens and body of the axis) (Stone *et al.*, 1979) (Figure 15.26).

Diagnosis: Extreme care should be taken when evaluating these animals to avoid exacerbating injuries due to vertebral instability. This can be accomplished by restraining the patient in a purpose built stretcher or by taping them to a rigid surface on

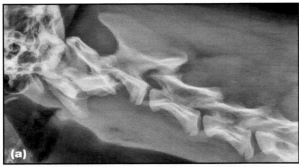
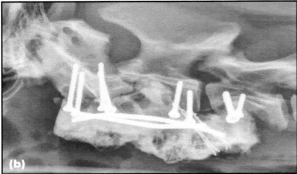

15.26 **(a)** Lateral cervical radiograph of a 7-month-old Dobermann that fell from a balcony. The body of C2 is fractured and displaced dorsally, causing severe compression of the overlying spinal cord. The fracture was reduced by traction wires placed around the heads of the two screws situated in the caudal body of C2. **(b)** Additional screws were placed in C1 and C3 and the construct was stabilized with polymethylmethacrylate cement.

presentation. Initial evaluation and management of the critical patient is covered in Chapter 20. A careful physical and neurological examination should be completed and systemic stabilization of the patient undertaken if indicated. Lateral survey radiographs of the entire spine should be obtained. If there is no evidence of a vertebral fracture or luxation on the lateral views, the animal can be placed carefully on its back to obtain a VD view of the spine (see Chapter 5), or horizontal beam views can be obtained. It is not uncommon for neurological deterioration to occur days after the traumatic incident as a result of instability secondary to a fracture (Hawthorne *et al.*, 1999). It is therefore important to obtain good quality cervical radiographs in any animal in which head and neck trauma is suspected (Olby *et al.*, 2002).

The timing and type of further imaging studies depends on the neurological status of the animal and the radiographic findings: myelography, CT and MRI may each be of benefit. Myelography or MRI is indicated if the clinical findings do not match the survey radiographic findings. CT of lesions identified on survey radiography is appropriate (if the radiographic and clinical findings are in agreement) to obtain good anatomical detail of the bone lesions and relative displacement of bone fragments. However, if the owner does not want spinal surgery to be performed (for financial or other reasons), further imaging will usually not help with case management. In addition, the animal may

have other medical problems that preclude anaesthesia at that time (e.g. cardiac arrhythmias secondary to myocardial trauma).

Treatment and prognosis: Treatment can be medical or surgical.

Medical management: Medical management includes placement of an external splint (in the case of unstable fractures or luxations), cage confinement, provision of analgesia and nursing care, and rehabilitation (see Chapter 25). Splints should be placed on animals with evidence of vertebral instability (see also Chapters 16 and 20) to prevent movement of the affected area. For cervical fractures, the caudal cervical spine and atlantoaxial junction must be included. Medical management is appropriate in cases with mild neurological deficits, minimally displaced fractures/luxations or no evidence of spinal cord compression.

Surgical management: Surgical management is indicated in cases with severe neurological deficits or pain and evidence of compression or vertebral instability on imaging. The aims of surgery are to realign and stabilize the spinal column as well as decompress the spinal cord and intervertebral foramina (to prevent persistent nerve root pain). Stabilization is usually achieved by the placement of screws or pins in the vertebral bodies with the application of polymethylmethacrylate cement around the protruding heads (see Figure 15.26) but plates can also used. A full discussion of surgical techniques is beyond the scope of this Manual and can be found in surgical texts (Wheeler and Sharp, 1994; Tobias and Johnson, 2011).

Prognosis: Prognostic factors have been evaluated in 56 dogs with cervical vertebral fractures (Hawthorne *et al.*, 1999). Non-ambulatory tetraparesis and a prolonged interval from trauma to referral (>5 days) were associated with a worse outcome. Prompt identification and referral of these cases is therefore important. Perioperative mortality was relatively high (4 of 11 dogs suffered cardiopulmonary arrest) in dogs undergoing surgery. This may reflect the need for ventilatory support in severely injured dogs, particularly if the surgery is associated with further iatrogenic damage. In the same study, 37 of 40 dogs managed conservatively recovered, indicating that the prognosis for recovery is good in dogs in which surgery is not indicated. Dogs with severe spinal cord injuries (tetraplegia) that require ventilatory support have a worse prognosis. Dogs with complete cervical spinal cord transection causing loss of nociception are unlikely to survive the initial injury.

Vascular diseases

Spinal haemorrhage

Clinical signs: Clinical signs reflect the location of the haemorrhage and can be extensive or multifocal depending on the underlying cause. Epidural haemorrhage is usually associated with pain, whilst intraparenchymal haemorrhage is rarely a painful condition.

Pathogenesis: Bleeding disorders can be inherited (e.g. von Willebrand's disease) or acquired secondary to rodenticide toxicity or infectious/inflammatory diseases (e.g. immune-mediated thrombocytopenia, disseminated intravascular coagulation, *Angiostrongylus vasorum* infection). It should be noted that tick-borne infectious causes of vasculitis and thrombocytopenia, such as Rocky Mountain spotted fever, are common in some parts of the world. Haemorrhage into the CNS can also occur with any bleeding disorder and, although unusual, can be the first manifestation of the systemic disease. For example, epidural haemorrhage causing spinal cord compression has been reported in Dobermanns with von Willebrand's disease (Applewhite *et al.*, 1999). The presence of petechiae, ecchymoses or prolonged bleeding following venepuncture should alert the veterinary surgeon to the possibility of a bleeding disorder. It is not unusual to find extensive extradural haemorrhage at the site of acute intervertebral disc herniations or vertebral fractures and luxations. These animals do not have an underlying coagulopathy; the haemorrhage has occurred as a direct result of disruption of the venous sinuses that overlie the disc.

Diagnosis: The history and clinical findings may be suggestive of a bleeding disorder. A buccal mucosal bleeding time (BMBT) test can be performed to evaluate platelet function by gently tying the upper lip back with gauze to expose the mucosa, and then making 1 mm deep, 5 mm long parallel cuts with a blade and noting the time taken for the bleeding to stop. Devices specifically designed to make these cuts are commercially available. Blood can be blotted away as it runs down the gum, but the incision should not be touched. Bleeding times >3 minutes are abnormal but there is a lot of individual variation (Christopherson *et al.*, 2011). If rodenticide toxicity is suspected, activated clotting time (ACT) should be measured. Values >120 seconds are supportive of a coagulopathy. Further evaluation of clotting function includes a manual platelet count, one stage prothrombin time (OSPT) and activated partial thromboplastin time (aPTT). The levels of individual clotting factors can be measured by specialist laboratories.

If a bleeding disorder is not suspected, a routine work-up for focal spinal cord signs should be undertaken. Survey radiographs are unremarkable and the CSF may be diffusely haemorrhagic if the haemorrhage is intraparenchymal. If the haemorrhage is extradural, it is visible as an extradural mass on myelography and is readily identifiable on CT if it has occurred in the preceding 24 hours. MRI can detect and differentiate both recent and old haemorrhage as the appearance changes with time (Thomas, 1996). If haemorrhage is suspected based on imaging, surgery should not be undertaken unless the coagulation profile is normal.

Treatment and prognosis: Treatment is specific to the cause (e.g. rodenticide toxicity can be treated with vitamin K1 at an initial dose of 2.5–5 mg/kg s.c. in several sites followed by 0.25–5 mg/kg orally q8–12h for 5 days to 5 weeks depending on the specific product ingested) and a plasma or whole blood transfusion is required if the patient is actively bleeding. Prognosis depends on the underlying aetiology and the severity of the neurological dysfunction caused.

Fibrocartilaginous embolism

Clinical signs: Fibrocartilaginous embolism (FCE) causes peracute onset of non-painful neurological deficits, most commonly in the lumbosacral intumescence (see Chapter 16) but can also occur in the brachial intumescence. Affected dogs are usually large, young, non-chondrodystrophoid breeds, which are engaged in exercise at the onset of signs. However, smaller breeds such as Shetland Sheepdogs, Miniature Schnauzers and Yorkshire Terriers can be affected and are more likely to have signs localized to the C6–T2 spinal cord segments. Cervical FCE is less common but has been reported in cats (Abramson *et al.*, 2002; Nakamoto *et al.*, 2010). Signs are often dramatically lateralized, resulting in hemiparesis. Involvement of the sympathetic tracts in the cervical spinal cord can result in Horner's syndrome and vasodilatation on the affected side. The vasodilatation can cause differential hyperthermia, which can be detected by comparing the temperature of the front feet or external pinnae (the affected side will be 'flushed') (Griffiths, 1970).

Pathogenesis: FCE is a syndrome in which fibrocartilage identical to that found in the nucleus pulposus embolizes to the spinal cord vasculature, causing an area of ischaemic necrosis centred on the spinal cord grey matter (Cauzinille and Kornegay, 1996). Signs are often lateralized as the embolus usually lodges in a distal arterial branch. For a full discussion of the aetiology of FCE, the reader is referred to Chapter 16.

Diagnosis: FCE should be suspected in animals presenting with peracute onset of lateralizing signs in the absence of spinal pain. Cervical disc herniations as a result of trauma can result in a similar syndrome with dramatic lateralization of signs and differential hyperthermia, but these animals usually have neck pain. Survey spinal radiographs are unremarkable and there is no evidence of spinal cord compression. On T2-weighted MR images, the infarcted area is visible as an intraparenchymal hyperintensity (Abramson *et al.*, 2005; De Risio *et al.*, 2007) (Figure 15.27). There may be more than one lesion visible (thought to reflect a shower of emboli) and CSF analysis may reveal a disproportionately elevated protein and neutrophilic pleocytosis.

Treatment and prognosis: Treatment is centred on successful rehabilitation of the animal (see Chapter

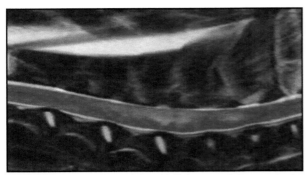

15.27 Sagittal T2-weighted MR image of the cervical spine of a 3-year-old Yorkshire Terrier. The dog suffered an acute onset of lateralizing signs localized to C6–T2. There is no evidence of a compressive lesion, but multifocal intraparenchymal hyperintensities are visible from C5–C7. These lesions did not enhance with contrast medium and CSF analysis was unremarkable. A presumptive diagnosis of FCE was made.

25). Improvement can be dramatic over the first 7 days and continues for 1–3 months following the injury. The extent of recovery depends on the extent of the injury (De Risio *et al.*, 2008), although there is some evidence that early intervention with rehabilitation aids recovery (Nakamoto *et al.*, 2008). If nociception is preserved in the thoracic and pelvic limbs on the affected side, the prognosis is good. If nociception is absent in one or more limbs, the prognosis is more guarded. Nociception should be monitored weekly, and its reappearance indicates the potential for recovery. The author has seen dogs that did not regain nociception or use of the thoracic limb on the affected side, but recovered full use of the other three legs and were able to ambulate without problem.

Miscellaneous vascular disease

Focal spinal cord deficits can be caused by emboli as a result of extreme hyperlipidaemia (inherited in Miniature Schnauzers or associated with hypothyroidism), vegetative valvular disease (secondary to endocarditis) and neoplasia. A variety of different focal neurological deficits have been reported with extreme polycythaemia and leukaemia as a result of sludging within the blood vessels. Vascular anomalies are a very rare cause of spinal cord disease that can be diagnosed by their characteristic appearance on MRI (MacKillop *et al.*, 2007).

Lower motor neuron diseases

The LMN diseases that cause tetraparesis are listed in Figure 15.28.

Degenerative diseases

Breed-specific neuropathy

Inherited and breed-related neuropathies are rare diseases that usually affect young animals, and can result in generalized motor, mixed motor and sensory, pure sensory and/or autonomic deficits (see Chapter 19 for information on dysautonomia) (Figure 15.29).

Mechanism of disease	Specific diseases
Degenerative	Inherited peripheral neuropathies (motor, sensorimotor, sensory) [15] Inherited myopathies [18] Inherited junctional disease [18] Distal denervating disease [15]
Anomalous	Congenital myasthenia gravis [18]
Metabolic/endocrine	Diabetes mellitus [15] Hypothyroidism [15, 18] Hyperthyroidism [18] Hypoadrenocorticism [18] Hyperadrenocorticism [15] Metabolic myopathies [18]
Neoplastic	Paraneoplastic (insulinoma, other) [15]
Inflammatory	Chronic inflammatory demyelinating polyneuropathy [15] Ganglioradiculitis [15] Myasthenia gravis [18] Polyradiculoneuritis: infectious (protozoal); immune-mediated [15] Polymyositis: infectious; immune-mediated [18]
Toxic	Botulism [15] Drug-induced [15] Tick paralysis [15]

15.28 LMN diseases that can cause tetraparesis. The numbers in square brackets denote the chapters in which the conditions are discussed in detail.

Breed	Disease
Dogs	
Alaskan Malamute; Dalmatian; Italian Spinone; Labrador Retriever; Leonberger; Podhale Shepherd; Pyrenean Mountain Dog; Rottweiler; Russian Black Terrier	Laryngeal paralysis polyneuropathy complex
Chesapeake Bay Retriever; Great Dane; Labrador Retriever; Newfoundland; Rottweiler; St Bernard	Distal sensorimotor polyneuropathy
Boxer	Progressive axonopathy (sensory)
Brittany Spaniel; Dobermann; English Pointer; German Shepherd Dog; Great Dane/Bloodhound or St Bernard cross; Griffon Briquet; Rottweiler; Saluki; Swedish Lapland Dog	Motor neuron disease
Cairn Terrier; West Highland White Terrier	Globoid cell leucodystrophy
Border Collie; English Pointer; English Spaniel; French Spaniel; Irish Setter; Longhaired Dachshund	Sensory neuropathy

15.29 Inherited peripheral neuropathies. (continues) ▶

Breed	Disease
Dogs (continued)	
Boxer; German Shepherd Dog	Giant axonal neuropathy
Golden Retriever	Sensory ataxic neuropathy
Tibetan Mastiff	Hypertrophic neuropathy
Cats	
Bengal	Demyelinating polyneuropathy
Birman	Distal polyneuropathy
Domestic Longhaired; Domestic Shorthaired; European; Himalayan; Persian; Siamese	Hyperchylomicronaemia
Domestic Shorthaired	Hyperoxaluria
Norwegian Forest	Glycogenosis (type IV)
Siamese	Niemann–Pick disease (subtype A)

15.29 (continued) Inherited peripheral neuropathies.

Motor and mixed sensorimotor neuropathies:
This group of diseases includes the motor neuron diseases (in which the motor neurons in the ventral horn of the spinal cord degenerate), axonopathies, demyelinating diseases and distal neuropathies. Typically, progressive LMN paresis develops, often affecting the pelvic limbs initially but eventually involving the thoracic limbs. The concurrent development of laryngeal paralysis and megaoesophagus is recognized as a syndrome called laryngeal paralysis polyneuropathy complex. This syndrome has been reported in young Rottweilers, Dalmatians, Leonbergers, white coated German Shepherd Dogs and Pyrenean Mountain Dogs amongst others (Braund, 2003; Granger, 2011). However, it is now recognized that older dogs with idiopathic laryngeal paralysis, in particular Labrador Retrievers, also suffer from a more generalized neuropathy that is likely to be hereditary (Thiemen *et al.*, 2010). Several different breeds of cat are also reported to have hereditary neuropathies (Bensfield *et al.*, 2011). Although many different breeds have been reported with these disorders (see Figure 15.29 and Appendix 1), most are extremely rare and are reviewed elsewhere (Braund, 2003; Granger, 2011).

Sensory neuropathies: Familial sensory neuropathies are particularly unusual but have been reported in English Pointers (Cummings *et al.*, 1981), English Springer Spaniels, French Spaniels (Paradis *et al.*, 2005), Border Collies (Vermeersch *et al.*, 2005) and Longhaired Dachshunds (Duncan and Griffiths, 1982) with sporadic reports in other dog breeds. Dachshunds present with nociceptive deficits, mild ataxia and loss of conscious proprioception. Male Dachshunds have been reported to self-mutilate their penis and dribble urine. The disease in English Pointers and French and English

Spaniels is more severe and more specific to nociception. They lose nociception in the distal limbs at approximately 3–8 months of age and as a result lick, chew and even autoamputate their digits. These dogs do not have conscious proprioceptive deficits. Treatment centres on prevention by using an Elizabethan collar to protect the feet and allow wounds to heal. If a paraesthesia is suspected, a drug such as gabapentin or pregabalin can be administered. A sensory ataxic neuropathy due to a mitochondrial mutation has also been described in Golden Retrievers (Jäderlund *et al.*, 2007; Baranowska *et al.*, 2009). Affected dogs exhibit a slowly progressive dysmetric ataxia due to a central and peripheral senorimotor axonopathy.

Inherited metabolic disorders: Certain storage diseases (e.g. Niemann–Pick disease in cats and globoid cell leucodystrophy in Cairn and West Highland White Terriers and Irish Setters) cause a peripheral neuropathy in addition to CNS signs (Fletcher *et al.*, 1966; Cuddon *et al.*, 1989; McDonnell *et al.*, 2000). Inherited metabolic disorders that cause generalized peripheral neuropathies in cats include hyperchylomicronaemia (Jones *et al.*, 1986) and hyperoxaluria (Blakemore *et al.*, 1988). Hyperchylomicronaemia has been reported in Siamese, Domestic Shorthaired and Longhaired, Persian and Himalayan cats. It occurs as a result of a mutation in the gene encoding the enzyme lipoprotein lipase and is inherited as an autosomal recessive trait (Watson *et al.*, 1992). The resultant fasting hyperchylomicronaemia is associated with the development of focal xanthomata. These are granulomatous masses believed to represent organizing haematomas and comprise macrophages, cholesterol and triglyceride crystals, haemosiderin and lipofuscin. They are more likely to develop over pressure points that are susceptible to trauma. Affected cats develop a variety of neuropathic signs as a result of compression of the peripheral nerves by the xanthomata. The specific neurological deficits vary between individuals, reflecting the location of the xanthomata, but typically include LMN monoparesis, paraparesis or tetraparesis and CN deficits. Signs usually develop after 8 months of age and can be reversed by feeding a low fat, high fibre diet.

Diagnosis: The diagnosis of these disorders is confirmed by recognition of typical breed, age of onset and presentation, and by ruling out other disorders via electrophysiological evaluation and nerve biopsy (see Chapter 3). Hyperchylomicronaemia in cats is diagnosed by the presence of fasting hyperlipidaemia, measurement of the lipid profile (elevated chylomicrons, cholesterol and triglycerides and a mild elevation in very low density lipoproteins) and measurement of lipoprotein lipase activity. Fundic examination sometimes reveals lipaemia retinalis. There is a genetic test for the mutation that causes globoid cell leucodystrophy in Irish Setters, West Highland White Terriers and Cairn Terriers (Victoria *et al.*, 1996; McDonnell *et al.*, 2000) as well as for the polyneuropathy seen in Leonbergers (see Appendix 1).

Treatment and prognosis: Therapy is limited to the management of clinical signs in most diseases, including laryngeal tie back in dogs with upper airway obstruction secondary to laryngeal paresis/ paralysis and physical therapy to maintain range of motion and muscle mass (see Chapter 25). One exception is hyperchylomicronaemia in cats which can be successfully treated by feeding a low fat, high fibre diet. It is important to recognize problems and diagnose the cause of clinical signs in animals used for breeding (see Figure 15.29 and the Appendix for reported syndromes).

Distal denervating disease

Distal denervating disease is reportedly a common peripheral neuropathy in the UK, although it has not be recognized elsewhere. The aetiology of this disease is unknown, but the terminal and intramuscular branches of the motor nerves degenerate resulting in progressive tetraparesis that is first evident in the pelvic limbs (Griffiths and Duncan, 1979). Weakness progresses over days to weeks, leading to LMN tetraplegia and dysphonia, and the development of severe muscle atrophy. Diagnosis is aided by electrophysiological studies (electromyography confirms denervation and that nerve conduction velocities are reduced). Biopsy is not helpful except to rule out other diseases as the lesion is usually distal to the biopsy site. Treatment involves supportive care and the prognosis is excellent if adequate nursing care can be given.

Metabolic diseases

Endocrine neuropathy

Endocrine diseases that are known or suspected to cause a peripheral neuropathy include diabetes mellitus, hypoglycaemia (most commonly as a result of insulinoma in dogs), hypothyroidism and hyperadrenocorticism.

Diabetes mellitus: Poorly controlled diabetes mellitus causes distal axonal degeneration with the longest peripheral nerves affected first. The most common manifestation of this problem is sciatic neuropathy in cats, which causes a plantigrade stance in the pelvic limbs both at rest and when walking (Kramek *et al.*, 1984) (Figure 15.30). Affected cats retain the ability to ambulate but hock flexion is reduced to absent when the withdrawal reflex is tested. As the signs progress, affected cats also develop a palmigrade stance. Although pathological changes and sporadic cases of neuropathy have been detected in diabetic dogs (Morgan *et al.*, 2008), it is usually a subclinical problem in this species. Diagnosis is strongly suspected in animals with poorly controlled diabetes and classic neurological findings. A definitive diagnosis is made by electrophysiological studies and nerve biopsy. Although axonal degeneration can be present in severely affected animals, the most common findings are abnormalities in the Schwann cells and myelin (Mizisin *et al.*, 2002). Prognosis for full recovery of peripheral nerve function is guarded, but

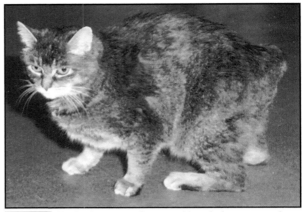

15.30 Typical stance of a cat with sciatic neuropathy associated with diabetes mellitus.

restoring normoglycaemia prevents progression and in mild cases may result in complete resolution of the neurological signs (Kramek *et al.*, 1984; Morgan *et al.*, 2008).

Hypothyroidism: This has been reported to be a cause of weakness in dogs as a result of a generalized neuropathy. In addition, idiopathic neuropathies such as facial or laryngeal paralysis, peripheral vestibular syndrome and megaoesophagus have been linked to hypothyroidism (Jaggy *et al.*, 1994). In general, these reports document resolution of signs with the correction of hypothyroidism. However, there is some controversy regarding whether hypothyroidism is truly associated with peripheral neuropathies, and a recent study with experimentally-induced hypothyroid dogs was unable to demonstrate any evidence of an associated generalized neuropathy, although myopathic changes were seen (Rossmiesl, 2010). An epidemiological study of acquired megaoesophagus was unable to demonstrate an association with hypothyroidism (Gaynor *et al.*, 1997). A diagnosis of hypothyroidism is made by measurement of the serum total and free T4 and thyroid-stimulating hormone (TSH) levels. Supplementation with thyroxine may reverse the signs of the generalized peripheral neuropathy over 2–3 months, but the laryngeal and oesophageal abnormalities usually persist.

Hyperadrenocorticism: A peripheral neuropathy has been reported in dogs with hyperadrenocorticism, but it is a rare complication of this disease, which is more commonly a subclinical disorder.

Neoplastic diseases

Insulinoma

Chronic, severe hypoglycaemia (<3.9 mmol/l) is almost invariably associated with insulinoma in dogs. The most common neurological signs result from the effects of hypoglycaemia on the CNS (seizures, weakness, exercise intolerance and collapse). However, persistent hypoglycaemia may also cause a distal peripheral neuropathy that manifests initially as a stiff gait, particularly in the pelvic limbs, but progresses to more obvious signs of a generalized peripheral neuropathy with prominent sciatic deficits (Chrisman, 1980; Braund *et al.*, 1987a). Treatment of the insulinoma may improve the gait, depending on the extent of the underlying disease.

Paraneoplastic neuropathy

Paraneoplastic peripheral neuropathies are well recognized in humans in association with particular types of cancer but are infrequently seen in dogs and cats. With the exception of the neuropathy associated with insulinomas in dogs, there are only sporadic reports of neuropathies associated with a variety of different cancers such as bronchogenic and mammary carcinoma and multiple myeloma (Braund *et al.*, 1987b; Villiers and Dobson, 1998; Mariani *et al.*, 1999). Treatment of the primary neoplasia may result in an improvement in signs due to the neuropathy.

Inflammatory diseases

Chronic inflammatory demyelinating polyneuropathy

Clinical signs: Chronic inflammatory demyelinating polyneuropathy causes slowly progressive LMN tetraparesis in adult dogs and cats with no gender or breed bias (Cummings and deLahunta, 1974; Shores *et al.*, 1987; Braund *et al.*, 1996; Cuddon, 2002). Signs can relapse intermittently and can progress to tetraplegia. Shifting lameness, a plantigrade stance and ventroflexion of the neck have all been described in cats, as well as megaoesophagus and regurgitation. Leg tremors and laryngeal and facial paralysis have been noted in dogs.

Pathogenesis: This is an apparently immune-mediated disease in which the inflammatory reaction is focused on the myelin sheaths of the peripheral nerves. The aetiology of the disease is unknown but it appears to be similar to chronic inflammatory demyelinating polyneuropathy in humans.

Diagnosis: The diagnosis is reached by a combination of electrophysiological studies and nerve biopsy. Typically, motor nerve conduction velocity is reduced. There is multifocal paranodal demyelination in teased nerve fibre preparations, and thinly myelinated fibres are visible on semi-thin sections. Electron microscopy reveals macrophages stripping myelin, and the presence of demyelinated and remyelinated fibres. There is also a mononuclear infiltrate.

Treatment and prognosis: Treatment consists of immunosuppression with prednisone (initial dose of 1 mg/kg orally q12h for 1–2 weeks followed by gradual tapering over a period of weeks). Most cases respond favourably to this regimen, although some eventually relapse and become steroid resistant.

Ganglioradiculitis

Ganglioradiculitis (also termed sensory neuronopathy, ganglionitis and sensory polyganglioradiculo-

neuritis) is a rare disease in which there is non-suppurative inflammation of the dorsal root and CN sensory ganglia (Cummings *et al.*, 1983).

Clinical signs: Affected dogs are usually mature and may have an apparent sudden onset in signs that are then slowly progressive over a period of months. The signs include ataxia, hypermetria and postural reaction deficits. Spinal reflexes may be reduced with good preservation of muscle mass and strength due to involvement of the sensory part of the spinal reflexes. CN deficits include head tilt, dysphonia and dysphagia, facial hypoalgesia and difficulty prehending food. Atrophy of the muscles of mastication may occur and self-mutilation is rarely reported. Ganglioradiculitis has been reported in a variety of different dog breeds, but the Siberian Husky appears to be over-represented.

Pathogenesis: The aetiology of this disease is unknown but it is speculated to be immune-mediated (Porter *et al.*, 2002). There is one report of a sensory neuronopathy that could have been the result of mercury toxicity (Jeffery *et al.*, 1993).

Diagnosis: Antemortem diagnosis is usually presumptive based on compatible clinical signs and decreased sensory nerve conduction velocity. CSF analysis is usually non-specific, although a mild increase in cellularity and protein levels is sometimes reported. As the inflammatory infiltrate is localized to the nerve ganglia, biopsy will not establish a specific diagnosis: biopsy of a dorsal root ganglion could be attempted.

Treatment and prognosis: There is currently no effective treatment and immunosuppression does not appear to alter the course of the disease.

Polyradiculoneuritis

Polyradiculoneuritis (inflammation of peripheral nerves and nerve roots) is probably the most common peripheral neuropathy of dogs and cats. It has been likened to the Guillain–Barré syndrome in humans.

Clinical signs: Affected dogs suffer from an ascending paralysis that progresses over 2–4 days to LMN tetraparesis or tetraplegia (see **Polyradiculoneuritis** clip on DVD). Spinal hyperaesthesia has been noted in some dogs and CNs can become involved, leading to dysphonia and facial weakness. Severe cases may suffer respiratory failure.

Pathogenesis: Signs are caused by an inflammatory reaction to axons and myelin sheaths, which is most intense at the level of the ventral nerve root (Cummings and Haas, 1966). Electrophysiological findings in dogs suggest that it is primarily a motor axonopathy (Cuddon, 1998). The disease can be further classified according to cause as Coonhound paralysis (seen in North America with onset of signs 7–10 days after raccoon bites), idiopathic polyradiculoneuritis or post-vaccinal polyradiculoneuritis (extremely rare). An important association in humans is concurrent infection with a specific sero-type of *Campylobacter jejuni* (Nachamkin *et al.*, 1998), but a variety of other infectious agents can also trigger the disease in humans, including *Toxoplasma gondii*. A recent study has shown that dogs with idiopathic acute polyradiculoneuritis are more likely to have positive titres for *Toxoplasma gondii* than control dogs (Holt *et al.*, 2011), suggesting that further investigation into the role of toxoplasmosis in polyradiculoneuritis is warranted in dogs.

Diagnosis: The number of diseases that cause acute onset LMN tetraparesis/tetraplegia is limited and polyradiculoneuritis should always be suspected when this clinical picture occurs. Other diseases to consider include botulism and tick paralysis (USA and Australia). Whilst rare, fulminant myasthenia gravis can present with similar clinical signs. Electromyography reveals spontaneous electrical activity consistent with denervation (fibrillation potentials and positive sharp waves); nerve conduction velocities are dispersed and reduced, with nerve roots more severely affected than the distal nerve (Cuddon, 1998). A definitive diagnosis is established with a nerve biopsy (see Chapter 6).

Treatment and prognosis: Treatment is centred on supportive care and rehabilitation. Corticosteroid administration is not beneficial (Cuddon, 2002). Humans are treated with plasmapheresis and intravenous immunoglobulins, but there are no reports of efficacy in canine polyradiculoneuritis as yet. The pulmonary function of recumbent animals must be monitored closely. If hypoventilation is suspected, an arterial blood gas analysis should be performed to determine whether mechanical ventilation is necessary. Animals should be turned and passive range of motion exercises and massage of limbs should be performed at least four times a day. Methods of maintaining muscle mass are discussed in Chapter 25. If pulmonary function is unaffected, with adequate supportive care, most animals recover over a period of 3–6 weeks. However, the need for mechanical ventilation, the presence of aspiration pneumonia and severe muscle atrophy with development of contractures all worsen the outcome.

Protozoal radiculoneuritis

Clinical signs: Clinical signs can be extremely variable as a result of infection of muscles, peripheral nerves and the CNS. Typically, the pelvic limbs are affected first and the combination of myositis and neuritis causes rigid extension of the limbs, with rapid development of severe muscle atrophy and contractures (Knowler and Wheeler, 1995). There is one report of a dog presenting with signs of cauda equina syndrome due to *Neospora caninum* (Saey *et al.*, 2010). However, multifocal CNS signs can be present and a cerebellar syndrome has also been reported (Garosi *et al.*, 2010) (see Chapter 11).

Pathogenesis: Infection with the protozoal organisms *Toxoplasma gondii* and *Neospora caninum* can cause an intense polyradiculoneuritis in dogs accompanied by myositis (Greene *et al.*, 1985; Dubey and Lindsay, 1996). Clinically significant protozoal infections affect young or immunocompromised dogs. Dogs are both definitive and intermediate hosts for *Neospora* (cattle, sheep, goats and other mammals also act as intermediate hosts). Cats are the definitive host for *Toxoplasma* with most mammals serving as intermediate hosts. Infection can occur transplacentally (common for *Neospora caninum*), by ingestion of protozoal cysts from infected secondary hosts, and by ingestion of oocytes shed in faeces (common for toxoplasmosis). *Neospora* is probably the most common protozoal infection in dogs, particularly as retrospective immunohistochemical evaluation of archived tissue samples confirmed that many animals previously diagnosed with toxoplasmosis were actually infected with *Neospora*.

Diagnosis: A definitive diagnosis can be made by identification of the organisms in muscle (Figure 15.31) or nerve biopsy samples, combined with serology. Serology alone can be confusing with a high rate of false-positive titres, particularly in the case of toxoplasmosis (see Chapter 11 for further details). Polymerase chain reaction (PCR) analysis of the CSF may provide a more specific diagnosis, but the sensitivity of this test is unknown (Schatzberg *et al.*, 2003).

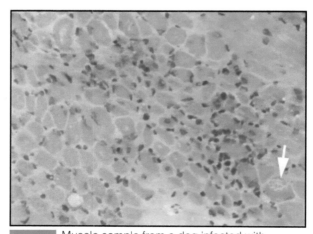

15.31 Muscle sample from a dog infected with *Neospora caninum*. A group of tachyzoites can be seen within a myocyte (arrowed). (H&E stain; original magnification X150)

Treatment and prognosis: Treatment of protozoal infections can be attempted using clindamycin. However, a combination of trimethoprim/sulfadiazine and pyremethamine is more effective at actually killing the organisms and penetrates the CNS well. Azithromycin can be added as it is effective at killing intracellular organisms. Animals on this protocol can be supplemented with folic acid. Prognosis depends on the severity of the clinical signs and the muscle contractures. Recovery of normal function is unlikely, although institution of treatment can prevent progression of signs. If treatment is initiated whilst the signs are mild, the prognosis is better, but relapses can occur as can increasing titres in the face of clinical normality.

Toxic diseases

Botulism

Clinical signs: Botulism causes LMN tetraparesis that originates in the pelvic limbs as mild weakness and can progress to tetraplegia in severe cases (see Botulism clip on DVD). CNs are often involved, resulting in facial paresis, dysphonia, megaoesophagus and regurgitation. Autonomic signs such as mydriasis and dry eye are variably present. The onset of signs usually occurs over 2–4 days and is often preceded by a history of dietary indiscretion (usually consuming spoiled meat) and vomiting or diarrhoea. Botulism has not been reported in cats.

Pathogenesis: Botulism is caused by absorption of the botulinum toxin following ingestion of spoiled carrion or raw meat. The botulinum toxin, produced by *Clostridium botulinum*, is taken up and prevents synaptic release of acetylcholine at the neuromuscular junction of cholinergic nerves. There are several forms of botulinum toxin, but botulinum C is the only form associated with canine disease (Coleman, 1998). Botulinum toxins, like other clostridial toxins, are zinc endopeptidases and botulinum C binds to the presynaptic protein SNAP 25 (Binz *et al.*, 2010).

Diagnosis: History and clinical signs are indicative of the disease. Electrophysiological studies may be supportive of the diagnosis (decreased amplitude of compound muscle action potentials). Reduced motor nerve conduction velocity has been reported suggesting that there is a concurrent neuropathy (van Nes and van der Most van Spijk, 1986). A definitive diagnosis is difficult to establish: the presence of the botulinum toxin in the serum, faeces or vomitus may be detected using a specific antitoxin to perform a neutralization test in mice, and use of an enzyme-linked immunosorbent assay (ELISA) has also been reported. These tests demonstrate an increase in serum titres to botulinum neurotoxin type C, 3 weeks after the onset of signs (Bruchim *et al.*, 2006). Typically, the toxin is no longer detectable by the time neurological signs are evident.

Treatment and prognosis: Treatment is supportive and recovery occurs over a period of approximately 3 weeks. Recumbent dogs should be turned regularly, kept clean and dry, and their bladder expressed if necessary. Megaoesophagus and regurgitation should be managed by intermittent suction of the oesophagus by means of a naso-oesophageal tube, antacids (e.g. famotidine) to decrease the acidity of the stomach contents, and

antibiotics for aspiration pneumonia if required. Ampicillin, aminoglycosides, erythromycin, ciprofloxacin and imipenem interfere with neuromuscular conduction and should be avoided. If megaoesophagus is present, the dog should be fed whilst held or propped with the head up, and this position should be maintained for approximately 30 minutes after feeding. Arterial blood gas analysis should be performed to check for hypoventilation in tetraplegic animals and in animals that may have aspirated their stomach contents. Passive range of motion exercises and massage should be performed every 6 hours whilst the animal is recumbent (see Chapter 25 for further details on rehabilitation). If pulmonary function is not adversely affected, dogs have a good prognosis with adequate nursing. If aspiration pneumonia or hypoventilation develop, the prognosis is grave, but recovery can occur if appropriate ventilatory support is provided.

Drug-induced toxic neuropathy

Drug-induced toxic neuropathies are rarely encountered in clinical practice. However, certain drugs and substances have the potential to cause peripheral neuropathies, including the chemotherapeutic drugs vincristine and cisplatin. One case of vincristine-induced neuropathy has been reported: the dog was given 16 weekly doses of vincristine at a dose rate of 0.5 mg/m^2 (Hamilton *et al.*, 1991). Signs improved following discontinuation of the drug. As radiation therapy becomes more routine for the treatment of neoplasia, radiation-induced neuropathies are likely to become more common. This can be a late effect and in an experimental study on intraoperative radiation in dogs, paraparesis developed between 1 and 19 months after radiation therapy if the dose exceeded 15 Gy (LeCouteur *et al.*, 1989; Johnstone *et al.*, 1995).

There are rare reports of organophosphate-induced delayed neuropathy occurring in cats with chronic exposure. Thallium toxicity, from ingestion of insecticides and rodenticides that contain this substance, has been reported in dogs and cats, but the banning of this substance has made this an extremely unlikely occurrence. In Europe there was an outbreak of a generalized peripheral neuropathy in cats, which was determined to be the result of contamination of their food with the ionophore salinomycin (van der Linde-Sipman, 1999). The cats developed tetraplegia and many died or were euthanased. Similar signs have been reported in dogs that ingested food contaminated with lasalocid (Safran *et al.*, 1993). Contamination of the food in both these instances occurred at the processing plant as ionophores are frequently added to ruminant or porcine feed as growth promoters.

Tick paralysis

Certain species of female ticks contain a toxin within their saliva that causes presynaptic blockade of acetylcholine release and a flaccid tetraplegia (Malik and Farrow, 1991). Signs appear after the tick has been attached for 3–5 days and progress over 1–3 days. They usually resolve within an equal period following removal of the tick (see **Tick paralysis** clip on DVD), except in the case of the Australian tick where signs can progress despite removal of the tick. The tick species responsible for this disease are not indigenous to the UK, so it is only a concern if the dog has recently travelled from Australia or the USA (Adamantos *et al.*, 2005). It is commonly encountered in the USA and more severe forms occur in Australia and Africa.

References and further reading

Available on accompanying DVD

DVD extras

- Botulism
- Caudal cervical spondylomyelopathy
- Cervical disc herniation
- Polyradiculoneuritis
- Tetanus
- Tick paralysis

16

Paraparesis

Joan R. Coates

Terminology

Paraparesis is a non-specific term for bilateral motor dysfunction of the pelvic limbs.

Paraparesis is a very common presentation in small animal veterinary practice and can be caused by orthopaedic, muscle, neuromuscular junction, nerve and spinal cord dysfunction. More rarely, systemic and metabolic disorders can present as episodic or progressive paraparesis (e.g. cardiac and pulmonary dysfunction, endocrine and electrolyte disturbances), and animals with drug-induced side effects (e.g. phenobarbital and potassium bromide) may show pelvic limb dysfunction manifest as general proprioceptive ataxia. Diseases of the thoracolumbar spinal cord are the most common cause of paraparesis and, as late or misdiagnosis of many of these disorders can have catastrophic consequences for the patient, it is important to understand fully how to evaluate and manage paraparetic patients.

Clinical signs

Clinical signs of thoracolumbar spinal cord disorders reflect sensory, motor and autonomic dysfunction of the pelvic limbs, tail, bladder and gastrointestinal tract (Figure 16.1). Depending upon the severity of the pelvic limb dysfunction, the paresis may be clinically evident.

Gait

Gait should be evaluated at a slow and fast pace and when walking up and down steps. Abnormal gait descriptions include:

- General proprioceptive ataxia – loss of general proprioception and incoordination
- Fatigability – one or more muscles become weaker with repetitive but normal use, and may imply neuromuscular dysfunction
- Paresis – reduced voluntary motor function
- Paralysis or paraplegia – absence of voluntary motor function
- Weakness – a non-specific term referring to an inability to carry out a desired movement with normal force because of a reduction in the strength of the muscles necessary to carry out the movement.

Ataxic gait

Animals with spinal cord disease have general proprioception and postural reaction deficits (specifically proprioceptive placing), resulting in general

Parameter	Spinal cord segments T3–L3	Spinal cord segments L4–S3
Mental status	Normal	Normal
Posture	Normal or pelvic limbs tucked under body and altered tail carriage	Normal or pelvic limbs tucked under body and altered tail carriage
Gait	Pelvic limb ataxia; symmetrical or asymmetrical paraparesis/paraplegia	Pelvic limb ataxia; symmetrical or asymmetrical (more often with cauda equina) paraparesis and/or paraplegia
Cranial nerves	Normal	Normal
Postural reactions	Mild to severe deficits or absent	Mild to severe deficits or absent
Spinal reflexes	Normal to hyperreflexic pelvic limb(s)	Hyporeflexia or areflexia; pseudo-hyperreflexia[a]
Spinal hyperaesthesia	Variable; dependent on disease process	Variable; dependent on disease process
Pain perception	Variable; dependent on disease severity	Variable; dependent on disease severity
Micturition	Usually affected with loss of motor function and detrusor muscle areflexia–sphincter hypertonia	None or mild to severe detrusor muscle areflexia; sphincter hypotonia

16.1 Clinical signs of thoracolumbar and lumbosacral spinal cord dysfunction. [a] Psuedo-hyperreflexia is only seen with the patella reflex when the sciatic nerve is dysfunctional, resulting in a lack of antagonism to the extensor function of the quadriceps muscles.

proprioceptive ataxia. Proprioceptive placing (paw replacement) is a non-weight-bearing test used to discriminate between orthopaedic and neurological lameness. Subtle proprioceptive loss and paresis may become apparent during postural reaction testing (i.e. hopping, extensor postural thrust and wheelbarrow reactions).

Stiff gait

A stiff or stilted gait is characteristic for an animal with orthopaedic, muscle or neuromuscular junction disease. In order to differentiate orthopaedic from neurological disease, the animal is often required to undergo strenuous exercise. In cases of neuromuscular disease this exacerbates the paraparesis, whereas clinical signs often improve with exercise in animals with orthopaedic disease.

Muscle tone

Paraparesis may be accompanied by changes in muscle tone that are elicited by passive movements, including:

- Flaccidity – the absence of normal muscle tone
- Spasticity (in quadrupeds) – a selective increase in extensor tone
- Rigidity – an increase in flexor and extensor tone.

Postural reactions

Asymmetry of neurological deficits is common with vascular, inflammatory and compressive myelopathies. Animals with orthopaedic disease do not have proprioceptive deficits, although the associated loss of strength with these conditions may make interpretation of test results difficult.

Spinal reflexes

Spinal, myotatic and withdrawal (flexor) reflexes can assist further with neuroanatomical lesion localization (see Chapter 1). The cutaneous trunci reflex can assist with localization and lateralization of a thoracolumbar lesion, but it is not always a reliable indicator.

Nociception

Assessment of pelvic limb nociception is extremely important in paraplegic animals as it provides critical prognostic information (see Chapters 1 and 20).

Schiff–Sherrington posture

Schiff–Sherrington posture is characterized by thoracic limb extension with normal to sometimes decreased tone in the pelvic limbs (Figure 16.2). Lesions located within the thoracolumbar spinal cord segments alter the ascending inhibitory pathways from the border cells in the lumbar grey matter (L2–L4). Axons from these cells cross to ascend in the contralateral fasciculus proprius to terminate in the cervical intumescence. Loss of this ascending inhibition to the thoracic limbs results in extension. In spite of the increase in extensor tone, the thoracic limbs are neurologically normal with respect to motor function and general proprioception. Schiff–Sherrington posture does not indicate that the spinal cord lesion is irreversible.

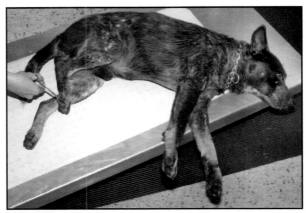

16.2 Schiff–Sherrington posture. Note the increased extensor muscle tone in the thoracic limbs and paralysis in the pelvic limbs. The absence of nociception is the most important prognostic indicator.

Neuromuscular diseases

Myopathic disease usually presents with generalized weakness and exercise intolerance, which can be episodic or persistent. Gait is usually stiff and stilted or 'bunny-hopping'. Exercise intolerance and episodic weakness are often not obvious until the animal is exercised. With myopathic diseases, the pelvic limbs are commonly affected first and more severely than the thoracic limbs; thus, animals may initially present with paraparesis (see Chapter 18 for further information). Muscle palpation may reveal severe atrophy or hypertrophy with or without tremors and/or fasciculations. In addition, myopathies (and polyneuropathies) can result in dysphagia, dyspnoea and dysphonia. Depending upon the severity of the atrophy, the range of joint movement may be limited. Pain may also be evident upon palpation of the muscles.

The neuromuscular junction disorder that is most often confused with other paraparetic conditions is generalized myasthenia gravis. Although rare, myasthenia gravis may manifest as episodic weakness with pelvic limb involvement only. The gait of affected animals can show a shortened stride or 'bunny-hop' that progresses to collapse. Strength returns with rest (see Chapter 18).

Neuropathies are characterized by flaccid paresis, postural reaction deficits and neurogenic muscle atrophy (see Chapter 15). Paraesthesia or analgesia may be evident with involvement of the sensory component of the nerve. Gait evaluation may reveal moderate to severe ataxia and a characteristic 'high-stepping' gait, usually due to lack of strength. The distal limbs may have a flaccid appearance. Muscle palpation reveals severe atrophy and in chronic cases muscle contractures. Muscle fasciculation may be present. Spinal reflexes are often decreased or absent. Neuropathies can be responsible for dysphagia, dysphonia and dyspnoea.

The presence of paraspinal hyperaesthesia also assists with the differential diagnoses (Figure 16.3). Paraspinal hyperaesthesia usually indicates a compressive and/or inflammatory cause. Pain-sensitive structures include the periosteum of the vertebrae,

Mechanism of disease	Specific diseases	Disease onset
No spinal hyperaesthesia		
Degenerative	Degenerative myelopathy (myelinopathy, spongy degenerative myelopathy, central and central–peripheral axonopathy, neuroaxonal dystrophy, multiple system degeneration); lysosomal storage diseases; spondylosis deformans; dural ossification	Chronic
Neoplasia	Primary: astrocytoma, ependymoma, oligodendroglioma	Chronic; may have acute manifestation
Vascular	Fibrocartilaginous embolic myelopathy; thrombosis; infarction	Acute
Spinal hyperaesthesia		
Degenerative	Calcinosis circumscripta; intervertebral disc disease; spinal extrasynovial cyst; mucopolysaccharidosis	Acute or chronic
Anomalous	Intra-arachnoid cysts; spinal dysraphism; syringo(hydro)myelia; vertebral malformations; spinal stenosis	Chronic
Metabolic	Hyperchylomicronaemia	Chronic
Neoplastic	Primary: extradural (vertebral, lymphoreticular); intradural–extramedullary (nerve sheath tumour, meningioma, nephroblastoma) Secondary: metastatic (mammary gland carcinoma, haemangiosarcoma)	Acute or chronic
Idiopathic	Diffuse idiopathic skeletal hyperostosis; calcinosis circumscripta	Usually chronic
Inflammatory	Infectious: meningitis/myelitis (viral, fungal, bacterial, protozoal, rickettsial, agal, spinal empyema); discospondylitis (bacterial, fungal); vertebral physitis Non-infectious: granulomatous meningoencephalomyelitis; steroid-responsive meningitis–arteritis; vasculitis	Usually acute
Trauma	Traumatic disc herniation; vertebral fractures/luxations	Acute
Vascular	Epidural haemorrhage	Acute

16.3 Disorders of the thoracolumbar spinal cord region by mechanism of disease and pain status.

meninges, nerve roots and intervertebral discs (see Chapter 14). Disorders that classically do not manifest paraspinal hyperaesthesia are degenerative spinal cord diseases, intramedullary neoplasia and fibrocartilaginous embolism (FCE) or ischaemic myelopathy.

Lesion localization

Thorough physical, orthopaedic and neurological examinations of the patient are crucial for localizing the clinical signs and avoiding unnecessary diagnostic testing and client expense. Patients with suspected orthopaedic diseases should undergo a neurological examination. It is important to remember that localization refers to spinal cord segments rather than vertebrae. Thus, a lesion that localizes to the L4–S3 spinal cord segments could lie anywhere caudal to the second lumbar vertebra (the approximate site of the L4 spinal cord segment) (see Chapter 2).

Neuroanatomical localization of paraparesis is specific to spinal cord segments T3–L3 or L4–S3 (Figure 16.4) based upon the signs of upper motor neuron (UMN) or lower motor neuron (LMN) limb weakness, respectively (see Chapters 1 and 2). UMN weakness refers to a lesion that interrupts the descending motor pathways from the supraspinal neurons that converge on the LMN pool. Clinical signs of UMN weakness manifest as paresis and/or plegia with normal to increased spinal reflexes (hyperreflexia) and muscular hypertonia. LMN weakness refers to a lesion of the ventral spinal cord grey matter and its axon coursing to the muscle through the spinal nerve roots and peripheral nerve. LMN weakness manifests as paresis and/or plegia, decreased to absent spinal reflexes (hyporeflexia to areflexia), decreased muscle tone (flaccidity) and muscle atrophy that is severe and rapid in onset. The sacral and coccygeal regions are localized according to LMN signs involving the perineal region, bladder function, urethral tone and tail tone (see Chapter 19).

A stiff or stilted gait, muscle atrophy and lack of proprioceptive deficits are suggestive of orthopaedic, junctional or myopathic disease. LMN signs relevant to the pelvic limbs, with a lack of involvement of the tail and bladder, should raise suspicion for a peripheral neuropathy rather than a process affecting the

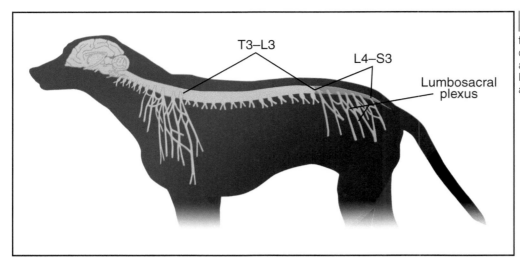

16.4 Lesion localization for paraparesis. Spinal cord segments T3–L3 and L4–S3, and the lumbosacral plexus are highlighted.

spinal cord or cauda equina. Neuropathies may be associated with signs of megaoesophagus.

Due to the multiplicity of anatomical dysfunctions that can result in clinically similar disorders, the clinician faces a diagnostic dilemma. Aged patients often have concurrent orthopaedic and neurological disorders, which further complicates the examination process. For example, in middle-aged, large-breed dogs, disorders that often mimic each other and coexist include:

- Degenerative lumbosacral stenosis
- Degenerative myelopathy
- Hansen type II intervertebral disc disease (IVDD)
- Degenerative joint disease as a result of hip dysplasia or rupture of the anterior cruciate ligament.

To complicate matters further, a specific ante-mortem diagnostic test is lacking for some diseases (e.g. degenerative myelopathy should always be considered as a cause of paraparesis in German Shepherd Dogs, even in the face of other aetiologies). It is important to note that signs of pelvic limb dysfunction can present prior to signs of thoracic limb paresis in some cases of cervical spinal cord disease (e.g. giant-breed Wobbler syndrome) and generalized peripheral neuropathies, junctionopathies and myopathies. These disorders are considered in more detail in Chapters 15 and 18.

Pathophysiology

The severity of the motor and sensory deficits associated with spinal cord disease is dependent upon the rapidity of disease onset, extent of spinal cord involvement and the area within the vertebral column that is affected. Spinal cord dysfunction can be a secondary consequence of extrinsic or intrinsic injuries to the spinal column. Traumatic aetiologies, such as vertebral fractures, luxation and penetrating injuries from missiles and animal bites, are examples of extrinsic injuries. Intrinsic injuries include embolization of the spinal cord

vasculature, extrusion of the nucleus pulposus and developmental anomalies. As with tetraparesis (see Chapter 15), disease processes affecting the spinal cord, nerves and muscles may be compressive (neoplasia, intervertebral disc herniation), concussive (traumatic), inflammatory, vascular, metabolic or degenerative.

Animals with acute, severe thoracolumbar spinal cord injuries may develop an unusual systemic complication known as neurogenic shock and a neurological dysfunction known as spinal shock.

- Neurogenic shock – associated with cervical or cranial thoracic injuries to the spinal column. It has been observed in humans and experimentally in dogs and cats, but is rarely evident in clinical patients. This syndrome results from sympathetic loss (decreased blood pressure and heart rate as a result of unopposed vagal tone) and continual vagal tone. Ultimately, there is loss of spinal cord blood flow regulation and subsequent ischaemia. Neurogenic shock resolves with fluid therapy and use of pressor agents.
- Spinal shock – usually manifests as flaccidity caudal to the lesion. Spinal reflexes are depressed to absent and the bladder may be flaccid with urine retention and sphincter hypotonia (Smith and Jeffery, 2005). The cause of spinal shock is unclear. A transient decrease in limb tone may be due to loss of descending supraspinal input to the alpha-motor neurons and interneurons, along with an increase in segmental inhibition. Spinal shock is important to recognize to prevent improper lesion localization. Spinal shock or ascending myelomalacia should be considered in animals with LMN paraplegia in which other clinical findings (e.g. hyperaesthesia; the point at which the cutaneous trunci reflex and line of analgesia are observed) are present cranial to the lumbosacral intumescence. It is not uncommon for spinal shock to cause reduced withdrawal reflexes in the hindlimbs, especially in small dogs following acute intervertebral disc herniation and FCE.

Neurodiagnostic investigation

The history and findings from physical and neuro-logical examinations help identify neurological problems and assist with neuroanatomical localization and consideration of the differential diagnoses. The onset (acute or chronic), rate of progression (rapid or gradual) and temporal relation (intermittent/episodic, stable or insidious) can be established. A recommended diagnostic approach to spinal cord diseases is as follows:

- Complete blood count (CBC), serum biochemistry and urinalysis
- Thoracic radiography in animals >5 years old and following trauma
- Survey spinal radiography can assist with recognition of obvious abnormalities such as discospondylitis, luxations and bone neoplasia. If an abnormality is not seen, advanced imaging and cerebrospinal fluid (CSF) analysis are indicated
- CSF collection (preferably from the cerebello-medullary cistern and caudal lumbar region)
- Myelography and epidurography are useful for the detection and characterization of compressive spinal cord lesions (extradural, intradural and intramedullary) and for determining the extent of the compression (Figure 16.5)
- Computed tomography (CT) is used as a primary method to evaluate the spine or assist with determining lesion extent following myelography
- Magnetic resonance imaging (MRI) is becoming more widely available to veterinary surgeons in general and specialty practice and is considered the standard for detection of lesions within the spinal cord
- Additional diagnostic procedures include electro-diagnostic evaluation (electromyography and nerve conduction studies), nerve and muscle biopsy, CSF protein electrophoresis, serology, polymerase chain reaction (PCR) and exploratory surgery.

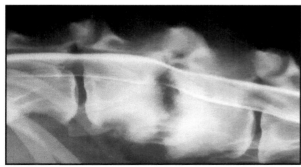

16.5 Lateral myelogram of the cranial lumbar spine showing extradural compression secondary to discospondylitis.

Differential diagnosis

The causes of paraparesis are summarized in Figure 16.6. The anatomical localization and distinguishing features of lesions that cause paraparesis are detailed in Figure 16.7.

Mechanism of disease	Specific diseases
Degenerative	Calcinosis circumscripta [16] Degenerative myelopathy [16] Dural ossification [16] Intervertebral disc disease (Hansen types I and II) [15, 16] Mucopolysaccharidosis [16] Spondylosis deformans [16, 19] Synovial cyst [15, 16]
Anomalous	Dermoid sinus [15, 16, 19] Osteochondromatosis [16] Syringo(hydro)myelia [15, 16] Vertebral and spinal cord anomalies [5, 14, 15, 16, 19] Intra-arachnoid cyst [15, 16]
Metabolic	Diabetes mellitus (neuropathy) [15]
Neoplastic	Extradural [16]: metastasis; vertebral tumours (sarcomas, plasma cell tumours); lymphomas Intradural–extramedullary [16]: meningiomas; nerve sheath tumours; spinal neuroepitheliomas (nephroblastomas); metastasis Intramedullary [16]: ependymomas; gliomas; metastasis; round cell tumours Insulinoma (paraneoplastic neuropathy) [15]
Nutritional	Hypervitaminosis A [15]
Inflammatory	Discospondylitis/osteomyelitis/physitis [16] Empyema [16] Vertebral physitis [16] Granulomatous meningoencephalomyelitis [11] Infectious meningoencephalomyelitis [11, 14, 15, 16] Steroid-responsive meningitis–arteritis [14]
Idiopathic	Diffuse idiopathic skeletal hyperostosis [16]
Traumatic	Fracture/luxation [16, 19, 20] Spinal cord contusion [15, 16, 20] Traumatic disc herniation [15, 16, 19, 20]
Toxic	Antiepileptic drugs [8, 15]
Vascular	Fibrocartilaginous embolism [15, 16, 19] Spinal cord/epidural haemorrhage [16] Thromboembolic disease [16]

16.6 Causes of thoracolumbar spinal cord and peripheral nerve disease. Numbers in brackets refer to the chapters in which diseases are discussed further.

Location	Distinguishing factors on examination
T3–L3	Paraparesis, ataxic gait, postural reaction and proprioceptive deficits (pelvic limbs); intact to increased spinal reflexes; ± focal spinal hyperaesthesia, faecal incontinence and urine retention
L4–S3	Paraparesis, postural reaction and proprioceptive deficits (pelvic limbs); decreased to absent spinal reflexes; ± change in tail carriage/tone, incontinence and focal spinal hyperaesthesia

16.7 Anatomical localization of lesions that can cause paraparesis. (continues) ▶

Location	Distinguishing factors on examination
Bilateral orthopaedic disease of pelvic limbs	Paraparesis but stilted gait; normal proprioception; abnormal findings on orthopaedic examination
C1–T2	As for T3–L3 plus subtle postural reaction or gait deficits in thoracic limbs; ± neck pain
Peripheral neuropathy	As for L4–S3 but no change in tail function or continence; ± laryngeal paralysis, megaoesophagus and thoracic limb involvement; decreased to absent spinal reflexes
Junctional disease	Often see paraparesis ± thoracic limb involvement which is exacerbated by exercise or activity; normal proprioception; spinal reflexes may be initially normal but decrease with repetition; no evidence of spinal pain ± laryngeal paralysis and/or megaoesophagus; no evidence of incontinence
Myopathic disease	Paraparesis or tetraparesis; episodic weakness exacerbated by exercise; normal proprioception; spinal reflexes usually intact but can be absent with some myopathies; ± muscle pain and megaoesophagus

16.7 (continued) Anatomical localization of lesions that can cause paraparesis.

Degenerative diseases

Degenerative myelopathy

Clinical signs

Dogs with degenerative myelopathy show an insidious, progressive ataxia and paresis of the pelvic limbs, ultimately leading to paraplegia and euthanasia (Averill, 1973). If pelvic limb hyporeflexia (reflecting nerve root involvement) is observed, the disease is sometimes termed canine degenerative radiculomyelopathy (Griffiths and Duncan, 1975). Although the German Shepherd Dog was the first recognized afflicted breed, degenerative myelopathy has since been reported in many other pure and mixed-breed dogs (Coates and Wininger, 2010). There is no sex predilection. In most breeds, the mean age of onset of neurological signs is 9 years old.

Progressive asymmetrical UMN paraparesis, pelvic limb general proprioceptive ataxia and lack of paraspinal hyperaesthesia are key clinical features of degenerative myelopathy (see **Degenerative myelopathy** clip on DVD). The clinical course of degenerative myelopathy is relatively uniform among breeds following a presumptive diagnosis. Pet owners usually elect for euthanasia when the animal can no longer support weight in its pelvic limbs and needs assistance to walk. Smaller dogs can be cared for by the owner for longer than larger dogs (Matthews, 1985). For example, the median disease duration in Pembroke Welsh Corgis in one study was 19 months (Coates et al., 2007). As a result of the longer survival time, affected Pembroke Welsh Corgis often have signs of thoracic limb paresis at the time of euthanasia.

Early-stage disease: The earliest clinical signs of degenerative myelopathy are general proprioceptive ataxia and mild spastic paresis in the pelvic limbs. Worn nails and asymmetrical pelvic limb weakness are apparent upon physical examination. Asymmetry of signs at disease onset is frequently reported (Averill, 1973; Kathmann et al., 2006; Coates et al., 2007). At the onset of disease, spinal reflex abnormalities are consistent with UMN paresis localized to the T3–L3 spinal cord segments. Patellar reflexes may be normal or exaggerated to clonic; however, hyporeflexia of the patellar reflex has also been described (Griffiths and Duncan, 1975). Flexor reflexes may also be normal or show crossed extension (suggestive of chronic UMN dysfunction). Most large-breed dogs progress to non-ambulatory paraparesis within 6 to 9 months following onset of clinical signs and are euthanased (Averill, 1973; Griffiths and Duncan, 1975; Braund and Vandevelde, 1978).

Late-stage disease: If the dog is not euthanased early in the course of the disease, clinical signs progress to LMN paraplegia and ascend to affect the thoracic limbs (Averill, 1973; Matthews, 1985; Kathmann et al., 2006; Coates et al., 2007). Flaccid tetraplegia ultimately occurs in dogs with advanced disease (Awano et al., 2009). The paresis becomes more symmetrical as the disease progresses. LMN signs (hyporeflexia of the patellar and withdrawal reflexes, flaccid paralysis and widespread muscle atrophy, beginning in the pelvic limbs) manifest as the dog becomes non-ambulatory. Widespread and severe loss of appendicular muscle mass occurs in the late stage of degenerative myelopathy. Most reports have attributed the loss of muscle mass to disuse (Averill, 1973; Griffiths and Duncan, 1975; Matthews, 1985; Coates et al., 2007), but flaccidity in dogs with protracted disease suggests denervation (Awano et al., 2009). Cranial nerve (CN) signs include swallowing difficulties and an inability to bark. Urinary and faecal continence are usually spared until the dog becomes paraplegic.

Pathogenesis

For many years, the aetiology of degenerative myelopathy was unknown. Immunological (Waxman et al., 1980ab; Barclay et al., 1994), metabolic and nutritional (Williams et al., 1983, 1984; Sheahan et al., 1991; Johnston et al., 2001; Fechner et al., 2003), oxidative stress (Coates et al., 2007); excitotoxic (Olby et al., 1999) and genetic mechanisms have all been explored as potentially underlying the pathogenesis of degenerative myelopathy. The uniformity of clinical signs, histopathology, age and breed predilections suggest an inherited basis for degenerative myelopathy. Segregation of degenerative myelopathy in families has been reported in the Siberian Husky (Bichsel, 1983), Pembroke Welsh Corgi (Coates et al., 2007) and Chesapeake Bay Retriever (Long et al., 2009).

In one study using genome wide association studies, a missense mutation in the superoxide dismutase 1 (*SOD1*) gene was determined (Awano et al., 2009). Mutations in the *SOD1* gene are an underlying cause of some forms of human amyo-trophic lateral sclerosis (ALS; Lou Gehrig's disease), an adult-onset fatal paralytic neurodegenerative disease. The disease derives its name from the combined degeneration of UMNs and LMNs project-ing from the brain and spinal cord. The Greek deri-vation of amyotrophy means 'muscle without nourishment'; lateral refers to the location of the axonal disease within the spinal cord; and sclerosis refers to 'hardening' with axons being replaced by astrogliosis. Canine degenerative myelopathy asso-ciated with this *SOD1* mutation resembles an UMN form of human ALS. Dogs that are homozygous for the mutation are at risk for developing degenera-tive myelopathy. However, some dogs are homo-zygous for the mutation but remain free of clinical signs, which suggests an age-related incomplete penetrance.

Although the clinical signs, disease progression and genetic analysis are provocative for considering degenerative myelopathy as a canine model of ALS, there remain significant pathological and clinical dif-ferences. These include neuronal cell body degen-eration or loss in the ventral horn of the spinal cord, and the involvement of the proprioceptive pathways as well as the UMN tracts in the axonopathy. Studies are underway to further describe the neu-ronal cell body and spinal nerve and nerve root pathology associated with degenerative myelopathy.

Diagnosis
A tentative antemortem diagnosis is based upon rul-ing out other diseases that can cause progressive myelopathy (Kneller *et al.*, 1975). Common differen-tial diagnoses include IVDD, inflammatory disease and spinal cord neoplasia. Hip dysplasia and degen-erative lumbosacral stenosis can often be confused with degenerative myelopathy; however, the neuro-logical findings are different if a careful examination is performed. It is not uncommon for dogs with degenerative myelopathy to have coexisting neuro-logical and orthopaedic diseases. Diagnostic testing is typically performed in the early stage of the dis-ease. The lack of abnormal findings on electrodiag-nostic testing, myelography or cross-sectional imaging (MRI and CT), along with a characteristic pattern of progression of the neurological signs and the presence of two copies of the *SOD1* mutation, support a presumptive diagnosis of degenerative myelopathy. Later in the disease course, electromyo-graphy and nerve conduction studies show abnor-malities associated with denervation atrophy and axonopathy/demyelination (Awano *et al.*, 2009).

A definitive diagnosis of degenerative myelo-pathy is determined postmortem by histopathologi-cal examination of the spinal cord (Figure 16.8). In general, neuropathological lesions involve the spinal cord myelin and axons in all funiculi, but are most severe in the dorsal portion of the lateral funiculus and medial portion of the dorsal funiculus. Histo-pathological changes, including degeneration and neuronal fibre loss of ascending sensory and descending motor pathways, are most severe in the mid to caudal thoracic spinal cord (Averill, 1973;

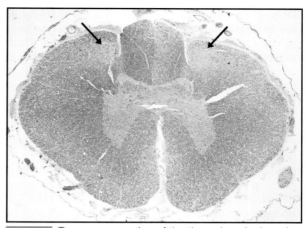

16.8 Transverse section of the thoracic spinal cord from a dog with degenerative myelopathy. Note the neuronal fibre loss, which is most prominent in the dorsal portion of the lateral funiculi (arrowed). (Luxol fast blue stain; original magnification X20) (Courtesy of Dr G Johnson)

Griffiths and Duncan, 1975; March *et al.*, 2009). In dogs with advanced degenerative myelopathy, nerve specimens show fibre loss as a result of axonal degeneration and secondary demyelination. Muscle samples reveal changes typical of denerva-tion atrophy (Awano *et al.*, 2009).

Treatment and prognosis
Treatment regimens have been empirical with a lack of evidence-based medicine approaches. Moreover, there is no prophylactic or curative treatment for human ALS. Aminocaproic acid (an anti-protease agent) has been advocated for the long-term man-agement of degenerative myelopathy (Clemmons, 1992); however, there have been no published data to support drug efficacy. Whilst the treatment of vita-min deficiencies can resolve neurological disease in some animals, therapy with parenteral cyanocobala-min or oral alpha-tocopherol did not affect neurologi-cal progression in a study of dogs with degenerative myelopathy (Johnston *et al.*, 2000, 2001; Williams, unpublished). Physical rehabilitation regimens have been advocated for the management of degenera-tive myelopathy (Kathmann *et al.*, 2006). Overall, long-term prognosis is considered poor.

Dural ossification
Dural ossification (also known as osseous metapla-sia) is a benign condition comprising bony plaques on the inner surface of the dura mater. This condi-tion is common in the cervical and lumbar regions of small and large-breed dogs >2 years of age (Morgan, 1969). These bony plaques are seen as radiopaque lines that outline the spinal cord and are best visualized at the intervertebral foramina. Dural ossification is rarely associated with clinical disease.

Hansen type I intervertebral disc disease

Clinical signs
The onset of neurological signs may be peracute (<1 hour), acute (<24 hours) or gradual (>24 hours).

Dogs presented with peracute or acute thoracolumbar disc extrusions may manifest clinical signs of spinal shock or Schiff–Sherrington postures. These indicate acute and severe spinal cord injury but do not determine prognosis. The degree of neurological dysfunction is variable and affects prognosis. Clinical signs vary from spinal hyperaesthesia only to paraplegia with or without nociception. Dogs with back pain only are usually reluctant to walk and may show kyphosis. These dogs often have myelographic evidence of substantial spinal cord compression. Dogs with paraplegia and a lack of nociception usually have acute and severe disc extrusions. This can lead to pannecrosis of the grey and white matter as a result of primary and secondary spinal cord injury mechanisms (Olby, 2010) (see Chapter 20). One potential end sequela of these processes is a syndrome of ascending/descending myelomalacia.

The incidence of ascending/descending haemorrhagic myelomalacia has been reported to be as high as 10% in dogs with acute thoracolumbar IVDD and loss of nociception (Scott and McKee, 1999; Olby *et al.*, 2003). Severe neurological dysfunction is also common with acute non-compressive disc extrusions (e.g. traumatic disc extrusion, high velocity low volume disc extrusion and missile disc extrusion, sometimes also referred to as type III disc herniation) where the extruded nucleus spreads along the epidural space and may completely surround or penetrate the dura mater (Sanders *et al.*, 2002; De Risio *et al.*, 2009) (Figure 16.9).

Neuroanatomical localization for thoracolumbar lesions is determined by intact (T3–L3) or hyporeflexive (L4–S3) spinal reflexes and the site of paraspinal hyperaesthesia. Asymmetrical neurological deficits may be less reliable for determining the side of the disc extrusion.

Pathogenesis

Hansen (1951) first classified IVDD as types I and II. Hansen type I IVDD is herniation of the nucleus pulposus through the annular fibres and extrusion of mineralized nuclear material into the spinal canal. Hansen type I IVDD is typically associated with chondroid disc degeneration. The disc extrudes through the dorsal annulus causing ventral, ventrolateral or circumferential compression of the spinal cord.

- Acute disc extrusion is characterized by the presence of soft disc material within the vertebral canal and extradural haemorrhage.
- Chronic disc extrusion is characterized by extradural fibrous adhesions around the herniated disc material, which often becomes a hard mineralized mass.

Hansen type I IVDD typically affects chondrodystrophic breeds and has an acute onset. However, large non-chondrodystrophic breeds of dog (such as the Dobermann and Labrador Retriever) may also be affected (Cudia and Duval, 1997). Hoerlein (1952) determined that IVDD accounted for 2.02% of all diseases diagnosed in dogs. The incidence of IVDD peaks at 4–6 years of age in chondrodystrophic breeds and at 6–8 years in non-chondrodystrophic breeds (Priester, 1976). The Dachshund had the highest incidence followed by the Pekingese, Welsh Corgi, Beagle, Lhaso Apso and Miniature Poodle (Hoerlein, 1987). In Dachshunds, severe disc degeneration denoted by the presence of mineralization on spinal radiography is highly heritable (Jensen and Christensen, 2000; Jensen and Arnbjerg, 2001). Further studies have determined an association between the number of mineralized intervertebral discs and the occurrence of disc herniation in Dachshunds (Jensen *et al.*, 2008).

Hansen type I IVDD most commonly occurs within the thoracolumbar region of chondrodystrophic breeds. The thoracolumbar junction (T12–T13 to L1–L2) accounts for the highest incidence of all disc lesions (Gage, 1975; Hoerlein, 1987). The incidence of thoracolumbar IVDD progressively decreases caudally from T12–T13. The most common site for Hansen type I IVDD in large, non-chondrodystrophic breeds is the interspace between L1 and L2 (Cudia and Duval, 1997).

Diagnosis

The initial diagnosis of thoracolumbar IVDD is obtained from the signalment, history and neurological examination. Differential diagnoses to consider include trauma, FCE, discospondylitis, neoplasia and (meningo)myelitis. The diagnosis of thoracolumbar disc extrusion and/or protrusion is confirmed by cross-sectional imaging and surgery.

Radiography: Survey spinal radiography can help determine the diagnosis and site of a thoracolumbar

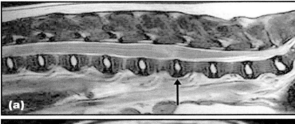
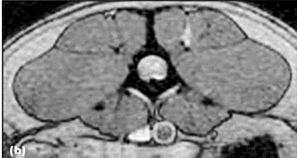

16.9 **(a)** Sagittal T2-weighted MR image of the lumbar spine of a 3-year-old Beagle. Note the hyperintensity in the spinal cord dorsal to the L4–L5 intervertebral disc space, reflecting spinal cord oedema caused by a high velocity disc extrusion. Note the dorsal displacement of the nucleus pulposus (arrowed). **(b)** Transverse T2-weighted MR image at the level of the L4–L5 spinal cord segment showing a hyperintensity associated with oedema of the spinal cord.

disc extrusion if the radiographic signs are well defined and consistent with the neuroanatomical localization (Figure 16.10) (see Chapter 5). Radiographic findings that should raise suspicion for intervertebral disc extrusion include:

- Narrowing of the intervertebral disc space
- Wedging of the disc space
- Narrowing of the intervertebral foramen
- Mineralized material in the spinal canal or superimposed over the intervertebral foramen.

Normal variants for the thoracolumbar spinal region include narrowing of the anticlinal disc space at T10–T11 and of the L4–L6 interspace (Widmer, 1998). Studies of dogs with surgically confirmed thoracolumbar IVDD showed that survey radiography had an accuracy of 68–72% for identifying the site of disc extrusion, but that the percentage accuracy was higher with myelography (Kirberger *et al.*, 1992; Olby *et al.*, 1994).

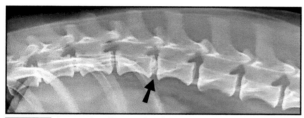

16.10 Lateral radiograph of the thoracolumbar spine showing opacity of the T11–T12, T12–T13 and L1–L2 intervertebral disc spaces. Note the narrowed intervertebral foramen and opacity in the spinal canal at the L1–L2 disc space (arrowed), which should raise suspicion for intervertebral disc herniation.

Myelography: As survey radiography identifies the correct site of disc extrusion in only approximately 70% of cases, further imaging studies with myelography, CT or MRI are recommended prior to surgery. The injection of contrast medium in the caudal lumbar region is preferred over the cerebellomedullary cistern for demonstrating thoracolumbar disc extrusion (Kirberger and Wrigley, 1993; Lamb, 1994) (see Chapter 5). Longitudinal lesion localization for thoracolumbar IVDD with myelography (Figure 16.11) varies in accuracy from 40–97%, but is usually close to 90% (Black, 1988; Kirberger and Wrigley, 1993; Olby *et al.*, 1994). Extensive

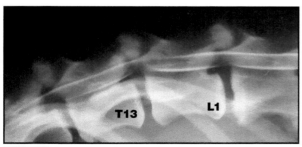

16.11 Lateral myelogram showing extradural compression on the ventral aspect of the spinal cord at the T13–L1 intervertebral disc interspace. This is suggestive of intervertebral disc extrusion.

attenuation of the subarachnoid space can occur with spinal cord oedema or extensive extradural haemorrhage and may obscure the site of the disc extrusion. Myelomalacia should be suspected if contrast medium is visible within the spinal cord parenchyma.

Computed tomography: CT or MRI are used alone or as an adjunct to myelography to more completely delineate lateralization of the extruded disc material and lesion extent. CT alone has been shown to be more accurate than myelography at identifying the major site of disc herniation and has the advantages of being a more rapid imaging modality with fewer side effects than myelography (Olby *et al.*, 1999). Mineralized disc material and acute haemorrhage can be identified in the vertebral canal using non-contrast enhanced CT. Acutely extruded disc material is typically visible as a heterogeneous hyperattenuating extradural mass (Figure 16.12). The attenuation of the disc material increases with the degree of mineralization. Chronically extruded disc material has a more homogeneous hyperattenuating appearance.

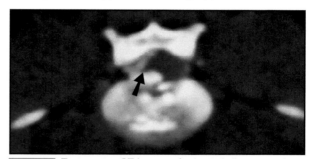

16.12 Transverse CT image of a lateral disc extrusion at the T12–T13 intervertebral disc interspace (arrowed).

Magnetic resonance imaging: MRI is a more sensitive technique for identifying spinal cord pathology (e.g. oedema and haemorrhage). It provides three-dimensional (3D) delineation of spinal cord compression, allowing an accurate surgical approach and the extent of decompression required to be determined (Figure 16.13). MRI is considered the best method for early recognition of *in situ* disc degeneration based on a decrease in signal intensity within the nucleus pulposus on T2-weighted images (Besalti *et al.*, 2006), and for determining the localization and extent of extruded disc material within the epidural space (Besalti *et al.*, 2005; Naude *et al.*, 2008). The hypointensity seen with degenerative disc disease is linked with changes in glycosaminoglycan concentrations. Focal signal voids within the intervertebral disc space or spinal canal may represent a free fragment of mineralized nucleus pulposus (Besalti *et al.*, 2005, 2006).

Acute pathologies of spinal cord tissues that may be seen as high signal intensities on T2-weighted images include necrosis, myelomalacia, intramedullary haemorrhage, inflammation and oedema. It is difficult to distinguish these specific types of pathology, but MRI may be better at identifying

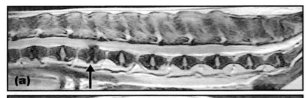

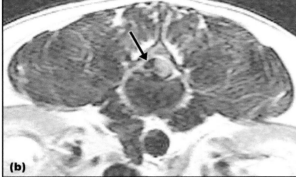

16.13 **(a)** Sagittal T2-weighted MR image of the thoracolumbar spine in a paraplegic 3-year-old Dachshund. Note the loss of hyperintensity (arrowed) in the L1–L2 intervertebral disc space, signifying degeneration of the nucleus pulposus. There is also a hypointense mass in the spinal canal at the level of the L1–L2 disc space, causing spinal cord compression and attenuation of the dorsal and ventral subarachnoid space. **(b)** Transverse T2-weighted MR image at the level of the L1–L2 intervertebral disc space. Note the hypointense mass (arrowed) compressing the spinal cord. A right-sided hemilaminectomy revealed extruded nucleus pulposus.

haemorrhage associated with intervertebral disc extrusion than other imaging techniques. However, timing of the MRI studies in relation to the onset of the lesion can confound interpretation of signal intensity, since rapid changes can occur within areas of haemorrhage in the early stages following injury. MRI studies of myelomalacia in dogs with intervertebral disc extrusion have demonstrated high signal intensity on T2-weighted images cranial and caudal to the compressive lesion (Ito *et al.*, 2005; Platt *et al.*, 2006). MRI may have diagnostic value in detecting myelomalacia. Findings from a recent study in dogs with intervertebral disc extrusion and lack of nociception suggest that an area of hyperintensity >6 times the length of L2 on sagittal T2-weighted images may allow for a presumptive diagnosis of myelomalacia (Okada *et al.*, 2010).

Treatment

Medical management: Indications for non-surgical management of thoracolumbar IVDD include first-time incident of spinal pain only, mild to moderate paraparesis, and the financial constraints of the client. The last indication is the only reason for non-surgical treatment of a recumbent patient, which should be considered a surgical candidate if possible. Dogs can be managed with strict cage rest for 4–6 weeks combined with pain relief using anti-inflammatory drugs, opioids and muscle relaxants. Gastrointestinal protectants may also be necessary

with the use of anti-inflammatory drugs. Acupuncture has also been advocated as a treatment for pain management (see Chapter 26).

> **WARNING**
> Never use non-steroidal anti-inflammatory drugs (NSAIDs) in combination with corticosteroids. This can cause gastric ulcers and in some cases may lead to the death of the animal.

Dogs should be monitored closely for deterioration of neurological status. If pain persists or the neurological status worsens, surgical management is recommended. Studies have shown that recovery rates in non-ambulatory dogs are lower and recurrence rates higher following medical rather than surgical treatment. Success rates for medical management of ambulatory dogs with pain only or mild paresis range from 82% to 100% (Funkquist, 1978; Davies and Sharp, 1983). More recent retrospective studies of medically managed dogs with thoracolumbar disc disease reported recurrence rates between 30% and 50% in dogs with minimally affected ambulatory status (Levine *et al.*, 2007; Mann *et al.*, 2007). Recurrence of spinal pain in dogs with thoracolumbar IVDD that are managed medically usually occurs within 6–12 months following onset of the initial clinical signs (Mann *et al.*, 2007).

Methylprednisolone sodium succinate (MPSS) has been advocated as an adjunctive treatment for acute disc herniations causing paraplegia and loss of nociception (see Chapter 20). Two trials with experimental models of canine spinal cord injury failed to demonstrate an effect with MPSS, but both of these studies were underpowered (Coates *et al.*, 1995; Rabinowitz *et al.*, 2008). A blinded, placebo-controlled study of MPSS in dogs with acute intervertebral disc herniation is currently underway and may help to resolve whether MPSS has any beneficial effects.

Surgical management: Indications for surgical management of thoracolumbar IVDD include spinal pain or paresis unresponsive to medical therapy, recurrence or progression of clinical signs, non-ambulatory paraparesis or paraplegia with intact nociception, and paraplegia without nociception for <24–48 hours. Prolonged loss of nociception (>48 hours) carries a poor prognosis and owners should be made aware of this prior to surgery. However, it is often difficult to know when nociception was lost. In addition, recovery has been observed in dogs that had surgery >5 days following the onset of paraplegia. Surgery includes spinal cord decompression by removal of the extruded disc material. Chronicity of disc extrusion at the time of surgery may influence the ease with which the extruded disc material can be removed.

Decompressive procedures for thoracolumbar IVDD include dorsal laminectomy (Funkquist, 1970; Prata, 1981), hemilaminectomy (Hoerlein, 1956) and pediculectomy (also known as mini-hemilaminectomy) (Braund, 1976; Bitetto and Thacher, 1987).

These approaches are described in Chapter 22. There are advantages and disadvantages to each decompressive technique. Hemilaminectomy significantly improves retrieval of extruded disc material with minimal spinal cord manipulation: a clear advantage over pediculectomy and dorsal laminectomy. Pediculectomy is the least invasive and destabilizing technique, but these advantages may not be clinically significant except in cases that require a bilateral approach to the vertebral canal. Unilateral facetectomy and fenestration do not significantly destabilize the spine in lateral bending, which suggests that the articular facets of the thoracolumbar spine are more important to stiffness in axial rotation and extension (Schulz *et al.*, 1996).

The type of decompressive procedure may not affect outcome; however, the ability to retrieve disc material depends on the decompressive procedure. The primary purpose of decompressive surgery is to provide adequate exposure to allow removal of disc material whilst minimizing spinal cord manipulation. Hemilaminectomy allows easier access to extruded disc material and a dorsolateral approach allows access to the disc spaces for fenestration. McKee (1992) reported retrieval of disc material in 93% of dogs that underwent a hemilaminectomy compared with 40% that underwent dorsal laminectomy, although the initial neurological recovery following hemilaminectomy was not significantly different compared with that following dorsal laminectomy. Radical dorsal laminectomy (removal of the lamina and pedicle – Funkquist A) has an increased risk of constrictive laminectomy membrane formation (Gage and Hoerlein, 1968).

Durotomy: In combination with decompression and removal of the extruded disc material, durotomy is often advocated in dogs with absence of nociception. Durotomy allows for visualization of the spinal cord parenchyma to determine the presence of myelomalacia. Durotomy is ineffective as a treatment for acute spinal cord trauma caused by IVDD (Loughin *et al.*, 2005). The absence of visual evidence of myelomalacia does not guarantee functional recovery; conversely, functional recovery may still occur despite the presence of focal myelomalacia.

Fenestration: First described by Olsson (1951), fenestration has been advocated as a treatment and prophylactic procedure for disc disease. Fenestration of the herniated disc at the time of surgical decompression is recommended to prevent continued extrusion of the remaining disc material. Surgical approaches for disc fenestration include dorsolateral, lateral and ventral incisions. The effectiveness of fenestration is related to the amount of nucleus pulposus removed (Shores *et al.*, 1985). Multiple disc fenestration is commonly performed at T11–T12 to L3–L4; however, the more commonly affected disc interspaces for extrusion are T12–T13 to L2–L3 (Brisson *et al.*, 2011).

Prognosis

The overall success rates following decompressive surgery range from 58.8% (Brown *et al.*, 1977) to 95% (Schulman and Lippincott, 1987). However, the success of a surgical approach may depend on what criteria are used to define it, how long following surgery the patient is assessed, and the outcome the owners are willing to accept. Surgical success may be improvement of the patient's pre-surgery neurological grade, but may not mean that the patient is functionally normal and the residual clinical signs (e.g. faecal incontinence) can be unacceptable to many owners. One study reported that approximately 40% of dogs that regained nociception continued to have faecal incontinence (Olby *et al.*, 2003). Recurrent urinary tract infection (UTI) is also common in dogs during recovery following acute intervertebral disc extrusion (Olby *et al.*, 2010).

The extent of spinal cord swelling seen with myelography may assist in establishing a prognosis. Dogs with loss of nociception have a significantly worse prognosis if the extent of the intramedullary swelling visible on myelography extends >5 times the length of L2 (Duval *et al.*, 1996). MRI can also identify parenchymal lesions, which may affect the prognosis. The extent of the intramedullary hyperintensity on sagittal and transverse T2-weighted MR images (Figure 16.14), and the detection of an intramedullary hypointensity on gradient-echo MR images, have been associated with outcome in several studies (Ito *et al.*, 2005; De Risio *et al.*, 2009). The success rates for surgical outcome have been reported (Ito *et al.*, 2005):

- Dogs with no areas of hyperintensity in the spinal cord = 100%
- Dogs with areas of hyperintensity in the spinal cord = 55%
- Dogs with areas of hyperintensity and loss of nociception = 31%
- Dogs with areas of hyperintensity >3 times the length of the L2 vertebral body and no nociception = 10%.

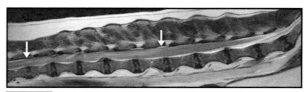

16.14 Sagittal T2-weighted MR image of the thoracolumbar spine of a 5-year-old Dachshund with loss of nociception. Note the loss of the dorsal subarachnoid space extending from the T11–T12 to the L5–L6 disc interspaces (arrowed). A hyperintensity in the spinal cord is visible extending from the T11–T12 to the L3–L4 interspaces. The extensive hyperintensity may be indicative of oedema, inflammation, malacia, haemorrhage and necrosis. Surgical decompression and durotomy revealed extensive myelomalacia.

The recovery rate of non-ambulatory dogs varies according to the severity of the neurological dysfunction (neurological grade), time interval from initial clinical signs to surgery, and the speed of onset of signs (Figure 16.15). The administration of corticosteroids or high-dose MPSS does not appear to

Neurological status and complications	Medical management	Surgical management
Pain, ataxia, paraparesis	75–85% (Funkquist, 1978; Davies and Sharp, 1983; Hoerlein, 1987); 55% (Levine et al., 2007)	96% (pain only) (Sukhiani, 1996); 96% (Schulman and Lippincott, 1987); >95% (Davies and Sharp, 1983; Forterre et al., 2008); 65–83% (Brown et al., 1977)
Paraplegia with superficial nociception	51% (Funkquist, 1970)	96% (Davies and Sharp, 1983); 91% (Brisson et al., 2004); 86% (Forterre et al., 2008); 82% (Ruddle et al., 2006); 81% (Funkquist, 1970); 79% (Schulman and Lippicott, 1987)
Paraplegia with deep nociception	50% (Davies, 1983)	89% (Gambaredella, 1980); 86% (Ferreira, 2002)
Absent deep nociception <12 hours	5–10% (Davies, 1983)	76% (Anderson et al., 1992); 69% (Ruddle et al., 2006); 62% (Scott, 1997); 60% (Loughin et al., 2005); 58% (Olby et al., 2003); 50% (Gambaredella, 1980); 47% (Brown et al., 1977)
Absent deep nociception >48 hours	5–10% (Davies, 1983)	33% (Scott and McKee, 1999); 6.7% (Loughin et al., 2005)
Recurrence rate	50% (Mann, 2007); 48% (Funkquist, 1978); 40% (Levine, 1984); 34% (Davies, 1983); 33% (Ferreira, 2002)	Without fenestration: 42% (Funkquist, 1970); 32% (McKee, 1992); 27% (Levine and Caywood, 1984); 23% (Black, 1988); 17% (Funkquist, 1978); 16% (Brisson et al., 2004); 15% (Necas, 1999); 6% (Dhupa et al., 1999; Olby et al., 2003); 5% (Muir, 1995); 3% (Brown et al., 1977) With single site fenestration: 15% (Ferreira, 2002); 13% (Scott, 1997) With multi-site fenestration: 24% (Knapp, 1990); 16% (Levine and Caywood, 1984); 6.25% (Olby et al., 2003); 7.5% (Brisson et al., 2011); 4% (McKee, 1992); 3.5% (Bartels, 2003); 0% (Black, 1988)

16.15 Success rates for medical *versus* surgical treatment in dogs with thoracolumbar intervertebral disc disease.

improve the outcome in dogs undergoing surgery for intervertebral disc extrusion, but has been associated with a higher prevalence of gastrointestinal and urinary tract complications, increased length of stay in hospital and greater owner expense (Boag et al., 2001; Levine et al., 2008).

Neurological grade: Nociception is considered the most important prognostic indicator for functional recovery. In general, the majority of dogs with intact nociception, whether paraplegic or paraparetic, have an excellent prognosis, particularly if treated surgically. Dogs with loss of nociception for >24–48 hours prior to surgery have a poorer prognosis for return of function. Without surgery, or with delayed surgery, dogs with absence of nociception have an extremely guarded prognosis; however, duration of absence of nociception prior to surgery as a prognostic indicator is controversial. Recovery rates for dogs with thoracolumbar IVDD and absent nociception range from 0–76%. A study of 87 dogs with loss of nociception reported that 58% of the animals regained nociception and the ability to walk (Olby et al., 2003). In summary, dogs with absence of nociception that have surgery within 12–36 hours have a better chance of more rapid and complete recovery than those with delayed surgery. In general, the prognosis is poor if nociception does not return within 2 to 4 weeks from the time of surgery (Scott and McKee, 1999; Olby et al., 2003; Laitinen and Puerto, 2005).

Time to ambulation: Dogs with more severe neurological dysfunction have a longer period of recovery to ambulation. In one study, the mean time from

post-surgery to ambulation varied from 10 days for dogs with pain only or paraparesis to 51.5 days for paraplegic dogs (Brown et al., 1977). Other long-term studies reported recovery times of 2–14 days for dogs that were either ambulatory or non-ambulatory with voluntary motor movement, and up to 4 weeks for paraplegic dogs (Yovich et al., 1994; Scott, 1997). The results from a study of 218 non-ambulatory dogs with intact deep nociception have been reported (Ruddle et al., 2006); 42% of the dogs were ambulatory by 2 weeks and 79% were ambulatory by 4 weeks following decompression. This study also reported that dogs with disc extrusions caudal to L3–L4 are likely to achieve ambulatory status sooner than dogs with disc extrusions between T10 and L3. Patient age and weight are also associated with the time required for the animal to become ambulatory (Olby et al., 2003). In addition, dogs that undergo physical rehabilitation may have shorter times to ambulation (Ruddle et al., 2006).

Onset and duration of clinical signs: There are many contradictory studies about the effect of the speed of clinical sign onset and the duration of the clinical signs prior to surgery on the time taken for recovery and final outcome. In general, it is agreed that rapid removal of extruded disc material facilitates a more complete and speedy recovery (McKee, 1992). Dogs with a shorter duration of clinical signs prior to surgery and a gradual onset of neurological dysfunction (<48 hours) have a quicker recovery (Brown et al., 1977; Gambardella, 1980).

However, a more recent study of 71 paraplegic dogs with intact nociception demonstrated that although a shorter duration of signs was associated with a shorter recovery time, the rate of onset of clinical signs did not influence the recovery time (Ferreira *et al.*, 2002). This study also reported that animals that showed clinical signs for >6 days took significantly longer to recover. Scott and McKee (1999) demonstrated that peracute onset of signs indicated a poorer prognosis for dogs with absent nociception. Knecht (1970) compared the outcome of dogs following hemilaminectomy with the duration of clinical signs and concluded that a delay prior to surgery does not influence the outcome in dogs with mild neurological dysfunction, but does affect functional recovery in paraplegic dogs. When performed within 12 hours of clinical sign onset, hemilaminectomy in paraplegic dogs had a higher success rate.

Recurrence: The recurrence of clinical signs following decompressive surgery in dogs with thoracolumbar IVDD is a common clinical entity with incidence rates reported from 2% to 42% (Funkquist, 1970; Brown *et al.*, 1977; Levine and Caywood, 1984; Black, 1988; McKee, 1992; Yovich *et al.*, 1994; Dhupa *et al.*, 1999) (see Figure 16.15). Risk factors determined for recurrence include the presence of mineralization of multiple discs on radiography at the time of initial surgery, and a breed predilection for Dachshunds (Dhupa *et al.*, 1999). The time for recurrence is usually between 1 month and 2 years following surgery. The recurrence of clinical signs within 1 month of surgery is likely to be related to the original herniated disc space. The recurrence of clinical signs >1 month following surgery is caused by disc herniation at a site distinct from the initial extrusion (Levine and Caywood, 1984; Dhupa *et al.*, 1999; Necas, 1999). Prognosis for functional recovery was not affected by a second surgical procedure (Dhupa *et al.*, 1999). Subclinical recurrence of disc herniation observed on MRI was reported to be as high as 60% in dogs following initial thoracolumbar decompression (Forterre *et al.*, 2008).

Dogs undergoing prophylactic fenestration tend to have lower recurrence rates. Published studies suggest recurrence rates of 0% to 24% with prophylactic fenestration, and 2.7% to 41.7% without prophylactic fenestration. One study determined a 4.7% recurrence rate following multiple disc fenestrations in 265 dogs, but noted that prophylactic fenestration could promote disc extrusion at an adjacent non-fenestrated disc (Brisson *et al.*, 2004). These findings provide further support for additional therapeutic interventions such as prophylactic fenestration (Brisson *et al.*, 2004, 2011) and disc ablative procedures (Bartels *et al.*, 2003; Forterre *et al.*, 2011).

Hansen type II intervertebral disc disease

Clinical signs

The clinical signs of Hansen type II IVDD include slowly progressive, pelvic limb general proprioceptive ataxia, weakness, reluctance to rise or jump on to furniture and difficulty climbing stairs. The onset of clinical signs is considered chronic and progressive, although acute exacerbation of signs is not uncommon. Localization is focal with asymmetrical or symmetrical weakness. Paraspinal hyperaesthesia may be present.

Pathogenesis

Hansen type II IVDD is annular protrusion caused by shifting of central nuclear material and is commonly associated with fibroid disc degeneration (see Chapter 15). The annulus fibrosus slowly protrudes into the spinal canal to cause spinal cord compression. The chronic compression can lead to focal ischaemic and other microvascular derangements of the spinal cord. Type II IVDD usually occurs at the mobile points of the spinal column and is more common in older non-chondrodystrophic breeds of dog. It is not uncommon to identify multiple affected disc spaces. Chronic spinal instability may give an underlying predisposition to type II IVDD.

Diagnosis

The diagnosis may be suspected on routine spinal radiographs that show the presence of degenerative changes in the spinal column, such as spondylosis. Myelography, CT myelography or MRI is necessary to locate the spinal cord compression.

Treatment and prognosis

Medical management: Medical therapy is indicated in animals with early-onset type II IVDD and mild deficits. It is also indicated in those animals that are concurrently affected with suspected degenerative myelopathy. Medical therapy involves the administration of NSAIDs or corticosteroids. The use of a muscle relaxant (e.g. diazepam or methocarbamol) should be considered in patients with spinal hyperaesthesia (see Chapter 14). Rehabilitation protocols may also be helpful. Clinical signs do not always respond to medical therapy and often return following discontinuation of treatment. Surgical decompression may offer a better long-term outcome.

Surgical management: The type of surgical decompression depends upon the location of the lesion. A hemilaminectomy is performed for lesions in the thoracic spine and lumbar spine cranial to L5. A dorsal laminectomy is performed if the lesion is located in the lumbosacral area. Typically, type II disc protrusions require more spinal cord manipulation to relieve the compression from the annulus. The protrusion is usually excised; however, decompression by laminectomy alone may also be adequate in cases where the disc material is irretrievable. Lateral corpectomy is an alternative method for decompression of ventral and lateroventral thoracolumbar disc disease (Moissonnier *et al.*, 2004, 2011).

The neurological status of the animal is often worse following surgery, but this is usually temporary. Surgery may not be beneficial for those dogs with severe clinical signs that have progressed over several months because of irreversible neuronal loss as a result of the chronic compression. Dogs with chronic clinical signs often have multiple intervertebral disc herniations, which complicates the surgical decision-making process.

If surgery is instituted early, the prognosis is usually fair to good when patients are considered refractory to medical therapy. If the disease has coursed for several months and is associated with severe neurological signs (e.g. paraplegia), the prognosis is considered guarded.

Feline intervertebral disc disease
Intervertebral disc extrusions in cats causing secondary clinical signs of cervical and thoracolumbar myelopathy have been documented. However, clinically significant IVDD degeneration in cats is rare compared with dogs.

Clinical signs
Clinically significant intervertebral disc extrusion has been reported in cats <5 years of age, but is more common in middle-aged to older animals (Bagley *et al.*, 1995; Knipe *et al.*, 2001; Muñana *et al.*, 2001). Clinical signs due to disc disease may reflect a painful transverse myelopathy at any region of the spinal cord, but the probability of clinically significant disc extrusion seems to be higher in the thoracolumbar and lumbar regions. The onset of Hansen type I IVDD in cats is usually acute (Muñana *et al.*, 2001). Clinical signs of thoracolumbar IVDD include paraspinal hyperaesthesia, paraparesis and incontinence (Muñana *et al.*, 2001; Rayward, 2002). Commonly reported signs for lumbosacral IVDD are reluctance to jump, low tail carriage, paraparesis, urinary incontinence and constipation (Harris and Dhupa, 2008).

Pathogenesis
Hansen types I and II IVDD have been observed in cats, with type II being the more common. However, these are usually discovered as incidental findings at necropsy (King and Smith, 1964). Ventral annular protrusions and degenerative changes were commonly observed, especially in the caudal thoracic and lumbar spinal regions (King and Smith, 1960). Age-related studies of disc degeneration in cats between 10 weeks and 18 years of age, that had no clinical signs of disc disease, showed that dorsal degenerative changes were most marked in the thoracic region followed by the cervical spinal region, and that ventral degenerative changes were more marked in the lumbar region. It was also shown that older cats with intervertebral disc protrusions had multiple lesions and that frequency increased with age. Hansen type I extrusions tended to predominate at the thoracolumbar junction (Rayward, 2002), although one study found the peak incidence at L4–L5 (Muñana *et al.*, 2001).

Diagnosis
Similar techniques for the diagnosis of disc disease in dogs apply for cats (see above).

Treatment and prognosis
Medical and surgical techniques for the treatment of disc disease in dogs also apply for cats, but there have been no large studies published that evaluate and compare the relative success of medical or surgical therapy in cats. The response to surgical treatment for type I IVDD can be excellent, although it is dependent on the severity of the initial injury (Knipe *et al.*, 2001; Muñana *et al.*, 2001; Rayward, 2002; Harris and Dhupa, 2008). Decompressive surgical techniques promote a more rapid and complete clinical recovery and definitively determine the diagnosis.

Spondylosis deformans

Clinical signs
Spondylosis rarely causes neurological signs (see Chapter 14).

Pathogenesis
Spondylosis deformans is characterized by the formation of bony growths and bridges at the intervertebral spaces. This condition is a common radiographic finding in older dogs along the thoracic and lumbar spine (Larsen and Selby, 1981; Kornegay, 1986). Spondylosis is most likely associated with degeneration of the annulus fibrosus of the intervertebral disc. The presence of spondylosis deformans has been associated with type II IVDD (Levine *et al.*, 2006) and degenerative lumbosacral stenosis; however, these diagnoses are often made independent of the presence of spondylosis.

Diagnosis
The lesion is radiographically characterized (Wright, 1980; Romatowski, 1986). The osteophyte formation does not usually compress the neural tissue or encroach within the vertebral canal (Figure 16.16).

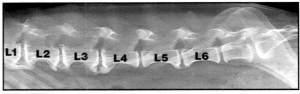

16.16 Lateral radiograph of the lumbar spine showing spondylosis at the L1–L2, L2–L3, L3–L4 and L5–L6 intervertebral disc spaces.

Treatment and prognosis
NSAIDs or corticosteroids have been reported to lessen spinal discomfort in animals with severe ankylosing spondylosis. Spondylosis deformans is usually an incidental finding and is rarely associated with clinical signs; therefore, the prognosis is good.

Spinal synovial cysts

Clinical signs
Clinical signs are consistent with a progressive myelopathy and include paraspinal hyperaesthesia.

Pathogenesis
Spinal synovial cysts occur in the cervical spine (see Chapter 15) of young large-breed dogs but more commonly involve the thoracolumbar region in

older large-breed dogs (Perez *et al.*, 2000; Dickinson *et al.*, 2001b). Spinal extradural synovial cysts and ganglion cysts arise from the articular facets. Some authors have referred to both structures as intraspinal cysts due to the confusion of tissue origin (Perez *et al.*, 2000). The pathogenesis of synovial cysts has been associated with degenerative disease and trauma. Increased mechanical stress and joint motion may predispose the thoracolumbar junction to osteoarthritis and synovial cyst formation. Histopathology of the cyst reveals fibrous connective tissue with a synovial cell lining.

Diagnosis
Radiographic findings include degenerative changes and remodelling of the articular processes. Myelography demonstrates spinal cord compression, especially on the ventrodorsal view, with attenuation of the contrast medium column medial to the articular processes. Attenuation of the ventral and dorsal contrast medium columns (giving an hourglass appearance) is also visible on lateral views. The lesion is better defined using CT myelography or MRI. Cysts appear as hyperintense lesions on both T2-weighted and STIR images. Albuminocytological dissociation is a consistent finding on lumbar CSF analysis.

Treatment and prognosis
Treatment often involves surgical decompression and excision of the cyst. Surgical intervention is indicated with severe neurological deficits and refractory pain. A hemilaminectomy is often performed if one side is affected. The cyst and any protruding disc material are removed. Marked improvements in gait and neurological deficits occur following surgery.

Calcinosis circumscripta
Calcinosis circumscripta (tumoral calcinosis) is an unusual disease that affects young dogs. Mineralization of the soft tissues of the spine (typically the ligamentum flavum) causes compression of the underlying spinal cord. The most common site for these lesions is dorsal to C1–C2. However, cranial thoracic lesions that cause spinal hyperaesthesia and paraparesis have been reported, particularly in German Shepherd Dogs. The reader is referred to Chapter 15 for a full discussion of this disease.

Mucopolysaccharidosis

Clinical signs
The major forms of mucopolysaccharidosis (MPS) seen in cats are types I, VI and VII and in dogs are types I, II, IIIA, IIIB and VII (March, 2001; Ellinwood *et al.*, 2004). These diseases are characterized by multi-systemic abnormalities, including skeletal, ocular, hepatic, splenic and CNS. The axial and appendicular skeletons are affected most severely, causing facial and limb deformities. MPS VI causes bony proliferative lesions of the thoracolumbar spine, leading to secondary compressive myelopathy, most commonly from T12 to L2 (Haskins *et al.*, 1980, 1983). Necropsy demonstrates bony fusion in the cervical, thoracic and lumbar vertebrae.

Pathogenesis
MPS comprises a group of lysosomal diseases that result from defects in metabolism of certain glycosaminoglycans or acidic mucopolysaccharides, which accumulate in the connective tissues and brain. The genetic defect associated with MPS in dogs and cats is considered to be autosomal recessive.

Diagnosis
A diagnosis of MPS is suspected based on clinical signs and signalment, Radiography of the spine reveals bony proliferation. The lesions are better defined by myelography and CT. A definitive diagnosis can be made by measuring lysosomal enzyme activity in leucocyte pellets, frozen liver, serum or cultured skin fibroblasts. DNA testing is available for some forms of MPS (Ray *et al.*, 1998; Ellinwood *et al.*, 2004) (see Appendix 1). The toluidine blue spot test for urinary sulphated glycosaminoglycans is positive. In some forms of MPS, circulating neutrophils contain metachromatic granules when stained with toluidine blue.

Treatment and prognosis
Surgical correction of the spinal cord compression is performed by dorsal or hemilaminectomy to ameliorate the signs of compressive myelopathy associated with MPS VI (Haskins *et al.*, 1980, 1983). Some forms of MPS have been partially corrected following heterologous bone marrow transplantation, viral vector or other gene transfer agent therapy, and enzyme replacement therapy (Ellinwood *et al.*, 2004; Vite, 2010). The prognosis is considered guarded for dogs and cats with spinal cord compression secondary to MPS.

Anomalous diseases

Osteochondromatosis

Clinical signs
Clinical signs are reflected as pain and loss of function during active bone growth. Progressive paraparesis is the most common neurological finding.

Pathogenesis
Osteochondromatosis (also known as multiple cartilaginous exostosis or multiple osteochondroma) has been described in young dogs, cats and horses (Finnie and Sinclair, 1981; Reidarson *et al.*, 1988). Bony growths arise in any bone formed by endochondral ossification. Outgrowths are related to the metaphysis of growing bones. Lesions are present in the axial and appendicular skeleton. Vertebral involvement is common in dogs.

Diagnosis
The bony lesions are characterized radiographically as variably sized circumscribed radiopaque densities with radiolucent areas (Figure 16.17) (see Chapter 5). CT and MRI can aid in the characterization of osteochondromas (Caporn and Read, 1996). A definitive diagnosis is made by histopathology.

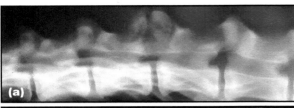

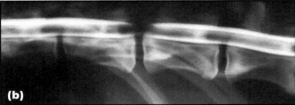

16.17 **(a)** Lateral radiograph at the level of the thoracolumbar junction showing osseous proliferation of the T13–L1 articular processes. **(b)** Lateral myelogram at the level of the thoracolumbar junction showing dorsal and ventral extradural compression cause by the osseous proliferation. Histopathology confirmed osteochrondroma of the articular processes. (Courtesy of Dr D P O'Brien)

Treatment and prognosis

The masses should be surgically excised if there is appendicular or neurological dysfunction (Caporn and Read, 1996). The prognosis is dependent on the severity of the neurological deficits at presentation. The exostoses usually stop growing after closure of the physes, so surgical removal of the masses, if spinal cord compression has occurred, can result in a successful outcome.

Spinal cord and vertebral column malformations

Dogs and cats with congenital spinal malformations often have abnormalities involving multiple areas of the CNS. Malformations associated with the spinal cord parenchyma are often referred to as spinal dysraphism (previously known as myelodysplasia) and involve defects in closure of the neural tube (associated with the mesodermal and ectodermal layers) (Dewey, 2003; Westworth and Sturges, 2010). Such defects may also involve the vertebral column.

In the veterinary literature, specific conditions affecting the vertebral column and/or spinal cord include spinal dysraphism, syringomyelia, dermoid sinus, spina bifida (± meningomyelocele) and caudal vertebral hypoplasia (Westworth and Sturges, 2010) (see also Chapters 15 and 19). These anomalies have been classified into two major groups based on embryological origin (Bailey, 1975) (Figure 16.18):

- Abnormalities originating in tissues of mesodermal origin – vertebrae and intervertebral discs
- Abnormalities originating in tissues of ectodermal origin – spinal cord and meninges.

Malformation	Abnormalities	Clinical signs
Vertebral body and intervertebral disc		
Embryonic phase of development		
Butterfly vertebrae	Sagittal cleft in the vertebral body due to the presence of notochordal remnants	Incidental finding; common in brachycephalic, screw-tailed breeds
Hemivertebrae or wedge vertebrae	Failure of ossification in part of the vertebral body with hypoplasia and lack of vascularization (mediolateral wedge vertebrae)	Scoliosis; compressive myelopathy; instability
Fetal phase of development (failure of segmentation)		
Vertebral body hypoplasia or aplasia	Centrum hypoplasia or aplasia (dorsoventral wedge vertebrae)	Kyphosis; compressive myelopathy; instability
Transitional vertebrae	Vertebrae with characteristics of adjacent divisions of vertebral column	Usually not clinically significant; sacralization of the lumbar vertebrae has been associated with lumbosacral stenosis
Block vertebrae	Lack of segmentation of somites and fusion of adjacent vertebrae	Rarely of clinical significance; may cause spinal stenosis
Spinal stenosis	Can occur with congenital anomalies	May cause compressive myelopathy
Spinal cord and meninges (spinal dysraphism)		
Spina bifida occulta	Defect involving only incomplete closure of one or more vertebral arches	Usually an incidental radiographic finding
Spina bifida manifesta, cystica or aperta	Defect in the vertebral arch with protrusion of meninges ± spinal cord structures	Manifesta – implies associated clinical signs Cystica – implies meningocele or meningomyelocele Aperta – lesion communicates with environment

16.18 Anomalous conditions of the vertebrae and spinal cord. (continues) ▶

Malformation	Abnormalities	Clinical signs
Spinal cord and meninges (spinal dysraphism) continued		
Meningocele	Herniation of meninges from the vertebral canal through the bony defect; spinal cord remains in the canal	Usually no neurological deficits; may cause tethering of filum terminale by fibrous tissue
Meningomyelocele	Meningeal sac contains the spinal cord	Usually associated with severe neurological deficits; may be identified as a dorsal midline mass
Sacrocaudal dysgenesis	Defective or absent formation of sacral or spinal cord segments	Associated with severe neurological impairment (typically at S1–S3)
Rachischisis	Entire length of the vertebral canal open; contents of spinal cord exposed	Often not compatible with life
Other dysraphic states (spinal cord lipoma, dermal sinus tract, dermoid and epidermoid cysts)	Tracts vary in extent of tissue involvement and may communicate with the skin or vertebrae or penetrate the dura	Usually no neurological deficits but communication between the skin and dura may predispose to meningitis
Other spinal cord malformations	Hydromyelia; syringomyelia causing fluid accumulations	Neurological impairment may be apparent

16.18 (continued) Anomalous conditions of the vertebrae and spinal cord.

Spinal dysraphism

Spinal dysraphisms (defects in closure of the neural tube) are further subdivided as open and closed. Open spinal dysraphism refers to when the neural tissue is exposed to the environment, with or without herniation of the meninges (meningocele) and spinal cord (meningomyelocele). Spinal dysraphism was first documented in the Weimaraner (McGrath, 1965) but has been described in many other breeds, including the Rottweiler (Shell *et al.*, 1988), Dalmatian (Neufeld and Little, 1974), Alaskan Malamute (Rishniw *et al.*, 1994), Chihuahua (Chesney, 1973) and Golden Retriever (Malik *et al.*, 1991).

Clinical signs: Characteristic clinical signs include a hopping gait, crouched stance, wide-based stance and reduced postural reactions. Head tilt, tail abnormalities and scoliosis have also been recognized in some dogs. Scoliosis is a reflection of denervation muscle atrophy subsequent to damage to the grey matter and associated LMN signs. Clinical signs are evident as early as 4–6 weeks of age. There is a poor correlation between severity of histopathological lesions and clinical signs. Clinical signs often remain static.

Pathogenesis: Spinal dysraphism is thought to be inherited in the Weimaraner as a co-dominant lethal gene: homozygotes die and heterozygotes are variably affected (Shelton, 1977). Histopathology of the spinal cord reveals asymmetry of the grey matter with neuronal ectopia and syringomyelia. Although dysraphisms are congenital defects that result from failure of the neural tube to close, no fusion defects have been documented.

Diagnosis: Survey spinal radiography may reveal evidence of scoliosis. Syringomyelia is detected on MRI. A definitive diagnosis is based on histopathology (Figure 16.19).

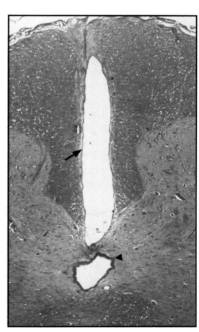

16.19 Transverse section of the spinal cord from a dog with syringomyelia (arrowed) and hydromyelia (arrowhead). (H&E stain; original magnification X40) (Courtesy of Dr GE Lees)

Treatment and prognosis: There is no treatment for this disorder. As the clinical signs often remain static, the prognosis depends on the functional capabilities of the dog for its resultant quality of life.

Syringo(hydro)myelia

Syringomyelia refers to a disease where a tubular cavitation filled with CSF extends through many spinal cord segments (Figures 16.19 and 16.20). Hydromyelia is characterized by the accumulation of CSF within an enlarged central canal of the spinal cord. These diseases occur most commonly (but not exclusively) in the cervical spinal cord and are described in full in Chapter 14.

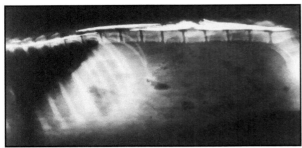

16.20 Lateral myelogram showing syringo(hydro) myelia in the lumbar spinal cord region. (Courtesy of Dr GE Lees)

Dermoid sinus tract

Dermoid sinus tract is an inherited neural tube defect in the Rhodesian Ridgeback (Gammie, 1986) but has also been reported in other dog breeds (Selcer *et al.*, 1984; Fatone *et al.*, 1995; Cornegliani *et al.*, 2001) and rarely in cats (Henderson *et al.*, 1993; Rochat *et al.*, 1996).

Clinical signs: Dermoid sinuses more often occur in the cervical region but can involve the thoracolumbar region (Selcer *et al.*, 1984; Fatone *et al.*, 1995). In the Rhodesian Ridgeback, the sinus tract is most commonly located in the cervical region, whereas in other breeds the most common location is the cranial to mid-thoracic region. The neurological examination is normal in the non-communicating form but neurological signs may occur if the sinus communicates with the dura or becomes infected (Selcer *et al.*, 1984). Neurological signs reflect the neuroanatomical localization of the sinus. Close inspection of the hair on the midline may reveal abnormal placement. The sinus can often be palpated as a thin fibrous cord under the skin.

Pathogenesis: The defect results from incomplete separation of the skin and neural tube during embryonic development (Bailey and Morgan, 1992; Westworth and Sturges, 2010). The sinus often extends from the skin to the supraspinous ligament as a closed sac filled with keratin debris. Communication with the subarachnoid space can predispose to meningomyelitis. An autosomal dominant mutation in the fibroblastic growth factor genes has been described in the Rhodesian Ridgeback (Salmon-Hillbertz *et al.*, 2007).

Diagnosis: The diagnosis is based on the physical examination. Radiography can be used to evaluate the extent of the sinus. Contrast radiography, using a non-ionic contrast medium (e.g. iohexol), determines whether the tract is closed and non-communicating or open and communicating with the spinal canal. Myelography demonstrates the amount of spinal cord displacement. MRI or CT may define other neural tube defects in a communicating dermoid sinus (Figure 16.21).

Treatment and prognosis: The treatment requires surgical excision (Gammie, 1986). A laminectomy is required for complete dissection of the sinus from

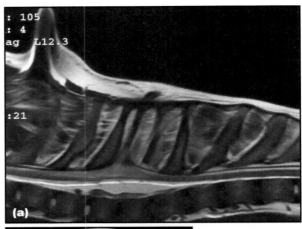

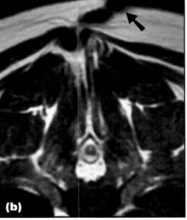

16.21 T2-weighted MR images of the thoracic spine of a 3-year-old male German Shepherd Dog with a dermoid sinus, spina bifida, meningocele and spinal dysraphism at T5–T6. **(a)** Sagittal view. There is widening of the vertebral canal with dorsal displacement of the spinal cord, which appears to be pulled against the roof of T5–T6. The dura is displaced dorsally and protrudes between the abnormal dorsal spinous processes of T5 (due to spina bifida) and continues as a thin hypointense column to the surface of the skin. **(b)** Transverse view. The displacement of the dura is also evident on this view. Note there is a depression in the surface of the skin where the dura makes contact (arrowed).

the involved dura. The prognosis is excellent in patients that have no neurological signs and no associated communication between the sinus and spinal cord. Residual neurological deficits may be present if the spinal cord is involved.

Vertebral column anomalies

Mesodermal anomalies involve defects in the formation of the vertebra and segmentation defects. Congenital anomalies of the vertebral column may be associated with the spinal cord (e.g. dysraphism) or other organ systems (e.g. cardiovascular or urogenital). Spina bifida can occur in the thoracic region but is more common in the caudal lumbar region of the vertebral column (see Chapter 19). Spina bifida is considered a form of spinal dysraphism (see above) and is characterized by failure of the vertebral arches to fuse, with or without protrusion of the spinal cord and meninges (Westworth and Sturges, 2010).

Clinical signs: Vertebral anomalies are often incidental findings and usually cause no clinical signs (Morgan, 1968; Westworth and Sturges, 2010). Malformations involving the spinal cord are more likely to cause neurological deficits, the nature of which is determined by the location of the abnormality.

Pathogenesis: Vertebral anomalies are common in brachycephalic and screw-tailed breeds of dog such as the Bulldog and Boston Terrier, and in the tailless Manx cat (see Chapter 19).

Diagnosis: The diagnosis is suspected based on the clinical signs, signalment and survey radiographic findings (Figure 16.22). Myelography and cross-sectional imaging are useful for determining the extent of compression, stenosis and other possible spinal cord and vertebral column deformities (Knecht *et al.*, 1979). MRI is more sensitive for determining spinal cord involvement and associated alterations in CSF flow (e.g. due to a cyst, syrinx or oedema) (see Chapter 5).

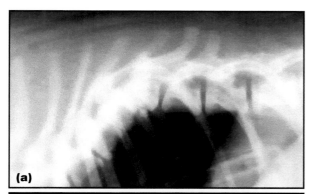
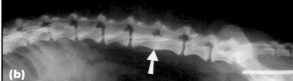

16.22 **(a)** Kyphosis and multiple vertebral anomalies of the thoracic region of the spine. **(b)** Block vertebral anomaly of the fourth and fifth lumbar vertebrae. (Courtesy of Dr M Walker)

Treatment and prognosis: If the clinical signs are non-progressive, medical management is recommended. Decompressive surgery is recommended with clinical signs of compressive myelopathy. Spinal instability and malalignment require vertebral stabilization techniques. The prognosis is considered guarded if signs of spinal cord dysfunction are present. Multiple anomalies may exist concurrently.

Transitional vertebrae

Transitional vertebrae are congenital anomalies that usually occur at the junctions or divisions of the vertebral column (e.g. cervicothoracic, thoracolumbar, lumbosacral and sacrocaudal). The condition most commonly involves the transitional processes or ribs and can be symmetrical or asymmetrical (see Chapters 5 and 19).

Spinal stenosis

Congenital spinal stenosis indicates a malformation of the spine present at birth and occurs as either a primary lesion or in association with other anomalies that predispose to stenosis (Bailey and Morgan, 1992).

Clinical signs: The neurological signs reflect the neuroanatomical localization of the stenosis. Onset in usually insidious and progressive.

Pathogenesis: Relative stenosis refers to canal narrowing that does not cause compression of the neural tissue, whereas absolute stenosis refers to stenosis that causes spinal cord compression (Bailey and Morgan, 1992). Dobermanns have a relative stenosis that most commonly involves the cranial thoracic vertebrae (T3–T6). There have also been reports of thoracic vertebral stenosis in Bullmastiffs, Great Danes, Basset Hounds, Dogues de Bordeaux and English Bulldogs (Knecht *et al.*, 1979; Stigen *et al.*, 1990; Stalin *et al.*, 2009; Westworth and Sturges, 2010).

Diagnosis: The diagnosis is based on survey radiography, which defines the associated vertebral anomalies, but myelography and/or cross-sectional imaging is required to determine the presence of stenosis. MRI of the spinal cord is recommended to further delineate associated neural tissue anomalies or abnormalities (Figure 16.23).

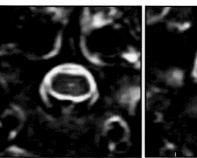
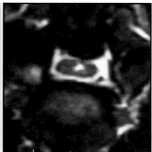

16.23 Transverse T2-weighted MR images of the thoracic spine showing a normal canal (left) and a stenotic canal (right). Note the deformation of the spinal cord as a result of dorsal compression.

Treatment and prognosis: Surgical decompression may relieve the compression; however, associated vertebral and spinal cord anomalies need to be taken into account. The prognosis is guarded due to chronicity and the presence of other anomalies. The lack of information available with regard to surgical follow-up makes it difficult to provide an accurate prognosis.

Intra-arachnoid cysts

Clinical signs

Clinical signs reflect a progressive T3–L3 myelopathy that usually lacks paraspinal hyperaesthesia. Incontinence may be a prominent clinical feature.

Pathogenesis

Intra-arachnoid cysts (also known as subarachnoid cysts, meningeal cysts, leptomeningeal cysts and arachnoid diverticula) can cause compression of the thoracolumbar spinal cord. Intra-arachnoid cysts occur in the intradural–extramedullary space. It is proposed that these cysts are actually diverticula in the intradural space (see also Chapter 15). Thoracolumbar intra-arachnoid cysts more commonly occur over the caudal thoracic vertebrae (T11–T13) and may expand over two vertebrae (Skeen et al., 2003). Dogs with thoracolumbar intra-arachnoid cysts are older at the age of onset than those animals with cervical cysts (Skeen et al., 2003). Pugs appear to be predisposed. Congenital forms may be associated with other neural tube defects and syringomyelia. Spinal intra-arachnoid cysts also occur in cats (Shamir et al., 1997; Vignoli et al., 1999).

Diagnosis

Myelography is useful for detecting the cysts within the intradural space. On MRI the cysts appear as focal, well circumscribed lesions that are isointense to the CSF both on T1-weighted and T2-weighted images (Figure 16.24). MRI is more sensitive than CT myelography for detecting associated intramedullary lesions such as syringomyelia (Galloway et al., 1999).

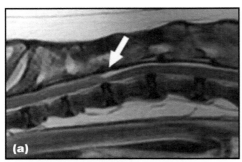

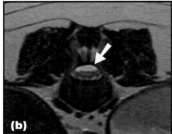

16.24 **(a)** Lateral and **(b)** transverse T2-weighted MR images of the thoracolumbar spine of a 5-year-old Shih Tzu with progressive paraparesis. The cyst is visible as a distension of the subarachnoid space dorsally (arrowed).

Treatment and prognosis

Surgical decompression of the spinal cord is the recommended treatment. Various surgical procedures involve spinal cord decompression and removal or drainage of the fluid-filled structure via fenestration or marsupialization of the dura mater (Rylander et al., 2002; Skeen et al., 2003). Dogs that undergo cyst marsupialization may have a better long-term outcome than those cases where the cyst is fenestrated (Skeen et al., 2003). Medical management is indicated in dogs with mild neurological deficits and includes anti-inflammatory doses of prednisolone and controlled exercise.

The prognosis is good for young dogs if treated soon after the onset of clinical signs (Rylander et al., 2002; Skeen et al., 2003). In one study, dogs that were >3 years of age, and had clinical signs for a duration of >4 months, were more likely to have a poor long-term outcome (Skeen et al., 2003). However, this finding was not statistically significant.

Metabolic diseases

Endocrine neuropathies

Diabetes mellitus can be associated with a peripheral neuropathy (predominantly in cats). This disease is described fully in Chapter 15, but it is important to note that the sciatic nerves tend to be affected first and most obviously, causing pelvic limb weakness and a plantigrade stance. The appearance of signs in the pelvic limbs first is also a feature of hypothyroid and insulinoma paraneoplastic neuropathy in dogs (see Chapter 15).

Neoplastic diseases

Certain spinal cord neoplasms have a predilection for the thoracolumbar spine. Tumours can involve the vertebral body causing secondary spinal cord compression. Tumours affecting the spinal cord are described as extradural, intradural–extramedullary and intramedullary based on their location (Luttgen et al., 1980; Gilmore, 1983; Waters and Hayden, 1990) (Figure 16.25; see also Chapter 14).

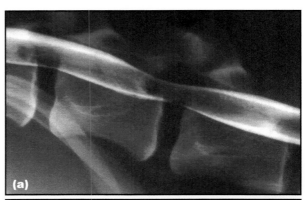

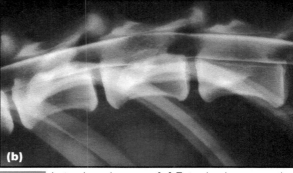

16.25 Lateral myelograms. **(a)** Extradural compression with ventral and dorsal compression of the contrast medium column. The diagnosis of an undifferentiated sarcoma was confirmed by surgery. **(b)** Intramedullary compression over the T13 vertebral body is suggestive of an intramedullary neoplasm.

- Extradural tumours include primary bone tumours, metastatic tumours and haemopoietic tumours (e.g. lymphomas and plasma cell tumours).
- Intradural–extramedullary tumours include meningiomas, neuroepitheliomas and nerve sheath tumours.
- Intramedullary tumours include gliomas (e.g. oligodendrogliomas and astrocytomas), ependymomas and metastatic tumours (e.g. lymphomas and haemangiosarcomas).

Spinal meningiomas

Clinical signs
Meningiomas of the spinal cord in dogs and cats tend to present with progressive paraparesis. The clinical signs represent the spinal cord region involved. Paraspinal pain may be present.

Pathogenesis
Spinal meningiomas are the most common primary spinal cord tumour in cats >8 years of age (Marioni-Henry *et al.*, 2004, 2008). The mean age of onset of spinal meningiomas in dogs is 9 years (Peterson *et al.*, 2008). Spinal meningiomas in dogs are most common in the cervical spinal cord but can occur in any region.

Diagnosis
Myelography typically reveals an intradural–extramedullary compressive lesion. On MRI, these tumours are isointense to hypointense on T1-weighted images and hyperintense on T2-weighted images. The lesions demonstrate strong, uniform contrast enhancement.

Treatment and prognosis
These tumours should be managed surgically because many meningiomas can be completely or partially removed and therefore may be associated with prolonged survival times following surgery (Fingeroth *et al.*, 1987; Levy *et al.*, 1997). Postoperative radiation therapy may be used adjunctively to prolong survival in dogs with incompletely excised tumours. Treatment with surgery and radiation therapy can result in an improved outcome and prevent recurrence (Peterson *et al.*, 2008). The surgical outcome is guarded when meningiomas are associated with an intumescence, have a ventral location or invade the neural parenchyma (McDonnell *et al.*, 2005).

Vertebral body tumours

Clinical signs
Clinical signs may be focal or multifocal depending upon the extension of the tumour. Signs include pain and paraparesis or paralysis. Pathological fractures of the vertebral body result in an acute onset of neurological deficits.

Pathogenesis
Vertebral body tumours are primary or metastatic tumours and are most frequently reported in large-

and giant-breed dogs. Commonly described tumours in dogs include osteosarcomas, fibrosarcomas, chondrosarcomas, haemangiosarcomas, plasma cell tumours, carcinomas, lymphomas and liposarcomas (Morgan *et al.*, 1980; Cooley and Waters, 1997; Levy *et al.*, 1997). Small-breed dogs have a higher rate of vertebral metastasis than large-breed dogs (Cooley and Waters, 1997). In cats, the most commonly described vertebral body tumour is osteosarcoma (Marioni-Henry *et al.*, 2008). Primary vertebral body tumours cause secondary myelopathy by compression or direct spinal cord invasion (Figure 16.26).

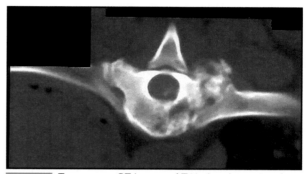

16.26 Transverse CT image of T11 showing extensive osteolysis of the vertebral body. The diagnosis of an osteosarcoma was confirmed by histopathology.

Diagnosis
The diagnosis is often based on survey radiographic findings (e.g. lysis) and pathological fractures secondary to tumour destruction of the bone. Other supportive diagnostic techniques, such as CT, MRI (Figure 16.27) and myelography, are used to determine lesion extent (see Chapter 5). MRI and scintigraphy can be used to detect multiple metastases. Fluoroscopic-guided needle aspiration or surgical biopsy can be used to obtain a definitive diagnosis.

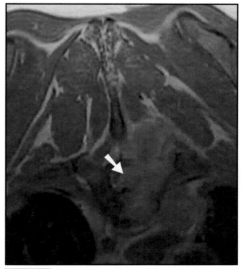

16.27 Transverse T2-weighted MR image of the thoracic spine of a neutered cross-breed bitch that presented with progressive paraparesis. Note the large mass extending from the vertebral body to occupy two-thirds of the vertebral canal (arrowed). The mass is causing severe spinal cord compression.

Treatment and prognosis

Palliative treatment options include surgery, radiation therapy, chemotherapy or various combinations of the three. A vertebrectomy with a bone allograft fusion has been used for the treatment of a primary vertebral neoplasm in a dog (Chauvet *et al.*, 1999). Decompression or stabilization techniques are used in patients that are rapidly deteriorating. The overall prognosis is considered guarded for dogs and cats with vertebral neoplasia. Survival time is not impacted greatly by various treatments but is often determined by the neurological deficits at the time of diagnosis (Dernell *et al.*, 2000).

Vertebral plasma cell tumours

Clinical signs

Paraspinal pain and neurological deficits related to the location of the neoplasm are common signs.

Pathogenesis

Plasma cell tumours have a predilection for the marrow of the axial skeleton. The two types of plasma cell tumour of the spine are the disseminated form (multiple myeloma) and the focal form (plasmacytoma) (Rusbridge *et al.*, 1999). Multiple myeloma is characterized by proliferation of plasma cells within the bone marrow, with or without other organ involvement (Vail, 2000). The neoplastic cells secrete paraproteins causing a monoclonal gammopathy. The disease is associated with other paraneoplastic syndromes. Solitary plasmacytomas have been described infrequently in dogs.

Diagnosis

Spinal radiography, CT myelography and MRI can assist with confirming a suspected diagnosis, localization and lesion extent (Figure 16.28). These tumour types are confirmed by cytology or histopathology. The diagnosis of multiple myeloma requires demonstration of two or more criteria (Vail, 2000):

- Radiographic or MRI evidence of osteolytic lesions
- A bone marrow biopsy with >5% plasma cells
- Monoclonal gammopathy in serum or urine
- Light chain (Bence–Jones) proteinuria
- Hypercalcaemia.

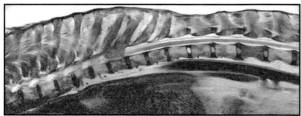

16.28 Sagittal T2-weighted MR image of the thoracic spine of a 9-year-old cross-breed dog with a mass extending from the T7 spinous process and overlapping the spinal cord segment of T7. Note the hyperintensity in multiple vertebral bodies. The diagnosis was confirmed as multiple myeloma. (Courtesy of Dr FA Wininger)

Immunoperoxidase staining for monoclonal immunoglobulin should be conducted on tissues from patients with non-secretory disease (Marks *et al.*, 1995). Diagnosis of a plasmacytoma requires: a biopsy-proven plasma cell tumour; a normal bone marrow biopsy; normal results of serum and urine protein electrophoresis; absence of other lesions on radiographs; and absence of blood dyscrasias.

Treatment and prognosis

Chemotherapy is the mainstay treatment for multiple myeloma. For solitary plasmacytomas, irradiation therapy with chemotherapy is the optimal treatment (Rusbridge *et al.*, 1999). Surgical excision may also be effective for management, but may be limited if it is incomplete.

Chemotherapy with radiation therapy has been shown to decrease metastasis and prolong survival time. Solitary plasmacytomas may represent an early state of multiple myeloma. Since these tumours are both chemosensitive and radiosensitive, long-term prognosis is considered better than for other secondary tumours (Rusbridge *et al.*, 1999).

Nephroblastoma

Clinical signs

Clinical signs of spinal nephroblastoma (thoracolumbar spinal tumour of young dogs) are related to the typical tumour location in the region of the thoracolumbar junction. The most common neurological findings include progressive asymmetrical T3–L3 paraparesis and ataxia.

Pathogenesis

Canine nephroblastoma is an intradural–extramedullary neoplasm seen in young dogs, located between T10 and L2 in the spinal cord. Occasionally these tumours are extradural or intramedullary. The origin of these tumours is unknown, but descriptions have included medulloepitheliomas, embryonal nephromas, nephroblastomas and Wilm's tumours. Primary spinal nephroblastomas are thought to arise from embryonic tissue trapped within the dura during fetal development. The histological appearance may vary. Usually, nephroblastomas involve one kidney or the spinal cord, but not both. Rarely, renal neuroepitheliomas secondarily metastasize to the spinal cord, bone marrow and spinal canal (Gasser *et al.*, 2003).

Diagnosis

Survey radiography of the spine shows no abnormalities. Myelography is useful for determining location and lesion extent. CT and MRI can better assess vertebral and spinal cord involvement (Figure 16.29) (McConnell *et al.*, 2003). Abdominal radiography and ultrasonography can evaluate primary renal involvement if present. Immunohistochemistry is used to identify the mesenchymal or epithelial components of the nephroblastoma. The results of staining with Wilm's tumour 1 (WT-1) antibody can support a diagnosis of nephroblastoma (Brewer *et al.*, 2011).

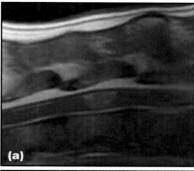

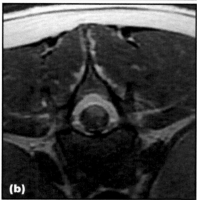

16.29 **(a)** Sagittal and **(b)** transverse T1-weighted MR images (post-contrast medium administration) of the thoracolumbar spine of a 3-year-old female neutered German Shepherd Dog with a 2-week history of progressive paraparesis, due to a nephroblastoma. The tumour is seen as a contrast-enhancing lesion compressing the parenchyma.

Treatment and prognosis

If detected early, surgical excision can result in long-term palliative therapy with limited morbidity (Moissonnier and Abbott, 1993; Macri *et al.*, 1997). Adjunct irradiation is considered when total surgical resection is not possible and may provide a good functional outcome (Dickinson *et al.*, 2001a; Brewer *et al.*, 2011).

The overall prognosis is uncertain because of the limited number of cases reported. Prognosis is considered guarded to poor because spinal cord involvement is often extensive by the time of diagnosis (Brewer *et al.*, 2011). Long-term prognosis is poor because of tumour recurrence.

Spinal lymphoma

Extradural lymphoma is the most common tumour to induce spinal cord dysfunction in cats (Marioni-Henry *et al.*, 2004, 2008) and occurs less commonly in dogs.

Clinical signs

Neurological signs are related to the location of the lymphoma and are often insidious, but there can be an acute exacerbation with rapid deterioration. Cats with lymphoma often have multifocal signs reflective of multiple lesions within the CNS. The most common initial clinical sign in cats is paraparesis, which may be associated with other non-specific abnormalities such as anorexia, lethargy, weight loss and respiratory tract infection (Marioni-Henry *et al.*, 2008).

Pathogenesis

Feline leukaemia virus (FeLV) has been implicated and is an important factor associated with lymphoma in young cats. Lymphoma in cats commonly is found in extraneural sites. Feline spinal lymphoma has a predilection for the thoracic and lumbar spinal cord. Most affected cats are <2 years of age, but older animals may also be affected (Spodnick *et al.*, 1992; Lane *et al.*, 1994; Marioni-Henry *et al.*, 2008). Renal lymphoma is likely to relapse in the CNS (Mooney *et al.*, 1987). Lymphoma is the most commonly diagnosed malignant tumour in dogs but involvement of the nervous system is relatively unusual. Involvement of the CNS is more common than the peripheral nervous system (PNS) in both dogs and cats.

Diagnosis

The safest and most reliable method of obtaining a diagnosis of lymphoma in the CNS may be by confirming the presence of lymphoma in other organ systems (Noonan *et al.*, 1997). The abdominal organs and bone marrow are commonly aspirated but may not be affected. CSF analysis may detect the presence of malignant lymphocytes, but lack of this finding cannot rule out CNS involvement. Survey spinal radiography may detect bone involvement. Myelography is useful for determining lesion extent and extradural, intradural–extramedullary or intramedullary involvement. Spinal lymphoma is detected most commonly as an extradural lesion. MRI may detect intramedullary lesions.

A definitive diagnosis can be determined from the cytological examination of fluoroscopic-guided fine-needle aspirates or surgical biopsy samples (Figure 16.30). In addition, PCR analysis for antigen receptor rearrangement can be used to confirm the presence of neoplastic lymphocytes in the CSF (Burnett *et al.*, 2003) (see Chapter 3).

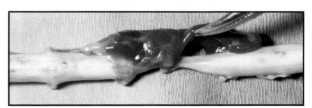

16.30 Necropsy finding of an extradural mass in a cat, causing severe spinal cord compression. The mass was confirmed by histopathology to be a lymphosarcoma.

Treatment and prognosis

Therapies used in combination or alone include surgical resection, focal irradiation and systemic chemotherapy (e.g. cytarabine or methotrexate and corticosteroids; see Chapter 23) (Noonan *et al.*, 1997). A laminectomy provides an accurate histological diagnosis and adequate decompression. Surgical treatment is necessary for cats that fail to respond rapidly to chemotherapy.

Duration and remission times vary between studies. Intramedullary lymphoma is difficult to treat because of the poor penetration across the blood–brain barrier of some chemotherapeutic agents. The effectiveness of chemotherapy for lymphoma with neural involvement still remains to be determined. In general, the prognosis for pelvic limb paresis or paralysis in cats is guarded to poor. The median duration of complete or partial remission in six cats with spinal lymphoma and severe neurological deficits, treated with vincristine sulphate, cyclophosphamide and prednisolone, has been reported as 14 weeks (range: 5–28 weeks) and 6 weeks (range: 4–10 weeks), respectively (Spodnick *et al.*, 1992).

Nutritional diseases

Hypervitaminosis A
Hypervitaminosis A is a rare cause of paraparesis in cats and is discussed in Chapter 14.

Inflammatory diseases

Discospondylitis
Discospondylitis refers to an infection of the intervertebral disc and its contiguous vertebrae. Involvement of the thoracolumbar spine is an important cause of paraparesis but as the most common initial sign is pain, discospondylitis is discussed in full in Chapter 14.

Spinal empyema

Clinical signs
Characteristic clinical signs include a high fever, acute progressive spinal hyperaesthesia and progressive myelopathy.

Pathogenesis
Spinal empyema is defined as an extensive accumulation of purulent material in the epidural space of the vertebral canal (Dewey *et al.*, 1998). This is an uncommon condition also reported in humans after spinal epidural anaesthesia, spinal surgery or haematogenous spread. Direct extension of osteomyelitis or discospondylitis is another cause of the infection.

Diagnosis
Haematology reveals an inflammatory leucogram. Blood cultures can be positive. *Staphylococcus* and *Streptococcus* species are commonly isolated. Radiography may reveal vertebral physitis or discospondylitis. Myelography, CT and MRI can identify extradural compression that extends over multiple spinal cord segments (Figure 16.31) (Dewey *et al.*, 1998; Lavely *et al.*, 2006; Destefani *et al.*, 2008; Holloway *et al.*, 2009). MRI is the most sensitive modality for assessing the severity and extent of the changes associated with infection of the paraspinal muscle and other soft tissue structures (Holloway *et al.*, 2009). Cross-sectional imaging can also help to guide surgery (Figure 16.32).

Treatment and prognosis
Effective treatment is rapid institution of an appropriate antimicrobial therapy and surgical

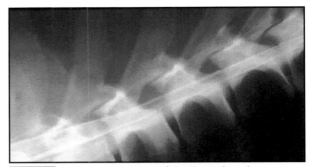

16.31 Lateral myelogram of the thoracic spine showing an extensive epidural compressive lesion dorsally, which was confirmed as spinal empyema. (Courtesy of Dr CW Dewey)

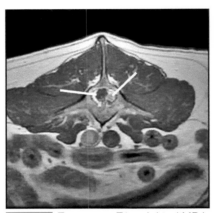

16.32 Transverse T1-weighted MR image of the lumbar spine of a cross-breed dog. The spinal cord is compressed by a lateralized mass of pus.

drainage of the epidural fluid (Jerram and Dewey, 1998). Surgery is the treatment of choice because it allows for spinal cord decompression, drainage of the infected material and direct culture of the organism. Dogs with spinal empyema have a good outcome when treated surgically, followed by appropriate long-term antimicrobial therapy based on culture and sensitivity testing (Lavely *et al.*, 2006; Destefani *et al.*, 2008).

Inflammatory spinal cord diseases
Inflammatory diseases of the meninges and CNS can also cause focal signs of paraparesis and plegia. Infectious diseases include feline coronavirus (the causative agent of feline infectious peritonitis, FIP), canine distemper virus (CDV), feline immunodeficiency virus (FIV), protozoal, rickettsial, algal and fungal diseases (see Chapter 11). Non-infectious inflammatory diseases include granulomatous meningoencephalomyelitis (GME) (see Chapter 11) and steroid-responsive meningitis–arteritis (see Chapter 14). The diagnosis of these disorders is supported by the clinical presentation, CSF analysis, serology and necropsy examination.

Canine distemper viral myelitis

Clinical signs: Respiratory, enteric, neurological and ocular manifestations have been described in naturally occurring disease (Appel, 1969; Tipold *et al.*, 1992; Thomas *et al.*, 1993). Respiratory and enteric forms of the disease are more common in puppies or severely immunosuppressed adult dogs. Neurological signs, whether acute or chronic, are usually progressive. Neurological signs vary with the area of the CNS infected but spinal cord signs can predominate. Clinical signs of CDV myelitis can be focal or diffuse and the T3–L3 spinal region is frequently involved. Paraspinal hyperaesthesia can occur as a result of meningeal inflammation. Myoclonus (involuntary twitching of muscles) can present without other neurological signs, but as the spinal cord disease progresses there may be UMN signs in the affected limbs.

Pathogenesis: Canine distemper is a *Morbillivirus* within the family Paramyxoviridae that can cause focal or diffuse lesions in both the grey and white matter of the CNS (Greene and Appel, 1998). Focal or diffuse demyelination can occur in the white matter of the spinal cord. Neurological forms often occur as the only clinical manifestation in dogs with intermediate levels of viral immunity. The type of lesion that arises in the CNS depends upon host immunity and the age and duration of the infection. The type of lesion ranges from acute polioencephalomyelopathy with glial and neuronal necrosis in immature or immunodeficient dogs, to more chronic leucoencephalomyelopathy with demyelination in older or immunosuppressed dogs (Appel, 1969; Krakowka and Koestner, 1976; Higgins *et al.*, 1982; Zurbriggen and Vandevelde, 1994). Demyelination is therefore a more prominent feature in the chronic stages of disease (Vandevelde and Zurbriggen, 2005).

Diagnosis: The diagnosis of CDV infection is based on the history and clinical signs. A definitive antemortem diagnosis of CDV infection is difficult to obtain. MRI may provide evidence of white matter involvement in the brain and spinal cord (Bathen-Noethen *et al.*, 2008). Clinical laboratory findings and CSF analysis are often non-specific. Immunofluorescent techniques for identifying CDV antigen in conjunctival tissues, CSF, urine, skin or blood can facilitate a diagnosis but lack sensitivity. Multiple methods of detection should increase the diagnostic suspicion of CDV infection. Determining the CSF-specific immunoglobulin G (IgG) levels and the CSF:serum ratio, as well as PCR analysis, can be used to detect chronic CDV infections.

Treatment and prognosis: The treatment of CDV myelitis is often unsuccessful. Corticosteroid therapy of short duration may provide some remedy. Clinical signs typically wax and wane over time, followed by a more rapid progression. The prognosis for recovery is considered poor.

Feline infectious peritonitis, myelitis and meningitis

Clinical signs: Most infected cats are <2 years old but animals of any age can be affected (Addie and Jarrett, 1998). Clinical signs are often insidious and present with a focal, diffuse or multifocal distribution. Signs are often vague and reflect multiple organ system involvement. Systemic signs include pyrexia, weight loss, dullness and anorexia. Commonly recognized spinal signs include pelvic limb or generalized ataxia and paraspinal hyperaesthesia (Legendre and Whitenack, 1975; Kline *et al.*, 1994). Pathology of spinal cord disease includes hydromyelia and myelitis. Other areas of the CNS are also involved; typically, these cases also present with intracranial signs (see Chapter 11).

Pathogenesis: FIP in cats is caused by the ubiquitous feline enteric coronavirus (Pedersen, 1995; Addie and Jarrett, 1998). FIP is an immune complex forming condition involving virus, antibodies and complement. Histological findings include granulomatous inflammation of the meninges, ependymal cells and choroid plexus (Kornegay, 1978). FIP occurs in two forms: non-effusive (dry) and effusive (wet). CNS involvement is seen most commonly with the dry form.

Diagnosis: Confirmation of FIP antemortem is very difficult. Biopsy confirmation of infected tissue is the only method to diagnose FIP definitively. CSF analysis is abnormal with an elevated total nucleated cell count and protein levels (Kline *et al.*, 1994). The white blood cell (WBC) differential often reflects a neutrophilic pleocytosis, but cellular distribution can be variable. CSF protein concentrations can be extremely elevated (1000–2000 mg/dl). Results of serological testing are difficult to interpret reliably. The most useful antemortem indicators of disease are a positive anti-coronavirus titre in the CSF, a high serum total protein concentration, and findings on imaging studies including periventricular enhancement, ventricular dilatation and hydrocephalus (Foley *et al.*, 1998).

Treatment and prognosis: FIP is an incurable condition. Clinical management is supportive and revolves around the provision of palliative care. The use of corticosteroids and other immunosuppressive drugs may slow the progression of the condition. Various other drugs such as antiviral and immunomodulating (interferon) drugs have been used, but none has been shown to be effective. The prognosis for cats with FIP is poor.

Feline leukaemia virus-associated myelopathy
This disease has been reported in cats chronically infected with FeLV (Carmichael *et al.*, 2002). Clinical signs consist of hyperaesthesia and progressive paraparesis and paralysis. Light microscopic examination identifies swollen axons and myelin sheaths in the brainstem and spinal cord of affected cats. Immunohistochemical staining of affected tissues reveals FeLV antigens in the neural tissue.

Protozoal myelitis
Neospora caninum and *Toxoplasma gondii* infections can cause a focal or disseminated myelopathy

in dogs and cats, respectively (Dubey and Lappin, 1998). Meningoencephalomyelitis and myositis are common lesions associated with *N. caninum* infection (Dubey *et al.*, 1988) (see also Chapter 11). Rapid ascending myelitis is more common with *N. caninum* infection (Ruehlmann *et al.*, 1995). Many previously reported cases of *T. gondii* are now thought to be due to *N. caninum*.

Clinical signs: The neurological signs of protozoal infection reflect disseminated or progressive multifocal disease. Dogs as young as 4 weeks of age may develop a progressive asymmetrical or symmetrical paraparesis as a result of infection with *T. gondii* or *N. caninum* (Core *et al.*, 1983; Hay *et al.*, 1990; Ruehlmann *et al.*, 1995). The organism infects the lumbosacral nerve roots and muscles and often causes a myelitis and/or meningitis (Cuddon *et al.*, 1992). These dogs may have a 'bunny-hopping' gait or present with severe rigid extension of the pelvic limbs. The limbs are rigid because of muscle fibrosis and tendon contracture. The patellar and withdrawal reflexes are lost and severe muscle atrophy often develops. Rarely, the disease progresses rapidly to tetraparesis and respiratory paralysis (Braund *et al.*, 1988; Cummings *et al.*, 1988; Ruehlmann *et al.*, 1995).

Pathogenesis: Infection can occur *in utero*, by ingestion of oocysts (due to faecal contamination) or by ingestion of bradyzoites (in muscle). Although subclinical infection is common, clinically significant protozoal infections tend to occur in immunocompromised or young animals and can affect the muscles, peripheral nerves and the CNS (see Chapters 11 and 15).

Diagnosis: The diagnosis is suspected based upon the history and clinical signs. Electromyography reveals diffuse fibrillation potentials and sharp waves in the lumbar paravertebral and pelvic limb musculature. CSF analysis shows a mixed cell or mononuclear pleocytosis and an elevated protein concentration. Histology of muscle samples and identification of the organism confirms the diagnosis. Serology for *T. gondii* and *N. caninum* is often positive and PCR analysis of the CSF can confirm the diagnosis (Schatzberg *et al.*, 2003).

Treatment and prognosis: Early treatment for 2–4 weeks with a combination of trimethoprim/sulfadiazine or ormetoprim sulfadimethoxine and clindamycin may improve clinical signs (Hay *et al.*, 1990; Mayhew *et al.*, 1991). Pyrimethamine may be added to the regimen but can cause bone marrow suppression in young animals.

Early antimicrobial treatment may improve clinical signs, but recovery is often incomplete. Poor prognostic indicators for the resolution of clinical signs include rapidly progressive disease, signs of multifocal CNS disease, pelvic limb hyperextension and a long time interval between the onset of clinical disease and treatment (Ruehlmann *et al.*, 1995).

Vertebral physitis

Clinical signs
Clinical signs include paraparesis, back pain and lethargy. A high incidence of UTIs has coincided with a diagnosis of vertebral physitis.

Pathogenesis
Vertebral physitis is a condition separate from discospondylitis in young dogs. Bone lysis is confined to the caudal physeal zone of the infected vertebrae. Infection appears most likely to become established in the highly vascular, slow-flowing metaphyseal and epiphyseal capillary beds (Jimenez and O'Callaghan, 1995). Establishment in the metaphyseal–physeal–epiphyseal area is more likely to lead to asymmetrical lesion distribution.

Diagnosis
Radiographic findings are usually confined to the lumbar vertebrae. Lesions initially occur at the caudal physis of the affected vertebral body. Radiographic findings include lucent widening of the caudal vertebral physis with loss of definition of the metaphyseal and epiphyseal margins of the physis, followed by increasing sclerosis in the cancellous bone, collapse of the physis and remodelling of the ventrocaudal aspect of the affected vertebra (Jimenez and O'Callaghan, 1995). Bacteria may be cultured from the blood and urine as well as aspirates taken from the lesion.

Treatment and prognosis
Identification of the organism with culture and sensitivity studies (e.g. of urine) is helpful for determining an appropriate antimicrobial regimen, which should be continued for 6–8 weeks. The prognosis is considered good to excellent if the organism is susceptible to the antimicrobial regimen.

Idiopathic diseases

Diffuse idiopathic skeletal hyperostosis
Diffuse idiopathic skeletal hyperostosis (DISH) refers to extensive ossification throughout the axial and appendicular skeleton, including the vertebrae, in dogs and cats (Morgan and Stavenborn, 1991; LeCouteur, 2000). This disorder is characterized by a proliferative bony response to minor stresses. Radiographic signs are characterized by a flowing ossification, primarily located at the ventrolateral aspect of the spine and extending for at least four contiguous vertebrae (Figure 16.33). The

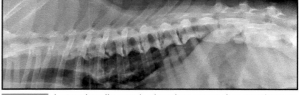

16.33 Lateral radiograph showing extensive contiguous bony proliferation in the thoracolumbar spine of a 10-year-old Boxer. These findings are suggestive of DISH.

interspinous ligaments and the extraspinal ligamentous attachments may also be ossified. Neural involvement is confirmed with the aid of advanced imaging. Clinical signs, such as gait abnormalities and decreased joint mobility, reflect the effects of periarticular involvement of the axial and appendicular skeleton. There is no known cure, although surgical decompression of the neural tissues may provide remission of the signs with likely recurrence. This disorder has a higher prevalence in the Boxer breed (Kraneburg *et al.*, 2010). For further information, the reader is referred to Chapters 5 and 14.

Traumatic diseases

Fractures and luxations of the thoracolumbar spine

Clinical signs
The neurological examination is unique with acute thoracolumbar injury and minimal manipulation is usually advised (see Chapter 20). The neurological signs are determined by the level at which any associated spinal cord damage has occurred. A Schiff–Sherrington posture is a common finding and indicates severe and acute injury of the thoracolumbar spinal cord region, but is not a prognostic indicator. Nociception is carefully assessed in paraplegic animals to assist with determining the prognosis.

Pathogenesis
Spinal fractures and luxations in dogs and cats are most commonly associated with severe external trauma and result in spinal cord dysfunction in approximately 6% of cases (Marioni-Henry *et al.*, 2004; Fluehmann *et al.*, 2006). Vehicle-related injury is the most common cause of exogenous trauma to the spine (Turner, 1987; Selcer *et al.*, 1991). The thoracolumbar junction is frequently injured in dogs and cats (Bruce *et al.*, 2008; Bali *et al.*, 2009). Fractures occur between T11 and L6 in 50–60% of patients following blunt trauma (Feeney and Oliver, 1980). Fractures in the thoracic spine may have little displacement because of the protection provided by the ribs, ligamentous support and epaxial musculature. Fractures and luxations of the thoracolumbar spine are often associated with other systemic injuries (e.g. pneumothorax, pulmonary contusions, orthopaedic injuries, urogenital injuries and diaphragmatic hernia). Approximately 20% of patients with thoracolumbar fractures have a second spinal column fracture/luxation (Feeney and Oliver, 1980). Primary mechanical injury to the neural tissues can subsequently lead to secondary biochemical injury (secondary injury theory; see Chapter 20). The degree of neural tissue injury is related to the rapidity and severity of the insult and the extent and duration of compression.

Diagnosis
The results of the neurological examination are used to determine the neuroanatomical localization and severity of the spinal cord injury. It is important to perform the neurological examination with care to prevent further injury and displacement of the spine. The neurological examination findings are most important in establishing the prognosis irrespective of radiographic findings.

Plain radiography of the entire spine should be performed. Two views should be obtained: lateral and ventrodorsal (patient movement should be minimized by obtaining the ventrodorsal view using a horizontal beam technique). Survey radiography is used to determine the precise lesion location(s) and extent, demonstrate multiple lesions and guide appropriate management (Figure 16.34). Myelography or cross-sectional imaging is performed when the radiographic findings do not correlate with the neurological examination, to evaluate spinal cord swelling in concussive injuries, and to assess further the severity of the spinal cord compression. CT (Figure 16.35) and MRI (Figure 16.36) are useful for evaluating bone and spinal cord tissues, respectively, and provide a 3D configuration of the fracture/luxation extent for assessment of spinal stability.

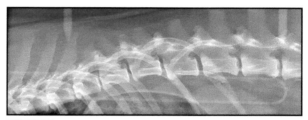

16.34 Lateral radiograph of the thoracolumbar spine of a 5-year-old Golden Retriever with spinal displacement at T12 and T13 after being hit by car.

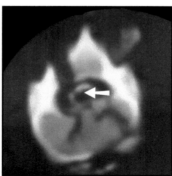

16.35 Transverse CT image showing a complete vertebral body fracture of T13 and displacement of all three compartments (dorsal, middle and ventral). The spinal cord is arrowed.

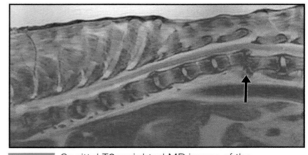

16.36 Sagittal T2-weighted MR image of the thoracolumbar spine showing displacement of the T12 and T13 vertebrae at the disc interspace (arrowed) and spinal cord compression. There is also disruption of the T12–T13 articular processes.

Treatment and prognosis

The critical factor in determining whether medical or surgical management of the spinal fracture and luxation is appropriate depends upon the presence of instability. Spinal stability is assessed using a three compartment theory (Shires *et al.*, 1991) (see Chapter 20 for further information).

Medical management: Priority is placed on the treatment of extraneural injuries, beginning with management of shock and haemorrhage (Jeffery, 2010). Management of an animal with spinal trauma focuses on the prevention of secondary injury to the spinal cord parenchyma (Olby, 2010). The principles of management of the acute spinal cord injury patient, including the use of methylprednisolone sodium succinate, are further addressed in Chapters 20 and 23.

The indications for non-surgical management include minimal neurological deficits, minimal vertebral displacement and lack of myelographic evidence of spinal cord compression. Medical management comprises appropriate confinement for 6–8 weeks and the use of external coaptation. The aim of external support is to immobilize the vertebral segments cranial and caudal to the damaged area (Bagley *et al.*, 1999). It is important to follow the principles of bandage care when using methods of external support. The patient needs to be turned regularly and kept clean and dry to prevent urine scalding (see Chapter 25).

Surgical management: This often provides a better chance for a more rapid and complete neurological recovery. However, the role of surgery for spinal trauma remains unclear. Indications include severe neurological deficits and deteriorating neurological status, imaging evidence of compression and damage to two or more vertebral compartments (Bagley, 2000). Timely surgical intervention is important to allow for maximal recovery. The objectives for surgical management of spinal trauma are decompression, realignment and stabilization (Sturges and LeCouteur, 2003). The decompressive procedure should be conservative so as not to disrupt further the integrity of the vertebrae, but large enough to allow removal of the compressive material (Schulz *et al.*, 1996).

Internal fixation methods are commonly used to stabilize spinal fractures. The method used is dependent upon the size of the patient, fracture type and surgeon preference (Sturges and LeCouteur, 2003; Jeffery, 2010). Common techniques used for internal stabilization include securing plastic plates to the dorsal spinous processes, vertebral body plating, pins and/or screws and polymethylmethacrylate (PMMA), articular process stabilizing and vertebral spinal stapling. Spinal stapling using pins and wire is a widely used technique in small-sized patients (Figure 16.37). PMMA and metallic implantation is the most popular method of fixation because of its flexibility in application to any vertebra (Figure 16.38). Pins or screws are used to anchor the PMMA to the bone (Blass and Seim,

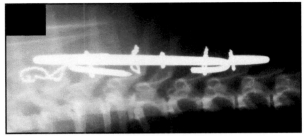

16.37 Lateral radiograph showing the spinal stapling technique used to stabilize a T6–T7 spinal fracture in a cat.

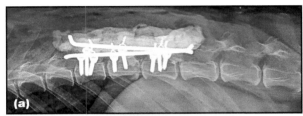

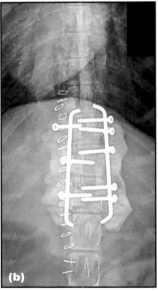

16.38 **(a)** Lateral and **(b)** ventrodorsal radiographs showing the use of PMMA and implants to stabilize a T12 fracture.

1984; Garcia *et al.*, 1994). A successful outcome following surgical fixation depends on the type and strength of the fixation, the skill of the surgeon and their knowledge of spinal anatomy, and the accuracy of vertebral column alignment.

Close attention to postoperative care is imperative for the wellbeing of the patient (Olby *et al.*, 2005; Millis, 2008). Potential complications include UTIs, decubital ulcers and implant failure. Physical rehabilitation is important in the recovery process (see Chapter 25).

The prognosis for animals with acute thoracolumbar injury is dependent upon the results of the neurological examination. The prognosis for recovery from a spinal fracture or luxation that results in paraplegia with loss of nociception is considered poor (Olby *et al.*, 2003). Patients that maintain nociception may still require months to recover and have residual neurological deficits, including urinary and/or faecal incontinence. Studies of thoracolumbar fractures and luxations have reported a 70–95%

recovery rate for medical management in selected cases (Carberry *et al.*, 1989; Bruce *et al.*, 2008). Although displacement can vary, results of spinal stabilization tend to be good if nociception remains intact (Bruce *et al.*, 2008; Bali *et al.*, 2009). Further discussion of traumatic diseases can be found in Chapters 15 and 20.

Toxic diseases

Most toxicities that cause paraparesis do so by having an effect on peripheral nerve function and often quickly progress to tetraparesis (see Chapter 15 for further information).

Antiepileptic drugs
High levels of antiepileptic drugs (e.g. phenobarbital and potassium bromide either used in isolation or in combination) in the blood may result in pelvic limb ataxia, which can progress to tetraparesis (Ross-meisl and Inzana, 2009). Regular serial monitoring of blood levels of these drugs is recommended in epileptic patients that are receiving treatment and have become paraparetic or ataxic.

Vascular diseases

Fibrocartilaginous embolism

Clinical signs
Neuroanatomical localization is often associated with the spinal cord intumescences but other spinal cord regions can be involved (Cauzinille and Kornegay, 1996). Thoracolumbar signs are more common than cervicothoracic. Clinical signs are usually associated with trauma or exercise. Asymmetrical lesion distribution (Figure 16.39) is a clinical feature due to the distribution of the blood vessels to the spinal cord parenchyma (Figure 16.40); however, the lesion can be symmetrical. Symmetrical lesions are more often associated with loss of nociception. Spinal hyperaesthesia can be present initially but is absent after the onset of ischaemia. Maximal neurological deficits

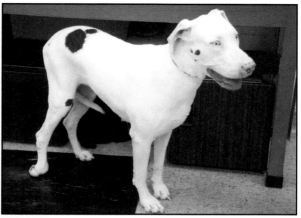

16.39 Great Dane with an asymmetrical spinal cord lesion suggestive of FCE. Note the conscious proprioceptive deficit and atrophy of the biceps femoris muscle in the right pelvic limb.

usually occur within the first 24 hours. Dogs with lumbosacral intumescence involvement more often have loss of nociception.

Pathogenesis
FCE is characterized by acute spinal cord infarction caused by embolism of fibrocartilage identical to that of the nucleus pulposus of the intervertebral disc (Griffiths, 1973). Many theories exist as to the pathophysiology of embolization (Penwick, 1989; Cauzinille, 1993; De Risio and Platt, 2010). Entry of disc material into the vascular system and embolization from the point of entry to the arteries and veins of the spinal cord has yet to be elucidated. The grey matter is more severely affected because of its higher metabolic demand.

Non-chondrodystrophoid breeds are predisposed, which may relate to the disc being more gelatinous and prone to cause microextrusion. FCE is frequently recognized in large- and giant-breed dogs but can also affect small- to medium-sized dogs (deLahunta and Alexander, 1976; Cauzinille and Kornegay, 1996). Certain pure-bred dogs have been documented with FCE including Miniature Schnauzers (Hawthorne *et al.*, 2001) (see **Fibrocartilaginous**

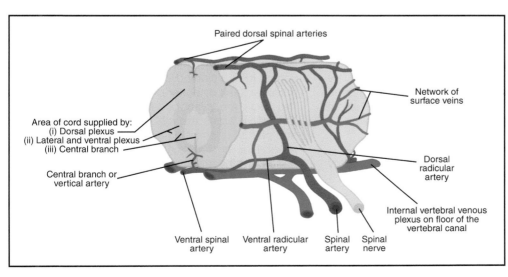

16.40 The spinal cord vascular supply showing the approximate regions of the parenchyma, which have differing arterial networks.

Paired dorsal spinal arteries

Network of surface veins

Area of cord supplied by:
(i) Dorsal plexus
(ii) Lateral and ventral plexus
(iii) Central branch

Central branch or vertical artery

Dorsal radicular artery

Ventral spinal artery

Ventral radicular artery

Spinal artery

Spinal nerve

Internal vertebral venous plexus on floor of the vertebral canal embolism clip on DVD), German Shepherd Dogs and Irish Wolfhounds (Junker *et al.*, 2001). FCE is rare in cats (Scott and O'Leary, 1996; Abramson *et al.*, 2002). In dogs, the male:female ratio varies between studies; the median age of onset in most studies is 5–6 years but there is a wide age range (De Risio and Platt, 2010). In cats, males and females are equally represented with most animals >7 years old at onset (De Risio and Platt, 2010).

Diagnosis

The diagnosis is based on the history, signalment and clinical signs. Early myelographic evidence of FCE is intramedullary spinal cord swelling (Gandini *et al.*, 2003). MRI is the preferred diagnostic imaging modality for the detection of intramedullary lesions and to make a presumptive diagnosis of FCE. MRI findings include a focal, sharply demarcated and often asymmetrical intramedullary lesion, which predominantly affects the grey matter (Abramson *et al*, 2005; De Risio *et al.*, 2007, 2008) (Figure 16.41).

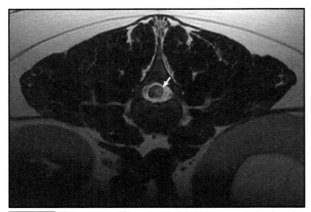

16.41 Transverse T2-weighted MR image at the level of L2 in a 4-year-old Labrador Retriever with acute-onset right pelvic limb plegia and a diagnosis of presumptive FCE. Note the hyperintense grey and white matter lesion on the right-hand side of the spinal cord (arrowed).

The signal intensity compared with the normal spinal cord is increased on T2-weighted images and isointense to hypointense on T1-weighted images. CSF analysis may reveal abnormalities in severe cases. Dogs that are ambulatory on presentation are more likely to have normal MRI findings (De Risio *et al.*, 2007). The severity of the neurological signs has been associated with longitudinal and transverse lesion extent on MRI (De Risio *et al.*, 2007). The diagnosis of FCE is confirmed by histopathology and documentation of nucleus pulposus in the spinal cord vasculature (Figure 16.42).

Treatment and prognosis

Treatment is with medical and supportive care. Early administration of methylprednisolone sodium succinate following the onset of FCE (≤8 hours) has been recommended. As for all spinal cord injuries, physical rehabilitation is important in the process of recovery (Gandini *et al.*, 2003).

Depending upon inclusion criteria, recovery rates range from 54% to 84% (Gilmore and deLahunta,

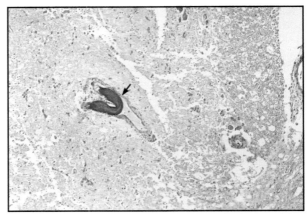

16.42 Transverse section of the dorsal funiculus of the sacral spinal cord. An artery is occluded by Alcian blue-positive material (arrowed), suggestive of a cartilaginous substance. Note the degeneration of the axons and myelin in the white matter of the spinal cord. (Courtesy of Dr BR Berridge)

1986; De Risio *et al.*, 2008). Partial or complete recovery is dependent upon the extent of the spinal cord damage. Negative indicators of prognosis have been correlated with involvement of the intumescences, symmetry of signs, severe neurological dysfunction, lack of improvement within 14 days and decreased nociception (Cauzinille and Kornegay, 1996; Gandini *et al.*, 2003; De Risio *et al.*, 2008; De Risio and Platt, 2010). The outcome has also been associated with the longitudinal and transverse extent of the ischaemic intramedullary lesion on MRI (De Risio *et al.*, 2008). However, no associations have been identified between recovery times and clinical or MRI variables (Gandini *et al.*, 2003; De Risio *et al.*, 2008). Dog size and the severity of the clinical signs contribute to owners electing for euthanasia (Cauzinille and Kornegay, 1996). Animals with functional recovery within 2 weeks have a better prognosis; however, recovery may not be complete (Gilmore and deLahunta, 1986; Cauzinille and Kornegay, 1996).

Aortic thrombosis

Clinical signs

Clinical signs consist of acute onset of an asymmetrical pelvic limb paresis and/or paralysis. Abyssinian, Birman, Ragdoll and male cats were over-represented in one study (Smith *et al.*, 2003). The femoral pulse is weak or absent. The limbs are cold and the nail beds are cyanotic and fail to bleed when cut. The pelvic limbs are stiff and the muscles are hard and painful upon palpation. Typically, there is loss of pelvic limb nociception distally. In one study, tachypnoea and hypothermia were seen in 91% and 66% of 127 cats, respectively (Smith *et al.*, 2003). Congestive heart failure and arrhythmias were each seen in >40% of cats in this study.

Pathogenesis

Aortic thromboembolism is also known as saddle thrombus. Cats with systemic thromboembolic disease have a thrombus that obstructs the terminal aorta (Flanders, 1986). The most frequent underlying disease in cats with thromboembolism is hypertrophic cardiomyopathy, but it can also occur with unclassified cardiomyopathies (Atkins *et al.*, 1992; Laste and Harpter, 1995; Rush *et al.*, 2002; Smith *et al.*, 2003). Thrombi form in the left atrium and dilatation of the left atrium is one of the greatest risk factors for aortic thromboembolism (Rush *et al.*, 2002). The three conditions that favour thrombus formation include blood stasis, hypercoagulability and endothelial damage. Once the thrombus has formed, it usually follows the path of least resistance and eventually lodges at the aortic trifurcation. The restriction of blood flow by the embolus and the release of vasoactive substances cause ischaemic injury to the nerves and muscles of the pelvic limbs.

Diagnosis

Aortic thromboembolism is suspected based upon the clinical signs. Common biochemical abnormalities in these cats include hyperglycaemia, hyperkalaemia, azotaemia and a markedly elevated creatine kinase concentration soon after the embolic episode. Evidence of cardiac disease is further supported by the physical examination findings, thoracic radiography and echocardiography. Doppler ultrasonography of the aorta and its trifurcation can sometimes identify thrombotic disease.

Treatment and prognosis

Initially therapy involves management of the cardiac disease and supportive care. Cats benefit from the administration of appropriate fluid therapy, acepromazine maleate, thromboembolism treatment and pain management. The use of acepromazine maleate is controversial; although it may improve collateral blood flow and decrease anxiety, it may also cause hypotension and current advice is to avoid its use. Specific therapies for the clot include surgical removal, anticoagulants and thrombolytic agents, but risks versus benefits need to be considered (Laste *et al.*, 1995; Moore *et al.*, 2000; Rush *et al.*, 2002; Welch *et al.*, 2010). Given time, the clot may undergo spontaneous thrombolysis.

The use of agents to prevent further clot formation is controversial. Therapies include use of warfarin, heparin, aspirin and thienopyridine derivatives (Hogan *et al.*, 2004; Smith *et al.*, 2004; Hamel-Jolette *et al.*, 2009). Low-dose aspirin (5 mg/cat q72h) has been shown to result in similar survival times and recurrence rates to high-dose aspirin (>25 mg/cat q72h), but with fewer side effects (Smith *et al.*, 2003).

The long-term prognosis for cats with aortic thromboembolism is guarded during the early recovery phase, but may improve if cats survive long enough to be discharged. Studies have shown that rates of survival to discharge range between 27% and 35% with various treatments (Laste *et al.*, 1995; Moore *et al.*, 2000; Smith *et al.*, 2003; Welch *et al.*, 2010). Survival times of cats following discharge range from 117–345 days (Laste *et al.*, 1995; Rush *et al.*, 2002; Smith *et al.*, 2003; Welch *et al.*, 2010). Cats with congestive heart failure tend to have significantly shorter survival times than cats without this problem.

Spinal haemorrhage

Bleeding disorders can cause focal signs of myelopathy (see Chapter 15 for further information).

References and further reading

Available on accompanying DVD

DVD extras
- Degenerative myelopathy
- Fibrocartilaginous embolism

17

Monoparesis

Sònia Añor

The term monoparesis denotes the presence of neurological deficits in one limb. However, monoparetic animals are frequently presented to the veterinary surgeon with the main complaint being lameness. True paresis and lameness of orthopaedic origin can be difficult to differentiate so complete and careful neurological and orthopaedic examinations are mandatory. A lame dog or cat without an obvious orthopaedic cause may well have a neurological lesion which, in many cases, can be resolved if detected early in the course of the disease, whereas a delayed diagnosis (i.e. nerve root neoplasia) may have devastating consequences.

Terminology

Terms that are commonly used include:

- Horner's syndrome – miosis, ptosis, enophthalmos and protrusion of the third eyelid
- Mononeuropathy – dysfunction of a single peripheral nerve
- Monoparesis – decreased voluntary motor function of one limb
- Monoplegia – absent voluntary function of one limb
- Nerve root signature – pain manifest as lameness due to nerve root irritation/compression
- Paraesthesia – abnormal sensation (itching or tingling) due to denervation, usually in the distal part of the limbs. Can lead to self-mutilation.

Clinical signs

The monoparetic animal shows motor dysfunction (usually manifest as weakness) and, frequently, sensory dysfunction (manifest as conscious proprioceptive deficits and areas of hypoaesthesia or anaesthesia) in one limb. Monoparesis is most commonly caused by dysfunction of the lower motor neurons (LMNs) innervating the affected limb. The lesion responsible for dysfunction may affect the motor neuron cell body in the ventral horn of the spinal cord grey matter, its axon (ventral nerve root, spinal nerve, peripheral nerve) or the neuromuscular junction (see Chapter 2). A lesion affecting either a single nerve or several nerves that lie in close proximity (i.e. in the brachial or lumbosacral plexi) can result in clinical monoparesis.

Thoracic limb monoparesis can present in conjunction with ipsilateral Horner's syndrome and/or a decrease or loss of the ipsilateral cutaneous trunci reflex (Figure 17.1) (see Chapters 1 and 2).

- Horner's syndrome is caused by a decrease or loss of sympathetic innervation to the eye. Lesions affecting the T1–T3 ventral nerve roots can injure the preganglionic sympathetic nerves exiting the spinal canal at this level and cause

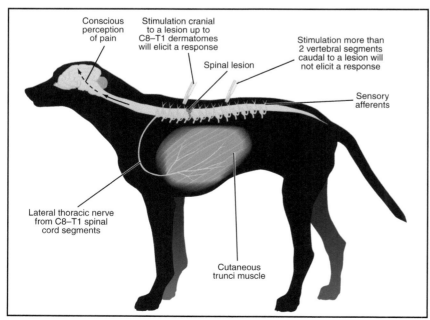

17.1 Neurological pathways responsible for the cutaneous trunci reflex. Cutaneous stimulation along the thoracolumbar region often elicits a twitching of the skin. The twitching is due to contraction of the cutaneous trunci muscle.

Conscious perception of pain

Stimulation cranial to a lesion up to C8–T1 dermatomes will elicit a response

Spinal lesion

Stimulation more than 2 vertebral segments caudal to a lesion will not elicit a response

Sensory afferents

Lateral thoracic nerve from C8–T1 spinal cord segments

Cutaneous trunci muscle

miosis (partial Horner's syndrome) of the ipsilateral pupil (see Chapter 10). Complete Horner's syndrome (miosis, ptosis, enophthalmos and protrusion of the third eyelid) rarely occurs with lesions in this location.

- A decrease or loss of the ipsilateral cutaneous trunci reflex occurs when the C8–T1 motor neuron cell bodies or ventral nerve roots forming the lateral thoracic nerve are injured, causing a subsequent decrease or loss of innervation of the ipsilateral cutaneous trunci muscle (see Figure 17.1).

Lateralized disc protrusions or extrusions localized to the caudal cervical spine commonly cause cervical pain in addition to motor dysfunction of one thoracic limb (monoparesis) or the ipsilateral thoracic and pelvic limbs (hemiparesis). Lateralized disc extrusions or protrusions localized to the caudal lumbar spine or lumbosacral junction can cause ipsilateral pelvic limb monoparesis with neurological deficits localized to the L4–S2 nerve roots (femoral and sciatic nerves).

Lesion localization

Lesion localization for monoparesis is summarized in Figure 17.2. Lesions causing monoparesis of the thoracic limbs are commonly located in the grey matter of spinal cord segments C6–T2, or in any anatomical region of the peripheral nerves forming the brachial plexus (Figure 17.3). Lesions affecting the spinal cord at this level can also cause ipsilateral hemiparesis if they affect the upper motor neurons (UMNs) to the ipsilateral pelvic limb. Unilateral spinal cord lesions (Figure 17.4) at C1–C5 more

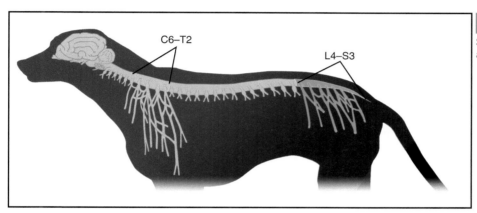

17.2 Lesion localization for monoparesis. Spinal cord segments C6–T2 and L4–S3 are highlighted.

Nerve	Spinal cord segments	Muscles innervated	Reflexes affected	Muscle function loss	Cutaneous sensation	Signs of dysfunction
Suprascapular	C6–C7	Supraspinatus; infraspinatus		Shoulder extension	Shoulder	Little/limited gait abnormality ± shoulder abduction
Musculocutaneous	C6–C8	Biceps brachii; brachialis	Biceps; withdrawal (flexor)	Elbow flexion	Medial antebrachium and first digit	Little/limited gait abnormality; weak elbow flexion
Radial	C7–T2	Triceps brachii; extensor carpi radialis; digital extensors	Triceps; extensor carpi radialis	Elbow extension; carpus extension; digit extension	Cranial antebrachium and foot	Loss of weight bearing; knuckling
Median and ulnar	C8–T2	Superficial and deep digital flexors; carpal flexors	Withdrawal (flexor)	Carpus flexion; digit flexion	Caudal antebrachium and foot; lateral aspect of the fifth digit	Little/limited gait abnormality; mild carpus hyperextension
Lateral thoracic	C8–T1	Cutaneous trunci	Cutaneous trunci	Cutaneous trunci		
Sympathetic nerves to head and neck	T1–T3	Dilator of pupil	Pupillary light	Pupil dilatation		Miosis (partial Horner's syndrome); ipsilateral peripheral vasodilatation causing elevated skin temperature

17.3 Origin and function of the peripheral nerves of the brachial plexus.

Spinal cord lesion localization	Signs in thoracic limbs	Signs in pelvic limbs	Other signs
C1–C5	UMN	UMN	
C6–T2	LMN	UMN	Horner's syndrome [10] Loss of ipsilateral cutaneous trunci reflex Possible self-mutilation of ipsilateral limb
T3–L3	Normal	UMN	
L4–S2	Normal	LMN	Incontinence [19] Flaccid tail Flaccid anus Possible self-mutilation of ipsilateral limb

17.4 Clinical signs caused by unilateral spinal cord lesions. (Numbers in square brackets denote chapters where these are discussed in detail.)

commonly cause ipsilateral UMN hemiparesis. UMN monoparesis of the pelvic limbs can be caused by unilateral T3–L3 spinal cord lesions, whereas lesions causing LMN monoparesis of the pelvic limbs are located in the L4–S2 spinal cord segments or the nerve roots of the cauda equina, or affect the peripheral nerves of the lumbosacral plexus (Figure 17.5). Ipsilateral partial Horner's syndrome and loss of the ipsilateral cutaneous trunci reflex indicate lesions affecting the C8–T2 spinal cord segments or respective nerve roots.

In order to localize a lesion causing monoparesis accurately, it is important to know the motor and sensory innervation of the thoracic and pelvic limbs (Figure 17.6). The cutaneous area innervated by a particular nerve is called the dermatome or cutaneous zone of that nerve. This area includes a peripheral zone (where there is overlap of several cutaneous zones) and a central autonomous zone innervated exclusively by that nerve (Bailey and Kitchell, 1987). Sensory dysfunction (decrease or loss of cutaneous sensation) in these specific autonomous zones can localize the lesion to one or more specific peripheral nerves or spinal cord segments (Figure 17.7).

Pathophysiology

Peripheral nerve injuries can be classified based on the degree of injury and the physical and functional integrity of the nerve trunk.

- Neurapraxia refers to interruption of nerve conduction without physical disruption of the axon. This type of injury is more commonly caused by transient loss of blood supply, blunt trauma or compression, which can sometimes cause demyelination without axonal discontinuity. Recovery is usually spontaneous and complete, and occurs within 1–2 weeks. If demyelination has occurred recovery may take a little longer (5–6 weeks).
- Axonotmesis refers to physical interruption of the axon, with separation of the axon from the neuronal cell body, which results in Wallerian-like degeneration and loss of conduction distal to the injury. The endoneurium and the Schwann cell sheath remain intact. Recovery, if possible, depends on the regrowth of axons, which usually occurs at a rate of 1–4 mm/day (Uchida *et al.*, 1993).

Nerve	Spinal cord segments	Muscles innervated	Reflexes affected	Muscle function loss	Cutaneous sensation	Signs of dysfunction
Obturator	L4–L6	Pectineus; gracilis		Hip adduction		Little/limited gait abnormality
Femoral	L4–L6	Quadriceps group; psoas group	Patellar	Stifle extension; hip flexion	Medial surface of limb and first digit	Loss of weight bearing
Sciatic	L6–S2	Biceps femoris; semimembranosus; semitendinosus; cranial tibial; gastrocnemius	Withdrawal (flexor); cranial tibial; gastrocnemius	Hip extension; stifle flexion; hock flexion and extension; digit flexion and extension	Entire limb, except medial aspect and first digit	Knuckling of paws but weight bearing present
Peroneal	L6–S2	Cranial tibial	Cranial tibial	Hock flexion; digit extension	Craniolateral surface of limb, distal to stifle	Hyperextended hock; knuckled paw
Tibial	L6–S2	Gastrocnemius	Gastrocnemius	Hock extension; digit flexion	Caudal surface of limb, distal to stifle	Dropped hock

17.5 Origin and function of the peripheral nerves of the lumbosacral plexus.

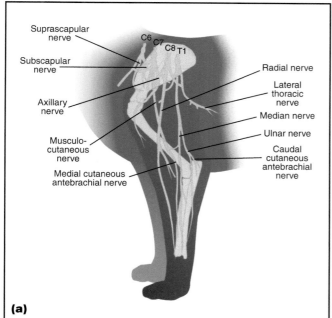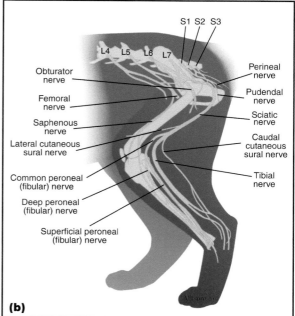

17.6 Peripheral nerve supply to **(a)** the thoracic limb and **(b)** the pelvic limb.

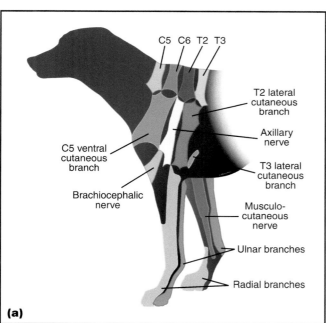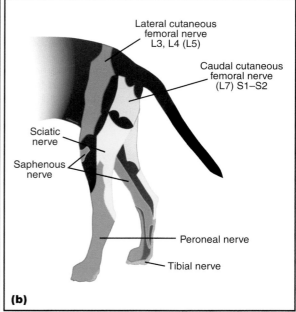

17.7 Cutaneous autonomous zones of innervation of **(a)** the thoracic limb and **(b)** the pelvic limb. (Based on Bailey and Kitchell, 1984 and 1987, respectively)

- Neurotmesis implies complete severance of the nerve trunk (axons, Schwann cells and supporting connective tissue). This is the most severe type of injury. Successful regeneration to the correct target is unlikely to occur and may result in neuroma formation.

Differential diagnosis

The main conditions causing acute non-progressive and chronic progressive monoparesis are listed in Figure 17.8.

Acute non-progressive

• Trauma [17]:
   – Brachial plexus avulsion
   – Radial nerve injury
   – Sciatic nerve injury
• Fibrocartilaginous embolism (FCE) [15, 16]
• Arterial thromboembolism [16, 17]

17.8 Differential diagnoses for clinical monoparesis. (Numbers in square brackets denote the chapters in which these are discussed in detail.) (continues) ▶

Chronic progressive

• Foraminal stenosis:
   – Disc disease [15, 16, 17]
• Neoplasia:
   – Nerve sheath tumours [17]
   – Spinal tumours [16]
• Inflammatory disease:
   – Myelitis/meningomyelitis [11]
   – Plexus neuritis [17]
• Peripheral neuropathy [15]

17.8 (continued) Differential diagnoses for clinical monoparesis. (Numbers in square brackets denote the chapters in which these are discussed in detail.)

Neurodiagnostic investigation

All the specific diagnostic tests to assess a monoparetic animal need to be performed under general anaesthesia (see Chapter 21). A minimum database of complete blood count (CBC), serum biochemistry, urinalysis, thoracic radiography and abdominal ultrasonography is indicated in any neurological patient. These tests are required to assess the general health status of the patient and rule out metastatic neoplasia or systemic disease. In addition, a comprehensive coagulation profile (activated clotting time (ACT), prothrombin time (PT), activated partial thromboplastin time (aPTT), fibrin degradation products (FDPs)) should be performed when vascular (haemorrhage, infarction) disease is suspected. Advanced testing in patients with vascular disease can also include thromboelastography (see Chapter 3).

Electrophysiology

Electrophysiological studies provide more accurate information about the integrity and function of the peripheral nerves (see Chapter 4). Electromyography allows detection of spontaneous electrical activity (fibrillation potentials and positive sharp waves) in denervated muscles 7–10 days after the nerve injury has occurred. If regeneration results in reinnervation, this can be detected by the presence of giant motor unit potentials on the electromyogram (EMG), so repeated studies to monitor progress after acute injuries are useful. Motor and sensory nerve conduction velocity (NCV) studies can be performed in specific peripheral nerves to assess function and integrity, and to determine the severity of the lesion. Cord dorsum potentials can also be recorded to assess dorsal nerve root function in cases of sensory nerve dysfunction (Cuddon et al., 1999). F wave studies allow assessment of ventral nerve root function in cases of proximal motor nerve injuries.

Diagnostic imaging

Radiography

Survey radiographs of the vertebral column may show signs of intervertebral disc disease, enlarged intervertebral foramina in cases of peripheral nerve sheath tumours, or proliferative and/or lytic changes indicative of other neoplasms.

Myelography

A myelogram can be helpful in cases of lateralized intervertebral disc extrusions and protrusions if there is disc material within the canal, as well as in cases of peripheral neoplasms that grow into the vertebral canal.

Computed tomography

Computed tomography (CT) can be useful to detect and better determine lateralization and extension of nerve root tumours, intervertebral disc disease, and some neoplastic conditions affecting the spinal cord.

Magnetic resonance imaging

Magnetic resonance imaging (MRI) is the technique of choice to visualize soft tissue changes and is particularly useful for examining the spinal cord parenchyma, as well as the nerve roots and/or spinal nerves. MR images provide highly valuable information regarding the extent and nature of many spinal cord lesions (e.g. neoplasms, vascular accidents, inflammatory and anomalous diseases), as well as the degree of spinal cord invasion or compression (e.g. intervertebral disc disease, neoplasia).

Degenerative diseases

Foraminal stenosis

Clinical signs

Animals with stenosis of the caudal cervical (vertebral level C5–C7), caudal lumbar (vertebral level L5–L7) or lumbosacral intervertebral foramina show LMN signs localized to one or more nerve roots. Sensory signs, such as proprioceptive placing deficits and regions of hypoaesthesia in the cutaneous areas of the affected nerve roots, can also be seen but are not common and are difficult to assess.

The caudal cervical and lumbosacral regions are the most mobile parts of the vertebral column. 'Nerve root signature' or pain upon manipulation or palpation of the affected limb is commonly seen when there is nerve root impingement secondary to foraminal stenosis, and excessive vertebral movement causes intermittent compression of the affected nerve root. Lameness of the affected limb due to irritation or compression of the nerve root is also frequently observed. The animal may hold the affected limb in flexion, close to the body wall and avoid bearing weight on it (see Chapter 14). This clinical sign may be constant, intermittent or exacerbated by exercise. The exacerbation of clinical signs during exercise, described as 'neurogenic intermittent claudication' (Lenehan et al., 1998), is believed to be caused by engorgement of nerve root (radicular) blood vessels, resulting in further compression and ischaemia of the nerve root in an already narrowed foramen (Jones et al., 1996).

The most common site of foraminal stenosis is the lumbosacral intervertebral foramen. Dogs with degenerative lumbosacral stenosis can develop (unilateral or bilateral) stenosis of the lumbosacral foramina due to degenerative changes, and subsequent compression of the L7 nerve root. These animals may show pelvic limb monoparesis or lameness as the only clinical sign (Figure 17.9). Other animals present with clinical signs indicative of sciatic nerve involvement (i.e. pelvic limb paresis, atrophy of flexor muscles, pelvic limb conscious proprioceptive deficits). Most affected dogs exhibit severe pain on manipulation of the lumbosacral joint or extension of the coxofemoral joint.

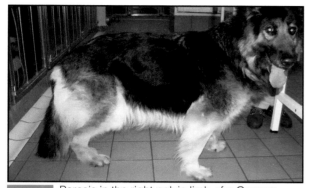

17.9 Paresis in the right pelvic limb of a German Shepherd Dog due to ipsilateral lumbosacral foraminal stenosis. (Courtesy of S Platt)

Foraminal stenosis affecting the caudal cervical area may cause ipsilateral thoracic limb monoparesis. In addition, atrophy of the infraspinatus and supraspinatus muscles, detected clinically as a prominent scapular spine, can also be seen when the suprascapular nerve roots (C6–C7) are affected.

Pathogenesis
Intervertebral foraminal stenosis is most commonly caused by lateralized disc protrusions or extrusions. Other less frequent causes of cervical foraminal stenosis include the formation of synovial cysts at the articular processes (Levitski *et al.*, 1999; Dickinson *et al.*, 2001) (see Chapter 15) or any other type of mass (i.e. neoplasm) growing inside the intervertebral foramina. Lumbar juxta-articular cysts have also been described as causing pelvic limb monoparesis in one dog (Bley *et al.*, 2007).

Diagnosis

Radiography: Plain radiographs of the vertebral column may show the presence of calcified disc material inside the intervertebral foramen in cases of lateralized disc extrusions, but are often unremarkable. Soft tissue opacities within the vertebral foramen may also be seen. Oblique plain radiographs of the cervical and lumbar spine allow better visualization of the intervertebral foramina and detection of any soft tissue or calcified mass in this location. Enlargement of the affected intervertebral foramen may also be observed.

Degenerative changes affecting the vertebrae in cases of lumbosacral degenerative stenosis or cervical stenosis may also be seen, including:

• Enlarged articular facets
• Increased density of articular facets

• Spondylosis deformans
• Endplate sclerosis.

Myelography: This may be useful in identifying disc material, degenerative soft tissue or neoplastic tissue growing inside the intervertebral foramen and extending into the vertebral canal. However, myelograms are normal if there is no encroachment into the canal.

Advanced imaging: CT and MRI are the most useful modalities for identifying intervertebral foraminal stenosis (Figure 17.10). Transverse sections at the level of the affected intervertebral foramina reveal any mass causing narrowing of the intervertebral foramen and nerve root entrapment. The abnormalities observed may be subtle, so careful assessment of the images, paying particular attention to any asymmetry (muscle mass, nerve root size, intervertebral foramen diameter), is essential. The findings should always be interpreted in light of the clinical signs and the veterinary surgeon should be aware that subclinical abnormalities may be found in normal dogs (Jones and Inzana, 2000).

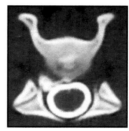

17.10 Transverse CT image showing a foraminal disc extrusion at the C6–C7 right intervertebral foramen. (Courtesy of Dr K Vernau)

Electromyography: This may demonstrate the presence of spontaneous electrical activity in the muscles innervated by the affected nerve root, thus confirming the neurological origin of the deficits and differentiating this from orthopaedic disease.

Treatment and prognosis

Medical management: Medical treatment with anti-inflammatory drugs (steroidal and non-steroidal) may help to temporarily alleviate signs of radicular pain. However, pain and paresis usually recur upon discontinuation of therapy. If anti-inflammatory therapy does not work, acupuncture can provide temporary pain relief (see Chapter 26) and foraminal injection of corticosteroids is gaining credibility.

Surgical management: Surgical removal of the extruded disc material or degenerative connective tissue causing narrowing of the intervertebral foramen is the only effective long-term treatment. Dorsal laminectomy and/or foraminotomy are indicated in cases of lumbosacral foraminal stenosis to relieve compression of the affected nerve root (see Chapter 22). In the cervical region, dorsal laminectomy and/or facetectomy should be performed to remove lateralized disc extrusions or articular synovial cysts (see Chapter 22). If there are signs of vertebral 'instability' (dynamic lesions), cervical or lumbo-sacral distraction and fusion techniques should be used to stabilize the affected vertebral segment and to avoid further progression of clinical signs (see Chapter 22).

Surgical removal of disc material or connective tissue from the intervertebral foramen is a difficult task and requires specialized neurosurgical skills. Endoscopic-assisted foraminotomy (Wood *et al.*, 2004) and a lateral approach to the lumbosacral joint (Gödde and Steffen, 2007; Carozzo *et al.*, 2008) have been described to relieve foraminal stenosis. Lateral approaches to the cervical spine to give good access to the cervical foramina have also been described (Lipsitz and Bailey, 1995; Rossmeisl *et al.*, 2005). When nerve root decompression is incomplete, radicular pain and lameness or paresis may persist. Thus, the prognosis depends on the ability to relieve the compression, in addition to the degree of damage to the nerve roots.

Anomalous diseases

Vertebral anomalies
Some vertebral anomalies can cause monoparesis (e.g. transitional lumbar vertebrae are associated with degenerative lumbosacral stenosis; see Chapter 16). Vertebral anomalies are covered in full in Chapters 15 and 16.

Neoplastic diseases

Nerve sheath tumours
Peripheral nerve sheath tumours are neoplasms that arise from cells surrounding the axons in the peripheral nerves or nerve roots, and can be divided into benign and malignant variants (Schulman *et al.*, 2009). Most peripheral nerve sheath tumours in dogs are anaplastic, have a high mitotic index and an aggressive biological behaviour, so are designated as malignant. Malignant nerve sheath tumours are common in dogs but rare in cats (Hayes *et al.*, 1975; Okada *et al.*, 2007; Schulman *et al.*, 2009). No sex or breed predilection has been reported for peripheral nerve sheath tumours in dogs. Most affected animals are adults >7 years old, but younger animals may also be affected.

Clinical signs
The predominant clinical signs are slowly progressive thoracic limb lameness or paresis, and muscle atrophy. In addition, pain upon palpation of the limb or axillary region may be encountered. A palpable axillary mass may be present in some cases but is not common. Enlargement of the affected limb has been described in one case (Brower *et al.*, 2005). As the clinical signs progress slowly, orthopaedic disease is often suspected before a definitive diagnosis is confirmed. As the peripheral nerve sheath tumour spreads proximally and compresses the spinal cord, neurological deficits may develop in the ipsilateral pelvic limb and progress to involve all four limbs. If the dorsal cervical nerve roots are affected, animals may also show cervical pain. Unilateral, partial or complete Horner's syndrome may arise if the cranial thoracic nerve roots are affected by the tumour itself or if there is cord compression at this point. Similarly, the ipsilateral cutaneous trunci reflex may be absent due to invasion of the C8–T1 ventral nerve roots or compression of these spinal cord segments.

Pathogenesis
Malignant peripheral nerve sheath tumours in dogs most commonly affect the caudal cervical (C6–C8) and the cranial thoracic (T1–T2) nerve roots (Carmichael and Griffiths, 1981; Brehm *et al.*, 1995), although nerve sheath tumours have also been described affecting the sciatic nerve (Abraham *et al.*, 2003) and femoral nerve (Harcourt-Brown *et al.*, 2009). These tumours may have their origin in the nerve roots, the brachial or lumbosacral plexi, or may arise from a more peripheral location in the nerves. Usually, the tumour spreads slowly, both distally and proximally, and may invade the vertebral canal causing spinal cord compression and associated neurological deficits. As the tumour grows proximally, it spreads to the neighbouring nerves in the plexus bundle, with a high percentage of dogs showing evidence of multiple nerve involvement at the time of diagnosis. Peripheral nerve sheath tumours are highly locally invasive, but rarely metastasize, although pulmonary metastasis in advanced cases has been described (Carmichael and Griffiths, 1981; Bradley *et al.*, 1982).

Diagnosis
Orthopaedic disease must be excluded by careful examination and radiography of the appropriate joints. A complete blood count, serum biochemistry, thoracic radiography and abdominal ultrasonography should be performed in any dog suspected of having a malignant peripheral nerve sheath tumour to rule out metastatic disease and assess general health status.

Radiography: Survey radiographs of the spine are often normal. Oblique views may reveal enlargement of the affected intervertebral foramen due to pressure atrophy, caused by the thickened nerve root. Occasionally, lysis of the affected vertebral bodies may be observed.

Myelography: This may be useful to detect spinal cord or nerve root compression once the tumour has reached this location. An intradural–extramedullary defect may be seen at the point where the nerve root exits from the spinal cord (Figure 17.11). However, the myelogram can frequently be normal in the presence of disease.

Computed tomography: CT allows visualization of some malignant peripheral nerve sheath tumours (Figure 17.12), and masses as small as 1.0 cm can be identified on contrast-enhanced images (Rudich *et al.*, 2004). Enhancement of the mass with iodinated

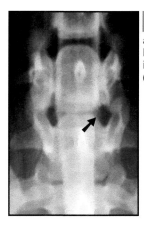

17.11 Ventrodorsal myelogram showing an intradural–extramedullary lesion at the C6–C7 intervertebral foramen (arrowed).

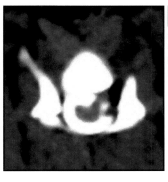

17.12 Transverse CT image showing enlargement of the ventral and dorsal nerve roots at the C6–C7 intervertebral foramen.

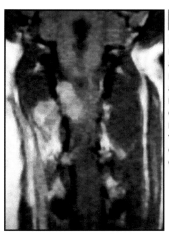

17.13 Dorsal T1-weighted MR image of a peripheral nerve sheath tumour arising from the C2 nerve root following intravenous administration of contrast medium. Note the extension of the neoplasm inside the vertebral canal (arrowed) causing secondary spinal cord compression.

contrast medium provides excellent views, helps differentiate vascular structures and allows subtle differences in soft tissue opacity created by the tumour vasculature to be seen (Niles *et al.*, 2001). Ring contrast enhancement is frequently noted, whilst enhancement within the mass is often non-uniform. However, it should be noted that whilst CT allows visualization of small masses, they may not be specifically associated with neuronal structures, making a definitive diagnosis difficult (Rudich *et al.*, 2004). In addition, many peripheral nerve sheath tumours are not clearly visible on CT images.

Magnetic resonance imaging: MRI of the brachial plexus or peripheral nerves provides excellent diagnostic images, but not all peripheral nerve sheath tumours can be detected using this modality early in the course of the disease. Peripheral nerve sheath tumours are usually hyperintense on T2-weighted images and isointense to the surrounding soft tissue structures on T1-weighted images. Contrast enhancement with paramagnetic contrast media may allow precise delineation of the tumour mass and detection of vertebral canal invasion (Platt *et al.*, 1999) (Figure 17.13). However, tumours may enhance minimally to mildly and many do so heterogeneously (Kraft *et al.*, 2007). In addition, caution should be taken since enlarged, contrast-enhanced nerve roots can also be seen in cases of trauma and focal hypertrophic neuritis. Transverse images with a large enough field of view to allow visualization of the axillae and vertebral canal are essential to detect lesions, and multi-planar, multi-pulse sequence MRI examinations are needed to detect tumours in challenging cases (Kraft *et al.*, 2007).

Ultrasonography: Ultrasound examination of the affected limb may allow visualization of large, hypoechogenic tubular masses that displace vessels and destroy normal architecture (Rose *et al.*, 2005). Ultrasound-guided fine-needle aspiration (FNA) of the mass may be required to reach a final diagnosis in some cases (da Costa *et al.*, 2008); however, it should be noted that FNA can be non-diagnostic.

Electromyography: This reveals abnormal, spontaneous electrical activity in the affected limb muscles and is of great assistance in differentiating neurological from orthopaedic disease (see Chapter 4).

Treatment and prognosis

There is usually no curative treatment for peripheral nerve sheath tumours. Complete surgical resection may be difficult due to the invasive nature of these tumours and the late detection of the disease in most cases.

Tumours within the brachial plexus or peripheral nerves are treated with local excision or amputation of the affected limb. Tumours located within the spinal canal necessitate a dorsal laminectomy or hemilaminectomy to be resected. Tumours originating in the spinal canal and extending peripherally or originating in the plexus and extending proximally can be approached both peripherally and through a laminectomy, and often require durotomy and rhizotomy (nerve root resection). Hemipelvectomy may be necessary to completely excise lumbar plexus lesions. Repeated surgical procedures may be needed as recurrences are common. In many instances, amputation of the limb is the only option.

In one report, there was a tendency for dogs with more proximally located tumours to respond less favourably to surgery and to relapse earlier (1 month for nerve root tumours and 7.5 months for plexus tumours) than those with peripherally located tumours (>9 months after surgery) (Brehm *et al.*, 1995). Incomplete resection is common, indicating that grossly visible margins at the time of surgery are frequently inaccurate indicators of tumour excision.

Early diagnosis and aggressive surgical intervention are recommended to maximize the possibility of complete tumour resection. Aggressive surgical resection at an early stage, if the tumour is peripheral, can be curative. Amputation is only advisable when the tumour is distal and there is no invasion of the spinal canal. In addition, amputation is performed in some cases to prevent or avoid self-mutilation and injuries to the limb in cases of loss of sensation or paraesthesia.

Surgery can be followed by a course of radiation therapy, but it is unclear whether this positively affects the prognosis, since these tumours are poorly responsive to radiation. Despite aggressive management, the overall prognosis is considered poor for most cases of malignant peripheral nerve sheath tumours.

Other neoplastic diseases

Any neoplastic condition affecting the spine, meninges or spinal cord can cause monoparesis of a pelvic limb if located laterally within the vertebral canal caudal to the third thoracic spinal cord segment. Meningiomas in particular can initially cause lateralized clinical signs. However, most spinal tumours cause bilateral disease.

Lymphoma

Lymphoma is the most common tumour that affects the spinal cord in cats. Affected cats are usually young (<5 years old) and are frequently infected with feline leukaemia virus (FeLV). Typically, there is an extradural mass causing spinal cord compression and signs of myelopathy. However, there are several reports of spinal lymphoma in which there was infiltration of the brachial plexus in cats, causing initial signs of monoparesis (Fox and Gutnick, 1972; Spodnick et al., 1992). This disease is described in full in Chapter 16.

Miscellaneous

Whenever a tumour grows adjacent to a nerve, it can cause compression of that nerve. Examples of tumours that behave in this way include:

- Vertebral tumours (see Chapter 16)
- Infiltrating liposarcomas and other sarcomas (Montoliu et al., 2008)
- Ganglioneuromas
- Malignant apocrine sweat glands (one reported case; Carmichael and Griffiths, 1981).

The clinical presentation mimics that of a peripheral nerve sheath tumour but a mass may be palpable and should be identifiable on CT or MRI.

Inflammatory diseases

Myelitis and meningomyelitis

Focal forms of myelitis and meningomyelitis of infectious or immune-mediated origin can cause monoparesis of the thoracic or pelvic limbs when the inflammatory focus is unilateral and located in the brachial (C6–T2) or lumbosacral (L4–S2) intumescences of the spinal cord. These diseases are described in detail in Chapter 11.

Plexus neuritis

Plexus neuritis is an uncommon inflammatory condition that can affect the brachial plexus of dogs (Cummings et al., 1973; Alexander et al., 1974) and cats (Bright et al., 1978; Garosi et al., 2006) (Figure 17.14). Reported cases describe an acute onset of thoracic limb paresis with decreased or absent spinal reflexes. A similar condition in humans (serum neuritis) has been described after the administration of certain vaccines (Miller et al., 2000) and is associated with specific viral infections (Fabian et al., 1997). The pathogenic mechanism is believed to have an immunoallergic basis that causes severe shoulder and upper arm pain followed by upper arm weakness.

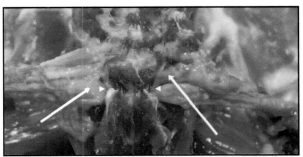

17.14 Brachial plexus neuritis with bilateral nerve root swelling in a 9-year-old Burmese cat. This post-mortem specimen shows the swollen nerves (arrowed) as they exit ventrally from the intervertebral foramina (arrowheads). (Courtesy of T Scase and L Garosi)

Some of the sporadic cases described in dogs and cats have been related to a purely horsemeat diet (one dog) and the administration of a modified-live rabies virus vaccine (one dog and one cat). A case of brachial plexus neuritis induced by a foreign body has been described (Walmsley et al., 2009). In many animals a definitive cause cannot be found.

Cerebrospinal fluid (CSF) analysis can be normal or reveal a severe increase in protein concentration and mild pleocytosis. MRI may show swelling of the affected spinal nerves, which are hyperintense on T2-weighted images and isointense on T1-weighted images. Mild contrast enhancement can be observed on T1-weighted images, especially at the periphery of the affected nerves (Garosi et al., 2006). Similar MRI findings may be seen in cases of lymphoma. Affected animals show diffuse EMG changes consistent with denervation in the thoracic limbs and neurogenic atrophy in all thoracic limb muscles. Pathological examination shows severe Wallerian-like degeneration of the brachial plexus nerves (most pronounced in the ventral nerve roots) together with a prominent inflammatory infiltration of mononuclear cells. Fibrosis may be evident in chronic cases.

Affected dogs may respond to corticosteroid treatment and/or a change to a poultry-based diet that contains no beef or horse products. Prognosis is guarded, since some animals may recover slowly (months) whilst others may remain non-ambulatory. One of the feline cases reported recovered spontaneously over a 3-week period, and the other had to be euthanased because of a lack of improvement.

Traumatic diseases

Brachial plexus avulsion

Traumatic injuries resulting in avulsion of the nerve roots of the brachial plexus are the most common cause of acute thoracic limb monoparesis or monoplegia in small animals. These injuries are usually the result of road traffic accidents or falls from a height, which cause abduction and simultaneous caudal displacement of the thoracic limbs.

Clinical signs

Signs are peracute in onset following the traumatic incident. Depending on which nerve roots are affected, avulsions are divided into three types:

- Cranial avulsions (C6–C8 nerve roots)
- Caudal avulsions (C8–T2 nerve roots)
- Complete avulsions (C6–T2 nerve roots).

Cranial avulsions are rare and result in few clinical signs. The elbow extensor muscles are not affected, so the animal can bear weight on the affected limb. There is loss of shoulder movement and elbow flexion, and atrophy of the supraspinatus and infraspinatus muscles usually occurs.

Caudal and complete avulsions are more common and cause severe clinical signs (Griffiths *et al.*, 1974). Both types of avulsion cause paralysis of the triceps brachii muscle, so the animal cannot extend the elbow or bear weight on the affected limb. Affected animals drag the limb knuckled over (Figures 17.15 and 17.16; see also **Right brachial plexus avulsion** clip on DVD). The thoracic limb

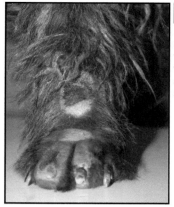

17.16 Brachial plexus avulsion. Excoriations are seen in the affected thoracic limb, secondary to dragging of the limb and decreased sensation.

muscles are hypotonic and severe neurogenic atrophy begins approximately 1 week following the injury. Spinal reflexes and postural reactions are lost (see **Partial brachial plexus avulsion** clip on DVD). If the elbow flexor muscles are spared (caudal avulsions), the animal can carry the limb flexed at this level and avoid contact with the floor.

Sensory signs are also common. The pattern of decreased or absent sensation in the affect limb allows better determination of the type of avulsion (Bailey and Kitchell, 1987) (Figure 17.17). Cutaneous sensation should be checked in the entire limb, but particular attention should be paid to nociception in the medial (radial and musculocutaneous) and lateral (radial and ulnar) digits, since this is essential in determining a prognosis.

A high percentage of patients with brachial plexus avulsions show partial Horner's syndrome and/or loss of the cutaneous trunci reflex ipsilateral to the side of the avulsion (Wheeler *et al.*, 1986). Avulsion of the T1 ventral nerve root causes injury to the pre-ganglionic sympathetic nerve fibres to the eye, resulting in ipsilateral miosis (partial Horner's syndrome). Loss of the cutaneous trunci reflex is caused by damage to the C8–T1 ventral spinal nerve roots that form the lateral thoracic nerve and innervate the cutaneous trunci muscle. The contralateral reflex is usually present after ipsilateral stimulation.

Pathogenesis

The site of root avulsion is usually intradural where the nerve roots arise from the spinal cord. At this point, nerve roots lack a well defined perineurium and constitute the weakest structure between the spinal cord and the peripheral nervous system (PNS). If the avulsion is severe enough, it may place traction over the spinal cord and damage the spinal cord pathways, causing ipsilateral pelvic limb neurological deficits. Both dorsal and ventral nerve roots can be affected, but the motor roots appear to be more susceptible to this type of trauma (Griffiths, 1974).

Diagnosis

A history of thoracic limb monoparesis after a traumatic incident should raise a high suspicion of brachial plexus avulsion. Every animal unable to use one thoracic limb following trauma should be

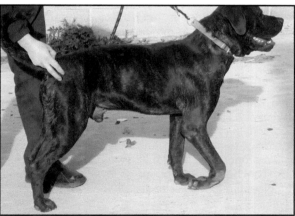

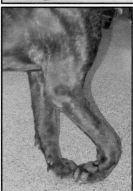

17.15 Brachial plexus avulsion caused by a road traffic accident in a 3-year-old male Mastiff. Note that only one limb is affected. The close-up of the affected limb demonstrates severe neurogenic atrophy.

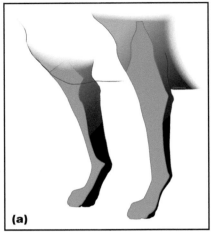 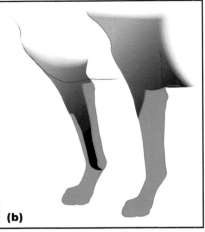 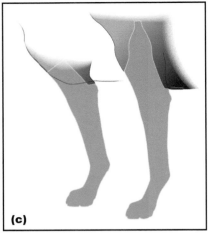

(a)   (b)   (c)

17.17 Sensory loss associated with brachial plexus avulsion. Shaded zones are dermatomes that lack sensation. (Based on Bailey, 1984). **(a)** Cranial plexus avulsion. **(b)** Caudal plexus avulsion. **(c)** Complete plexus avulsion.

examined carefully to detect orthopaedic as well as neurological abnormalities. MRI of the affected plexus may provide information on the degree of nerve and associated soft tissue trauma.

Electromyography allows detection of spontaneous electrical activity in the denervated muscles 7–10 days after the injury (Steinberg, 1979). NCV studies of the radial and ulnar nerves allow determination of the degree of injury (see Chapter 4). Since the radial nerve is commonly injured in brachial plexus avulsions, serial electrodiagnostic evaluations of this nerve may provide useful diagnostic and prognostic information.

Treatment and prognosis
There is no effective treatment for this type of injury. The degree of recovery depends only on the severity of the nerve lesion at the time of injury. The outcome is often good for animals with cranial plexus avulsions that are able to bear weight on the affected limb and maintain normal sensation over the distal part of the limb. Animals with caudal and complete brachial plexus avulsions have a poor to guarded prognosis if neurotmesis has occurred. Only those with neurapraxic injuries show improvement and recover completely. Most animals do not improve but go on to show severe limb atrophy, and eventually develop serious complications, including:

- Trophic ulcers
- Joint contractures and self-mutilation as a result of paraesthesia
- Abnormal sensation in the affected areas as a result of regeneration of sensory nerves (Sharo, 1995).

When the proximal branches of the radial and musculocutaneous nerves are spared (i.e. the elbow flexor and extensor muscles are not denervated), corrective surgery can be performed to provide carpal extension and prevent the distal part of the limb from collapsing (Steinberg, 1988). Tendon transplantation or carpal arthrodesis procedures can be performed.

- Muscle tendon transplantation can be successful with partial avulsions.
- Carpal fusion may be useful in animals with adequate triceps muscle function that walk knuckling over their carpus.

In addition, experimental studies in dogs have demonstrated that ventral root reimplantation can promote successful reinnervation (Moissonnier *et al.*, 1998, 2001). However, before performing any type of surgery, it is essential to perform electromyography to determine whether the elbow extensor muscles or the muscles to be transplanted have normal function and are not denervated. Amputation may be necessary if sensation has been lost and self-mutilation secondary to paraesthesia has developed. The reader is referred to standard surgical texts for further information on these procedures.

Decreased radial NCV at the onset of clinical signs is a poor prognostic indicator (Faissler *et al.*, 2002). If this remains unchanged after 4 weeks, with concurrent severe EMG changes in the triceps muscle, there is virtually no chance of spontaneous recovery. However, the presence of giant motor unit potentials in any of the affected muscles is an indicator of reinnervation and may represent a favourable prognostic sign (Griffiths and Duncan, 1978).

The best predictor for recovery appears to be nociception (Faissler *et al.*, 2002).

- If nociception is present in the medial and lateral digits, the prognosis for recovery is good and aggressive physiotherapy should be recommended to the owner (see Chapter 25).
- If nociception is absent, the prognosis depends on the severity of the axonal injury (being good for neurapraxic lesions, but guarded to poor for axonotometic and neurotmetic lesions). Pure axonotmesis occurs rarely, so the potential for recovery, although present, is low and the prognosis is poor.

Supportive treatment is essential during the recovery time to prevent contractures and excoriations from dragging the limb. Keeping the limb clean and dry, treating any wounds that may develop, and covering the foot with boots or bandages are all important therapeutic measures. At the same time, performing physical therapy (flexion and extension movements) several times a day is crucial to lessen muscle atrophy as well as to prevent muscle contractures and joint fusions (see Chapter 25).

However, if no improvement is seen during the first 2 months, recovery is unlikely to occur. In a study of 53 cases (36 dogs and 17 cats) of unilateral brachial plexus trauma, absence of nociception, ipsilateral loss of the cutaneous trunci reflex, partial Horner's syndrome and a poor response to magnetic motor stimulation were related to a poor clinical outcome in 29 dogs and 13 cats. An inability to evoke magnetic motor potentials was associated with an unsuccessful outcome in all animals (Van Soens *et al.*, 2009).

Peripheral nerve injury

Clinical signs
Clinical signs reflect the site of injury and the function of the injured nerve.

Diagnosis
The diagnosis of traumatic peripheral neuropathies is based on the history and clinical signs. Electromyography can help determine which muscles are affected, differentiating proximal lumbosacral injuries caused by pelvic trauma, from proximal sciatic nerve injuries. Nerve integrity may be assessed by NCV studies, stimulating regions both proximal and distal to the site of injury. Electromyographic abnormalities are evident from 5–7 days following the injury, thus in order to avoid false-negative results electrodiagnostic studies should not be performed until after this time.

Treatment and prognosis
Treatment involves supportive measures to protect the foot from injury (e.g. boots or bandages) and physical therapy to preserve joint motion and delay muscle atrophy. Exploratory surgery to evaluate nerve damage, and neurorrhaphy (anastomoses) or neurolysis (debridement of inflammatory adhesions) may be indicated when there is severe nerve damage.

Serial EMGs and NCV studies of the affected limb help to determine the prognosis. If these tests are not available, serial neurological examinations should be performed monthly for at least 4 months. If no improvement is seen within 4–6 months, recovery is unlikely and amputation of the affected limb should be considered.

The prognosis is guarded with peripheral nerve injuries. Axonotmetic and neurapraxis lesions have a better prognosis than neurotmetic lesions. If nociception is present, there is a chance of recovery (see above). Neuropraxic lesions recover within days to weeks, depending on the severity of the initial injury. With axonotmetic lesions, axon regrowth occurs at a rate of 1–4 mm per day; however, after

6 months shrinkage of the nerve sheath may impede further growth. Thus, the closer the nerve injury is to the muscle to be reinnervated, the better the prognosis.

Radial nerve injury
The radial nerve can be injured proximally by fractures of the first rib or distally by humeral fractures. Fractures of the humerus can cause radial nerve injury at sites both proximal and distal to the branches that supply the triceps muscle.

- If the lesion is proximal to these branches, the elbow, carpal and digital joints cannot extend, resulting in the elbow being 'dropped', and the animal walks with the carpus and digits knuckled over and cannot bear weight on that limb.
- If the lesion is distal to these branches, the animal can extend the elbow but the carpus still knuckles over when the animal walks due to paralysis of the carpal and digital extensor muscles.

Unless there is complete severance of the nerve, most animals recover completely within a few months. However, if neurotmesis has occurred, cutaneous sensation is lost in the cranial aspect of the limb distal to the injury and nociception is absent in the lateral digit. This may lead to the development of paraesthesia and subsequently self-mutilation. In these cases, prognosis for recovery is poor.

Lumbosacral plexus trauma
Traumatic injuries to the lumbosacral plexus, resulting in pelvic limb monoparesis, most often affect the sciatic truck or nerve.

Caudal lumbar vertebrae and lumbosacral junction trauma
The sciatic nerve originates from spinal cord segments L6–S2. These segments lie cranially inside the vertebral canal, approximately over the L4–L5 vertebral bodies (see Chapter 2). After exiting the spinal cord, the nerve roots run caudally in the vertebral canal until they exit through the corresponding intervertebral foramina. Within the vertebral canal, nerve fibres forming the sciatic nerve can be injured by any type of trauma (e.g. fractures and luxations) affecting the caudal lumbar vertebrae or lumbosacral junction. However, traumatic injuries to these areas more often affect the nerve roots forming the pudendal, pelvic and caudal nerves, which run inside the vertebral canal together with the sciatic nerve fibres at this level. Thus, most injuries to this area do not cause true monoparesis, and neurological deficits related to dysfunction of the other nerves will also be present (see Chapter 19). In addition, most vertebral injuries cause bilateral deficits. Foraminal stenosis of the lumbosacral junction secondary to degenerative lumbosacral stenosis may cause a true sciatic monoparesis (see above).

Pelvic trauma
Traumatic injuries to the pelvic area, causing fractures of the shaft of the ilium or acetabulum or

sacroiliac fracture/luxation, are a common cause of proximal sciatic nerve injury or injury to the lumbo-sacral plexus. For a more complete discussion on the classification and specific management of sacral and pelvic fractures, the reader is referred to standard surgical texts and the *BSAVA Manual of Small Animal Fracture Repair and Management*.

Proximal sciatic nerve dysfunction causes severe pelvic limb monoparesis. The affected animal should be able to bear weight on the affected limb, but will walk with the paw knuckled over, the stifle joint will not flex, and the tarsus and digits will not flex or extend. In addition, the hock is usually 'dropped'. Sensation is affected in the entire limb except for the medial aspect (and medial digit) which is supplied by the saphenous branch of the femoral nerve (see **Left sciatic nerve neuropathy** clip on DVD). The flexor reflex is severely affected due to the inability of the patient to flex its stifle, hock or digits. If the medial digit is stimulated, a mild flexion of the hip (femoral nerve) can be observed. Nociception should be checked in all digits to assess the severity of the lesion. A lack of nociception in the digits innervated by the sciatic nerve indicates severe injury (neuro-tmesis) and a poor prognosis for recovery.

Pelvic fractures can cause compression or lacer-ation of the sciatic nerve or lumbosacral plexus. Surgical exploration and decompression of the nerve plus internal fixation is indicated if the animal shows moderate to severe signs of peripheral nerve injury (nociception preserved) and severe pain, to relieve nerve entrapment, avoid further damage by unstable fractures and assess prognosis (Jacobson and Schrader, 1987). If no improvement is seen within 3–4 months, prognosis is poor and amputa-tion of the limb is recommended to avoid excoria-tions and self-mutilation.

Proximal sciatic nerve injury
The proximal segment of the sciatic nerve is often injured by entrapment caused by muscle or fibrous tissue that can develop secondary to:

- Femoral fractures
- Ischial fractures
- Acetabular fractures
- Femoral head and neck excision surgical procedures
- Triple pelvic osteotomy
- Surgery of the coxofemoral joint
- Intramuscular injections
- Pinning of the femur.

The more common injuries result from retrograde intramedullary pinning of the femur (Fanton *et al.*, 1983), from ischial and acetabular fractures (Cham-bers and Hardie, 1986) and from intramuscular injections of various agents into the caudal thigh. In a report on 27 sciatic nerve injuries, the majority (25) resulted from surgery (sacroiliac luxation repair, intramedullary pinning, other orthopaedic proce-dures and perineal herniorrhaphy). Immediate surgi-cal treatment of entrapped or injured nerves (removal of nails, cement or entrapping suture)

resulted in complete recovery of approximately 50% of dogs, and in clinical improvement of about 25% of dogs (Forterre *et al.*, 2007).

Retrograde intramedullary pinning of the femur may injure the sciatic nerve directly via pin insertion or secondarily as a result of scar formation around the nerve due to excessive pin length. Acetabular or ischial fractures can damage the sciatic nerve directly or by entrapment secondary to progressive fibrosis at the fracture site. Intramuscular injections in the caudal thigh may cause direct laceration of the sciatic nerve due to needle placement or injec-tion of the substance into the nerve. Injury second-ary to the formation of scar tissue around the nerve may also been seen. The degree of nerve damage varies with the agent injected (penicillin, diazepam, chlorpromazine and some steroids, especially hydrocortisone and triamcinolone acetonide, cause severe damage), the amount of drug injected and the site of injection (intrafascicular injections cause more severe damage than extrafascicular injec-tions). To avoid this type of injury, intramuscular injections should be given in other muscle groups (e.g. quadriceps or lumbar muscles).

Prognosis for this type of injury depends on the severity of the nerve damage, with loss of nociception in the digits innervated by the sciatic nerve indicating a poor prognosis. If nociception is preserved, early fixation of fractures, nerve decompression and aggressive physical therapy should be instituted to avoid further nerve damage and promote recovery of nerve and muscle function.

Peroneal and tibial nerve injury
The peroneal nerve is exposed to traumatic injury as it crosses the lateral aspect of the stifle. The more common causes of injury at this site include intramuscular injections, pressure from orthopaedic casts and surgery of the stifle joint (cruciate liga-ment repair).

Isolated tibial nerve lesions are rare, but may occur following intramuscular injection into the thigh muscles. In most animals, tibial nerve lesions occur in association with peroneal or higher (main trunk) sciatic nerve injuries. Pure peroneal or tibial nerve signs (Figure 17.18; see also **Peroneal nerve paral-ysis** clip on DVD) are not common.

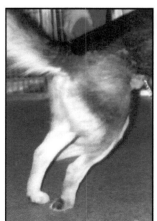

17.18 Sciatic nerve dysfunction in a young male Siberian Husky. There were severe conscious proprioception deficits with loss of tone in the distal limb.

Femoral nerve injury

Spinal cord segments L4–L6 and femoral nerve roots within the vertebral canal can be affected by several disease conditions (e.g. disc disease, trauma, neoplasia). In these cases, bilateral disease is more common; true femoral monoparesis is a rare occurrence.

Peripheral femoral nerve injuries are uncommon because the nerve and its roots are well protected by the sublumbar musculature. However, extreme extension of the hip causing iliopsoas muscle tears can damage the femoral nerve, resulting in femoral neuropathy (Stepnik *et al.*, 2006). Other lesions that occur within this muscle group (such as neoplasms, haematomas) can also injure the femoral nerve fibres that run within the psoas muscle group after they exit the spinal canal.

Dysfunction of the femoral nerve causes monoparesis with severe gait abnormalities. The patient cannot bear weight on the affected limb and carries it flexed at the stifle (Figure 17.19). There is little hip flexion and the patellar reflex is severely decreased or lost. Neurogenic atrophy of the quadriceps muscle usually develops. With severe lesions there is anaesthesia over the medial aspect of the pelvic limb and medial digit. Nociception should be checked in the medial digit to assess the severity of the injury.

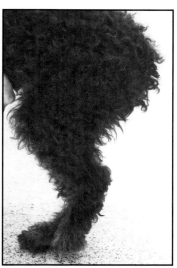

17.19 Femoral nerve dysfunction in a 9-year-old male mixed-breed dog. The inability to bear weight is profound with the affected limb carried flexed at the stifle.

Toxic diseases

Tetanus

Tetanus usually causes generalized signs of increased extensor rigidity and is described in full in Chapter 15. However, signs can be limited to a single limb, causing monoparesis associated with extensor rigidity. A wound can usually be found on the distal extremity of the affected limb. This syndrome has been reported in humans and occurs when the patient has either pre-existing anti-tetanus antibodies or an extremely small injury. Local tetanus has been reported most commonly in cats, but can occur in dogs (Malik *et al.*, 1989; Polizopoulou *et al.*, 2002).

Vascular diseases

Fibrocartilaginous embolism

Unilateral infarctions affecting the ventral grey matter of the C6–T2 or the L4–S2 spinal cord segments, or affecting the white matter of the T3–L3 spinal cord segments, may cause acute monoparesis of the thoracic (C6–T2) or pelvic (T3–L3 and L4–S2) limbs. The paretic pelvic limb shows UMN deficits if the infarct occurs in the T3–L3 segments, and LMN deficits if the infarct occurs in the L4–S2 spinal cord segments. The clinical signs, diagnosis, treatment and prognosis of this type of injury are discussed in detail in Chapter 16.

Arterial thromboembolism

The acute onset of monoparesis in cats may be associated with arterial thromboembolism (in the thoracic limbs due to brachial artery embolism; in the pelvic limbs due to aortic or iliac embolism). The long-term prognosis is very poor as many cats have a severe underlying cardiovascular disease. Aortic thromboembolism has also been reported in 13 dogs causing pelvic limb monoparesis (Gonçalves *et al.*, 2008). Further details on this condition can be found in Chapter 16.

References and further reading

Available on accompanying DVD

DVD extras

- Left sciatic nerve neuropathy
- Partial brachial plexus avulsion
- Peroneal nerve paralysis
- Right brachial plexus avulsion

18

Exercise intolerance and collapse

Simon Platt and G. Diane Shelton

Exercise intolerance, which may also be considered as activity-related weakness, occurs with walking or running and dissipates with rest. It is recognized as early fatigue with mild activity, although in some cases more vigorous or prolonged exercise may be needed to induce the problem. It may be associated with episodic muscle cramps (prolonged, involuntary, painful muscle contractions).

Collapse of an acute nature may take one of three major forms: seizure, syncope or narcolepsy–cataplexy. All are clinical syndromes with more than one cause. Seizures are addressed in Chapter 8. Syncope due to cardiovascular disease is beyond the scope of this manual and readers are referred to the *BSAVA Manual of Canine and Feline Cardiorespiratory Medicine* for further information. Narcolepsy–cataplexy is discussed in Chapter 13. Collapse may also occur as a result of acute or chronic, progressive neuromuscular diseases, which are discussed here.

Clinical signs

Signs of activity-related motor weakness include an intermittent paretic gait (often manifest as a stiff stride that becomes progressively shorter with accompanying ventroflexion of the neck), reluctance to walk or run, lying down and collapse (see **Exercise intolerance** clip on DVD). Ataxia, suggestive of upper motor neuron (UMN) or sensory deficits, is usually not present with neuromuscular junction disorders and myopathies. The animal may be alert or depressed and may pant excessively. Progression of the underlying disease can rapidly lead to severe respiratory compromise due to loss of diaphragmatic and intercostal muscle strength (see **Neuromuscular disease** clip on DVD). General muscle strength can greatly improve following rest.

- Generalized weakness
- Exercise intolerance
- Stiff, stilted gait
- Localized or generalized muscle atrophy or hypertrophy
- Pain on palpation (myalgia)
- Contractures with chronic disease
- Ventroflexion of the head and neck (especially in cats)
- Regurgitation if the oesophagus is involved

18.1 Principal clinical signs of muscle disease.

In between the episodes of weakness, the animal may be completely normal or may have clinical signs of muscle (Figure 18.1) or nerve disease (see Chapter 15).

Lesion localization

A thorough history and physical and neurological examinations are essential to localize the lesion. It may be possible only to isolate a system (Figure 18.2), or a lesion may be suspected in the brain, spinal cord/nerve root, peripheral nerve, neuromuscular junction or muscle (Figure 18.3).

Pathophysiology

Knowledge of the normal physiology of nerve and muscle function is essential. The basic physiology of the central nervous system (CNS) and peripheral nervous system (PNS) is discussed in Chapters 9, 15 and 16. In addition to an understanding of muscle function during exercise and rest, the function of other organs that support muscle metabolism during exercise must be considered. Primary muscle disease can cause activity-related or continuous weakness if the process of normal muscle contraction is targeted by the disease.

In the normal animal, skeletal muscle fibres are stimulated to contract by the lower motor neurons (LMNs). The coupling of neuronal impulses to the activation of muscle contractile proteins requires the sequential activation of a variety of ion channels. Electrical activity in the form of action potentials is generated along the nerve cell membranes by the movement of sodium and potassium ions and is influenced by calcium. Therefore, diseases that cause electrolyte imbalances may result in weakness that waxes and wanes as their primary clinical manifestation (Figure 18.4).

Electrical activity is transmitted from the axons to the muscle fibres at the neuromuscular junction (motor endplate; Figure 18.5) via the release of the neurotransmitter acetylcholine. The release of acetylcholine is modulated by calcium ions and the neurotransmitter itself is inactivated by acetylcholinesterase. Thus, disturbances of calcium homeostasis or disorders that affect the activity of acetylcholine (e.g. organophosphate toxicity) or

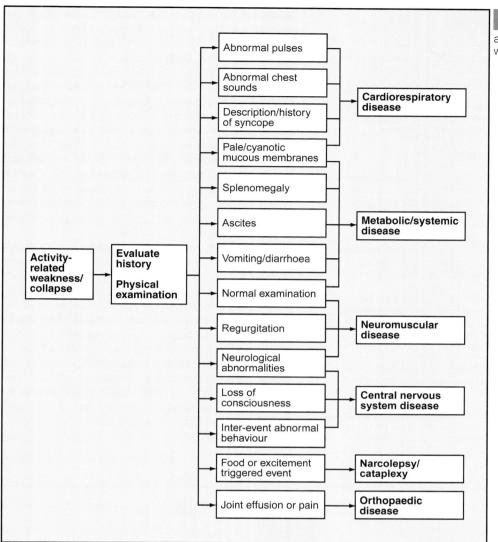

18.2 An approach to the work-up of animals with episodic weakness and collapse.

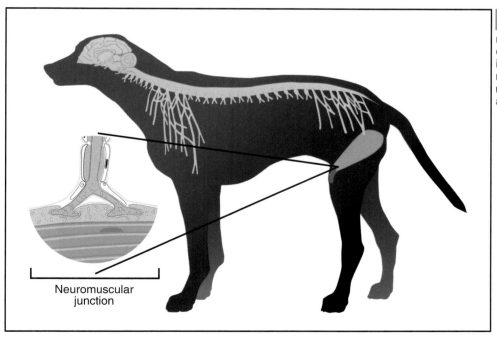

18.3 Lesion localization for neuromuscular causes of collapse. Possible sites include the peripheral nerves, the neuro-muscular junction (inset) and the skeletal muscles.

Electrolyte abnormality	Primary causes	Clinical signs
Hypokalaemia	Renal loss; intestinal loss; metabolic alkalosis	Muscle weakness; hypovolaemia
Hyperkalaemia	Acute renal failure; hypoadrenocorticism; potassium-sparing diuretics; metabolic acidosis; iatrogenic	Muscle weakness; irregular cardiac rhythm
Hypocalcaemia	Primary hypoparathyroidism; hyperphosphataemia; eclampsia; iatrogenic	Muscle weakness; tetany; mental depression; seizures
Hypercalcaemia	Malignant tumours; primary hyperparathyroidism; hypervitaminosis D	Muscle weakness; mental depression; polydipsia/polyuria; constipation
Hyponatraemia	Intestinal loss; hypoadrenocorticism; inappropriate antidiuretic hormone secretion; iatrogenic	Muscle weakness; lethargy; seizures; coma
Hypernatraemia	Water deprivation; excess salt gain; pure water loss	Muscle weakness; muscle rigidity; tremors; seizures/ coma

18.4 Electrolyte abnormalities that can lead (directly or indirectly) to neuromuscular weakness.

postsynaptic cholinergic receptor function (e.g. myasthenia gravis) may adversely affect neuromuscular transmission and can lead to weakness or tetraparesis (see Chapter 15).

Activation of the acetylcholine receptors initiates an action potential. The action potential conducts along the myofibre and spreads into the cell via a series of membranous tubules (T tubules), where it stimulates the release of calcium ions stored within the sarcoplasmic reticulum. The calcium ions then stimulate contraction of the myofibrils and are subsequently responsible for relaxation as they are sequestered back into the sacroplasmic reticulum; therefore, the concentration of calcium ions within the body is critical for normal muscle contraction and relaxation.

The energy needed for muscle contraction is derived chiefly from the metabolism of carbohydrates and fats. During anaerobic exercise, the primary source of energy is muscle glycogen. Muscle glycogen can be rapidly depleted during exercise, and blood glucose then becomes the primary energy source. In hypoglycaemic conditions with a lack of this energy source, episodic weakness may occur. If the supply of oxygen is adequate, aerobic (oxidative) processes prevail. Lipid fuels in the form of fatty acids predominate and glucose is conserved. Disorders of oxidative metabolism of lipids or carbohydrates also result in episodic weakness.

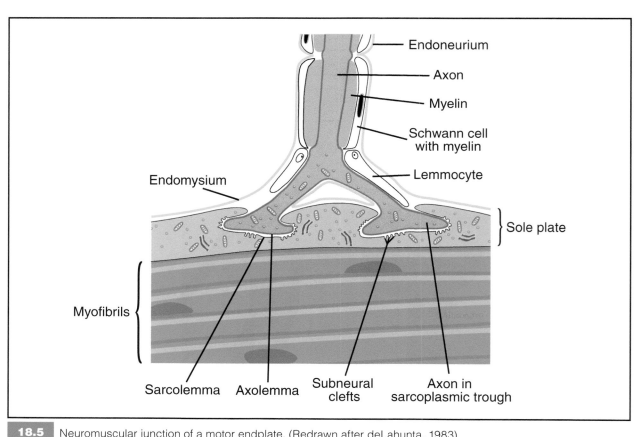

18.5 Neuromuscular junction of a motor endplate. (Redrawn after deLahunta, 1983)

Differential diagnosis

The differential diagnosis depends on the precise lesion localization. The differential diagnoses for metabolic and systemic diseases (Figure 18.6) and cardiorespiratory diseases (Figure 18.7) are discussed in internal medicine texts and appropriate BSAVA Manuals. The differential diagnoses for each of the neuromuscular lesion localizations are listed in Figure 18.8. In young animals, primary considerations should be inherited, breed-associated (see Appendix 1) and infectious diseases. The differential diagnoses for seizure activity are discussed in Chapter 8.

Neurodiagnostic investigation

The diagnostic plan is dependent on the localization of the clinical signs, as well as the suspected underlying disease process. As some problems are episodic, the frequency of occurrence must also be taken into account, and it should be recognized that many tests need to be performed at the time of an 'episode'. However, most neuromuscular diseases result in continual signs, which may vary in severity based on the level of activity. The following tests should be considered for all cases of weakness or collapse, particularly if a neuromuscular disorder is suspected.

Video footage

If the episodes are so infrequent that they are not observed by the clinician, the owners should attempt to capture the event on videotape. Observation of the event is critical to the diagnosis. Without observation, the nature of the event must be surmised by listening to the 'eye-witness' description offered by the owner.

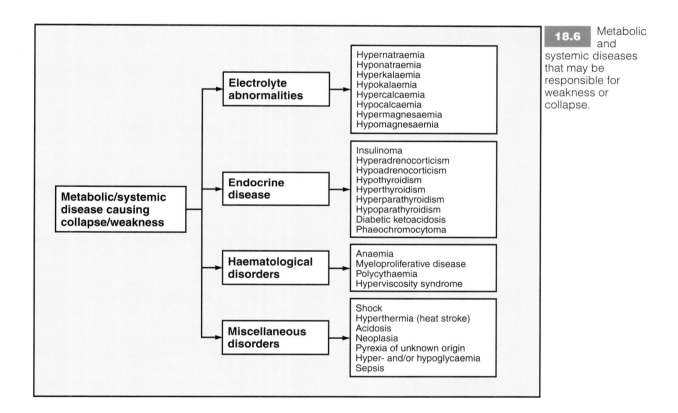

18.6 Metabolic and systemic diseases that may be responsible for weakness or collapse.

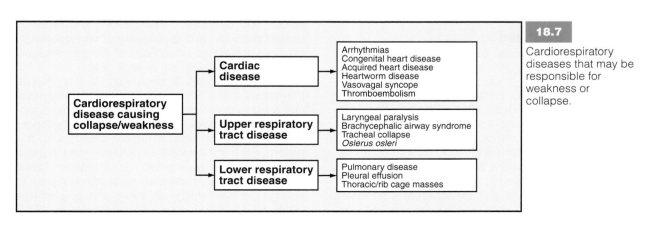

18.7 Cardiorespiratory diseases that may be responsible for weakness or collapse.

Non-inflammatory myopathies
• Acquired:
– Toxic
– Metabolic (endocrine)
• Inherited:
– Central core myopathy
– Muscular dystrophy
– Myotonia
– Metabolic myopathies [a]
– Centronuclear myopathy
Inflammatory myopathies
• Infectious:
– Viral
– Bacterial
– Rickettsial
– Protozoal
• Immune-mediated:
– Dermatomyositis
– Polymyositis
• Paraneoplastic
• Nutritional
Idiopathic myopathies
• Exercise-induced collapse in Labrador Retrievers
• Fibrotic myopathy
• Exertional rhabdomyolysis
Neuromuscular transmission disease
• Myasthenia gravis
• Botulism [b]
• Tick paralysis [b]
• Snake bite
• Toxicity
Neuropathies [c]
• Degenerative
• Metabolic
• Infectious
• Paraneoplastic
• Idiopathic
• Traumatic
• Toxic
• Vascular

18.8 Categories of differential diagnoses that should be considered for neuromuscular diseases.
[a] Although most metabolic myopathies are not confirmed as inherited, it is likely that many could be classified as inborn errors that are degenerative rather than inflammatory. [b] See Chapter 15 for a full description of these diseases. [c] See Figure 18.12 and Chapter 15.

Minimum database

The minimum essential database (see Chapter 3) should comprise comprehensive haematology, serum biochemistry (including creatine kinase, lactate and electrolytes), urinalysis, faecal examination, resting electrocardiogram (ECG), thoracic radiography and abdominal ultrasonography. A thyroid panel and an adrenocorticotropic hormone (ACTH) stimulation test should also be considered as neuromuscular disease may be the first and only manifestation of endocrine disorders. Resting blood pressure measurements should also be obtained if there are any concerns about cardiorespiratory disease, and peripheral vascular pulses should be palpated to evaluate for compromise.

Creatine kinase

Creatine kinase, a specific enzyme marker for myofibre damage, is frequently used in the diagnosis of muscular diseases. Creatine kinase levels are often increased with necrotizing, inflammatory and dystrophic myopathies, and are usually normal with muscular diseases in which necrosis is not a feature (e.g. myotonia) (Shelton, 2010). The enzyme is very labile and so is non-specific; however, as the half-life is only about 2 hours, the magnitude and persistence of the increased creatine kinase level is an indication of the severity and activity of the underlying muscle disease. This enzyme can also be elevated following intramuscular injections, surgery, prolonged recumbency and even anorexia in cats. Conversely, muscle disease should never be ruled out based upon a normal creatine kinase level.

Troponin I

Troponin is located in myofibrils and is the regulatory protein of contractile skeletal and cardiac muscle. Cardiac muscle can be affected by generalized myopathies, including muscular dystrophy, mitochondrial myopathies and necrotizing myopathies (Shelton, 2010). Although cardiac troponin concentrations are not affected by non-specific types of skeletal muscle damage, generalized muscle disease affecting the myocardium could elevate this enzyme. This may be potentially helpful in the future as a prognostic marker based on the extent of the disease.

Lactate and pyruvate analysis

Lactate concentrations increase in normal animals following strenuous anaerobic exercise. Resting lactic acidaemia or lactate elevations that are disproportionate to the degree of exercise performed may be an indication of an underlying disorder of muscle metabolism. Lactic acid is the product of anaerobic glucose metabolism, and lactic acidosis can result from a defect in the anabolic metabolism of pyruvate. Lactic acidaemia develops in association with deficiencies in pyruvate dehydrogenase or pyruvate carboxylase, defects in the mitochondrial respiratory chain, or defects in the Krebs cycle involving ketoglutarate dehydrogenase complex (Figure 18.9).

In human patients, documentation of high serum lactate and pyruvate concentrations with a normal lactate:pyruvate ratio is consistent with a defect in pyruvate dehydrogenase or one of the gluconeogenic enzymes. Lactic acidosis in association with a high lactate:pyruvate ratio is seen with defects involving the mitochondrial electron transport chain, pyruvate carboxylase deficiency or other mitochondrial myopathies. When evaluating post-exercise lactate concentrations in dogs with exercise intolerance, it is essential to compare values obtained from the patient with those from appropriate control dogs. Lactate concentrations after exercise vary depending on the duration and intensity of the exercise performed (Platt, 2002). Spurious elevations in plasma lactate

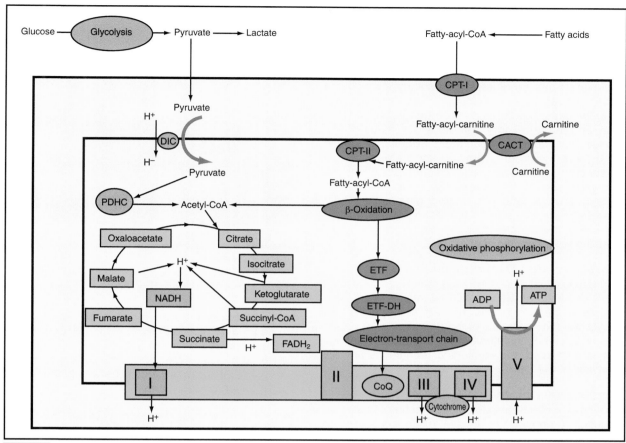

18.9 An overview of selected metabolic pathways in the mitochondria. ADP = adenosine diphosphate; ATP = adenosine triphosphate; CACT = carnitine translocase; CoA = coenzyme A; CoQ = coenzyme Q; CPT = carnitine palmitoyltransferase; DIC = dicarboxylate carrier; ETF = electron transfer flavoprotein; ETF-DH = electron transfer dehydrogenase; FAD = flavin adenine dinucleotide; FADH₂ = reduced FAD; NADH = reduced nicotinamide adenine dinucleotide; PDHC = pyruvate dehydrogenase complex; TCA = tricarboxylic acid.

can occur if the animal is agitated during blood collection and due to poor venepuncture technique. Fasted samples should be submitted as increased pyruvate levels can be seen following a meal.

Blood for lactate measurements should be collected into sodium fluoride/potassium oxalate tubes. The plasma should then be separated and stored at –20°C until analysis. Paired blood samples for pyruvate analysis should be mixed 1:1 with 8–10% perchloric acid for deproteinization, centrifuged, and the supernatant removed and frozen at –20°C. Samples should be submitted to laboratories on dry ice. Samples for both lactate and pyruvate analysis should be evaluated within 30 days.

Amino acid analysis
Mitochondrial disease can cause alanine abnormalities, as well as changes in the concentrations of proline, glycine and sarcosine. These amino acids are best measured in plasma samples, which should be submitted to a specialized laboratory for analysis.

Carnitine analysis
Primary mitochondrial diseases affecting the muscles can be associated with carnitine deficiencies. Carnitine is a 'shuttle' for free fatty acids into the

mitochondria and buffers potentially toxic coenzyme A esters (Shelton, 2010). Total, free and esterified carnitine concentrations in the plasma, urine and muscle can help identify primary amino acidaemias, organic acidaemias and fatty acid oxidation defects, as well as carnitine deficiency syndromes.

Organic acid analysis
Urine should be submitted for organic acid measurements in animals that have clinical evidence of concurrent neuromuscular and CNS disease, particularly young, pure-breed animals. Organic acids are byproducts of protein, carbohydrate and fat catabolism (Shelton, 2010). Specialized laboratories are required to analyse and interpret the results (Shelton et al., 1998).

Myoglobin
Myoglobin present in the urine (myoglobinuria) usually indicates severe muscle damage, frequently as a result of rhabdomyolysis following trauma, toxins, infections and malignant hyperthermia. However, a correlation does not exist between serum creatine kinase levels and myoglobinuria and so it is considered an insensitive test. Recurrent myoglobinuria may be detected in inherited metabolic myopathies and in muscular dystrophy (Shelton, 2010).

Serology

Investigation of infectious diseases may require extensive serological tests and their interpretation may be difficult but, depending on the potential for exposure, serology should be performed for all possible infectious candidates (particularly *Toxoplasma gondii, Neospora caninum, Hepatozoon* and *Leishmania* spp.), depending on geographical location and travel history. Serology for autoimmune conditions such as rheumatoid arthritis, systemic lupus and myasthenia gravis may be warranted if suspected. Antibodies against the acetylcholine receptor should be measured in all dogs with acquired megaoesophagus and dysphagia. Polymerase chain reaction (PCR) testing of blood samples for these infections is likely to be more sensitive and specific, if available.

Cerebrospinal fluid analysis

A cerebrospinal fluid (CSF) tap may help to rule out CNS diseases as well as diffuse inflammatory conditions of the nerve roots, but it is non-specific and rarely helpful in cases of neuromuscular collapse (see Chapter 3). Evaluation for infectious diseases can be achieved with serological techniques or PCR analysis of the CSF.

Electrophysiology

Extensive electrophysiological testing may be required to confirm the precise lesion localization of the disease if a neuromuscular abnormality is suspected (see Chapter 4). An abbreviated needle electromyogram (EMG) may be worthwhile in the initial investigations, as it can quickly aid identification of an axonal or muscular disease. This is particularly helpful in cases with obvious muscle hypertrophy or atrophy. Repetitive nerve stimulation and single fibre EMGs should be considered for neuromuscular junction assessment (see Chapter 4).

Advanced imaging

Unless a CNS abnormality is suspected, it may not be necessary to consider spinal radiography, computed tomography (CT) or magnetic resonance imaging (MRI). Thoracic radiographs can assist with the diagnosis of megaoesophagus and associated aspiration pneumonia. Fluoroscopy or contrast-enhanced radiography (Figure 18.10) may be helpful to evaluate the function of the oesophagus if enlargement is not obvious on plain survey radiographs and swallowing if dysphagia is present. Cardiac ultrasonography may be required if a cardiorespiratory condition is suspected.

MRI (Figure 18.11) and CT have recently been utilized to document the presence of muscle pathology, particularly on post-contrast images (Platt *et al.*, 2006; Reiter and Schwarz, 2007; Thibaud *et al.*, 2007; Bishop *et al.*, 2008). The location of the contrast medium uptake within the muscles, as detected on MRI and CT, can assist with choosing suitable areas to obtain high yield biopsy samples, which is important in early onset localized or patchy myopathies. Although the clinical use of MRI phosphorus spectroscopy has not yet been documented in veter-

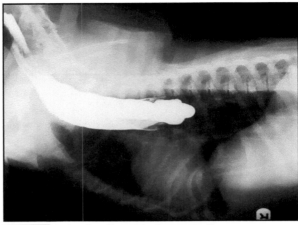

18.10 Lateral radiograph demonstrating an abnormally large oesophagus (megaoesophagus) with the aid of barium contrast medium. When performing such studies, the risk of aspiration pneumonia should be considered.

inary medicine, it has been described experimentally in dogs with muscular dystrophy (McCully *et al.*, 1991). This type of imaging study may become useful for the determination of the extent of muscle injury or pathology and could be a valuable marker for the response to treatment.

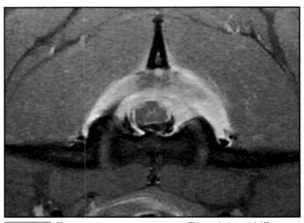

18.11 Transverse, post-contrast T1-weighted MR image of the cranial cervical spine in a dog with focal myositis, presenting with neck pain. A well defined muscle hyperintensity is visible.

Muscle and nerve biopsy

If a neuromuscular disease is suspected, a muscle or nerve biopsy can provide a specific diagnosis of the underlying cause (see Chapter 6). Since a peripheral nerve can react in only a limited number of ways to a variety of insults, the biopsy in most instances just confirms the presence of axonal degeneration, demyelination, abnormalities of the supporting structures, inflammation and infiltrative neoplasia. However, a nerve biopsy can provide information on regeneration, remyelination and the degree of fibre depletion and fibrosis, which are important for prognosis. A muscle biopsy is of utmost importance for the diagnosis of most muscle diseases, particularly those which are inherited.

Peripheral neuropathies

Figure 18.12 lists the acute and chronic peripheral neuropathies that should be considered for cases of episodic weakness or collapse (Chapter 15 provides a complete review of these disorders). In general, these diseases cause continuous rather than intermittent signs, but exercise intolerance or activity-related weakness often feature.

Mechanism of disease	Specific neuropathy
Degenerative	Motor neuron diseases Breed-specific neuropathies or laryngeal paralysis polyneuropathy complex
Metabolic	Diabetes mellitus Hypothyroidism Insulinoma or hypoglycaemia Hyperlipidaemia or hyperproteinaemia
Neoplasia	Lymphoma Paraneoplastic
Infectious	Polyradiculoneuritis (*Toxoplasma, Neospora*)
Idiopathic	Idiopathic polyradiculoneuritis (Coonhound paralysis) Chronic inflammatory demyelinating polyneuropathy Distal denervating disease Ganglioradiculoneuritis
Toxic	Vincristine Cisplatin Organophosphates and carbamates
Vascular	Ischaemic neuromyopathy

18.12 Peripheral neuropathies responsible for episodic weakness and collapse (see Chapter 15 for a complete discussion of these diseases).

Disorders of neuromuscular transmission

Specific diseases affect neuromuscular transmission (see Figure 18.8), resulting in clinical signs that may be very similar to those of peripheral neuropathies or myopathies. Apart from the majority of cases with immune-mediated myasthenia gravis, these diseases often cause an acute onset of ascending weakness, progressing from the pelvic limbs to the thoracic limbs. Myasthenia gravis is discussed below; Chapter 15 gives a complete review of other disorders, including botulism and tick paralysis.

Immune-mediated myasthenia gravis

Immune-mediated myasthenia gravis is a relatively common neuromuscular disease affecting dogs and occasionally cats (Shelton, 2002). Acquired myasthenia gravis has been observed in dogs >3 months old of all breeds, but German Shepherd Dogs, Golden Retrievers and Labrador Retrievers appear to be predisposed. In one report, the relative risk of acquired myasthenia gravis in different breeds of dog was highest in Akitas (Shelton *et al.*, 1997). Newfoundlands (Lipsitz *et al.*, 1999) and Great Danes (Kent *et al.*, 2008) may be predisposed to a familial form of acquired myasthenia gravis. In fact, recent preliminary data suggest that there is a strong association with a specific *DRB1* allele among Newfoundlands affected with myasthenia gravis (King *et al.*, 2010). A bimodal age of onset (<5 years and >7 years) has also been reported in affected dogs, and neutered bitches may have a heightened risk. In one review of cats with acquired myasthenia gravis, Abyssinians and the closely related Somalis seemed to be over-represented and gender was not a risk factor (Shelton *et al.*, 2000a).

Clinical signs

Several forms of myasthenia gravis have been described in dogs (Dewey *et al.*, 1997), including:

- Focal myasthenia gravis – the only clinical signs are regurgitation, megaoesophagus and dysphagia. The incidence ranges from 26% to 43% of all cases of myasthenia gravis
- Generalized myasthenia gravis – associated with severe exercise intolerance and megaoesophagus. Reported in up to 57% of dogs with myasthenia gravis
- Acute fulminating form of generalized myasthenia gravis – associated with a rapid onset of paralysis and megaoesophagus.

Thus, up to 43% of dogs with myasthenia gravis may not have clinically detectable limb muscle weakness (Shelton *et al.*, 1997). Approximately 7% of dogs with myasthenia gravis have generalized weakness without oesophageal or pharyngeal dysfunction. Generalized weakness without megaoesophagus or dysphagia occurs in approximately 30% and 20% of feline cases, respectively. Generalized weakness associated with thymoma occurs in approximately 26% of cats with myasthenia gravis, whilst focal forms of myasthenia gravis, including megaoesophagus and dysphagia, without signs of generalized weakness occur in approximately 15% of affected cats.

Affected dogs may develop a stiff choppy gait, in which the stride shortens until they crouch in sternal recumbency and rest their head on their forepaws. Cats with myasthenia gravis are usually hypotonic, 'floppy' and reluctant to walk (see **Myasthenia gravis** clip on DVD). After rest, dogs walk normally for a short period before repeating the cycle. Many animals have facial weakness; repeated stimulation of the palpebral reflex causes it to diminish. Many dogs and cats are unable to close their eyelids (accompanied by lack of menace response and absent palpebral reflex). The third eyelids may be protruded. Neurological examination may reveal normal sensation and intact tendon reflexes but diminished withdrawal reflexes, poor postural reactions and proprioceptive deficits. There is a greater incidence of mediastinal thymoma in cats with myasthenia gravis (25.7%) than in dogs (3.4%) (Shelton, 2002).

Thymoma-associated myasthenia gravis can also be considered a clinical form of the disease. All dogs and cats with a cranial mediastinal mass should be tested for the presence of acetylcholine receptor antibodies prior to surgical removal of the mass, as weakness can become apparent following the procedure. Complete removal of the tumour can be associated with normalization of the acetylcholine receptor antibody titre and resolution of clinical signs. Incomplete removal of the mass is associated with tumour regrowth and persistence of antibodies (Shelton, 2002).

Pathophysiology

Myasthenia gravis is characterized by failure of neuromuscular transmission due to a reduction in the number of functional nicotinic acetylcholine receptors on the postsynaptic membrane of the neuromuscular junction. This deficiency of functional receptors reduces the sensitivity of the postsynaptic membrane to acetylcholine (Shelton, 2002). Acquired canine myasthenia gravis is an immune-mediated disease caused by the production of autoantibodies (predominantly immunoglobulin G) directed against muscle acetylcholine receptors at the neuromuscular junction. Based on experimental and human clinical studies, myasthenia gravis involves both B and T cells. Complement-mediated destruction of the postsynaptic membrane of the neuromuscular junction and antibody-induced blockade of acetylcholine receptor function occur (Richman and Agius, 1994).

Diagnosis

A presumptive diagnosis of myasthenia gravis may be made following the resolution of muscle weakness as a result of an intravenous injection of edrophonium chloride (dogs: 0.1 mg/kg to a maximum dose of 5 mg; cats: 0.2–1.0 mg total). This test may be useful in diagnosing focal myasthenia gravis if a decreased or absent palpebral reflex responds to edrophonium. A negative test does not rule out focal or generalized myasthenia gravis. Occasionally this test causes a cholinergic crisis (bradycardia, profuse salivation, miosis, dyspnoea, cyanosis and limb tremors) which can be reversed with atropine (0.05 mg/kg i.v.).

The diagnosis is confirmed by demonstrating the presence of circulating acetylcholine receptor antibodies in a serum sample. Reactive antibodies are found in approximately 98% of dogs with acquired myasthenia gravis and in most affected cats. Antibody elevations are specific for myasthenia gravis, whether it is acquired, paraneoplastic or concurrent with another autoimmune disease. In the absence of immunosuppressive therapy, there is a good correlation in dogs between the clinical course of myasthenia gravis and the acetylcholine receptor antibody titre. Immunosuppressive therapy for longer than 7–10 days lowers antibody titres, so a thorough history is important to establish prior medication administration (Shelton, 2010).

Antibody titres may be negative early during the course of the disease, so re-testing is suggested if the clinical signs are recent in onset. Seronegative myasthenia gravis may occur if low titre, high affinity antibodies are bound to muscle acetylcholine receptors in a range undetectable by the standard serum assay. Most human seronegative myasthenia gravis patients have autoantibodies against muscle-specific tyrosine kinase (MuSK) receptors; antibodies against MuSK receptors have been identified in one seronegative myasthenia gravis dog (Shelton, 2010).

Antibodies reactive with muscle striations and other autoantibodies (ryanodine receptor) may co-exist with a high titre of acetylcholine receptor antibodies in the presence of a thymoma or with older onset myasthenia gravis in dogs. A thorough examination for other autoimmune diseases that can occur concurrently with myasthenia gravis (e.g. autoimmune haemolytic anaemia, thrombocytopenia and inflammatory bowel disease) should be undertaken.

In dogs, acquired myasthenia gravis has been reported in association with tumours, including cholangiocellular carcinomas, osteogenic sarcomas, anal sac adenocarcinomas and non-epitheliotropic cutaneous lymphomas; therefore, investigation for these tumours is warranted. Acquired myasthenia gravis has also been reported in dogs with hypothyroidism and in hyperthyroid cats receiving methimazole therapy. Chest radiographs should always be evaluated for a cranial mediastinal mass (such as thymoma), aspiration pneumonia and megaoesophagus (Wray and Sparkes, 2006).

Electrodiagnostics in the form of repetitive stimulation and single fibre electromyography can assist in the diagnosis, although the tests lack sensitivity and specificity (see Chapter 4). However, lengthy anaesthesia is necessary and this may be contraindicated in a critical patient.

Treatment and prognosis

Treatment should begin with oral anticholinesterase drugs (pyridostigimine bromide at a dose of 0.5–3 mg/kg q8–12h). The drug dosage should be started at the low end to avoid cholinergic crisis, and can then be modified based on response. If oral treatment is not possible due to severe regurgitation, injectable neostigmine can be given (0.04 mg/kg i.m. q6h).

If limb muscle strength has not returned to normal following anticholinesterase treatment or if intolerable side-effects of cholinergic excess are noted, and if there is no evidence of aspiration pneumonia, alternate day, low dose corticosteroid therapy should be initiated (0.5 mg/kg orally q24h). Immunosuppressive dosages of corticosteroids should be avoided early in the disease as this can exacerbate weakness. However, the steroid dose can be increased every 2 weeks up to an immunosuppressive daily dose (2 mg/kg) if necessary. Once a state of clinical remission is achieved, the dose is reduced by 50% every 2–4 weeks, whilst monitoring carefully for relapse. If there is no response to immunosuppressive doses of corticosteroids, azathioprine can be added to the regimen (2 mg/kg orally q24h) (Dewey et al., 1999). A regimen of mycophenolate mofetil added to pyridostigmine was recently evaluated in dogs with myasthenia gravis. The rationale for using mycophenolate mofetil is that its relative sparing of neutrophil function allows initiation of immunosuppression in the face of aspiration pneumonia. The results did not support the routine use of this drug, with no additional benefit noted over the use of pyridostigmine alone in the long term (Dewey *et al.*, 2010). However, this was a retrospective study and it was noted that treatment with mycophenolate was reserved for the more severely affected cases. Mycophenolate mofetil may be useful early in the course of myasthenia gravis when treatment may be most difficult. Further studies are warranted.

Treatment of acute human myasthenia gravis or a myasthenia gravis crisis involves plasmapheresis (plasma exchange) or the administration of intravenous immunoglobulin. Recent comparative analysis of these treatments revealed that they have similar efficacy and complication profiles (Mandawatt *et al.*, 2010), although delaying plasmapheresis for more than 48 hours following admission was associated with higher mortality rates (Mandawat *et al.*, 2011). A preliminary report has described the successful short-term outcome in 3 dogs with severe myasthenia gravis treated with plasmapheresis (Palm *et al.*, 2011). A prospective study performed in 10 dogs established the potential role of vaccination against acetylcholine receptor-specific T and B cell antigen receptors (Galin *et al.*, 2007). The vaccination was seen to increase the proportion of dogs that went into remission (compared with historical controls) from 17% to 75%. The vaccines also accelerated the rate of decline in acetylcholine receptor antibody titres, resulting in a three-fold decrease in the time to achieve remission. However, care must be taken in the interpretation of this study as an appropriate control group was not included.

Supportive care includes the elevation of food and water, or placement of a percutaneous endoscopic gastrostomy (PEG) tube. Many dogs can be fed with food presented as small balls; the animal is then kept in a vertical position for 10–20 minutes to assist with the passage of food into the stomach. Water must also be offered, in reduced quantities, on a more frequent basis and from an elevated position. Construction of a 'vertical feeding' system (e.g. a Bailey chair) has been described by owners of dogs with myasthenia gravis. These maintain the dog in an upright position during and following eating (Figure 18.13).

Famotidine administered orally or via a PEG tube (0.5–1.0 mg/kg q12h) may reduce the nausea and gastrointestinal irritation caused by pyridostigmine. These side effects may also be prevented by diluting liquid pyridostigmine 50:50 with water. In addition, famotidine helps to reduce oesophagitis due to acid reflux. Concurrent hypothyroidism is treated with levothyroxine sodium (0.02 mg/kg orally q12h). Surgical removal of a cranial mediastinal mass is suggested if the animal is clinically unstable. Antibiotic therapy is essential if there is suspicion of concurrent aspiration pneumonia. Care must be

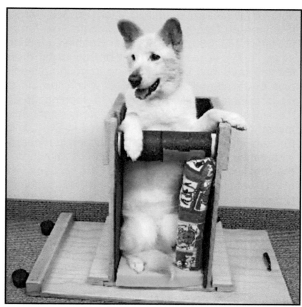

18.13 A Bailey chair used to aid in feeding dogs with megaoesophagus. (Courtesy of Roxie's Mega Mission)

taken to select an appropriate antibiotic that does not interfere with neuromuscular transmission.

The natural course of the disease in dogs, in the absence of underlying neoplasia and without concurrent aspiration pneumonia, is clinical and immunological remission (Shelton and Lindstrom, 2001). Although surgical stress can exacerbate myasthenia gravis, oestrous cycles in bitches may make it difficult to control, thus intact animals should be neutered. In addition, vaccinations have been shown to increase antibody titres and exacerbate weakness in dogs already diagnosed with immune-mediated myasthenia gravis (Shelton and Lindstrom, 2001).

Periodic testing of acetylcholine receptor antibody titres should guide the course of therapy, and treatment may be discontinued once the clinical signs have resolved (including radiographic confirmation of the resolution of megaoesophagus) and the antibody titre is within the reference range. Myasthenia gravis can recur once remission is achieved; therefore, the prognosis in the early stages of the disease is still guarded. In one report, up to 50% of dogs admitted to a referral hospital with myasthenia gravis died or were euthanased within 2 weeks, often due to the poor response to therapy and aspiration pneumonia (Dewey *et al.*, 1997). The 1-year mortality rate for dogs with myasthenia gravis, previously estimated to be 40%, may be greatly improved through early and accurate diagnosis, avoidance of immunosuppressive doses of prednisolone at the onset of the disease, and initiation of appropriate therapy.

Congenital myasthenia gravis

Congenital myasthenic syndromes with an onset at 6–8 weeks of age are rarely seen in dogs and cats. Congenital myasthenia gravis is thought to be an autosomal recessive trait in Jack Russell Terriers (Palmer and Goodyear, 1978), Smooth Fox Terriers (Miller *et al.*, 1983) and Springer Spaniels (Johnson *et al.*, 1975). A reversible form of congenital myasthenia gravis has been identified in young Smooth-haired Miniature Dachshunds, in which the clinical signs spontaneously resolve by 6 months of age (Dickinson *et al.*, 2005). Presynaptic congenital myasthenia gravis has been reported in Old Danish Pointers (12–16 weeks old) with autosomal recessive inheritance (Flagstad *et al.*, 1989). A mutation in the choline acetyltransferase (*CHAT*) gene has been identified as the cause of this syndrome (Proschowsky *et al.*, 2007). Congenital myasthenia gravis has also been reported in several cats, including a Siamese (5 months of age) and Domestic Shorthaired cats (4 and 7 months of age) (Joseph *et al.*, 1988).

The diagnosis is confirmed by the presence of exercise-related weakness in very young dogs for which muscle biopsy does not indicate a congenital muscle or peripheral nerve disease. The response to intravenous edrophonium is variable with an increase in muscle strength and a decremental response of the muscle action potential following repetitive nerve stimulation seen in animals with postsynaptic deficits, or no response seen in animals with presynaptic deficits. Biochemical quantification of acetylcholine receptor concentration in an external intercostal muscle specimen can be performed at a few research centres. As this is not an immune-mediated disease, testing for acetylcholine receptor antibodies is not indicated. Animals with postsynaptic defects may be maintained on oral anticholinesterase drugs for months to years, although drug resistance may develop over time. Acetylcholinesterase-inhibitor therapy has been reported to improve clinical signs and reduce crises in humans with congenital presynaptic myasthenic syndromes (Schara *et al.*, 2010).

Organophosphate and carbamate toxicity

Organophosphate and carbamate compounds are frequently used for external parasite control in dogs and cats, and for the control of insects in the home and garden. Both compounds inhibit acetylcholinesterase; the inhibition is irreversible in the case of organophosphates whilst carbamates cause a reversible inhibition. Cats are considered relatively susceptible to acute toxicosis by the organophosphate compound chlorpyrifos. Both topical exposure and ingestion can result in clinical signs.

Clinical signs

Organophosphate and carbamate compounds result in the build-up of acetylcholine, which leads to overstimulation of the receptors. Clinical signs can be related to:

- Cholinergic muscarinic crisis – excessive parasympathetic stimulation causing salivation, lacrimation, urination, defecation, miosis, bronchospasm, bronchoconstriction and bradycardia

- Cholinergic nicotinic crisis – skeletal muscle stimulation resulting in muscle twitching and tremors with a stiff gait, leading to weakness and paralysis in some cases
- Central stimulation leading to seizures, anxiety and restlessness.

Clinical signs vary with the compound involved and the susceptibility of the individual (e.g. fenthion toxicity usually results in nicotinic signs, leading to activity-related collapse).

Diagnosis

The diagnosis is suggested by the clinical signs and a history of exposure, and can be confirmed by measurement of blood cholinesterase levels (see Chapter 3). Levels reduced by ≥25% confirm exposure in dogs; marked reductions (>50%) need to be documented to confirm the diagnosis in cats.

Treatment and prognosis

Prompt treatment with atropine and symptomatic support is often required. The administration of atropine (0.2–0.4 mg/kg slow i.v. over 5 minutes) results in rapid resolution of the muscarinic signs (e.g. salivation) and may need to be repeated at a lower dose if the signs recur. Atropine does not affect the nicotinic actions of acetylcholine on the skeletal muscle. These can be improved in cases of organophosphate toxicity with the prompt administration of pralidoxime chloride (2-PAM) (dilute to a 10% solution and administer at a dose of 40 mg/kg for dogs or 10–20 mg/kg for cats i.m., s.c., or slow i.v. over 30 minutes, q8h if needed). Organophosphates combine with 2-PAM, resulting in a non-toxic compound that is excreted in the urine, and the reactivation of acetylcholinesterase. It is only effective if given within 24–48 hours of exposure, before the enzyme/organophosphate complex has aged to a non-reactive form. As it does not enter the CNS, 2-PAM does not affect CNS signs of toxicity. This drug is not effective against carbamate toxicity and may cause clinical deterioration. Diphenhydramine has been used to treat refractory cases at a dose of 4 mg/kg orally, i.v., i.m. (i.m. only in cats) q4–8h as it has both anti-nicotinic and muscarinic effects.

Drug toxicity

Several drugs have been shown to reduce the safety margin of neuromuscular transmission, including aminoglycoside antibiotics, antiarrhythmic agents, phenothiazines and magnesium. These agents should be avoided in any patient with neurological weakness, particularly if associated with a disorder of neuromuscular transmission.

Myopathies

Non-inflammatory myopathies: acquired

Nutritional myopathies

Vitamin E (alpha tocopherol) deficiency has been reported to cause a myopathy in large animals, but is rare in cats and dogs. Myalgia, weakness and sudden death may result, due the effects on the heart. Once the deficiency has been addressed, the myopathic signs may resolve.

Endocrine myopathies: disorders of steroid metabolism

Steroid myopathy: Steroid myopathy may be overlooked in patients receiving steroid treatment for disorders that result in weakness, such as inflammatory myopathies or CNS diseases.

Clinical signs: Chronic corticosteroid therapy may result in dramatic muscle atrophy and weakness (see **Steroid myopathy** clip on DVD), particularly in dogs (Platt, 2002). Patients with steroid myopathy commonly have other clinical signs of glucocorticoid excess; skin and hair coat changes are typical (Figure 18.14). Patients rarely develop severe clinical weakness with <4 weeks of steroid administration. Muscle atrophy, particularly of the masticatory muscles, may occur with 2 weeks of steroid therapy (Shelton, unpublished). It has been reported that steroid myopathy is more common following the administration of fluorinated corticosteroids such as triamcinolone, betamethasone and dexamethasone (Platt, 2002).

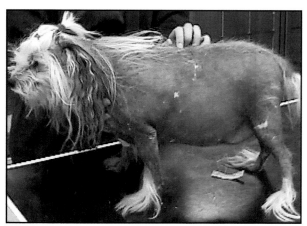

18.14 A 9-year-old Chinese Crested dog with a pendulous abdomen and thin skin due to hyperadrenocorticism. Alopecia was obviously difficult for the owner to detect in this breed and so the condition progressed to loss of muscle mass and pelvic limb weakness.

Pathophysiology: The major actions of glucocorticoids are to increase muscle protein catabolism and inhibit synthesis of myofibrillar proteins. Protein synthesis is inhibited primarily in type II muscle fibres, thus net protein loss is greatest in these fibres. Inhibition of protein synthesis is dependent on the dose of steroids administered. Steroid myopathy is also associated with alterations in muscle carbohydrate metabolism, due in part to steroid-induced insulin resistance.

Diagnosis: The diagnosis necessitates exclusion of other causes of generalized muscle disease, in addition to evidence of long-term steroid administration,

and is confirmed by muscle biopsy. The typical pattern of type II fibre atrophy may be identified early in the disease course with examination of muscle biopsy samples.

Treatment and prognosis: The treatment of choice for iatrogenic steroid myopathy is steroid dose reduction. However, this can only be achieved if the condition that warranted treatment with cortico0steroids is safely controlled. Conversion to a nonfluorinated steroid preparation and alternate-day treatment are recommended. Improvement may be seen but can take many weeks or longer. Due to the catabolic effect of corticosteroids, optimizing nutritional status is important. Protein supplementation for patients with loss of muscle mass is recommended. Physical therapy or mild exercise may be useful in the prevention and treatment of muscle weakness and wasting in patients receiving glucocorticoids. Androgens can partially antagonize the catabolic actions of glucocorticoids.

Cushing's myopathy: A myopathy has been described in dogs with spontaneous hyperadrenocorticism (Greene *et al.*, 1979). Pseudomyotonia is most often seen.

Clinical signs: Most affected dogs are middle-aged with bitches being predisposed. Poodles and smaller breeds are also over-represented. Affected dogs often have characteristic signs of hyperadrenocorticism, in addition to generalized muscle atrophy, but with a stiff gait and hypertrophy of the proximal appendicular muscles. Of the cats reported with hyperadrenocorticism, the majority are middle-aged or older (average 10–11 years old) and are usually of mixed breeding. Approximately 70% of affected cats are queens. No distinct myopathy has been reported in these cats, but muscle wasting is a prominent finding.

Pathophysiology: The myopathy seen in association with hyperadrenocorticism has been attributed to glucocorticoid excess (as described for steroid myopathy). It has been suggested that elevated levels of ACTH may also be myopathic.

Diagnosis: The diagnosis necessitates exclusion of other causes of generalized muscle disease, in addition to biochemical confirmation of hyperadrenocorticism and evidence of type II myofibre atrophy on muscle biopsy samples. There may be a mild serum creatine kinase elevation in some dogs. Electromyography often reveals complex repetitive discharges, most consistently in the proximal appendicular groups, which has led to this disease being labelled as a pseudomyotonia. Unlike myotonic discharges, there is no waxing or waning of these discharges. The associated pathological changes have been described as dystrophic (Duncan *et al.*, 1975). The most obvious features include a rounding of the myofibres on cross-section and variation in fibre size with numerous internal nuclei, many of which can be seen to form chains.

Degeneration and regeneration have been seen with a slight increase in perimysial and endomysial connective tissue. Enzyme histochemistry has failed to demonstrate any selective type I fibre atrophy in pseudomyotonic cases; however, type II fibre atrophy is a consistent finding (Duncan *et al.*, 1975).

Treatment and prognosis: Signs can resolve in some dogs over a period of months when they are treated for the primary disease, but deficits can persist. Improvement in motor function appears unlikely, but may be inversely related to the duration of disease prior to therapy. Dietary modification and rehabilitation should also be instituted (as for steroid myopathy).

Adrenal insufficiency:

Clinical signs: Muscle weakness, including reversible megaoesophagus and dysphagia, frequently occurs in association with hypoadrenocorticism (Addison's disease) in cats and dogs. Painful episodic cramping affecting all four limbs has been reported in two Standard Poodles with hypoadrenocorticism (Saito *et al.*, 2002). The dogs were neurologically normal between episodes.

Pathophysiology: Adrenal insufficiency impairs muscle carbohydrate metabolism, water and electrolyte balance, muscle blood flow and adrenergic sensitivity, which all contribute to the weakness associated with hypoadrenocorticism. Hyperkalaemia develops with depletion of muscle intracellular potassium, decreased membrane sodium (Na^+)/potassium (K^+) adenosine triphosphatase (ATPase) activity, and diminished adrenergic stimulation of the Na^+/K^+ pump.

Diagnosis: The diagnosis is made by exclusion of other causes of weakness and biochemical confirmation of hypoadrenocorticism.

Treatment and prognosis: The weakness and fatigue are usually rapidly corrected with glucocorticoid replacement. The prognosis is good with correction of the underlying endocrine disorder.

Endocrine myopathies: disorders of thyroid metabolism

Hypothyroid myopathy: A myopathy occurs in dogs associated with spontaneous (Braund *et al.*, 1981) or experimentally induced (Rossmeisl *et al.*, 2009) hypothyroidism.

Clinical signs: Neuromuscular signs including stiffness, weakness, reluctance to move and muscle wasting may be the first indication of an underlying endocrine disorder. Typical signs of hypothyroidism, including lethargy, weight gain, seborrhoea and alopecia, may be clinically evident.

Pathophysiology: In general, hypothyroidism affects carbohydrate, protein and lipid metabolism within muscle. Muscle glycogenolysis is impaired, protein synthesis and degradation are decreased (causing net protein catabolism), and muscle uptake of triglycerides is reduced. Thyroid hormone imbalance has been determined to contribute to abnormalities of cellular energy generation in striated muscle through multiple carnitine-dependent mitochondrial biochemical pathways, supported in part by the fact that chronic hypothyroidism in dogs is associated with a marked reduction of skeletal muscle free carnitine (Rossmeisl *et al.*, 2009).

Diagnosis: Serum creatine kinase concentrations may be normal (especially in the first 6 months of the disease) or significantly elevated. Aspartate aminotransferase (AST) and lactate dehydrogenase levels can also be elevated. Prominent histopathological alterations include variation in muscle fibre size with type II fibre atrophy and an increased population of type I fibres (Figure 18.15), and multifocal nemaline rod inclusions. Subsarcolemmal accumulations of abnormal mitochondria can also be seen. Increased insertional activity, diffuse and variably severe fibrillations, positive sharp waves and complex repetitive discharges can be detected in some dogs using electromyography.

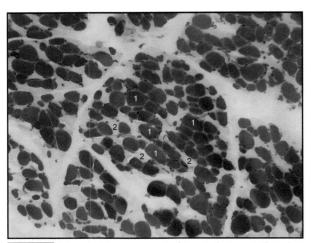

18.15 Muscle biopsy sample from a dog revealing the classic appearance of hypothyroid myopathy. The type I fibres are larger than the atrophied type II fibres. (Myofibrillar ATPase reaction at pH 4.3 stain; original magnification X100)

Treatment and prognosis: The only effective treatment is to restore the patient to a euthyroid state. Once this is achieved, the prognosis for recovery can be good and may be accomplished within a few weeks (Panciera, 1994). It is reasonable to institute physical therapy to limit disuse atrophy and joint contractures. There is no evidence that dietary manipulation improves muscle function in this disease.

Hyperthyroid myopathy in cats: Although specific pathological changes are lacking in the muscles of hyperthyroid patients, there is a good correlation between severity of hyperthyroidism and clinical muscle weakness. In a study of 202 hyperthyroid cats, it was noted that 12% were reported as weak by the owners but only 1% exhibited a ventral neck flexion characteristic of muscle weakness in cats (Broussard *et al.*, 1995). With more advanced disease, owners report a decreased ability to jump and fatigue associated with physical exertion such that cats may lie down or rest when moving from one place to another, with breathlessness not uncommon. Hypokalaemia may be a complicating factor in cats with extreme weakness, known as thyrotoxic periodic paralysis in humans. In this condition, patients can have recurrent attacks of weakness, which can be precipitated by a carbohydrate challenge or rest after exercise. Muscle weakness should rapidly resolve following achievement of a euthyroid state.

Non-inflammatory myopathies: dystrophic

Muscular dystrophy

Muscular dystrophies are a heterogeneous group of inherited, degenerative, mostly non-inflammatory disorders characterized by progressive muscle weakness, muscle atrophy or hypertrophy, gait abnormalities and muscle contractures beginning within the first few months of life. Whilst over 30 muscular dystrophies have been identified to date in humans, only a small number have been characterized in dogs and cats.

Muscular dystrophies were originally characterized based on phenotypic features such as pattern of inheritance and the distribution of muscle involvement. With the advent of the molecular age, most have been shown to occur due to mutations in the genes that code for proteins in the dystrophin–glycoprotein (DAG) complex (Figure 18.16) which spans the muscle cell membrane. Dystrophin and its associated glycoproteins connect the contractile apparatus in the muscle to the sarcolemma, providing mechanical stability. Dystroglycan (a widely expressed transmembrane protein) and sarcoglycans (which have a more restricted distribution) form part of the DAG complex, linking the intracellular actin cytoskeleton with the extracellular matrix. When dystrophin is absent, the dystrophin-associated proteins at the sarcolemma are often also reduced or absent. Laminin is a structural component of the basement membrane, the specialized extracellular matrix that immediately abuts and surrounds each muscle fibre. Laminin $\alpha2$ in the muscle is linked to dystrophin via dystroglycan.

The dystrophin gene is one of the largest in the human genome and thousands of mutations have been recorded. However, 70% of human dystrophin deficient patients have gene deletions in a mutation rich area or 'hot spot' in the central genomic region. A mutation in a comparable region has been reported in dystrophin deficient Cavalier King Charles Spaniels (Walmsley *et al.*, 2010). A mutation identified as a long interspersed repetitive element-1 (LINE-1) insertion in intron 13 has recently been confirmed in Corgis (Smith *et al.*, 2011). These now represent the most valid 'models' for gene therapy for muscular dystrophy. Currently, there are no specific clinical therapies available and the general prognosis is poor. Affected animals should not be used in breeding programmes.

Dystrophin deficiency: Muscular dystrophy associated with dystrophin deficiency is the most common and best studied of the dystrophies in humans (also termed Duchenne muscular dystrophy), dogs and cats (Valentine *et al.*, 1992; Shelton and Engvall, 2005). It has been documented in several breeds of dog, including the Golden Retriever, Rottweiler, German Shorthaired Pointer, Irish Terrier, Groenendaeler Shepherd, Japanese Spitz, Samoyed, Miniature Schnauzer, Brittany Spaniel, Rat Terrier, Old English Sheepdog, Pembroke Welsh Corgi, Cavalier King Charles Spaniel, Weimaraner, Alaskan Malamute and Labrador Retriever, as well as the Domestic Shorthaired cat. In some cases, dystrophin

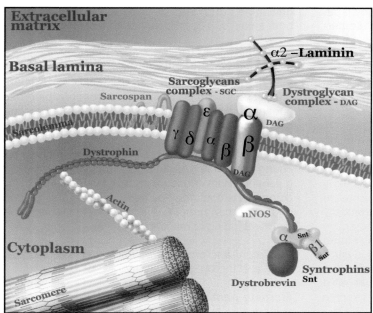

18.16 Dystrophin–glycoprotein (DAG) complex and its relationship with the muscle membrane and contractile units.

is present but abnormal. In humans, partial dystrophin deficiencies are classified as Becker muscular dystrophy. This disease generally has a milder clinical presentation (localized weakness, high creatine kinase level, myalgia, cramps and cardiomyopathy) and progression. A Becker-type muscular dystrophy with truncated dystrophin has been described in Japanese Spitz dogs (Jones *et al.*, 2004).

Clinical signs: Clinical signs usually develop within the first 6 months of life and are rapidly progressive, although a slower disease course has been documented in some dogs (Baltzer *et al.*, 2007). Affected dogs may demonstrate remarkable phenotypic variation with some animals dying within the first few days following birth whilst others live well into adulthood (Olby *et al.*, 2011). As an X-linked disease, it is seen predominantly in males. Typically, dystrophin deficiency causes diffuse muscle atrophy and hypertrophy of certain muscle groups (cranial sartorius, semimembranosus, semitendinosus and tongue muscles) in dogs and generalized muscle hypertrophy or atrophy in cats (Kornegay *et al.*, 2003; Shelton and Engvall, 2005).

Affected animals can be weak from birth and ineffectual sucklers, necessitating nutritional supplementation. As affected animals age, exercise intolerance becomes increasingly evident. Dogs have a characteristic plantigrade stance with the paws laterally rotated and the tarsi held close together. Whilst walking they may advance the pelvic limbs simultaneously ('bunny hop') and abduct the thoracic limbs (see **Muscular dystrophy** clip on DVD). Dysphagia, regurgitation and dyspnoea may occur as a result of hypertrophy of the lingual, pharyngeal and oesophageal musculature and diaphragm. Cardiomyopathy may result in heart failure.

Pathophysiology: Dystrophin links the myofibre cytoskeleton to the extracellular matrix and is crucial in stabilization of the muscle fibre membrane during contraction. The gene for dystrophin is located on the X-chromosome, thus dystrophin deficiency is an X-linked recessive trait transmitted by a female carrier. Females may be heterozygous (either asymptomatic or expressing clinical signs) or homozygous for the disease. Homozygous females have elevated creatine kinase levels and comparable histological lesions to those seen in affected males (Shelton *et al.*, 2001).

Diagnosis: The serum creatine kinase concentration is usually markedly elevated (10,000–100,000 IU/l). Electromyography reveals complex repetitive discharges. A dystrophic phenotype, characterized early in the course of the disease by small group muscle fibre necrosis and regeneration, and more chronically by fibrosis and fatty deposition, is typically seen on histopathology of muscle biopsy specimens (Figure 18.17). An absence, or decreased level, of dystrophin on immunohistochemistry and immunoblotting of muscle specimens confirms the diagnosis. MRI has also been used to characterize dystrophic muscle (Thibaud *et al.*, 2007; Kobayashi *et al.*, 2009).

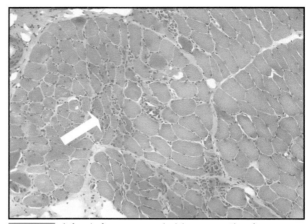

18.17 A fresh-frozen muscle biopsy section from a young dog with muscular dystrophy showing necrotic fibres undergoing phagocytosis, clusters of basophilic regenerating fibres (arrowed) and endomysial fibrosis. Immunohistochemistry is needed to confirm the absence of dystrophin and associated glycoproteins. (H&E stain; original magnification X100)

Treatment and prognosis: There is no specific treatment. Prednisone therapy for Duchenne muscular dystrophy slows disease progression and has become the standard of care. By extrapolation, prednisone (at a dose of 0.5 mg/kg orally q24h) could also be beneficial in dogs. However, this has not been substantiated by clinical studies. If steroids are used, they should be combined with physical therapy. The prognosis is poor.

Sarcoglycan deficiency: Muscular dystrophy associated with sarcoglycan deficiency has been reported in a few breeds, including the Boston Terrier, Cocker Spaniel and Chihuahua (Schatzberg and Shelton, 2004; Deitz *et al.*, 2008). Muscular dystrophy associated with reduced β-sarcoglycan has also been reported in a cat (Salvadori *et al.*, 2009).

Clinical signs: The clinical presentation is indistinguishable from that of dystrophin deficiency, but both sexes can be affected at equal rates.

Pathophysiology: The sarcoglycan complex consists of four transmembrane glycoproteins, which form a subcomplex within the DAG complex. In humans, mutations in sarcoglycans are responsible for a subset of autosomal recessive limb girdle muscular dystrophies.

Diagnosis: The laboratory findings and pathological changes seen in muscle biopsy samples are indistinguishable from those of dystrophin deficiency. The diagnosis is confirmed by demonstrating the absence of sarcoglycan protein on immunohistochemistry and immunoblotting of muscle biopsy specimens.

Treatment and prognosis: There is no specific treatment and the prognosis is poor.

Merosin (laminin α2) deficiency: Congenital muscular dystrophy associated with laminin α2 deficiency has been described in a young Brittany Spaniel x Springer Spaniel mixed-breed dog (Shelton *et al.*, 2001b) and in four unrelated cats, including a young Flame-point Siamese, two young Domestic Short-haired queens and a Maine Coon (O'Brien *et al.*, 2001; Poncelet *et al.*, 2003).

Clinical signs: Gait abnormalities and generalized weakness from 8 weeks of age have been reported in laminin α2 deficient dogs. Clinical signs in cats vary from muscle weakness and atrophy to severe contractures with limb rigidity.

Pathophysiology: Laminin α2 is the major component of the basal lamina which surrounds each muscle fibre and is one of the extracellular ligands that links dystrophin to the extracellular matrix, contributing to the stability of the muscle basement membrane. Laminin α2 deficiency is associated with autosomal recessive congenital muscular dystrophy in humans.

Diagnosis: Serum creatine kinase levels are moderately elevated (10 times normal) compared with marked elevations seen with dystrophin deficiency (may be 100 times normal). A dystrophic phenotype with endomysial fibrosis should be evident on evaluation of muscle biopsy samples. An absence of laminin α2 on immunohistological analysis of muscle biopsy specimens confirms the diagnosis.

Treatment and prognosis: These are as for dystrophin deficiency.

Dystroglycan deficiency: A form of muscular dystrophy associated with loss of α-dystroglycan has been identified in young Sphinx and Devon Rex cats (Martin *et al.*, 2008).

Clinical signs: Clinical signs of generalized and progressive weakness are evident at 10–16 weeks of age. Physical findings include an inability to jump, passive ventroflexion of the head and neck, difficulty swallowing, dorsal protrusion of the scapulae, decreased muscle mass and fatigability that occur following short periods of activity.

Pathophysiology: Dystroglycan is a central part of the DAG complex and plays an important role in maintaining membrane integrity in skeletal muscle. α-Dystroglycan is an extracellular membrane associated protein that binds to a variety of extracellular matrix proteins, including laminin α2.

Diagnosis: Serum creatine kinase levels are normal or only mildly increased. A mildly myopathic phenotype is found on histopathology and histochemistry of muscle biopsy samples. The diagnosis is confirmed by demonstrating decreased levels of α-dystroglycan on immunohistochemistry and immunoblotting.

Treatment and prognosis: No specific treatment is available and the prognosis for recovery is poor.

Non-inflammatory myopathies: non-dystrophic congenital myopathies

Non-dystrophic congenital myopathies are defined by distinctive morphological abnormalities seen on examination of skeletal muscle biopsy samples. These myopathies include:

- Centronuclear myopathy
- X-linked myotubular myopathy
- Inherited myopathy of Great Danes
- Protein accumulation myopathy (including nemaline rod and myofibrillar myopathies).

The genetic basis for some of these myopathies is known in dogs.

Centronuclear myopathy

Centronuclear myopathies in humans are heterogeneous forms of inherited muscle disorders which share common clinical and histological features (Pele *et al.*, 2005). Hallmarks of the disease include generalized muscle weakness, ptosis, ophthalmoplegia externa, absence of the patellar reflex (Labrador Retrievers), muscular atrophy predominately affecting type I myofibres, nuclear centralization and pale central zones with variably staining granules. A centronuclear myopathy was first described in 1976 in Labrador Retrievers as a form of hereditary myopathy (Shelton, 2007a), and was previously known as Labrador Retriever myopathy, type II fibre deficiency and autosomal recessive muscular dystrophy.

Clinical signs: This autosomal recessive myopathy affects yellow, chocolate and black Labrador Retrievers from 8 weeks to 11 months of age, causing a stiff 'bunny hop' gait with an abnormal 'low' head and neck posture and exercise intolerance. Tendon reflexes are absent or reduced. The signs are exacerbated by a cold ambient temperature, exercise and excitement but tend to stabilize at 1 year of age. Affected dogs often have a reduced muscle mass and poor conformation. Working dogs are over-represented.

Pathophysiology: Historically, this disorder has been referred to as a polyneuropathy, muscular dystrophy, myotonia and a hereditary myopathy. The precise aetiology was unknown and there was much debate about whether it represented a myopathy or neuropathy, as characteristics of both disorders were observed. Investigation of chronic pathological changes in a group of Labrador Retrievers with a similar phenotype demonstrated that the muscle pathology became more obviously myopathic with time and that central nuclei were evident (Blot, 2003). The term centronuclear myopathy was proposed for this disease as the majority of muscle fibres had centrally placed nuclei, with disorganized sarcoplasmic architecture over the long term. In 2005, a short interspersed repetitive element (SINE) exonic insertion in the *PTPLA* gene was identified, which results in multiple splicing defects, and confirmed that this myopathy was a member of the centronuclear/myotubular family of myopathies (Pele *et al.*, 2005). Recently, the frequency of the allelic variant of the *PTPLA* gene responsible for centronuclear myopathy in Labrador Retrievers was assessed to be approximately 1 in 20,000 at risk (Gentilini *et al.*, 2011).

Diagnosis: Serum creatine kinase levels are normal or mildly elevated. Electromyography reveals fibrillation potentials, positive sharp waves and complex repetitive discharges. Nerve conduction studies are normal. Pathological changes within muscle biopsy specimens are variable and can include both neuropathic and myopathic abnormalities (McKerrell and Braund, 1986). There is usually dramatic variation in myofibre size with small and large group atrophy. A few fibres have centrally placed nuclei and this percentage increases over the long term. A type II fibre deficiency has been described. Genetic testing provides a definitive diagnosis and a DNA-based test is now available for identification of affected dogs and carriers (see **Useful websites** on DVD).

Treatment and prognosis: Supportive therapy and avoiding cold ambient temperatures are advised until the condition stabilizes. The disease itself is not fatal and so the prognosis is fair, but affected dogs have reduced exercise tolerance and are not able to perform as working dogs.

X-linked myotubular myopathy
In humans this disease is a well defined subgroup of centronuclear myopathies characterized by early onset and the presence of uniformly small muscle fibres with centrally located nuclei resembling fetal myotubes. An X-linked myotubular myopathy has been identified in a family of Labrador Retrievers (Beggs *et al.*, 2010) and a family of Manchester Terriers.

Clinical signs: The clinical presentation in young male Labrador Retrievers with X-linked myotubular myopathy is virtually indistinguishable from that seen with centronuclear myopathy, although the clinical signs are more severe. Affected male Manchester Terriers are presented at 2 months of age for severe weakness and failure to thrive.

Pathophysiology: In several species X-linked myotubular myopathy is associated with an absence of the protein myotubularin. Myotubularin plays a critical role in establishing or maintaining structural and functional integrity of the membranous structures at the muscle triads. A defect of excitation–contraction coupling may be a primary cause of the weakness and hypotonia seen with this condition.

Diagnosis: The serum creatine kinase level is normal or mildly elevated. A diagnosis of myotubular myopathy can be made from histopathology of muscle biopsy specimens. Gene sequencing of *MTM1* from affected Labrador Retrievers has revealed a unique exon 7 variant causing a non-conservative missense change. A specific mutation has not yet been identified in Manchester Terriers.

Treatment and prognosis: No specific treatments are available and the prognosis is poor.

Inherited myopathy of Great Danes
A hereditary, non-inflammatory myopathy with distinct histological myopathic features has been described in young Great Danes of both sexes (Targett *et al.*, 1994; Lujan Feliu-Pascual *et al.*, 2006). Originally described as a central core (or core-like) myopathy, the histochemical characteristics differ from this disease in humans (Shelton, 2007b), and the disease is now termed 'inherited myopathy of Great Danes' (potentially until an underlying cause is identified). An autosomal recessive mode of inheritance is most likely. Recent unpublished studies have confirmed that this myopathy belongs in the centronuclear/myotubular group of myopathies (Shelton, unpublished).

Clinical signs: Clinical dysfunction can be seen to affect both males and females from 6–19 months of age (median age at onset is 7 months) and comprises progressive muscle wasting, exercise intolerance, general body tremors and collapse, which can be exacerbated by excitement or exercise (Lujan Feliu-Pascual *et al.*, 2006). All affected dogs have fawn or brindle coat coloration. Affected dogs are usually stunted compared with their littermates. The generalized muscle atrophy is typically mild to moderate and particularly affects the biceps femoris, quadriceps, temporalis, gluteal, supraspinatus and infraspinatus muscles. Dogs 'tuck' their legs under their abdomen and have an extended tail carriage; when they walk or run they have a short stride with a stiff pelvic limb gait and begin to 'bunny hop' as they move faster (see **Inherited myopathy** clip on DVD). Tremors are present at rest and get worse with movement or excitement. The neurological examination is unremarkable but some dogs have been described with reduced reflexes. Myalgia has not been described in any dogs.

Diagnosis: Serum creatine kinase levels are normal or increased (up to 26-fold). Electromyography reveals fibrillations and positive sharp waves in all muscles. The diagnosis is easily confirmed by examination of muscle biopsy specimens, which show well defined central cytoarchitectural changes highlighted by localization of oxidative enzyme activity (Figure 18.18).

Treatment and prognosis: There is no known treatment at present and the disease is usually progressive and fatal (Targett *et al.*, 1994), although survival for up to 55 months has been described (Lujan Feliu-Pascual *et al.*, 2006).

Miscellaneous congenital myopathies
A few congenital myopathies associated with protein accumulations in muscle have been described in dogs and cats. Nemaline rod myopathy has been described in a Border Collie (Delauche *et al.*, 1998) and in cats (Cooper *et al.*, 1986; Kube *et al.*, 2006).

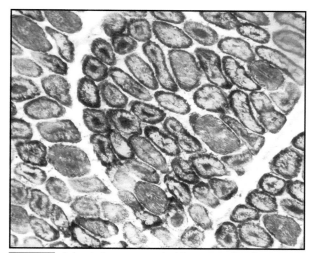

18.18 A fresh-frozen muscle biopsy section from a young Great Dane with progressive muscle wasting and exercise intolerance. Note the well defined central areas within several myofibres. (NADH dehydrogenase reaction; original magnification X100)

Myofibrillar myopathy with desmin accumulation has been described in a young Australian Shepherd Dog (Shelton *et al.*, 2004). A deficiency of myostatin in Whippets with gross muscle hypertrophy has been described and a mutation identified (Mosher *et al.*, 2007; Shelton and Engvall, 2007).

Metabolic myopathies

Metabolic myopathies are a group of muscle disorders caused by a biochemical defect of the skeletal muscle energy system, resulting in inefficient muscle performance. Although the metabolic myopathies reported in dogs have not all proved to be inherited, the suspicion is that they are at least 'inborn'. A number of specific metabolic myopathies have been recognized in veterinary patients; however, they are generally considered rare conditions.

Mitochondrial myopathies

Very few confirmed cases of mitochondrial myopathy have been reported in dogs and cats, although mitochondrial dysfunction has been suspected in larger numbers. The combination of muscle and brain disease occurring in an animal should alert the clinician to the potential diagnosis of a mitochondrial disorder.

Clinical signs: A mitochondrial myopathy associated with pyruvate dehydrogenase deficiency has been described in Clumber (Herrtage and Houlton, 1979) and Sussex (Houlton and Herrtage, 1980; Abramson *et al.*, 2004) Spaniels from the UK and USA. The disease is characterized by poor exercise tolerance with development of severe metabolic acidosis, and lactic and pyruvic acidaemia. A mitochondrial myopathy with altered cytochrome c oxidase activity and reduced mitochondrial mRNA has been described in Old English Sheepdog littermates with exercise intolerance (Vijayasarathy *et al.*, 1994). A Jack Russell Terrier presenting with progressive exercise intolerance and elevated blood lactate and pyruvate concentrations has been reported with a tentative diagnosis of mitochondrial myopathy (Olby *et al.*, 1997).

Diagnosis: Evaluation of mitochondrial disorders requires analysis of resting and post-exercise lactate and pyruvate concentrations, blood gas analysis and specific assays of the enzymes involved in oxidative phosphorylation. Light and electron microscopic evaluation of mitochondria within muscle biopsy sections can be helpful in identifying structural abnormalities and accumulations, although such changes are non-specific. A classic finding is massive proliferation or enlargement of muscle mitochondria with subsarcolemmal accumulation, represented pathologically as 'ragged-red' fibres with the Gomori trichrome stain (Figure 18.19) and highlighted by oxidative enzyme localization (Platt, 2002). Biochemical analysis in the Sussex Spaniel from the UK and Clumber Spaniel from the USA demonstrated a defect in pyruvate oxidation (Shelton *et al.*, 2000b). For both Clumber and Sussex Spaniels, a null mutation has been identified in the *PDP1* gene, encoding the phosphatase enzyme that activates the pyruvate dehydrogenase complex (Cameron *et al.*, 2007, 2009). Of the current Clumber and Sussex Spaniel populations, 20% are carriers for the mutated *PDP1* gene. Homozygous animals have severe exercise intolerance. A genetic test is available for both breeds (see **Useful websites** on DVD).

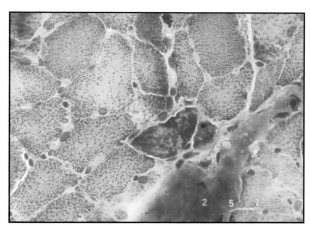

18.19 Modified Gomori trichrome-stained muscle biopsy specimen from a dog with suspected mitochondrial myopathy. Subsarcolemmal and intermyofibrillar deposits of membranous material stains red with the trichrome stain, and represents the accumulation of mitochondria. Myofibres with the staining pattern are called ragged-red fibres. (Original magnification X400)

Treatment and prognosis: At present there is no cure for disorders of mitochondrial metabolism and any treatment should be supportive, with a reduced daily level of activity. Treatment with L-carnitine, conenzyme Q10 and riboflavin may be attempted (Figure 18.20) and can result in temporary stabilization of some forms of mitochondrial disease (Abramson *et al.*, 2004).

Supplement	Dose regimen
Riboflavin	100 mg orally q24h
Coenzyme Q10	100 mg orally q24h
L-Carnitine	50 mg/kg orally q12h

18.20 Recommendations for treatment of mitochondrial and lipid storage myopathies.

Defects of glycogen metabolism

Glycogen storage diseases resulting from inborn errors of glycolysis or glycogen metabolism are rare myopathic disorders in dogs and cats (see Figure 18.17). The enzyme defect results in inadequate glycogen utilization, frequently fasting hypoglycaemia and the accumulation of glycogen-like material within muscles and other tissues. Clinical signs include muscular weakness, exercise intolerance, collapse and occasionally seizures. Glycogen storage disease type IIIa has been reported in Curly-Coated Retrievers and is caused by a mutation of the glycogen debranching enzyme gene (Gregory *et al.*, 2007). Affected dogs present with episodic exercise intolerance, collapse and lethargy. The disease is autosomal recessive and a DNA sequence-based carrier test has been developed. This test is currently available at centres in the UK and USA (see **Useful websites** on DVD). Carriers have been identified in the USA, New Zealand, Australia and Finland.

Lipid storage myopathy

Clinical signs: Dogs with abnormalities of lipid metabolism generally have chronic progressive signs of muscle weakness, atrophy and myalgia (Platt *et al.*, 1999).

Pathophysiology: Mitochondrial fatty acid oxidation is a vital source of energy production in all cells, especially skeletal and cardiac muscle. This complex pathway involves up to 20 individual steps, resulting in the formation of acetyl coenzyme A, which enters the citric acid cycle (Krebs cycle, tricarboxylic acid cycle, TCA cycle) and ultimately results in the production of ATP necessary for muscle contraction. The fundamental steps in lipid metabolism are (see Figure 18.9):

1. Transportation of fatty acids into skeletal muscle.
2. Carnitine transport of fatty acids across the mitochondrial membrane.
3. β-Oxidation.

Other than secondary defects of carnitine metabolism, specific defects of β-oxidation have not yet been identified in dogs.

Diagnosis: The diagnosis of a lipid storage disorder is made by demonstrating the presence of excessive droplets of neutral triglycerides in muscle biopsy specimens using Oil Red O staining (Figure 18.21). In addition to evaluation of a muscle biopsy

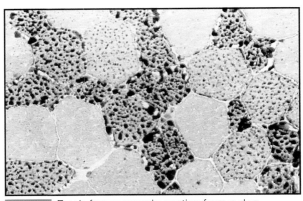

18.21 Fresh-frozen muscle section from a dog presented with exercise-related weakness and myalgia. The multiple large lipid droplets are indicative of a lipid storage myopathy. (Oil Red O stain; original magnification X400)

sample, blood lactate and pyruvate concentrations, urinary organic acid and plasma amino acid levels, and plasma and muscle carnitine concentrations should be measured (Shelton *et al.*, 1998).

Treatment and prognosis: Whilst no specific therapy is yet available for these disorders, treatment with L-carnitine, coenzyme Q10 and riboflavin (see Figure 18.20) may result in improvement in muscle strength and resolution of pain. The prognosis is fair to guarded.

Hypokalaemic myopathy

Clinical signs: In cats, clinical signs of muscle weakness become evident with any cause of potassium depletion and include generalized weakness and ventroflexion of the neck (Figure 18.22). The most severely affected patients exhibit profound exercise intolerance accompanied by collapse. The weakness can ultimately result in paralysis and is progressive until the potassium deficit is corrected. The neurological examination is within normal limits.

- Hyperthyroidism
- Polymyositis
- Hypokalaemic myopathy
- Organophosphate toxicity
- Thiamine deficiency
- Hereditary myopathies (e.g. Devon Rex myopathy)

18.22 Causes of neck ventroflexion in the cat.

Pathophysiology: Hypokalaemic myopathy is seen in cats and very rarely in dogs. It can result from:

- Reduced potassium intake
- Increased potassium entry into the cells
- Increased potassium loss from the body
- Familial disorder of electrolyte regulation (e.g. as seen in Burmese kittens).

Hypokalaemia significantly affects muscle membrane activity and thus muscle function (Fettman,

1989). The myocyte becomes increasingly refractory to depolarization in a hypokalaemic environment. Eventually, the muscle cell membrane suddenly becomes permeable to sodium ions and membrane hypopolarization occurs, inducing an acute onset of severe weakness.

Diagnosis: The serum levels of potassium and creatine kinase are often 1.5–3.5 mEq/l and 500–10,000 IU/l, respectively. Chronic renal failure with urinary loss of potassium should be ruled out using serum biochemistry and urinalysis, in conjunction with imaging studies to assess the structure and function of the kidney. The dietary potassium content should be investigated (diets should be at least 0.6% rich in potassium). Hyperthyroidism should be ruled out. Electrophysiological findings may be normal, or fibrillations and positive sharp waves may be seen (see Chapter 4). Histological examination of muscle biopsy samples may be normal or show muscle fibre necrosis with little or no evidence of inflammation.

Treatment and prognosis: Potassium gluconate (2–4 mEq orally q12h) may be used in all animals. The dosage is adjusted until the serum potassium levels are normal. Dietary modification may be all that is required if insufficient potassium was the inciting cause, but potassium supplementation may be needed for life in cats with renal disease. Severely affected cats may be treated with intravenous potassium chloride (0.2–0.4 mEq/kg/h diluted in intravenous fluids) with constant cardiac monitoring. The prognosis can be good if the potassium levels can be regulated or supplemented.

Potassium-aggravated muscle stiffness

An intermittent activity or stress-induced muscle stiffness has recently been described in cats (Kiesewetter *et al.*, 2011). The cats were normal at rest and all clinicopathological tests performed were normal, including muscle and nerve pathology. Consumption of a potassium-enriched diet caused severe aggravation of the signs. A similar myotonic disorder has been described in humans arising from a sodium channelopathy, and it has been suggested that this is the cause of the syndrome seen in cats.

Congenital myotonia

Myotonia is defined as prolonged contraction or delayed relaxation of a muscle following a voluntary movement or after mechanical or electrical stimulation. Congenital myotonia has been described in the Chow Chow (suspected autosomal recessive; Jones *et al.*, 1977), Miniature Schnauzer (autosomal recessive; Vite *et al.*, 1999), Australian Cattle Dog (Finnigan *et al.*, 2007), Jack Russell Terrier (Lobetti, 2009) and in a series of related kittens. Single cases have been reported in a Great Dane, Staffordshire Terrier and Cocker Spaniel.

Clinical signs: Myotonia is characterized by muscle stiffness without cramping and muscle dimpling after palpation. In dogs, clinical signs of muscle stiffness

are progressive and evident at the time of first ambulation (Figure 18.23). Signs can improve with exercise. Myotonia is accompanied by difficulty in rising, splaying of the limbs, a 'bunny-hopping' gait, muscle hypertrophy, regurgitation and stridor. Dental and craniofacial abnormalities have been seen in affected Miniature Schnauzers. Palpation of hypertrophied skeletal muscles does not elicit a pain response. Similar clinical signs have been documented in cats.

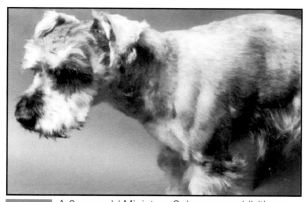

18.23 A 2-year-old Miniature Schnauzer exhibiting a stiff neck posture and marked prominence of the muscles over the proximal thoracic limb and neck. The dog was diagnosed with congenital myotonia. (Courtesy of C Vite)

Pathophysiology: Congenital myotonia is commonly due to diminished chloride conductance across the muscle membrane. As the chloride channel contributes approximately two-thirds of the resting membrane conductance, a decrease in chloride channel conductance significantly comprises the resting membrane potential. During normal muscle activation–depolarization, potassium ions accumulate in the sarcoplasmic reticulum and increase the probability of further depolarizations, which is 'buffered' in the presence of normal high chloride conductance. Loss of conductance tips the balance towards potassium-induced depolarization bursts that manifest as myotonia (Raja Rayan and Hanna, 2010). In some cases this is due to genetic defects in the skeletal muscle ion channels (Vite *et al.*, 1998; Bhalereao *et al.*, 2002). Sodium, calcium and potassium channel abnormalities have all been documented in humans with similar muscle dysfunction and likely exist in veterinary medicine (Raja Rayan and Hanna, 2010).

Diagnosis: Routine laboratory evaluations, including serum creatine kinase concentration, are usually normal. Electrophysiological findings are characterized by waxing and waning myotonic discharges (which sound like a 'revving' motorcycle). Muscle biopsy specimen evaluation may reveal muscle hypertrophy or a type I fibre predominance without inflammation. A DNA-based test on whole blood has been developed for the detection of the mutant allele in affected and carrier Miniature Schnauzers and is available at the University of Pennsylvania (Bhalerao *et al.*, 2002; see Appendix 1). A novel mutation of the *CLCN1* gene associated with hereditary myotonia has also been identified in the Australian Cattle Dog and a DNA test is now available (see **Useful websites** on DVD).

Treatment and prognosis: Treatment is directed at decreasing the repetitive activity in the muscle using antagonists to the voltage-gated sodium channels. These drugs include extended-release procainamide (40–50 mg/kg orally q8–12h), quinidine, phenytoin and mexilitine (8.3 mg/kg orally q8h). Treatment has been reported to improve but not normalize the condition; therefore, the prognosis depends on the severity of the clinical signs in the individual animal (Vite, 2002).

Inflammatory myopathies: infectious

Clinical signs
Clinical signs seen in these patients are not specific but represent diffuse muscle disease and include marked weight loss, weakness, exercise intolerance, generalized muscle atrophy, muscle pain (myalgia) and, in the late stages of disease, contractures and recumbency (Figure 18.24).

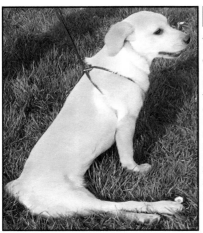

18.24 A 7-month-old Labrador Retriever exhibiting profound hyperextension of the pelvic limbs due to *Toxoplasma* infection of the muscles and nerve roots of the lumbar plexus. Such contractures are often permanent.

Pathophysiology
Inflammatory myopathies have been associated with protozoal, viral, rickettsial and, rarely, bacterial infections (Figure 18.25). Infections causing myopathies in dogs and cats are usually multisystemic. Protozoal and viral infections often become clinical in young immunocompromised animals. Older animals may have concurrent infections or neoplastic diseases affecting local immunocompetence.

Diagnosis
Diagnosis of an inflammatory myopathy necessitates muscle biopsy. Elevations in serum creatine kinase and an abnormal needle EMG can be nonspecific findings. A definitive aetiological diagnosis may be difficult as it relies upon identification of the organisms within the tissues, specifically using molecular or immunohistochemical methods. However, *Toxoplasma* and *Neospora* spp. are often seen in muscle biopsy samples. The interpretation of serological titres is particularly difficult during the acute stages of disease because a single positive result only implies exposure to the disease rather than clinical infection.

Treatment and prognosis
The prognosis for most infectious inflammatory myopathies is guarded, but partial function may remain if treatment is initiated early in the course of the disease. Clindamycin is recommended for protozoal myositis. However, it should be noted that although this has been reported to be successful, it may require months of administration (Crookshanks *et al.*, 2007). If CNS infection is suspected, additional antimicrobials (such as trimethoprim-sulpha drugs) should be considered. If treatment is not initiated until the disease has reached a state of recumbency, it is unlikely that the patient will walk again. Intense physiotherapy may be needed, in addition to specific antibiotics, especially in young patients that are continuing to grow in the face of severe muscle contractures.

Type of infection	Specific agent(s)	Clinical signs	Diagnostic tests [a]	Treatment
Bacterial	*Leptospira australis* and *L. icterohaemorrhagiae*	Fever, renal and hepatic disease in association with myopathy	Serology Urine culture	Management of renal failure Penicillin (25–40,000 IU/kg i.v. q12–24h for 14 days) Doxycycline (5–10 mg/kg orally q12h for further 14 days)
	Clostridium	Severe focal or multifocal muscle pain. Infection associated with a previous muscle injury, surgery or injection	Gram stain Tissue/blood culture	Surgical debridgement Metronidazole (dogs: 10 mg/kg orally q12h; cats: 62.5 mg orally q12h for 7 days) Clavulanated amoxicillin (22 mg/kg orally q12h for 7 days)
Rickettsial	*Ehrlichia canis*	Diffuse muscle atrophy during acute phase of systemic disease	Serology	Doxycycline (5–10 mg/kg orally q12h for 14 days)
Viral	Feline immunodeficiency virus	Can be asymptomatic but with periodic elevations of creatine kinase	Serology Western blot	Zidovudine (AZT) Protease inhibitors

18.25 Infectious causes of polymyositis. [a] Diagnostic tests required in addition to a minimum database, electrophysiology and muscle biopsy. (continues) ▶

Type of infection	Specific agent(s)	Clinical signs	Diagnostic tests [a]	Treatment
Protozoal	*Toxoplasma gondii* *Neospora caninum*	Often accompanied by diffuse nerve root disease (polyradiculoneuritis) causing severe muscle atrophy and rigid pelvic limb hyperextension	Serology	Trimethoprim/sulfadiazine (15 mg/kg orally q12h for 4 weeks) Clindamycin (10 mg/kg orally q8h for 4 weeks) Pyrimethamine (1 mg/kg orally q24h for 2 weeks in dogs)
	Leishmania infantum	Bilateral masticatory muscle pain and atrophy without loss of jaw function. Variable elevations of creatine kinase	Identification of amastigotes in Giemsa-stained lymph node or bone marrow aspirates	Antimonials Allopurinol (7–15 mg/kg orally q12h for 26 weeks)
	Hepatozoon canis and *H. americanum*	Weight loss, fever, anaemia, neutrophilic leucocytosis	Identification of tissue stages in fixed muscle	Trimethoprim/sulfadiazine (15 mg/kg orally q12h for 4 weeks) Clindamycin (10 mg/kg orally q8h for 4 weeks) Pyrimethamine (0.25 mg/kg orally q24h for 2 weeks in dogs) Decoquinate (10–20 mg/kg orally q12h indefinitely)
	Trypanosoma cruzi (Chagas' disease)	Heart disease as well as generalized myopathy	Organism isolation Cytology of blood smear Serology	Benzimidazole (5 mg/kg orally q24h for 8 weeks)

18.25 (continued) Infectious causes of polymyositis. [a] Diagnostic tests required in addition to a minimum database, electrophysiology and muscle biopsy.

Inflammatory myopathies: immune-mediated

Idiopathic polymyositis

Clinical signs: Progressive exercise intolerance with acute exacerbation of weakness can occur, but the disease may initially be episodic. Marked weight loss is often reported by the owner (Figure 18.26). A stiff, uncomfortable gait in all limbs is usually accompanied by an arched thoracolumbar spine (kyphosis) and a ventroflexed neck. Commonly, multiple skeletal muscles are affected, but it can manifest as a focal disease affecting the pharyngeal, laryngeal, oesophageal or tongue (infrequently) muscle groups, causing dysphagia, dysphonia and stridor or regurgitation. Masticatory and extraocular myositis are covered in Chapters 12 and 10, respectively. Myalgia may be present but this is not a consistent finding (Evans *et al.*, 2004). Pyrexia may be a feature of the disease or a consequence of aspiration pneumonia. Any age and breed of dog or cat can be affected. However, breed-specific variants of polymyositis affect Newfoundlands, Boxers, Pembroke Welsh Corgis and Hungarian Vizslas (Evans *et al.*, 2004; Toyoda *et al.*, 2010; Haley *et al.*, 2011). The disease affecting Vizslas is characterized by pharyngeal dysphagia, megaoesophagus and masticatory muscle atrophy, although exercise intolerance has also been described. Dysphagia and megaoesophagus are commonly seen in Newfoundlands with inflammatory myopathies. Corgis present with severe tongue atrophy, facial muscular atrophy and occasional gait abnormalities (Toyada *et al.*, 2010).

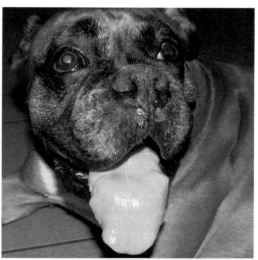
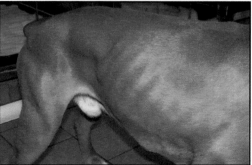

18.26 Polymyositis in a 10-year-old Boxer with marked generalized muscle atrophy. The dog initially presented with a complaint of dysphagia due to tongue dysfunction. The flaccid dysfunctional tongue was also affected by the inflammatory process.

Pathophysiology: Idiopathic polymyositis is a generalized inflammatory myopathy affecting dogs and less commonly cats, which is not associated with any other systemic connective tissue disease or infection. Tissue inflammation arises due to immune-mediated damage by CD8+ T lymphocytes (Pumarola *et al.*, 2004). Several genes involved with innate and adaptive immunity are up-regulated in this disease, as are those involved in pro-inflammatory and anti-inflammatory pathways (Shelton *et al.*, 2006).

Circulating autoantibodies against an unidentified sarcolemmal antigen supporting a humoral immune component have been reported in Newfoundlands and Boxers (Evans *et al.*, 2004; Hankel *et al.*, 2006). Autoantibodies to a 42 kDa molecule in striated muscle have been documented in the Pembroke Welsh Corgi (Toyoda *et al.*, 2010).

Diagnosis: The diagnosis is based on identification of at least three of the following (Podell, 2002):

- Appropriate clinical signs
- Elevated serum creatine kinase concentration (at least 5–10 times the upper reference range) (creatine kinase levels can be low with end-stage disease). Creatine kinase concentrations are not always elevated during active muscle disease; this seems to depend upon the distribution of cellular infiltrates and the degree of muscle damage
- Compatible electrophysiological findings (see Chapter 4)
- Negative infectious disease titres
- Muscle biopsy sample showing signs of inflammation (confirms the diagnosis), including mononuclear cell infiltration into muscle and invasion of cells into apparently non-necrotic fibres (Pumarola *et al.*, 2004).

Treatment and prognosis: Early and aggressive institution of immunosuppressive therapy is essential for a good clinical outcome (Figure 18.27). The prognosis can be good unless there is concurrent megaoesophagus or pharyngeal dysfunction, or if therapy is not initiated until after there has been severe myofibre loss or fibrosis. Robust muscle regeneration has been documented in the face of significant inflammation and fibrosis, suggesting that muscle can survive if treatment is initiated prior to the regenerative capacity of the muscle being exhausted (Salvadori *et al.*, 2005). Long-term treatment is usually required. The serum creatine kinase concentration should be monitored and immunosuppressive therapy continued until the level has returned to within the reference range and the clinical signs have resolved.

Dermatomyositis

Dermatomyositis is a familial autosomal dominant inflammatory disease of striated muscles, skin and blood vessels seen in young collies, Shetland Sheepdogs and, less commonly, collie cross-breed dogs. An autoimmune pathogenesis is suspected (Wahl *et al.*, 2008). Dogs <6 months old are most

Antibiotic therapy if aspiration pneumonia is suspected or infectious cause cannot be ruled out. Depending on the condition of the patient, this should be instituted first and for up to 3 days prior to the use of corticosteroids
Prednisolone: • **Dogs** 2 mg/kg **Cats** 3 mg/kg orally q12h for 14 days   • **Dogs** 2 mg/kg **Cats** 3 mg/kg orally q24h for 14 days   • **Dogs** 1 mg/kg **Cats** 2 mg/kg orally q24h for 14 days   • **Dogs** 1 mg/kg **Cats** 2 mg/kg orally q48h for 14 days   Taper to effect
Fentanyl patch for pain relief (25–75 µg/h) for first 3 days
If megaoesophagus, feed accordingly to avoid aspiration pneumonia
Azathioprine (if relapse or failure to respond) at a dose of 2 mg/kg orally q24h until remission, then 0.5–2 mg/kg orally q48h

18.27 Treatment regimen for idiopathic polymyositis.

commonly affected and demonstrate a range of skin lesions on the face, ears, tail and distal extremities concurrent with clinical signs similar to those seen with polymyositis. The temporalis and distal appendicular muscle groups are most commonly involved. Diagnosis requires histopathological evaluation of skin and muscle specimens. Treatment is for both the inflammatory myopathy and the skin lesion. The prognosis depends on the severity of the initial clinical signs.

Inflammatory myopathies: paraneoplastic

A paraneoplastic polymyositis, sometimes associated with myasthenia gravis, has been described in dogs and cats diagnosed with thymoma. Myositis has also been diagnosed in dogs with malignant neoplasia (e.g. myeloid leukaemia and carcinomas). Several Boxers have been reported to have developed lymphoma within 1 year of an initial diagnosis of polymyositis (Evans *et al.*, 2003). Lymphoma-associated polymyositis affecting two dogs has recently been described in detail in the literature (Neravanda *et al.*, 2009). Other neoplasms that affect muscle (e.g. haemangiosarcomas) are usually focal and are associated with a poor prognosis (Shiu *et al.*, 2011).

Necrotizing myopathies

Necrotizing myopathies are associated with myonecrosis in the absence of lymphocytic infiltrates. Inflammatory cells are limited to macrophages clearing necrotic debris (phagocytosis). Necrotizing myopathies may result from numerous causes, including inherited metabolic diseases, muscular dystrophies, myotoxins (e.g. snake venom) and idiopathic conditions (Shelton, 2007b). In humans, several drugs including statins have been documented to cause severe necrotizing myopathies. There have been sporadic reports of a severe necrotizing myopathy in dogs associated with ingestion of dog food contaminated with monensin, a coccidiostat and feed additive used for chickens and cattle (Wilson, 1980).

Rhabdomyolsis and myoglobinuria are often associated with severe myonecrosis, which can induce renal failure (Williamson *et al.*, 2011) and cardio-myopathy (Wells *et al.*, 2009). The creatine kinase level is markedly elevated in the few reported cases, and may be higher than elevations associated with dystrophic dogs. MRI has been used to evaluate a severe focal case affecting the serratus ventralis, subscapularis, supraspinatus and rhomboideus muscles (De Risio *et al.*, 2009). Depending on the underlying cause, some of these dogs recover with supportive care over a 2–3 week period.

Vacuolar myopathies

Sporadic inclusion body myositis is the most common myopathy in humans over the age of 50, but had not been reported until recently in dogs. This disease is characterized by blue-rimmed vacuoles in muscle fibres that may have a central or subsarcolemmal location. Similar vacuoles and congophilic intracellular inclusions were identified in an 11-year-old dog with a 2-year history of progressive weakness and atrophy (King *et al.*, 2009). Humans with this disease respond poorly to immunosuppressive therapies.

Miscellaneous myopathies and causes of collapse

Exercise-induced collapse in Labrador Retrievers

Clinical signs: A syndrome of exercise intolerance and collapse has been observed in young adult Labrador Retrievers (often 7 months to 2 years of age) of both sexes and all colours, especially those used in field trials. Affected dogs are normal at rest and with normal activity. They usually have well defined muscles, and are athletic and excitable. The earliest gait abnormalities seen in exercising dogs include a 'rocking' or forced gait with a wide-based limb stance (Taylor *et al.*, 2009). Dogs that can still walk after exercise exhibit a characteristic crouched pelvic limb gait with long strides and a wide-based posture when turning. Ataxia is usually noted after 5–15 minutes of strenuous activity, often followed by an episode of collapse, panting and distress (see **Exercise-induced collapse** clip on DVD). Patellar reflexes are lost during this time and this may persist beyond recovery to a normal gait. The dogs usually return to normal after 10–20 minutes of rest, especially if passive cooling actions (e.g. fans) are used.

A small percentage of dogs have died during the exercise period. Although dramatic elevations in body temperature after exercise (to >41.5°C) have been reported, normal Labrador Retrievers demonstrate similar elevations without collapse (Matwichuk *et al.*, 1999). Affected dogs are significantly tachycardic and have severe respiratory alkalosis following exercise compared with normal dogs (Taylor, 2009). Although a few dogs with exercise-induced collapse have been reported with mild elevations in serum creatine kinase levels following exercise, they are not compatible with those seen with dystrophic or myonecrotic muscle. Muscle biopsy sample characteristics and sequential lactate and pyruvate

concentrations are normal when evaluated. A similar syndrome has been seen in working Border Collies, Golden Retrievers and Australian Shepherd Dogs, although it is likely that a different genetic mutation is responsible.

Pathophysiology: After many years of investigation, the puzzle of this interesting disorder has been solved, and the causative mutation has been identified in the dynamin 1 *(DNM1)* gene (Patterson *et al.*, 2008). Dynamin 1 is expressed almost exclusively in the brain and spinal cord, where it plays a key role in synaptic vesicle endocytosis at the presynaptic terminal membrane. The mutant protein results in a temperature-dependent reversible loss of motor function. It appears that this is an autosomal recessive disease (Taylor *et al.*, 2008).

Diagnosis: Apart from severe alkalosis on arterial blood gas analysis, all clinicopathological tests, electrophysiological and histopathological tests are normal. A genetic test is now available for Labrador Retrievers, Chesapeake Bay Retrievers and Curly-Coated Retrievers to identify affected and carrier animals (see **Useful websites** on DVD).

Treatment and prognosis: The condition is not progressive and so a normal lifespan should be expected if the dogs are not heavily exercised. Exercise restriction (especially when ambient temperatures are high) is the only advice given at this time regarding treatment. Hunting dogs may be less affected in cold weather. Genetic testing can be used to guide breeding programmes.

Fibrotic myopathy

Fibrotic myopathy, an acquired, usually non-painful disorder associated with a fibrous band within a muscle, has been reported sporadically in dogs. Specific muscle groups, including the medial thigh (gracilis, semimembranosus and semitendinosus), sartorius, infraspinatus and iliopsoas muscles are often affected. This disorder is most commonly seen in male German Shepherd Dogs aged between 8 months and 9 years (Lewis *et al.*, 1997). A similar disorder has been reported in Dobermanns, Rottweilers, St Bernards, Boxers and Old English Sheepdogs. Fibrotic myopathy of the semitendinosus muscle has been reported in a cat (Lewis, 1988).

Clinical signs: Fibrotic myopathy may be a unilateral or bilateral disease and the clinical signs depend on the muscle groups involved. Whilst the onset in some dogs is acute, the gait deficit appears to be insidious in most animals and is best seen when dogs are 'trotting'.

Gracilis muscle myopathy: In dogs with gracilis and/or semimembranosus or semitendinosus muscle involvement, the hindlimb gait is characterized by a shortened stride with a rapid medial rotation of the paw, external rotation of the hock, and internal rotation of the stifle during the mid-to-late swing phase of the stride, resulting in the paw being slapped to the ground prematurely (see **Gracilis muscle myopathy** clip on DVD). The gait anomaly results from restricted abduction of the coxofemoral joint and reduced extension of the stifle and hock.

Iliopsoas muscle fibrotic myopathy: This has been associated with chronic progressive lameness, flexion contracture of the coxofemoral joints, severe pain and decreased femoral reflexes (Ragetly *et al.*, 2009).

Infraspinatus muscle myopathy: Fibrotic contracture of the infraspinatus muscle (a rare musculotendinous disorder mainly affecting hunting dogs) arises as acute onset, painful, non-weight bearing lameness. The initial pain and lameness improve over a period of 1–4 weeks, after which a characteristic circumducted gait abnormality develops in the forelimb accompanied by elbow adduction with external rotation of the distal part of both front limbs (Devor and Sorby, 2006; Franch *et al.*, 2009).

Pathophysiology: Fibrotic myopathy has been called gracilis or semitendinosus muscle myopathy, although any of the hamstring muscles can be affected, and a similar disease has been described affecting the infraspinatus, sartorius and iliopsoas muscles (Devor and Sorby, 2006; Spadari *et al.*, 2008; da Silva *et al.*, 2009; Franch *et al.*, 2009; Ragetly *et al.*, 2009; Laksito *et al.*, 2011). A fibrous band can be palpated within the affected muscle belly and can extend the length of the muscle. Active dogs seem to be susceptible to this disorder and studies suggest that the fibrotic myopathy may be related to muscle injury caused by excessive activity (including jumping and sprinting). It is proposed that muscle strain causes inflammation, oedema and localized haemorrhage, which leads to fibrosis (Steiss, 2002). Increased angulation (flexion) at the stifle in normal German Shepherd Dogs may predispose these dogs to increased hamstring stress during physical activity, explaining their over-representation.

Diagnosis: The gait is characteristic of the disease and the neurological examination is usually normal. Tight fibrous cords are palpable in affected muscles. Atrophy or swelling may be associated with this disease if it affects the infraspinatus muscles. Serum creatine kinase levels may be normal or moderately elevated in some animals. The absence of myoelectrical activity in the band on EMG evaluation is consistent with total replacement of muscle fibres with dense connective tissue. Ultrasonography, CT and MRI can all be useful for diagnosing muscle fibrosis in the specific muscles affected by this disease.

Treatment and prognosis: Prognosis is guarded to poor, since the condition in dogs tends to recur within several months following surgical resection of the fibrous band, or transection, partial excision or complete resection of the affected muscle. However, tenectomy has been described to improve gait and

provide pain relief for both iliopsoas and bilateral infraspinatus muscle contractures (Franch *et al.*, 2009). Non-surgical treatment (e.g. corticosteroids, non-steroidal anti-inflammatory drugs, acupuncture) is usually ineffective. Non-surgical rehabilitation, including therapeutic ultrasonography and cross-fibre friction massage, has resulted in a mild improvement (slight increase in range of motion of the stifle and less crossing over of the pelvic limbs) in several dogs. Gracilis and semitendinosus fibrosis does not appear to be painful but simply causes a gait deficit: dogs can live with these diseases without a problem.

Rhabdomyolysis and malignant hyperthermia
Rhabdomyolysis is a clinical syndrome comprising acute muscle necrosis with swollen painful muscles, resulting in weakness and collapse. With the exception of racing Greyhounds and sled dogs, exertional rhabdomyolysis is rare. Malignant hyperthermia is a hereditary disorder of skeletal muscle, with collapse episodes triggered by exposure to halothane, depolarizing muscle relaxants and, occasionally, stress or exercise (Brunson and Hogan, 2004). Malignant hyperthermia has been reported in various breeds, including St Bernards, Border Collies, Labrador Retrievers, pointers, spaniels, Greyhounds and Dobermann cross-breeds (Vite, 2003). Immature and adult dogs can be affected.

Clinical signs: Clinical signs of exertional rhabdomyolysis may occur during or within 24–48 hours following a race or trial and are characterized by extreme distress, hyperpnoea and generalized muscle pain, especially over the back and hindquarters, which may appear swollen and firm (Piercy *et al.*, 2001). Limbs may be rigidly tonic and affected dogs may have a 'hunchback' appearance and refuse to walk. Myoglobinuria and death within 48 hours are common in severe, acute cases (Shelton, 2004). Typical manifestations of collapse associated with malignant hyperthermia include a rapidly progressive elevation in body temperature, tachycardia, hypercarbia and rhabdomyolysis.

Pathophysiology: In racing Greyhounds exhibiting exertional rhabdomyolysis, severe lactic acidosis leading to muscle cell swelling, local ischaemia, muscle cell necrosis and myoglobinuria with nephropathy has been proposed as a likely sequence of events (Bjotvedt *et al.*, 1983). The final step in the process, as a result of direct injury to the sarcolemma or failure of energy supply to the muscle, is an uncontrolled rise in the free intracellular calcium concentration and activation of the calcium-dependent proteases (Shelton, 2004). These abnormalities result in the destruction of the myofibres and lysosomal digestion of the muscle fibre contents (myonecrosis). With malignant hyperthermia, the underlying defect in calcium homeostasis occurs at the level of the skeletal muscle sarcoplasmic reticulum, where there is hypersensitive and heightened ligand-gating of the calcium release channel. Most variants of malignant hyperthermia are known to be

Systemic complication	Pathogenesis	Treatment
Acute tubular necrosis	Myoglobin toxicity; hypotension	Intravenous volume expansion
Hyperkalaemia	Muscle breakdown; renal failure	Diuresis; calcium gluconate if severe
Hypocalcaemia	Hyperphosphataemia; decreased renal 1,25-dihydroxycholecalciferol formation	Replacement therapy
Hypercalcaemia	Release of calcium from muscle binding sites; renal insufficiency	Diuresis
Hyperphosphataemia	Release of organic and inorganic phosphates	Diuresis
Hypovolaemia and hypoalbuminaemia	Massive intramuscular capillary destruction with leakage of intravascular contents	Intravenous volume expansion
Disseminated intravascular coagulation	Release of tissue thromboplastins	Transfusion of whole blood or plasma products

18.28 Systemic complications of rhabdomyolysis. (Modified from Shelton, 2004)

caused by a mutation in the gene on chromosome 1 encoding the skeletal muscle calcium release channel (ryanodine receptor 1, *RYR1*) (Roberts *et al.*, 2001). Rhabdomyolysis may also occur sporadically in dogs as a complication of prolonged convulsive seizures (and extreme muscle exertion), infections (e.g. babesiosis and neosporosis), heat stroke and malignant hyperthermia. Rhabdomyolysis has also been reported following various intoxications and envenomations, and as an idiopathic disorder in dogs (Wells *et al.*, 2009).

Diagnosis: Clinical signs associated with an acute episode of exertion should prompt suspicion. Serum creatine kinase levels may be markedly elevated. Urinalysis should be performed to rule out subsequent myoglobinuria. Electromyography findings are normal with acute muscle disease. Muscle biopsy confirms rhabdomyolysis but, as time is of the essence for the treatment of this disease, it is rarely advised.

Treatment and prognosis: Treatment for rhabdomyolysis is mainly supportive with intensive fluid therapy being necessary to maintain normal renal function. The systemic complications of rhabdomyolysis should be identified and individually addressed (Figure 18.28). Multimodal drug therapy, including dantrolene, analgesics, antibiotics and mannitol, has been described with beneficial effects (Wells *et al.*, 2009). Frequent blood gas analysis, biochemistry and urinalysis are advised to monitor systemic acid–base status as well as kidney function. The prognosis is guarded.

It is essential to remove triggering agents in the treatment of malignant hyperthermia; this should be combined with symptomatic treatment. Stomach lavage with iced water, body surface cooling and the intravenous administration of a cold isotonic saline solution may be beneficial. Dantrolene can prevent a malignant hyperthermia crisis or reverse anaesthetic-induced malignant hyperthermia if administered early enough (3–5 mg/kg i.v.). As for rhabdomyolysis, the prognosis is guarded.

References and further reading

Available on accompanying DVD

DVD extras

- **Exercise-induced collapse**
- **Exercise intolerance**
- **Gracilis muscle myopathy**
- **Inherited myopathy**
- **Muscular dystrophy**
- **Myasthenia gravis**
- **Neuromuscular disease**
- **Steroid myopathy**

19

Tail, anal and bladder dysfunction

Joan R. Coates

Lesions that cause tail, anal and bladder dysfunction can involve the S1 to caudal (also known as coccygeal) spinal cord segments and nerve roots; together with the L7 nerve roots these structures form the cauda equina. The sacral spinal cord segments (S1–S3) innervate the detrusor muscle of the bladder (pelvic nerves) and the external anal and urethral sphincters (pudendal nerve). Neurons from the S1 spinal cord segment also contribute to the sciatic nerve. The caudal spinal cord segments provide motor and sensory innervation of the tail (via the caudal or coccygeal nerves). Due to the potential for causing incontinence, diseases affecting these structures can have extremely serious ramifications for both the patient and the owner.

Clinical signs

Clinical signs of sacrocaudal spinal cord dysfunction, also referred to as cauda equina syndrome, reflect sensory, motor and autonomic disturbances.

- Gait is affected if the sciatic nerve is involved; lameness, ataxia (loss of proprioception) and paresis (weakness) can occur. The femoral nerve is unaffected by lesions in this location; therefore, pelvic limb paralysis (or paraplegia) should not ensue.
- The pelvic limbs may show decreased withdrawal reflexes and muscle tone (Figure 19.1).
- Radicular pain or nerve root signature characterized by flexion and limited weight-bearing of the affected pelvic limb can occur.
- Signs of tail dysfunction include low carriage, loss of 'wag', reduced tone and reduced to absent sensation (Figure 19.2).
- With sacral nerve dysfunction, the perineal reflex is reduced or absent and anal sphincter tone is reduced on digital rectal palpation. This can result in faecal incontinence. Sensory disturbances are characterized by reduced or absent perineal sensation.
- Paraspinal hyperaesthesia may be elicited upon palpation of the lumbosacral region or upon tail manipulation (Figure 19.3).
- The bladder is usually easily expressed if the urethral tone is reduced. The detrusor reflex may be lost, and urine dribbling results from overflow of a full bladder. (Normal and abnormal micturition is addressed below.)

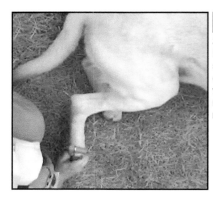

19.1 Pelvic limb of a 3-year-old Labrador Retriever showing decreased withdrawal reflexes and muscle tone.

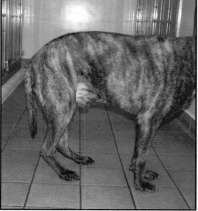

19.2 A dog showing signs of tail dysfunction and loss of 'wag'.

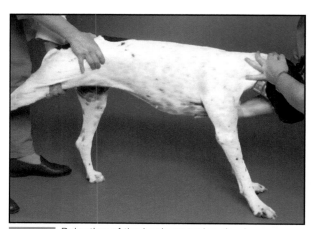

19.3 Palpation of the lumbosacral region in a 10-year-old neutered German Shorthaired Pointer bitch to elicit paraspinal hyperaesthesia.

Lesion localization

The first to third sacral, and the caudal spinal cord segments are responsible for innervation of the tail, anus and bladder. The sacral segments are invariably located over the body of the fifth lumbar vertebra and the five caudal segments are located over the sixth lumbar vertebra in dogs (Figure 19.4). In cats they are situated further caudally. The sacral nerves arising from these spinal segments pass over the seventh lumbar vertebra and the lumbosacral junction (as the cauda equina) before exiting through foramina in the sacrum and between the caudal vertebrae.

It is important to be aware that lesions between L7 and S1 of the vertebral canal can affect all or part of the sacral and caudal nerves, in addition to the seventh lumbar spinal nerve, which exits through the L7–S1 intervertebral foramen. Lesion localization for bladder dysfunction is addressed in the section on Normal and abnormal micturition.

Pathophysiology

As for spinal cord diseases, lesions of the sacrocaudal region can be anomalous, compressive, concussive, inflammatory or vascular. However, this region is distinct from other areas of the vertebral column because it contains the peripheral nerve roots of the cauda equina, rather than the spinal cord. Peripheral nerves are more resistant to injury than neurons in the central nervous system (CNS) and have a robust regenerative response (see Chapter 17).

Although the nerve roots found in the canal are more sensitive than the nerves themselves, they can be manipulated carefully during surgery without detrimental effect, and traumatic luxations of the lumbosacral junction can occur without permanent nerve damage.

An additional consideration is that the lumbosacral area is prone to disease because the lumbosacral junction is a mobile part of the spine

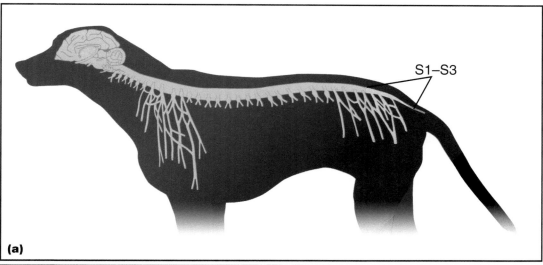

(a)

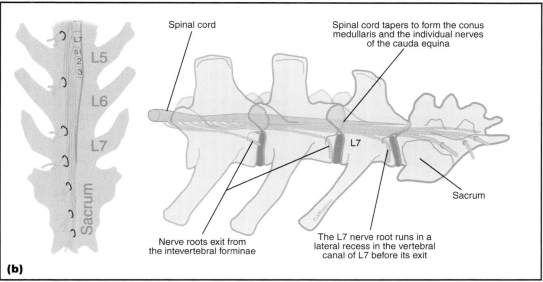

(b)

19.4 **(a)** Lesion localization for disorders of the tail, anus and bladder; the sacral spinal cord segments and associated nerves (S1–S3) are highlighted. **(b)** Dorsal (left) and lateral (right) overviews of the caudal lumbar and lumbosacral vertebrae and associated nerve tissue.

responsible for transmitting the propulsive force of the pelvic limbs to the rest of the spine, and also because of its developmental complexity.

Neurodiagnostic investigation

History and signalment are important when determining the differential diagnoses associated with tail, anal and bladder dysfunction. Urinary and faecal incontinence are established and characterized by determining the frequency and animal's awareness of voiding, along with an accurate description of urination and defecation. For example: does the animal strain to defecate and does the process appear painful to the animal? A history of trauma is important as tail, anal and bladder disorders are also associated with traumatic events such as animal bites and road traffic injuries.

A recommended diagnostic approach to sacro-caudal spinal cord diseases includes:

- Complete blood count (CBC), serum biochemistry profile and urinalysis to detect other systemic illnesses
- Cerebrospinal fluid (CSF) collection, preferably from the caudal lumbar region, to identify localized inflammatory diseases
- Electrodiagnostics (e.g. electromyography to detect muscle abnormalities secondary to denervation and nerve conduction velocity studies to evaluate specific nerves; see Chapter 4)
- Thoracic radiography in animals >5 years of age and following trauma
- Abdominal radiography and ultrasonography to detect sublumbar masses and abnormalities of the caudal abdomen
- Survey spinal radiography of the lumbosacral spine to identify vertebral lesions such as discospondylitis, fractures, vertebral anomalies and vertebral neoplasia
- Epidurography to outline the cauda equina, but images can be difficult to interpret (see Chapter 5)
- Myelography is less useful to diagnose compressive spinal cord disease in the lumbosacral region because the subarachnoid space (and therefore the contrast medium) may not descend far enough caudally to outline the cauda equina, particularly in large dogs
- Computed tomography (CT) and magnetic resonance imaging (MRI) are the most useful imaging modalities to delineate bone and soft tissue structures associated with the cauda equina.

Additional diagnostic procedures include urine culture, culture of disc aspirates, CSF protein electrophoresis, serology and exploratory surgery.

Disorders of the tail, anus and bladder

The causes of tail, anal and bladder dysfunction are summarized in Figure 19.5.

Mechanism of disease	Specific diseases
Degenerative	Degenerative lumbosacral stenosis [19] Intervertebral disc disease (Hansen types I and II) [15, 16, 19] Spondylosis deformans [16]
Anomalous	Vertebral and spinal cord anomalies [5, 14, 16, 19] Vertebral: sacrocaudal dysgenesis [19] Primary vertebral anomaly with associated cord abnormalities: spina bifida [16, 19]
Neoplastic	Extradural: chordomas [19], metastasis, vertebral tumours (sarcomas, plasma cell tumours), lymphomas [16] Intradural–extramedullary: meningiomas [16], nerve sheath tumours [17], lipomas [19] Intramedullary: ependymomas, gliomas, metastasis, round cell tumours [16]
Inflammatory	Discospondylitis/osteomyelitis/physitis [14, 16] Tail abscessation [19] Granulomatous meningoencephalomyelitis [11] Infectious meningoencephalomyelitis [11, 14] Steroid-responsive meningitis–arteritis [14]
Idiopathic	Diffuse idiopathic skeletal hyperostosis [16] Dysautonomia [19]
Traumatic	Lumbosacral fracture/luxation [19] Sacrocaudal luxation [19] Sacral fractures [19]
Vascular	Fibrocartilaginous embolism [15, 16, 19] Limber tail [19]

19.5 Causes of tail, anal and bladder dysfunction. Note the numbers in square brackets indicate the chapter in which the disease is discussed in detail.

Degenerative diseases

Degenerative lumbosacral stenosis

Clinical signs: Neuroanatomical localization to the lumbosacral region is determined by the neurological examination based on signs related to sensory, motor and autonomic dysfunction. Non-specific observations include reluctance to rise and pelvic limb lameness. Neurological signs commonly include pain and motor dysfunction as a result of lower motor neuron (LMN) weakness (sciatic, pudendal, caudal nerves) (see **Degenerative lumbosacral stenosis** clip on DVD.)

Pain is the most consistent clinical sign and reflective of compressive or inflammatory processes affecting pain-sensitive structures (nerve root, meninges, periosteum and joints) (see Chapter 14). It is the opinion of the author that the pain primarily originates from nerve root (radicular pain) compression (particularly L7; Figure 19.6). The affected patient often stands with the pelvic limbs tucked under the caudal abdomen to flex the spine and lessen the nerve root compression (Figure 19.7).

Pain is manifest by hyperaesthesia and/or paraesthesia.

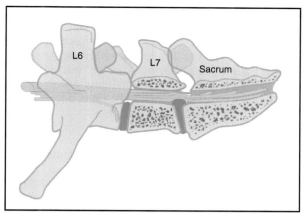

19.6 Sagittal section of the L7 vertebra, the intervertebral disc space and the sacrum demonstrating disc protrusion and nerve root compression.

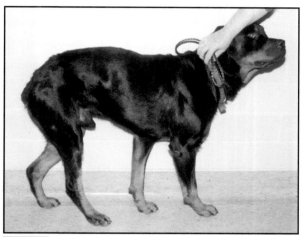

19.7 A 6-year-old Rottweiler with degenerative lumbosacral stenosis. Note that the pelvic limbs are tucked under the caudal abdomen in order to flex the spine and lessen the nerve root compression.

- Hyperaesthesia is elicited upon palpation of the lumbosacral joint or by hyperextension of the pelvic limbs and tail, causing lordosis of the lumbar spine. This accentuates canal stenosis and nerve root compression, causing pain.
- Paraesthesia is caused by irritation of the nerve roots without an external stimulus. Clinical signs include biting at the tail, rump and feet. Pain of lumbosacral origin is also exacerbated by exercise and presents as asymmetrical lameness, which is termed neurogenic intermittent claudication.

Motor dysfunction varies in severity. The patient may have mild to severe gait and postural reaction deficits. The gait is frequently short-strided or shuffled. Postural reaction deficits are often asymmetrical, depending upon the degree of cauda equina involvement.

Reflex dysfunction of the limbs commonly involves those muscles innervated by the sciatic nerve (L6–S1 nerve roots but L7 and S1 provide the major contribution), particularly the flexor and extensor muscles of the hock. The patellar reflex may appear hyperreflexic due to loss of antagonism from the flexor muscles (pseudo-hyperreflexia). The cranial tibial and gastrocnemius reflexes may be hyporeflexic. The withdrawal reflexes are reduced in the stifle and hock joints. Less commonly, the pudendal and caudal nerves may be involved. The pudendal nerve (S1, S2 and S3) innervates the perineal region, including the external anal and urethral sphincters. The caudal nerves innervate the tail. Decreased tail tone is assessed upon palpation and inability to wag.

Other less common clinical signs include faecal and urinary incontinence. If micturition dysfunction is suspected it is important to evaluate closely sensation of the perineal region and the anal reflex. A digital rectal examination assesses rectal tone, the urethra and the prostate gland.

Pathogenesis: Lumbosacral stenosis (cauda equina syndrome, lumbosacral malarticulation and malformation, lumbosacral instability, lumbosacral spondylopathy) is common in middle- to old-aged, large-breed dogs and represents a plethora of orthopaedic abnormalities associated with the lumbosacral anatomy (De Risio *et al.*, 2000; Meij and Bergknut, 2010). Degenerative lumbosacral stenosis is also being recognized with increasing frequency in the cat (Newitt *et al.*, 2009). Neurological abnormalities occur coincident with tissue (joint capsule, interarcuate ligament, disc, bone, fibrous adhesions) impingement on the cauda equina, the nerve roots at the level of the foramina, or the vascular supply. The pathological process begins with Hansen type II intervertebral disc degeneration followed by osteophyte formation of the L7–S1 endplates and articular processes (Chambers, 1989). The syndrome is characterized by stenosis of the spinal canal from vertebral subluxation and/or stenotic intervertebral foramina. Concurrent with compressive disease, underlying instability may further accentuate the clinical signs, especially in active dogs.

Diagnosis: A diagnosis of lumbosacral syndrome is suspected from the neurological examination. Definitive diagnosis of degenerative lumbosacral stenosis is difficult because no one test has 100% specificity and sensitivity, leading to false-positive and false-negative results. Dynamic imaging is important to investigate the mobility of the joint and concurrent changes in neural tissue compression. Diagnostic procedures to test for degenerative lumbosacral stenosis include electrophysiology, survey and contrast radiography, CT and MRI.

Electrophysiology: Electromyography is used to evaluate spontaneous activity (fibrillation and positive sharp waves) in the following muscle groups: limbs; lumbosacral and caudal paraspinal; external anal sphincter; and pelvic diaphragm muscles (Oliver *et al.*, 1978; Sisson *et al.*, 1989). Abnormal findings support pathology but negative findings do not rule out lumbosacral lesions. Sciatic nerve conduction velocity studies and sensory evoked potentials may also be abnormal (Meij *et al.*, 2006).

Survey radiography: This is useful to rule out other causes of cauda equina syndrome. Abnormal findings associated with degenerative lumbosacral stenosis (Figure 19.8) include:

- Osteochondrosis of the sacral endplate (Lang *et al.*, 1992; Hanna, 2001)
- Transitional vertebrae (Morgan *et al.*, 1993)
- Spondylosis (Wright, 1980)
- Subluxation
- Sclerosis of the endplates
- Bony proliferation of the articular processes (Steffen *et al.*, 2007).

Transitional vertebrae have been identified as a predisposing cause of cauda equina syndrome in German Shepherd Dogs (Morgan *et al.*, 1993) and other breeds (Damur-Djuric *et al.*, 2006; Flückiger *et al.*, 2006). Stress radiography (extension and flexion views) has been used to identify underlying 'instability' of the lumbosacral junction; however, it should be noted that normal dogs may also have evidence of such 'instability'. MRI is superior to radiography for demonstrating dynamic compression of the neural tissues (Gradner *et al.*, 2007).

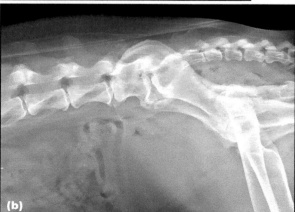

19.8 **(a)** Neutral and **(b)** extended lateral radiographs of a 7-year-old German Shepherd Dog with degenerative lumbosacral stenosis. Note the ventral spondylosis, proliferation of the articular processes and tunnelling of the dorsal lamina, which is accentuated on extension of the pelvis.

Myelography: This contrast procedure is mainly used to rule out other causes of compressive myelopathies cranial to L4. Although myelography may be used to assess the lumbosacral region (Lang, 1988), due to early termination of the dural sac, the contrast medium column may not cross the lumbosacral junction in large-breed dogs. Myelography is not now recommended.

Epidurography: This is a contrast procedure used to evaluate dynamic and compressive lumbosacral lesions (Selcer *et al.*, 1988). The contrast medium should be injected between S3 and Cd1, or more caudally. Radiographic exposure should occur during the contrast medium injection; lateral (neutral, flexion and extension) and ventrodorsal views should be obtained. A normal epidurogram occurs when contrast medium fills the epidural space and the ventral column is visible on the vertebral canal. Abnormal findings include narrowing, elevation, deviation or obstruction of the contrast medium column involving >50% of the vertebral canal diameter (Figure 19.9). Involvement of <50% of the canal diameter makes the diagnosis less certain. Diagnostic sensitivities vary between 75 and 80%.

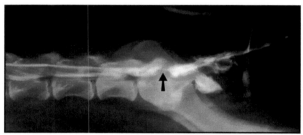

19.9 Abnormal epidurogram showing >50% compression of the epidural space.

Discography: This is a contrast procedure used to evaluate for evidence of disc protrusion at the lumbosacral space (Sisson *et al.*, 1992; Barthez *et al.*, 1994). The technique consists of injecting contrast medium into the nucleus pulposus of the disc.

Computed tomography: CT has the advantage of better soft tissue and bone resolution (Jones *et al.*, 1995). Cross-sectional, dorsal and sagittal images allow determination of lesion extent (Figure 19.10). The articular processes, intervertebral discs and foramina can be evaluated (Jones *et al.*, 2008). CT imaging studies should be performed prior to injecting contrast medium into the vertebral canal or subarachnoid space. Abnormalities detected by CT include loss of epidural fat, increased soft tissue opacity in the intervertebral foramen, bulging of the intervertebral disc, thecal sac displacement, spondylosis, narrowed vertebral canal, thickened articular processes and osteophyte formation of the articular processes in the intervertebral foramen (Jones *et al.*, 1996, 1999). CT has a higher sensitivity for the diagnosis of degenerative lumbosacral stenosis than does either epidurography or discography.

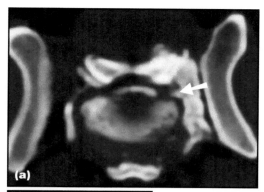

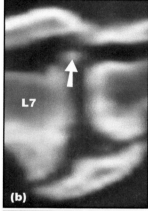

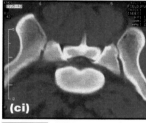
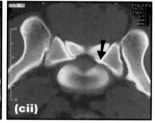

19.10 CT images of degenerative lumbosacral stenosis. **(a)** Transverse view of proliferative bony changes (arrowed). **(b)** Sagittal view showing dramatic disc protrusion (arrowed). **(c)** Serial transverse views demonstrating canal and foraminal stenosis (arrowed).

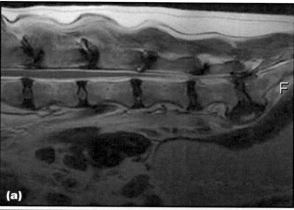

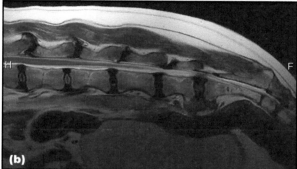

19.11 Sagittal T2-weighted **(a)** neutral and **(b)** flexed MR images of a 7-year-old German Shepherd Dog with lumbosacral pain and dysuria. There is marked ventral compression of the nerve roots due to disc protrusion at L6–L7 and L7–S1 with loss of epidural fat and attenuation of the thecal sac. In addition, there is dorsal compression due to ligamentous hypertrophy at L6–L7 and L7–S1. On the flexion view, note the improvement in impingement by the ligamentous structures. This provides evidence of dynamic compression at the lumbosacral joint. The dog underwent surgery for dorsal decompression of L6–L7 and L7–S1 as well as stabilization of the lumbosacral joint.

Magnetic resonance imaging: MRI is superior to CT with regard to soft tissue definition (de Haan *et al.*, 1993). The spinal cord, CSF, intervertebral discs, ligaments and nerve roots can be directly visualized (Figure 19.11). MRI may allow early recognition of intervertebral disc degeneration and a more accurate assessment of epidural fat displacement, although this is open to over-interpretation. Parasagittal and transverse views can provide evidence of stenosis within the L7–S1 intervertebral foramina (Suwankong *et al.*, 2006; Godde and Steffen, 2007). As with radiography, extension and flexion views of the lumbosacral spine can provide evidence of dynamic disease. Importantly, CT and MRI findings may not correlate with the severity of the clinical signs, and thus should not be used to predict surgical outcomes or determine the prognosis (Jones *et al.*, 2000).

Treatment and prognosis: Degenerative lumbosacral stenosis can be managed medically or surgically.

Medical management: Indications for medical management include the first episode of clinical signs or intermittent pain. Management consists of strict confinement for 8–14 weeks, anti-inflammatory medication using low-dose prednisolone or non-steroidal anti-inflammatory drugs (NSAIDs) and weight loss. The recovery rate for medical management is between 24 and 50% (De Risio *et al.*, 2001). A recent report described the use of methylprednisolone sodium acetate (40 mg/ml) injections into the lumbosacral epidural space at a dose of 1 mg/kg (Janssens *et al.*, 2009). The treatment resulted in clinical improvement in 79% and complete resolution of clinical signs in 53% of dogs mildly affected by degenerative lumbosacral stenosis. The protocol included injections at 0, 2 and 6 weeks, with additional injections as needed.

Surgical management: Indications for surgical management include failure of medical management, severe pain and moderate to severe neurological deficits (in particular incontinence). Surgical techniques include decompression and excision of the proliferative tissue, and fixation and fusion of the lumbosacral junction. Surgical decompression is the most common treatment, although distraction–fusion techniques may also be used if indicated (Chambers *et al.*, 1988).

Dorsal laminectomy allows decompression and visualization of the cauda equina. The nerve roots can be retracted laterally for visualization of the disc for annular fenestration. A foraminotomy, using a dorsal or lateral approach, can be performed using a bone curette or pneumatic drill (Godde and Steffan, 2007; Carozzo *et al.*, 2008). It is important to preserve the articular processes because sacrifice of these structures may destabilize the lumbosacral joint (Smith *et al.*, 2003). Short-term success with decompressive laminectomy ranges from 73 to 93% (Chambers *et al.*, 1988; Danielsson and Sjostrom, 1999; De Risio *et al.*, 2001; Linn *et al.*, 2003).

Stabilization procedures include distraction–fusion, fusion, lag screw of facets, Kirschner techniques and pedicle screw–rod fixation (Slocum and Devine, 1986, 1989; Auger *et al.*, 2000; Meij *et al.*, 2007; Hankin *et al.*, 2012; Molders *et al.*, 2012). The purpose of the distraction–fusion technique is to enlarge the collapsed disc space and foramina. The lag screw technique has the potential to further weaken and fracture the articular processes. If there is potential for instability, the author prefers placement of cancellous bone screws in the articular processes of L7–S1 along with autogenic or allogenic bone grafts (Figure 19.12). Long-term outcomes remain to be determined with the various procedures.

The most crucial aspect of postoperative care is strict cage confinement for 8–12 weeks and a gradual return to fitness. It is important to use controlled exercise as part of the physical rehabilitation programme. In addition, bladder management involves proper monitoring of bladder emptying to avoid urinary tract infections (UTIs).

Prognosis: If the clinical signs resolve with surgery, then the prognosis is fair to good. Dogs with severe neurological deficits and urinary and faecal incontinence for more than a few weeks prior to surgery have a guarded to poor prognosis (De Risio *et al.*, 2000; Linn *et al.*, 2003; Suwankong *et al.*, 2008). Rates of postoperative improvement range from 41 to 95% (Danielsson and Sjostrom, 1999; Janssens *et al.*, 2009; Jones *et al.*, 2000; De Risio *et al.*, 2001; Godde and Steffen, 2007; Linn *et al.*, 2003). A large retrospective study of 156 dogs reported postoperative improvement in 79% of dogs (Suwankong *et al.*, 2008).

Expectations of outcome differ between the owners of pet and active/working dogs. In working dogs, postoperative improvement rates range from 66 to 79% and recurrence rates vary between 3 and 18% following decompression surgery alone (Danielsson and Sjostrom, 1999; Jones *et al.*, 2000; De Risio *et al.*, 2001; Linn *et al.*, 2003). It is possible that a subset of the dogs for which treatment is unsuccessful may also have lumbosacral instability or dynamic disease. Currently,

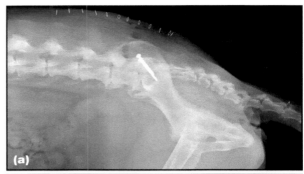
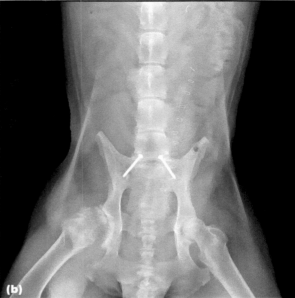

19.12 Postoperative **(a)** lateral and **(b)** ventrodorsal radiographs of a 7-year-old German Shepherd Dog with degenerative lumbosacral stenosis following dorsal decompression and articular process stabilization and fusion using an autogenous bone graft.

recommendations for management of degenerative lumbosacral stenosis are based on experience and opinion, which are considered of low evidentiary value (Cook and Cook, 2010). Standardized and validated outcome measures are needed to compare cohorts of dogs using tailored treatment approaches (Suwankong *et al.*, 2007; Meij and Bergknut, 2010).

Intervertebral disc disease

Hansen type II intervertebral disc herniation is an important component of degenerative lumbosacral stenosis (see above). Hansen type I herniation of mineralized disc material is much more unusual at this site but can occur (see Chapters 15 and 16 for further information).

Anomalous diseases

Transitional vertebrae

Transitional vertebrae are relatively common at the lumbosacral junction and have been shown to predispose to degenerative lumbosacral stenosis in German Shepherd Dogs (Figure 19.13).

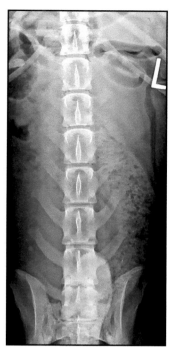

19.13 Ventrodorsal radiograph of a 5-year-old German Shepherd Dog with lumbosacral pain and evidence of sacralization of L7. Note the absence of the left transverse process of L7.

Spina bifida

Clinical signs: Spina bifida occurs most commonly in the caudal lumbar region, but can occur in the thoracic region (Westworth and Sturges, 2010) (Figure 19.14). Physical examination at the site of the lesion may reveal abnormal directions of hair growth, a skin dimple or an open tract draining CSF. More severe lesions have protruding cysts or open regions of the spinal canal (Fingeroth *et al.*, 1989). Clinical signs are reflective of a myelopathy from the L4 to S3 spinal cord region. The severity of the clinical signs varies with the degree of meningeal and spinal cord involvement. Tethered cord syndrome can contribute to the progression of the condition as the animal matures. Spinal cord tethering is defined as caudal displacement of the spinal cord associated with one or more abnormality (e.g. meningocele). Affected animals may have ambulatory difficulties

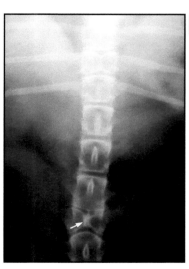

19.14 A young male Bulldog with spina bifida affecting the 12th thoracic vertebra. Note the butterfly vertebra at L4 (arrowed).

and faecal or urinary incontinence. Animals with spina bifida occulta usually have no neurological deficits related to the malformation.

Pathogenesis: Spina bifida, a form of spinal dysraphism, is characterized by failure of the vertebral arches to fuse, with or without protrusion of the spinal cord and meninges (Bailey and Morgan, 1992; Kroll and Constantinescu, 1994; Westworth and Sturges, 2010). Spina bifida occulta or closed spinal dysraphism is characterized by an absence of the vertebral arches, with a normal spinal cord and meninges. More severe forms or open spinal dysraphism include protrusion of the meninges (meningocele) and/or spinal cord (meningomyelocele) through the defect (see also Chapter 16).

Spina bifida occurs in both dogs and cats and there is a high incidence in the Bulldog and Manx cats (see below), which may suggest a heritable cause (Kitchen *et al.*, 1972; Wilson, 1982). Teratogenic compounds, nutritional deficiencies and environmental factors may be associated with spina bifida (Khera, 1973; Scott *et al.*, 1975). A combination of genetic predisposition and environmental factors may also be responsible.

Diagnosis: Survey spinal radiography can detect failure of the dorsal spinous processes to fuse, especially on the ventrodorsal view (Figure 19.15). Spina bifida is usually an incidental finding. Cross-sectional imaging and myelography can detect a meningocele. MRI may further delineate other spinal cord abnormalities.

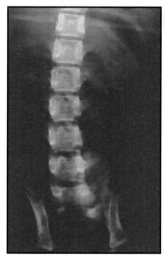

19.15 Ventrodorsal radiograph of a 12-week-old Pug with paraparesis, flaccid anus with anaesthesia of the perineal region, and urinary and faecal incontinence. The dorsal spinous process of L7 is missing and the sacrum is hypoplastic.

Treatment and prognosis: Treatment of spina bifida occulta is rarely needed. Meningoceles may be amenable to surgery, but associated spinal cord abnormalities need to be taken into account. The filum terminale is severed to promote subsequent release of the tether (Fingeroth *et al.*, 1989; Plummer *et al.*, 1993). The prognosis is considered good if there are minimal clinical signs and spina bifida is the only abnormality. If the animal has faecal or urinary incontinence and an absence of perineal sensation, the prognosis is poor.

Sacrocaudal dysgenesis in Manx cats

Clinical signs: Affected Manx cats have a 'bunny-hopping' gait but can manifest more severe signs of paresis and urinary and faecal incontinence. Sensory abnormalities include hypoaesthesia or analgesia of the perineal region. Malformations of the sacral or caudal vertebrae may be palpable. A dimple in the skin may indicate a meningocele. Innervation of the anus and bladder is often absent, resulting in urinary and faecal incontinence. The urinary bladder may be easily expressed. Postural reactions and spinal reflexes are decreased in the pelvic limbs. A fistulous meningocele can cause hypochloraemia and hyponatraemia subsequent to CSF drainage (Hall *et al.*, 1988).

Pathogenesis: The autosomal dominant trait in Manx cats lends itself to the absence of a tail but also to numerous sacral related anomalies (Kitchen *et al.*, 1972; Yeatts, 1998). The Manx gene is considered semi-lethal with homozygotes not surviving. Manx tail types are classified into four phenotypic groups (Davidson, 1986):

- Rumpy (no caudal vertebrae)
- Rumpy-riser (several caudal vertebrae fused)
- Stumpy (several mobile caudal vertebrae)
- Longie ('normal' tail).

Neurological deficits are often found in animals with the rumpy phenotype. The 'rumpies' can exhibit an absence of sacral and even lumbar vertebrae with increased associated spinal cord dysgenesis. Deficits sometimes develop over weeks to months as the cat matures. These deficits are due to the failure of cranial migration or 'tethering' of the spinal cord as the caudal end of the spinal cord and dural sac fail to stretch normally (Dorn and Joiner, 1976; Plummer *et al.*, 1993). Spina bifida is usually present. Other concurrent spinal abnormalities include meningocele, myelomeningocele, syringomyelia, diastematomyelia and spinal dysraphism (see Chapter 16).

Diagnosis: Survey radiography of the lumbosacral spine demonstrates bony defects. The spinal defects can be detected with CT, myelography or MRI. Intraspinal changes such as syringomyelia are only evident on MRI. Electrophysiology can be used to confirm the extent of denervation.

Treatment and prognosis: Early surgical intervention is recommended if signs of spinal cord tethering are suspected. The filum terminale is transected or freed from the abnormal meningeal attachments. Any fistulous tract that exists between the skin and subarachnoid space should be dissected free and completely resected to prevent infection and loss of CSF (Dorn and Joiner, 1976; Plummer *et al.*, 1993) (Figure 19.16). The bladder needs to be frequently expressed. Bladder infections are treated with appropriate antibiotics. When the clinical signs are due to an absent or severely affected nerve supply,

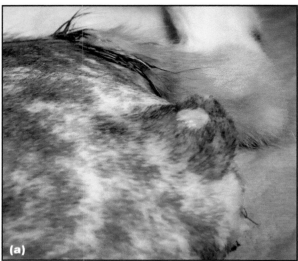

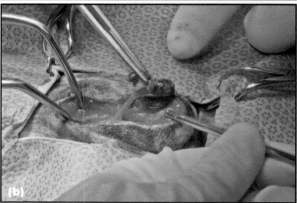

19.16 **(a)** A 12-week-old Manx kitten with a meningocele on the tail. The meningocele was covered with a thin layer of epithelium and intermittently leaked CSF. The cat was normal on neurological examination. **(b)** Intraoperative photograph showing the fistulous tract that extended into the thecal sac. The sacral and coccygeal nerves were unaffected.

the prognosis for functional improvement is grave. If the clinical signs are secondary to spinal cord tethering, the prognosis can be good with early surgical intervention.

Neoplastic diseases

See Chapter 16 for a description of all neoplastic diseases that affect the spinal cord and Chapter 17 for a description of peripheral nerve sheath tumours. Tumours specific to the cauda equina are addressed here.

Chordomas

Chordomas have been recognized in humans, dogs and cats. Most chordomas develop in the sacrocaudal region, but can occur in other parts of the CNS (Williams *et al.*, 1993; Pease *et al.*, 2002). Chordomas most likely originate from notochordal remnants. The notochord normally remains as the nucleus pulposus within the intervertebral disc. Residual notochord outside the intervertebral discs lies close to the base of the skull and sacrum.

Chordomas may occur at the site of a previous tail docking (Munday *et al.*, 2003). Tail amputation may displace the notochord cells, which subsequently undergo neoplastic transformation. Chordomas are slow growing with low metastatic potential. Routine histology of an excisional biopsy sample allows for a presumptive diagnosis based on the characteristic histological and immunohistochemical appearance. Prognosis is good with complete surgical excision.

Lipomas

Intradural lipomas are recognized in humans with tethered spinal cord syndrome. There are reports of intradural lipomas in a young Manx-type cat associated with a meningocele (Plummer *et al.*, 1993) and in a dog (Morgan *et al.*, 2007).

Inflammatory diseases

The sacrocaudal nerves can be involved in multifocal or diffuse inflammatory diseases (see Chapters 9 and 11). The involvement of these nerves may imply a poor prognosis for the patient due to the possibility of permanent incontinence. Specific inflammatory diseases of the tail, anus and bladder are discussed here.

Tail abscessation

Clinical signs: Abscessation of the tail causes severe pain, paresis or paralysis of the tail and, depending on the extent of the lesion, can spread to involve the sacral and sciatic nerves causing incontinence and paraparesis. A wound is usually visible on the tail.

Pathogenesis: Trauma, bite wounds or surgery to the rump may disrupt innervation to the tail, anus and bladder (Ndikuwera *et al.*, 1987). A focal bacterial abscess develops in the area of the tail head or involves the cauda equina. This is most common in cats.

Diagnosis: Cytology and culture of the abscess confirm the diagnosis.

Treatment and prognosis: Antibiotics are selected based upon culture and antimicrobial drug sensitivity test results, and should be administered for 6–8 weeks. Depending on the response to therapy and the severity of the neurological deficits, a dorsal laminectomy may be necessary for decompression and removal of the abscess. The prognosis for recovery can be good, but is dependent on the severity of the neurological deficits at the time of presentation.

Discospondylitis

Discospondylitis refers to infection (usually bacterial) of the intervertebral disc and adjacent vertebral endplates. The L7–S1 disc space and vertebrae are regularly involved (Figure 19.17) causing severe lumbosacral pain and cauda equina syndrome (see Chapter 14 for more details).

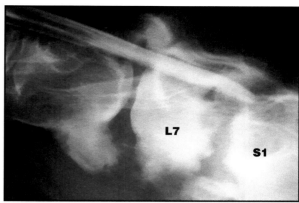

19.17 Infection of the L7 and sacral endplates (discospondylitis) and the associated vertebral bodies.

Idiopathic diseases

Feline dysautonomia

Dysautonomia in cats was initially described by Key and Gaskell in 1982 (Griffiths *et al.*, 1982; Sharp *et al.*, 1984). The incidence of this disease in the UK and Scandinavia between 1982 and 1986 reached near-epidemic proportions; the frequency has since spontaneously decreased. The disease has been rarely reported in the Midwestern USA (Kidder *et al.*, 2008).

Clinical signs: There is no breed, gender, age or environmental predisposition in cats affected by dysautonomia; however, young cats are most often affected (Sharp *et al.*, 1984; Kidder *et al.*, 2008). Onset of clinical signs is acute or insidious. The most consistent clinical findings include anorexia, weight loss and lethargy (Rochlitz, 1984; Kidder *et al.*, 2008). Common clinical signs reflective of autonomic dysfunction include dilated pupils, constipation, dry mucous membranes, reduced tear production, regurgitation and protruded third eyelid (see **Feline dysautonomia** clip on DVD).

Pathogenesis: The aetiology of feline dysautonomia is unknown despite extensive efforts to establish an association. Ingestion of botulism spores has been proposed as a toxicoinfectious cause, but evidence is scant (Nunn *et al.*, 2004). The disease is histologically characterized by chromatolysis of the sympathetic and parasympathetic ganglia with less severe changes in the ventral horn grey matter and motor nuclei of the oculomotor, trigeminal, facial, vagus and hypoglossal nerves (Sharp *et al.*, 1984).

Diagnosis: A presumptive diagnosis is made based on the clinical signs in fulminant cases of dysautonomia. Radiography, ocular examination and pharmacological testing confirm loss of autonomic function. Radiography may detect megaoesophagus or signs of gastrointestinal stasis (Novellas *et al.*, 2010). Ophthalmic examination reveals mid-range to dilated pupils, a prolapsed nictitating membrane and a reduced Schirmer tear test (Figure 19.18). In a study by Guilford *et al.* (1988) a dilute (0.1%) pilocarpine

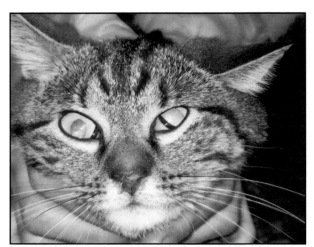

19.18 Ophthalmic examination of a Domestic Shorthaired cat with feline dysautonomia. Note the dried nasal mucosa, the prolapsed nictitating membrane and the dilated pupil of the left eye. The pupil of the right eye is miotic following treatment with 0.1% pilocarpine.

solution (a direct-acting cholinergic agonist) was applied topically to one eye of an affected cat and to one eye of a normal cat. The pupil of the affected cat produced a miotic response within 20–40 minutes, suggesting denervation supersensitivity. These ocular signs combined with signs of generalized parasympathetic and sympathetic failure are highly suggestive of feline dysautonomia. The intradermal histamine test (see below) is not reliable in cats (Guilford *et al.*, 1988). A definitive diagnosis is obtained by histological evaluation of the autonomic ganglia (Kelly, 1987).

Treatment and prognosis: Management of feline dysautonomia is achieved with supportive care. Adequate nutrition is maintained by alimentary or parenteral feeding methods. Artificial tears and nebulization are used to reduce irritation from dried mucous membranes. Pilocarpine is used to ameliorate ocular abnormalities. Low-dose bethanechol chloride may aid in urination (see Figure 19.30). Antiemetics such as metoclopramide may offer some relief in cats with severe vomiting. Supportive treatment offers palliation of clinical signs and time for some cats to recover neurological function (McNulty *et al.*, 1999).

Owners should be informed about the length of convalescence and the amount of care required. Recovery usually begins several months after the onset of clinical signs and may take a year or longer. Some animals never regain function. Cats that are more severely affected have longer and less complete recoveries. Complications such as untreatable vomiting and urinary incontinence may necessitate euthanasia.

Canine dysautonomia

Clinical signs: The onset of clinical signs is considered acute and progressive. Clinical signs reflect severe autonomic nervous system damage (Longshore *et al.*, 1996; Harkin *et al.*, 2002). Common

clinical signs include depression, dilated or mid-range pupils with no pupillary light reflex, dysuria, dry mucous membranes, gastrointestinal signs (dysphagia, regurgitation or vomiting), elevated third eyelids and a decreased anal reflex (Figure 19.19). The severity and type of clinical signs vary in dogs affected by dysautonomia. The disease usually affects young dogs.

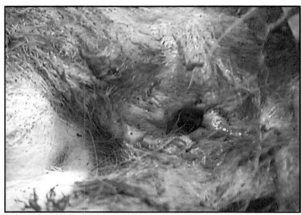

19.19 A young male mixed-breed dog with canine dysautonomia demonstrating a dilated anus. (Courtesy Dr D O'Brien)

Pathogenesis: Canine dysautonomia was first reported in the UK in 1983 (Rochlitz and Bennett, 1983). The aetiology of the disease is unknown but is characterized by widespread degeneration of the neurons and ganglia of the autonomic nervous system (Pollin and Sullivan, 1986; Pollin and Griffiths, 1992). Progressive dysfunction of the gastrointestinal, urinary and other autonomic dependent systems leads to severe physical deterioration and death. In the USA, dogs are the predominately affected species and most cases described in the literature originate from the Midwestern states (Berghaus *et al.*, 2002). Risk factors include a rural environment and dogs spending >50% of their time outdoors (Berghaus *et al.*, 2001). Seasonal risk is highest between February and April (Harkin *et al.*, 2002).

Diagnosis: A presumptive diagnosis is based on clinical signs, signalment, history and pharmacological testing. Pharmacological testing provides supportive evidence for a diagnosis. The responses to ocular instillation of dilute (0.05–0.1%) pilocarpine drops and subcutaneous injection of low-dose bethanechol chloride (0.04 mg/kg bodyweight) have been used to rule out the inability of the iris and detrusor muscles to contract and thus suggest denervation hypersensitivity (Longshore *et al.*, 1996). A negative test response does not rule out dysautonomia as Harkin *et al.* (2002) demonstrated that 10–15% of dogs with histologically confirmed dysautonomia do not respond to dilute pilocarpine.

The intradermal histamine test elicits a wheal and flare response. The flare response is dependent upon the sympathetic neuron reflex to develop. The wheal is dependent upon the direct actions of histamine on the blood vessels, which should be intact in dogs with dysautonomia. Sympathetic dysfunction results in a variable wheal response but no flare at the site of the histamine injection (Harkin *et al.*, 2002). A definitive diagnosis of dysautonomia is made by histological examination of the autonomic ganglia (Figure 19.20).

Radiographic findings supportive of dysautonomia include aspiration pneumonia, megaoesophagus and/or a distended stomach, small bowel or urinary bladder (Detweiler *et al.*, 2001). Echocardiography reveals altered systolic cardiac function in affected dogs (Harkin *et al.*, 2009).

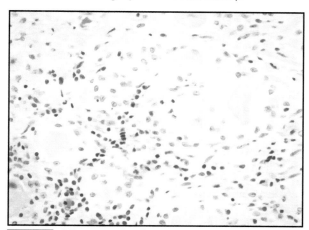

19.20 Ciliary ganglion from a dog with dysautonomia. Note the neuronal death. (H&E stain; original magnification X560) (Courtesy of Dr G Johnson)

Treatment and prognosis: Treatment is considered palliative. Autonomic dysfunction can be treated specifically with low-dose pilocarpine and bethanechol chloride to improve signs of dysuria; however, over time the response to therapy decreases. The prognosis is grave unless dogs are mildly affected with dysuria and do not have gastrointestinal signs (Harkin *et al.*, 2002).

Traumatic diseases

Fractures and luxations of the caudal lumbar and sacral vertebrae

Clinical signs: Luxations at L7–S1 can cause severe compression of the L7 nerve roots, resulting in severe pain and a dramatic nerve root signature. Neurological signs reflect damage to the sciatic, sacral and caudal nerves.

Pathogenesis: Fractures of L6 and L7 are common, with the caudal part of the vertebrae often cranioventrally displaced. Since the spinal cord terminates cranial to these vertebrae only the nerve roots (the cauda equina) occupy this region (Turner, 1987).

Diagnosis: The diagnosis is based on the radiographic findings (Figure 19.21). Myelography or CT/MRI may be necessary to further establish spinal cord compression or damage. Spinal instability is assessed based upon the degree of vertebral damage (Shires *et al.*, 1991) (see Chapter 20).

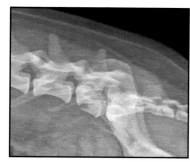

19.21 Lateral radiograph of a Golden Retriever that was hit by a trolley and presented with a decreased perineal reflex and tail tone. Note the L7 fracture with ventral displacement of the caudal fragment.

Treatment and prognosis: Fractures and luxations are managed either medically or surgically.

Medical management: For information on the medical treatment of fractures and luxations of the caudal lumbar and sacral vertebrae, see Chapter 16.

Surgical management: Treatment usually requires surgical stabilization. Several surgical techniques for internal spinal fixation of caudal lumbar fractures have been reported (Swaim, 1971; Blass and Seirn, 1984; Ullman and Boudrieau, 1993; Bagley *et al.*, 2000). Techniques often involve pins or screws and polymethylmethacrylate (PMMA) (Beaver *et al.*, 1996; Sturges and LeCouteur, 2003; Weh and Kraus, 2007). The advantages of using screws or pins with PMMA compared with other techniques (e.g. spinal stapling) are minimized tissue dissection and shorter segments of the vertebral column being immobilized. A dorsal laminectomy may also be indicated to evaluate the cauda equina for compression and nerve root integrity. External spinal fixation has been used to successfully facilitate stability and healing (Shores *et al.*, 1989; Lanz *et al.*, 2000). Postoperative management focuses on avoiding complications of recumbency with physical therapy and bladder care (Bagley *et al.*, 2000; Tefend and Dewey, 2003) (see Chapter 25).

Although considerable displacement may occur, the results of stabilization tend to be good if nociception is intact in the tail and lateral digits of the pelvic limbs and perineal sensation is present (as an indicator of the severity of injury to the sacral segments). Transection of the sacral nerves usually results in permanent faecal and urinary incontinence.

Sacral fractures

Sacral fractures (Figure 19.22) occur frequently following vehicular-related trauma. The sacrum contains the nerve roots that contribute to the pelvic and pudendal nerves. The caudal nerves also course through the sacral canal. Sacral fractures may result in faecal and urinary incontinence and neurological deficits associated with the pelvic limbs, perineum and tail. Fractures medial to the sacral foramina (axial) cause significantly more severe deficits but the prognosis for recovery does not differ from fractures lateral (abaxial) to the foramina (Kuntz *et al.*, 1995). Axial sacral fractures most frequently result in urinary and/or faecal incontinence, loss of perineal sensation and tail analgesia. Abaxial fractures are more frequently associated with pelvic limb deficits.

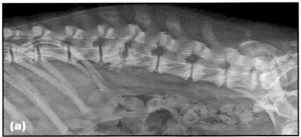

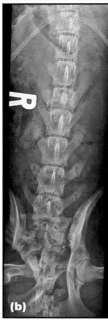

19.22 **(a)** Lateral and **(b)** ventrodorsal radiographs of a mixed-breed dog with multiple fractures of the right pelvis and sacrum, luxation of the right sacroiliac joint, a compression fracture of the L3 vertebral body and fractures of the L3, L4 and L5 spinal processes. The dog was able to support weight on the left pelvic limb. The spine maintained alignment during flexion and extension on fluoroscopic evaluation. The sacral and pelvic fractures were repaired whilst the spinal fracture was managed medically.

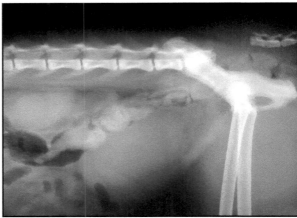

19.23 Radiographic confirmation of a complete caudal vertebral luxation in a cat with avulsion of the tail.

Sacrocaudal fractures/luxations and tail avulsions

Clinical signs: Sacrocaudal fractures/luxations and tail avulsions occur most commonly in cats (Smeak and Olmstead, 1985). Affected cats usually have a paralysed tail with complete anaesthesia. Depending upon the extent of the injury, these cats may also have urinary and faecal incontinence and partial loss of sciatic nerve function.

Pathogenesis: The degree of displacement following sacrocaudal fracture and/or luxation varies considerably. Damage to the nerve roots and associated spinal cord is caused by traction, resulting in injury to the more cranial lumbosacral intumescence.

Diagnosis: The diagnosis is suggested by the history and clinical signs, and confirmed by radiography (Figure 19.23). In rare instances there is no evidence of a fracture or luxation but the signs and history are consistent with a traction injury.

Treatment and prognosis: Fractures of the caudal vertebrae should be stabilized as soon as possible to prevent further traction injuries to the lumbosacral spinal cord. If stabilization of the caudal vertebrae is not possible, tail amputation is a viable option. The bladder must be manually expressed or catheterized until function is regained (see Chapter 25).

The prognosis for the return of urinary continence is good if anal tone and perineal sensation are present on initial examination. Cats that do not become continent within 1 month usually fail to regain urinary function (Smeak and Olmstead, 1985).

Vascular diseases

Coccygeal muscle injury

Clinical signs: Coccygeal muscle injury or 'limber tail' is a term used to describe a condition seen in hunting dogs (Steiss *et al.*, 1999). Pointer breeds and Labrador Retrievers are most commonly affected but it can occur in other breeds. Tail carriage is affected to varying degrees and the tail can appear flaccid. The hair on the proximal tail is raised and dogs may resent palpation. Dogs exhibiting this type of tail carriage are usually withdrawn from competition.

Pathogenesis: Prolonged transportation in cages, underconditioning or overexertion, and changes in climate are factors known to predispose to this condition. Pathology is associated with ischaemic damage to the coccygeal muscles, which is confirmed by histology, and is suggested to be related to compartment syndrome. Compartment syndrome is characterized by pain, swelling, lack of arterial pulses and paralysis in muscle groups that are adjacent to the bone and enclosed by thick fascial layers.

Diagnosis: The diagnosis is based upon the history and clinical signs, with trauma as a primary differential. The diagnosis can be substantiated by detecting an elevated serum creatine kinase concentration early in the course of the disease or by thermography. Biopsy of the tail is not recommended because the muscle groups are small and the nerves are located in close proximity. Abnormal spontaneous activity has been detected on electromyography.

Treatment and prognosis: Most dogs recover spontaneously within a few days to weeks. Anti-inflammatory drugs administered at the onset of clinical signs may hasten the recovery process. Prognosis is good and <50% of the cases have been known to recur.

Fibrocartilaginous embolism
Embolization of fibrocartilage into the spinal cord vasculature commonly affects the lumbosacral intumescence. When the embolic episode is limited to the sacral spinal cord it causes mild paresis with sciatic deficits, and severe urinary and faecal incontinence, with variable involvement of the tail. This syndrome of embolization of nuclear disc material is described in full in Chapters 15 and 16.

Normal and abnormal micturition

The micturition process includes both the storage and emptying phases of bladder function, whereas urination refers to just the voiding phase. Normal bladder and urethral function is required for micturition to occur. The normal micturition process involves passive filling of the bladder (which uses mechanisms that maintain continence) and active bladder emptying (which requires relaxation of the sphincters in conjunction with a coordinated voluntary bladder contraction) (de Groat and Booth, 1980). The process is under the control of the CNS, which integrates the autonomic and somatic nervous systems (Fowler *et al.*, 2008).

Functional neuroanatomy
A basic knowledge of the anatomy and physiology of micturition is necessary to evaluate and manage disorders (O'Brien, 1990; Fowler *et al.*, 2008; Lorenz *et al.*, 2011). The lower urinary tract comprises a detrusor (bladder) muscle (smooth muscle) and two sphincters: the internal smooth muscle sphincter at the proximal urethra and bladder neck, and the external skeletal muscle sphincter that encompasses the membranous urethra (Augsburger

et al., 1993). These structures are innervated by the autonomic (smooth muscle) and somatic (skeletal muscle) nervous systems.

Detrusor muscle innervation
Beta-adrenergic (hypogastric nerve; spinal cord segments L1–L4 in the dog and L2–L5 in the cat) and cholinergic/muscarinic (pelvic nerve; spinal cord segments S1–S3) receptors coordinate bladder filling and evacuation, respectively (Figure 19.24). Sensory receptors in the wall of the bladder include:

* Stretch receptors innervated by afferent fibres of the pelvic nerve
* Pain receptors innervated by afferent fibres transmitted via the pelvic and hypogastric (primarily) nerves.

Urethral innervation
The smooth muscle portion of the urethra is innervated by the hypogastric nerve (alpha-adrenergic receptors), which causes constriction and internal sphincter closure. The skeletal muscle portion of the urethra is innervated by the pudendal nerve (nicotinic cholinergic receptors) whose cell bodies are located in the sacral spinal cord (S1–S2). There are also sensory receptors in the wall of the urethra that detect stretch, pain and urine flow. These receptors are primarily innervated by the afferent nerves of the pudendal nerve; although, nociceptors are innervated by afferent fibres of the hypogastric nerve.

Central integration
The brainstem micturition centre in the pons receives sensory input from the bladder stretch and pain receptors. The centre is responsible for coordinating sphincter relaxation with detrusor muscle contraction. The cerebral cortex, basal nuclei, thalamus and cerebellum have an inhibitory influence on the micturition process and are ultimately responsible for its voluntary control.

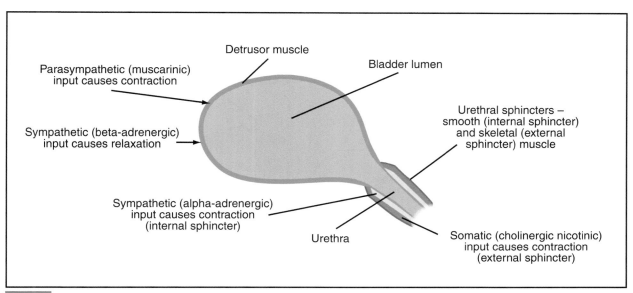

19.24 Anatomy of the bladder and urethra.

Storage phase of micturition

1. During the storage phase of micturition, the detrusor muscle is innervated by the sympathetic nervous system (SNS; beta-adrenergic receptors) via the hypogastric nerve (Oliver *et al.*, 1969; Purinton and Oliver, 1979) (Figure 19.25). The SNS facilitates urine storage via bladder wall relaxation via the influence of noradrenaline (norepinephrine) on the beta-adrenergic receptors.
2. The bladder trigone (neck) and proximal smooth muscle of the urethra are innervated by the SNS (also via the hypogastric nerve), mediated via the alpha-adrenergic receptors, resulting in sphincter contraction.
3. The striated muscle of the urethra is innervated by the somatic nervous system via the pudendal nerve with acetylcholine binding to nicotinic receptors (Bradley *et al.*, 1973). The function of the pudendal nerve during the storage phase is to provide tonic sphincter contraction.
4. Supraspinal organization of the micturition reflex (micturition centre in the pons) supplies descending pathways to mediate sympathetic, parasympathetic and somatic activities during the storage and voiding phases of urination. Urine storage involves coordinated relaxation of the detrusor muscle and contraction of the sphincter muscles. (SNS activities predominate – an easy way to commit this concept to memory is that the SNS provides the 'fight' or 'flight' mechanism and 'when you are fleeing, you shouldn't be peeing'.)
5. As the volume of urine and bladder pressure increase, stretch receptors in the urinary bladder are activated and project afferent sensory

information to the brainstem and cerebral cortex via the pelvic nerve and pathways within the dorsal funiculus. Painful stimuli within the bladder mucosa are transmitted via the hypogastric nerve and associated sympathetic pathways and spinothalamic tracts.

Voiding phase of micturition

1. During the voiding phase of micturition, the detrusor muscle is innervated by the parasympathetic nervous system (PNS; cholinergic receptors) via the pelvic nerve (Oliver *et al.*, 1969; Purinton and Oliver, 1979) (Figure 19.26). The pelvic nerve facilitates contraction of the detrusor muscle via the action of acetylcholine on the muscarinic/cholinergic receptors.
2. Urine voiding involves coordinated contraction of the detrusor muscle and relaxation of the sphincter muscles.
3. When stretch receptors within the bladder wall are stimulated, afferent impulses are transmitted via the pelvic nerve to the sacral spinal cord and ascend to the pontine reticular formation in the brainstem (micturition centre) and the cerebral cortex.
4. The micturition centre coordinates urethral sphincter relaxation and initiates and sustains detrusor muscle contraction during voiding. Coordination of urination from the reflex arc involving the spinal cord and brainstem is also known as the detrusor reflex and does not require input from the cerebral cortex.
5. During detrusor muscle contraction, afferent impulses also enter the sacral spinal cord to inhibit the cell bodies of the pudendal nerve and

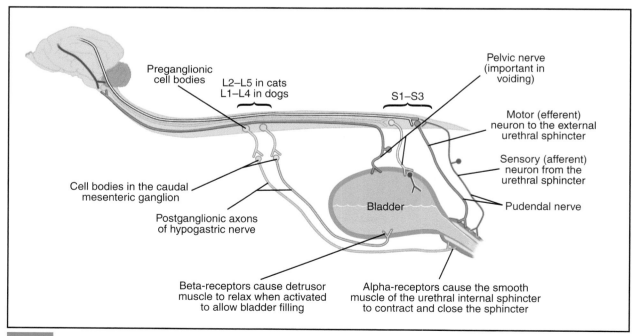

19.25 Overview of the neuroanatomy of the storage phase of micturition.

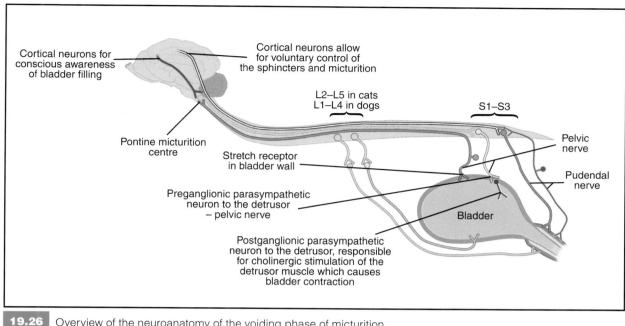

19.26 Overview of the neuroanatomy of the voiding phase of micturition.

ascend to inhibit the cell bodies of the hypogastric nerve. Thus, initiation of detrusor muscle contraction results in inhibition of contraction of the urethral sphincters.

6. Voluntary control originates from the cerebral cortex and projects to the pons and reticular spinal tract of the spinal cord (Bradley and Timm, 1974). This control is primarily inhibitory and prevents involuntary bladder contraction. In addition, voluntary inhibition of the somatic discharge to the external sphincter decreases urethral outlet resistance. The pons is modulated by the cerebral cortex, which coordinates this activity to allow normal voiding with decreased urethral sphincter resistance.

Diagnosis

History and physical examination
A thorough history and physical examination need to be performed in all cases of micturition dysfunction (Lane, 2000, 2003). The external genitalia should be examined for masses, abnormal conformation and urine scalding. In cases of urinary incontinence, the physical examination may reveal evidence of urine scalding around the genitalia and caudal thigh region. A pool of urine may be found where the animal has been lying down or sleeping. Abdominal palpation may reveal bladder size, wall thickness and the presence of any masses. In cases of urinary retention the bladder is often enlarged. The bladder tends to be large, firm and difficult to express with upper motor neuron (UMN) lesions, whereas it is large, flaccid and easily (but not completely) expressed with LMN lesions. Manual expression of the bladder can be performed to assess urethral sphincter tone. Digital rectal palpation can be undertaken to assess the pelvic urethra and prostate gland.

Character of urination
Urination is evaluated for duration, stream character, dysuria and haematuria.

Storage disorders
Storage disorders are characterized by involuntary leakage of small amounts of urine in conjunction with a normal to small sized bladder.

Voiding disorders
Voiding disorders are characterized by dysuria, stranguria and urine retention. Once urination is complete, the bladder should be palpated and catheterized to determine the volume of residual urine (normal range is <10 ml for dogs and <2 ml for cats). Urethral bladder catheterization simultaneously assesses for obstructive lesions.

Neurological examination
A neurological examination ascertains the presence of neurological disease and the neuroanatomical localization (Lorenz et al., 2011) (Figure 19.27). Reflexes associated with the pudendal nerve are particularly important to evaluate.

- Anal sphincter tone is evaluated by digital rectal examination.
- The bulbocavernosus reflex is a sharp contraction of the anal sphincter and tail in response to a squeeze of the bulb of the penis or clitoris.
- The perineal reflex is a contraction of the anal sphincter in response to a pinch of the perineal region. Sensory perception is simultaneously evaluated.
- Urethral sphincter tone is assessed by manual bladder expression.

Lesion localization	Conscious voiding attempts	Bladder expression/ size	Residual urine volume	Perineal reflex	Type of micturition dysfunction
Cerebral cortex to brainstem	Absent	Difficult/small	Small	Present	Inappropriate urination
Cerebellum	Normal; increased frequency	Difficult/small	Small	Present	Detrusor muscle hyperreflexia
Brainstem to L7	Absent; dyssynergia	Difficult/large; tapering stream; small spurts of urination	Moderate to large	Present	Failure to eliminate urine; reflex incontinence; overflow incontinence
Sacral spinal cord	Absent; may attempt but limited success	Easy; leakage; may have some resistance/ large	Large	Reduced to absent	Urethral incompetence; detrusor muscle atony; overflow incontinence
Disruption of tight junctions to the detrusor muscle	Absent	Some resistance; bladder is flaccid/large	Large	Present	Overflow incontinence

19.27 Localization and clinical signs of micturition dysfunction.

Urinalysis and urine culture

Urinalysis and urine culture are performed to identify obvious pathological processes such as UTIs and neoplasia. An animal with neurogenic bladder dysfunction often has a UTI. The urine specific gravity should be informative in dogs with polyuria.

Imaging

Survey abdominal radiography, ultrasonography, contrast cystography and urethrography can further delineate masses or anatomical obstructive lesions.

Urodynamic testing

Urodynamic testing can assist with anatomical localization.

- A cystometrogram monitors bladder pressure during filling and emptying (Oliver and Young, 1973).
- Urethral pressure profilometry (UPP) can assess for decreased urethral tone (decreased mean urethral closure pressure) and functional urethral length (Rosin et al., 1980). UPP measures pressure at points along the length of the urethra using a small catheter connected to a pressure transducer, which is slowly withdrawn.
- Leak point pressure testing is a functional technique used to stimulate urethral compliance associated with an external abdominal press (Rawlings et al., 1999).
- Electromyography to assess pudendal nerve function is performed using a recording electrode on the perineum and external sphincter (Bradley et al., 1975).

Although urodynamic testing can be performed at some university referral hospitals, similar information can often be acquired by closely observing the animal during urination, measuring residual volume and determining whether there is any resistance during catheterization.

Causes of micturition dysfunction

Disturbances of micturition can be classified into two categories (O'Brien, 1988; Lane, 2000; Coates and Kerl, 2008; Lorenz et al., 2011):

- Failure to store urine
- Failure to eliminate urine.

Structural and neurogenic lesions that primarily or secondarily affect the bladder and urethra cause abnormalities in micturition.

Failure to store urine

Failure to store urine can result from either urinary bladder dysfunction or urethral sphincter incompetence. Incontinence must be distinguished from inappropriate urination since both abnormalities appear similar to the owner. Inappropriate urination is the act of voiding urine at the wrong time and in the wrong place, but it is still under the voluntary control of the animal. History and direct observation of the patient will distinguish inappropriate urination from incontinence. Underlying disorders of inappropriate urination in dogs include senility, forebrain disease and lack of willingness or difficulty in reaching an acceptable place to urinate. Forebrain (cerebral cortex and diencephalon) lesions also typically cause behavioural changes and other sensory and motor deficits.

Bladder storage dysfunction: Bladder storage dysfunction relates to poor bladder compliance and/or elasticity during the filling phase or involuntary voiding at low bladder volumes and pressures.

Urge incontinence is commonly associated with this type of dysfunction. Non-neurogenic causes include UTIs, chronic inflammatory processes, infiltrative diseases (e.g. neoplasia) and idiopathic hypercontractility. Neurogenic causes of bladder storage dysfunction include detrusor muscle hyperreflexic conditions that occur with cerebellar disorders (degenerative, neoplastic, inflammatory/infectious) and chronic UMN spinal cord diseases (detrusor muscle–sphincter dyssynergia or overflow incontinence). Overflow incontinence occurs when detrusor muscle pressure exceeds urethral sphincter resistance.

Urethral incompetence: Urethral incompetence is a result of weakened responses of urethral smooth or skeletal muscles, which allows urine leakage during the storage phase of micturition. Non-neurogenic causes include UTIs, neoplasia, ectopic ureters, prostate gland disorders, hormone-responsive urethral incompetence and metabolic disorders. Polyuric disorders secondary to metabolic disturbances can intensify an underlying incontinence problem when an increase in urine volume further stresses an incompetent urethra. Causes of polyuria include renal failure, diabetes insipidus, diabetes mellitus, hypercalcaemia, electrolyte disturbances, hyperadrenocorticism, hypoadrenocorticism, thyroid disorders, hepatic failure, medications (e.g. glucocorticoids, anticonvulsants, diuretics), prostatic abscesses and pyometra. Neurogenic causes for urethral incompetence include those disorders affecting the sacral spinal cord (Figure 19.28).

Disease category	Specific diseases
Degenerative	Compressive myelopathy – intervertebral disc disease, lumbosacral syndrome, lumbosacral stenosis Non-compressive myelopathy – degenerative myelopathy (late stages)
Anomalous	Sacrocaudal dysgenesis; myelodysplasia; stenosis
Neoplastic	Primary – osteosarcoma, chondrosarcoma, fibrosarcoma, nerve sheath tumour, meningioma, chordoma Metastatic (common) – prostatic adenocarcinoma, perianal gland adenocarcinoma, lymphoma
Infectious	Discospondylitis (*Staphlococcus intermedius*, *Brucella canis* and *Escherichia coli*)
Inflammatory	Immune-mediated peripheral neuropathies; polyradiculoneuritis; myasthenia gravis (detrusor muscle atony, secondary overflow)
Idiopathic	Dysautonomia
Traumatic	Lumbosacral luxation; traction spinal cord injury
Toxic	Botulism
Vascular	Fibrocartilaginous embolism

19.28 Sacral spinal cord lesions causing micturition dysfunction.

Hormone-responsive urethral incompetence is the most common cause, especially in bitches. Urine leakage frequently occurs when the animal is at rest, but voluntary control is present when the animal is alert. A strong correlation exists between bodyweight and the incidence of incontinence. The onset of incontinence following neutering varies between immediately and 10 years, with an average of 3 years after surgery. A diagnosis of hormone-responsive urethral incompetence should be made only after all other causes of acquired incontinence have been ruled out.

Failure to eliminate urine
Failure to eliminate (urinary retention) can result from either incomplete or absent bladder contraction, or urethral outflow obstruction (anatomical or functional).

Incomplete or absent bladder contraction: The most common cause of voiding dysfunction associated with urinary retention is considered to be neurogenic failure. UMN dysfunction occurs with lesions between the pons and the L7 spinal cord segment. UMN bladder dysfunction is a common sequela to T3–L3 myelopathies. Both the motor and sensory pathways of the detrusor reflex are affected. The bladder becomes large and firm and urethral sphincter tone is increased. The bladder is difficult to express manually. Secondary overflow incontinence occurs when the bladder pressure exceeds the urethral pressure.

LMN bladder dysfunction occurs with lesions located in the sacral spinal cord and nerve roots and/or the pelvic plexus. Lesions in this area abolish the detrusor reflex. The detrusor muscle becomes flaccid (detrusor muscle atony) as a result of over-distension secondary to absent detrusor muscle contraction and external sphincter tone is lost. The internal sphincter, innervated by the hypogastric nerve, remains intact. This may make bladder expression difficult. Animals with LMN bladder dysfunction also lose sensation and the perineal reflex. Trauma is the most common cause for this type of dysfunction.

Bladder atony from over-distension can result from non-neurogenic or neurogenic causes. Non-neurogenic bladder atony is secondary to urinary obstruction and disruption of the tight junctions of the detrusor myofibres. Over-distension can also result from pain (e.g. following pelvic fractures) and recumbency. Disorders associated with generalized weakness, such as myopathic, neuropathic and neuromuscular junction disorders, can also result in over-distension (Figure 19.29). Dysautonomia may initially present with urination dysfunction (usually an over-distended bladder that is flaccid and easily expressed).

Urethral obstruction: The most common cause of outflow obstruction is an anatomical blockage of the urethra. Causes include urolithiasis, neoplasia, prostatic disease and urethral inflammation. Urethral catheterization is often difficult.

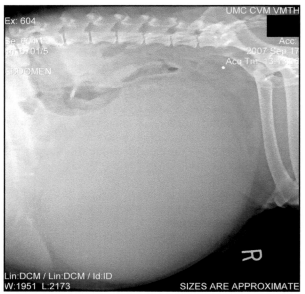

19.29 Lateral abdominal radiograph of a well house-trained dog with osteoarthritis that was unable to ambulate outside. Note the over-distension of the bladder, which was presumed to be the result of detrusor muscle atony. The urinary bladder was catheterized and emptied for several days before the detrusor muscle regained function.

Functional urethral obstruction results from neurogenic or non-neurogenic causes (Lane, 2003). UMN lesions result in uninhibited urethral sphincter tone and increased urethral resistance, making voiding and manual expression difficult. This condition is often related to detrusor muscle–sphincter dyssynergia (reflex dyssynergia), which refers to loss of coordination between the bladder and the sphincter muscles. It is commonly encountered in animals with spinal cord injury (Oliver, 1983; Barsanti et al., 1996). Dyssynergia is characterized by the simultaneous contraction of muscles whose activity is opposite in direction. Mechanisms for dyssynergia of smooth and skeletal muscle sphincters are mediated by loss of the inhibitory reticulospinal pathways (from the micturition centre) to the sympathetic and somatic (pudendal) efferents, respectively. Affected animals usually have large volumes of residual urine, primarily as a result of urethral sphincter spasticity. Cauda equina lesions can also cause uncoordinated sphincter activity, which results in dyssynergic-like voiding patterns and urinary retention (Coates, 1999). Non-neurogenic causes of functional urethral obstruction are related to a lack of coordination between detrusor muscle contraction and urethral relaxation (e.g. idiopathic detrusor muscle–urethral dyssynergia) or an increase in urethral resistance.

Treatment

Successful management of micturition dysfunction depends on identification and treatment of the underlying disorder. Storage and voiding disorders can be treated either medically or surgically. Medical therapy includes control of secondary complicating UTIs and management of the bladder and urethral dysfunction. Pharmacological therapies for urethral and bladder disorders are summarized in Figure 19.30. It is important to understand mechanisms of action, side-effects and contraindications of these drugs. The detrusor muscle should not be stimulated to contract unless the bladder is easily manually expressed.

Surgical management is used to treat urethral incompetence in cases that are refractory to medical therapy. Several methods have been described, including mesh and sling procedures,

Desired effect	Drug	Mechanism of action	Dosage [a]	Side effects
Stimulate detrusor muscle contraction	Bethanechol	Cholinergic stimulation	Dogs: 2.5–25 mg orally q8h Cats: 1.25–5 mg/cat orally q8–12h	Increased GI motility; vomiting; diarrhoea; hypersalivation; hypotension; bradycardia; dyspnoea
	Cisapride	Increase acetylcholine release	Dogs: 0.5 mg/kg orally q8h Cats: 1.25–5 mg/cat orally q8–12h	Diarrhoea; abdominal pain
Decrease detrusor muscle hyperreflexia	Propantheline bromide	Anticholinergic; antispasmodic	5–30 mg orally q8h or 0.25–0.5 mg/kg orally q8h	Pupillary dilatation; decreased GI motility; constipation; dry mucous membranes
	Oxbutynin chloride	Direct antispasmodic	2–5 mg orally q8–12h	Urine retention; vomiting; constipation; tachycardia
Increase urethral tone	Phenylpropanolamine	Alpha-adrenergic agonist	5–50 mg orally q8h or 1.5 mg/kg orally q8h	CNS stimulation; tachycardia; urine retention
	Imipramine	Alpha- and beta-adrenergic stimulation	5–15 mg orally q12h	Seizures; tremors; hyperexcitability

19.30 Medical management of micturition disorders. [a] Dose for dogs unless otherwise stated. CNS = central nervous system; GI = gastrointestinal. (continues) ▶

Desired effect	Drug	Mechanism of action	Dosage [a]	Side effects
Increase urethral tone (continued)	Diethylstilboestrol	Increase sphincter sensitivity to noradrenaline	0.1–1.0 mg orally for 3–5 days then 1.0 mg weekly	Bone marrow suppression; oestrus
	Testosterone	Unknown	2.2 mg/kg i.m. q30days	Prostatic hypertrophy; behavioural changes
Decrease urethral tone	Phenoxybenzamine	Alpha-adrenergic antagonist	0.25–0.5 mg/kg orally q12–24h	Hypotension; tachycardia
	Prazosin	Alpha-adrenergic antagonist	Dogs: 1 mg/15 kg orally q8–24h, administer 30 minutes prior to bladder expression attempts Cats: 0.25–0.5 mg orally q12–24h	Hypotension; tachycardia
	Diazepam	Centrally acting skeletal muscle relaxant	Dogs: 2–10 mg orally q6–8h Cats: 1–2.5 mg orally q8–12h	Hepatotoxicity in cats; sedation; excitement
	Dantrolene	Skeletal muscle relaxant	Dogs: 1–5 mg orally q8–12h Cats: 0.5–2 mg/kg orally q8h	Weakness; GI upset; sedation; hepatotoxicity

19.30 (continued) Medical management of micturition disorders. [a] Dose for dogs unless otherwise stated. CNS = central nervous system; GI = gastrointestinal.

Teflon injections and colposuspension. Cysto-urethropexy and colposuspension procedures have been performed with variable success (Gregory and Holt, 1994; Rawlings *et al.*, 2000). Colposuspension is a surgical technique that moves the bladder neck from an intrapelvic to an intra-abdominal position and restores continence by increasing pressure transmission to the proximal urethra and bladder neck.

Basic principles need to be followed to prevent bladder over-distension in animals with urinary retention. When urethral tone is increased, manual bladder expression alone is usually not effective and sometimes dangerous. Aseptic urethral/bladder catheterization is required, but long-term indwelling catheters should be avoided if possible (Bubenik and Hosgood, 2008). Intermittent urinary catheterization is often indicated and has a lower risk of inducing a UTI than continuous urinary catheterization techniques (Bubenik *et al.*, 2007; Bubenik and Hosgood, 2008). Manual expression is indicated if the bladder can be easily expressed but residual urine volumes should be periodically monitored by ultrasonography or urinary catheterization. Large residual urine volumes predispose to UTIs (Stiffler *et al.*, 2006; Bubenik *et al.*, 2007; Olby *et al.*, 2010). Urine culture should be periodically performed.

Prognosis

The prognosis depends on the underlying disorder of micturition. If the underlying disorder is reversible and correctly diagnosed, the prognosis is generally good. Chronic disorders with associated micturition dysfunction have a less favourable or more guarded prognosis. Some disorders may require life-long monitoring and medical management. UTIs pose the most serious complication of micturition dysfunction.

References and further reading

Available on accompanying DVD

DVD extras

- **Degenerative lumbosacral stenosis**
- **Feline dysautonomia**

20

Neurological emergencies

Simon Platt and Natasha Olby

Neurological emergencies require rapid and accurate decision making and treatment. Inappropriate management in the early stages of disease can have catastrophic consequences for the animal. Studies on acute head injury and status epilepticus in humans show that having an emergency protocol in place improves the outcome (Brain Trauma Foundation, 2000, 2007). Thus, to ensure optimal treatment in an emergency situation, it is recommended that emergency protocols that take into account the availability of staff and equipment for each clinic are developed pre-emptively.

Acute spinal cord injury

Acute onset of non-ambulatory paraparesis, hemiparesis or tetraparesis should be considered an emergency.

Aetiology
The most common causes of acute spinal cord injury include (Figure 20.1):

- Acute intervertebral disc herniation – both Hansen type I and acute non-compressive nucleus pulposus extrusions (De Risio et al., 2009)

Disease	Type of spinal cord injury
Intervertebral disc disease [15, 16]	Contusion; compression
Vertebral fractures/luxations [15, 16, 20, 22]	Contusion; compression; laceration; ongoing instability
Fibrocartilaginous embolism [15, 16]	Ischaemia
Haemorrhage [15, 16]	Ischaemia; compression
Congenital instability (e.g. atlantoaxial subluxation) [15]	Contusion; compression; ± laceration; ongoing instability
Neoplasia [14, 15, 16]	Compression; ± vertebral fractures
Discospondylitis [14, 15, 16]	Compression; inflammation; ± vertebral fractures; ongoing instability
Myelitis [11, 16]	Inflammation

20.1 Types of spinal cord injury associated with different diseases. Square brackets refer to the chapters in which diseases are discussed further.

- Vertebral fractures and luxations
- Vascular diseases – fibrocartilaginous embolism (FCE) and haemorrhage
- Cervical spondylomyelopathy (Wobbler syndrome)
- Congenital malformation causing instability – atlantoaxial subluxation.

Many chronic diseases, such as neoplasia, discospondylitis and inflammatory or infectious spinal cord diseases, can also present acutely as a result of the sudden development of associated pathology (i.e. vertebral fractures due to vertebral neoplasia or discospondylitis, or intraparenchymal haemorrhage due to haemangiosarcoma and vasculitis). These diseases are described in Chapters 15 to 17.

Pathophysiology
Acute onset of spinal cord dysfunction is most commonly caused by a combination of one or more events, including contusion, compression, ischaemia and laceration of the spinal cord.

Contusion
Contusion of the spinal cord is commonly caused by intervertebral disc extrusion, as well as vertebral fractures and luxations. Repeated contusion may occur in some diseases due to vertebral instability. Acute contusion of the spinal cord initiates a series of biochemical and metabolic events that expand the primary zone of tissue necrosis. The majority of this secondary damage occurs within 24 hours of injury and, although cellular apoptosis continues for weeks to months (Crowe et al., 1997), it is not common for clinical signs of deterioration to be evident much beyond 72 hours following the injury. The detrimental events are initiated by the mechanical insult, which causes the release of neurotransmitters, damage to glial and neuronal cell membranes and damage to the local vasculature. This causes energy failure and increased cell membrane permeability, which leads to a cascade of events including destruction of the microvascular bed, leading to a progressive reduction in perfusion of the injured area, an increase in intracellular calcium concentration, and free-radical production. Many of these factors interact leading to a cycle of destructive events. The end result is an expanding zone of cellular necrosis and apoptosis (Figure 20.2) (Dumont et al., 2001; Olby, 2010).

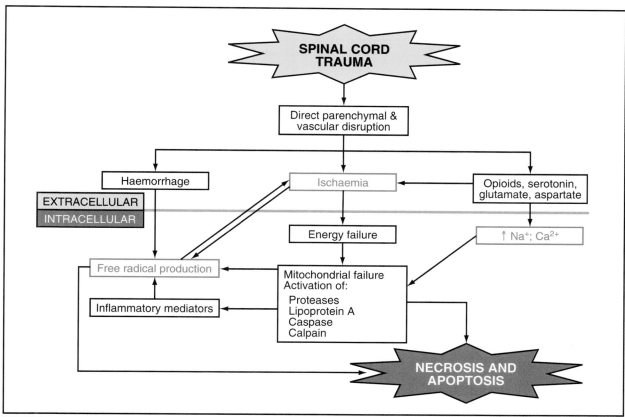

20.2 Overview of the pathophysiology of spinal cord trauma showing the underlying vasculature and biochemical components of secondary injury.

Ischaemia

Primary ischaemic injuries (e.g. FCE) initiate a similar biochemical and metabolic cascade but the injury is centred on the zone of the embolized blood vessel, often resulting in asymmetrical and focal signs (see Chapters 15 and 16).

Compression

Compression of the spinal cord is commonly due to intervertebral disc protrusion or extrusion, neoplasia, and malalignment of the vertebral canal secondary to fractures, luxations or congenital defects. Compression interferes directly with axonal ion channel function, myelin sheath integrity (Shi and Blight, 1996; Ouyang *et al.*, 2011) and vascular perfusion of the affected area (Griffiths *et al.*, 1978; Milhorat *et al.*, 1996) causing demyelination and eventually axonal, glial and neuronal necrosis.

Laceration

Laceration of the spinal cord by external objects (e.g. gunshot wounds) or internally (luxation of the vertebrae) not only interrupts the blood supply and contuses and compresses the spinal cord, but also causes axonal transection. As the central nervous system (CNS) axons do not regenerate effectively, the consequences of this are extremely serious.

Patient assessment

An approach to the assessment and management of spinal injury is given in Figure 20.3.

Primary assessment

On admission, the first aim is to stabilize the patient by assessing the airway, breathing and circulation ('ABC') and treating abnormalities where necessary. Complete routine blood work and urinalysis should be performed if possible; otherwise a packed cell volume (PCV), total protein level, blood urea nitrogen (BUN) assessment, and glucose and electrolyte levels should be ascertained. Cardiovascular stability should be investigated with the aid of an electrocardiogram (ECG) and blood pressure measurements. The important systemic parameters to monitor, the suggested reference values following trauma and the management protocols are similar to those following head trauma and are detailed later (see Figure 20.13).

Secondary assessment

A thorough physical and orthopaedic examination can follow the initial patient evaluation and stabilization. Consideration should also be given to obtaining a coagulation panel, a buccal mucosal bleeding time (BMBT) and a platelet count if there has been associated haemorrhage. A patient that has experienced blood loss, or that is expected to do so during surgery, should be blood-typed or cross-matched and appropriate blood products should be obtained.

Neurological assessment

The neurological examination should be aimed at localizing the lesion and determining its severity (see Chapters 2, 14 and 15). Thoracolumbar spinal

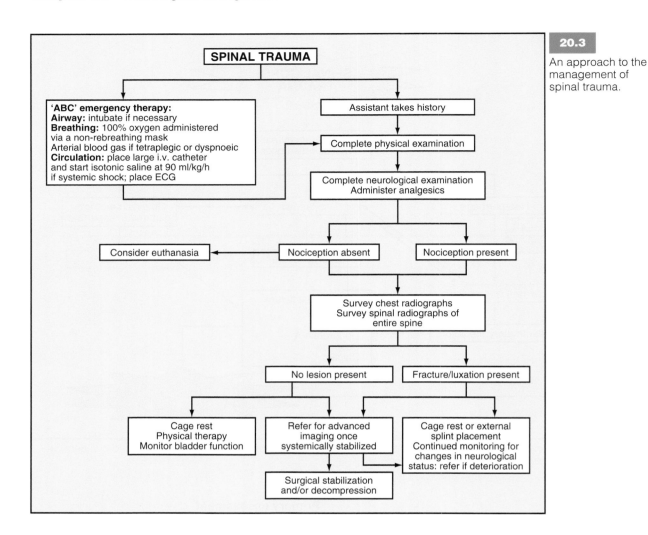

20.3

An approach to the management of spinal trauma.

(Flowchart contents:)

SPINAL TRAUMA

'ABC' emergency therapy:
Airway: intubate if necessary
Breathing: 100% oxygen administered via a non-rebreathing mask
Arterial blood gas if tetraplegic or dyspnoeic
Circulation: place large i.v. catheter and start isotonic saline at 90 ml/kg/h if systemic shock; place ECG

Assistant takes history

Complete physical examination

Complete neurological examination
Administer analgesics

Nociception absent → Consider euthanasia

Nociception present

Survey chest radiographs
Survey spinal radiographs of entire spine

No lesion present

Fracture/luxation present

Cage rest
Physical therapy
Monitor bladder function

Refer for advanced imaging once systemically stabilized

Cage rest or external splint placement
Continued monitoring for changes in neurological status: refer if deterioration

Surgical stabilization and/or decompression

---

cord injury severity is commonly graded as follows (Griffiths, 1982):

0 – Normal.
1 – Painful.
2 – Conscious proprioceptive deficits, ataxia and paraparesis.
3 – Non-ambulatory paraparesis.
4 – Paraplegia with intact nociception.
5 – Paraplegia with loss of nociception.

Lack of nociception is not as relevant in tetraparesis; however, special attention should be paid to the respiratory rate and pattern in any non-ambulatory tetraparetic or tetraplegic patient with a view to detecting hypoventilation. The presence of hypoventilation indicates the need for ventilatory support and immediate diagnostic workup.

Diagnostic imaging

Survey radiography: Thoracic radiographs should be obtained following significant trauma to look for pleural effusions, contusions, pneumomediastinum and pneumothorax, as well as the possibility of pericardial effusion and diaphragmatic herniation. If a vertebral injury is suspected, it is recommended that survey lateral radiographs are taken of the entire spine prior to additional manipulation of the animal. Sites particularly predisposed to fracture and luxation include the atlantoaxial junction, the thoracolumbar junction and the lumbar and lumbosacral spine. As some fractures can be subtle, good quality and well positioned radiographs from two orthogonal planes are necessary (Figure 20.4). This may be accomplished with the animal conscious but immobilized; however, analgesia may be required. Poor radiographic technique resulting in rotation of the spine (especially in the cervical area) can make assessment for unstable and malaligned vertebral segments difficult. Extreme care should be taken when positioning the animal for ventrodorsal views: horizontal beam radiographs can be obtained if the equipment is available.

Sedation may be necessary to achieve accurate positioning for radiography in some animals. This should not be performed if the examiner is unsure of the physical diagnosis, as sedation often influences the results of the neurological examination. In addition, sedation or anaesthesia results in the loss of voluntary paraspinal muscle contraction, and unstable vertebral segments may be more likely to subluxate (Bagley, 2000). It is important to remember that radiographs provide a static record of the location of the vertebrae at the time of the study, but they do not allow assessment of how extensive the displacement

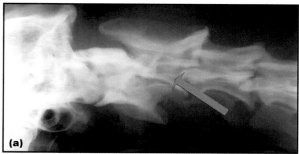

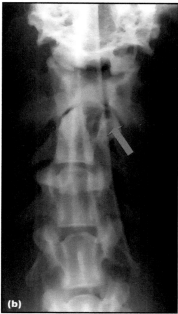

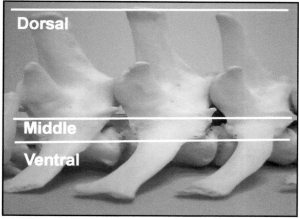

20.5 The three-compartment theory of assessment of spinal trauma. The dorsal compartment contains the spinous processes and supporting ligamentous structures, in addition to the articular facets, laminae and pedicles. The dorsal longitudinal ligament, the dorsal vertebral body and the dorsal annulus of the disc are contained within the middle compartment. The ventral compartment contains the rest of the vertebral body, the lateral and ventral aspects of the annulus of the disc, the nucleus pulposus and the ventral longitudinal ligament. If two or more compartments are damaged, the fracture is considered unstable, whereas damage to just one compartment may indicate a stable fracture. This does not take into account associated compression of the spinal cord, which may occur with damage to just one of the compartments.

20.4 Radiographs of the cranial cervical spine of a 2-year-old German Shepherd Dog following a traumatic accident. **(a)** Lateral radiograph showing a comminuted fracture of C2 (arrowed) as well as evident dorsal subluxation of this vertebra with respect to C1. **(b)** Ventrodorsal radiograph showing lateral displacement of the C2 vertebra (arrowed) with respect to C1.

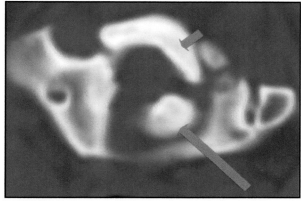

20.6 Transverse CT image (bone window) of C1 and C2 in a 16-month-old German Shepherd Dog with neck pain following a traumatic incident. The dens (long arrow) can be seen within the vertebral canal but is displaced laterally. The dorsal lamina of C1 (short arrow) can be identified and is misshapen as a result of a congenital malformation (see Figure 20.7). (Courtesy of F McConnell)

of the vertebrae was at the time of the injury and prior to imaging. As a result of the strong paraspinal musculature, vertebrae can be significantly displaced acutely at the time of injury but then subsequently pulled back into a more normal position. A scheme has been devised for predicting spinal instability in human patients based upon the degree of vertebral damage, which has been modified for use in animals (Shores, 1992). In this model the vertebrae are divided into three compartments (Figure 20.5). Damage to more than one compartment indicates a need for internal or external stabilization (see Chapter 16).

Advanced imaging: Myelography or other advanced imaging techniques such as computed tomography (CT) or magnetic resonance imaging (MRI) are needed to evaluate spinal cord compression and ensure that additional lesions unidentifiable on survey radiography are not present. CT is invaluable in identifying bone defects that may not be apparent on survey radiography (Figure 20.6). A three-dimensional (3D) reconstruction from CT

images may provide additional anatomical information regarding bone contour for surgical planning (Figure 20.7). There is a mounting body of evidence that MRI can provide prognostic information for acute intervertebral disc herniation (Ito *et al.*, 2005; De Risio *et al.*, 2009) and can identify complete physical disruption of the spinal cord. MRI has the distinct advantage that it enables visualization of the intramedullary spinal cord structure and soft tissue injuries as well as multiplanar images, but it does not provide as good bone detail as CT (Figure 20.8).

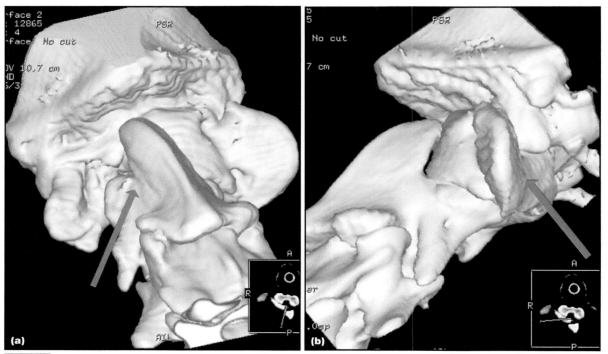

20.7 A 3D reconstruction of the case described in Figure 20.6. **(a)** Dorsal oblique view. C1 is malformed with partial absence of the right neural arch and a misshapen wing. C2 is arrowed. **(b)** Ventrolateral view. The arrow indicates the ventral surface of C1, which is fused to the occipital bone. (Courtesy of F McConnell)

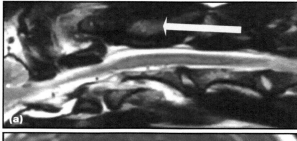

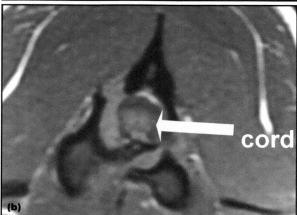

20.8 MR images of the German Shepherd Dog in Figure 20.4. **(a)** Sagittal T2-weighted MR image of the cervical vertebrae and spinal cord. Although the degree of bone definition is not as good as that seen with CT, the effects of injury (spinal cord and parenchymal compression) can be assessed accurately in three views. The arrow indicates the dorsal arch of C2. **(b)** Transverse T2-weighted MR image of C2. Note that there is no evident compression of the cord, despite the comminuted nature of the fracture of the vertebra.

Urinary tract assessment

In addition to blood urea and creatinine values and urine specific gravity levels, urethral catheterization may be required in patients that have undergone severe concurrent abdominal or pelvic trauma in order that urine production may be assessed over the subsequent 72 hours. This will also be of value in those patients with systemic shock due to the traumatic event. Abdominal ultrasonography may be required to evaluate the bladder wall and kidneys, and to detect the presence of free abdominal fluid; contrast-enhanced imaging of the urinary tract may provide further information on the function and form of the individual structures.

Treatment

The treatment of spinal fractures and luxations is considered in more detail in Chapter 16.

Medical management

Medical treatment of acute spinal cord contusion and ischaemia is aimed at limiting the final extent of the secondary tissue damage. Minimizing secondary injury is generally achieved by ensuring adequate perfusion and oxygenation of the animal. The ultimate aim is to identify an effective neuroprotective agent that could be given, but this has proven elusive (Olby, 2010), making it all the more important to focus on maintenance of perfusion and oxygenation. Treatment must be initiated as soon as possible following the injury, as the majority of secondary tissue damage occurs within 24 hours of the primary injury.

Stabilization: The first considerations are systemic blood pressure and oxygenation, particularly in the trauma victim. In the normal spinal cord, perfusion is maintained in the face of changes in systemic blood pressure by an autoregulatory process. Autoregulation is lost in the injured spinal cord, and hypotension results in a further decrease in the already compromised perfusion of the injured segment. Hypoxaemia exacerbates the local energy failure. Hypotension should be treated with the administration of appropriate fluids (see Head trauma below) and oxygen supplementation provided by facemask or with a nasopharyngeal or transtracheal catheter if necessary.

An effective means of restoring perfusion to the injured CNS is to perform a durotomy. This approach has been investigated in dogs in experimental models of spinal cord injury (Parker and Smith, 1975) and retrospectively in cases with acute intervertebral disc herniations (Loughlin *et al.*, 2005). Both studies failed to show a benefit but were likely underpowered to detect one and, given the success of cerebrospinal fluid (CSF) drainage in the management of head trauma and in aortic aneurysm surgery, this approach deserves further evaluation. An alternative is to place a lumbar intrathecal catheter and drain the CSF. While this practice has been shown to be safe in humans (Kwon *et al.*, 2009), data on efficacy are still not available.

Neuroprotection: Unfortunately there is little (if any) objective information available on the most effective treatment for acute spinal cord injury in dogs, and so treatment protocols for humans with acute spinal cord injuries have been adopted by veterinary surgeons. It should be emphasized that the efficacy of these protocols has not been established in dogs with spontaneous spinal cord injuries.

Although many different therapeutic agents, including opioid antagonists and agonists, calcium and sodium channel blockers and glutamate receptor antagonists, have been shown to be protective experimentally (for a more complete review, see Olby, 2010), the only drugs shown to be of benefit in randomized prospective human clinical trials are methylprednisolone sodium succinate (MPSS) and its derivative, tirilizad (Bracken *et al.*, 1985, 1997; Bracken and Holford, 1993), both being used for their free-radical scavenging properties rather than any anti-inflammatory effect (Hall *et al.*, 1995). However, many question the validity of these results and the use of MPSS remains controversial in human medicine (Nesathurai, 1998; Coleman *et al.*, 2000; Hurlbert, 2000). The authors do not recommend the use of MPSS in dogs or cats with acute spinal injury.

MPSS use has been reported in experimental models of canine spinal cord injury and a benefit has not been seen (Coates *et al.*, 1995; Rabinowitz *et al.*, 2008), although both studies were underpowered. Suggested protocols have been extrapolated from human medicine (Figure 20.9). Delaying the initiation of treatment for >8 hours has a detrimental effect on outcome in humans (Bracken and Holford, 1993). As MPSS has both glucocorticoid and free-radical scavenging effects, it is postulated that delaying

treatment until after the majority of free-radical-induced damage has occurred is more likely to result in glucocorticoid-induced side effects. Although there continues to be widespread use of glucocorticoids such as dexamethasone to treat acute spinal cord injuries in veterinary practice, there is no good evidence that such drugs are beneficial in experimental studies (Parker and Smith, 1976; Arias, 1987) or retrospective analyses of clinical cases (Ruddle *et al.*, 2006; Levine *et al.*, 2008) and the side effects have been well documented (Toombs *et al.*, 1980).

Time elapsed since injury	Suggested MPSS protocol
<3 hours	30 mg/kg i.v. followed by 5.4 mg/kg/h continuous rate infusion (CRI) for 24 hours OR followed by 15 mg/kg i.v. at 2 and 6 hours after the initial injection then 2.5 mg/kg CRI for 18 hours
3–8 hours	30 mg/kg i.v. followed by 5.4 mg/kg/h CRI for 48 hours OR followed by 15 mg/kg i.v. at 2 and 6 hours after the initial injection then 2.5 mg/kg CRI for 42 hours
>8 hours	MPSS contraindicated

20.9 Suggested protocols for MPSS administration in patients with acute spinal cord injuries taken from human clinical trials (Bracken et al., 1997).

Polyethylene glycol has been advocated as an effective therapy for canine spinal cord injury and has been evaluated in a pilot clinical trial in dogs with acute disc herniations that suffered the most severe grade of injury (paraplegia with loss of nociception) (Laverty *et al.*, 2004). This polymer has surfactant properties and targets and fuses damaged membranes following intravenous administration, thus interrupting the injury cascade. The treatment protocol was as follows: 3500 Da polyethylene glycol as a 30% w/w solution in sterile saline administered at a dose rate of 2 ml/kg as soon as possible after the injury and repeated once 4–6 hours later. The published study did not encounter any adverse effects and reported recovery of ambulation in 13 of 19 dogs (68%). However, this is comparable with other reports of recovery of ambulation in this population of dogs when treated with surgical decompression alone (see Figure 20.10). There is currently no approved medical grade preparation of this compound.

Non-surgical treatment of spinal fractures and luxations is dependent on whether the injury is determined to be unstable based on the three-compartment model (see Figure 20.5). If there is no instability, cage rest for 6 weeks is adequate (Carberry *et al.*, 1989). If the fracture/luxation is determined to be unstable, and the owners decline surgery, an external splint can be placed in such a manner that the damaged area of the spine is immobilized (Selcer *et al.*, 1991; Patterson and Smith, 1992) (see also Chapters 14 and 15 for further details). If the animal has significant skin, abdominal or thoracic injuries, splint placement may be contraindicated, in which case the animal should be strictly cage rested for 6 weeks.

Surgical management

Animals with compressive lesions or spinal instability should ideally undergo surgical decompression and stabilization as soon as possible. The surgical treatment of intervertebral disc disease (IVDD) is addressed in Chapters 16 and 22, that of Wobbler syndrome and atlantoaxial subluxation in Chapters 15 and 22, and that of spinal fractures and luxations in Chapters 15, 16 and 22.

Prognosis

Factors influencing the prognosis of the acutely paralysed animal include the nature of the underlying disease, the severity of the neurological signs, the duration of the signs and the resources of the owner.

Severity of neurological signs

Nociception in affected limbs is the single most important prognostic indicator of injury severity that can be obtained from the neurological examination. Nociception is tested by applying heavy pressure to the bones of the digits with large haemostatic forceps such that pressure is applied to the underlying periosteum. Nociception is present if the animal displays a conscious awareness of the stimulus rather than simply a reflex withdrawal of the limb (see Chapter 1). Typically, both the medial and lateral digits of each paralysed limb and the tail is tested. Lack of nociception implies functional spinal cord or peripheral nerve transection at the time of testing and provides useful prognostic information. As a general rule, animals with intact nociception have the potential to recover motor function if the underlying disease process can be prevented from progressing.

The prognosis for paraplegic animals that lack nociception in the pelvic limbs varies with the cause (Figure 20.10) and is generally worse with longer duration of the signs. It is unusual to be presented with a tetraplegic animal that lacks nociception as functional cervical spinal cord transection causes paralysis of the respiratory muscles. In addition, the sympathetic nervous system (SNS) is interrupted as it runs down the cervical spinal cord, resulting in

Disease	Prognosis for recovery
Acute intervertebral disc herniation	50–75% chance of recovery with surgery within 24 hours (Anderson *et al.*, 1991; Duval *et al.*, 1996; Scott and McKee, 1999; Olby *et al.*, 2003)
Spinal fracture/luxation	<5% with displaced vertebrae; <25% if no displacement (Olby *et al.*, 2003)
Fibrocartilaginous embolism	No information available. If no recovery of nociception within 2 weeks, prognosis is guarded
Haemorrhage (bleeding disorder for rodenticide)	Guarded
Neoplasia	Guarded

20.10 Prognosis for paraplegic animals with loss of pelvic limb nociception as a result of various diseases.

pronounced bradycardia. As a result, animals with extremely severe cervical spinal cord injuries die rapidly of hypoventilation and cardiac arrest.

Head trauma

Severe head trauma is associated with high mortality rates in humans and animals. Although there is no standard of care for head trauma in human medicine, a series of guidelines have been developed, centred around maintaining adequate cerebral perfusion (Brain Trauma Foundation, 2000, 2007). The appropriate therapy for head trauma patients remains controversial in veterinary medicine due to a lack of objective information. However, treatment of affected animals must be immediate to increase the chance of recovery to a level that is both functional and acceptable to the owner. Many dogs and cats can recover from severe brain injuries, if the systemic and neurological abnormalities that can be treated are identified early enough.

Aetiology

Common causes of head injuries in cats and dogs include road traffic accidents, falls, kicks, gunshot or pellet wounds, and bites from larger animals. Traumatic injuries to the brain may result from blunt or penetrating insults: most canine head trauma results from blunt vehicular injury, whilst most feline head trauma is associated with crush injury (Syring *et al.*, 2001).

Pathophysiology

Head trauma pathophysiology can be divided into primary and secondary injury. Primary injury to the brain cannot be reversed, occurs immediately and describes the physical disruption of brain tissue. This can be caused by contusions, haematomas, lacerations and diffuse axonal injury, leading to vasogenic oedema (Sande and West, 2010). The underlying vascular and cellular pathophysiology of head trauma is similar to that described for spinal cord trauma, but is complicated by elevations in intracranial pressure (ICP) (Figure 20.11). This secondary injury is delayed and progressive, potentially providing targets for treatment. In addition to excitatory neurotransmitter release, adenosine triphosphate (ATP) depletion resulting in cytotoxic oedema, intracellular calcium accumulation causing activation of the intracellular enzyme systems and oxygen radical production leading to lipid peroxidation, traumatic brain injury is associated with a marked inflammatory response (Ramlackhansingh *et al.*, 2011). The inflammatory response perpetuates secondary brain injury by inducing nitric oxide production and activating the arachidonic acid cascades. The secondary injury 'cascade' is exacerbated by systemic abnormalities in the patient, including hypotension, hypoxia, hypoglycaemia or hyperglycaemia, hypocapnia or hypercapnia, and hyperthermia (Sande and West, 2010).

Following head trauma, the volume of the brain tissue compartment increases, usually due to

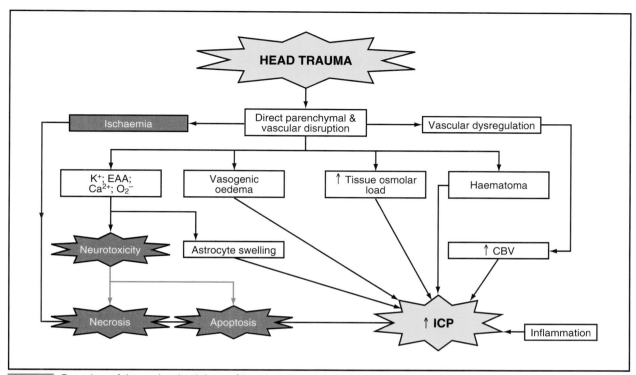

20.11 Overview of the pathophysiology of head trauma as it relates to the increase in intracranial pressure (ICP), showing the underlying vasculature and biochemical components of secondary injury. CBV = cerebral blood flow; EAA = excitatory amino acids.

oedema or haemorrhage (Bagley, 1996). As the brain tissue compartment increases, the CSF and blood compartments must decrease or ICP will increase (see Chapter 21). Compensation for increased brain tissue volume initially involves the translocation of CSF out of the skull; this is followed by decreased production of CSF and, eventually, decreased cerebral blood flow (Dewey, 2000). These compensatory mechanisms prevent an increase in ICP for an undetermined period. Once the ability for compensation is exhausted, a further small increase in intracranial volume results in dramatic elevations of ICP, with the immediate onset of clinical signs (see Chapter 21).

ICP is of enormous importance because of its effect on cerebral perfusion. Cerebral perfusion pressure is equal to systemic blood pressure minus ICP, and so elevations in ICP result in decreased perfusion of the brain (see Chapter 21). Thus, increases in ICP are often responsible for clinical decline after head trauma. Marked increases in ICP can trigger an ischaemic response or Cushing reflex: the increased pressure causes decreased cerebral blood flow leading to an elevation in carbon dioxide (CO_2) levels, which is detected at the vasomotor centre in the brainstem. A subsequent SNS response causes an elevation in mean arterial blood pressure detected by baroreceptors in the walls of the carotid arteries and aortic arch, resulting in reflex bradycardia. In addition to a drop in heart rate coupled with an elevated mean arterial blood pressure, other clinical manifestations of ICP elevation include anisocoria, miosis, mydriasis,

altered mentation and loss of motor function with the development of vertical nystagmus and extensor rigidity toward the end stages.

Patient assessment

Primary assessment
As with all types of acute injury, the 'ABC' (airway, breathing, circulation) of emergency care is extremely important (Figure 20.12). The initial physical assessment of the severely brain-injured patient focuses on imminently life-threatening abnormalities. The major parameters that need to be initially and continuously assessed are listed in Figure 20.13. It is important not to focus first on the neurological status of the patient, as many animals will be in a state of hypotensive shock following a head injury, which can exacerbate a depressed mentation. Hypotension and hypoxaemia need to be recognized and addressed immediately. In addition, a minimum essential database (including PCV, total protein level, blood urea level, glucose and electrolyte levels as well as urine specific gravity) should be performed. A continuous ECG evaluation is also recommended when monitoring head trauma patients (Haley *et al.*, 2010).

Respiratory system dysfunction can be common after head injury. The most dramatic respiratory abnormality seen following head injury is neurogenic pulmonary oedema. Neurogenic pulmonary oedema may result from sympathoadrenal overstimulation, causing marked peripheral vasoconstriction and increased venous return. This results

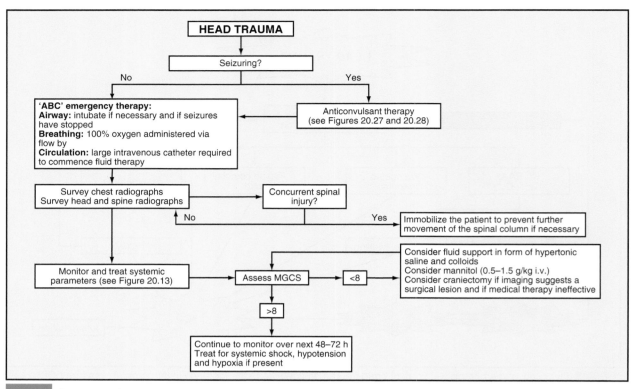

20.12 An approach to management of head trauma. MGCS = modified Glasgow coma score.

Monitoring parameter	Suggested goal	Suggested treatment
Neurological examination	Modified Glasgow coma score >15	Ensure head elevation (30 degrees); ensure all points below are addressed; consider mannitol (see text); consider surgery (see text)
Blood pressure	Mean arterial blood pressure 80–120 mmHg	Adjust fluid therapy; pressor support (dopamine 2–10 µg/kg)
Blood gases	P_aO_2 ≥80 mmHg P_aCO_2 <35–40 mmHg	Oxygen supplementation; consider mechanical ventilation
Pulse oximetry	S_pO_2 ≥95%	Oxygen supplementation; consider mechanical ventilation
Heart rate and rhythm	Avoid tachycardia and bradycardia; avoid arrhythmia	Adjust fluid therapy; treat for pain; express bladder frequently; address intracranial pressure; treat arrhythmias specifically
Central venous pressure	5–12 cmH$_2$O	Adjust fluid therapy
Respiratory rate and rhythm	10–25 breaths/min	Ventilate if necessary
Body temperature	37–38.5 °C	Passive warming or cooling; non-steroidal anti-inflammatory drugs if pyrexic
Electrolytes	(See laboratory normal values)	Adjust fluid therapy; supplement fluids accordingly
Blood glucose	4–6 mmol/l	Adjust fluid therapy; consider dextrose administration
Intracranial pressure	5–12 mmHg	Ensure head elevation (30 degrees); ensure all points above are addressed; consider mannitol (see text); consider surgery (see text)

20.13 The monitoring parameters and suggested goals of treatment for patients with head trauma. (Modified from Johnson and Murtaugh, 2000)

in an increased left ventricular afterload with a rise in pulmonary capillary hypertension, leading to oedema. The oedema is usually self-limiting (if the patient survives) and resolves in a matter of hours to days, but can cause severe dyspnoea, tachypnoea and hypoxaemia. Hypoxaemia exacerbates

the development of secondary tissue damage. Other causes of respiratory system dysfunction may include pneumothorax, haemothorax, rib fractures and pulmonary contusions. The patterns of ventilation seen with cerebral diseases such as head trauma are described in Chapter 9. Breathing patterns reflect lesion localization in humans, but to date there is no consensus regarding a clinical localizing value to specific breathing patterns in veterinary patients.

Secondary assessment

Once normotension, normovolaemia and appropriate oxygenation and ventilation are established (see below), the patient should be thoroughly assessed for traumatic injuries. These include skull, vertebral and long bone fractures, as well as splenic torsion and a ruptured bladder and ureters. The neurological examination, cranial imaging and ICP measurement can then be considered.

Neurological assessment

The neurological assessment should be repeated every 30–60 minutes in patients with severe head injuries to assess for deterioration and to monitor the efficacy of any therapies administered. This requires an objective mechanism to 'score' the patient so that logical treatment decisions can be made.

Modified Glasgow coma scoring system: In humans, traumatic brain injury is graded as mild, moderate or severe on the basis of an objective scoring system: the Glasgow coma scale (GCS). A modification of the GCS has been proposed for use in veterinary medicine (Shores, 1989) (Figure 20.14). The scoring system enables grading of the initial neurological status and serial monitoring of the patient. The modified scoring system incorporates three categories of the examination (level of consciousness; motor activity; brainstem reflexes), which are assigned a score from 1 to 6, providing a total score of 3 to 18. Such a system can facilitate assessment of prognosis (the higher the score, the better the prognosis; Figure 20.15), which is crucial information for both the veterinary surgeon and owner (Platt *et al.*, 2001).

Motor activity	Score
Normal gait, normal spinal reflexes	6
Hemiparesis, tetraparesis or decerebrate rigidity	5
Recumbent, intermittent extensor rigidity	4
Recumbent, constant extensor rigidity	3
Recumbent, constant extensor rigidity with opisthotonus	2
Recumbent, hypotonia of muscles, depressed or absent spinal reflexes	1
Brainstem reflexes	
Normal pupillary light reflexes and oculocephalic reflexes	6
Slow pupillary light reflexes and normal to reduced oculocephalic reflexes	5
Bilateral unresponsive miosis with normal to reduced oculocephalic reflexes	4

20.14 Modified Glasgow coma scale. (continues) ▶

Brainstem reflexes continued	
Pinpoint pupils with reduced to absent oculocephalic reflexes	3
Unilateral, unresponsive mydriasis with reduced to absent oculocephalic reflexes	2
Bilateral, unresponsive mydriasis with reduced to absent oculocephalic reflexes	1
Level of consciousness	
Occasional periods of alertness and responsive to environment	6
Depression or delirium, capable of responding but response may be inappropriate	5
Semi-comatose, responsive to visual stimuli	4
Semi-comatose, responsive to auditory stimuli	3
Semi-comatose, responsive only to repeated noxious stimuli	2
Comatose, unresponsive to repeated noxious stimuli	1

20.14 (continued) Modified Glasgow coma scale.

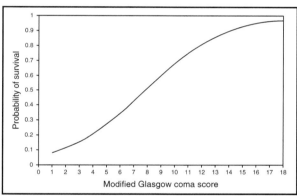

20.15 Probability of survival of the head trauma patient during the first 48 hours after admission, expressed as a function of the modified Glasgow coma score. (Reproduced from Platt *et al.*, 2001 with permission from the *Journal of Veterinary Internal Medicine*)

Diagnostic imaging

Radiography: Imaging of the patient's head is often indicated, especially in animals that fail to respond to aggressive medical therapy or deteriorate after an initial response. Skull radiographs are unlikely to reveal clinically useful information about the brain injury, but may occasionally reveal evidence of calvarial fractures (Figure 20.16). Cervical spinal radiography is also advised at the time of skull imaging to rule out concurrent spinal lesions (Olby *et al.*, 2001). As for spinal trauma, thoracic radiography helps to evaluate for evidence of thoracic and cardiac trauma.

Advanced imaging: CT is the preferred modality in cases of severe head injury associated with fractures.

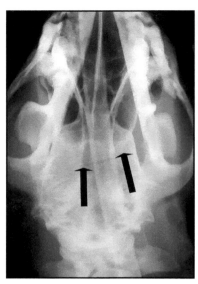

20.16
Dorsoventral skull radiograph of a 6-year-old Hungarian Vizla following an incident causing head trauma. Note the large linear calvarial fracture (arrowed). Such images do not provide any useful information about associated parenchymal damage or haematomas. (Courtesy of J Penderis)

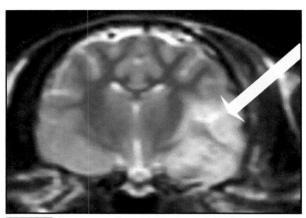

20.18 Transverse T2-weighted cranial MR image of a 1-year-old Domestic Shorthaired cat that was hit by a car. It is difficult to appreciate the damage to the calvaria on MRI but the associated parenchymal damage is visible (arrowed).

Even animals with 'mild' head trauma can exhibit abnormalities on CT, so the initial decision to image the patient's head should not be based on the neurological examination alone (Platt *et al.*, 2002). CT image acquisition time is faster and often less expensive than MRI, and CT also demonstrates bone detail better than MRI (Figure 20.17). However, MRI has been shown to provide key information relevant to the prognosis based upon its ability to detect subtle parenchymal damage not evident on CT (Figure 20.18). The detection of a midline parenchymal shift and ventricular obliteration on MR images are associated with a poor prognosis for survival based on one canine study (Platt *et al.*, 2007). Furthermore, intracranial lesions that may benefit from surgery (such as haematomas and pneumocephalus) can be accurately identified using advanced imaging (Haley and Abramson, 2009).

Intracranial pressure monitoring

Medical and surgical decisions based on ICP measurements rather than on gross neurological findings have decreased morbidity and mortality in human head trauma victims. ICP monitoring is a standard procedure for human head trauma management but has only recently been investigated in dogs and cats. Unfortunately, the extremely high cost of the fibreoptic system needed is likely to limit its use in veterinary medicine, but other systems may become available to enable ICP monitoring to be an integral part of head trauma management in dogs and cats (Figure 20.19). For example, transcranial Doppler ultrasonography can be used to measure the resistive index of blood flow in the basilar artery. This has been shown to be an indirect measure of ICP in dogs (Fukushima *et al.*, 2000) and to correlate with the severity of neurological signs in hydrocephalic dogs (Saito *et al.*, 2003).

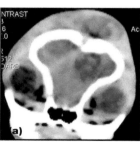
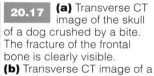
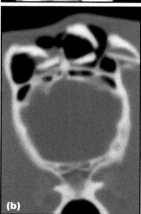

20.17 **(a)** Transverse CT image of the skull of a dog crushed by a bite. The fracture of the frontal bone is clearly visible. **(b)** Transverse CT image of a skull of a dog with a frontal sinus fracture. CT was advantageous in this case as it confirmed that the skull fracture did not affect the inner table of the frontal sinus and therefore had no notable effect on the brain.

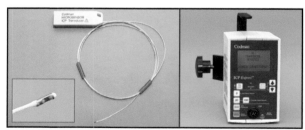

20.19 Intracranial pressure monitoring system with a fibreoptic catheter.

Urinary tract assessment

Urinary output should be monitored and if it is elevated (>2–3 ml/kg/h) for at least 2 consecutive hours, central diabetes insipidus should be considered, as it can result from severe damage to the hypothalamic area of the brain. The diagnosis is based upon the presence of high serum sodium as well as low urine sodium levels and low urine osmolality. Polyuria due to fluid overload, hyperglycaemia and therapeutic osmotic diuresis must be excluded. Oliguria (in the absence of hypovolaemia) may indicate inappropriate antidiuretic hormone secretion, if it is accompanied by hyponatraemia and an elevated urine sodium concentration; however, hypotension, pain and even stress can cause a similar situation.

Treatment

The most important factor with head injuries is maintenance of cerebral perfusion by treating the hypotension and elevated ICP. The considerations for management of head trauma cases are outlined in Figures 20.12 and 20.13. As well as ensuring adequate cerebral perfusion, head injury management is aimed at measures to prevent and limit the development of secondary nervous system damage.

Medical management

Minimizing increases in intracranial pressure:
Simple precautions can be taken in positioning the animal, with its head elevated at a 30-degree angle from the horizontal to maximize arterial supply to, and venous drainage from, the brain (Dewey, 2000). It is also important to ensure that there is no constrictive collar obstructing the jugular veins, as this would immediately elevate ICP.

Fluid therapy: The basic goal of fluid management in head trauma cases is to maintain a normovolaemic to slightly hypervolaemic state to ensure an adequate cerebral perfusion pressure. There is no support for attempting to dehydrate the patient in an attempt to reduce cerebral oedema and this is now recognized to be deleterious to cerebral metabolism. In contrast, immediate restoration of blood volume is imperative to ensure normotension and adequate cerebral perfusion pressure (see Chapter 21).

Initial resuscitation usually involves intravenous administration of hypertonic saline and/or synthetic colloids (Figure 20.20). Use of these solutions allows rapid restoration of blood volume and pressure whilst limiting the volume of fluid administered. In contrast, crystalloids extravasate into the interstitium within an hour of administration and thus larger volumes are required for restoration of blood volume. This could lead to exacerbation of oedema in head trauma patients, although the benefits

obtained by restoring the cerebral perfusion pressure with any type of fluid initially outweigh this potential risk. If isotonic crystalloids are chosen for administration (appropriate in mild head trauma), an aliquot of the shock dose (90 ml/kg in the dog and 60 ml/kg in the cat) can be given rapidly and repeated until improved tissue perfusion is achieved. Improved perfusion is evident based upon normal heart rate, mucous membrane colour, capillary refill time and blood pressure (Syring, 2005).

Hypertonic saline administration (4–5 ml/kg i.v. over 2–5 minutes; 4 ml/kg of 7.5% or 5.3 ml/kg of 3% solution) draws fluid from the interstitial and intracellular spaces into the intravascular space, which improves systemic blood pressure and cerebral blood pressure and flow, with a subsequent decrease in ICP (Proulx and Dhupa, 1998; Qureshi et al., 2002). Hypertonic saline solutions have also been shown to decrease brain excitotoxicity by promoting re-uptake of glutamate into the intracellular space (Doyle et al., 2001). However, this should be avoided in the presence of systemic dehydration or hypernatraemia and it should be noted that the volume expansion effects of this fluid only last between 15 and 75 minutes (Sande and West, 2010), although the beneficial effects on ICP are maintained far longer (Qureshi and Suarez, 2000). Hypertonic solutions act to dehydrate the tissues; thus it is essential that crystalloid solutions are subsequently administered (at a rate to account for the patient's maintenance demands and insensible losses) to ensure that systemic dehydration does not occur. In addition, hypertonic saline may aggravate pulmonary oedema or contusion in patients, with underlying cardiac or respiratory pathology which should be considered in the polytrauma case.

Colloid solutions can be administered after hypertonic saline to maintain the intravascular volume, possibly due to the retention of fluids within the intravascular compartments maintaining an intravascular oncotic gradient (Qureshi and Suarez, 2000). The sole use of colloids does not prevent dehydration. In addition, the co-administration of hypertonic solutions and colloids is more effective at restoring blood volume than either alone. A total dose of 4 ml/kg of a 1:2 combination of 23.4% hypertonic saline with 6% Hetastarch has been recommended (Sande and West, 2010).

Osmotic diuretics: Osmotic diuretics are very useful in the treatment of intracranial hypertension. Many studies confirm that hypertonic saline (see above) is superior to the effects of another potent osmotic diuretic, mannitol, in reducing ICP and doing so for a more sustained period of time (Qureshi et al., 1999; Battison et al., 2005). However, the use of mannitol is recommended once the vascular volume has been stabilized. Mannitol has an immediate plasma-expanding effect that reduces blood viscosity, leading to increased cerebral blood flow and oxygen delivery. This results in vasoconstriction within a few minutes, causing an almost immediate decrease in ICP. The better known osmotic effect of mannitol reverses the blood–brain osmotic gradient, thereby reducing

Fluid	Half-life (hours)	Average molecular weight (Daltons)	Dose
Oxypolygelatin	2.5	30,000	Maximum daily dose 20 ml/kg Rates: Dog: up to 10–20 ml/kg/h Cat: up to 5–10 ml/kg/h (preferably with CVP monitoring to ensure volume overload does not occur)
Succinylated gelatin	2–4	35,000	
Pentastarch	2.5	280,000	
Hetastarch	25	450,000	
Dextran 40	2.5	40,000	
Dextran 70	25	70,000	

20.20 Colloid type, characteristics and dose for use in the head trauma patient.

extracellular fluid volume in both normal and damaged brain tissue.

Mannitol should be administered as a bolus over a 15-minute period (rather than as an infusion) in order to obtain the plasma-expanding effect; its effect on brain oedema takes approximately 15–30 minutes to establish and lasts between 2 and 8 hours (Dewey, 2000; Sande and West, 2010). Doses of 0.5–1.5 g/kg appear to be equally effective in lowering ICP, but the duration of effect is shorter with lower doses. Repeated administration of mannitol can cause an accompanying diuresis, which may result in volume contraction, intracellular dehydration and the concomitant risk of hypotension and ischaemia. It is therefore recommended that mannitol is reserved for the critical patient (GCS <8) or the deteriorating patient. There has been no clinical evidence to prove the theory that mannitol is contraindicated in the presence of intracranial haemorrhage, which has been a frequently raised concern. The concept of reverse osmotic shift has also been reported as a drawback of mannitol treatment. This process may occur with repeated bolus administrations of mannitol, whereby the extravascular accumulations can lead to brain oedema. The risk of this process has been reported to be low when mannitol is used at appropriate doses (Sande and West, 2010).

There is evidence that the combination of mannitol with furosemide (0.7 mg/kg) may lower ICP in a synergistic fashion, especially if furosemide is given first (Bagley 1996); however, recent work disputes the additive effect of administering furosemide and so it is no longer recommended for the treatment of traumatic brain injury (Brain Trauma Foundation, 2007).

Oxygenation and ventilation: Oxygen supplementation is recommended for most animals with acute brain injuries. The partial pressure of oxygen in the arterial blood (P_aO_2) should be maintained as close to normal as possible (≥80 mmHg). Other monitoring parameters include respiratory rate and depth, mucous membrane and tongue colour, and thoracic auscultation. Pulse oximetry is one method for determining oxygenation status. Oxyhaemoglobin saturation (S_pO_2) values from pulse oximeters >95% are considered normal and reflect a P_aO_2 of at least 80 mmHg (Sande and West, 2010). An S_pO_2 value <89% (P_aO_2 <60 mmHg) is compatible with a serious degree of hypoxaemia.

Supplemental oxygen should be administered initially via flow by, as oxygen cages are usually ineffective because constant monitoring of the patient does not allow for a closed system. As soon as possible, nasal oxygen catheters or transtracheal oxygen catheters should be used to supply a 40% inspired oxygen concentration with flow rates of 100 ml/kg/min or 50 ml/kg/min, respectively. The method of oxygen delivery must be tolerable to the patient to avoid stress or anxiety causing an increase in ICP. If the patient is in a coma, immediate intubation and ventilation may be needed if this is indicated by blood gas measurements. A tracheostomy tube may be warranted in some patients for assisted ventilation (Dewey, 2000).

Hyperventilation has traditionally been known as a means of lowering abnormally high ICP through a hypocapnic cerebral vasoconstrictive effect. However, hyperventilation is a 'double-edged sword'. Besides reducing the ICP, it induces potentially detrimental reductions in the cerebral circulation if the P_aCO_2 level is <30–35 mmHg. The major difficulty with hyperventilation is the inability to monitor the presence and effects of ischaemia on the brain. It is important that animals do not hypoventilate, and such animals should be ventilated to maintain a P_aCO_2 of 30–40 mmHg. Aggressive hyperventilation can be used for short periods in deteriorating or critical animals. In intubated patients end-tidal CO_2 measurement is a useful tool but can underestimate the actual P_aCO_2 level.

Arterial blood pressure support: The presence of arterial hypotension despite fluid resuscitation may require administration of vasoactive agents such as dopamine (2–10 µg/kg/min i.v.). Conversely, arterial hypertensive episodes ('Cushing's response') may be managed with calcium channel blockers such as amlodipine (0.625–1.25 mg/cat orally q24h; 0.05–0.1 mg/kg orally q24h in dogs). However, the authors recommend treating increased ICP aggressively before using drugs to assist blood pressure regulation.

Ancillary treatment

Seizure prophylaxis: Although the role of prophylactic anticonvulsants in preventing post-traumatic epileptic disorders remains unclear, seizure activity greatly exacerbates intracranial hypertension in the head injury patient. For this reason, it is recommended that all seizure activity in these patients should be treated aggressively. As most cases need to be treated parenterally, diazepam (0.5–2.0 mg/kg i.v.), phenobarbital (2 mg/kg i.m. or i.v. q6–8h) or levetiracetam (20–60 mg/kg i.m. or i.v q8h) is recommended. Oral phenobarbital or levetiracetam can be continued for 3–6 months following the trauma and can then be slowly tapered off if there have been no further seizures. Phenobarbital has the additional benefit of reducing cerebral metabolic demands and therefore acts as a cerebral protectant, but the clinician should be cautious of the sedative and respiratory depression side effects with these drugs.

Corticosteroids: These have been studied extensively in cases of head injury. Human clinical trials have not shown a beneficial effect of corticosteroids, including MPSS, in the treatment of head injury. In addition, they have been associated with an increased risk of infection, are immunosuppressive, cause hyperglycaemia leading to cerebral acidosis, and have other significant effects on metabolism. Their use is not recommended.

Nutritional support and glycaemic control: Nutritional support is essential as brain injury results in a hypermetabolic and catabolic state. The metabolic changes in these patients are in part attributable to an increase in cytokines and counter-regulatory hormones including cortisol, adrenaline (epinephrine), noradrenaline (norepinephrine) and glucagon (Vizzini and Aranda-Michel, 2011). Such support has been shown to improve the neurological recovery, as well as shorten the time to recovery, as long as it is initiated within 72 hours following the head injury. On a short-term basis, a nasogastric tube can be used to deliver peptide-rich compounds. Caution should be used when placing and maintaining these tubes as they may cause sneezing, which can elevate ICP. For medium- to long-term management, pharyngostomy or oeso-phagostomy tubes should be used. If there is brain-stem damage, a gastrostomy tube should be inserted in case there is poor oesophageal function.

Care should be taken to avoid hyperglycaemia, which may promote cerebral acidosis in brain-damaged individuals (Johnson and Murtaugh, 2000). Hyperglycaemia has been associated with increased mortality and morbidity in humans and animals with head trauma. It has been associated with the severity of head trauma in dogs and cats (Syring *et al.*, 2001), although not with outcome. However, whether hyperglycaemia represents severe brain injury or is the cause of a worse secondary injury is a contentious issue in the human literature. Hyperglycaemia results from a sympathoadrenal response to the trauma and so could just be a consequence of the injury to the brain. However, hyperglycaemia is known to potentiate neurological injury, increase free-radical production, glutamate release and cerebral oedema, and alter the cerebral vasculature (Sande and West, 2010).

Hypothermia: This was thought to decrease the metabolic demands of the brain, but it is currently thought to be beneficial for the reduction of glutamate and inhibition of the post-traumatic inflammatory response (Schreckinger and Marion, 2009). Human patients cooled to 32–34°C (using cooling blankets and nasogastric lavage with iced saline for 24–48 hours) have demonstrated variable outcomes. A large meta-analysis concluded that hypothermic therapy constitutes a beneficial treatment in some head trauma cases (Peterson *et al.*, 2008). However, the recent National Acute Brain Injury Study did not confirm the utility of hypothermia as a primary neuroprotective strategy in patients with severe traumatic brain injury (Clifton *et al.*, 2011). As such, hypothermia is recommended with reservations in the most current Brain Trauma Foundation guidelines (Brain Trauma Foundation, 2007). The use of hypothermia has been documented recently in a veterinary case with head trauma (Hayes, 2009); however, at this time, the use of hypothermia in veterinary brain trauma cases cannot be advocated as a routine therapy.

Pain management: Pain control may be essential in the head trauma patient, particularly if there are other systems involved and musculoskeletal injuries. Appropriate pain relief may also help reduce the

ICP. Although opioids are associated with respiratory depression and hypotension, they are safe first-line analgesics if titrated to effect. Fentanyl can be administered as a constant rate infusion (CRI: 2–6 µg/kg/h), which keeps the analgesia consistent (Sande and West, 2010). Butorphanol can also be considered for these patients as it causes less respiratory and cardiovascular depression, although it may need to be repeated every 2 hours. For further information on analgesia, the reader is directed to Chapter 21.

Barbiturates: These drugs can lower the energy requirement of the brain, decreasing oxygen demand and effectively resulting in decreased blood flow to the brain, in turn reducing the ICP. However, the use of these drugs to induce comas in humans has been associated with poor outcomes, although it is documented to be of benefit when used as a last resort measure. The Brain Trauma Foundation recommends the use of high-dose barbiturates to control elevated ICP refractory to maximum standard medical and surgical treatment as long as haemo-dynamic stability has been attained (Brain Trauma Foundation, 2007). There are no reports of this therapy in veterinary medicine and as such it cannot currently be recommended as a routine approach.

Progesterone: Current clinical evidence in human medicine indicates that progesterone may improve the neurological outcome of patients suffering from traumatic brain injuries (Junpeng *et al.*, 2011). Progesterone and its metabolites have demonstrated neuroprotective properties in a variety of brain injury models. It is now well documented that neurosteroids have neurotrophic, anti-inflammatory and anti-apoptotic properties, all of which contribute to reducing the extent of injury and preserving neural and vascular integrity early in the injury cascade that inevitably accompanies traumatic brain injury (Stein, 2011). Progesterone has been shown to reduce both vasogenic and cytotoxic oedema following traumatic brain injury, although the mechanisms by which this happens are unclear. No treatment recommendations currently exist in veterinary medicine and it must be noted that synthetic and proprietary hormones such as medroxyprogesterone acetate may have different effects from those of natural progesterone in post-injury treatment (Stein, 2008).

Hyperbaric oxygen therapy: Recent studies have suggested that hyperbaric oxygen therapy may have a role in the treatment of brain injury (Lin *et al.*, 2008; Meyer *et al.*, 2010). In a hyperbaric oxygen environment (Figure 20.21), several physiological effects have been described, including improved oxygenation, vasoconstriction (resulting in reduced vasogenic oedema), modulation of inflammation, immune function and angiogenesis (Edwards, 2010). Post-trauma, the only recognized contra-indication for hyperbaric oxygen therapy is pneumothorax. This type of treatment is in its infancy in veterinary medicine and supportive evidence for

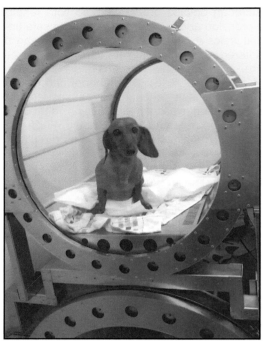

20.21 A Daschund receiving postoperative treatment inside a hyperbaric chamber.

its role in head trauma is lacking, although it has a promising potential.

Surgical management

A description of the surgical techniques for intracranial surgery can be found elsewhere. Although it is rare that surgery is indicated in head injury cases, there are several specific abnormalities that can be associated with an episode of head trauma which may warrant the consideration of surgical treatment.

Calvarial fractures: A skull fracture *per se* may have significant implications for patient management. Skull fractures are typically differentiated based upon:

* Pattern (depressed, comminuted, linear) (Figure 20.22)
* Location
* Type (open, closed).

A fracture is generally classed as depressed if the inner table of the bone is driven in to a depth equivalent to the width of the skull. All but the most contaminated, comminuted and cosmetically deforming depressed fractures can be managed without surgical intervention (Figure 20.23).

Acute extra-axial haematomas: Generous craniotomies are generally indicated once these abnormalities have been diagnosed with imaging (Dewey *et al.*, 1993). If the haematoma is due to a fracture across a venous sinus, there may be profuse bleeding associated with surgical intervention. The need for blood transfusions should be expected. Haematoma removal also increases the risk of bleeding from previously compressed vessels.

Acute intraparenchymal haematomas: In contrast to acute extra-axial haematomas, acute intraparenchymal clots may be managed medically, unless subacute enlargement of initially small intraparenchymal clots is identified with repeat imaging.

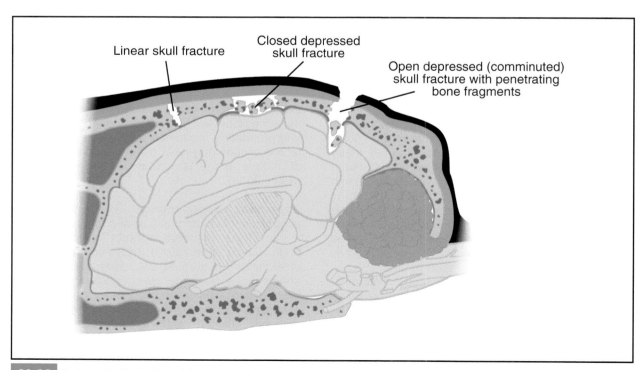

Linear skull fracture

Closed depressed skull fracture

Open depressed (comminuted) skull fracture with penetrating bone fragments

20.22 Schematic illustration of three categories of skull fracture.

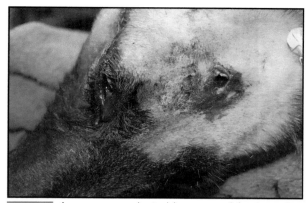

20.23 An open comminuted (compound) fracture of the skull can be seen in this German Shepherd Dog, which had been kicked in the head by a horse.

Haemorrhagic parenchymal contusions: Most haemorrhagic contusions do not require surgical management. The main indication for surgery with these types of lesions is limited to cerebellar contusions with compression of the fourth ventricle and brainstem. The aims of surgery are to reduce the potential for further compression and herniation, which can develop over the initial 24–48 hours following surgery.

Intracranial hypertension: Benefit can be found when decompressive procedures (craniectomy and durectomy) are performed prior to the development of irreversible bilateral pupillary dilatation (Bagley, 1996). However, 'prophylactic' decompressive surgery seems inappropriate before non-surgical management of elevated intracranial hypertension has been carefully maximized. Although there are currently no veterinary studies on this topic, a randomized controlled decompressive craniectomy (DECRA) trial testing the efficacy bifrontotemporoparietal decompressive craniectomy has been reported recently in humans (Cooper *et al.*, 2011). Although patients undergoing this surgery had lower ICP, there was no effect on the 6-month mortality rate. The 2006 Cochrane review of humans with head trauma found that decompressive craniectomy reduced the risk of death and unfavourable outcome in paediatric patients, but no evidence was found to support its use in adults (Sahuquillo and Arikan, 2006).

Status epilepticus and cluster seizures

Status epilepticus (SE) can be defined as continuous seizure activity lasting for 30 minutes or longer, or repeated seizures with failure to return to normality within 30 minutes (Engel, 1989). This definition is based upon the time after which there are serious changes in brain metabolism and function. A more practical 'operational' definition of SE is continuous or repeated seizure activity for more than 5 minutes without recovery of consciousness (Alldredge *et al.*, 2001). Cluster seizures describe the occurrence of multiple seizure events (usually >3) within a 24-hour period.

SE and severe cluster seizures can cause permanent neurological sequelae or even death. Immediate treatment is necessary. There is some evidence to suggest that early aggressive treatment of prolonged seizures results in their termination, with smaller doses of medication and less overall risk to the patient than would be incurred by delaying therapy. In humans, a seizure duration of >1 hour has been associated with a mortality rate of 32–39% compared with a mortality rate of 2.7% for a seizure duration of <1 hour (Neligan and Shorvon, 2011). In addition, profound haemodynamic and metabolic abnormalities commonly occur during seizures and may cause significant morbidity despite appropriate treatment of the seizures. Management of SE requires a prompt, comprehensive and dynamic approach and should be individualized, depending on the clinical status of the animal (Boothe, 1998) (Figure 20.24).

Aetiology
The causes of SE are listed in Figure 20.25.

The prevalence of SE in a veterinary referral hospital has been estimated to be up to 0.7% of all cases (Bateman and Parent, 1999). SE can occur as the first seizure in 44–58% of dogs without any prior history (Platt and Haag, 2002). Risk factors for SE and cluster seizures in veterinary patients are not well documented; however, increased bodyweight has been established as a significant variable between dogs that have SE and those that do not (Saito *et al.*, 2001). In addition, neutered females and German Shepherd Dogs have been shown to have an increased risk of developing SE (Zimmermann *et al.*, 2009).

Studies evaluating SE and cluster seizures in dogs admitted to hospital have not revealed a specific cause for the seizures in 25–28% of cases (Bateman and Parent, 1999; Platt and Haag, 2002). Approximately 28–37.5% of cases are diagnosed with primary (genetic or idiopathic) epilepsy. Up to 59% of dogs with primary epilepsy experience at least one episode of SE during their life (Hulsmeyer *et al.*, 2010). Secondary or symptomatic epilepsy (dogs with an identifiable structural cause within the brain) causes seizures in 32–40% of cases (Podell *et al.*, 1995), whilst reactive epileptic seizures are seen in 7–22% of cases (Zimmermann *et al.*, 2009). However, reactive epileptic seizures were reported as being responsible for up to 50% of SE cases in one study (Gandini *et al.*, 2003). When individual causes are separated out from these three broad classifications, it appears that toxicity is the most significant risk factor for developing SE, particularly in dogs without any prior history of seizures (Zimmermann *et al.*, 2009).

Chronic processes that cause SE include preexisting epilepsy, in which SE is caused by breakthrough seizures or the discontinuation of antiepileptic drugs. CSF abnormalities have been documented in up to 73.5% of dogs with either SE or cluster seizures, and neuroimaging (MRI or CT)

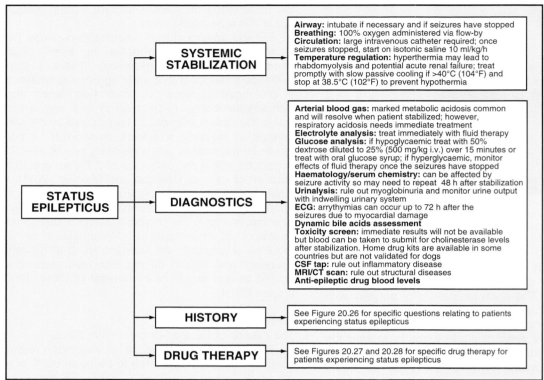

Approach to systemic stabilization and management of the status epilepticus patient.

Class of epilepsy	Mechanism of disease	Specific diseases
Primary	Idiopathic	Breed-related; familial
Secondary	Degenerative	Storage diseases
	Anomalous	Hydrocephalus
	Neoplasia (primary or metastatic)	Meningioma; glial cell tumour; choroid plexus papilloma; lymphoma
	Inflammatory: infectious	Viral; rickettsial; bacterial; fungal; parasitic
	Inflammatory: sterile	Granulomatous meningoencephalitis; breed-specific encephalitides
	Trauma	Acute; chronic
	Vascular	Infarction; haemorrhage
Reactive seizures	Metabolic	Hepatic encephalopathy; hypoglycaemia; hypocalcaemia; electrolyte imbalances
	Toxic	Organophosphate; lead; metaldehyde
Other	Low anticonvulsant concentrations	

20.25 Classification and causes of status epilepticus.

can be abnormal in up to 46% of SE cases (Platt and Haag, 2002). The survival time of dogs with SE differs between the aetiological groups, with secondary or symptomatic epilepsy cases having a shorter survival time than dogs with idiopathic and reactive epilepsy (Zimmermann *et al.*, 2009).

Pathophysiology

The emergence of SE requires a 'pool' of neurons capable of initiating and sustaining abnormal firing. This abnormal discharge is facilitated by the loss of inhibitory synaptic transmission mediated by gamma-amino butyric acid (GABA) and sustained by excitatory transmission mediated by glutamate. The abnormal neuronal discharges, together with increased cerebral and muscle blood flow and metabolism, mediate the acute pathophysiological changes. During the early stages of SE, the seizures can be accompanied by increased autonomic discharge, the systemic manifestations of which include tachycardia, hypertension and hyperglycaemia. After approximately 30 minutes, physiological deterioration can ensue, with the patient developing hypotension, hypoglycaemia, hyperthermia and hypoxia (Russo, 1981). Incessant skeletal muscle contractions and impaired ventilation may lead to lactic acidosis, hyperkalaemia, hypoxia, hypercarbia and hyperthermia. In addition, severe myoglobinuria (resulting from hyperthermia-induced rhabdomyolysis) may cause impairment of renal function, especially when accompanied by systemic hypotension.

Treatment

Guidelines for the management of SE are outlined in Figure 20.24. A team approach to patients in SE is beneficial in accomplishing emergency stabilization, therapeutic intervention and diagnostic investigation simultaneously. Although immediate anticonvulsant therapy and systemic stabilization are warranted, concurrent history-taking (Figure 20.26), physical examination and diagnostic tests may also be useful.

1. When did the episode start?
2. Is there a pre-existing seizure disorder?
3. Has the patient had status epilepticus or cluster seizure events before?
4. Have there been any systemic health problems within the last 4 months?
5. Has there been any change in the patient's personality or behaviour within the last 4 months?
6. Is the patient on any medication, including anticonvulsant therapy?
7. Which anticonvulsants are being given; what is the dose; when was the last dose?
8. How long has the patient been on anticonvulsants?
9. Have recent serum anticonvulsant measurements been performed?
10. Is there any recent trauma, travel history or toxin exposure?
11. Has the patient eaten a meal within the last few hours?

20.26 Important questions to ask about the patient in status epilepticus.

Systemic stabilization

The initial care of a patient in SE involves basic medical emergency measures ('ABC': airway, breathing, circulation) but also includes oxygenation, attention to electrolyte, glucose and BUN levels and acid–base status, obtaining intravenous access, and temperature regulation (see Figure 20.13). In patients with pre-existing seizures that are already on antiepileptic drugs, blood samples for drug level measurement should be taken at the initial evaluation.

Drug treatment regimens for initial management

Due to the relative lack of objective information to guide veterinary surgeons in the choice of the optimal treatment regimen, a wide range of treatment practices has been adopted. Recommendations are outlined in Figure 20.27.

Benzodiazepines: These drugs (e.g. diazepam) are potent, fast-acting anticonvulsants and the preferred initial therapy for SE (Boothe, 1998). Braund (2003) recommends the use of 0.5–2.0 mg/kg i.v., up to a maximum dose of 20 mg, in dogs and cats. This dose can be repeated to effect two or three times (see Figure 20.27). Probably the most common and dangerous error made in the management of SE is to treat repeated seizures with repeated doses of intravenous diazepam without administering an adequate loading dose of a longer-acting antiepileptic drug. Rectal administration of diazepam may be considered at a dose of 0.5–2.0 mg/kg (Wagner *et al.*, 1998). It may be necessary to use the higher dose in dogs receiving long-term phenobarbital therapy.

Intranasal or buccal instillation of benzodiazepines is widely used in human SE, particularly for at-home treatment. Intranasal diazepam and a novel intranasal midazolam gel formulation have been pharmacokinetically evaluated in dogs (Platt *et al.*,

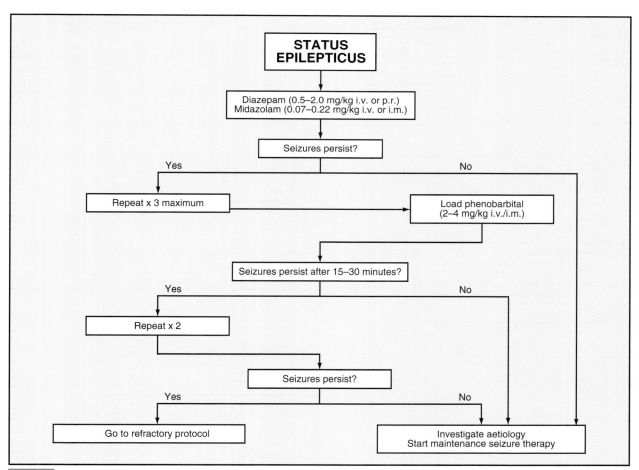

20.27 Approach to the initial pharmacological management of the status epilepticus patient.

2000; Eagleson *et al.*, 2012). This type of administration results in a faster attainment of peak plasma levels and greater bioavailability than that seen with rectal administration. There is a reasonable evidence base supporting the use of buccal midazolam in human SE, stopping seizure activity in half the time compared with rectal dosing (Shorvon, 2011). A midazolam maleate preparation specifically indicated for buccal administration in human SE is marketed in Europe.

Phenobarbital: This is a safe, inexpensive drug that may be administered orally, intravenously or intramuscularly. Distribution of phenobarbital to the CNS may take up to 30 minutes (Boothe, 1998). The recommended dose can initially be 2–4 mg/kg i.v., repeated every 20–30 minutes to effect, to a maximum total 24-hour dose of 24 mg/kg (see Figure 20.28). The parenteral form can also be given by the intramuscular route, which is recommended if diazepam has already been administered. This may avoid the potentiation of profound respiratory and cardiovascular depression.

Drug treatment regimen for refractory patients
SE that does not respond to a benzodiazepine or phenobarbital is considered refractory and requires more aggressive treatment. Potential reasons for resistant seizure activity include inadequate anti-convulsant doses, an uncorrected metabolic abnormality, a cerebral mass (such as a tumour) or encephalitis (e.g. Pug dog encephalitis). If the seizure activity can be stopped for 12 hours with one of the approaches below, none of which has been prospectively evaluated in veterinary medicine, drug doses can be gradually reduced over a further 12 hours. If seizures recur then this cycle may need to be repeated.

Levetiracetam: This is an effective oral maintenance anticonvulsant in dogs with minimal side effects (Volk *et al.*, 2008; see Chapter 8 for further details). Parenteral levetiracetam is well tolerated and appears safe following intramuscular and intravenous administration in dogs (20 mg/kg). In one study, the half-life of the drug was determined to be approximately 3 hours and the mean time to peak concentration following intramuscular injection was 40 minutes (Patterson *et al.*, 2008). This drug can be administered repeatedly up to 60 mg/kg q8h, with the only side effect noted being sedation. If seizures can be controlled using parenteral levetiracetam, oral maintenance therapy with the same drug can be continued. In humans this drug has been shown to be an effective adjunctive treatment for SE, especially when given early on in the course of the seizures (Aiguabella *et al.*, 2011). A prospective double-blinded placebo-controlled study of

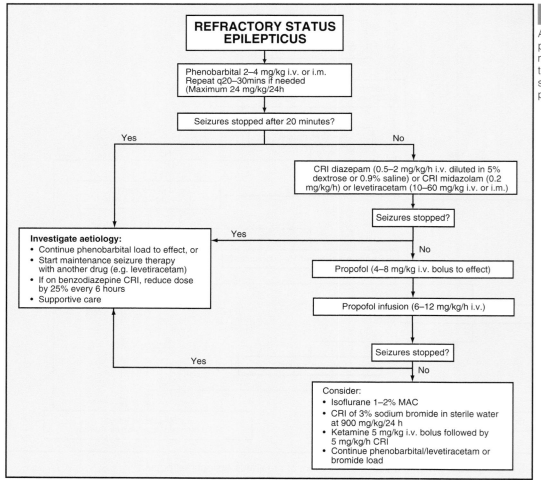

20.28 Approach to the pharmacological management of the refractory status epilepticus patient.

intravenous levetiracetam for SE in dogs is under way and early results show promise (Leppik *et al.*, 2009).

Propofol: This has barbiturate- and benzodiazepine-like effects and can suppress CNS metabolic activity. Propofol can be administered by intravenous bolus (4–8 mg/kg, to effect) or by constant rate infusion (0.1–0.6 mg/kg/min or 6–12 mg/kg/h) (Heldmann *et al.*, 1999). However, this drug should be used with caution, preferably in settings where definitive airway control and haemodynamic support are possible, as hypoxaemia secondary to apnoea is a primary side effect, as is myocardial depression. The use of propofol has been a matter of controversy in both human and veterinary medicine because of the documented anticonvulsive and proconvulsive effects. However, the use of propofol in combination with phenobarbital has been described in dogs for the successful treatment of SE (Gommeren *et al.*, 2010).

Benzodiazepines: A CRI of benzodiazepines such as diazepam and midazolam can be useful to induce sedation or anaesthesia in a patient that requires time for the longer acting anticonvulsants to take effect (e.g. phenobarbital) or to metabolize systemic toxicities. This has been shown to be an effective mode of therapy for refractory SE in both human and veterinary patients (Singhi *et al.*, 1998). In one study, diazepam was administered as a CRI in 124 of 186 (66.8%) dogs with severe seizures (Bateman and Parent, 1999); however, the efficacy of this treatment could not be determined. The authors stated that continuous infusions of diazepam may be underused in the management of dogs with seizures. The dose should be calculated hourly (0.1–0.5 mg/kg/h) and is usually diluted in saline in 5% dextrose in water (D5W). The volume used is equal to the maintenance fluid requirement over the hour and can be delivered with an infusion pump. There is some concern regarding the infusion of diazepam because of its poor aqueous solubility, formation of a deposit and absorption on polyvinyl chloride. Midazolam is completely water-soluble and has been shown to be an effective and safe therapeutic approach in paediatric cases of SE but has not been evaluated in veterinary medicine. If the seizures stop when using a CRI, the infusion can be decreased by 25% every 6 hours.

Barbiturates: Thiopental and pentobarbital have potential, although unproven, cerebral protective effects in the management of SE. These drugs almost always control the physical manifestations of seizures but with negligible anticonvulsant properties. Pentobarbital should be given to effect rather than at a specific dose (2–15 mg/kg i.v.) as there is tremendous individual variation in response (Indrieri, 1989). The limited worldwide availability of a sterile pentobarbital preparation has now reduced the potential of this option, with other methods being preferred to induce an anaesthetic coma.

Inhalational anaesthetics: These are recommended only as a last resort in cases of resistant SE (Platt and McDonnell, 2000). Isoflurane, an inhalational general anaesthetic agent, may be efficacious in the treatment of resistant SE but may need to be used for an extensive period of time. Isoflurane decreases the synchronization of neuronal activity, mainly through enhancing GABAergic inhibition by influencing chloride conductance. In addition, isoflurane therapy necessitates ventilation and intensive care monitoring, and hypotension may occur during therapy.

Bromide: A small study on the use of loading doses of potassium bromide administered intrarectally (100 mg/kg q4h for 24 hours) indicates that this drug is both well absorbed and safe when used in this manner (Dewey *et al.*, 1999). The clinical effect of this regimen has yet to be evaluated. Sodium bromide can be administered intravenously and a CRI of a 3% solution mixed in sterile water can be successful for the treatment of refractory SE when used at a dose of 900 mg/kg over 24 hours. Sedation is the major side effect expected and oral maintenance therapy should be considered in most patients once the 24-hour infusion is complete (see Chapter 8 for further details).

Ketamine: Experimental studies have indicated that *N*-methyl-D-aspartate (NMDA) glutamate receptor antagonists (e.g. ketamine) may be used to treat the condition self-sustaining status epilepticus (SSSE). This type of SE exists after approximately 10 minutes to 1 hour and may have a different underlying pathophysiology to the initial SE, in that the NMDA receptors may be over-stimulated by the excessive glutamate concentrations. Ketamine has been used in humans with refractory SE or SSSE and has been shown to be effective in a dog with SSSE when administered at a dose of 5 mg/kg i.v. followed by a CRI of 5 mg/kg/h (Serrano *et al.*, 2006).

Fosphenytoin: Fosphenytoin sodium is a phosphate ester prodrug of phenytoin, developed as a refinement of parenteral phenytoin (Morton *et al.*, 1997). Following administration, phenytoin is cleaved from the prodrug by phosphatases in the blood and several other organs. However, fosphenytoin is freely soluble in aqueous solutions and is rapidly absorbed by the intramuscular route. Recent work has evaluated the pharmacokinetics and tolerability of this drug in dogs when given intravenously, although no specific data exist on its efficacy for the treatment of SE in veterinary medicine (Craft 2011). If this drug proves to be efficacious, its main drawbacks may be the associated sedation and cardiorespiratory depression.

Lacosamide: This is a new anticonvulsant for seizure control in humans, which is available as an intravenous preparation and was initially developed for use in SE (Shorvon, 2011). Lacosamide selectively enhances slow inactivation of voltage-gated sodium channels without affecting fast inactivation.

It did not inhibit or induce a wide variety of cytochrome P450 enzymes at therapeutic concentrations in experimental animals. In safety pharmacology and toxicology studies conducted in dogs lacosamide was well tolerated (Beyreuther *et al.*, 2007). Either none or only minor side effects were observed in safety studies involving the CNS, respiratory, gastrointestinal and renal systems. Repeated dose toxicity studies demonstrated that following either intravenous or oral administration of lacosamide, the adverse events were reversible and consisted mostly of exaggerated pharmacodynamic effects on the CNS. Although the drug shows considerable promise in human clinical trials, there are no clinical data available as yet in veterinary medicine.

Electroencephalography

Five phases of electroencephalogram (EEG) pattern have been described in the temporal evolution of true SE, although they may not all be present in one patient (Nandhagopal, 2006). These include:

- Intermittent discrete seizure discharges with interictal background slowing
- Waxing and waning of seizure discharges
- Continuous discharges ± intervening flat periods
- Periodic epileptiform discharges.

Continuous monitoring serves as a useful guide for the titration of anticonvulsants beyond the cessation of clinical SE, to ensure that the EEG patterns indicating continued subclinical SE or non-convulsive SE are not present. Non-convulsive SE can continue to cause brain damage if undetected and therefore untreated. A recent report on the use of continuous EEG in the clinical management of veterinary patients with SE detailed how it served as a monitoring guide to recognize and suppress seizures when clinical signs of seizure activity had abated (Raith *et al.*, 2010). However, further study is required to address the question of whether persistent EEG patterns of SE during treatment is a poor prognostic sign.

The impracticality of utilizing EEG during seizure activity, in addition to the artefacts which can hinder objective interpretation in regular EEG recording in animals, have prevented this diagnostic modality from playing as big a part in SE treatment in veterinary medicine as it does in human medicine. However, recent work using the NeuroVista Seizure Advisory System, which utilizes subdural electrodes, has demonstrated that continuous real-time intracranial electroencephalography can be safely performed and will potentially be tremendously beneficial in the future for the treatment and monitoring of SE in animals (Sturges *et al.*, 2010).

References and further reading

Available on accompanying DVD

21

Anaesthesia and analgesia

Anthea L. Raisis and Gabrielle C. Musk

Patients with neurological disease may require anaesthesia for diagnostic or therapeutic procedures. The manifestations of the neurological condition determine the inherent risk of anaesthesia and whether or not an analgesic plan is required. A balanced anaesthetic approach for patients with neurological disease requires an understanding of the physiology and pathophysiology of the underlying disease process. Every technique should aim to achieve unconsciousness, antinociception and muscle relaxation.

Physiological considerations

The aims of anaesthesia in animals with central nervous system (CNS) disease are the preservation of neuronal function and prevention of secondary neuronal injury. Neuronal function is dependent on adequate blood flow.

Blood flow in the CNS
Blood flow to the CNS is altered by anaesthesia and disease. To minimize the effect of anaesthesia on CNS blood flow, it is essential to understand the physiology of blood flow regulation within the CNS and how it is altered by anaesthesia and disease. Many references describe the regulation of cerebral blood flow, and the same concepts apply to the regulation of spinal cord blood flow.

Cerebral blood flow (CBF) = cerebral perfusion pressure (CPP) / cerebral vascular resistance (CVR)

Where CPP = mean arterial pressure (MAP) – intracranial pressure (ICP)

Thus, CBF = (MAP – ICP) / CVR

There are local mechanisms that regulate blood flow within the CNS. These mechanisms act by altering the resistance within the cerebral vasculature and include:

- Autoregulation
- Flow metabolism coupling
- Chemical regulation
- Neurogenic regulation
- Response to changes in blood viscosity.

Autoregulation
Autoregulation, or myogenic regulation, is a reflex that maintains constant blood flow by altering the

vascular resistance in response to changes in perfusion pressure. Increased perfusion pressure results in reflex vasoconstriction; conversely, decreased perfusion pressure results in vasodilatation.

In most organs perfusion pressure is defined as the difference between arterial and venous blood pressure. In the CNS, perfusion pressure is determined by the difference between MAP and ICP, except when central venous pressure (CVP) is higher than the ICP. When this occurs, perfusion pressure is determined by the difference between MAP and CVP. Pathology within the CNS and many anaesthetic agents alter the normal myogenic response to changes in perfusion pressure. As a result, CBF can become directly related to changes in systemic arterial pressure.

Normal autoregulation operates between a CPP of 50 and 150 mmHg, provided that fluctuations within this range are not rapid. Outside this physiological range CBF changes linearly with CPP (Figure 21.1).

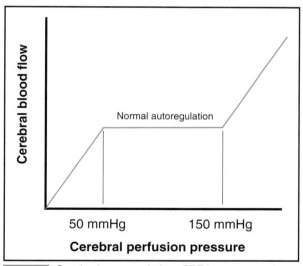

21.1 Cerebral autoregulation. CBF is constant when CPP is between 50 and 150 mmHg.

Flow metabolism coupling
Flow metabolism coupling describes the linear relation between CBF and cerebral metabolic rate (CMR). Increases in CMR result in an increased consumption of glucose and oxygen, and an increased production of local tissue metabolites such

as adenosine and potassium. These metabolites dilate the cerebral arterioles and increase CBF. Conversely, decreases in CMR result in decreased CBF and cerebral blood volume, due to arteriolar constriction. Intracranial pathology and some anaesthetic agents can alter the relationship between metabolism and flow, resulting in a non-linear relation. The volatile agents, particularly halothane, disrupt the relationship between CMR and CBF. Thus, for a given decrease in CMR, there will be a relatively smaller decrease in CBF and cerebral blood volume when compared with anaesthetic agents that maintain the relationship between blood flow and metabolism (e.g. propofol).

Chemical regulation

Chemical regulation of cerebral blood flow is mediated via changes in carbon dioxide and oxygen.

Carbon dioxide is a potent arterial vasodilator in the CNS. Increased arterial CO_2 tension (P_aCO_2) causes vasodilatation of the cerebral vasculature and an associated increase in blood flow. Conversely, decreases in P_aCO_2 promote cerebral vasoconstriction, increased CVR and associated decreases in CBF (Figure 21.2).

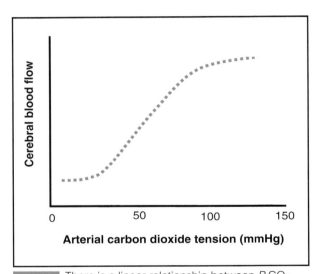

21.2 There is a linear relationship between P_aCO_2 and CBF except at the extremes, as the vessels are maximally constricted or dilated.

It should be noted that chronic increases in P_aCO_2 result in compensatory changes that normalize the pH of the cerebrospinal fluid (CSF). This may be important in animals with chronic airway disease (e.g. dogs with brachycephalic airway syndrome that results in chronic hypercapnia; Figure 21.3).

The responsiveness of vessels to P_aCO_2 may be altered by disease or pharmacological agents. This can result in development of the following phenomena:

- Intracerebral steal syndrome: if P_aCO_2 increases, dilatation of vessels within the normal CNS will increase blood flow to the normal tissues. Blood is shunted away from the diseased tissues, resulting in expansion of the abnormal area

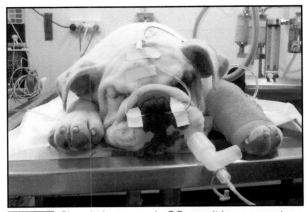

21.3 Chronic increases in CO_2 result in comensatory changes that normalize the pH of the CSF. This may be important in dogs with brachycephalic airway syndrome, such as this English Bulldog.

- Robin Hood phenomenon: decreased P_aCO_2 (e.g. due to mechanical ventilation) will cause vasoconstriction within the normal CNS tissue, but not in the diseased tissue. This will result in preferential blood flow to the diseased area and ischaemia of the normal CNS tissue
- Luxury perfusion: vessels in the tissues surrounding tumours and infarcts become maximally dilated, presumably due to the acidic environment that develops. This results in maximum CBF. These vessels do not respond normally to changes in P_aCO_2.

Arterial oxygen also influences CBF. Decreases in arterial oxygen tension (P_aO_2) cause arterial vasodilatation and, thus, increases in CBF.

Neurogenic reflexes

Neurogenic reflexes are mediated by sympathomimetic receptors within the cerebral vasculature. Beta-1 adrenoreceptors mediate vasodilatation and alpha-2 adrenoreceptors mediate vasoconstriction in response to circulating catecholamines. High concentrations of catecholamines, such as those that occur during haemorrhagic shock, will cause predominantly alpha-2 adrenoreceptor stimulation and marked cerebral vasoconstriction, predisposing to ischaemia.

Changes in blood viscosity

Increases in packed cell volume (PCV) due to haemoconcentration (e.g. dehydration) result in vasodilatation and increased blood flow within the CNS. A reduced red blood cell count results in vasoconstriction. In human patients, the PCV associated with optimal oxygen delivery has been observed to be 30–34%.

Cerebral perfusion pressure

CPP is determined by the difference between systemic MAP and ICP (see above). A direct or linear relation exists between CBF and CPP under a variety of physiological and pathological conditions, which include:

- When CPP is outside the normal autoregulatory range
- When there is a sudden marked increase in blood pressure
- When autoregulation is abnormal due to anaesthesia or disease.

The regulation of systemic blood pressure is complex and a full discussion is beyond the scope of this chapter. The main factors that influence MAP can, however, be described by the following formula:

Mean arterial pressure (MAP) = CO × SVR
$$= HR \times SV \times SVR$$
Where: CO = cardiac output, HR = heart rate, SV = stroke volume, SVR = systemic vascular resistance.

Decreased MAP (hypotension) may be due to:

- Reduced SVR (e.g. vasodilatation)
- Reduced SV (e.g. myocardial depression, dehydration and haemorrhage, marked tachycardia and reduced filling time)
- Reduced HR (e.g. bradycardia).

Anaesthetic agents can reduce blood pressure by many of these mechanisms, including vasodilatation (e.g. isoflurane, propofol), myocardial depression (e.g. halothane) and bradycardia (e.g. opioids).

Conversely, increased MAP may be due to increased SVR (vasoconstriction), increased HR and SV (increased sympathetic nervous system activity due to disease, pain and stress). Anaesthetic agents that increase MAP include ketamine (increased SVR and HR) and anticholinergics (increased HR).

Intracranial pressure

Increased ICP occurs when pathological increases in intracranial tissue volume exceed the compensatory decreases in other intracranial tissues. The result is decreased CPP, which causes neuronal ischaemia, dysfunction and, ultimately, neuronal death (Bagley, 1996).

The CNS is surrounded by rigid bony structures. As a result, the volume of the intracranial tissues is fixed. The intracranial contents consist of solid tissues, tissue water, CSF and blood. Increases in any of these must be accompanied by a compensatory decrease in the volume of one of the other components to prevent an increase in ICP (Figure 21.4). The ability for compensatory mechanisms to maintain a consistent ICP varies with disease process. In acute disease (e.g. head trauma) compensatory mechanisms may not occur rapidly enough to cope with the rise in CNS volume, and increased ICP is likely. In chronic disease, compensatory mechanisms may be able to prevent increases in ICP initially; however, if a lesion continues to increase in size, compensatory mechanisms will eventually fail and further small increases in intracranial volume will dramatically increase ICP. Clinically it is not possible to determine the amount of compensation remaining; thus, any animal with intracranial disease should be managed to prevent any further increases in ICP.

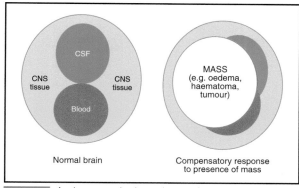

21.4 An increase in the volume of one tissue component within the skull requires a compensatory decrease in the volume of the other tissues to prevent an increase in ICP.

Increases in ICP during anaesthesia are typically associated with increases in blood volume (both arterial and venous). As the venous circulation forms the greatest proportion of blood volume within the CNS, changes in venous volume have marked effects on ICP.

Causes of increased cerebral *venous* blood volume include:

- Obstruction of the jugular veins (catheters, neck bandages, leads, venepuncture)
- Head down positioning
- Increased intrathoracic pressure during intermittent positive pressure ventilation (IPPV)
- Excessive intravenous fluid administration.

Causes of increased cerebral *arterial* blood volume include:

- Increased MAP in excess of normal autoregulatory range
- Increased MAP when autoregulation is altered (disease or anaesthetic agents)
- Increased P_aCO_2 (inadequate ventilation)
- Decreased P_aO_2 (ventilation/perfusion inequality, decreased oxygen uptake (pneumonia, pulmonary oedema))
- Increased CMR (hyperthermia, ketamine)
- Altered flow metabolism coupling (inhalant anaesthetic agents)
- Increased PCV (dehydration, diuretics).

Prior to anaesthesia, pre-existing increases in ICP should be reduced as much as possible.

Anaesthesia of patients with intracranial disease

The main aims during anaesthesia of animals with intracranial disease are to maintain cerebral blood flow and to prevent life-threatening increases in ICP that could lead to herniation (Figure 21.5).

Understanding the regulation of cerebral blood flow and factors that increase ICP enables the development of safe anaesthetic protocols. The

Aim	Management
Cerebral blood flow: cerebral vascular resistance	
Maintain local regulation	Select anaesthetic agents that minimally affect local regulatory mechanism; avoid sudden or excessive increases in MAP that impair autoregulation
Avoid excessive increase in CVR	Do not hyperventilate: decrease in P_aCO_2 (<30–35 mmHg) causes excessive cerebral vasoconstriction; prevent increased sympathetic stimulation due to stress/anxiety and pain
Cerebral blood flow: mean arterial pressure	
Maintain MAP at 70–80 mmHg	Use balanced anaesthesia to reduce doses of anaesthetic agents that decrease blood pressure
Intracranial pressure: arterial blood volume	
Avoid increases in MAP outside the normal autoregulatory range	Minimize stress and anxiety; maintain adequate pain relief
Avoid sudden increases in MAP	Minimize response to intubation, extubation and surgical stimulus; provide good analgesia
Maintain normal P_aCO_2	Mechanical ventilation; use short-acting anaesthetic agents to ensure rapid return to normal ventilation in the recovery period
Maintain adequate oxygenation	Preoxygenate prior to induction; use high inspired O_2 percentage during anaesthesia; give supplemental O_2 in the recovery period
Avoid increases in CMR	**Do not use agents that increase CMR** (e.g. ketamine); maintain normal body temperature; reduce seizure activity; use anaesthetic agents that decrease CMR (e.g. propofol)
Avoid dehydration and haemoconcentration	Adequate fluid therapy
Maintain relationship between CMR and CBF	**Do not use halothane**; careful use of newer volatile agents
Intracranial pressure: venous blood volume	
Avoid jugular compression	Take blood samples from peripheral veins; use harnesses (not neck leads) when walking dogs; place central venous catheters in peripheral vein for monitoring CVP
Avoid over-hydration	Excessive fluid therapy increases CVP and decreases venous drainage from the CNS; if CVP exceeds ICP, then CPP becomes dependent on the difference between MAP and CVP
Avoid excessive increases in intrathoracic pressure	Careful mechanical ventilation; avoid coughing during intubation and extubation; avoid vomiting; avoid sneezing

21.5 Considerations for patients with intracranial disease. PICC = peripherally inserted central catheter.

following description demonstrates how the above considerations can be applied to an anaesthetic technique.

Stabilization prior to anaesthesia

The overall aim before anaesthetizing a patient with intracranial disease is to establish an airway, ensure breathing (and oxygenation), support the circulation (i.e. ABC), and reduce ICP.

Airway, breathing and circulation

The amount of pulmonary and cardiovascular support required prior to anaesthesia will depend on the severity of the neurological disease and other concurrent injury/disease. Mildly affected animals and animals without concurrent disease may only require minimal supportive care in the form of oxygen supplementation and intravenous fluid therapy. Severely affected animals (severe mental depression/obtundation) may require additional stabilization, including tracheal intubation to protect the airway and facilitate ventilation.

Intracranial pressure

Any patient with increased ICP, regardless of the cause, requires stabilization before considering anaesthesia.

Initial emergency treatment of increased ICP should always include correction of hypoxaemia, hypercapnia and poor perfusion. Specific management of increased ICP is indicated if deterioration of neurological status occurs rapidly or continues despite normal oxygenation, ventilation and perfusion.

Osmotic diuretics are extremely effective in reducing ICP and are usually the first line of treatment for stabilizing patients with increased ICP. Administration of corticosteroids can be beneficial in reducing vasogenic cerebral oedema associated with neoplasia or encephalitis, but do not appear to reduce ICP in other disease states. In the event of impending herniation, intubation and hyperventilation may be necessary to prevent death.

Diuretics:

> Mannitol is administered at 0.5–1.5 g/kg i.v. over 10–15 minutes. Peak effect occurs within 60 minutes of administration. Repeated dosing q4h can be performed if neurological deterioration recurs despite appropriate management of initial cause and continued supportive care.

Mannitol decreases ICP partly by increasing the osmotic gradient between the intravascular and extravascular fluid compartments, causing fluid to move out of the tissues into the blood for a mean period of 3.5 hours and for up to 8 hours (Sande and West, 2010; Sakellaridis *et al.*, 2011). The increase in blood volume also contributes to the decrease in ICP due to the dilutional effects and resultant decrease in blood viscosity. Decreased blood viscosity improves oxygen delivery, which ultimately stimulates cerebral vasoconstriction and decreased cerebral blood volume (Bagley, 1996). The osmotic effects of repeated doses of mannitol on ICP are effective for 16–48 hours, after which the brain tissue alters its osmolality to match the continued increase in serum osmolality. The use of hypertonic saline to reduce ICP is gaining acceptance and there is some evidence that it is superior to mannitol (see Chapter 20 for full details).

Furosemide is a loop diuretic that inhibits the sodium/potassium/chloride ion pump in the thick ascending loop of Henle, resulting in decreased sodium and water resorption. Previously, administration of furosemide at 0.7 mg/kg i.v. was reported to be synergistic with mannitol for reducing ICP (Bagley, 1996) but this is now contentious and combination therapy is no longer recommended in human medicine (Todd *et al.*, 2006). Furosemide on its own has a rapid onset of action and may be useful for emergency management of increases in ICP that are expected to progress rapidly to herniation and death. If furosemide is used, it must be remembered that the effect is prolonged and that diuresis may continue for 6–8 hours after administration.

Adverse effects of diuretics: All diuretics increase urine output and fluid loss from the body. Fluid restriction after mannitol therapy has been associated with poor outcome in human patients (Clifton *et al.*, 2002); thus it is imperative that replacement fluid therapy is performed to prevent dehydration and haemoconcentration following the use of diuretics. Increased PCV and blood viscosity associated with haemoconcentration can trigger cerebral vasodilatation and lead to increased ICP.

Electrolyte abnormalities are also observed following diuretic therapy. Due to relatively greater water loss associated with the administration of mannitol, hypernatraemia can occur. Loop diuretics cause the loss of large amounts of potassium. Thus electrolyte balance needs to be monitored closely if

these agents are used, and abnormalities should be corrected prior to anaesthesia.

Hyperventilation

> Hyperventilation and lowering P_aCO_2 to 30–35 mmHg can be used for stabilization of acute, transient increases in ICP, particularly when herniation is imminent (Barbacia and Williams, 2001).

Hyperventilation decreases ICP by causing respiratory alkalosis, which stimulates constriction of the cerebral arterioles. Hyperventilation may lead to ischaemia in normal brain tissue. It is recommended that this method of reducing ICP is reserved for emergency situations and is not used for prolonged periods; P_aCO_2 should not drop below 30 mmHg, in order to minimize ischaemia in the normal regions of the brain. Hyperventilation requires the delivery of higher than normal respiratory rates and tidal volumes. This increase in minute volume may interfere with blood flow to the heart and increase the risk of hypotension. This will further increase the risk of cerebral ischaemia. Close monitoring of cardiovascular and respiratory function should be performed in ventilated animals.

Sedation or premedication

The aims of premedication are to:

- Provide analgesia
- Reduce stress and anxiety
- Reduce the dose of agents used for induction and maintenance of anaesthesia.

Figure 21.6 provides examples of common premedicants used in small animals. The table is divided into agents that can be used with care and agents that should be avoided in patients with intracranial disease.

Agent	Comments
Use (with care)	

Opioids:
Stable animal requiring analgesia:
  Methadone 0.2–0.4 mg/kg i.m.
Stable animal not requiring analgesia:
  Butorphanol 0.2–0.4 mg/kg i.m.
Unstable animals:
  Fentanyl 1–5 µg/kg i.m./i.v., 2–5 µg/kg/h by i.v. infusion
  Remifentanil 2–5 µg/kg/h by i.v. infusion
	Sole agent or in combination with other agents. Do not alter CBF regulation nor increase ICP. Minimal respiratory and cardiovascular depression at lower clinical doses. Note: Use short-acting agents that can be titrated to effect in unstable animals

21.6 Drugs for premedication of dogs and cats. The doses provided are those used in clinically normal small animals. However, disruption of the blood–brain barrier and mental depression in animals with intracranial disease increases the response to these agents, thus use of doses smaller than those routinely used in normal clinical patients is recommended. (continues) ▶

Agent	Comments
***Use (with care)* continued**	
Benzodiazepines: Diazepam 0.1–0.2 mg/kg i.v. Midazolam 0.1–0.2 mg/kg i.v.; 0.2–0.4 mg/kg i.m.	Can be useful as anxiolytics. Can cause unpredictable behaviour, excitement, dysphoria and dysinhibition in mentally alert animals, particularly when used alone. Combining benzodiazepines and opioids can provide good sedation in the anxious, sick or old animal
Phenobarbital 2–3 mg/kg i.m.	The authors have found that phenobarbital can be useful for premedication in some anxious dogs, when administered in conjunction with an opioid such as methadone
Agents best avoided	
Acepromazine 0.02–0.05 mg/kg i.m.	Anxiolytic commonly used in healthy animals. Risk of seizures in animals with intracranial pathology [a]. Systemic vasodilatation predisposes to hypotension. Cerebral vasodilatation may increase ICP
Alpha-2 agonists: Medetomidine 2–5 μg/kg i.m. (Dexmedetomidine: due to higher potency the dose of dexmedetomidine used should be half that of medetomidine)	Marked sedation and significant cardiopulmonary dysfunction (Pypendop and Verstegen, 1998; Murrell and Hellebrekers, 2005). Increased MAP and accompanying bradycardia can simulate Cushing reflex. Vomiting is common in cats
Ketamine (cats only) 2–5 mg/kg i.m.	Increased MAP. Increased CMR and ICP. Increased incidence of seizures [a]

21.6 (continued) Drugs for premedication of dogs and cats. The doses provided are those used in clinically normal small animals. However, disruption of the blood–brain barrier and mental depression in animals with intracranial disease increases the response to these agents, thus use of doses smaller than those routinely used in normal clinical patients is recommended. [a] Recent clinical studies question the validity of this statement in some cases. There are currently no definitive prospective studies. Thus, authors recommend continued caution with this agent in animals with intracranial disease.

Induction of anaesthesia and endotracheal intubation

Pre-oxygenation for 5–10 minutes prior to induction of anaesthesia and the delivery of oxygen during this period is recommended to prevent hypoxaemia. Oxygen can be delivered via a mask; however, many conscious animals object to a mask being placed over their face. To minimize stress, 'flow-by' oxygen can be provided (Figure 21.7).

Titration of short-acting agents carefully to effect (e.g. propofol) can help maintain normal ventilation during induction. Manual ventilation with a close-fitting mask can help prevent hypercapnia if ventilation is depressed or abolished during induction

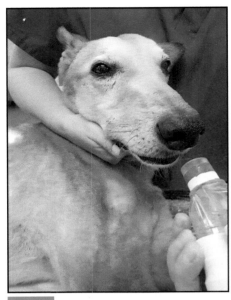

21.7 Administering 'flow-by' oxygen.

(Figure 21.8). It should be noted that ventilation using a mask predisposes to gastric distension, which will impair ventilation. Gastric decompression using a nasogastric tube can be performed once adequate anaesthetic depth and intubation has been achieved.

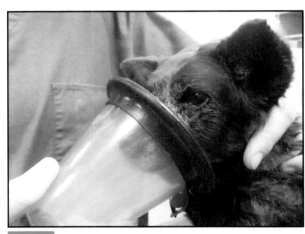

21.8 Manual ventilation with a close-fitting facemask.

Induction of anaesthesia is performed using intravenous agents to facilitate endotracheal intubation without stimulating a response.

Co-induction agents

Co-induction agents are sedative and/or analgesic agents that are administered immediately prior to the induction agent. Use of co-induction agents can help reduce the dose of the induction agent and associated side effects. This is particularly useful in animals that have received no or minimal premedication. Some co-induction agents can also help reduce coughing during intubation. Co-induction agents used by the authors in animals with intracranial disease are listed in Figure 21.9.

Agent	Comments
Benzodiazepines: Diazepam 0.1–0.2 mg/kg i.v. Midazolam 0.1–0.2 mg/kg i.v.	No effect on CBF or ICP. Reduce seizure activity. No cardiovascular depression. Can potentiate respiratory depression of induction agents and may warrant use of ventilation during induction
Fentanyl 1–5 µg/kg i.v.	No effect on CBF or ICP. Larger doses can result in bradycardia ± respiratory depression
Butorphanol 0.1–0.2 mg/kg i.v.	Very effective antitussive. Useful for non-painful procedures such as imaging
Lidocaine 1–2 mg/kg i.v. (dogs only)	No effect on CBF or ICP. Reduces seizure activity (at low doses). May decrease laryngeal sensitivity (Raisis *et al.*, 2003). No respiratory depression. Can decrease MAP

21.9 Common co-induction agents used in animals with intracranial disease.

Induction agents

Figure 21.10 lists agents commonly used for induction of anaesthesia in animals with intracranial disease. The agents are divided into those that should be used with caution and those that should be avoided.

Agent	Comment
Use carefully	
Propofol Dogs: 2–4 mg/kg i.v. Cats: 4–6 mg/kg i.v.	Maintains regulation of CBF. Decreases ICP (due to decreased CMR). Dose- and rate-dependent cardiovascular and respiratory depression. Dose required and side effects can be minimized by administration of co-induction agent. Slow administration to effect will also reduce depressant effects of cardiovascular and pulmonary systems. NB: Handling patient around nose can elicit sneezing if inadequately anaesthetized
Alfaxalone 1–2 mg/kg i.v.	Based on studies on alfaxalone/alfadalone, this drug should have minimal detrimental effects of CBF. However, conclusive studies with alfaxalone have not been performed
Thiopental 10 mg/kg i.v.	Intravenous agents provide smooth induction with minimal struggling and rapid control of the airway. Slow administration in minimally sedated/mentally alert animals can cause excitement. Residual mental depression present after recovery may delay return to completely normal ventilation and behaviour
Avoid	
Ketamine (usually used with another agent such as diazepam)	Increased risk of seizures. Increased CMR (and ICP). Sympathetic stimulation can cause hypertension

21.10 Considerations for choosing agents for induction of anesthesia in animals with intracranial disease.

To prevent coughing during tracheal intubation it is essential to achieve an adequate depth of anaesthesia before attempting to intubate. Coughing can also be minimized by the administration of agents with potent antitussive effects, e.g. opioids (especially butorphanol), either as premedicants or co-induction agents. Spraying the larynx with lidocaine can also reduce coughing on intubation in both cats and dogs (Figure 21.11).

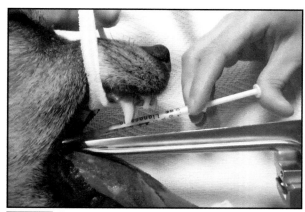

21.11 Topical lidocaine spray applied to the larynx prior to intubation will inhibit the response to intubation.

Maintenance of anaesthesia

Due to species differences in the metabolism of agents commonly used for maintenance of anaesthesia in dogs and cats with intracranial disease, maintenance of anaesthesia in these species will be discussed separately.

Dogs

Stable animals: Inhalation anaesthesia is still the most common method of maintaining anaesthesia in stable animals requiring diagnostic procedures. Figure 21.12 notes inhalation agents that should be used with care, and agents that are best avoided. The detrimental effects of these agents can be minimized by the concurrent administration of opioids to

Agent	Comment
Use with care	
Isoflurane	Causes a slight increase in ICP. Useful for short procedures when used with care. Anecdotal report of increased swelling and greater chance of postoperative dysphoria in dogs following craniectomy; this is not as notable as that seen with halothane
Sevoflurane	Smallest increase in ICP of all inhalation agents. No increase in ICP reported in human patients when administered at 1 x MAC. Recent evidence that may cause seizure activity during anaesthesia in human patients. Used successfully by the authors in dogs and cats

21.12 Inhalational anaesthetic agents and the considerations for their use in patients with intracranial disease. (continues) ▶

Agent	Comment
Use with care continued	
Nitrous oxide	Frequently recommended that N₂O be avoided due to increases in ICP associated with its use. Recent review of recovery in human patients found no evidence of harmful effects (Pasternak and Lanier, 2010). No clinical studies on use in animal neuroanaesthesia exist
Avoid	
Halothane	Marked increase in ICP
Desflurane	Marked increase in ICP

21.12 (continued) Inhalational anaesthetic agents and the considerations for their use in patients with intracranial disease.

reduce the dose of volatile agent used. Ventilating these animals to normocapnia also reduces the detrimental effects of inhalation agents.

Unstable animals or those requiring surgery: In this group total intravenous anaesthesia (TIVA), using a combined infusion of propofol and a short-acting opioid such as fentanyl or remifentanil, is advised. The rationale for the use of TIVA is based on the beneficial effects of propofol on cerebral perfusion and on its pharmacokinetics, which allow propofol to be administered by a continuous infusion without accumulation and prolonged recovery.

Concurrent infusions of opioids such as remifentanil are used to decrease the dose of propofol and thus reduce the effects of propofol on systemic cardiovascular function (Padfield, 2000). In addition, continuous infusions of opioids help to minimize sympathetic nervous system stimulation and haemodynamic responses to surgery, which can cause marked increases in MAP and accompanying increases in CBF and ICP.

Cats

Due to the slower metabolism of propofol in cats, accumulation and prolonged recoveries are likely if this agent is administered as an infusion. While this does not preclude the use of propofol in this species, the need for a longer duration of ventilation and supportive care should be expected and provided.

Inhalation anaesthesia with agents such as isoflurane or sevoflurane is still more common for maintenance of anaesthesia in the cat. It is important to remember that, although recoveries are more rapid using volatile agents, there is a greater risk of increasing ICP and herniation in the immediate perioperative period.

Whichever maintenance agent is used, the side effects can be minimized by reducing the dose. Continuous infusion of short-acting opioids such as fentanyl and remifentanil can also be used in cats to provide analgesia and reduce required doses of maintenance agent.

Supportive care

IPPV (see later) is essential during anaesthesia of animals with intracranial disease to ensure normocapnia (P_aCO_2 35–45 mmHg).

Fluid therapy is also essential during anaesthesia to ensure normal blood volume and electrolyte balance. Water restriction was previously thought to cause a decrease in brain water; however, it is now known that the adverse effects on blood viscosity result in decreased oxygen delivery, which stimulates vasodilatation and increases CBV and ICP (Cornick, 1992). Excessive fluid therapy should be avoided, however, as increases in venous pressure may predispose to increased ICP. For more information on types and rates of fluids used in neurological disease, see later.

It is important to maintain a normal body temperature in animals with CNS disease. Hypothermia decreases CMR and has been used in human patients as a form of neuroprotection; however, the benefits of controlled hypothermia in veterinary patients are still being investigated. As the adverse effects of hypothermia (including increased risk of infection, increased surgical blood loss, shivering and increased oxygen consumption during recovery) could cause serious complications in the neurological patient, this technique is best avoided at this time. Hyperthermia increases CMR, which increases CBF and can lead to increases in ICP and further reductions in CPP.

Mild head elevation is recommended to ensure venous drainage and prevent increases in ICP. Positioning of the patient during surgery is important. Craniectomy and imaging (CT and/or MRI) is performed with the animal positioned in sternal recumbency. It is important to ensure that the jugular veins are not occluded when the animal is placed in this position (Figure 21.13).

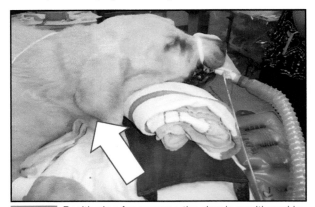

21.13 Positioning for surgery: the dog is positioned in sternal recumbency with the head level with the spine. Careful positioning and padding is essential to prevent occlusion of the jugular veins (arrowed).

Monitoring

Monitoring of arterial blood pressure is important to ensure that adequate MAP and CPP are maintained. Monitoring of CVP is important to ensure that venous return is not impaired and hydration is adequate.

For surgical procedures, invasive monitoring of ABP and CVP is recommended. In patients with increased ICP, it is recommended that MAP is maintained between 80 and 100 mmHg to ensure adequate CPP. CVP should normally be between 0–4 mmHg in spontaneously breathing animals; higher values are expected in animals that are being mechanically ventilated. High CVP (>10 mmHg) associated with overhydration, decreased cardiac function or excessive pressures during ventilation should be avoided.

> Monitoring of pulmonary function is essential to ensure normocapnia (P_aCO_2 35–45 mmHg) and adequate oxygenation (P_aO_2 >80 mmHg). Capnography and pulse oximetry can be used as a guide to the adequacy of pulmonary function. However, in critically ill animals, or during neurosurgery, direct measurement of arterial blood gases is recommended.

For details on techniques used for monitoring cardiovascular and respiratory function see later.

Recovery and postoperative analgesia

Aims during the anaesthetic recovery period are to:

- Minimize excitement and agitation by ensuring adequate analgesia and recovery in a quiet, warm, dimly lit environment
- Ensure normal ventilation and maintenance of normocapnia before extubation
- Minimize or avoid coughing during extubation.

Return to spontaneous breathing

The timing of extubation of animals with intracranial disease is a compromise between ensuring that the animal is able to ventilate adequately and maintain normocapnia, and preventing excessive stimulation that could lead to hypertension and coughing.

Guidelines to extubation: dogs with normal airways

1. Move the patient to a quiet, warm environment with minimal noise and stimulation before discontinuing the anaesthetic.
2. Prepare for extubation: untie the endotracheal tube (ETT); have cuff syringe available to deflate the cuff; have additional ETT and anaesthetic agents ready for re-intubation if necessary.
3. Discontinue anaesthetic and monitor closely for clinical signs suggesting reducing depth of anaesthesia: return of palpebral reflex, increasing heart rate and arterial blood pressure.
4. Attempt a short period of trial apnoea (<1 minute). Do not allow end-tidal CO_2 ($ETCO_2$) to exceed 45 mmHg.
5. If spontaneous breathing does not return, continue ventilation.
6. Continue to repeat short periods of apnoea intermittently until spontaneous ventilation returns.
7. Once spontaneous ventilation returns, use capnography to monitor adequacy. If $ETCO_2$ >45 mmHg, resume ventilation. If $ETCO_2$ is maintained below 45 mmHg, extubate.
8. Monitor for patency of airway and continued ventilation.

Management of hypertension

Persistent hypertension despite adequate analgesia can be treated by the administration of beta receptor antagonists, or calcium channel blockers. Agents that have been used in human patients with head trauma include esmolol (beta-blocker), labetalol (mixed alpha- and beta-blocker) and nicardipine (calcium channel blocker). Use of these agents in small animal neurological patients has not been reported. Esmolol is commonly used to treat tachyarrhythmias in small animals, and labetolol has been described for the use in hypertensive crisis. Nicardipine is not used clinically in small animals at present; however, amlodipine is a calcium channel blocker used in small animals with cardiovascular disease and may be a suitable alternative (Hopper and Silverstein, 2009).

Management of dysphoria and agitation

Management of dysphoria in animals with forebrain disease can be a challenge. It is essential to ensure that the behavioural change is not due to pain. It is also important to differentiate dysphoria from forebrain disease with agitation and anxiety that can occur in animals with vestibular–cerebellar dysfunction that are unable to stand or lie down without circling, falling or rolling.

Provision of adequate analgesia will eliminate pain as a cause of agitation. Maintaining a quiet warm dimly lit environment and calming the animal with gentle voice and touch is also useful. This may be the only treatment required in mild to moderate agitation. For animals that have cerebella dysfunction, agitation can be minimized by careful nursing and positioning. Many animals that are prone to circling will have a preferred side they lie on.

If agitation and/or vocalizing is severe and persists despite adequate analgesia, other treatments may be warranted. Most of the sedative drugs that are useful for controlling extremely agitated animals have potentially detrimental effects on cardiovascular function, cerebral perfusion and ICP. However, these animals are at risk of injuring themselves, particularly if thrashing occurs. In addition, vocalizing and agitated behaviour may also lead to increases in ICP. In these situations, provided the animal is normovolaemic, normally hydrated and has normal cardiovascular function, the benefits of using sedative agents such as acepromazine or the new alpha-2 agonists (medetomidine or dexmedetomidine) may outweigh the risks (Figure 21.14).

To reduce the potential for side effects associated with the administration of sedatives, it is recommended that low doses are used initially and that the agent is administered intramuscularly. If intravenous administration is preferred it is recommended that the calculated dose of the agent is diluted and the dose is subsequently titrated, allowing sufficient time between doses to determine effect of each dose (at least 5 minutes for acepromazine and 1–2 minutes for medetomidine or dexmeditomidine). Once the animal is calm, monitoring of the cardiovascular and pulmonary systems should be performed to detect any potential adverse effects associated with administration of these agents.

Agent	Advantages	Disadvantages
Acepromazine 5 µg/kg i.m.; 5 µg/kg i.v. (dilute and give ¼ dose every 5–10 minutes)	Sedation relatively less profound when administered carefully. Cardiovascular effects can be decreased by low doses and ensuring normovolaemia	Longer onset. Prolonged effect No specific antagonist. Increases seizure activity and ICP
Medetomidine 1–3 µg/kg i.m.; 0.5-1 µg/kg i.v. (dilute and give ¼ dose every 1–2 minutes); 0.5–1 µg/kg/h, titrated to effect	Can be infused. Can be reversed	Profound sedation and inability to protect airway observed with overdose. Marked cardiovascular changes observed at low clinical doses and during infusions. Can cause vomiting after rapid i.v. injection. Diuresis can cause fluid loss that is masked by vasoconstriction. Reduced HR and increased BP can mimic the Cushing reflex
Dexmedetomidine (half dose of medetomidine)		

21.14 Sedative drugs for management of animals with dysphoria.

Anaesthesia of patients with spinal disease

The main aims during anaesthesia of animals with spinal disease are focused on preventing further injury to the spine. This is achieved by maintaining spinal cord perfusion and using careful handling and restraint. Appropriate analgesia is also essential. Considerations for anaesthesia of patients with spinal disease are given in Figure 21.15.

Stabilization prior to anaesthesia
The amount of respiratory and cardiovascular support required prior to anaesthesia will depend on the severity of the spinal disease and other concurrent injury/disease. Animals that have not suffered concurrent trauma and/or have mild spinal disease may not require stabilization prior to induction of anaesthesia, or may simply require fluid therapy to correct pre-existing dehydration. Severely affected animals (concurrent trauma, cervical lesions interfering with ventilation) may require additional stabilization

including oxygen supplementation or intubation and ventilation. For more details on these treatments see Supportive care, later.

Sedation or premedication
The aims of premedication are the same as for patients with intracranial disease. Premedication of patients with spinal disease usually includes opioids with or without agents with sedative or anxiolytic properties. Agents commonly used for premedicating these patients are noted in Figure 21.16.

Induction of anaesthesia and endotracheal intubation
Preventing further injury to the spine is essential during induction of anaesthesia of patients with spinal disease. A calm and controlled environment will facilitate this aim, as will a balanced anaesthetic technique that minimizes cardiovascular depression. Induction of anaesthesia is performed with intravenous agents to ensure a rapid, controlled induction with minimal struggling; a fitted mask delivering

Aim	Management
Prevent further injury to spine; Maintain spinal perfusion	
Avoid hypovolaemia: absolute hypovolaemia may occur due to dehydration or blood loss; relative hypovolaemia may be due to vasodilatation from anaesthetic drugs or autonomic imbalance caused by cervical lesions	Correct fluid and electrolyte abnormalities before anaesthesia. Use balanced anaesthesia techniques to reduce anaesthetic-related cardiovascular depression. Avoid hypothermia as this leads to increased surgical bleeding and cardiovascular instability
Maintain regulation of spinal cord perfusion	Use agents that minimally depress local regulation of spinal perfusion (see intracranial disease)
Minimize increases in spinal cord pressure	Maintain normal ventilation, oxygenation and stable blood pressure (see intracranial disease)
Prevent further injury to spine; Careful handling and restraint	
Minimize risk of further disc prolapse. Avoid excessive/ inappropriate movement in animals with mechanical instability, e.g. spinal fracture, cervical malformation, atlanto-axial subluxation	Careful moving and positioning of animal. Support the neck during tracheal intubation. Do not overextend or hyperflex the neck during tracheal intubation. Avoid agents that cause vomiting
Provide adequate analgesia	
Many spinal lesions are painful: intervertebral disc disease, spinal fractures, tremors	Opioids; muscle relaxants (stable lesions only); lidocaine; ketamine (care in trauma)

21.15 Considerations for anaesthesia of patients with spinal disease.

Drugs	Comments
Useful	
Opioids: Methadone 0.2–0.4 mg/kg i.m. Fentanyl 2–5 µg/kg i.v., i.m. Fentanyl 2–5 µg/kg/h by i.v. infusion Remifentanil 2–5 µg/kg/h by i.v. infusion	Good analgesia. Mild sedation. Minimal cardiovascular and pulmonary depression at lower clinical doses. Use shorter-acting agents in unstable animals
Use with care	
Acepromazine 0.02–0.05 mg/kg i.m.	Extremely useful in anxious animals. Paretic and paralysed animals are frequently extremely anxious. Marked vasodilator: DO NOT USE in dehydrated, hypovolaemic animals
Benzodiazepines: Midazolam 0.2–0.4 mg/kg i.m. Diazepam 0.2–0.4 mg/kg i.v.	Good sedation in old/young or compromised animals. Can cause agitation in mentally alert animals due to paradoxical disinhibition. Skeletal muscle relaxant: DO NOT USE in conditions associated with mechanical instability
Medetomidine Dogs 2–5 µg/kg i.m. Cats 5–20 µg/kg i.m. Dexmedetomidine (1/2 dose of medetomidine)	Marked depression of cardiovascular system. Only use in healthy animals. Skeletal muscle relaxant: DO NOT USE in conditions associated with mechanical instability
Ketamine 2–5 mg/kg i.m. (cats only)	May provide additional analgesia in neuropathic pain. Pain on injection can elicit violent physical reaction which increases the potential for exacerbation of unstable lesions. NEVER use alone: combine with opioids ± acepromazine or benzodiazepine

21.16 Premedication and considerations for use in small animal patients with spinal disease.

inhalant anaesthetic and oxygen can be stressful and increases the risk of struggling and further injury. Appropriate premedication will help ensure an uneventful induction. Selection of an appropriate induction agent is based on similar principles to those described for animals with intracranial disease. Common intravenous induction agents used in small animals are described in Figure 21.17. Induction agents are divided into those that are suitable for all animals with spinal disease and those that should only be used in animals that have no concurrent abnormalities (e.g. trauma, dehydration).

Tracheal intubation should be performed carefully with adequate support of the head and neck, particularly in animals with cervical column injury. The animal should be placed on a flat surface with the head and neck supported. Intubation is facilitated by the use of a laryngoscope (Figure 21.18). Excessive neck extension should be avoided in dogs with caudal cervical lesions, while excessive neck flexion should be avoided in animals with atlantoaxial subluxation or other cervical fractures.

Agent	Comment
Suitable for all animals	
Propofol Dogs 2–4 mg/kg i.v. Cats 4–6 mg/kg i.v.	Can be titrated slowly to effect with minimal to no excitement in lightly sedated or unsedated animals. Dose- and rate-dependent cardiovascular and respiratory depression. Can be minimized by slow administration and use of a balanced approach. Note: handling around nose can elicit sneezing when inadequately anaesthetized
Alfaxalone 1–2 mg/kg i.v.	Can be titrated slowly to effect with minimal to no excitement in lightly sedated or unsedated animals. Dose- and rate-dependent cardiovascular and respiratory depression. Can be minimized by slow administration and use of balanced approach
Suitable for healthy animals	
Thiopental 10 mg/kg i.v.	Can cause excitement on induction in minimally sedated animals. Careful use in animals with concurrent trauma and cardiovascular abnormalities
Ketamine (usually given with diazepam to offset muscle rigidity)	Advantages in animals with neuropathic pain (chronic spinal disease). Careful use in animals with concurrent trauma and cardiovascular abnormalities

21.17 Intravenous agents used for induction of anaesthesia in patients with spinal disease. Nearly all induction agents cause alterations in cardiovascular function in a dose-dependent manner. By reducing the dose of these agents, alterations in cardiovascular function can be minimized. This helps maintain spinal perfusion. Adequate premedication will help reduce doses of intravenous and maintenance agents. When the physical condition of the animal precludes use of sedatives as part of the premedication, co-induction agents (fentanyl and/or benzodiazepines) can be used to reduce the induction agent.

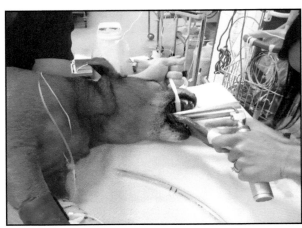

21.18 Endotracheal intubation with adequate support of the head and neck is essential for patients with cervical spinal lesions.

Maintenance of anaesthesia

Maintenance of anaesthesia for patients with spinal disease should focus on the provision of a balanced technique to minimize the dose of agents that alter cardiovascular function. This will in turn minimize alterations to spinal cord blood flow. Targeting normocapnia is also important, and appropriate analgesia must be provided. Routine spinal surgery is still commonly performed using inhalation agents without any reported untoward effects. As autoregulation and chemoreceptor responses to carbon dioxide are maintained better with isoflurane and sevoflurane than with halothane, the former agents are preferred.

There are certain conditions affecting the spinal cord in which the authors prefer to maintain anaesthesia using TIVA. These include:

- Animals with severe cervical cord compression resulting in impaired ventilation
- Animals with cranial cervical instability, e.g. atlantoaxial instability, fracture.

Surgery in these animals has the potential to cause life-threatening complications such as respiratory failure. TIVA is preferred to help minimize further neurological damage. A description of TIVA is given earlier in this chapter.

Intraoperative infusions of short-acting pure mu agonist opioids such as fentanyl, alfentanil and remifentanil not only provide good analgesia but, at higher doses, reduce the dose of inhalation agent required to maintain anaesthesia. This helps to maintain systemic blood pressure and spinal cord perfusion, particularly in animals with concurrent abnormalities in hydration or blood volume status, or cardiovascular function.

Supportive care

IPPV is recommended during anaesthesia in the spinal patient for several reasons:

- Increased P_aCO_2 may increase spinal compression due to increased blood flow and blood volume within the spinal column

- Surgical access requires that the animal is positioned in sternal recumbency; this interferes with diaphragmatic excursions and impairs ventilation
- The dose of opioids required to reduce the dose of inhalation agents used for maintenance of anaesthesia generally cause respiratory depression.

For more details on techniques for ventilating animals with neurological disease, see later.

Intravenous fluid therapy is essential during anaesthesia to maintain blood volume and pressure. Blood loss can be surprisingly high during spinal surgery; thus the amount of blood on swabs and in suction bottles should be monitored throughout anaesthesia. A blood transfusion is indicated when blood loss exceeds 20% of the circulating blood volume or haemoglobin concentration is <8 g/dl. Smaller amounts of blood loss associated with hypotension can be managed with administration of colloids such as hetastarch (maximum dose 20 ml/kg/24h).

Passive warming is recommended in all anaesthetized animals. In animals with spinal disease, heat loss can be increased, particularly when spinal cord injury causes sympathetic nervous system imbalance and peripheral vasodilatation. Monitoring of temperature should be performed during anaesthesia. Warming can be provided during anaesthesia by use of warm water beds or air blowers.

Monitoring

During diagnostic imaging and surgery in animals with spinal disease, non-invasive monitoring of cardiopulmonary function with electrocardiography, oscillometric blood pressure measurement, capnography and pulse oximetry is generally adequate. In animals where cardiopulmonary dysfunction (e.g. cranial cervical surgery, trauma involving multiple organ systems) or excessive blood loss is expected, invasive monitoring is recommended. Monitoring techniques are discussed in detail later in the chapter.

Recovery and postoperative analgesia

To minimize injury to the spine in the postoperative period, the recovery room must be quiet, dimly lit and comfortable. Adequate analgesia is paramount and judicious sedation may be required. In some cases, it may be advisable to move the patient before anaesthesia is discontinued or very soon thereafter. This will reduce the risk of the animal suddenly waking up during transit.

Bedding should be sufficiently padded to provide comfort to the animal (Figure 21.19) but not excessively padded as this can make it difficult for the animal to obtain solid footing when trying to stand. The cage size should also not be too large, to ensure that animals do not gain too much momentum when trying to stand as this may lead to injury. A non-slip mat should also be considered when the animal begins to bear weight.

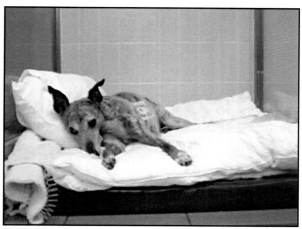

21.19 Comfortable and supportive bedding in the intensive care unit or recovery ward is important.

It is essential that the administration of analgesia is continued throughout the postoperative period to ensure a calm, pain-free recovery. Analgesia in the immediate postoperative period can be provided by incremental administration or infusion of pure mu opioid agonists. These can be used alone or combined with a variety of other agents including lidocaine, ketamine and medetomidine (see later). In some cases the use of low-dose sedatives such as acepromazine (0.01 mg/kg i.v.) or medetomidine (1 µg/kg i.v.) may be required in extremely stressed or agitated animals.

Diagnostic procedures: myelography and MRI

Considerations for anaesthesia of patients with spinal disease requiring myelography or MRI are given in Figures 21.20 and 21.21.

Problem	Anaesthetic management
Side effects of contrast medium injection	
Seizures	Avoid anaesthetic agents that decrease seizure threshold (acepromazine, ketamine, tramadol (?)). Seizures in recovery can be treated with diazepam 0.5 mg/kg i.v. or CRI
Cardiopulmonary depression (apnoea, tachypnoea, bradycardia, tachycardia, arrhythmias hypotension and hypertension (Court *et al.*, 1990; Barone *et al.*, 2002))	Close monitoring of cardiovascular and pulmonary function. Minimized by slow injection rate and ensuring an adequate depth of anaesthesia during injection
Cisternal injection	
Neck flexion during injection	Monitor with capnography for obstruction of ETT. Complete obstruction will prevent ventilation. If unable to ventilate, the procedure should be aborted and the head and neck repositioned; or a different ETT placed. Partial obstruction of the ETT may necessitate higher inspiratory pressures to ensure adequate ventilation. Reinforced ETTs will reduce the risk of occlusion
Cervical lesions	
Extubation may be required for radiographs of the cervical spine	Be prepared to maintain anaesthesia intravenously. Have equipment for re-intubation to hand

21.20 Considerations for anaesthesia of patients with spinal disease requiring myelography.

Problem	Management
Magnetic field	
Ferromagnetic objects become projectile within the magnetic field	Ferromagnetic objects must remain outside the 5g line. Metallic objects such as anaesthetic machines must be made of non-ferrous metal if required to be within the magnetic field
ECG leads within magnetic field can induce current and cause burns	Use insulated ECG leads; avoid large loops of wire; apply sensors away from imaged area
Distant monitoring	
Preferable for staff to remain outside magnetic field	Use specialized MRI-compatible equipment that can be viewed from outside the magnetic field. Increase length of sampling lines so monitors can be positioned outside the magnetic field (oscillometric blood pressure, capnography)

21.21 Considerations for the anaesthesia of patients with spinal disease requiring MRI.

Anaesthesia of patients with peripheral nervous system disease

Animals with peripheral nervous system disease usually present with paresis or weakness, which may be localized or generalized. These animals are at risk of laryngeal, pharyngeal and intercostal muscle weakness. Considerations for these patients are outlined in Figure 21.22.

In contrast, tetanus is a toxicoinfectious disease affecting the CNS and lower motor neurons and causing muscle rigidity.

Sedation or premedication

As weakness is a feature of peripheral neuromuscular disease, heavy sedation or premedication is best avoided and is usually unnecessary. Light sedation with an anxiolytic such as acepromazine (0.01–0.02 mg/kg i.m.) may be helpful. The usual contraindications to the administration of acepromazine apply (hypovolaemia, hypotension, anaemia, a history of seizures). Other sedative agents such as benzodiazepines and alpha-2 adrenoreceptor agonists produce skeletal muscle relaxation, which may compromise respiratory muscle function and upper airway protective mechanisms.

Patients with tetanus may also require muscle relaxation (even though the infection acts primarily on the CNS) and so these drugs can also be used (midazolam 0.2–0.5 mg/kg i.v. or medetomidine 1–10 µg/kg i.m. or i.v.). In addition, acepromazine is extremely useful for reducing responsiveness of these animals to environmental stimulation (noise) and handling, which lead to muscle spasms.

Opioids can be administered for analgesia and sedation but care should be taken to avoid high doses and the associated respiratory depression. Methadone (0.1–0.3 mg/kg i.m) or fentanyl by infusion (0.1–0.4 µg/kg/min i.v.) should be considered.

Induction of anaesthesia and endotracheal intubation

Preoxygenation with 100% oxygen by facemask should be performed in every neuromuscular case. The administration of oxygen will increase the alveolar PO_2 and delay desaturation if intubation of the trachea is difficult (Figure 21.23).

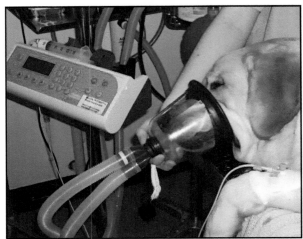

21.23 Preoxygenation prior to induction of anaesthesia in a patient with neuromuscular disease.

Consideration	Causes	Management
Dehydration	Weakness and recumbency may prevent normal food and water intake. Regurgitation may increase fluid loss	Correct fluid and electrolyte imbalances prior to anaesthesia
Aspiration	Dysphagia. Megaoesophagus. Laryngeal dysfunction	Rapid sequence induction: minimal sedation, bolus administration of induction agents in sternal recumbency with neck extended and head elevated, cricoid pressure, intubation with a cuffed endotracheal tube
Pneumonia	Aspiration. Recumbency	Preoperative treatment with antibiotics. Preoxygenation prior to induction of anaesthesia
Hypoventilation	Respiratory muscle weakness	Manual or mechanical IPPV. Appropriate monitoring (capnography and arterial blood gas analyses)
Upper respiratory tract obstruction	Laryngeal paralysis or spasm	Anaesthesia and tracheal intubation. Tracheostomy may be required
Hypoxaemia	Hypoventilation. Pneumonia. Lung collapse (atelectasis)	Preoxygenation prior to induction of anaesthesia; 100% oxygen during anaesthesia. Appropriate monitoring (pulse oximetry and arterial blood gas analyses). Oxygen supplementation during the recovery period (nasal tubes, oxygen cage or oxygen by mask)
Hypothermia	Inability to shiver	Passive warming in cold environments: warm intravenous fluids, warm air blankets, heat lamps, heat pads. Close monitoring of core body temperature
Hyperthermia	Inability to pant effectively	Passive cooling in warm environments: fans. Close monitoring of core body temperature

21.22 Considerations for anaesthesia of patients with peripheral nervous system disease.

A rapid sequence induction, using drugs that have a rapid onset of action, facilitates rapid control of the airway. Animals should be positioned in sternal recumbency, with the neck extended and the head held high. Pressure applied to the cricoid cartilage will minimize the risk of aspiration in the event of regurgitation. This pressure should be maintained until the cuff of the ETT has been inflated. The pharynx and oesophagus should also be suctioned at this point to prevent aspiration at the end of the procedure (Figure 21.24).

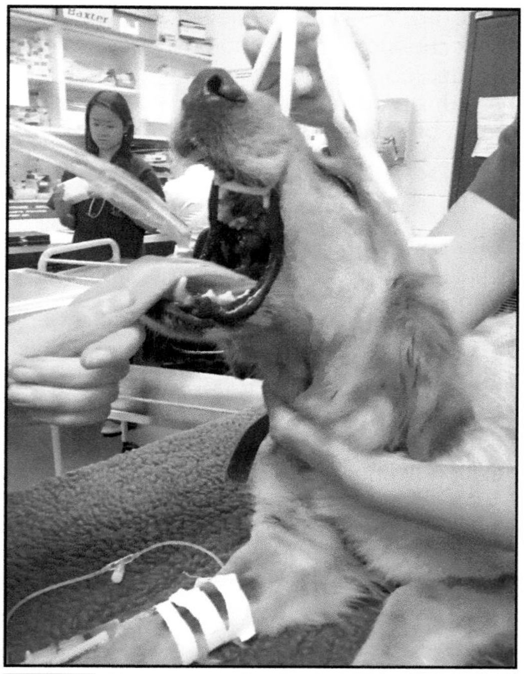

21.24 Pressure applied to the cricoid cartilage during a rapid sequence induction of anaesthesia.

Maintenance of anaesthesia

Anaesthesia can be maintained with an inhalant anaesthetic delivered in 100% oxygen or a mixture of oxygen and nitrous oxide. Either isoflurane or sevoflurane is appropriate. IPPV may be required (see later). Comprehensive monitoring during anaesthesia should also be performed (see later).

Recovery and postoperative analgesia

Towards the end of anaesthesia, suction of the pharynx and oesophagus is prudent. Removing stomach contents from these areas will minimize the risk of aspiration once the ETT has been removed. If there is concern about aspiration it may be safer to extubate the trachea carefully with the cuff partially inflated. This will pull any fluid that may have accumulated above the cuff out of the trachea. The patient should be positioned in sternal recumbency to encourage efficient spontaneous ventilation. If vomiting or regurgitation occurs at this time, the patient's head should be lowered to allow passive drainage. Repeat suctioning should be considered if the patient will tolerate it. These patients should never be extubated until there is convincing resumption of upper airway reflexes.

Patients with peripheral nervous system disease are unlikely to be in pain (an exception is polyradiculoneuritis) but the procedures to which they are subjected may cause pain. Muscle biopsy, nerve biopsy and nerve conduction studies may necessitate the administration of opioid analgesic drugs. Morphine may cause vomiting and so is best avoided in these patients.

Diagnostic procedures: electromyography and nerve conduction studies

Electrodiagnostic testing may be necessary in patients with peripheral nervous system disease. There are no specific considerations for this procedure in these patients above and beyond those detailed above. Mechanical ventilation may be required and so careful monitoring of adequacy of ventilation should be performed using capnography.

Intermittent positive pressure ventilation

Terminology

- PIP = peak inspiratory pressure; P_{max} = maximum inflation pressure – Peak or maximum pressure achieved at the end of inspiration. PIP should not exceed 20–25 cmH_2O in patients with normal healthy lungs
- PEEP = positive end-expiratory pressure – The pressure applied by the ventilator at the end of expiration to 'splint' the lung open and prevent alveolar collapse. Increasing the PEEP will help stabilize recruited alveoli but may have adverse haemodynamic effects. PEEP should be set between 1 and 5 cmH_2O in patients with normal healthy lungs
- I:E ratio = inspiratory:expiratory time ratio – The ratio of time spent during inspiration compared to expiration. During spontaneous ventilation it is usually 1:2.5 or 1:3. Relatively more time is spent in expiration as it is a passive process. Gas trapping is possible if the I:E ratio approaches 1:1
- t_i = inspiratory time – The actual time in seconds spent on inspiration. Altering t_i will alter the I:E ratio if the respiratory rate stays the same. A longer t_i may be indicated if slower inflation of alveoli is required, and less time will be spent at PIP. A shorter t_i will deliver the breath faster and expand the alveoli more rapidly. This may be more injurious. t_i of 0.2–0.4 seconds is common
- V_T = tidal volume – The volume of gas delivered in one breath. Normal V_T is 10–15 ml/kg. The V_T is a function of compliance and PIP. The more compliant the lung, the higher the V_T delivered for a set PIP

Manual or mechanical ventilation can be performed in patients with neurological disease as long as the haemodynamic and respiratory consequences are considered. Indications for manual or mechanical ventilation include maintenance of normocapnia (P_aCO_2 35–45 mmHg or 4.7–6 kP_a), management of hypoxaemia, and performance of neuromuscular blockade. Manual IPPV is best performed using a breathing system that has a manometer in the inspiratory or expiratory limb, so that inflation pressures can be monitored (Figure 21.25). Alternatively, a spirometer will measure the tidal volume of each breath and is helpful to standardize the size of each breath. The normal tidal volume of a patient is 10–15 ml/kg but the overall aim is to target the desired

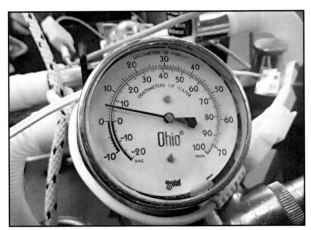

21.25 Airway pressure monitored during inspiration. Do not exceed 20 cmH$_2$O unless the respiratory and cardiovascular impact of ventilation can be assessed accurately and continuously.

P_aCO$_2$. The best non-invasive assessment of P_aCO$_2$ is the end-tidal CO$_2$ measured by a capnograph.

There is a plethora of mechanical ventilators available with a range of options (and terminology). The basis of most strategies is either volume or pressure cycling between breaths. This means that the breath is terminated when a set volume or pressure is reached.

During IPPV the lungs are inflated by applying positive pressure periodically to the upper airways through a tight-fitting mask or through an ETT or tracheostomy tube. The most efficient ventilation is achieved with the latter two. Changes in airway resistance and lung compliance can be overcome by manipulating the inspiratory flow and peak inspiratory pressure during IPPV. Mechanical ventilators will periodically create a pressure gradient between the machine circuit and alveoli that results in inspiratory gas flow. Exhalation is usually passive. The major disadvantages of IPPV are altered ventilation and perfusion relationships, potentially adverse circulatory effects and the risk of pulmonary barotrauma and volutrauma (see below).

Furthermore, IPPV will increase physiological dead space because gas flow is directed preferentially to the more compliant, non-dependent areas of the lungs while blood flow favours dependent areas. This may be offset to a degree by the use of positive end-expiratory pressure (PEEP). In patients with high ICP, PEEP should be used with extreme caution, if at all.

Haemodynamic consequences

The pressure changes during IPPV will impact upon venous return and cardiac output, and the extent of compromise to blood flow will depend upon the pressure generated, the duration of exposure to that pressure, the volume status of the patient, and the performance of the myocardium. Furthermore, the increased intrathoracic pressure created during IPPV will increase ICP.

Arterial blood pressure (ABP) should be monitored during IPPV. The gold standard for blood pressure monitoring is invasive, via a transducer connected to a catheter positioned in a peripheral artery. Non-invasive blood pressure measurement is suitable for cases where intermittent information is sufficient. Monitoring CVP will help determine whether the volume status of the patient is normal and the heart can pump the venous return effectively. If CVP decreases during IPPV, inflation pressures should be lowered.

Respiratory consequences

Non-invasive assessment of the respiratory consequences of IPPV can be achieved with pulse oximetry and capnography. In some cases, invasive methods are more appropriate and arterial blood samples can be collected for analysis. Decreasing S_pO$_2$ should be investigated. Causes of hypoxaemia include:

- Delivery of a hypoxic gas mix (<21% oxygen)
- Profound hypoventilation
- Ventilation and perfusion mismatch
- Shunting of blood through the lungs
- Pulmonary parenchymal disease inhibiting gaseous diffusion across the alveolar membrane.

For short procedures, monitoring the adequacy of ventilation with capnography is sufficient. For longer procedures, arterial blood gas analyses should be performed periodically to check the accuracy of the non-invasive techniques. Further details about pulse oximetry and capnography are given later in the chapter.

Ventilator-induced lung injury

Ventilator-induced lung injury may occur as a result of trauma to the lungs from the size, frequency, duration or pressure of delivered breaths. During prolonged procedures, or when ventilation is required for prolonged periods of time, ventilator-induced lung injury can be minimized with judicious monitoring. Careful decisions should be made regarding inflation pressures, tidal volumes and inspired oxygen concentration.

Barotrauma is lung injury resulting from high peak inflation pressures. Diseased lungs are more vulnerable to barotrauma and particular care must be taken when setting the peak inspiratory pressure (PIP). A maximum PIP of 20 cmH$_2$O is usually 'safe' in healthy lungs. In extreme cases of barotrauma, gas from overdistended ruptured alveoli leads to interstitial pulmonary emphysema and tracks along the adventitia to intrapulmonary blood vessels. Eventually the gas bubbles coalesce as they migrate centrally and mediastinal emphysema occurs. If this process persists, a pneumothorax may develop.

Volutrauma occurs as a result of the repeated opening and closing of normal or diseased lungs. Shearing forces injure the lung and exudative pulmonary oedema may form as a result of increased alveolar permeability. Lung compliance will then deteriorate and the tidal volume is displaced to more compliant areas, and injury is propagated.

High inspired oxygen concentrations will exacerbate the insult.

Close monitoring of oxygenation will allow titration of the inspired oxygen concentration (F_iO_2) to ensure the minimum is delivered. High inspired oxygen concentrations will promote alveolar collapse and, while this is unlikely to be problematic for short-term ventilation, it is recommended that mixing the inspired gas mix with medical air is performed to minimize the F_iO_2.

Volume-cycled IPPV

Volume-cycled ventilators terminate inspiration when a preselected tidal volume (V_T) is delivered. Most of these ventilators will alarm or terminate delivery of the V_T if inspiratory pressure exceeds a pressure limit. A percentage of V_T will be lost to the compliance of the breathing system during inspiration. The higher the lung compliance, the more is lost to the equipment. To assess V_T accurately, a spirometer must be placed between the ETT and the breathing system. Some volume-cycled ventilators do not terminate delivery of the V_T at a particular pressure (although an alarm will be triggered); patients must therefore be monitored continuously.

Pressure-cycled IPPV

Pressure-cycled ventilators cycle into the expiratory phase when airway pressure reaches a predetermined level. Both V_T and inspiratory time (t_i) vary according to airway resistance and lung and equipment compliance. A significant leak in the system will prevent the necessary rise in circuit pressure and therefore cycling between inspiration and expiration. Conversely, a sudden increase in circuit pressure (e.g. kinked tube or obstruction with blood or mucus) will cause rapid cycling between inspiration and expiration, and the delivery of smaller tidal volumes. Pressure-cycled ventilators are useful for small and paediatric patients and are arguably associated with less barotrauma than volume-cycled ventilators if appropriate pressures are set. It is useful to assess V_T during ventilation to appreciate lung compliance.

Perioperative patient monitoring

Pulse oximetry

Pulse oximetry provides a non-invasive beat-by-beat assessment of the amount of oxygen carried by haemoglobin within the arterial blood. This can provide information on the adequacy of oxygen exchange within the lungs. Pulse oximetry has a variety of limitations, particularly in anaesthetized animals, which need to be considered when interpreting measurements. These limitations include:

- Shape of the oxygen–haemoglobin dissociation curve: small changes in oxyhaemoglobin saturation (S_pO_2) are associated with large changes in arterial oxygen tension (P_aO_2). Mild hypoxaemia (P_aO_2 ~80 mmHg; 10.7 kPa) corresponds to 95% saturation; severe

hypoxaemia (P_aO_2 <60 mmHg; 8 kPa) corresponds to <90% saturation (Figure 21.26)
- Inspiration of high inspired oxygen (>30%) during anaesthesia:
  - Haemoglobin is almost 100% saturated when animals with normal lungs breathe room air (F_iO_2 0.21). When animals are breathing higher inspired concentrations no further saturation of haemoglobin will occur (Figure 21.27)
  - The adequacy of alveolar ventilation cannot be assessed using pulse oximetry. In animals breathing room air, increases in alveolar CO_2 will decrease alveolar oxygen available for diffusion into the circulation. This can lead to hypoxaemia and hypoxia. In animals breathing a high F_iO_2, increases in CO_2 will not significantly decrease the alveolar oxygen tension. This means that severe hypercapnia can be present in animals with normal S_pO_2 readings
- Pulse oximeters do not provide information on the total amount of oxygen carried by the blood. The oxygen content of blood is dependent on

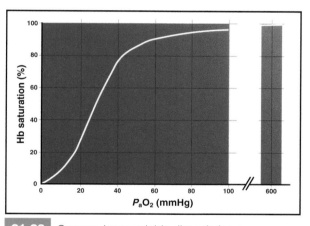

21.26 Oxygen–haemoglobin dissociation curve.

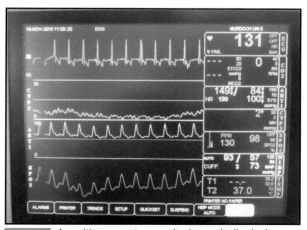

21.27 A multi-parameter monitoring unit displaying (from top): electrocardiogram; CVP waveform and measurement; invasive ABP waveform and measurements; and a plethysomograph with pulse rate and oxyhaemoglobin saturation (S_pO_2).

haemoglobin concentration and inspired oxygen concentration. This is particularly important in anaemic animals. In these cases, red cell count and haemoglobin and thus oxygen-carrying capacity is reduced, but haemoglobin can be fully saturated. Therefore, oxygen saturation may be normal even when oxygen delivery is decreased

- The accuracy of pulse oximetry is influenced by perfusion. A reduction in peripheral perfusion due to low blood pressure and perfusion pressure or vasoconstriction can result in inaccuracies in $S_pO_2\%$
- Accuracy of pulse oximetry is also influenced by ambient light. Exposure of the probe to high levels of light will artefactually increase the S_pO_2.

Due to these limitations it is recommended that intermittent arterial blood gas analysis is performed in the following situations:

- Animals that are having surgery, particularly intracranial surgery
- Animals with concurrent pulmonary and/or cardiovascular disease
- Animals requiring long-term ventilation.

Capnography

Capnography measures the changes in inspired and expired gases over time. The CO_2 pressure at the end of expiration is the end-tidal CO_2 ($ETCO_2$) (Figure 21.28), which approximates the CO_2 tension in the alveoli (P_ACO_2). In animals with normal cardio-pulmonary function the alveolar gases should be in equilibrium with arterial blood, thus $ETCO_2$ should approximate P_aCO_2. In normal animals under anaes-thesia $ETCO_2$ is equal to, or slightly lower than, P_aCO_2. In animals with reduced pulmonary blood flow (e.g. low cardiac output, pulmonary embolus), a proportion of alveoli will not be perfused (physiologi-cal deadspace) and thus gas exchange will not occur. As a result these alveoli will not contain CO_2. During expiration, the gas from these alveoli will dilute the gases from perfused alveoli, resulting in $ETCO_2$ that is lower than P_aCO_2. The magnitude of

the difference between arterial and $ETCO_2$ will depend on the proportion of alveoli being perfused and on the magnitude of reduction in pulmonary blood flow.

In any animal where maintenance of normocap-nia is essential (e.g. intracranial disease), arterial blood gas analysis should be performed intermit-tently to determine whether $ETCO_2$ is an accurate estimate of P_aCO_2. Where discrepancies occur, adjustments to ventilator settings should be based on arterial CO_2 tension only. Adjustment based on $ETCO_2$ may result in development of hypercapnia.

Arterial blood gas analysis

Collection of arterial blood for blood gas analysis should be performed in any animal where accurate assessment of P_aCO_2 and P_aO_2 is required. Blood can be collected via a needle or from a catheter placed in a peripheral artery; the latter is preferable as this allows repeated samples to be collected easily and also allows concurrent measurement of arterial blood pressure.

The most common site for collection of blood and/or arterial catheter placement in small animals is the dorsal pedal artery (Figure 21.29). Blood can also be collected from the femoral artery. However, there is a greater risk of haemorrhage from the fem-oral artery as this site cannot be bandaged. If the femoral artery is used for sampling, a small gauge needle (25 G) is recommended and firm digital pres-sure must be applied immediately over the puncture site and maintained for 1–2 minutes.

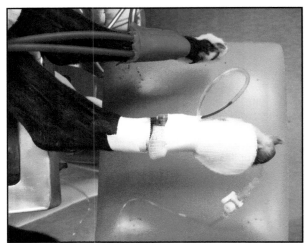

21.29 A catheter in the dorsal pedal artery of a dog for invasive blood pressure measurement (foreground) and a non-invasive blood pressure cuff in position for non-invasive blood pressure measurement (background).

The alveolar oxygen tension (P_AO_2) can be cal-culated from results of arterial blood gas analysis. This determines the amount of oxygen that should be available in the alveoli for gas exchange.

$$P_AO_2 = F_iO_2 (P_{atmos} - PH_2O) - (P_aCO_2/R)$$

Where: P_{atmos} = atmospheric pressure = 760 mmHg; PH_2O = water vapour pressure = 147 mmHg; R (respiratory quotient) = 0.8–1.

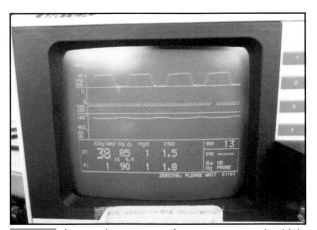

21.28 A normal capnogram from a capnograph which measures inspired (Fi) and expired (ET) CO_2, O_2, N_2O and inhalant anaesthetic.

Calculating the P_AO_2 enables determination of the effect of hypercapnia on oxygen availability. Marked increases in arterial and therefore alveolar CO_2 can significantly decrease the amount of oxygen available for gas exchange, especially in animals breathing room air. Furthermore, the difference between P_AO_2 and P_aO_2 can be calculated. The greater the difference, the more shunting of blood is occurring through the lungs. This may occur during non-cardiogenic pulmonary oedema or ventilator-induced lung injury or as a result of atelectasis from anaesthesia or recumbency.

Oxygen content (C_aO_2) is calculated as the sum of oxygen bound to haemoglobin and oxygen dissolved in the plasma.

$$C_aO_2 = (S_pO_2 \times [Hb] \times 1.34) + (0.003 \times P_aO_2 \, mmHg)$$

Calculating the C_aO_2 provides a more accurate assessment of the amount of oxygen available to the tissues, particularly in anaemic animals. S_pO_2 and P_aO_2 may be normal in these animals despite marked decreases in haemoglobin concentration and thus oxygen available for delivery to the tissues.

Oxygen delivery (DO_2) to tissues is a product of cardiac output (CO) and arterial oxygen content.

$$DO_2 = CO \times C_aO_2$$

Calculation of DO_2 is the ultimate measure of adequacy of tissue oxygenation as it determines the adequacy of the blood delivery to the tissues as well as the amount of oxygen in the blood. Calculation of DO_2 emphasizes the fact that simply maintaining C_aO_2 does not ensure adequate oxygen delivery if blood volume and cardiac output are inadequate. Specialist equipment is required for the measurement of CO, so it is usually limited to referral institutions. In clinical practice, due to the relationship between CO and MAP ($MAP = CO \times SVR$), MAP can provide an indirect indicator of adequacy of CO.

Electrocardiography

Electrocardiography is recommended in animals with neurological disease. The electrocardiogram (ECG) provides continuous measurement of heart rate and also provides important information about heart rhythm. While the ECG only gives information about electrical activity of the heart, it is useful for detection of changes in rate and rhythm that can alter cardiac output and perfusion of the tissues. Furthermore, changes in rate and rhythm can help with early detection of brain herniation in anaesthetized patients. As the brainstem starts to herniate, the increase in sympathetic activity may manifest as a tachyarrhythmia. This is followed by bradycardia in response to the increase in blood pressure that also occurs (Cushing reflex).

Arterial blood pressure

Monitoring of arterial blood pressure (ABP) is essential for ensuring adequate perfusion pressure of CNS tissue and other vital organs (kidney, heart) during anaesthesia. ABP can be measured non-invasively using oscillometric or Doppler techniques or invasively via an arterial catheter connected to a transducer.

Oscillometric techniques are useful for measuring blood pressure in stable animals and animals undergoing short periods of anaesthesia such as imaging or other diagnostic procedures. Many of the commercial systems available are unreliable in very small animals such as cats and animals with low blood pressure, bradycardia and irregular heart rates. However, the accuracy in these situations is improving, with newer equipment becoming more readily available.

The Doppler technique is a useful non-invasive technique for measurement of blood pressure in animals that are very small (cats and small dogs) and animals that have low blood pressure or low heart rates. The main limitation of this technique is that it only measures systolic arterial blood pressure (SAP).

Invasive measurements of ABP are performed via an arterial catheter connected to a fluid-filled line and a transducer which converts the pressure signal to an electronic signal that is subsequently displayed on the monitor. The advantages of invasive blood pressure measurement include the greater accuracy of diastolic, mean and systolic blood pressure values, the continuous nature of the measurement and the production of a waveform (which itself provides useful information about cardiovascular performance).

Catheters are most commonly placed in the dorsal pedal artery in small animals (see Figure 21.29). Arterial blood gas samples can also be obtained from the arterial catheter, allowing accurate assessment of pulmonary function and oxygen delivery (see above). Invasive techniques are recommended over non-invasive techniques in unstable animals, animals having intracranial surgery, animals expected to suffer marked blood loss during surgery and chronically ventilated animals.

Central venous pressure

CVP provides a measurement of the pressure within the compliant vessels supplying the right atrium. It is measured via a catheter inserted into a central vein such as the cranial or caudal vena cava. The catheter is then connected by a fluid-filled line to a water manometer or transducer. The most common site for central venous catheter placement is the jugular vein. However, in animals with intracranial disease, placement of the catheter in the jugular vein may increase the risk of disturbance to venous return and increased ICP. An alternative is to place a catheter via a peripheral vein such as the medial saphenous vein into the caudal vena cava (peripherally inserted central catheter, PICC). When this is not possible, the catheter can be placed via the jugular vein provided care is taken not to occlude the jugular during placement (surgical exposure may be required) and a small diameter catheter is used so that interference with venous return is minimized. The use of neck bandages over these catheters is also discouraged in animals with intracranial disease.

Measurement of CVP is useful in the following scenarios:

- Volume overload: CVP measurement is recommended in animals that are prone to volume overload (cardiac disease, renal disease) or in animals where volume overload may have detrimental effects on CNS function (intracranial disease). In these animals CVP can provide information on the adequacy of the rate and volume of fluid that has been administered
- Risk of hypovolaemia: CVP is more sensitive to changes in blood volume than blood pressure. To minimize secondary neurological injury due to volume loss, CVP is recommended in animals where haemorrhage during surgery is considered a major risk
- Detrimental effects of IPPV: Measurement of CVP is helpful to determine whether IPPV is interfering with venous return and potentially contributing to increases in intracranial blood volume and ICP. Mean and peak intrathoracic pressures used during mechanical ventilation can be adjusted if detrimental increases in CVP are observed.

The volume and pressure within the central veins are influenced by blood volume and cardiac function. Increases in CVP may be due to increased blood volume or poor cardiac function. Typically, increased blood volume would also be associated with normal/high ABP. In contrast, poor cardiac function will cause low ABP. As the normal range for CVP is relatively large (0–8 cm H_2O), changes in CVP are more useful than the absolute value. For example, in animals with low blood volume and normal cardiac function, rapid administration of fluids will produce gradual increase in CVP as volume is restored. By contrast, in animals with poor cardiac function, increased rates of fluid therapy may not be tolerated and rapid increases in CVP are observed. In these cases the rate of fluid administration is reduced until rapid/marked increases in CVP are no longer seen.

Body temperature

Monitoring of body temperature is important in all anaesthetized animals as hypothermia is associated with numerous side effects including prolonged recovery, reduced anaesthetic requirement, reduced immunity and increased risk of infection, poor healing, increased blood loss and reduced cardiovascular function.

Analgesia

Patients with CNS disease are more likely to be in pain if they have spinal disease as opposed to intracranial disease. The exceptions are traumatic injury causing intracranial lesions and surgery for intracranial disease. Patients with spinal disease may require aggressive analgesic therapy based on an opioid with non-steroidal anti-inflammatory drugs, ketamine, alpha-2 adrenoreceptor agonists, tramadol, gabapentin and amantadine as adjunctive therapies. With the exception of polyradiculoneuritis, peripheral nervous system disease is unlikely to be painful and so analgesia is unlikely to be required unless the procedure to which the patient has been subjected causes tissue trauma (e.g. nerve or muscle biopsy).

In each and every case, assessment of pain is essential to ensure appropriate pain management. Pain assessment is very difficult in animals and is arguably more difficult in patients with neurological disease. Despite these difficulties, application of a scoring system such as the visual analogue scale or a simple descriptive scale is important. A composite scoring system is ideal and the short form of the Glasgow Composite Pain Scale (Murrell *et al.*, 2008) may be useful. Following the administration of analgesic drugs or efforts to provide comfort (positioning, bedding, and environment), regular review to ensure the desired effect is achieved is essential (Figure 21.30).

Indication	Drug	Doses	Advantages	Side effects
Perioperative analgesia and anaesthetic sparing	Morphine	0.1–0.4 mg/kg i.m. or i.v. q4h 0.1 mg/kg/h by i.v. infusion	Analgesia Sedation ↓ Anaesthetic requirements	↓ Heart rate Respiratory depression Nausea and vomiting
	Methadone	0.1–0.4 mg/kg i.m. or i.v. q4–6h	Analgesia ↓ Anaesthetic requirements	↓ Heart rate Respiratory depression Mild sedation
	Pethidine	2–5 mg/kg i.m. q1–2h	Short duration Analgesia	Histamine release if given i.v. Painful by i.m. injection
	Fentanyl	Intraoperatively 2–5 µg/kg i.v. q20min 0.1-0.4 µg/kg/min i.v. infusion Pre/postoperatively 2–5 µg/kg/h 2–5 µg/kg transcutaneous (patch)	Analgesia ↓ Anaesthetic requirements Short duration makes it suitable for infusion	↓ Heart rate Respiratory depression

21.30 Analgesic drugs for perioperative pain management in dogs and cats with neurological disease. Where a dose range is given, the lower dose is recommended for intravenous administration and intramuscular injection, and in less stable animals; higher doses are recommended for intramuscular administration in alert animals or those in pain. The dose interval may be longer in cats. (continues) ▶

Indication	Drug	Doses	Advantages	Side effects
Perioperative analgesia and anaesthetic sparing (continued)	Remifentanil	Intraoperative 0.1–0.4 µg/kg/min i.v. infusion	Analgesia ↓ Anaesthetic requirements Short duration makes it suitable for infusion	↓ Heart rate Respiratory depression No analgesia persists once infusion stopped
Analgesia for moderate pain	Buprenorphine	0.01–0.02 mg/kg i.m or s.c. q6–8h	Moderate analgesia Long duration	Prolonged onset of action (~45 min)
Sedation	Butorphanol	0.05–0.4 mg/kg i.m. or i.v.	Good sedation Antitussive	Poor analgesia Antagonizes pure mu agonists (morphine, methadone, pethidine and fentanyl)
Inflammatory pain	Carprofen	4 mg/kg s.c. or i.v. loading dose then 2 mg/kg orally or s.c. q24h	Effective analgesia for inflammatory pain	Renal damage and gastrointestinal ulceration may occur in animals with poor organ perfusion
	Meloxicam	0.2 mg/kg s.c. or i.v. loading dose then 0.1 mg/kg orally or s.c. q24h	Effective analgesia for inflammatory pain	Renal damage and gastrointestinal ulceration may occur in animals with poor organ perfusion
Sedation and analgesia	Medetomidine	1–20 µg/kg i.m. or i.v.	Analgesia at very low microdoses Sedation at moderate to high doses Reversible ↓ Anaesthetic requirements	Sedation Bradyarrhythmias Vasoconstriction Hypotension
Central or peripheral sensitization	Ketamine	1–10 mg/kg i.m. or i.v. 5–10 µg/kg/min infusion	Adjunctive analgesia for direct nerve trauma or chronic pain ↓ Anaesthetic requirements	↑ ICP ↑ Intraocular pressure Dissociative effects Tachyarrhythmias
	Lidocaine	20–40 µg/kg/min infusion	Adjunctive analgesia for direct nerve trauma or chronic pain ↓ Anaesthetic requirements	Hypotension due to direct myocardial depression and bradycardia
	Gabapentin	Titrate dose from 2mg/kg up to 10–20 mg/kg orally q8–12h	Adjunctive analgesia for direct nerve trauma or chronic pain	Oral form only; thus not ideal in perianaesthetic period Use in animals not well studied
Other analgesic agents with opioid activity	Tramadol	1–2 mg/kg s.c., i.m. or i.v q8–12h	Analgesia	Few at clinical doses Effectiveness in cats is uncertain Seizures reported in small number of human patients (Le Roux, 2000)
Muscle relaxation	Midazolam	0.1–0.4 mg/kg i.m. or i.v. q15–20 min 0.1–0.4 mg/kg/h infusion	Muscle relaxation may be useful in animals with pain associated with spinal disease	DO NOT use in animals with unstable spinal lesions Few side effects Paradoxical excitation possible

21.30 (continued) Analgesic drugs for perioperative pain management in dogs and cats with neurological disease. Where a dose range is given, the lower dose is recommended for intravenous administration and intramuscular injection, and in less stable animals; higher doses are recommended for intramuscular administration in alert animals or those in pain. The dose interval may be longer in cats.

Fluid therapy

Fluid therapy is indicated in the perianaesthetic period:

- Preoperative fluid therapy:
    - To replace fluid deficit (e.g. dehydration, traumatic blood loss, diuretic therapy)
- Intraoperative fluid therapy:
    - To maintain normal hydration and fluid volume during anaesthesia
    - To manage intraoperative hypotension
    - To replace surgical losses that may occur
- Postoperative fluid therapy:
    - To maintain hydration and electrolyte balance until the animal is eating and drinking adequately.

Preoperative fluid therapy

To minimize the risk of hypotension and reduced perfusion of the CNS, fluid deficits should be corrected before anaesthesia whenever possible. Numerous types of fluid and electrolyte abnormalities may be present in neurological animals. The management of each of these is beyond the scope of this chapter and the reader is referred to Di Bartola (2006).

As a general rule, fluid deficits are replaced with the type of fluid that resembles the fluid lost. The rate of replacement of the fluid deficit depends on loss of blood volume *versus* loss of total body water.

- Reduction in blood volume (e.g. haemorrhage, severe dehydration >12% bodyweight) affects blood pressure and tissue perfusion, and losses should be replaced quickly (1–2 hours).
- Loss of total body water that does not significantly reduce blood volume (<10% bodyweight) and is not associated with sodium abnormalities can be replaced at a slower rate (12–24 hours).
- Presence of sodium abnormalities for more than 2–3 days necessitates slow correction of sodium concentration to prevent neurological damage. Thus any concurrent fluid deficit needs to be replaced very carefully (2–3 days) once any deficit in blood volume has been corrected.

Note: When anaesthesia for diagnosis and treatment is required urgently to maximize recovery of neurological function (e.g. in spinal compression with absence of nociception, with ingested neurotoxin such as metaldehyde requiring gastric lavage for elimination of the toxin from body), replacement of the deficit may need to be performed quickly and completed during anaesthesia.

Intraoperative fluid therapy

Normotensive patients

Administration of fluids during surgery is essential to ensure maintenance of blood volume and pressure. Fluid administration is indicated during anaesthesia to:

- Fill the vascular space that has been increased by the vasodilatory effects of anaesthetic agents (i.e. manage anaesthetic-induced relative hypovolaemia)
- Replace fluid lost during surgery, such as evaporative losses from exposed tissues and losses from the respiratory tract that occur when cold and dry anaesthetic gases are inspired.

Typically polyionic isotonic fluids are administered. The initial rate is generally 10 ml/kg/h.

Hypotensive patients

Low blood pressure is typically defined as MAP <60 mmHg, SAP <80 mmHg. In animals with intracranial disease it is recommended that MAP be maintained >70 mmHg, and SAP >100 mmHg. Causes of hypotension under anaesthesia include:

- Relative hypovolaemia associated with drug-induced vasodilatation (e.g. propofol, isoflurane)
- Pre-existing unmanaged fluid deficit
- Volume loss during surgery.

Fluid therapy is indicated for management of low blood pressure when reduction in anaesthetic depth does not resolve hypotension rapidly (<10 minutes).

The type and rate of fluid therapy will depend on the severity and duration of hypotension and accompanying changes in PCV and total protein. Figure 21.31 provides some guidelines for selection of fluid type and rates for the correction of hypotension during anaesthesia.

Concurrent abnormalities	Fluid type	Fluid rates (i.v.)
Normal PCV/ total protein	Polyionic, isotonic crystalloids	Dogs: 20–80 ml/kg/h Cats: 20–50 ml/kg/h
Normal PCV/ total protein and increased ICP	Synthetic colloids	Dogs: 5–20 ml/kg/h Cats: 5–10 ml/kg/h
	Hypertonic saline	2–4 ml/kg over 10 minutes
Decreased total protein	Synthetic colloids	Dogs: 5–20 ml/kg/h Cats: 5–10 ml/kg/h
Decreased total protein and PCV	Whole blood	2–20 ml/kg/h

21.31 Fluid therapy for the management of hypotension. Regardless of the type of fluid used to correct hypotension, the response to fluid therapy should be assessed regularly. As soon as the target blood pressure is achieved, the rate of fluid administration may be decreased to minimize potential complications.

Blood loss: Loss of blood during surgery is not uncommon, especially during spinal surgery. Close monitoring of blood lost from the surgical site should be performed by weighing swabs or measuring the volume of blood in suction bottles.

When blood loss is minor (<20% of blood volume), the volume deficit can be replaced with crystalloids as long as oxygen-carrying capacity and colloid oncotic pressure (COP) remain adequate (PCV >30%; Hb >8 g/l; COP >15 mmHg). The volume of crystalloid required is three to four times the estimated remaining deficit in blood volume as only one-quarter to one-third of the crystalloid remains within the vascular space after approximately an hour. In the authors' experience, animals with intracranial disease can be less tolerant of blood loss than other animals. In these cases replacement of the volume deficit with blood products may be considered for smaller losses of blood (10–20% of blood volume).

The rate of replacement is influenced by accompanying changes in clinical signs of perfusion (heart rate, blood pressure, mucous membrane colour and mentation on recovery). A slower than expected recovery in an animal that has suffered loss of blood may support the need for replacement of the blood volume deficit with blood products to increase oxygen delivery to the brain. NB Close monitoring of blood pressure and PCV/total protein is still required as overtransfusion will also adversely affect CNS perfusion.

When the volume of blood lost is >20% of blood volume, the deficit needs to be replaced in part with blood products to prevent a reduction in red cell count or COP. Whenever blood loss during surgery is considered likely, cross-matching and/or blood typing should be performed to minimize any adverse reaction to the donor blood, especially in cats. In emergencies this may not always be possible. In dogs that have not had a previous blood transfusion or had puppies, there is minimal risk associated with administration of blood for the first time.

Blood loss associated with surgery generally occurs rapidly and is associated with clinical signs of surgical shock. Thus the blood volume deficit needs to be replaced rapidly (dogs 10–20 ml/kg/h; cats 5–10 ml/kg/h).

Replacement of the entire deficit in blood volume with blood products is not necessary and may be harmful. Overtransfusion can be detrimental in animals with intracranial disease due to resultant increases in viscosity that will decrease cerebral perfusion. In human patients with intracranial disease, the ideal PCV is 30% as this provides adequate oxygen-carrying capacity and also produces beneficial rheological properties that enhance cerebral perfusion.

As a general guideline, blood products are administered until <20 % of the deficit is remaining or PCV is 30%. The remaining deficit can be replaced with crystalloids as described above.

Postoperative fluid therapy

Fluid therapy should be continued into the postoperative period to provide maintenance fluid requirements and to replace any ongoing fluid deficits. Normal maintenance rates are 2 ml/kg/h (~50 ml/kg/day). However, higher maintenance requirements are required in animals receiving corticosteroids and osmotic diuretics and those with increased body temperature or that are panting. The cornerstone of

fluid therapy in the postoperative period is formed by isotonic crystalloids. In inappetent animals, supplementation of potassium chloride is also recommended until the animal is eating. Supplementation of other electrolytes (phosphorus, magnesium) should be guided by analysis of serum biochemistry. The type and rate of other fluids administered will depend on concurrent abnormalities that are present in the postoperative period. Examples of postoperative fluid therapy are provided in Figure 21.32.

Concurrent abnormalities	Fluid type	Fluid rates (i.v.)
Normal PCV/ total protein; no ongoing deficits	Polyionic isotonic crystalloids + KCl 20 mmol/l	2 ml/kg/h + estimated losses/h
Normal PCV and ongoing decrease in total protein	Polyionic isotonic crystalloids + KCl 20 mmol/l	2 ml/kg/h + estimated losses/h
	Synthetic colloids	20 ml/kg/day; rate will depend on presence of concurrent blood volume/pressure measurement
Ongoing deficit in blood volume	Polyionic isotonic crystalloids + KCl 20 mmol/l	2 ml/kg/h + estimated losses/h
	Crystalloids (remaining blood volume deficit <20%)	Add 3 x volume in crystalloids to maintenance for first 6–12 hours
	Whole blood/PRBC + colloid (remaining blood volume deficit >20%)	Administer remaining deficit over <6 hours (maximum hang time of blood bag)

21.32 Postoperative fluid therapy. The rate of administration of potassium chloride should not exceed 0.5 mmol/kg/h. PRBC = packed red blood cells.

References and further reading

Available on accompanying DVD

22

Principles of neurosurgery

Beverly K. Sturges and Peter J. Dickinson

Competency in the neurosurgical management of animals with nervous system disease is based on an understanding of a wide variety of clinical and basic science topics, in addition to the neurosurgical procedures themselves. A comprehensive knowledge of functional neuroanatomy and physiology is essential for competent surgical technique and well informed decision-making when surgical plans need to be modified and/or complications managed.

The value of cadaver dissections and ready access to skull and vertebral column preparations cannot be overemphasized. Every aspiring neurosurgeon should have his/her own collection of skulls and vertebrae to study and use as references before and during neurosurgical procedures. An authentic three-dimensional (3D) knowledge of the anatomical structures of the central nervous system (CNS), both superficial and deep, is developed by observing the anatomy of the brain and spinal cord from many different angles.

To design a rational treatment plan for any patient, the surgeon must first identify the underlying disease process and the likely course of events without (surgical) intervention. The potential risks and benefits of the various medical and surgical therapies available to the veterinary surgeon should be evaluated and weighed against the natural history of the disease. An evidence-based approach to treatment planning requires generalization of experimental and/or statistical clinical data to the individual patient. As yet, this information is lacking in veterinary medicine, particularly with respect to the field of neurosurgery. Anecdotal information and techniques prevent surgeons from predicting with confidence the best approach in many situations.

The purpose of this chapter is to provide an overview of the common neurosurgical procedures, the general and specific indications for their use and the complications that may result. A detailed description of specific neurosurgical procedures is beyond the scope of this chapter and the reader is directed to the following texts for more detailed reviews: Wheeler and Sharp (1994), Seim (1997), Sharp (2002) and Tobias and Johnston (2011). Procedures for treating vertebral fractures and luxations are described and illustrated in the BSAVA Manual of Small Animal Fracture Repair and Management.

Indications for neurosurgery

General indications
General indications for neurosurgery include:

- The surgical procedure has been shown to have a significantly better clinical outcome than medical treatment alone
- The disease is unresponsive or no longer responsive to medical therapy
- The clinical signs are severe or rapidly progressive
- There is vertebral column instability
- Diagnostic confirmation when this cannot be determined by other techniques.

The clinical response to medical versus surgical treatment varies over time and must be considered when deciding whether or not to perform surgery. Palliation of clinical signs with medical treatment may be effective in the short term but surgical intervention, such as resection or debulking of tumours, may result in an improved long-term outcome. The risks and benefits of surgery, together with the effects of delaying surgery to pursue medical treatment, must be assessed for each individual case.

When deciding whether or not to pursue surgery, it is essential to have an accurate neuroanatomical localization prior to conducting diagnostic procedures. Lesions identified outside the region of localization may not be clinically significant, and surgery may not be indicated. Lesions located within the region of localization should be defined as completely as possible to allow precise surgical planning.

Neurosurgical emergencies
Indications for emergency surgical referral are based on the presence of severe and/or progressively deteriorating neurological signs. For appropriate medical treatment prior to referral (e.g. cardiovascular stabilization, oxygen therapy, hyperosmolar treatment), the reader is referred to Chapter 20 and the BSAVA Manual of Canine and Feline Emergency and Critical Care. The most common neurological conditions that may require emergency surgery include acute spinal cord and brain injury.

Acute spinal cord injury
Causes of acute spinal cord injury include:

- Vertebral fracture/luxation
- Acute disc herniation

- Haemorrhage/haematoma
- Decompensating neoplasia.

The presence of any or all of the following clinical signs may warrant the need for immediate surgical intervention with acute spinal cord injury:

- Rapid progression from paresis to paralysis
- Acute onset of paralysis
- Loss of nociception
- Hypoventilation
- Suspected vertebral column instability.

Acute brain injury
Causes of acute brain injury include:

- Intracranial haemorrhage/haematoma
- Depressed skull fractures
- Decompensating neoplasia
- Rapidly progressing intracranial hypertension
- Acute cerebrospinal fluid (CSF) outflow obstruction.

The presence of any or all of the following clinical signs may warrant the need for immediate surgical intervention:

- Progressive deterioration in mental status (e.g. obtundation progressing to stupor or coma)
- Progressive loss of brainstem reflexes
- Decerebrate or decerebellate posture
- Abnormal ventilation patterns (not caused by pulmonary disease).

Common neurosurgical procedures

- Decompression involves removal of part of the bony calvaria or vertebra ± removal of space-occupying masses to alleviate ongoing compression of the neural tissue.
- Fenestration is the creation of an opening in the intervertebral disc by removal of a section of the annulus fibrosus to allow the removal of nucleus pulposus (pulpectomy).
- Realignment, stabilization and/or fusion of one or more vertebrae is indicated when vertebral column instability is present secondary to fracture, luxation or malformation/malarticulation.
- Mass resection may involve the removal of any infiltrative or compressive tissue, including neoplasia, inflammatory/infectious granulomas, haematomas, bony proliferation and hypertrophied soft tissues.
- Exploratory surgery and biopsy is indicated when a definitive diagnosis cannot be determined by other neurodiagnostics. Biopsy may also be undertaken as part of decompressive or excisional procedures, and can provide valuable information relating to drug sensitivity in infectious conditions such as discospondylitis. It is commonly used to determine the aetiology of peripheral nerve and muscle disorders. Minimally invasive stereotactic

image-guided biopsy procedures (see Chapter 6) are specifically indicated when definitive treatment plans are required and open surgical procedures are not indicated.

Selection of a neurosurgical procedure
Factors to consider when selecting a neurosurgical procedure include:

- Neuroanatomical location of the lesion along the neuraxis as well as the exact location of the pathological process (e.g. whether compression is situated ventral, lateral or dorsal to the spinal cord)
- Intended goal (decompression, excision, biopsy)
- Regional anatomy and neuroanatomy (e.g. vascular structures)
- Extent of the lesion and the amount of exposure needed
- Extent of removable bone and the impact this may have on regional biomechanical function and stability (especially if preoperative instability is present)
- Neurological status of the patient.

Considerations prior to neurosurgery

Preoperative patient assessment and management
A thorough history and physical and neurological examinations are fundamental in these cases. Following neuroanatomical localization and the generation of an appropriate list of differential diagnoses, further diagnostic tests should be considered, including a complete blood count (CBC), serum chemistry, urinalysis, thoracic radiography and abdominal ultrasonography.

It is also important to determine whether there are any concurrent diseases that may directly result in neurological disease or significantly impact either the decision to proceed with the surgical procedure or lead to complications during or after the surgery. For example, in a recent study of dogs with brain tumours, 23% had other neoplastic lesions unrelated to the primary tumour and approximately 20% had significant disease on thoracic radiographs (Snyder *et al.*, 2006). This is especially important in older animals and in breeds with predilections for specific conditions (e.g. cervical spondylomyelopathy in Mastiffs, Great Danes and Dobermanns).

The use of non-steroidal anti-inflammatory drugs (NSAIDs), particularly aspirin, should be avoided for several days prior to surgery due to their ability to cause platelet dysfunction. Although the use of the buccal mucosal bleeding time (BMBT) test as a screening tool for predicting the occurrence of intraoperative bleeding tendency is not recommended in humans (Chee *et al.*, 2008), two small case series in veterinary medicine suggest that preoperative BMBT may be correlated with intraoperative blood loss (Jergens *et al.*, 1987; Lee *et al.*, 2006).

Any animals with a history or clinical examination suggestive of anticoagulant intoxication should be assessed using coagulation tests (e.g. prothrombin time, partial thromboplastin time and activated clotting time) prior to undergoing neurosurgical procedures.

The use of corticosteroids following acute trauma to the CNS and as a preoperative prophylactic measure is controversial in both human and veterinary neurological practice. The only corticosteroid that may have a beneficial effect in selected human cases is methylprednisolone sodium succinate (MPSS), although this is not widely accepted by the human medical community. There is no clinical evidence to support the preoperative use of high dose MPSS in veterinary neurosurgery, and corticosteroid use is specifically contraindicated in humans with head trauma. However, anti-inflammatory doses of prednisone are often beneficial in reducing the associated oedema, CSF production and/or inflammation in intracranial disease where trauma is not the underlying cause (e.g. peritumoural oedema). Controlled studies demonstrating the benefit of this treatment have not been performed, and the potential side effects associated with the use of prednisone must be considered. Use of other presurgical medications such as vitamin E and inorganic polymers (e.g. polyethylene glycol) is also unproven, but appears to have fewer adverse effects.

Perioperative antibiotic prophylaxis is recommended for all neurosurgical procedures. A broad-spectrum bactericidal drug such as a cephalosporin or penicillin derivative is generally used. Neither preoperative nor postoperative administration is indicated unless there is an ongoing infection (e.g. a urinary tract infection) or there is potential compromise of the normal barriers to infection (e.g. surgical approach through the frontal sinuses).

Surgical equipment

Surgical instruments that are used for neurosurgery should be kept strictly for this purpose. The removal of bone during laminectomy or craniotomy is generally achieved using a high speed electrical or pneumatic drill. Other neurosurgical instruments such as titanium microdissectors and neurosurgical bayonette forceps/scissors are valuable for fine procedures such as the resection of tumours. Ultrasonic aspirators and lasers are particularly useful for more advanced neurosurgical procedures such as the removal of intra-axial neoplasms. Magnification is recommended for most neurological procedures. Operating loupes are generally sufficient; however, an operating microscope, exoscope or endoscope can be useful in certain circumstances. A head-mounted fibreoptic light source is also useful.

The key to success in many neurosurgical procedures is being able to avoid or adequately control haemorrhage at the surgical site. Monopolar cautery systems may be used for incising and cauterizing the more superficial tissues and muscles, but bipolar cautery must be used when working close to the neural tissues. Haemostatic sponges (e.g. Gelfoam®, compressed gelatine) and bone wax are ideal for controlling haemorrhage from cancellous bone and venous sinuses and are often left *in situ*. There are other absorbable haemostatic materials available (e.g. Surgicel®, oxidized regenerated cellulose), which are generally removed following control of the bleeding. Autogenous muscle or fat is also useful to aid in haemostasis. Postoperative swelling and subsequent compression can result when any haemostatic material used is left in proximity to the nervous system. Standard anaesthetic and physiological monitoring equipment is required to monitor body temperature, heart rate and rhythm, blood pressure, blood gases and urine production.

Basic surgical principles such as sterile draping, appropriate soft tissue handling and irrigation of soft tissues to prevent desiccation (particularly of neural tissue) are the same as for soft tissue and orthopaedic surgery.

Anaesthesia

Close communication between the neurosurgeon and the anaesthetist (including discussion of the potential intraoperative complications related to specific procedures) is essential for a successful surgical outcome. Surgeons should be present during the induction of anaesthesia in patients where inappropriate manipulation could be detrimental (e.g. animals with atlantoaxial instability or vertebral fractures/luxations). The choice of anaesthetic drugs depends on many factors, including the effects on cerebral/spinal cord blood flow, alterations in intracranial pressure (ICP) during surgery, ease of administration, effects at induction and recovery, and the anaesthetist's own comfort level with the anaesthetic protocol (see Chapter 21).

Patient positioning

This aspect of surgical preparation may be overlooked, although it is often critical to a successful outcome. Individual surgeons may have a preference for specific surgical procedures, however consistency is important. An extra few minutes spent ensuring that a patient undergoing a ventral slot procedure is perfectly aligned and fixed in place can make the difference between a satisfying surgery and a frustrating battle with venous plexus haemorrhage. Appropriate placement of pins or screws into vertebral bodies is much more challenging in a patient that is not symmetrically positioned. It is also important to consider limb and vertebral column position with regard to potential neurological injury and desired outcome following fixation/stabilization techniques.

In addition, compression of venous outflow caused by pressure on the abdomen or jugular veins has a deleterious effect on intraoperative bleeding, particularly from the venous sinuses. With respect to intracranial surgery specifically, jugular vein compression is contraindicated and must be avoided. The head should be kept in an elevated position to ensure that the brain is above the level of the heart and that jugular vein outflow is not compromised. It is also important to protect the tongue from compression, which may lead to postoperative swelling and potential airway obstruction during recovery.

Postoperative monitoring and care

Frequent monitoring of neurological status is of prime importance in all patients following surgery. Animals undergoing routine vertebral column procedures generally do not require intensive monitoring following anaesthetic recovery. Controlling pain as well as preventing anxiety and movement that might cause undue stress/torque on the vertebral column are immediate concerns. These patients should be recovered and rehabilitated in a space that is kept clean, dry and well padded at all times. In recumbent animals, regular repositioning is needed to minimize the chance of aspiration pneumonia, to keep the patient comfortable and to prevent complications involving the skin, joints and muscles. Bladder management is of prime importance when nursing animals with myelopathy and is discussed in detail in Chapter 25. Patients undergoing more advanced vertebral column procedures, where complications are anticipated, such as ongoing haemorrhage, inability to ventilate adequately (cervical myelopathy) or profound postoperative pain, may require intense postoperative monitoring.

Following intracranial procedures, animals should be recovered and monitored in an intensive or critical care unit for 24–72 hours. This allows optimal management of any pathophysiological sequelae to the brain injury and ensures that signs of neurological deterioration are closely monitored. The goal for postoperative monitoring of the brain is centred on maintaining adequate cerebral blood flow without compromising the systemic organs. Thus, physiological monitoring including body temperature, respiratory rate/character, electrocardiography, mean arterial blood pressure, blood gases, and fluid and electrolyte balance should be standard care.

Vertebral column surgery

Terminology

The terms commonly used in vertebral column surgery include:

- Continuous dorsal laminectomy – extension of the dorsal laminectomy cranially or caudally to include multiple vertebral arches
- Deep dorsal laminectomy – extension of the dorsal laminectomy ventrally to include the articular processes unilaterally or bilaterally, with or without pediculectomy
- Dorsal laminectomy – removal of the spinous process and the laminae of the vertebral arch
- Facetectomy – removal of an articular process/facet
- Fenestration – surgical creation of an opening in the intervertebral disc (annulus)
- Foramenotomy – enlargement of an intervertebral foramen
- Hemilaminectomy – removal of one-half of the vertebral arch
- Laminectomy – the excision of lamina or the dorsal portion of the vertebral arch
- Laminectomy membrane – a constrictive, fibrotic, usually hypertrophied, cicatricial tissue covering the region of a previous laminectomy site
- Spinal stabilization – the process of removing all motion between adjacent vertebrae by the application of various metallic/synthetic implants, bone cement and/or bone grafts
- Ventral slot – slot-like opening created ventrally through the intervertebral disc and cranial and caudal vertebrae endplates in the cervical region.

Vertebral anatomy is illustrated in Figure 22.1.

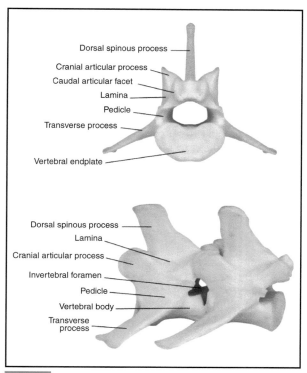

Dorsal spinous process
Cranial articular process
Caudal articular facet
Lamina
Pedicle
Transverse process
Vertebral endplate

Dorsal spinous process
Lamina
Cranial articular process
Invertebral foramen
Pedicle
Vertebral body
Transverse process

22.1 Vertebral anatomy.

Indications
The most common indications for vertebral column surgery in dogs and cats include:

- Degenerative disc disease
- Cervical spondylomyelopathy
- Degenerative lumbosacral stenosis
- Trauma
- Neoplasia.

Less commonly encountered indications for vertebral column surgery are:

- Congenital/acquired malformations (atlantoaxial instability, synovial cysts, intra-arachnoid cysts, scoliosis)
- Infectious disease (empyema, abscess, discospondylitis)
- Epidural/intradural haemorrhage.

General complications
The major technical complications associated with vertebral column surgery are:

- Iatrogenic trauma to the neural tissues
- Intraoperative haemorrhage (resulting in hypotension, anaemia or haematoma)
- Spinal cord vasculature compromise
- Vertebral column instability
- Excessive scar formation ('laminectomy scar').

The majority of these complications can be treated if they are recognized as they occur and appropriate measures are taken promptly. However, iatrogenic trauma to the neural tissues and compromise of the local vasculature are complications that are not easily rectified. Meticulous surgical technique and a thorough knowledge of regional anatomy are essential to a positive outcome.

In the immediate postoperative period (24–48 hours), inadequate patient confinement can lead to ongoing haemorrhage, haematoma/seroma formation and compression of neural elements. This also is the time when recumbent patients, especially those on opioid drugs, can develop aspiration pneumonia. In addition to postoperative pain, the neurological status of most patients is often temporarily worse following surgery.

Exuberant bone regrowth, leading to compression of the neural structures and the recurrence of neurological signs, is a complication of laminectomy performed in immature animals. This commonly occurs with continuous dorsal cervical laminectomy procedures performed in immature dogs, but may also occur when undue biomechanical stress or true instability occurs following laminectomy (Figure 22.2). When compressive bony regrowth occurs, another operation may be indicated if conservative treatment is ineffective and the patient continues to deteriorate.

Similar potential complications may occur following multiple procedures in the same region. In addition, altered anatomy, muscle fibrosis and scar tissue in the region of the previous surgical site can be problematic. By virtue of the fact that the neural tissue has sustained a second injury, the potential for recovery may not be as complete as with the initial event.

Bladder dysfunction and urinary tract infection are common problems in any patient with neurological disease, particularly those with spinal cord dysfunction. Appropriate bladder management, together with excellent nursing care, frequent patient assessment and physical therapy, is paramount to a positive outcome following neurological surgery (see Chapter 25).

Cervical vertebral column surgery

In most cases, the purpose of cervical vertebral column surgery is to decompress the spinal cord. This is most commonly achieved by direct decompression of the affected area (i.e. removal of the overlying bone and any soft tissues). However, in some situations, such as the treatment of dynamic lesions affecting the cervical spinal cord in large-breed dogs, indirect decompression of the spinal cord (i.e. cervical distraction and/or fusion) is warranted.

Ventral decompression (ventral slot)

The main indications for a ventral approach to the cervical spinal cord include removal of herniated disc material, cervical disc fenestration/biopsy and cervical vertebral column stabilization. There is minimal soft tissue and bony dissection with this approach, resulting in minimal postoperative morbidity and an early return to comfort and function (Figure 22.3). The window or slot created by the surgeon is directly on the midline and is particularly useful for removing disc material located in the ventral aspect of the vertebral canal. Removal of larger ventral extradural masses, intradural/intramedullary masses or lesions not primarily on the ventral midline should not be attempted because exposure of the spinal cord is very limited due to the anatomy of the internal ventral vertebral venous plexus and complications are potentially life-threatening. Ventral slot procedures may be combined with cervical vertebral stabilization (fusion) and distraction when dynamic instability is present.

The primary disadvantage of the ventral slot procedure is the limited exposure the surgeon has to the vertebral canal. If disc material or other space-occupying masses are located lateral to the midline, full decompression is generally not achieved without creating an excessively wide opening and predisposing the patient to vertebral column instability and subluxation (Lemarie et al., 2000). Ventral slots in adjacent vertebrae may also predispose to instability.

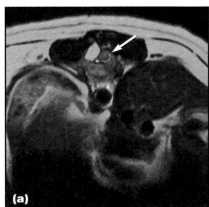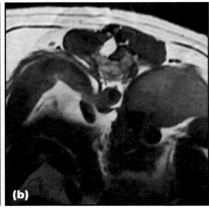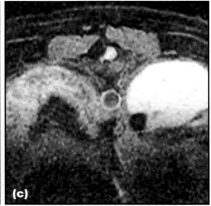

22.2 Transverse **(a)** T2-weighted, **(b)** T1-weighted and **(c)** fat suppressed MR images at the level of T11–T12 of a 10-year-old neutered Maltese cross-breed bitch showing compression of the spinal cord (arrowed) by fat. A hemilaminectomy had been performed at this site 2 years earlier. These images were taken 1 week after the progressive recurrence of clinical signs. The mass is hyperintense on the T1-weighted and T2-weighted images and hypointense on the fat suppressed image. Expansion of the surgical fat graft appeared to be caused by secondary revascularization and the active deposition of fat.

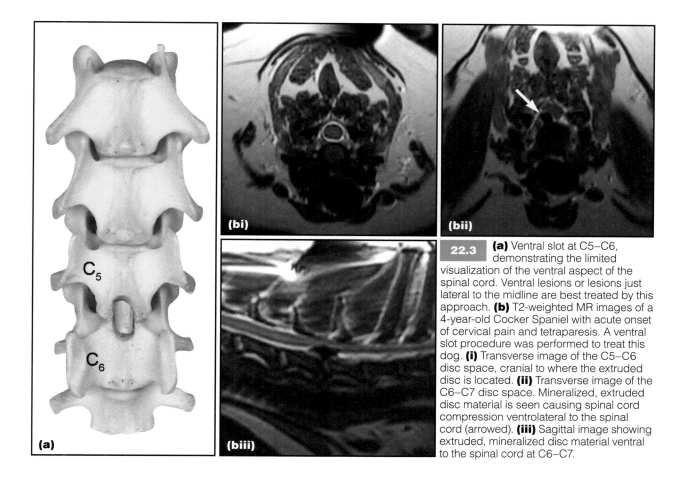

22.3 **(a)** Ventral slot at C5–C6, demonstrating the limited visualization of the ventral aspect of the spinal cord. Ventral lesions or lesions just lateral to the midline are best treated by this approach. **(b)** T2-weighted MR images of a 4-year-old Cocker Spaniel with acute onset of cervical pain and tetraparesis. A ventral slot procedure was performed to treat this dog. **(i)** Transverse image of the C5–C6 disc space, cranial to where the extruded disc is located. **(ii)** Transverse image of the C6–C7 disc space. Mineralized, extruded disc material is seen causing spinal cord compression ventrolateral to the spinal cord (arrowed). **(iii)** Sagittal image showing extruded, mineralized disc material ventral to the spinal cord at C6–C7.

Complications:

- Profuse haemorrhage due to laceration of the internal vertebral venous plexus
- Iatrogenic spinal cord trauma
- Collapse of the intervertebral disc space
- Vertebral column instability
- Surgery on the incorrect intervertebral disc space.

These complications may manifest as worsening neurological signs, cervical pain and/or thoracic limb lameness. Cardiac arrhythmias, respiratory compromise, hypotension and Horner's syndrome are uncommonly reported complications of cervical spinal cord injury and surgery (Clark, 1986; Stauffer *et al.*, 1988; Beal *et al.*, 2001). Damage to the recurrent laryngeal nerve, carotid artery, vagosympathetic trunk and vertebral arteries may also occur during tissue retraction, which is required to expose the ventral aspect of the cervical spine. Retraction and trauma to the trachea, although uncommon, may result in subsequent tracheal collapse, particularly in animals with underlying clinical or subclinical tracheal disease prior to surgery.

Dorsal laminectomy

This approach is indicated when exposure of the vertebral canal and/or spinal cord is required dorsally, dorsolaterally or laterally to the level of the intervertebral foramen. It is particularly useful when:

- Single or multiple, osseous or soft tissue, stenoses are present in the dorsolateral cervical vertebral column
- Multiple ventral compressive lesions are present
- Acute disc extrusion (i.e. disc and/or haemorrhage predominantly lateral (or dorsal) to the spinal cord) is present
- Intramedullary tumours and congenital or acquired conditions (e.g. syringomyelia and dorsal spinal intra-arachnoid cysts) need to be approached for biopsy, resection or marsupialization
- Nerve root tumours are present
- Spinal cord and vertebral column tumours are present.

Preservation of the articular processes is needed to maintain as much vertebral column integrity as possible. The laminectomy can be extended cranially and/or caudally in a continuous fashion over several vertebrae. Careful palpation of the floor of the vertebral canal is possible from this approach. Dorsal laminectomy at C1 is possible; however, hemidorsal laminectomy is preferred at C2 and C2–C3 in order to maintain the integrity of the attachment of the nuchal ligament (Figure 22.4) and to prevent instability from occurring at C2–C3. Sufficient surgical access may require extension of the laminectomy laterally and/or ventrally (including partial facetectomy) and/or enlargement of the

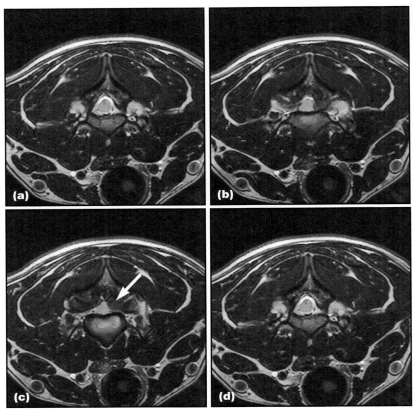

22.4 Sequential transverse T2-weighted MR images of a 5-month-old Great Dane with congenital spinal stenosis causing ataxia and tetraparesis. The vertebral canal is stenotic in all images but is most severe at the level of the C2–C3 articular processes. This dog was treated with a hemidorsal laminectomy, which allowed decompression of the spinal cord whilst preserving the attachment of the nuchal ligament and maintaining stability of the vertebral column. **(a)** Cranial C2. Hyperintense epidural fat surrounds the spinal cord where compression is minimal. **(b–c)** Cranial and caudal aspects of the C2–C3 articulation. Compression of the spinal cord is circumferential due to the bony encroachment (arrowed). **(d)** Caudal C2. Epidural fat again surrounds the spinal cord.

intervertebral foramen (foraminotomy). In addition, osseous and soft tissue stenoses (such as those created by synovial cysts) may be effectively removed by drilling away the inner lamina, leaving the outer side of the lamina intact. The resultant widening of the vertebral canal also allows for decompression of the neural tissue.

The main disadvantage of this approach is the extensive soft tissue dissection needed to gain access to the dorsal aspect of the vertebral column, especially in large- and giant-breed dogs, where the depth of the surgical field adds to the difficulty in visualization.

Complications:

- Profuse haemorrhage can result from soft tissue dissection as well as laceration of the internal ventral vertebral venous plexus. This can be potentially life-threatening, especially when operating in the rostral cervical region (C1–C3) where dorsal anastomosis of the venous plexus is common.
- Ongoing postoperative haemorrhage, haematoma formation leading to secondary spinal cord compression and hypoventilation are serious complications that may require further surgery and/or mechanical ventilation.
- Longer operating times (especially with continuous dorsal laminectomies), damage to the underlying spinal cord and/or nerve roots and a slower return to function compared with ventral cervical procedures are also considerations.

- Potential vertebral column instability, epidural scarring and the development of a clinically significant laminectomy membrane are potential long-term complications, leading to the recurrence of neurological signs.
- Extensive soft tissue dissection predisposes to postoperative seroma formation, particularly in active patients.

Lateral laminectomy

This approach to the cervical spinal cord provides the best visualization of the lateral aspect of the vertebral canal (Lipsitz and Bailey, 1995). The structures visualized are:

- Intervertebral disc
- Spinal cord
- Nerve root
- Proximal portion of the peripheral nerve as it exits the intervertebral foramen.

This is a technically challenging approach and should only be attempted by experienced neurosurgeons. Lateral cervical laminectomy is the best approach for resecting peripheral nerve tumours that have invaded the spinal cord, especially in conjunction with amputation of the affected thoracic limb. This approach is also useful for resecting spinal cord tumours (e.g. meningiomas) that exit the intervertebral foramen alongside the vertebral artery, vein and nerve, removing laterally herniated disc material and biopsying peripheral nerves and nerve roots (Rossmeisl et al., 2005).

Complications:

- Incorrect lesion localization at surgery.
- Profuse haemorrhage from vertebral arteries and/or internal vertebral venous plexus disruption.
- Severe postoperative pain during recovery.

Cervical vertebral column stabilization

The primary indications for cervical vertebral column stabilization are:

- Repair of cervical vertebral fracture/luxations
- Cervical vertebral fusion with or without distraction for the treatment of 'dynamic' forms of cervical spondylomyelopathy
- Atlantoaxial instability.

Implants placed in the vertebral bodies via a ventral approach provide superior stiffness compared with implants applied to the spinous processes or articular processes/facets (dorsally). The use of pins or screws and polymethylmethacrylate (PMMA) is the authors' technique of choice for stabilizing cervical vertebral fracture/luxations because of the versatility of these implants, low cost and stiffness of the construct. However, this is technically difficult to perform. Multiple implants (screws, pins) placed in the transverse processes of the cervical vertebrae (using a ventral approach), with or without Steinman pins embedded in PMMA, are also widely used to stabilize this region. Whilst this approach is technically easier and safer to perform, it is biomechanically less desirable.

Many surgical procedures have been described to accomplish distraction and stabilization of dynamic compressive lesions in cervical spondylomyelopathy, including:

- Regularly used procedures:
  - Ventral slot procedure (partial or complete) with or without stabilization using pins and PMMA or locking plates
  - Vertebral body plating using dynamic compression plates, locking plates and limited contact dynamic compression plates
  - PMMA vertebral body plugs
- Less commonly used or obsolete procedures:
  - Metal washers and screws
  - Polyvinylidine vertebral plates
  - Harrington rods
  - External fixators.

The ventral approach to the cervical spinal cord provides good visualization of the cervical vertebral bodies for accurate realignment with minimal trauma to the soft tissues. Surgical stabilization may also be indicated following a ventral slot procedure in situations where the slot is excessively large or instability following the slot procedure is anticipated (e.g. large- or giant-breed dogs) (Figure 22.5). Many dorsal and ventral approaches for the repair and stabilization of the atlantoaxial joint have been described

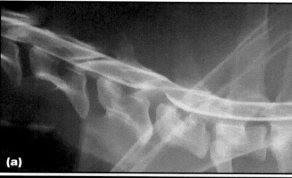

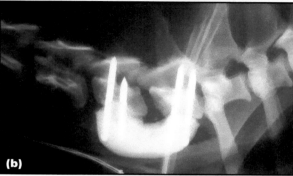

22.5 **(a)** Lateral cervical myelogram of a 5-year-old Dobermann with a chronic history of cervical pain, ataxia, pelvic limb paresis and thoracic limb lameness. A narrowed disc space and ventral extradural compression are seen at C6–C7, consistent with chronic disc herniation. The compression resolved completely when traction was applied to the vertebral column. **(b)** Lateral radiograph showing the pins and PMMA used to distract and stabilize C6–C7 and achieve decompression of the spinal cord.

in the literature. However, most surgeons agree that ventral repair results in superior fixation.

Complications: Complications unique to the application of implants to the cervical vertebral bodies may result from a lack of visualization of the spinal cord and nerve roots during placement. The surgeon must be comfortable with 3D visualization of these structures, based on the landmarks on the ventral aspect of each cervical vertebra. The most common complications are:

- Laceration of vertebral arteries and spinal nerves/nerve roots
- Iatrogenic spinal cord trauma
- Implant failure due to:
  - Pin migration or inadequate size of implants/PMMA (note: this is not a known complication when using positive profile threaded pins)
  - Inadequate placement of screws/plate (locking plates)
  - Endplate fracture (cement plugs, metal washers)
- Infection of the implant
- 'Domino' lesions may develop in the disc spaces adjacent to the fused disc space, especially in the caudal cervical region of Dobermanns and other large-breed dogs (Jeffery and McKee, 2001; da Costa, 2010).

Complications unique to atlantoaxial stabilization vary considerably depending on the approach/technique used and the expertise of the surgeon:

- Improper pin placement due to the lack of visualization of the neural structures and fracture of the vertebrae during pin/screw placement are potential complications of atlantoaxial stabilization, especially in miniature breeds, which frequently have congenitally malformed vertebrae
- Placement of pins into the cranial spinal cord, brainstem, atlanto-occipital joint or C1 spinal nerves causes serious complications that can lead to vestibular signs, respiratory compromise (requiring assisted ventilation), severe neck pain and/or permanent paralysis (Figure 22.6)
- Dorsal fixation techniques have been associated with an increased incidence of implant failure and respiratory compromise.

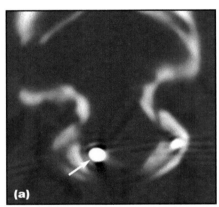

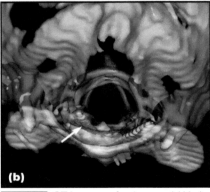

22.6 CT images of a 1-year-old Yorkshire Terrier that was referred for continued cervical pain 8 weeks after surgical stabilization for atlantoaxial instability. The pins and cement were removed. Arthrodesis had developed since the pins were placed at C1–C2 and the dog's pain resolved. **(a)** Transverse CT image showing that one of the pins is in the vertebral canal (arrowed) and the other pin is in the atlanto-occipital joint. **(b)** 3D CT reconstruction showing the pin in the vertebral canal (arrowed).

Cervical disc fenestration

Chondrodystrophic breeds with degenerative disc disease benefit from cervical disc fenestration. This may be performed at the time of decompressive surgery or may be undertaken prophylactically when there is radiographic or MRI evidence of degenera-tive disc disease. Generally, cervical disc fenestration is not recommended in medium- and large-breed dogs with degenerative disc disease because of the possibility of creating vertebral instability and/or spinal cord compression secondary to disc collapse, and theoretical 'buckling' of the dorsal longitudinal ligament resulting in spinal cord compression.

Thoracolumbar vertebral column surgery

Hemilaminectomy

This is the best approach for most pathological conditions affecting the thoracolumbar vertebral column, spinal cord and nerve roots. It is essential that the laterality of the lesion is known prior to this surgical procedure since the contralateral aspects of the spinal cord, nerve roots, and ligamentous and osseous structures are not visualized from this approach. Hemilaminectomy allows good visualization of the ventral and lateral aspects of the spinal cord and nerve roots (Figure 22.7). The stability of the vertebral column is not significantly affected since the spinous process and associated ligamentous structures, as well as the contralateral articulations, are maintained.

- The majority of clinically significant acute and chronic disc protrusions and extrusions are best treated in this manner.

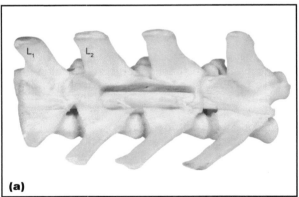

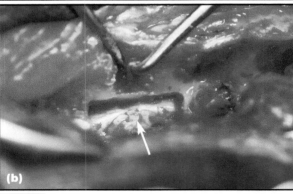

22.7 **(a)** Thoracolumbar hemilaminectomy illustrating the visualization of the lateral aspect of the spinal cord. Lesions located ventrally, laterally and dorsolaterally are best treated by this approach. **(b)** Intraoperative view of acute disc extrusion at L2–L3 (arrowed).

- This approach also allows easy access to the lateral aspect of the disc for fenestration.
- Extradural and intradural space-occupying lesions in the ventral and lateral aspects of the cord are also best approached by hemilaminectomy, which can be extended cranially, caudally or dorsally to allow for more complete visualization and/or excision of the mass.
- Progressive swelling of the spinal cord can be addressed quickly by extension of the laminectomy cranially and caudally.
- Removal of bony fragments and haematomas secondary to trauma (vertebral fracture/luxations) and migrating foreign bodies (grass seeds, bullets), as well as exploratory surgery/biopsy of the lateral or ventral spinal cord and nerve roots, are also routinely performed via hemilaminectomy.

Complications: Complications associated with thoracolumbar hemilaminectomy are uncommon, but can include:

- Iatrogenic spinal cord injury
- Nerve root trauma
- Haemorrhage/haematoma
- Vertebral column instability (note: although hemilaminectomies extending for >3 adjacent vertebrae are considered at risk for instability, there is little evidence-based data to support this idea. Furthermore, hemilaminectomies have been performed on >3 adjacent vertebrae without complications)
- Fracture of the spinous processes if the laminectomy is extended too far dorsally.

Dorsal laminectomy

Indications for dorsal laminectomy in the thoracolumbar region of the vertebral column are the same as those for the cervical region. Occasionally, fractures in the thoracolumbar region are approached via dorsal laminectomy, allowing fragment removal and decompression. Instability is a particular concern following dorsal laminectomy of the thoracic vertebrae. Bilateral loss of the articular facets and/or loss of the interspinous ligament can result in significant vertebral column instability and subsequent luxation.

Thoracolumbar vertebral column stabilization

Vertebral alignment and stabilization is indicated whenever vertebral instability is suspected clinically or when it is documented with dynamic imaging. The most common neurological conditions requiring stabilization in the thoracolumbar region are vertebral fractures and luxations. Surgical treatment of vertebral fractures and luxations includes vertebral realignment, decompression and stabilization. Occasionally, neoplastic and infectious diseases causing vertebral instability, malalignment or malarticulation (e.g. discospondylitis) may require surgical decompression, debulking and stabilization (Figure 22.8). Degenerative and/or congenital disease in the thoracolumbar region,

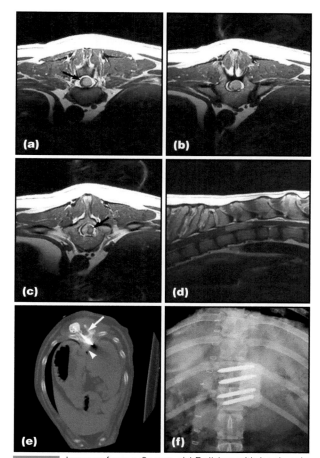

22.8 Images from a 2-year-old Bulldog with back pain and pelvic limb paresis. The dog survived 15 months following surgical resection and radiation therapy before becoming non-ambulatory from presumed recurrence of a nephroblastoma (intradural–extramedullary tumour of young dogs). **(a–c)** Sequential post-contrast T1-weighted MR images showing a contrast-enhanced mass occupying the majority of the cross-sectional diameter of the spinal cord, crossing over from the left side to the right side. A small crescent of spinal cord can be seen in (a) and (c) (arrowed). **(d)** Sagittal post-contrast T1-weighted MR image of the mass. **(e)** Postoperative transverse CT image following a dorsal laminectomy that was performed to remove the mass. Pins and PMMA were placed to help maintain stability of the vertebral column since the articulations were compromised bilaterally. The arrow denotes the spinal cord in the vertebral canal at the level of the dorsal laminectomy. The aorta can be seen at the tip of the arrowhead. **(f)** Postoperative radiograph showing the position of pins placed in the thoracic vertebral column.

leading to stenosis of the vertebral canal (e.g. synovial cysts, congenital vertebral anomalies and scoliosis), is often treated by stabilization in conjunction with a decompressive laminectomy.

Vertebral pins/screws and PMMA and vertebral body bone plates provide excellent rigid fixation in this region, and permit the accurate anatomical alignment of the vertebral column. Locking plates may also be used to stabilize lumbar vertebrae (Figure 22.9), but it is challenging to place the screws so that they are adequately engaged in the vertebral body and not in the vertebral canal (causing spinal cord injury), disc space or exiting below

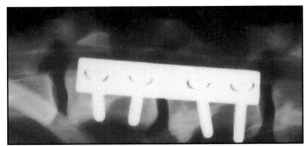

22.9 Dynamic compression plate used to treat a vertebral luxation at L2–L3.

the vertebral body (i.e. not adequately engaged in the cortical bone). The ribs, rib heads and the shape of thoracic vertebrae make it almost impossible to apply locking plates in this region. As in the cervical vertebral column, multiple implants (screws, pins) placed in the transverse processes and embedded in PMMA, with or without Steinman pins to 're-inforce' the PMMA, can also be used to stabilize the thoracolumbar vertebrae. Whilst this may prove to be technically easier, the stiffness of the implant may be inferior to other methods utilizing the vertebral body.

Complications: Intraoperative complications usually result from poor visualization of spinal cord and nerve roots during implant placement and can lead to iatrogenic damage to the neural tissues or vasculature lying ventral to the vertebral bodies (Figure 22.10). Iatrogenic vertebral fractures, implant migration and failure, as well as infection, are less common postoperative complications.

Thoracolumbar disc fenestration

Whilst debate surrounds the role of thoracolumbar annular disc fenestration with nuclear pulpectomy, most clinicians agree that fenestration of the affected disc space is essential to prevent further herniation/extrusion of disc material (Forterre *et al.*, 2008, 2011; Brisson *et al.*, 2011). It is the authors' opinion that this procedure is indicated for all at-risk intervertebral disc spaces (T11–L3) in chondrodystrophic breeds with degenerative disc disease. Since a dorsal midline approach is generally used to perform the hemilaminectomy preceding disc fenestration, discs are usually fenestrated from the dorsolateral aspect. A dorsolateral or lateral approach to the vertebral column may be taken when disc fenestration is not performed at the same time as a hemilaminectomy. These alternative approaches allow better visualization and an easier working angle, and may allow a more aggressive fenestration to be performed safely. Power-assisted fenestration, using a high-speed pneumatic drill and burr, is preferred by some neurosurgeons and may facilitate more complete removal of the nucleus pulposus.

Thoracolumbar lateral corpectomy

Lateral corpectomy is an alternative technique for the treatment of lateralized thoracolumbar chronic (type II) disc disease in dogs (Moissonnier *et al.*, 2004). A lateral slot is drilled under the protruding disc material and through the intervertebral disc and the vertebral epiphyses of the two adjacent vertebral bodies. This allows excision of the protruding portion of the disc and spinal cord decompression without manipulation of the spinal cord.

Complications: Although not reported to date, potential complications include spinal nerve injury, haemorrhage and pneumothorax (in the thoracic region). In addition, during the final phases of drilling there are risks of venous sinus bleeding, dura laceration and spinal cord/nerve injury (Flegel *et al.*, 2011).

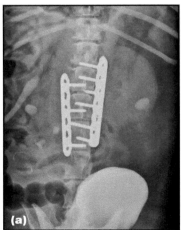
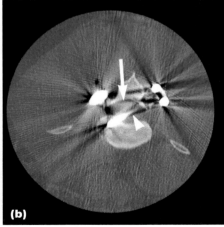
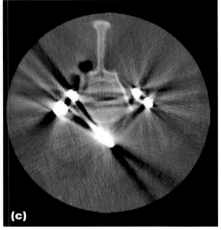

22.10 Suboptimal fixation in a dog referred following vertebral column stabilization using locking plates. Although locking plates have inherent biomechanical advantages over standard dynamic compression plates, the trajectories and positioning of the screws are fixed, and ideal placement in the vertebral bodies is technically challenging. This often results in the screws being biomechanically inferiorly placed in the transverse processes, disc spaces and, in extreme circumstances, into the vertebral canal. **(a)** Postoperative ventrodorsal radiograph showing the bilateral placement of the locking plates. Screws in the L2–L3 and L3–L4 disc spaces on the left are unlikely to provide significant mechanical advantage. **(b)** Transverse CT image of the most distal left screw entering the vertebral canal (arrowhead) and displacing the spinal cord (arrowed). **(c)** Transverse CT image showing the placement of screws through the transverse processes rather than through the vertebral body on both plates. This also reduced the biomechanical stiffness of the fixation.

Foramenotomy and/or pediculectomy

Enlargement of the intervertebral foramen may be achieved with or without removal of a portion of the pedicle. This provides access to masses within the intervertebral foramen and ventral aspect of the vertebral canal. This approach has the advantage of maintaining the integrity of the articular facets, and may be particularly useful when bilateral procedures are indicated.

Lumbosacral vertebral column surgery

Dorsal laminectomy

Compression of the cauda equina may result from malarticulation/malformation, instability and vertebral canal stenosis causing secondary degenerative joint disease, ligamentous hypertrophy and/or disc de-generation at the lumbosacral junction. Excellent visualization of the cauda equina, L7–S1 dorsal annulus, articular facets and surrounding soft tissues is possible following dorsal laminectomy at the lumbosacral junction. The cauda equina may be retracted gently to visualize underlying structures, such as the dorsal annulus, as well as to assess the L7 nerve root as it enters the intervertebral foramen. Nerve roots of the cauda equina may be easily biopsied from this approach, which also facilitates extradural as well as intradural mass excision. Secondary compressive osteoarthritis, ligamentous hypertrophy and disc protrusion may be treated by decompressive dorsal laminectomy with or without stabilization.

Complications: Complications associated with lumbosacral vertebral surgery are uncommon.

- Intraoperative haemorrhage around, and iatrogenic trauma to, the nerve roots can cause pain and worsening of lower motor neuron (LMN) signs (to the tail, bladder, anal sphincter and sciatic nerve).
- Seroma formation at the surgical site can occur, especially in animals not strictly confined in the immediate postoperative period.
- Extensive removal of the articular facets and pedicles may encourage the formation of a clinically significant laminectomy membrane, although this is not often seen until weeks or months following surgery.
- Discectomy performed in conjunction with dorsal compression may predispose the patient to discospondylitis and/or instability at the lumbosacral junction (Figure 22.11).

Foramenotomy/facetectomy

Entrapment of the L7 nerve root is a common occurrence with many conditions resulting in lumbosacral stenosis. Foramenotomy in conjunction with dorsal laminectomy may be performed to relieve compression of the nerve roots and associated apparent pain and/or dysfunction. Complete facetectomy is rarely indicated. Lateral foraminotomy is an alternative approach that may be used for decompression of the L7 nerve root in dogs with foraminal stenosis. The technique may be undertaken unilaterally or bilaterally and provides better access to the lateralized intraforaminal compressions of L7, whilst minimizing postoperative instability and possible facet fracture (Godde and Steffen, 2007).

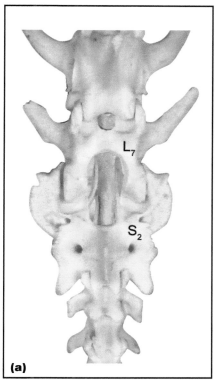

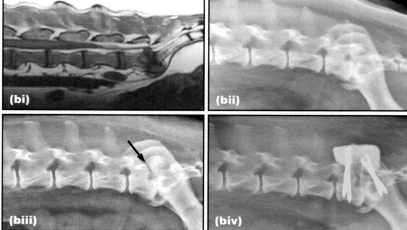

22.11 **(a)** Dorsal laminectomy at the lumbosacral junction. There is good visualization of the conus medullaris and nerve roots of the cauda equina. With gentle traction of these structures laterally, the dorsal annulus of the intervertebral disc can be seen and the L7–S1 intervertebral foramen explored. **(b)(i)** Sagittal T2-weighted MR image of a 4-year-old Pit Bull Terrier with degenerative lumbosacral stenosis. **(ii)** Lateral radiograph taken immediately prior to dorsal laminectomy, which was performed to decompress the cauda equina. **(iii)** Lateral radiograph taken when the dog was experiencing acute pain 4 days following surgery. Bilateral fracture of the L7 caudal articular processes was found (arrowed). This is a documented complication of dorsal laminectomy. **(iv)** Lateral radiograph showing surgical stabilization of L7–S1 with pins and PMMA.

Lumbosacral vertebral column stabilization

Lumbosacral vertebral column stabilization is controversial. Indications for stabilization of the lumbosacral joint have not been uniformly agreed upon. In general, stabilization of the lumbosacral joint may be indicated when there is strong evidence of excessive movement in the joint, based on dynamic imaging studies. Decisions are complicated by:

- Variations in normal and abnormal anatomy within and between breeds
- Variations in imaging techniques and positioning
- A paucity of biomechanical data relating to the lumbosacral joint.

Techniques using transarticular pins or screws, and pedicle screws have been described (Slocum and Devine, 1986; Hankin *et al.*, 2012; Smolders *et al.*, 2012); however, the authors' preferred technique for internal fixation of the lumbosacral joint involves the use of PMMA and pins placed in the L7 and S1 vertebral bodies (Sharp, 2002). This is accomplished accurately following decompressive dorsal laminectomy.

Complications: Pin/screw placement may cause fracture of the L7–S1 facets during stabilization. There is also the potential for implant failure and migration.

Cranial surgery

Competency in neurosurgical management of animals with brain disease is based not only on a thorough neurological assessment and the neurosurgical procedures themselves, but on a variety of related topics, including knowledge of intracranial anatomy, experience in interpreting neuroimaging studies and an understanding of the underlying pathophysiological processes associated with intracranial disease. Such knowledge enables the clinician to determine the most appropriate treatment for each individual patient during the entire perioperative period.

Terminology

Terms commonly used in cranial surgery include:

- Craniectomy – removal of part of the cranium
- Craniotomy – any operation on or incision into the cranium (usually implies replacement of bone at the end of the procedure)
- Caudal fossa craniectomy – removal of the caudal portion of the occipital bone and underlying osseous tentorium cerebelli with occlusion of the transverse sinus to allow access to the cerebellopontine angle and caudal occipital bone
- Rostrotentorial craniotomy – removal of the parietal/occipital bones to expose the frontal, parietal, occipital and temporal lobes of the brain
- Suboccipital craniotomy – entry into the caudal aspect of the occipital bones to allow access to the caudal cerebellum/brainstem
- Transfrontal craniotomy – entry into the cranial vault by removal of the frontal bones overlying the frontal sinus as well as the inner bony table to allow access to the olfactory bulb and frontal lobe.

Acquired brain injury may cause life-threatening intracranial hypertension, whether it is due to head trauma, brain disease (tumours, meningoencephalitis, hypoxic injury), metabolic derangements, prolonged seizures or surgical trauma. In addition to the physical destruction of neurons (primary injury), pathophysiological sequelae associated with brain disease include metabolic alterations in the neurons/glial cells, impairment of vascular supply to the normal tissues, impairment of homeostatic mechanisms, haemorrhage/haematoma formation, seizure generation, obstruction of CSF flow (hydrocephalus), oedema formation and production of physiologically active substances. These conditions all have the potential to cause secondary injury to the brain tissue. This may lead to increased intracranial pressure (ICP) beyond acceptable limits, which may seriously affect the outcome if it is not recognized early on and appropriately managed.

Although ICP monitoring is usually subjective (repeated neurological examinations), several systems have been described for use in dogs and cats, and the advantages and disadvantages of each have been reported. In general, ICP monitoring is useful for:

- Assessment of actual ICP and overall trends in ICP
- Optimization of cerebral perfusion pressure (CPP)-guided therapy
- Early intervention with treatment strategies
- Reducing indiscriminate treatment of elevated ICP
- Neurological assessment of the effects of treatment of elevated ICP
- Assessment in anaesthetized and comatose animals.

The disadvantages of ICP monitoring include:

- Expense of the monitoring system
- Additional surgery time required for placement of the ICP monitor
- Potential for iatrogenic brain injury.

Indications

Intracranial surgery is performed most frequently to:

- Remove intracranial masses (tumour, haematoma, foreign body)
- Biopsy intracranial lesions (open or stereotactic)
- Drain/evacuate intracranial granulomas or abscesses
- Treat cranial trauma (remove depressed skull fractures, evacuate haematomas, control haemorrhage, debride necrotic tissue)
- Place ventriculoperitoneal shunts
- Stabilize elevated ICP (decompressive craniectomy)
- Treat congenital anomalies (fenestration of intracranial intra-arachnoid cysts).

Intracranial surgery also has the potential to treat refractory epilepsy in the future (based on studies in human medicine). The clinical response to medical *versus* surgical treatment varies over time. Palliation of the clinical signs with medical therapy may be effective in the short term; however, surgical intervention may result in an improved long-term outcome (e.g. resection/debulking of tumours). The risks and benefits of surgery, together with the effects of delaying surgery to pursue medical treatment, must be assessed for each individual case.

Patient positioning

A head-holding frame is extremely helpful for positioning dogs and cats undergoing craniotomy and craniectomy procedures (Figure 22.12). It ensures that the patient's head is kept elevated above the level of the heart and that the jugular veins are not compromised. In addition, it allows for intraoperative rotation, as well as angulation, of the head and neck to facilitate visualization and ease of the operation.

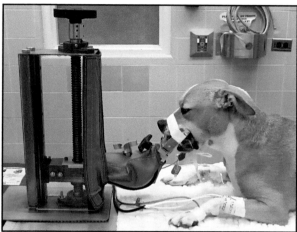

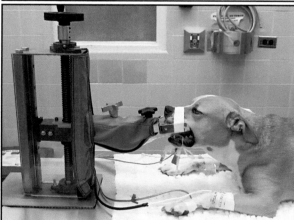

22.12 Surgical head-holding frame showing the versatility of head and neck positions into which the patient can be placed. An individualized bite mould is used to stabilize the upper jaw.

Surgical approach

Surgical anatomical approaches to intracranial lesions are based upon:

- Location of the lesion
- Size and extent of the lesion
- Vital structures in the vicinity of the lesion

- Suspected type of lesion (neoplastic *versus* inflammatory *versus* infectious)
- Purpose for approaching the lesion (biopsy *versus* excision)
- Potential for complications (brain swelling/ herniation)
- Instruments available (endoscope *versus* suction *versus* ultrasonic aspirator)
- Suspected nature of the lesion (fluid *versus* solid; friable *versus* fibrous).

A surgical corridor should be created that allows sufficient visualization and removal of tissues, as well as comfortable use of equipment in the surgical site. In general, maximum exposure of the lesions is important with intracranial surgery to avoid excessive brain manipulation, which might predispose the patient to iatrogenic brain injury and associated complications such as brain swelling and haemorrhage. Large approaches are usually needed for mass removals, ongoing haemorrhage, decompressive craniectomy (for the treatment of intracranial hypertension), foreign body removal, removal of depressed skull fragments and ventrally located lesions. Ultimately, large surgical approaches often consist of a combination of standard approaches in order to accomplish the intended goals. More conservative approaches may be sufficient for tissue biopsy, haematoma evaluation, and shunt or ICP monitor placement.

Rostral approach: transfrontal craniotomy

Lesions involving the olfactory and rostrolateral portions of the frontal lobes are best approached through a bilateral transfrontal craniotomy/craniectomy (Kostolich and Dulisch, 1987; Glass *et al.*, 2000) (Figure 22.13). Olfactory bulb/frontal lobe neoplasms, abscesses or granulomas secondary to foreign body migration, fungal granulomas and nasal tumours invading through the cribriform plate are the most common conditions for which this approach is indicated.

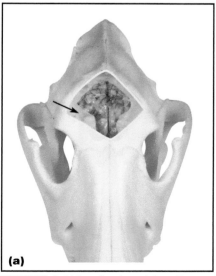

(a)

22.13 **(a)** Visualization of the olfactory/frontal lobes of the brain via a transfrontal craniotomy. The large air-filled frontal sinus lies between the frontal bone and the inner table of the cranial vault (arrowed). (continues) ▶

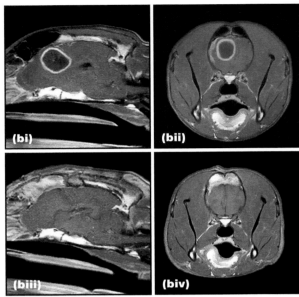

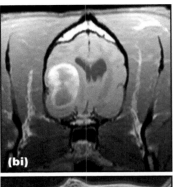

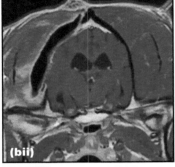

22.13 (continued) **(b)** Post-contrast MR images from a 2-year-old Dalmatian presented for progressive mental deterioration. **(i)** Sagittal and **(ii)** transverse images showing a well circumscribed, contrast-enhancing mass lesion in the right frontal lobe of the brain. Enhancement of the adjacent meninges is also visible. Postoperative **(iii)** sagittal and **(iv)** transverse images. The mass lesion, an intraparenchymal abscess, was removed via a transfrontal approach to the brain. *Streptococcus* was cultured from the abscess. A dural flap, using fascia from the temporalis muscle, was used to close the skull defect. The dog recovered well from surgery and had no recurrence of the infection.

22.14 (continued) **(b)** Transverse post-contrast T1-weighted MR images from a 7-year-old Boxer with a history of generalized seizures. **(i)** Preoperative image at the level of the parietal lobe showing a heterogeneously contrast-enhancing mass, consistent with a glial cell neoplasm. **(ii)** Postoperative image at the same level after the tumour was removed via a rostrotentorial craniectomy. A grade III oligodroglioma was diagnosed. A PMMA skull cap was used to cover the craniotomy defect.

Lateral and dorsal approaches: rostrotentorial craniotomy and transverse sinus occlusion

Lesions involving the lateral aspect of the parietal, temporal and occipital lobes of the cerebrum may be exposed by a rostrotentorial approach (Oliver, 1968; Niebauer *et al.*, 1991) (Figure 22.14). The most common clinical indications are resection/debulking of cerebral convexity or intraparenchymal masses and craniectomy for the stabilization of elevated ICP.

The transverse sinus may be occluded unilaterally for more caudolateral exposure of the brain (Bagley *et al.*, 1997) (Figure 22.15). This allows access to the cerebellomedullary angle, tentorial region and lateral aspect of the cerebellum. A bilateral rostrotentorial craniotomy/craniectomy also allows access to the dorsal aspects of the frontal, parietal and occipital lobes. However, complete occlusion of patent transverse sinuses bilaterally or of the caudal third of the dorsal sagittal sinus usually results in life-threatening circulatory compromise, and following surgery the patient requires at least artificial ventilation.

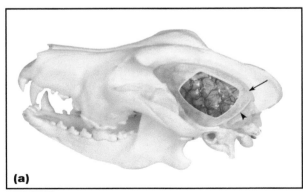

22.14 **(a)** Visualization of the parietal/occipital lobes of the brain via a unilateral rostrotentorial craniotomy. The caudal extent of the craniotomy is limited by the transverse sinus (arrowhead), which receives venous blood from the dorsal sagittal sinus (arrowed). (continues) ▶

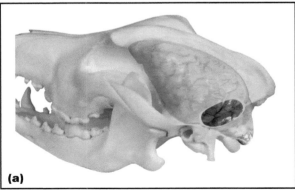

22.15 **(a)** Visualization of the caudolateral occipital lobe and cerebellum after occlusion of the transverse sinus. This approach is best used to treat mass lesions in the cerebellomedullary angle, caudal occipital lobe and lateral cerebellum. It is often combined with a unilateral rostrotentorial craniotomy and/or suboccipital craniotomy for removal of tentorial, brainstem and fourth ventricular masses. (continues) ▶

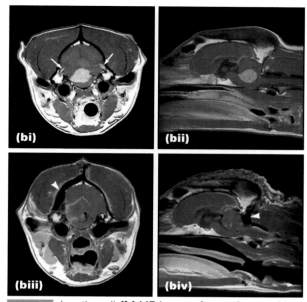

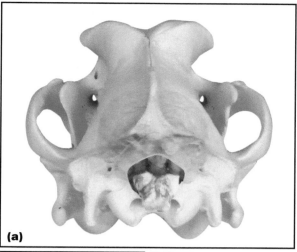

22.15 (continued) **(b)** MR images from a 6-year-old male neutered Basenji cross-breed dog with a fourth ventricular mass. A combined approach, including occlusion of the transverse sinus, was used to remove the mass, which was diagnosed as a choroid plexus tumour. **(i)** Transverse and **(ii)** sagittal post-contrast T1-weighted images showing a uniformly contrast-enhancing mass within the fourth ventricle, extending up to the caudal aspect of the midbrain. The transverse sinuses can be seen laterally on the transverse image (arrowed). Postoperative **(iii)** transverse and **(iv)** sagittal post-contrast T1-weighted images following tumour resection. Since complete removal of the mass required an extensive craniectomy, reconstruction using a PMMA skullcap was undertaken (arrowheads).

Caudal approach: suboccipital craniectomy

A suboccipital approach allows access to the caudal cerebellum, caudodorsal brainstem and craniodorsal spinal cord (Oliver, 1968; Niebauer *et al.*, 1991) (Figure 22.16). Decompression and excision of mass lesions, and treatment of syringomyelia located in the caudal brainstem/rostral cervical cord are achieved via this approach.

Ventral approaches

Access to the pituitary gland for resection of microadenomas is achieved by transsphenoidal hypophysectomy (Meij *et al.*, 1998). A ventral approach to the caudal brainstem is also possible; however, the surgery is technically challenging and exposure is extremely limited (Oliver, 1968; Klopp *et al.*, 2000).

Neuroendoscopy

Neurosurgical procedures using endoscopy as a primary tool (neuroendoscopy) or as an adjunct to microneurosurgery have become popular in human neurosurgery and have been documented in dogs and cats (Klopp and Rao, 2009). Neuroendoscopy has the distinct advantages of small incision site with minimal trauma to the brain and a shorter convalescent time. Although experience, dexterity and expensive equipment are needed to perform minimally invasive cranial surgery, it is likely to become more common in the future.

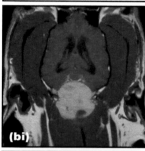
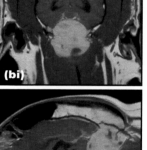
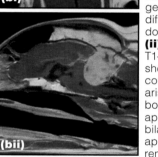
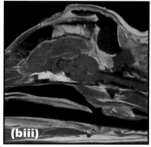

22.16 **(a)** Visualization of the caudal cerebellum and rostral brainstem via a suboccipital craniotomy. The location of the craniotomy is defined by the dorsal sagittal and transverse sinuses. **(b)** MR images from an 8-year-old Golden Retriever with progressive generalized ataxia and difficulty going up and down stairs. **(i)** Dorsal and **(ii)** sagittal post-contrast T1-weighted images showing a heterogeneously contrast-enhancing mass arising from the occipital bone. A suboccipital approach combined with a bilateral caudal fossa approach was used to remove this mass. **(iii)** Postoperative sagittal post-contrast T1-weighted image showing that the cerebellum and third ventricle have assumed their normal size and shape.

Common neurosurgical procedures

Brain biopsy

Advanced imaging techniques such as magnetic resonance imaging (MRI) and computed tomography (CT) allow the identification of intracranial lesions and the determination of a list of differential diagnoses. Whilst many lesions may be 'typical' when viewed in the context of case populations, definitive diagnosis and optimal treatment of the individual case is dependent on histopathological assessment of tissue samples. Biopsy of intracranial lesions may be achieved via standard surgical approaches or stereotactic brain biopsy (see Chapter 6). The decision to biopsy and what technique to use depends on many factors, including imaging characteristics, location, likely treatment options for the major differential diagnoses, and cost.

Closed stereotactic biopsy procedures rely on the generation of 3D coordinates identifying the location of the lesion using either MRI or CT (Figure 22.17). These coordinates are used to guide a biopsy needle and obtain tissue samples for analysis. Several stereotactic systems have been described for use in the dog and cat. All systems require a reference frame attached to the head of the animal (either directly to the skull or indirectly using mouthpieces and similar devices). The biopsy needle is inserted through a small drill hole (approximately 2 mm) in the skull, and the trajectory is planned to avoid critical structures (e.g. the dorsal sagittal sinus and ventricles) and minimize trauma to the normal brain tissue. Penetration of the dura prior to biopsy needle insertion is critical to avoid tearing the dura and potential haemorrhage.

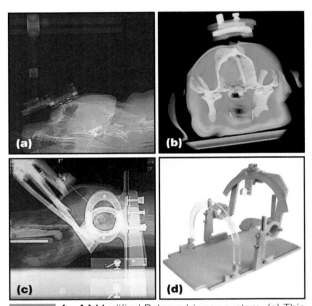

22.17 **(a–b)** Modified Pelorus biopsy system. (a) This CT-guided system requires the biopsy hardware to be fixed directly to the skull of the patient. (b) The biopsy needle can be seen targeting a ventral piriform location in the 3D reconstruction. The choice of trajectory is limited with this type of system.
(c–d) Center-of-arc biopsy system. This CT-guided system uses a mouth mould and ear bars to fix the head of the animal relative to the reference (fiducial) markers in the perspex arch. Once the lesion has been positioned in the centre of the arc, the biopsy needle can be rotated to any desired trajectory.

The most commonly used biopsy needle is a side-cutting Nashold needle, and 2–3 tissue samples are usually obtained (Figure 22.18). Intraoperative analysis of biopsy tissue specimens using rapid air-dried or alcohol-fixed techniques is essential to determine whether additional samples are needed (e.g. for culture) or whether repositioning is required. With experience, the diagnostic yield is usually >90%, particularly for neoplastic lesions.

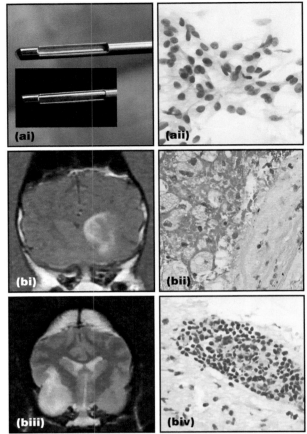

22.18 **(a) (i)** A typical side-cutting Nashold brain biopsy needle. Biopsy openings are typically 8–10 mm in length. **(ii)** Intraoperative alcohol-fixed smear preparation confirming biopsy of the lesion, in this case a meningioma. Sample processing time is approximately 20–25 minutes. **(b)** Two intra-axial lesions provisionally diagnosed as neoplastic disease on MR images. Analysis of biopsy tissue samples confirmed that the lesions were in fact **(i, ii)** a vascular infarct and **(iii, iv)** an inflammatory lesion.

Biopsy and diagnosis of inflammatory and infectious diseases may be more problematic, as it can be difficult to determine whether representative tissue samples have been obtained.

Complications: The major complications of brain biopsy include haemorrhage and failure to obtain diagnostic samples. All animals should be assessed prior to biopsy for coagulation parameters, and imaging studies should be performed following the procedure to determine whether haemorrhage is present. Complications resulting in significant morbidity or mortality are generally low (<5%); however, biopsy of the brainstem or caudal fossa structures, and biopsy in neurologically unstable animals, can result in higher complication rates.

Intraventricular shunt placement
Surgical management of congenital or acquired hydrocephalus refractory to medical management usually involves diversion of CSF from the ventricles within the brain to an extracranial site. Implantation of a ventriculoperitoneal shunt is preferred, with a fenestrated catheter, usually placed

into the lateral ventricle, connected to a pressure valve system, and a distal catheter placed into the abdomen (Figure 22.19). Although ventriculoperitoneal shunts are used commonly in human medicine, there are only a handful of peer-reviewed reports in the veterinary literature. These reports provide some evidence supporting the use of ventriculoperitoneal shunts in veterinary patients (de Stefani *et al.*, 2011); however objective data supporting their long-term efficacy and use in specific conditions are not available. Ventriculoatrial shunts are occasionally used in humans and their use has been reported in small animals.

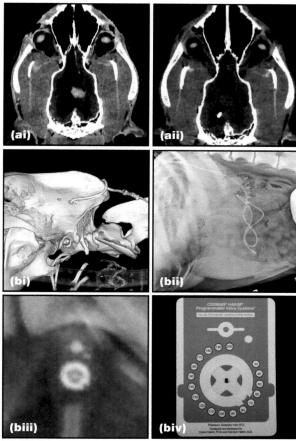

22.19 **(a)** Intraventricular shunt placement in a dog with a contrast-enhanced mass lesion in the third ventricle causing obstructive hydrocephalus and marked dilatation of the left lateral ventricle. Amelioration of progressive neurological signs (obtundation, circling and pacing) was necessary to allow for the delayed (several weeks) effects of stereotactic radiosurgery and treatment of the primary problem to occur. **(i)** Dorsal plane post-contrast CT image prior to shunt placement. **(ii)** Postoperative image showing the shunt tip (hyperattenuating) in a more appropriately sized lateral ventricle. **(b)** Placement of a Codman Hakimâ programmable shunt. **(i)** 3D CT reconstruction showing shunt placement in the brain. The second burr hole (craniotomy) just rostral to the shunt was used to place an indwelling ICP monitoring catheter. **(ii)** Drainage of CSF into the peritoneal cavity was achieved following placement of a distal catheter. **(iii, iv)** The opening pressure setting on the programmable valve can be confirmed by radiography and changed as necessary following placement. An opening pressure of 70 cmH₂O was chosen in this case.

Complications: Complication rates with this procedure approach 30%. Complications associated with ventriculoperitoneal shunt placement include iatrogenic brain trauma, infection, over-shunting resulting in 'brain collapse' and subdural accumulation of fluid, and under-shunting or shunt failure due to shunt blockage. The choice of valve with a specific opening pressure (low: <70 mmH$_2$O; medium: 70–120 mmH$_2$O; high: >120 mmH$_2$O) may be critical in determining both efficacy and likelihood of adverse events following placement. Use of newer and programmable valve systems that allow alterations in opening pressure following placement may help to alleviate some of these problems; however, shunt patency, particularly in conditions where there is active infection or inflammation, is still a major concern.

Complications

The incidence of perioperative complications associated with a poor long-term outcome from intracranial surgery involves many factors, including:

- Preoperative neurological status
- Location and size of mass
- Histological diagnosis
- Concurrent medical conditions
- Patient age.

Patients should be assessed on an individual basis when contemplating surgery. Serious common postoperative complications of craniotomy/craniectomy can be divided into neurological and non-neurological causes:

- Neurological complications generally result from iatrogenic injury to the brain and intracranial hypertension
- Non-neurological complications consist primarily of hypoventilation secondary to pneumonia or brainstem dysfunction.

Neurological complications

Iatrogenic brain injury leading to haemorrhage and/or cerebral oedema, ischaemia and progressive intracranial hypertension is apparent in the immediate postoperative period and reflected by deteriorating neurological status and possible brain herniation (Figure 22.20). Iatrogenic intracranial infection is rare in dogs and cats and usually not clinically apparent for at least 36–72 hours (Kostolich and Dulisch, 1987; Niebauer *et al.*, 1991). Exposure of the brain to the frontal sinus following transfrontal craniotomy may increase the risk of postoperative infection; however, clinical incidence is low. Infection is more likely to occur following reconstruction of large skull defects with prosthetic material such as PMMA (Bryant *et al.*, 2003).

Intraventricular pneumocephalus is a rarely reported complication following transfrontal craniotomy (Garosi *et al.*, 2002). The risk of both infection and pneumocephalus may be reduced by closure of dural defects using fascial transplants or synthetic dura. Further short-term complications of transfrontal craniotomy include ipsilateral epistaxis and subcutaneous emphysema.

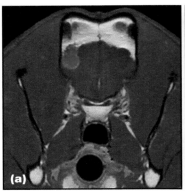
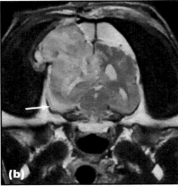

22.20 Peracute complication following craniectomy. Pre- and post-craniectomy MR images of a dog referred for lack of recovery from anaesthesia following resection of a frontal lobe mass. **(a)** Preoperative transverse post-contrast T1-weighted image showing a uniformly contrast-enhanced extra-axial mass consistent with a meningioma. **(b)** Postoperative transverse T2-weighted image obtained following referral showing an extensive mixed hyperintensity throughout the left cerebrum with cerebral herniation. Swelling and herniation appear to be secondary to ongoing haemorrhage, evidence of which can be seen as an area of extra-axial hyperintensity (arrowed).

Iatrogenic generation of seizure foci following lesion resection, nervous tissue retraction or post-operative haemorrhage and scarring is a significant potential complication (Kostolich and Dulisch, 1987). Extensive craniectomy without reconstruction, particularly involving lateral/dorsal approaches, may result in compression of the cortical tissue by the overlying musculature (Figure 22.21). The incidence of long-term sequelae is unknown; however, cortical atrophy and acquired seizure disorders may occur.

The neurological status of many patients deteriorates immediately following surgery. This is often most evident following procedures involving the cerebellum and caudal brainstem, although long-term compensation is generally good. Specific postoperative complications have been reported following transsphenoidal hypophysectomy (Meij *et al.*, 1998), including:

- Decreased tear production
- Hypothyroidism
- Hypernatraemia
- Diabetes insipidus.

However, it should be noted that hypernatraemia and diabetes insipidus may be associated with a variety of intracranial diseases and/or neurosurgical procedures.

Non-neurological complications

Aspiration pneumonia with secondary bacterial infection and/or chemical pneumonitis is the most common complication in craniotomy patients during the first 24–36 hours following surgery. The risk factors for aspiration appear to be multiple (Bagley *et al.*, 1997; Fransson *et al.*, 2001) and may include:

- Length of anaesthesia
- Regurgitation and vomiting
- Depressed pharyngeal/laryngeal function
- Seizures.

Fever, leucocytosis and tachypnoea are the first clinical signs seen, with radiographic changes occurring soon after. Aggressive treatment including tracheal wash and culture, intravenous antibiotic therapy, oxygen therapy, nebulization, coupage and mechanical ventilation may be necessary.

Stereotactic radiosurgery

Stereotactic radiosurgery is a radiation therapy technique whereby high doses of highly focused ionizing radiation are delivered to a target area in a single fraction. Whilst no physical surgery takes place with this procedure, the radiation dose given is high enough to ablate the area being treated, hence the use of the word 'surgery'. Gamma radiation or photons are most commonly used in stereotactic radiosurgery, although protons or other particles can be used.

Linear accelerator based radiotherapy uses a standard linear accelerator fitted with either stereotactic cones or a micro-multi leaf collimator to shape the field and it requires the use of a head frame (Figure 22.22). The Cyberknife® is a compact 6 MV

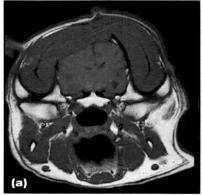
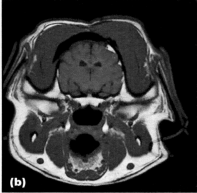

22.21 Chronic complication following craniectomy. Failure to reconstruct large craniectomy defects, particularly following a rostrotentorial approach, can result in compression of the neural tissue by the large overlying temporalis muscles. **(a)** Resection of the tumour *en bloc* resulted in a large skull defect and continued compression of the brain by the overlying musculature. **(b)** Resolution of the compression following subsequent skull reconstruction using PMMA.

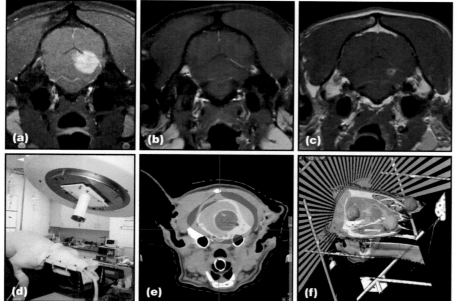

22.22 Linear accelerator based stereotactic radiosurgery system used to treat a dog with a caudal fossa mass. **(a–c)** Transverse post-contrast T1-weighted MR images obtained (a) before, (b) 3 months following and (c) 6 months following radiosurgery. **(d)** Patient undergoing stereotactic treatment. The restraining head frame and modified linear accelerator fitted with stereotactic cones can be seen. **(e–f)** Stereotactic radiosurgery planning based on fused MR and CT images. Highly conformal delivery to the mass (pink) is achieved using multiple beam trajectories in a single treatment plan. Delivery of radiation to critical structures, such as the eyes (red and green) and middle/inner ear (yellow and cyan), is avoided. (Courtesy of Dr M Kent, University of California, Davis)

linear accelerator mounted on a jointed robotic arm, allowing six degrees of freedom, and due to the real-time imaging system does not require a patient frame like other systems. A Gamma Knife® unit is a machine with over 200 cobalt-60 sources in a hemispherical array, allowing all beams to cross at a single point. There are currently no veterinary facilities using a Gamma Knife® to treat patients.

Potential advantages of stereotactic radiosurgery include lower morbidity and shorter hospital stays compared with conventional surgery. However, beneficial clinical effects may not be seen for several weeks or months (problematic in decompensating patients), and the technique is generally not suitable for treating large masses (>3 cm). In humans, stereotactic radiosurgery has been used to treat malignant and benign tumours, primary and metastatic lesions, and both single and multiple lesions. Benign lesions treated in humans include arteriovenous malformations, Parkinson's disease, trigeminal neuralgia and refractory obsessive–compulsive disorder. To date, there are only a small number of published papers in the veterinary literature reporting the clinical use of stereotactic radiosurgery, including one on the treatment of brain masses in three dogs (Lester *et al.*, 2001) and one on the treatment of pituitary tumours in 11 cats (Sellon *et al.*, 2009). Data on the efficacy of these types of treatments are still preliminary, but show promise.

References and further reading

Available on accompanying DVD

23

Drug therapy for diseases of the central nervous system

Mark G. Papich

Drug therapy for diseases of the central nervous system (CNS) involves the complicating factors of drug penetration across the blood–brain barrier (BBB), the therapeutic effect on the CNS, and the potential for adverse effects. Drug efficacy for CNS disorders depends on the extent of penetration across the BBB after systemic administration. However, once a drug penetrates the BBB it may cause an undesirable effect unrelated to the drug's therapeutic effect. For example, antibiotics and antiparasitic drugs can produce adverse CNS effects that are not relevant to the drug's therapeutic action. This chapter will not review all aspects of CNS drug therapy or toxicity but will focus on important issues of drug penetration, antimicrobial therapy, anti-inflammatory therapy, anticancer therapy and adverse drug reactions. Readers are referred to chapters on anticonvulsant therapy (see Chapter 8), treatment of traumatic CNS injury (see Chapter 20), and anaesthesia and analgesia (see Chapter 21) for more in-depth discussion on specific topics.

Drug entry to the brain

For a drug to elicit an effect on the CNS, either the drug or a metabolite of the drug must penetrate the BBB. An exception to this is drug-induced vomiting. The area of the brain that stimulates vomiting, the chemoreceptor trigger zone (CRTZ), is adjacent to the brain's fourth ventricle, outside the BBB and thus exposed to circulating toxins and drugs.

Blood–brain barrier

There have been some excellent reviews of drug penetration across the BBB (Demeule *et al.*, 2002; Wolka *et al.*, 2003; Shen *et al.*, 2004; Pardridge, 2012). These reviews provide more detail and examples than can be expressed in this chapter and the reader is referred to them for more in-depth coverage of the biology of the BBB. In most tissues of the body there is free drug movement from the plasma into the interstitial tissue through fenestrations in capillaries and between the gaps (junctions) in capillary endothelial cells. However, the BBB is more restrictive; here, capillary endothelial cells have tight junctions and a continuous basement membrane without fenestrations (Figure 23.1). The physiological function of the BBB is to maintain brain homeostasis by regulating brain interstitial

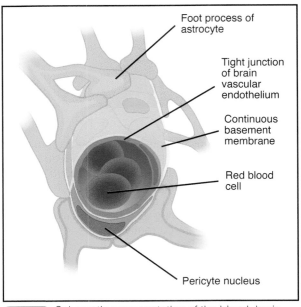

23.1 Schematic representation of the blood–brain barrier at the level of a cerebral capillary.

Labels: Foot process of astrocyte; Tight junction of brain vascular endothelium; Continuous basement membrane; Red blood cell; Pericyte nucleus

fluid independent of fluctuations in the peripheral circulation (Wolka *et al.*, 2003). In a review of thousands of drugs, fewer than 5% effectively penetrate the CNS (Pardridge, 2003). As described by Pardridge (2006), 'limited penetration of drugs into the brain is the rule, not the exception'. Drugs that are capable of penetrating the BBB, are primarily compounds used to treat depression, schizophrenia and insomnia. Most of these drugs are either of very small molecular weight or have high lipophilicity, which facilitates penetration across the BBB. There are conflicting views on BBB permeability, however. Fagerholm (2007) proposes that the BBB is actually much more permeable than previously thought and estimates for low penetration are exaggerated. Fagerholm further proposed that if drugs exhibit sufficiently good intestinal uptake and no, or minor, BBB efflux, there should be no problems to entering the brain readily, but the limiting factor is the short transit time through the circulation in the brain (~5 seconds), rather than permeability.

There are data for 150 drugs that correlate the penetrability from the blood to the brain with other factors such as drug molecular size and lipophilicity (Platts *et al.*, 2001). In addition, Shen *et al.* (2004)

examined the characteristics of 104 drugs for which data on blood–CSF penetration were available. These data, as well as the concepts presented in the reviews cited above, reveal the primary factors that determine the ability of drugs to penetrate the BBB. These studies have been performed on humans, laboratory animals and dogs and cats. There is relatively good correlation that allows extrapolation of data from animals to humans, and *vice versa* (Shen *et al.*, 2004).

Before continuing further into this discussion, it is important to note that drug diffusion into the CSF, and CSF:blood concentration ratios do not indicate that a drug will penetrate the brain. Drug entry into CSF *is not* a measure of BBB permeability (Pardridge, 2011). This has been a false assumption by neurologists and pharmacologists for many years. The blood–CSF barrier is more permeable than is the BBB. Virtually all administered drugs are capable of penetrating the blood–CSF barrier, but a much smaller proportion penetrate the BBB. Drugs enter the interstitial fluid of the brain not from CSF but from circulating blood. Studies in dogs demonstrated that a compound administered directly into the CSF is first taken up into the systemic circulation, then enters the brain via general circulation similar to a drug administered intravenously (Christy and Fishman, 1961). Drugs that enter the CSF may be transported out quickly via absorption by the arachnoid villi. Sampling of the CSF is relatively easy compared to measuring drug concentrations in the brain, which has led to generation of data of CSF:brain concentration ratios. However, these data can be misleading. Therefore, although CSF concentrations have been used as a surrogate marker for brain penetration, it may not necessarily be a strong correlation. Studies using a more elaborate approach beyond simply sampling the CSF are needed to fully characterize the ability of a drug to penetrate the brain.

Drug penetration across the BBB occurs via these processes:

- Simple diffusion through endothelial cells
- Carrier-mediated transport
- Receptor-mediated transport.

Factors that are most important to drug penetration to the CNS are:

- The drug's lipid solubility
- The size of the molecule
- Protein binding in plasma (fraction unbound)
- Number of hydrogen bonds.

Small protein-unbound lipid-soluble compounds can penetrate endothelial cells via simple diffusion. Unfortunately, not many drugs fit into this category. Passive diffusion correlates with the blood–brain drug concentration gradient and the lipid solubility of the drug, but is inversely correlated with the drug's extent of ionization and molecular weight (Jolliet-Riant and Tillement, 1999). In other words, if the

drug has a large blood to brain concentration gradient, is lipophilic or non-ionized, it can potentially cross the BBB. For drugs that are less lipophilic it may be necessary to attain a very high concentration gradient between plasma and brain in order to produce penetration into the brain. For example, even though the concentration of most antibiotics in CSF is less than 5–10%, high plasma concentrations may produce CSF concentrations that are sufficient for antibacterial effects. It is a misconception that inflammation of the CNS tissues will increase BBB penetration of drugs not ordinarily transported across this barrier. There is only a small transient increase in penetration across inflamed meninges for systemically administered antibiotics.

Factors affecting drug entry into the brain

Ionization

Drug ionization affects the lipophilicity of a drug and its ability to enter the CNS. Only neutral (uncharged) drugs enter the CNS to a high enough extent to produce therapeutic or adverse effects. There are several examples of drugs for which the degree of ionization influences CNS effects. Of the antimuscarinic drugs the tertiary amines atropine and butylscopolamine can produce CNS changes, such as excitement. These drugs are uncharged and cross the BBB readily. However, the quaternary amines of this group of drugs have a charged nitrogen atom that limits the ability to diffuse across the BBB. The quaternary amines, such as methylscopolamine, isopropamide, propantheline bromide and glycopyrronium bromide, are not associated with the same risk of CNS effects observed with tertiary amines. The opioid antagonist naloxone can readily cross the BBB to reverse effects of opioids but the more polar opioid antagonist methylnaltrexone does not cross the BBB in effective amounts and can reverse opioid-induced constipation in the gastrointestinal tract without decreasing the beneficial CNS effects of opioid analgesics.

Lipophilicity and hydrogen bonding

Small lipophilic drugs cross the BBB more easily than larger or more hydrophilic drugs. Minor changes in structure can drastically change a drug's lipophilicity and ability to cross the BBB. Increasing the number of hydrogen bonds tends to make a compound more polar, which restricts its penetration across the BBB. A few examples illustrate these chemical effects on BBB penetration:

- Morphine has two hydroxyl groups and crosses the BBB slowly. The hydroxyl groups are acetylated in heroin (diacetylmorphine), which greatly increases the BBB penetration and intensifies the immediate euphoric effect from an intravenous injection
- Diazepam has an additional methyl group compared with other benzodiazepines, which causes it to cross the BBB more rapidly and makes it the preferred drug for treating status epilepticus

- Enrofloxacin crosses the BBB and blood–ocular barrier more easily than ciprofloxacin because the addition of an ethyl group makes it more lipophilic. Enrofloxacin is known to produce a greater likelihood of CNS adverse reactions and ocular toxicity than ciprofloxacin. For example, ciprofloxacin at high doses does not produce ocular toxicity in cats, but enrofloxacin at doses above 5 mg/kg can cause retinal degeneration (Ford et al., 2007).

Molecular size
The molecular size of the drug affects penetration across the BBB. The molecular mass threshold for drugs active in the CNS appears to be <400–500 Daltons. Most therapeutic drugs have a molecular weight below this threshold but large molecules and proteins are restricted. Likewise, highly protein-bound drugs are restricted from penetrating the BBB.

Carrier-mediated transport
Carrier-mediated transport (CMT) can occur via facilitated diffusion or active transport, and allows carrier systems to transport nutrients from the blood to the brain. Such transport systems include the glucose transporter, the lactate transporter, the cationic amino acid transporter and the large amino acid transporter (LAT). The role of carrier-mediated diffusion for drug transport into the brain is minor except for a few drugs. One such example of a drug that utilizes CMT is dopamine. Dopamine as the parent drug does not penetrate the BBB after systemic administration. However, when converted to the alpha-amino acid derivative levodopa (L-dopa), it utilizes the LAT to be transported across the BBB. Once in the brain, levodopa is metabolized to dopamine, where it is helpful for treatment of Parkinson's disease.

CMT can also transport anticonvulsant drugs. Gabapentin is a gamma-amino acid used to treat epilepsy. It mimics an alpha-amino acid and utilizes the LAT to penetrate the brain.

Membrane efflux systems (P-glycoprotein)
A transmembrane protein coded by the multi-drug resistance (MDR) gene *ABCB1* (ATP-binding cassette transporters subform B, formerly called the *MDR1* gene) is present in the BBB to 'pump' drugs out of the CNS. This protein is called P-glycoprotein (P-gp), and is the most studied of several efflux transporters that can affect CNS drug concentrations.

P-gp is also found in the gastrointestinal tract, liver, placenta and kidneys, and in other organs (Preiss, 1998; Demeule et al., 2002). Detailed reviews have been published that describe the important role of P-gp in the functional BBB (Demeule et al., 2002; Sun et al., 2003). It is regarded as an integral part of the functional BBB and an important determinant of drug penetration into the CNS. P-gp may exclude important drugs, such as dexamethasone, antiviral (anti-HIV) drugs, antibiotics, anticancer drugs (used for treating brain tumours) and anticonvulsants. For example, this difference in corticosteroid penetration into the CNS

between normal dogs and P-gp-deficient dogs may produce an altered response to stress in deficient dogs. Suppression of the hypothalamic–pituitary–adrenal (HPA) axis in deficient dogs allows greater corticosteroid penetration into the CNS, which produces chronic suppression of the HPA axis (Mealey et al., 2007). Resistance to anticonvulsant drugs may be related to polymorphism of the gene that codes for P-gp. In some clinical cases refractory to anticonvulsant drugs, the membrane pump is upregulated, thus impairing drug penetration to an epileptogenic region of the brain (Pedley and Hirano, 2003). However, in a study of anticonvulsant drugs used in dogs, they were either weak substrates or were not substrates for canine P-gp (West and Mealey, 2007); those authors concluded that it seems unlikely that efficacy of anticonvulsant drugs is affected by the P-gp expression in the BBB of dogs. There has, however, been contradictory evidence. Alves et al. (2011) examined epileptic Border Collies resistant to phenobarbital treatment and identified a mutation in the P-gp gene that may upregulate this protein, resulting in overexpression that reduces phenobarbital penetration to the CNS. Pekcec et al. (2009) also provided evidence that overexpression of P-gp may be responsible for refractoriness of anticonvulsant treatment in dogs. In an attempt to inhibit P-gp in refractory canine epileptics, Jambroszyk et al. (2011) added verapamil (a putative P-gp inhibitor) to phenobarbital treatment in dogs; the results indicated that inhibiting P-gp with verapamil did not improve seizure control (it actually was associated with deterioration in some dogs). Those results leave many questions: phenobarbital may not be a substrate for P-gp in canine epileptics, verapamil at the doses used is not an effective P-gp inhibitor in dogs, or other actions of verapamil may be responsible for worsening of seizure control in dogs. Jambroszyk et al. also measured plasma and CSF phenobarbital concentrations, which were unchanged when verapamil was added to the treatment but, as discussed earlier in this chapter, CSF concentration of drugs is a poor indicator of BBB penetration.

P-gp participates in neuroprotection of the brain by regulating drug entry (Lechardeur et al., 1996) and acting as a 'guardian' of the CNS by preventing the accumulation of drugs in the brain (Demeule et al., 2002). Deficiency in BBB P-gp explains why some collies and related breeds are susceptible to adverse effects of therapeutic doses of ivermectin and similar drugs (discussed in more detail below). Inhibitors of P-gp that are of veterinary importance include ketoconazole, ciclosporin, calcium-channel blockers (diltiazem), erythromycin and antiarrhythmics (lidocaine and quinidine). Drug interactions caused by these inhibitors have allowed increased penetration of drugs that are normally excluded from the brain. For example, quinidine can increase the CNS effects of loperamide and of digoxin, which are ordinarily excluded from the brain (Sadeque et al., 2000; Lin 2003). Administration of ketoconazole to dogs is known to increase concentrations of ivermectin, which can result in adverse neurological effects.

Anti-infectious drug therapy

Activity and efficacy of antibiotics for treatment of CNS infections in small animals have not been critically evaluated. There are no documented clinical studies that have examined the efficacy of various antibiotics for CNS infections in veterinary patients and thus data continue to be extrapolated from human studies. Fortunately, primary bacterial infections of the CNS and meninges are uncommon in small animal medicine. However, bacterial infections of the CNS can arise as a complication from other primary diseases, such as otitis media (Spangler and Dewey, 2000; Sturges *et al.*, 2006), migration from nasal cavity infections, or due to contamination from surgery or other invasive techniques, such as epidural puncture. Other infectious agents, including fungi, protozoans, rickettsial agents and viruses may all infect the CNS. Therapeutic guidelines have been developed from the experience of veterinary specialists or extrapolated from experience in humans and laboratory animal studies.

This section of the chapter will focus on antibacterial, antifungal and antiprotozoal drugs. Antiviral drugs, although important in people, have not been evaluated for treatment of small animal nervous system infections, even though these infections do indeed occur (Leschnik *et al.*, 2002; Yanai *et al.*, 2003). There are no published references to guide antiviral treatment of CNS infections in small animals, except for a few accounts of the use of aciclovir or famciclovir for treating herpesvirus and FIV dementia in cats.

Antibacterial drugs

Treatment principles in animals generally follow the principles used for treatment in humans (Quagliarello and Scheld, 1997). Meningitis in people is usually caused by *Haemophilus influenzae*, *Streptoccus pneumoniae* or *Neisseria meningitidis*. Enteric Gram-negative bacteria (e.g. *Escherichia coli*) may be opportunistic pathogens in severely immunocompromised patients or as a complication of neurosurgery. Reports of CNS infections are few in veterinary literature, and the three most common bacterial pathogens in humans are not even listed as CNS pathogens for small animals. When bacterial infections of the CNS occur in animals, it is anticipated that the most common organisms will include *Streptococcus* spp., *Staphylococcus* spp. and enteric Gram-negative bacilli, such as *E. coli* and *Klebsiella pneumoniae*. In a retrospective review of 23 cases of bacterial meningoencephalomyelitis in dogs, *E. coli*, *Streptococcus* and *Klebsiella* were the most common isolates (Radaelli and Platt, 2002). Unfortunately these bacteria were all identified from post-mortem examination of nervous tissues (18 of 23 dogs). In only one of the 23 dogs was there a positive culture of the CSF *ante mortem*. The study did not evaluate effectiveness of antibacterial treatments. In the study cited earlier, (Sturges *et al.*, 2006) bacteria isolated from intracranial infection arising from ear disease (11 cats and 4 dogs) included *Staphylococcus*, *Streptococcus*, *E. coli*,

Enterococcus and *Pasteurella multocida*. The infection in these cases was successfully managed with surgery and treatment with antibiotics.

As discussed previously, the BBB prevents many antibiotics accessing the CNS. This presents a problem with achieving adequate bactericidal drug concentrations in the CSF. Here, more than in other tissues, high bactericidal drug concentrations are needed because of the limited natural bactericidal ability of the CNS. This deficiency of CNS defence mechanisms is attributed to the low protein content, low antibody levels and few phagocytic cells (Täuber *et al.*, 1984). The most common drugs used in veterinary medicine include cephalosporins, penicillins (and derivatives such as amoxicillin and ampicillin), and aminoglycosides. Because these antibiotics are hydrophilic polar molecules, they do not penetrate the BBB well.

For these drugs, high doses should be administered in order to produce an adequate concentration gradient between the systemic circulation and the brain, to facilitate diffusion into the CNS. When selecting an antibiotic from this list, one should use a third-generation cephalosporin over a first-generation cephalosporin. Other antibiotics that can be recommended for CNS infections include metronidazole (high lipophilicity), carbapenems (low molecular weight and high activity) and trimethoprim (high lipophilicity).

Cephalosporins

The third-generation cephalosporins are more active against Gram-negative bacteria, especially enteric organisms, than are the first-generation cephalosporins. Cephalosporins are relatively polar antibiotics that are minimally lipid-soluble and have poor intracellular penetration. Ordinarily they have poor distribution to the CNS. The rationale for selecting a third-generation cephalosporin is that because of their greater activity against Gram-negative bacilli, the minimum inhibitory concentration (MIC) is lower and even low BBB penetration may be effective. Cefotaxime, ceftazidime, ceftizoxime and ceftriaxone are capable of achieving drug concentrations in the CSF that are considered bactericidal for most Gram-negative bacteria. Therefore, these are the preferred drugs for treating serious bacterial infections of the CNS.

When an injectable third-generation cephalosporin is needed, cefotaxime is the preferred drug for small animals because it is active against Gram-negative enteric bacteria and *Streptococcus* spp. Even though it is a registered human drug, it is the one that veterinary surgeons have the most experience with. Although there are no published studies that evaluate the use of cefotaxime in veterinary patients, clinicians have relied on some published pharmacokinetic studies to guide dosing. The pharmacokinetics in dogs and humans are similar enough that doses, as well as clinical uses, have been extrapolated from human medicine. Generally, cefotaxime is administered intravenously, intramuscularly or subcutaneously to dogs and cats at a dose of 30 mg/kg q8h. When administered subcutaneously to dogs and intramuscularly to cats it was found that the absorption rates were high (Guerrini et al., 1986; McElroy et al., 1986) but that intramuscular and subcutaneous injections can cause pain.

Ceftazidime is the most active cephalosporin for treatment of *Pseudomonas aeruginosa* infection. Other cephalosporins, except cefoperazone, have little or no activity against the pathogen. Ceftazidime has been studied in dogs (Acred, 1983; Matsui et al., 1984; Moore et al., 2000); it has a short half-life (<1 hour) and a volume of distribution similar to that in humans. Dosages have ranged from 20–30 mg/kg q12h for *Enterobacteriaceae* to 30 mg/kg q4h for *Pseudomonas* (Moore et al., 2000).

Ceftiofur has been used extensively in cattle and is also approved for use in horses and dogs. However, at the doses at which it is currently registered for dogs (2.2 mg/kg s.c. q24h) it is *not* expected to attain concentrations in the CNS that are high enough to treat Gram-negative infections. Higher doses are not recommended because high doses of ceftiofur have caused bone marrow suppression in dogs.

The most commonly used oral third-generation cephalosporin in small animals is cefpodoxime proxetil. It is an inactive ester that is well absorbed orally. It is converted to the active metabolite in the intestinal wall and produces effective concentrations in the interstitial fluid for 24 hours (Papich et al., 2010). The only studies available of cefpodoxime concentrations in CSF were performed in pigs (Abdel-Rahman et al., 2000). In that study, the CSF:plasma concentration ratio demonstrated a penetration of only 5%. Despite this low penetration, the concentrations produced in CSF from this dose (10 mg/kg orally) approached or exceeded the MIC_{90} for many bacterial pathogens considered susceptible to cefpodoxime.

Penicillins

Penicillins include penicillin G, ampicillin and amoxicillin. The penetration of these drugs into the CNS is poor. Except for sensitive *Streptococcus* spp. (which have low MIC values) these drugs should not be used for treating infections of the CNS. There are no published reports of successful use in small animals.

An exception is in the treatment of tetanus. The organism that causes tetanus (*Clostridium tetani*) is highly susceptible to penicillins. The organism elaborates a toxin (tetanospasmin) that produces excitation by blocking inhibitory neurotransmission in the CNS. When treating tetanus, drug penetration into the CNS is not necessary because it is a peripheral infection, even though the toxin produces CNS effects.

Carbapenems

The carbapenems include imipenem–cilastatin, doripenem and meropenem. These drugs are the most active of any currently available antibiotics against a broad spectrum of bacteria. Imipenem has been associated with CNS adverse effects, including seizures, especially in human patients with meningitis. It is a small molecule and penetrates the BBB more effectively than the larger drugs of this class. However, to avoid CNS reactions, meropenem should be used instead when a highly active drug is needed, especially to treat infections that may be resistant to other drugs (Edwards and Betts, 2000). Small volumes can be administered subcutaneously with almost complete absorption. Based on pharmacokinetic experiments (Bidgood and Papich, 2002) the recommended dose for meropenem is 12 mg/kg s.c. q8h.

Trimethoprim/sulphonamides

Sulphonamides have been used alone in veterinary medicine for many years. Combination products that contain trimethoprim are more effective for systemic use. Examples of available formulations include both trimethoprim/sulfadiazine and trimethoprim/sulfamethoxazole. Sulfamethoxazole is more lipophilic than is sulfadiazine; this would presumably produce differences in CNS penetration, but a comparison between these drugs has not been performed.

Trimethoprim/sulphonamides are characterized by their good distribution to most tissues in the body. However, trimethoprim is more widely distributed than sulphonamides, especially to tissues such as the CNS. For treatment of CNS protozoan infections in horses, pyrimethamine combined with a sulfadiazine is used.

Trimethoprim/sulphonamides have activity against both bacteria and protozoans. It is difficult to correlate plasma drug levels (and plasma elimination rates) with clinical efficacy and dosing intervals because trimethoprim persists longer in some tissues than in the plasma. The optimum dosing regimen depends on the underlying disease. The recommended dose for CNS infections in dogs and cats is 15–30 mg/kg q12h.

Chloramphenicol

Chloramphenicol is a rather old drug (first introduced in 1947) but has seen recent increased use because of its activity against resistant bacteria in animals – specifically meticillin-resistant *Staphylococcus* and resistant strains of *Enterococcus* spp. It has been recommended for treatment of bacterial CNS infections because of its high lipophilicity. However, at the doses administered, the penetration across the BBB does not attain the level necessary for effectiveness against Gram-negative bacteria in infections of the CNS (Rahal and Simberkoff, 1979; Cherubin et al., 1984). Increasing the dose to improve the concentrations is not recommended because at high doses chloramphenicol can be toxic to dogs and cats.

Metronidazole

Metronidazole is indicated for treatment of CNS infections caused by anaerobic bacteria, particularly *Bacteroides fragilis* or its relatives. Metronidazole is lipophilic and penetrates the CNS. Dose recommendations have varied but effective concentrations can be attained with a dose of 10–15 mg/kg orally q12h. The dose in cats often is one-quarter of a 250 mg tablet per cat, which is equivalent to 62.5 mg. The most significant adverse effect is neurotoxicity, which is obviously a drawback if metronidazole is selected for treating CNS infections (see Chapter 11). The reactions observed are hypothesized to be caused by inhibition of the gamma-aminobutyric acid (GABA) neurotransmitter. These effects appear to be dose-related, but have been associated with high doses of 67–129 mg/kg/day (Dow *et al.*, 1989), as well as moderate doses of 33–83 mg/kg/day (Evans *et al.*, 2003). Metronidazole has caused cerebellar and vestibular ataxia, lethargy, paresis, proprioceptive deficits, nystagmus, tremors and seizure-like signs in dogs and seizures in cats (see Chapter 13). Dogs recover if drug administration is discontinued but recovery may take 1–2 weeks (Dow *et al.*, 1989). However, when diazepam was administered as a treatment (0.2–0.69 mg/kg i.v. or orally q8h for 3 days) recovery was faster (Evans *et al.*, 2003).

Fluoroquinolones

Fluoroquinolones include enrofloxacin, marbofloxacin, difloxacin and orbifloxacin. All of these are approved for use in dogs in the UK and the USA; orbifloxacin, marbofloxacin and enrofloxacin are approved for cats. Despite the high volumes of distribution, and otherwise good tissue penetration, these drugs do not reach therapeutic concentrations in the CNS. There are no documented indications for using fluoroquinolones to treat CNS infections in animals (Papich and Riviere, 2009). Potential adverse effects are discussed below.

Antifungal drugs

Occasionally, fungal meningoencephalitis is identified in small animal patients. There are few studies to document efficacy of treatment for these infections. However, treatment options are available using drugs registered for human medicine, which can be extrapolated to animals. The most common use of antifungal drugs for treating infections of the CNS is to treat *Cryptococcus* infection. Success of treating infections in dogs and cats depends a lot on the location; where there is CNS involvement with *Cryptococcus*, the outcome has been mixed. In a retrospective study (Sykes *et al.*, 2010) of dogs and cats with CNS cryptococcosis presented to the University of California, the success rate following treatment with antifungal drugs was only 32%. Where infection is non-CNS, the outcome is much better (84%) (O'Brien *et al.*, 2006). The current recommended regimen for treatment of cryptococcosis is fluconazole as an initial choice (O'Brien *et al.*, 2006; Trivedi *et al.*, 2011), although some isolates are resistant to fluconazole. In more severe cases, amphotericin B is administered (in combination with 5-flucytosine in cats but alone in dogs). Some cases can also be treated with itraconazole but there is no evidence that itraconazole is more effective than fluconazole and it may be associated with a higher incidence of toxicity. If treatment with amphotericin B is initiated, it should be continued until there are no clinical signs or antibody titres have dropped; follow-up treatment with an azole (usually either itraconazole or fluconazole) is then continued for 6–12 months (O'Brien *et al.*, 2006).

Amphotericin B

Amphotericin B is a polyene macrolide antibiotic with fungicidal antifungal activity. It has no effect on bacteria but is effective on some protozoans (e.g. *Leishmania*) and has been a valuable drug for the treatment of serious systemic fungal infections. However, it is tremendously toxic and requires careful administration and patient monitoring. Penetration of amphotericin B into the CNS is limited. Nevertheless, it has been used for the systemic treatment of cryptococcal meningitis and of meningoencephalitis caused by other fungi such as *Coccidioides immitis*, *Candida* and *Aspergillus*.

The most important feature of amphotericin B is that it is fungicidal. The other common antifungal drugs (azoles) are fungistatic and require long-term continuous treatment. One of the most important drawbacks to amphotericin B is nephrotoxicosis; individual daily doses produce acute reversible nephrotoxicosis, but permanent nephrotoxicosis can occur from the total cumulative dose. Assessments of renal function should be carefully monitored throughout treatment and it may become necessary to abandon therapy with amphotericin if there is persistent azotaemia. Other adverse effects that may be observed include vomiting, tremors, pyrexia and anorexia. These effects may be associated with each daily treatment and are somewhat alleviated by premedication with antihistamine drugs and antiemetics. Phlebitis is expected with intravenous administration; therefore, the sites for catheter administration are usually alternated.

A reference on this topic should be consulted before attempting to treat any patient with amphotericin B (Davis *et al.*, 2009). Nephrotoxicity is reduced if patients are pre-treated with fluid therapy (NaCl) and receive the infusion at a slow rate (over 4–6 hours). A recommended dose is 0.25 mg/kg for the first treatment, then 0.5–1.0 mg/kg administered every other day until a total cumulative dose of 4–8 mg/kg has been given. (Higher cumulative doses have been tolerated with subcutaneous administration – see later.) The total cumulative dose is limited by nephrotoxicosis. In the report by O'Brien *et al.* (2006) on the outcome of dogs and cats with cryptococcosis they observed that dogs were more tolerant of amphotericin B-induced nephrotoxicity than cats. In cats, but not dogs, administration of 5-flucytosine (5-FC) is recommended during initial treatment for cryptococcosis. Dogs predictably develop cutaneous lesions from 5-FC and it is not recommended.

Subcutaneous administration: Malik *et al.* (1996) have reported on the subcutaneous administration of amphotericin B for cryptococcosis. In their report, amphotericin B was administered to dogs and cats subcutaneously at cumulative doses of 8–26 mg/kg. Except for local irritation, the injections were well tolerated and, unlike intravenous injections, higher doses were administered without producing azotaemia. A follow-up study by O'Brien *et al.* (2006) demonstrated the effectiveness of this route of administration. It was administered at a dose of 0.5–0.75 mg/kg diluted in 350 ml of 0.45% saline and 2.5% dextrose, once, twice or three times a week. Cumulative doses of 23 mg/kg in cats and 60 mg/kg in dogs were achieved without permanent nephrotoxicity – although reversible nephrotoxicity was observed.

Intrathecal administration: Because of poor penetration of amphotericin B across the BBB, intrathecal administration has been performed. For this type of administration the conventional formulation of amphotericin B should be used. The intravenous formulation of 5 mg/ml may be further diluted to 0.25 mg/ml by mixing 1 ml of the solution (5 mg) with 19 ml of 5% dextrose solution. Typically the dose for the animal is diluted with CSF in the syringe. It is important to note that some dextrose solutions have a pH of <4.2 and the pH should be increased if necessary prior to intrathecal administration. For small animals a dose of 0.01–0.1 mg (total dose of base) should be administered every 48–72 hours. If the dose is tolerated it may be increased to 0.25 mg. This is a risky procedure and should be performed only as a last resort.

Lipid formulations: The lipid formulations of amphotericin B are used in humans but there is limited experience in their use in veterinary medicine due to their high cost. Three of these formulations are currently available (Plotnick, 2000):

- Amphotericin B lipid complex
- Amphotericin B cholesteryl sulphate complex
- Amphotericin B liposomal complex encapsulated in a lipid bilayer.

Amphotericin B lipid complex is a suspension of amphotericin B complexed with two phospholipids. This has been the most extensively evaluated formulation in dogs; it is the least expensive and was shown in one study to be safe and effective in dogs at a cumulative dose of 8–12 mg/kg. Amphotericin B lipid complex is the form used most frequently by veterinary surgeons in North America.

Amphotericin B cholesteryl sulphate complex is a colloidal dispersion, also called ABCD (amphotericin B colloidal dispersion).

The amphotericin B liposomal complex encapsulated in a lipid bilayer has been used successfully to treat a German Shepherd Dog with discospondylitis due to disseminated *Aspergillus* infection (personal communication, N. Olby).

The advantage of these lipid and cholesteryl formulations of amphotericin B is that, in comparison with the conventional formulation of amphotericin B (amphotericin B deoxycholate), these can be given at higher doses to produce greater efficacy with less toxicity (Hiemenz and Walsh, 1996). Amphotericin B lipid complex is 8–10 times less nephrotoxic in

dogs than the conventional formulation. These lipid complex formulations of amphotericin B have been administered at a dose of 3 mg/kg or more, compared with 0.25–0.5 mg/kg of the conventional formulation (Walsh *et al.*, 1999). Decreased toxicity is attributed to a selective transfer of the lipid complex amphotericin B, releasing the drug directly to the fungal cell membrane and sparing the mammalian cell membranes. Reduced drug concentrations in the kidneys and diminished release of inflammatory cytokines from the amphotericin B lipid complex compared with the conventional formulation may also prevent adverse reactions. Improved efficacy is attributed to the higher doses that can be administered, selective delivery of the drug to fungal cell membranes, and the concentration of the drug in inflammatory cells, which can deliver the drug directly to the site of infection.

Azole antifungal drugs

The only two oral azole antifungal drugs that should be used for systemic treatment of meningitis or meningoencephalitis caused by fungi are itraconazole and fluconazole. Ketoconazole has poor penetration into the CNS and should not be used for this indication. Posaconazole and voriconazole are new human drugs that are used for disseminated fungal infections. They have not been shown to be better than either itraconazole or fluconazole for treating cryptococcosis. Both drugs are very expensive at this time. Voriconazole has caused neurotoxicity in cats (Quimby *et al.*, 2010) and is not recommended until a safe dose can be established. Enilconazole (which has also been called imazalil) has been used to treat nasal aspergillosis in dogs. It is reported to have a vapour effect and, if instilled into the nasal cavity of dogs, will control fungal growth (Sharp *et al.*, 1991). It has been used successfully to treat sinonasal aspergillosis in dogs, therefore preventing more serious invasion into the CNS (Zonderland *et al.*, 2002).

Itraconazole: Itraconazole is usually used to treat systemic fungal infections or yeast infections, but may also be indicated to treat cryptococcal meningoencephalitis. It is highly lipophilic and attains high concentrations in tissues (Van Cauteren *et al.*, 1987). Even though the concentrations in aqueous fluids, such as aqueous humour and CSF, are low (this drug is not water-soluble), as discussed earlier, the drug concentrations in CSF may not represent the concentrations in the brain parenchyma. Therefore, the levels in the tissues are high enough for treatment of CNS infections (Denning *et al.*, 1989; Medleau *et al.*, 1995). Although specific tissue concentration studies are not available for dogs or cats, itraconazole may attain high enough tissue concentrations for effectiveness against CNS fungi (Perfect *et al.*, 1986).

In cats itraconazole has been used at a dose of 10 mg/kg q24h. The most common adverse effect is anorexia and hepatotoxicity that is cumulative and dose-related but reversible. Affected cats will initially have decreased appetite but will eventually develop increases in liver enzymes. In an evaluation of 35 cats with confirmed *Cryptocococcus neoformans* infection, cats were treated with itraconazole at a dose of either 50 mg/day or 100 mg/day (Medleau *et al.*, 1995). This dose was also used in the study by O'Brien *et al.* (2006). Adverse effects were observed in 26% of the cats, most of them in the high-dose group, and included increased liver enzymes, anorexia and weight loss. Successful outcome was observed in 57% of the cats (average dose 13.8 mg/kg/day) and improvement was observed in 29% of the cats. Median duration of treatment was 8.5 months.

Dosages used in dogs have been 2.5–5 mg/kg/day and as high as 5–10 mg/kg/day for the treatment of blastomycosis; 5 mg/kg/day is the most commonly recommended dose (Legendre, 1995) and may be as effective as high doses with less toxicity. Presumably, this dose would also be considered for CNS infections. If adverse effects are observed (e.g. anorexia) the dose should be lowered or a switch made to fluconazole or amphotericin B. According to Legendre (1995) about 10% of dogs receiving the recommended doses of itraconazole develop hepatic toxicosis. Liver enzyme elevations may occur in 10–15% of dogs. Anorexia may occur as a complication of treatment, especially with high drug doses and high drug serum concentrations. Anorexia usually develops in the second month of therapy in dogs.

Itraconazole is available as 100 mg capsules. The granules in these capsules may be added to food for convenience. It is better absorbed with food and should not be administered with an antacid or acid-suppressing drug (e.g. famotidine, omeprazole) because high stomach pH will decrease absorption. It is also available as a 10 mg/ml cherry-flavoured oral liquid formulation (Willems *et al.*, 2001). The oral solution formulation is a combination of the drug with cyclodextrins. Cyclodextrins are permeability enhancers made up of oligosaccharides with a hydrophilic outer surface and a lipophilic inner surface. They form complexes with highly insoluble drugs, allowing them to remain soluble in solution. Since dissolution is the rate-limiting step in the absorption of most orally administered drugs, the liquid formulation has a higher absorption rate and is less dependent on feeding than the capsule formulation. In a study in cats, itraconazole oral solution appeared to be much better absorbed than a capsule (Boothe *et al.*, 1997) even when cats were given food with each administration of the capsule. The long half-life of itraconazole in the cats of this study supports once-daily dosing.

Fluconazole: Fluconazole is usually the first choice for treatment of fungal meningoencephalitis, rather than itraconazole. It is less expensive (generic form available in North America), better tolerated, and better absorbed orally. It has been shown to attain effective drug concentrations in the CSF. The spectrum of activity is similar to that of other azoles, except that it has poor activity against *Aspergillus*. It has been the most commonly used oral drug for cryptococcal meningitis. Fluconazole has no effect on endocrine activity and has less tendency than itraconazole to cause drug interactions.

Fluconazole has different solubility characteristics compared with both ketoconazole and itraconazole and is absorbed well, regardless of other factors (such as feeding). It is available in tablets, oral suspension or as an intravenous injection. Fluconazole tablets and an oral suspension of 10 mg/ml are absorbed well; the oral dose is similar to the intravenous dose. Fluconazole is more water-soluble than itraconazole. Itraconazole does not dissolve in aqueous solutions and therefore fluconazole attains higher CSF concentrations than ketoconazole or itraconazole. Some clinicians have used this evidence to indicate that fluconazole is preferred for treating mycotic meningitis but superior efficacy of fluconazole over itraconazole has not been established clinically or experimentally (Perfect *et al.*, 1986; Sykes *et al.*, 2010). Higher CSF concentrations for fluconazole should not necessarily be interpreted as being equivalent to concentrations in CNS tissues (see above).

Fluconazole has a long half-life (25 hours) in cats, with good absorption and distribution to the CSF and aqueous humour (Vaden *et al.*, 1997). In humans the half-life is about 30 hours. For cats with systemic cryptococcosis, clinical studies have shown a benefit from a dose of 100 mg/cat/day in one or two divided doses. Other reported doses are 2.5–5 mg/kg q24h (Hill *et al.*, 1995). Pharmacokinetic studies support a dose of 50 mg/cat per day (Vaden *et al.*, 1997). Malik *et al.* (1992) treated 29 cats with cryptococcosis. The average dose of fluconazole was 50 mg/cat orally q12h and cats were treated for 2–6.5 months. The study by O'Brien *et al.* (2006) used a dose of 33–50 mg/cat orally q12h. Fluconazole was well tolerated, except for some anorexia, and all but one cat had clinical resolution. In dogs the dose is 10–12 mg/kg/day orally. However, in one case report (Tiches *et al.*, 1998) a dog treated for CNS cryptococcosis developed adverse effects at a dose of 9.1 mg/kg/day and the dose had to be lowered.

Flucytosine: As mentioned previously, in cats, but not dogs, administration of 5-flucytosine (5-FC) is recommended during initial treatment for cryptococcosis. Flucytosine inhibits fungal nucleic acid synthesis via a specific enzyme that converts 5-FC to 5-fluorouracil (5-FU) in fungal cells. It is synergistic when used with amphotericin B. If used as single agent treatment (monotherapy) resistance develops quickly, necessitating its combination with other drugs. The adverse effects from 5-FC are bone marrow suppression, especially when it accumulates in patients with renal insufficiency. Flucytosine clearance mimics creatinine clearance. It has been associated with cutaneous drug eruptions in dogs and is not recommended. For reasons that are unclear, cats do not appear to develop these lesions. A disadvantage of 5-FC is the rapid clearance, which necessitates frequent administration. A dose of 30 mg/kg orally q6h or 50 mg/kg orally q8h has been used in cats.

Antiprotozoal drugs

Pyrimethamine

Pyrimethamine is a diaminopyrimidine that is structurally related to trimethoprim, and acts via a similar mechanism. The major difference is that pyrimethamine is more potent than trimethoprim in terms of inhibition of the dihydrofolate reductase enzyme of protozoans and has therefore been used to treat protozoal infections in people, horses, dogs and cats.

Pyrimethamine is often administered in combination with a sulphonamide for treatment of protozoal infections as the drugs act synergistically. In dogs this combination has been used to treat *Neospora caninum* infection and in cats it has been used for treatment of *Toxoplasma gondii*, although efficacy has not been established in cats. The formulations available are either pyrimethamine alone in a 25 mg tablet, pyrimethamine 25 mg with sulfadoxine 500 mg, or pyrimethamine 12.5 mg/ml in combination with sulfadiazine 250 mg/ml in an equine formulation.

Pyrimethamine is well absorbed after oral administration. The dose used for cats (to treat toxoplasmosis) is 1 mg/kg q24h plus sulfadiazine at a rate of 25 mg/kg orally q12h (for 14–28 days). The pyrimethamine dose for dogs is 1 mg/kg q24h plus sulfadiazine at a rate of 12.5 mg/kg q12h (for 14–21 days).

Adverse effects from pyrimethamine administration have included signs of folate deficiency, i.e. agranulocytosis, anaemia and thrombocytopenia. Although many veterinary surgeons provide oral folic acid or folinic acid supplements during treatment to prevent adverse effects associated with folate deficiency, effectiveness of this supplementation has never been established (Castles *et al.*, 1971). It is advised to monitor patients (e.g. complete blood count (CBC) periodically) for signs of folate deficiency during treatment.

Clindamycin

Clindamycin in high doses has been used to treat toxoplasmosis in dogs and cats. Clindamycin has *in vitro* activity against *Toxoplasma gondii* but clinical results of efficacy for treating toxoplasmosis are conflicting. The effective doses used are higher than those administered for bacterial infections. Appropriate doses are 12–25 mg/kg orally q12h (Dubey and Yeary, 1977; Greene *et al.*, 1985; Lappin *et al.*, 1989). Treatment duration is typically 2 weeks. At these doses adverse effects of diarrhoea, vomiting and reduced appetite are possible (Greene *et al.*, 1992). In addition, the efficacy of clindamycin at these doses has been questioned. It may not be effective at clearing organisms from the CNS of chronically infected animals (Greene *et al.*, 1985; Lappin *et al.*, 1989); some studies of efficacy have only evaluated acute infections. In addition, clindamycin may not be effective for ocular forms of the disease (Lappin *et al.*, 1992; Davidson *et al.*, 1996). In one study (Davidson *et al.*, 1996) there was actually increased morbidity and mortality from clindamycin treatment compared to control groups. In human medicine clindamycin has been combined with pyrimethamine for treatment of toxoplasmosis. Except for a few reports of successful use of this combination in cats for toxoplasmosis (Foster and Martin, 2011), the effect of this combination requires further evaluation in dogs and cats.

Other antiprotozoal drugs

Trimethoprim/sulphonamides, discussed above, are sometimes used to treat protozoal infections.

Anti-inflammatory therapy

Anti-inflammatory therapy is indicated for CNS infection and as an adjunct treatment for vasogenic oedema in diseases such as neoplasia. Corticosteroids are the most valuable anti-inflammatory drugs for CNS disease. Their anti-inflammatory properties have been reviewed elsewhere (Franklin, 1984; Papich and Davis, 1989; Barnes and Adcock, 1993). They reduce CNS oedema via their action on blood vessels, and they produce anti-inflammatory effects via their action on neutrophils and inhibition of cytokine synthesis. For acute indications the drugs used should be rapid-acting and formulated for intravenous administration. The forms most often used are dexamethasone sodium phosphate, prednisolone sodium succinate and methylprednisolone sodium succinate (MPSS). These formulations have substitutions on the 17-alpha carbon (e.g. sodium succinate, sodium phosphate) to make them soluble in aqueous solutions. Formulations that are not in aqueous solutions (e.g. dexamethasone solution 2 mg/ml in polyethylene glycol) should not be administered rapidly intravenously to neurological patients because of the risk of adverse effects. On the other hand, aqueous solutions can be administered with intravenous fluids or given intravenously at high doses. For more chronic therapy, oral treatments of prednisolone/prednisone and dexamethasone have been used.

Corticosteroid use in CNS infections

In the treatment of CNS infection, cellular debris (particularly bacterial cell wall material) is liberated owing to the bactericidal effect of the antibiotics. Bacteriolysis promotes a cascade of inflammatory events, releasing tumour necrosis factor-alpha (TNF-α), interleukins (IL1, IL6) and other cytokines. These mediators damage the CNS tissues, produce oedema and promote a further, more serious, inflammatory cascade. Similar inflammatory reactions are seen when treating fungal infections. In addition to bactericidal or fungicidal drugs, anti-inflammatory drugs should be employed as early as possible in the course of therapy when treating bacterial or fungal meningoencephalomyelitis.

The most common corticosteroid used during treatment of bacterial CNS infections in humans has been dexamethasone, although no comparisons have been made with prednisolone. Dexamethasone administered early in the treatment of bacterial meningitis decreases the inflammatory response associated with release of bacterial cell material (DeGans and van de Beek, 2002; Tunkel and Scheld, 2002; Lutsar *et al.*, 2003). Dexamethasone should be instituted early in therapy; if treatment is delayed, benefits diminish. The dose most often recommended is 0.15 mg/kg of dexamethasone sodium phosphate (approximate anti-inflammatory equivalent is 1 mg/kg of prednisolone), administered intravenously every 6 hours for 2–4 days. Because bacterial meningoencephalitis is rare in small animals, a definitive diagnosis should be reached prior to administering corticosteroids to patients with inflammatory CNS disease.

Non-steroidal anti-inflammatory drugs (NSAIDs) have been considered alternatives to corticosteroids for anti-inflammatory treatment of the CNS. However, there is little published evidence either to support or to refute the use of these drugs for CNS disease. In one report, piroxicam was used as an adjunct to fluconazole when treating cryptococcal meningoencephalitis in a dog (Tiches *et al.*, 1998). Neurological improvement was noted in the report but other drugs were also administered.

Corticosteroid use in spinal trauma

Corticosteroids, specifically MPSS, have been administered to prevent further injury to the spinal cord caused by ischaemia and inflammation from trauma. The review by Olby (1999) provided an excellent summary of the studies in experimental animals and the human clinical trials that have evaluated the potential benefit of corticosteroids for this indication. Treatment of spinal cord trauma is discussed in this book more extensively in Chapter 20.

The action of corticosteroids was reviewed by Hall (1992) and by Brown and Hall (1992). The action of corticosteroids that appears to be most important for protection of spinal cord tissue from injury following trauma is that of inhibition of lipid peroxidation of membranes caused by oxygen-derived free radicals (Brown and Hall, 1992; Hall, 1992). This action is unrelated to the hormone effects of these drugs. High doses of MPSS (30 mg/kg) are required (see Chapter 20 for full details of recommended dosing protocols for MPSS in spinal cord injury). These doses far exceed the dose necessary to produce a typical corticosteroid effect from binding to glucocorticosteroid cellular receptors.

Lower doses are not effective for treating spinal cord trauma, even though at those doses all the corticosteroid receptors are probably occupied. A secondary beneficial effect may occur through the ability of corticosteroids to inhibit synthesis of inflammatory cytokines and suppress generation of arachidonic acid products (vasoactive prostaglandins), which may cause ischaemia of the neural tissue. MPSS is not as effective if treatment is delayed for more than 8 hours, and may actually be harmful. Administration of high doses of MPSS has been associated with side effects (see Corticosteroid use for immunosuppression, below); therefore, its use is not recommended unless the animal has complete loss of voluntary motor function, as paretic animals have a good prognosis.

Current recommendations support the use of MPSS as the superior corticosteroid for spinal cord trauma rather than prednisolone or dexamethasone. MPSS is a hemisuccinate ester, which is converted to a sodium salt to make it more water-soluble. Hydrocortisone is much less active, or even ineffective, at doses of 120 mg/kg (Hall, 1985). The 1,2 double bond of prednisolone (which is lacking in hydrocortisone) appears to be a requirement for the anti-lipid peroxidation effect. There is also evidence that dexamethasone is not as effective as methylprednisolone for preventing lipid peroxidation (Hoerlein *et al.*, 1985). It is not recommended to increase the dose of dexamethasone to achieve the desired effect because this would likely increase the risk of adverse effects. Intestinal perforation has been reported from administration of high doses of dexamethasone for treating spinal cord trauma (see Adverse reactions from corticosteroids, later). However, the efficacy of MPSS is questioned and there is no current evidence that it is beneficial in the treatment of canine spinal cord injury (see Chapter 20).

Corticosteroid use for immunosuppression

Corticosteroids (glucocorticoids) are usually the primary drugs used to treat or manage immune-mediated disorders of the CNS, including corticosteroid-responsive meningitis and meningomyelitis (Tipold, 2000) characterized by inflammation of the CNS without evidence of infection. Even though prednisolone or prednisone have been administered to dogs as the primary treatment for meningoencephalomyelitis of unknown origin (MUO), treatment results have not been encouraging. Complete clinical remission for MUO is uncommon, survival time is short, and prognosis is poor (see Chapter 11). Most patients die or are euthanased within a few months of diagnosis due to disease progression (Muñana *et al.*, 1998). Therefore, other adjunctive medications are often added to treatment; these are discussed below. Clinical features and other aspects of management of corticosteroid-responsive meningitis and corticosteroid-responsive meningomyelitis are discussed in Chapters 11 and 14.

During immunosuppressive therapy, glucocorticoids exert their action by binding to intracellular receptors, translocating to the nucleus and binding to receptor sites that regulate gene expression (e.g. expression of cytokines and immune function) (Boumpas *et al.*, 1993). Glucocorticoids decrease neutrophil migration and egress into inflammatory tissue. This effect is attributed to suppressed expression of adhesion molecules, decreased adherence of granulocytes to the vessel endothelium and decreased diapedesis from the vessels. As a result, there is decreased movement of polymorphonuclear cells (PMNs) into the tissues in response to chemotactic stimuli. Glucocorticoids inhibit the normal functions of macrophages (including phagocytosis) inhibit the release of inflammatory cytokines from macrophages (e.g. IL-1, TNF-α and prostaglandins) and decrease expression of cytokines from lymphocytes (e.g. IL-2).

As reviewed by Cohn (1991) corticosteroids suppress the ability of macrophages to engulf cells and process antigens that are necessary to stimulate an immune response. Corticosteroids also profoundly affect lymphocytes. A complex series of interactions between antigens, macrophages, T-cells and cytokines is important for immune expression. Glucocorticosteroids appear to have the most effect on T lymphocytes. Therefore, effects can be seen from suppression of helper cells to cell-mediated immunity. Direct effects on antibody synthesis are not observed.

In clinical veterinary medicine the action of glucocorticoids is dose-dependent. The lowest doses (using prednisolone as an example) produce physiological effects (0.25 mg/kg/day); higher doses produce anti-inflammatory effects (1.0 mg/kg/day); and still higher doses are considered immunosuppressive (for dogs 2–4 mg/kg/day). High doses are used for immunosuppressive therapy of the CNS.

Clinical use
As illustrated in the list of doses above, for immune-mediated disorders, dosages of corticosteroids are higher than are necessary for anti-inflammatory therapy (by at least 2x). These doses are usually administered initially on an every-day basis; after remission of clinical signs, every-other-day administration is attempted in order to reduce adverse effects and other complications from corticosteroids. There is no evidence from a well controlled study in animals to show that one glucocorticoid is superior to another when comparing efficacy, nor is there any documentation to show that injectable therapy is more effective than oral treatment. The choice of corticosteroid becomes a practical one: dexamethasone sodium phosphate is the most common injectable formulation in veterinary hospitals, and prednisolone (or prednisone) tablets are the most common oral forms. For long-term therapy, intermediate-acting steroids (i.e. prednisolone) should be used to reduce adverse effects. During short-term treatment, dexamethasone can be used.

Initial (induction) dosage regimens employed are in the range of daily doses of 2.2–4.4 mg/kg (prednisolone). A commonly used immunosuppressive dose of prednisolone for dogs is 2 mg/kg orally q12h. During the initial induction period the daily dose can be divided into a twice-daily dose to lessen (but not eliminate) some of the acute effects, such as gastrointestinal problems or behavioural changes. After the induction treatment phase the dose interval can be extended to once daily for another period of time until it is determined that the animal's disease is stable. If this is possible, the long-term maintenance dose should be 0.5–1 mg/kg every other day. The optimal dose that balances adverse effects and clinical response should be determined by titration. Immune-mediated diseases can vary greatly with respect to the level of glucocorticoids necessary to control clinical signs. Maintenance doses of 0.5–1 mg/kg q48h are possible in some patients but higher doses or the addition of other drugs may be necessary in patients that are more refractory. Cats often require higher dosages, sometimes twice as much as dogs. Although prednisone and prednisolone are considered equivalent in dogs because of efficient conversion of prednisone to prednisolone, the conversion is not as efficient in cats and prednisolone should be used for oral treatment.

Adverse reactions from corticosteroids
The two adverse effects most likely to occur in humans from administration of corticosteroids (used to treat CNS trauma) are secondary infection (e.g. pneumonia) and gastrointestinal injury. An additional effect that may be important is the hyperglycaemic action of corticosteroids, which increase glucose concentrations in the CNS with secondary increases in lactic acid resulting in CNS injury. The clinical relevance of this latter effect in veterinary patients has not been established.

The gastrointestinal complications are the most serious consequence in animals (Toombs et al., 1980; Moore and Withrow, 1982; Hanson et al., 1997; Culbert et al., 1998; Rohrer et al., 1999a). The adverse effects associated with high doses of corticosteroids include vomiting, gastrointestinal bleeding, ulcers, perforating ulcers and diarrhoea. The proposed mechanisms involved in gastrointestinal injury from corticosteroids were reviewed by Toombs et al. (1986) and were also discussed in the papers by Neiger et al. (2000) and Rohrer et al. (1999a). These effects of corticosteroids are a result of a complex relationship between sympathetic–parasympathetic imbalance, increased gastric acid secretion, stress, decreased synthesis of mucosal protective mechanisms and gastrointestinal ischaemia. Although these complications can be serious, most can be managed clinically by veterinary surgeons who practice conservative use of corticosteroids. Despite their widespread use, neither omeprazole, misoprostol, gastric protectants (sucralfate) nor H2-receptor blockers (cimetidine, ranitidine, famotidine) appear to prevent gastrointestinal problems associated with corticosteroids when they are used in surgery or to treat CNS trauma in dogs (Hanson et al., 1997; Rohrer et al., 1999b; Neiger et al., 2000). This suggests that neither increased acid secretion nor inhibition of prostaglandin synthesis plays an important role in gastrointestinal injury from corticosteroids.

Other immunosuppressive drugs
Occasionally some anticancer agents, such as methotrexate, cyclophosphamide and cytarabine, are used for their immunosuppressive effects. The anticancer drugs will be discussed later.

Mycophenolate
Mycophenolate mofetil is an ester pro-drug that is rapidly converted to the active compound mycophenolic acid (MPA). T and B lymphocytes are critically dependent on de novo synthesis of purine nucleotides and MPA is a potent inhibitor of inosine monophosphate dehydrogenate (IMPDH),

an enzyme important for *de novo* synthesis of purines in lymphocytes. Therefore, it effectively suppresses lymphocyte proliferation and decreases antibody synthesis by B-cells.

Mycophenolate is usually used in combination with glucocorticoids and/or ciclosporin. Effective doses have not been established but have ranged from 10 to 20 mg/kg orally q12h. There are only a few clinical studies that have reported the use of mycophenolate in veterinary medicine for treatment of immune-mediated diseases. After early promising reports of treatment of myasthenia in a dog (Dewey *et al.*, 2000) and some experience with treating skin diseases (Byrne and Morris, 2001), a more extensive retrospective study was reported (Dewey *et al.*, 2010). In that study, 27 dogs with acquired myasthenia gravis were treated with either pyridostigmine or a combination of pyridostigmine plus mycophenolate. There was no significant benefit detected by the addition of mycophenolate to the therapy. However, in a report of intravenous treatment with mycophenolate to three dogs that were unresponsive to other drugs, there were signs of clinical remission within 48 hours (Abelson *et al.*, 2009). These authors advocated intravenous administration of mycophenolate to dogs with generalized myasthenia gravis refractory to other treatments. More discussion on treatment of myasthenia gravis is provided in Chapter 18.

According to pharmacokinetic studies with mycophenolate in dogs conducted by veterinary investigators, the elimination rate was rapid (half-life <1 hour), limiting its usefulness for continuous therapy. However, in the study by Lange *et al.* (2008) the half-life was longer, but variable. At 20 mg/kg, the median half-life was 2.9 hours. These authors found that at 10 or 20 mg/kg orally q12h in dogs, mycophenolate did not maintain adequate concentrations for immunosuppression and higher doses of 30 mg/kg produced adverse effects. Therefore, the authors recommended 20 mg/kg orally q8h daily for dogs. Adverse effects include nausea, vomiting and diarrhoea, which are dose-related.

Thiopurines

Thiopurines have been used as a first-line therapy or as an alternative to nitrogen mustard alkylating agents for the treatment of immune-mediated disease. The most common drug used for this purpose is azathioprine. It is metabolized in the liver to the active metabolite 6-mercaptopurine (6-MP). *In vitro* studies indicate that some metabolism may occur at target cells responsible for immune effects. Azathioprine interferes with the *de novo* synthesis of purine nucleotides that are important for lymphocyte proliferation. 6-MP inhibits T-cell function and helper cell effects on antibody synthesis, with little direct effect on B-cells. In humans it has been suggested that azathioprine is more effective for IgG-mediated disease, whereas cyclophosphamide is more effective for IgM-mediated disease. This theory has not been tested in veterinary patients.

Clinical use: In veterinary medicine, azathioprine has been used for immune-mediated anaemia, colitis, immune-mediated skin disease, acquired myasthenia gravis and other immune-mediated diseases, but published controlled studies proving efficacy for these diseases are lacking. Response for treating MUO has been encouraging. A retrospective case study (Wong *et al.*, 2010) found that of 40 dogs, 60% had a complete response and 40% had a partial response to a combination of azathioprine and prednisone.

Azathioprine is available as 50 mg tablets. A dose of 2 mg/kg orally q24h is the typical starting dose, which is switched to q48h after 2 weeks if there is a positive response. Long-term therapy is administered at a dose of 0.5–1.0 mg/kg every other day, with prednisolone administered on the alternate days. In veterinary medicine the lag period from treatment to therapeutic effect is probably shorter than the 2–8 months recognized in humans, and therapeutic benefits have been observed after only 3–5 weeks. In the only published report of treatment of acquired myasthenia gravis in dogs with azathioprine (Dewey et al., 1999), there was encouraging, but not absolute, evidence of a beneficial outcome. There were only 5 dogs in the report: 3 dogs responded quickly; 4 had a decline in acetylcholine receptor antibody concentrations associated with clinical improvement.

Because cats may be at risk of bone marrow suppression from administration of azathioprine, current recommended doses are as low as 0.3 mg/kg q24h or q48h; however, dose regimens of 6.25 mg (1/8 tablet) or 1–2.2 mg/kg every other day have been documented (Caciolo *et al.*, 1984; Beale *et al.*, 1992; Helton-Rhodes, 1995). Careful monitoring of CBC is recommended during treatment.

Adverse effects: Bone marrow suppression is a concern in all animals. Leucopenia and thrombocytopenia can be serious, and gastrointestinal toxicity and hepatotoxicity are also possible. Monitoring CBC periodically will provide the clinician with evidence of bone marrow suppression. Gastrointestinal effects, such as nausea and diarrhoea, may only be temporary and so may subside after several days of therapy. There has been association (though not well documented) between the administration of azathioprine plus prednisolone and the development of acute pancreatitis in dogs. It has been suggested that this effect is caused by azathioprine decreasing pancreatic secretion in animals.

Metabolism: After azathioprine is converted to 6-MP, it is further metabolized by three routes. One metabolic route is via xanthine oxidase to inactive metabolites. Allopurinol will decrease this route because it inhibits xanthine oxidase. Another metabolic route is via thiopurine methyltransferase (TPMT), which is responsible for the conversion of 6MP to non-toxic 6-MP nucleotides. In humans there is a genetic polymorphism that determines high or low levels of TPMT. Humans with low TPMT activity are more responsive to therapy but have a high incidence of toxicity (myelosuppression); humans with high levels of TPMT activity have a low incidence of toxicity but lower drug efficacy (Lennard *et al.*, 1989). Most of the human population has high TPMT activity but about 11% have low levels and are more prone to toxicity. In humans with low TPMT activity, the dose of azathioprine must be lowered.

It appears that in dogs TMPT levels are highly variable in the population (Kidd *et al.*, 2004). TPMT activity varied 9-fold in a population of 177 dogs (Kidd *et al.*, 2004). Another study with fewer dogs indicated that 90% showed normal TPMT activity and 10% had low levels (White *et al.*, 1998). Cats have low TPMT activity and are highly susceptible to adverse effects (Foster *et al.*, 2000). It is possible that variations in TPMT activity among animals could account for azathioprine drug toxicity. However, Rodriguez *et al.* (2004) found that variations in TPMT activity in dogs were not associated with susceptibility to azathioprine-induced myelotoxicity. Therefore, further evidence is needed to document the causes of this idiosyncratic toxicity in dogs. Animals that are treated with azathioprine should have their bone marrow function monitored during initial therapy to identify those that may have low TPMT activity so doses can be adjusted accordingly. If there is any evidence of hepatic injury (e.g. loss of appetite, abdominal discomfort, nausea) liver enzymes should be monitored to rule out drug-induced hepatotoxicity.

Ciclosporin

Ciclosporin is an immunosuppressive agent that also has anti-inflammatory properties. It is a fat-soluble cyclic polypeptide fungal product with immunosuppressive activity. It has been an important drug used in human medicine, used primarily to produce immunosuppression in organ transplant patients. In 2003 the veterinary formulation Atopica was introduced; this is the same formulation as Neoral (microemulsion) and absorption, kinetics and dissolution are the same but there are more capsule sizes available (10, 25, 50 and 100 mg). There are also human generic versions of ciclosporin.

Ciclosporin binds to a specific cellular receptor on calcineurin and inhibits the T-cell receptor-activated signal transduction pathway by suppressing nuclear factor of activated T-cells (NFAT). Particularly important are its effects to suppress IL-2 and other cytokines and block proliferation of activated T-lymphocytes. The action of ciclosporin is more specific for T-cells compared to B-cells. One important advantage in comparison to other immunosuppressive drugs is that it does not cause significant myelosuppression or suppress non-specific immunity. It also does not typically cause renal or hepatic toxicity.

Clinical use: The most common clinical use of ciclosporin is for the treatment of dermatological disorders but it is also used to treat neurological disease. Anecdotal case reports and clinical trials using ciclosporin to treat MUO in dogs have been reported (Adamo and O'Brien, 2004; Gnirs, 2006; Adamo *et al.*, 2007; Jung *et al.*, 2007; Behr *et al.*, 2009; Pakozdy *et al.*, 2009). The rationale for using ciclosporin is that the inflammation in the brains of these patients features infiltration of lymphocytes in perivascular lesions, suggesting T-cell-mediated delayed-type hypersensitivity (Kipar *et al.*, 1998). Pakazdy *et al.* (2009), Adamo *et al.* (2007) and Jung *et al.* (2007) documented a significantly greater survival time when ciclosporin was added to corticosteroid therapy. The addition of ciclosporin has also allowed for a greater reduction in the corticosteroid dose. Doses of ciclosporin used in these studies are in the range of 5–6 mg/kg per day, but are sometimes higher. Ciclosporin is not detected in the CSF of treated dogs (Adamo and O'Brien, 2004) but, as mentioned earlier, CSF drug concentrations should not be used to determine brain concentrations.

The pharmacokinetics of ciclosporin in treated animals has been examined (Steffan *et al.*, 2004). Ciclosporin is metabolized in the intestine and liver to several metabolites: 25–30 such metabolites have been identified. The pre-hepatic intestinal enzymes account for significant metabolism of ciclosporin (Wu *et al.*, 1995), and systemic absorption in dogs is only 20–30% (Myre *et al.*, 1991). The intestinal metabolism by cytochrome P-450 enzymes (CYP) and the efflux caused by intestinal P-gp account for most of the loss in systemic availability after oral administration. Drug enzyme inhibitors such as ketoconazole, diltiazem or the flavonoids in grapefruit juice can inhibit the pre-systemic metabolism and produce a profound increase in systemic availability of ciclosporin. For example, 5–10 mg/kg of ketoconazole daily can decrease the dose of ciclosporin because clearance is reduced by 85% (Myre *et al.*, 1991). In some clinical studies, ketoconazole has been added to increase blood concentrations of ciclosporin with a reduced dose (Adamo *et al.*, 2007).

Adverse effects and precautions: Ciclosporin can cause vomiting, diarrhoea, anorexia, secondary infections and gingival hyperplasia. It may increase the risk of CNS infections (Galgut *et al.*, 2010). Hyperplastic skin lesions have occasionally developed in dogs treated with ciclosporin. Papillomavirus can be detected in some skin lesions. Tremors or shaking have been observed in dogs that have received high doses. These events are rare and are not usually a problem as long as doses are kept within accepted limits.

Gastrointestinal problems are the most common clinical side effect in dogs (Steffan *et al.*, 2003, 2005, 2006). Vomiting, anorexia and diarrhoea have been reported. When anorexia and vomiting are reported, veterinary surgeons have tried various interventions, such as lowering the dose or administering the dose with some food. Feeding will reduce the amount of ciclosporin absorbed in dogs by 15–20%, but it is unlikely that this decrease will be severe enough to affect efficacy. Nephrotoxicity, once a problem with older forms, is rare with current formulations. Secondary malignancies are a possible complication to long-term therapy but have not been reported in dogs or cats.

In cats, the most common adverse effects are anorexia, vomiting and refusal to eat food if it is mixed with ciclosporin. Toxoplasmosis has been reported in cats treated with ciclosporin, presumably due to the immunosuppression.

Leflunomide

Leflunomide has been used for immunosuppression in patients that have become refractory to other agents, or that cannot tolerate other medications. After oral administration, leflunomide is rapidly metabolized to the active metabolite A77-1726 (teriflunomide). Two mechanisms of action have been described for the active metabolite (Bartlett *et al.*, 1991; Cherwinski *et al.*, 1995; Fox *et al.*, 1999; Xu *et al.*, 1997):

- An enzyme involved in pyrimidine synthesis (dihydroorotate dehydrogenase) is inhibited, thereby arresting lymphocyte activation and expansion
- Tyrosine kinases involved in cellular differentiation and signal transduction are inhibited.

Leflunomide has been used as an adjunctive therapy for dogs refractory to traditional immunosuppressive therapy and to prevent anti-allograft immune responses (McChesney *et al.*, 1994; Lirtzman *et al.*, 1996; Gregory *et al.*, 1998; Affolter and Moore, 2000; Jin *et al.*, 2002; Kyles *et al.*, 2003; Bianco and Hardy, 2009; Colopy *et al.*, 2010). Information on the use of leflunomide for treatment of CNS diseases is only anecdotal and there are no published reports to indicate that it is effective.

The optimum dose and interval are uncertain in dogs (no information is available for cats). Although doses ≤4 mg/kg/day have been used in dogs with no reported adverse effects, anaemia and anorexia have been observed at doses >4 mg/kg/day (McChesney *et al.*, 1994; Lirtzman *et al.*, 1996; Gregory *et al.*, 1998; Bianco and Hardy, 2009; Colopy *et al.*, 2010). Pharmacokinetic studies reported in humans show that the active metabolite A77-1726 has a very long half-life (7–10 days) (Li *et al.*, 2002; Rozman, 2002; Chan *et al.*, 2004; van Roon *et al.*, 2004), which allows for consistent and sustained steady-state concentrations from repeated administration. However, in a recent study in dogs (Singer *et al.*, 2011), the plasma half-life was much shorter than in humans. At a dose of 4 mg/kg orally, the half-life was only 21.3 hours (±1.9); therefore, it may be difficult to maintain concentrations of the active metabolite as high as in humans. The protein binding for teriflunomide was high (99%), as it is in humans. High protein binding may prevent high penetration across the BBB.

Conversion of lefluonomide to teriflunomide in the human liver is mediated by the hepatic cytochrome P450 enzymes CYP1A2 and CYP2C19 (Bohanec Grabar *et al.*, 2008). Perhaps differences in human and canine P450 metabolism could account for the differences in activation and elimination between these species. Alternatively, differences in gastrointestinal absorption or membrane transporters may affect drug absorption.

Anticancer chemotherapy of the nervous system

Although CNS cancer is common in companion animals, treatment of CNS tumours with chemotherapy is unusual in veterinary medicine. There is little information on treatment outcomes because there are no controlled studies in which anticancer treatments have been evaluated. Therapeutic protocols, such as those available for other forms of cancer (Kitchell and Dhaliwal, 1999), are not established for CNS tumours; there are just a few case reports and anecdotal experience. In a review paper on treatment of CNS tumours, only brief mention is made of specific anticancer drugs (Moore *et al.*, 1996). Some reports of treating CNS tumours in animals make no mention of specific anticancer agents (Kraus and McDonnell, 1996).

Much of the medical therapy of CNS tumours involves palliation to control secondary problems, such as seizures or inflammation. Most often, anticonvulsant drugs are used to control seizures (see Chapter 8) and anti-inflammatory drugs (corticosteroids) are used to control oedema and inflammation caused by the tumour.

One of the challenges of applying cancer chemotherapy to CNS tumours is that most of these drugs do not penetrate the BBB well enough to achieve effective concentrations in the tumour. For example, doxorubicin, a popular anticancer drug for lymphoma and other tumours, does not cross the BBB and is not useful for treating CNS cancer. Cisplatin, another important anticancer drug, is over 90% bound to plasma proteins and also does not cross the BBB. On the other hand, drugs that penetrate the BBB have a high potential for causing adverse neurological effects. The risk of adverse CNS effects is higher in dogs that have a deficiency of P-gp owing to a mutation in the *ABCB1* gene (Mealey *et al.*, 2003).

Alkylating agents

The major alkylating agents are the nitrogen mustards and the nitrosoureas. These drugs covalently alkylate various cellular constituents. Most importantly for cancer treatment, alkylation occurs between the bases of DNA molecules of rapidly dividing cancer cells. This reaction cross-links the bases of DNA, causing cessation of DNA synthesis and cell death. Alkylation of the DNA molecule also causes abnormal base pairing, misreading of the genetic code and excision of bases, which prevents DNA transcription and RNA synthesis.

These drugs are more active on growing cells in the cell cycle than on dormant cells. However, they can act at any point of the cell cycle and therefore are non-cycle-specific. They are most active when DNA is dividing, such as in the G1 and S phases. As a consequence, in addition to their effect on cancer cells, they will also affect rapidly growing normal cells such as bone marrow cells and gastrointestinal mucosa.

Nitrosoureas

The nitrosoureas have received the most attention for treating tumours of the brain, in particular gliomas. These drugs are more lipophilic and have small molecular weights and are therefore more capable of penetrating the BBB than are other anticancer drugs. Concentrations in CSF exceed the plasma concentration by a 3-fold margin. Two nitrosoureas commonly used are lomustine (also known as CCNU) and carmustine (also known as BCNU). A third nitrosourea, temozolomide, is administered as the standard of care for the treatment of human gliomas but there are no published reports of its use to treat gliomas in veterinary medicine as yet, due in part to its cost.

These drugs act as alkylating agents. Following oral absorption, they are metabolized spontaneously to alkylating and carbamoylating compounds. The binding occurs preferentially at the O-6 of guanine and results in bifunctional interstrand cross-linking, which is responsible for cytotoxicity. Because oral absorption is high, these drugs can be administered effectively as tablets rather than by injection.

Clinical use: Lomustine has been used more often than carmustine. It has been administered to small animals at doses of 70 mg/m^2 to 90 mg/m^2 orally q4wk. For brain tumours, protocols of 60–80 mg/m^2 orally q6–8wk have also been cited (Fulton and Steinberg, 1990). These protocols are quite different from those for humans, where a dose of as much as 150–200 mg/m^2 is recommended. While there are no published reports of temozolomide use in dogs or cats to treat CNS neoplasia, it has been used as a rescue therapy of canine lymphoma and was well tolerated at doses of up to 100 mg/m^2 q3wk (Dervisis *et al.*, 2007).

The other clinical use of lomustine is for treating granulomatous meningoencephalomyelitis and necrotizing encephalitis in dogs. The effect in both diseases is attributed to suppression of B and T lymphocytes. In a retrospective study, lomustine at a dose of 60 mg/m^2 orally q6wk, plus prednisolone, was compared to prednisolone treatment alone (Flegel *et al.*, 2011). Dogs with granulomatous meningoencephalomyelitis and necrotizing encephalitis had similar efficacy from both treatments, but dosages of prednisolone were reduced significantly in the group that also received lomustine.

Adverse effects: The adverse effects of lomustine are primarily attributable to bone marrow effects. In humans the time to nadir of bone marrow activity

can be as long as 4–6 weeks, with slow recovery rates. In dogs maximal bone marrow effects (leucopenia) are generally seen 6–7 days after dosing. The doses cited above have been used to minimize the bone marrow effects. At higher doses (e.g. 100 mg/m^2) myelosuppression has been reported. Thrombocytopenia as a cumulative effect has also been reported from lomustine administration (Heading *et al.*, 2011).

The other adverse effects from nitrosoureas in dogs are gastrointestinal toxicity and hepatotoxicosis. In one report 6.1% of 179 treated dogs developed hepatotoxicity (Kristal *et al.*, 2004). The doses administered were 50–110 mg/m^2, at a minimum of q3wk, which are higher than doses that have been used for meningoencephalitis. When used to treat canine lymphoma at higher doses than used for meningoencephalitis, lomustine produced myelosuppression in up to 29% of the dogs, gastrointestinal signs in up to 22% and liver enzyme increases in up to 86% (Williams *et al.*, 2006). Signs of hepatic injury may be delayed for several weeks and may be related to cumulative dose. The hepatic damage may be irreversible in dogs. In humans carmustine has been associated with a higher rate of hepatic injury than lomustine, but there are currently no reports of carmustine administration being used for treating tumours in dogs. In cats, lomustine has been used for treating tumours but there is no record of treatment for CNS tumours. Lomustine has been well tolerated at a dose of 30–60 mg/m^2 orally q3–6wk (approximately 10 mg/cat) (Fan *et al.*, 2002; Rassnick *et al.*, 2008). In cats, maximum bone marrow toxicity, which consists of neutropenia and thrombocytopenia, occurs at 2–4 weeks.

Cytarabine

Cytarabine is a compound isolated from a sea sponge; it has also been referred to as cytosine arabinoside and Ara-C. Cytarabine is metabolized to an active drug that inhibits DNA synthesis. It was once thought that its action was via inhibition of the enzyme DNA polymerase, but the exact mechanism of action may not be known. The most common use of cytarabine is for the treatment of lymphoma and myelogenous leukaemia. Cytarabine is one of the drugs used in combination chemotherapy by veterinary oncologists (COAP protocols; see the *BSAVA Manual of Canine and Feline Oncology*).

One of the uses of cytarabine in small animal neurology is for treatment of MUO. It is often administered in combination with corticosteroids (prednisone or prednisolone) for this disease (Zarfoss *et al.*, 2006; Menaut *et al.*, 2008; Behr *et al.*, 2009). Doses and routes of administration of cytarabine for treatment of MUO are not firmly established. Some protocols use subcutaneous administration of 50 mg/m^2 given four times over 2 days (200 mg/m^2 total dose), and others use continuous rate intravenous administration (CRI) at 25 mg/m^2 for 8 hours (200 mg/m^2 total dose). These regimens are repeated every 3 weeks (Nuhsbaum *et al.*, 2002). These doses are lower than those used in the treatment of neoplasia (400–600 mg/m^2 i.v. or s.c. over

48–96 hours). In a recent study, data showed that the CRI protocol delivered over 8 hours was superior to the subcutaneous protocol (50 mg/m² s.c.) for producing sustained plasma concentrations (Crook *et al.*, 2012). The half-life after a subcutaneous injection in dogs was only 1–2 hours after rapid absorption from the injection site. Sustained plasma concentrations at steady state, which can only be maintained with a constant rate infusion, are important for producing the best conditions for BBB penetration. Maintaining consistently high plasma concentrations to produce diffusion into the CNS appears unlikely from concentrations that peak quickly and decline rapidly, such as with a rapid intravenous bolus or subcutaneous injection. If adequate plasma concentrations are attained, cytarabine can diffuse into the CSF; in a study of healthy dogs, after administration of 600 mg/m² i.v. the CSF:plasma concentration ratio was 0.62 (±0.14) (Scott-Moncrieff *et al.*, 1991). It is not known how well the CSF drug concentration correlates with concentrations in brain tissue, but these levels may be high enough to treat some tumours of the CNS.

Cytarabine can markedly suppress bone marrow and can cause granulocytopenia. In addition it may cause nausea and vomiting.

Methotrexate

Methotrexate is considered an antimetabolite anticancer drug. It is primarily active in the S phase of the cell cycle. Like other antimetabolites, methotrexate interferes with the biochemical reactions necessary for proper cell function, regulation or division. The structure of methotrexate is similar to that of folic acid. Subsequently, methotrexate binds and inhibits the dihydrofolate reductase enzyme (DHFR). The DHFR enzyme is a reducing enzyme necessary for purine synthesis. The reduced form of folic acid (tetrahydrofolate, FH4) acts as an important coenzyme for biochemical reactions, particularly DNA, RNA and protein synthesis. Methotrexate is used in some combination chemotherapy protocols, mostly for lymphoreticular neoplasia and osteosarcoma.

The action of methotrexate on CNS tumours is limited because, like other antimetabolites, methotrexate is most effective when tumour cells are in the logarithmic phase of growth; many CNS tumours can be slow-growing. Penetration across the BBB is also a problem because folic acid analogues are polar molecules and cross the BBB poorly. In humans (data not available for dogs) the CSF drug concentrations are only 3% of the corresponding plasma concentration. Intrathecal administration has been used in humans as a last resort. Another approach used in humans is the systemic administration of very high doses of methotrexate (>1.5 g/m²) with the intent of achieving high enough concentrations in the CNS to be effective. This can be compared with the usual doses given to dogs, of 2.5 mg/m² q48h or 0.5–0.8 mg/kg every 7–14 days. At the doses administered for CNS tumours in humans, systemic toxicity is high and rescue therapy with calcium folinate (leukovorin) must be used. Leukovorin is used because it is an antagonist of the action of methotrexate on the DHFR enzyme and therefore decreases the risk of toxicity.

In humans methotrexate also has been used as an immunosuppressive agent to treat diseases such as rheumatoid arthritis, and as an abortifacient. Its major adverse effects in animals are anorexia, nausea, myelosuppression and vomiting.

Hydroxycarbamide

Hydroxycarbamide (also called hydroxyurea) is used to treat human meningiomas that are not amenable to surgery and its use has been adopted to treat canine menigiomas at a dose rate of 30 mg/kg orally three times a week (Tamora *et al.*, 2007). The benefit is the relative safety of the drug; however, there are no data on efficacy available at this time.

Adverse CNS reactions caused by drugs

Antibiotics

Antibiotics are probably the most common group of drugs administered to animals, so it is not surprising that this class is frequently associated with adverse reactions in the CNS. The antibiotics implicated include primarily the beta-lactams but also fluoroquinolones (e.g. enrofloxacin) and metronidazole. There is an excellent review of antibiotic-associated convulsions by Wallace (1997), which explains the mechanisms and incidence in humans. The mechanism by which penicillins, cephalosporins, carbapenems and fluoroquinolones induce seizures is to inhibit binding of GABA to the GABA$_A$ receptor (Chow *et al.*, 2004). GABA ordinarily acts as an inhibitory CNS neurotransmitter, increasing chloride conductance.

The most important predisposing factor for antibiotics to cause seizures is renal insufficiency (Chow *et al.*, 2004); this is best documented for the beta-lactams (penicillins, cephalosporins, carbapenems). The increased risk of seizures is either related to an increase in the ability of these drugs to cross the BBB, caused by uraemia or decreased protein binding, or simply because these drugs accumulate to high concentrations in renal failure because they are not effectively excreted by the kidneys. The latter mechanism is probably more likely. The resultant high plasma concentration increases BBB penetration; indeed brain tissue fluid penicillin levels were higher in uraemic animals than normal controls (Chow *et al.*, 2004). In a patient with renal failure the veterinary surgeon should observe animals for CNS toxicity after administration of any antibiotics, particularly beta-lactams. Dose intervals should be increased in accordance with the degree of compromised renal function. If CNS adverse effects are observed, the antibiotics should be discontinued or the dose interval increased.

Despite the low CNS concentrations of fluoroquinolone antimicrobials (enrofloxacin, difloxacin, orbifloxacin, marbofloxacin), one of the adverse effects is CNS toxicity. CNS adverse effects (including seizures) have been associated with either high doses or intravenous doses given rapidly. This effect has lead to a warning on package inserts to use this class of drug with caution in animals with CNS disease. In clinical practice adverse CNS effects have been rare when these drugs are used according to label instructions. These reactions are also known to occur with fluoroquinolones in humans, although other CNS disorders may be a predisposing factor (Wallace, 1997). To avoid reactions in animals, rapid intravenous injections of quinolones should be avoided in seizure-prone animals. (Only one quinolone, enrofloxacin, is registered in an injectable form for small animals in the USA; marbofloxacin is registered as an injectable in Europe.)

Ivermectin and related drugs

The adverse CNS effects of ivermectin, and similarly acting drugs such as moxidectin and milbemycin, are well documented in the veterinary literature (Lovell, 1990; Dorman, 1995). The avermectin and milbemycin classes of parasiticides are neurotoxic to parasites through potentiating their glutamate-gated chloride ion channels. Paralysis and death of the parasite is caused by increased permeability to chloride ions and hyperpolarization of nerve cells. These drugs also potentiate other chloride channels, including ones gated by GABA. Mammals are not usually affected because they lack glutamate-gated chloride channels and there is a lower affinity for other mammalian chloride channels. Because these drugs ordinarily do not penetrate the BBB, GABA-gated channels in the CNS of mammals are not affected. However, when these drugs are administered to certain canine breeds that permit them to cross the BBB, CNS toxicity results. Collies, Shetland Sheepdogs, English Sheepdogs, Australian Shepherd Dogs and perhaps other breeds have this susceptibility (Mealey and Meurs, 2008). It is now recognized that dogs susceptible to ivermectin toxicosis have a deficiency in the P-gp transmembrane efflux pump coded by the multidrug resistance (MDR) gene *ABCB1* (formerly called the *MDR1* gene). This protein is ordinarily present in the BBB to 'pump' drugs out of the CNS (Nelson *et al.*, 2003; Roulet *et al.*, 2003; Mealey, 2004, 2008; Martinez *et al.*, 2008). The adverse CNS effects of ivermectin are most likely caused by accumulation of the drug in the brain because P-gp, which would normally transport the drug out of the brain through the BBB, is deficient or inhibited. In mice deficient in expression of P-gp (CF-1 mice) the doses of ivermectin necessary to produce CNS toxicity are 100 times lower than doses that produce toxicity in other strains of mice (Lankas *et al.*, 1997).

Approximately 30–50% of collies are susceptible. Single doses of ivermectin >1000 µg/kg have been administered to other canine breeds but doses of 100–500 µg/kg administered to susceptible collies have produced toxicity. Intoxication in dogs and cats has also been the result of administering concentrated equine or bovine formulations at excessively high doses, or even following consumption of equine faeces. Most reactions have been observed

with ivermectin because it has been available for the longest time. However, reactions to other related drugs moxidectin and milbemycin also have been reported in dogs (Tranquilli *et al.*, 1991; Beal *et al.*, 1999; Mealey, 2008). Toxic effects from milbemycin at 20 times the recommended dose were shorter in duration than signs caused by ivermectin at 20 times the recommended dose (Tranquilli *et al.*, 1991).

Clinical signs in affected dogs include incoordination, ataxia, mydriasis, tremors, depression, behavioural changes, seizures (rare), blindness, coma and even death (Lovell, 1990). Reduced or absent cranial nerve reflexes have also been reported. In some dogs that have recovered, permanent behavioural changes have persisted. Many animals recover with supportive treatment but recovery may take up to 10 days or longer (60 days in one account) depending on the dose administered. There is no effective antidote for ivermectin-induced CNS adverse effects. Physostigmine, a cholinesterase inhibitor, has been used to alleviate some signs but it must be administered frequently (e.g. every 60–90 minutes) and is not recommended for routine treatment. Picrotoxin, a GABA antagonist, has also been used in isolated cases for treatment but is not recommended routinely because it can cause seizures.

Other substrates for P-glycoprotein

The consequences of a deletion mutation in the *MDR1* gene that codes for P-gp may extend to other groups of drugs (Mealey 2004; Martinez *et al.*, 2008). The antidiarrhoeal drug loperamide ordinarily does not cause CNS effects after oral administration because it does not cross the BBB (Sadeque *et al.*, 2000). However, it has been reported that collies are at a higher risk of CNS toxicity from loperamide (Hugnet *et al.*, 1996; Sartor *et al.*, 2004). An *ABCB1* deletion mutation in a collie was associated with toxicity from loperamide. Signs of toxicity included lethargy, rear limb weakness, disorientation and ataxia.

ABCB1 mutations or inhibition of BBB P-gp can also potentially lead to CNS toxicity from other drugs. Toxicity caused by anticancer chemotherapeutic agents in a dog was attributed to an *ABCB1* deletion mutation that led to increased penetration across the BBB (Mealey *et al.*, 2003).

Antihistamines can also be substrates for P-gp. First-generation antihistamines cause sedation and behavioural changes as unwanted side effects. First-generation drugs include chlorphenamine, diphenhydramine, clemastine and hydroxyzine. Some of the tricyclic antidepressant drugs, such as doxepin, produce some sedative effects through antihistamine action. The second-generation antihistamines are not associated with these effects, which explains their popularity in human medicine (Papich, 1999). Such second-generation drugs include terfenadine, fexofenadine, astemizole, loratadine and cetirizine. Terfenadine and astemizole are no longer marketed because of cardiovascular effects.

The first-generation drugs produce their sedative effects by binding to the H1 receptor, which is

Drug	Clinical use and comments	Recommended dose
Azathioprine	Used to treat immune-mediated diseases. Use cautiously and at much lower doses in cats	Dogs: 2 mg/kg orally q24h, followed by long-term therapy with 0.5–1.0 mg/kg orally q48h
Cefotaxime	Used for infections caused by *Enterobacteriaceae* that are resistant to other drugs and *Streptococcus* spp. Penetrates the CNS better than other cephalosporins	Dogs and cats: 30 mg/kg i.v., i.m. or s.c. q8h
Ceftazidime	Used for infections caused by *Enterobacteriaceae* or *Pseudomonas* spp. that are resistant to other drugs and *Streptococcus* spp. Penetrates the CNS better than other cephalosporins	Dogs and cats: 20–30 mg/kg i.v. q12h
Chloramphenicol	Used for some infections of the CNS. However, the activity against Gram-negative bacilli not good enough for treatment of infections caused by these bacteria	Dogs: 50 mg/kg orally q8h Cats: 50 mg/cat orally q8h
Clindamycin	Used to treat protozoal infections. However, efficacy has not been established	Dogs and cats: 11 mg/kg q12h or 22 mg/kg orally q24h
Cytarabine	Used to treat CNS lymphoma and MUO	Dogs and cats: 50 mg/m^2 s.c. q12h for 2 days. Repeat every 3 weeks
Dexamethasone sodium phosphate	Used to treat CNS oedema and inflammation	Dogs and cats: 0.15 mg/kg i.v. q6h for 2–4 days
Fluconazole	Used to treat fungal infections of the CNS	Dogs: 10–12 mg/kg orally q24h Cats: 50 mg/cat orally q12h or q24h
Itraconazole	Used to treat fungal infections of the CNS	Dogs and cats: 5–10 mg/kg orally q24h
Lomustine	Used to treat tumours of the CNS, particularly gliomas and MUO	Dogs and cats: 60–80 mg/m^2 orally q6–8wk
Meropenem	Used for infections of the CNS. Use for cases in which resistant bacteria may be suspected. Does not have the risk of CNS toxicity compared with imipenem	Dogs and cats: 5.5–11 mg/kg i.v. q12h
Methylprednisolone sodium succinate	Used to treat acute spinal cord trauma, though efficacy has not been demonstrated in dogs	Dogs and cats: <3h since injury: 30 mg/kg i.v. injection followed by 5.4 mg/kg/h CRI for 24 hours. If a CRI is not available then treat initially with 30 mg/kg i.v. within the first 8 hours of trauma, followed by 15 mg/kg i.v. at 2 and 6 hours after the initial injection. Thereafter 15 mg/kg i.v. q6h for 48 hours
Metronidazole	Treatment of CNS infections caused by *Bacteroides* (anaerobe). Caution that metronidazole can cause adverse CNS effects	Dogs and cats: 10–20 mg/kg orally q8h (most common is 15 mg/kg q12h)
Prednisolone	Used to treat inflammation of the CNS	Start with 2 mg/kg orally q12h. Gradually taper to lower doses until goal of 0.5 mg/kg orally q48h is achieved
Pyrimethamine	Treatment of protozoal infections of the CNS. Usually used in combination with sulfadiazine or other sulphonamide	Dogs and cats: 1 mg/kg orally q24h. Used with sulphonamide concurrently at a dose of 25 mg/kg orally q12–24h
Trimethoprim/ sulphonamide	Used to treat protozoal infections	Dogs and cats: 15–30 mg/kg orally q12h

23.2 Clinical use of drugs for CNS disorders in dogs and cats. CRI = constant-rate infusion.

associated with wakefulness. Second-generation drugs lack the CNS effects because of a difference in the ability of the drug to cross the BBB (Timmerman, 1999). Whether or not an antihistamine penetrates the CNS depends on its ionization, hydrogen-binding capacity and substrate affinity for P-gp. Some antihistamines enter the brain via a carrier-mediated system.

Summary

Figure 23.2 summarizes the drugs used to treat CNS disorders in dogs and cats.

References and further reading

Available on accompanying DVD

24

Radiation therapy of the nervous system

Amy Pruitt and Donald E. Thrall

With the common use of computed tomography (CT) and magnetic resonance imaging (MRI) for assessing brain and spinal cord disease, more informed decisions can be made regarding potential therapeutic interventions. Surgery has been, and will probably remain, the mainstay of cancer treatment methods in dogs and cats, especially as it can also serve as a diagnostic procedure. However, tumours affecting the brain and spinal cord are often invasive and, given the anatomical complexity of the affected areas, the critical functions performed by the tissues involved and the lack of intraoperative imaging in most facilities, the extent of surgical resection is limited and rarely allows tumour-free margins to be obtained. In addition, some intracranial masses are located in regions where surgical intervention is not feasible without great risk of secondary complications (e.g. on the floor of the cranial cavity). Thus, radiation therapy, either alone or in combination with surgery, is considered regularly for patients with brain or spinal cord neoplasia.

Prescribing a radiation dose

When radiation is administered to a tumour, an area of adjacent normal tissue is also irradiated. This is necessary because of the aim to include all peripheral margins of the tumour, including presumed microscopic extensions into normal tissue. It is the response of this adjacent normal tissue that limits the amount of radiation that can be administered. Radiation doses are selected based on the philosophy that treatment of the tumour must be aggressive; therefore, some finite but small (≤5%) probability of serious normal tissue complication is acceptable.

Once a radiation dose prescription has been decided upon, that dose is not given as one large exposure. Rather, it is divided into smaller doses called fractions that are administered, preferably on a daily basis (Monday to Friday), until the total prescribed dose has been delivered. Intuitively, the risk that serious central nervous system (CNS) complications will develop is directly related to the total dose of radiation. However, it is also affected by the size of each of the fractions, the volume of tissue irradiated and, to a much lesser extent, the overall time wherein the total dose is administered.

Radiobiology of the nervous system

The unique aspects of the neural tissues necessitate some basic understanding of neural tissue radiobiology by those considering radiation therapy for a CNS tumour. Normal tissues can be divided into two basic types based on their response to radiation:

- Acutely responding tissues
- Late responding tissues.

Acutely responding tissues

Tissues that divide regularly, such as skin and mucosa, are classified as acutely responding tissues. Complications that arise in regularly dividing tissues as a result of radiation therapy, such as desquamation or mucositis, occur during or shortly after treatment. Their development is directly related to the radiation dose intensity.

Radiation dose intensity is the amount of radiation administered per unit time. An increased radiation dose intensity can arise from the use of larger doses per fraction and/or decreasing the time between fractions. As the radiation dose intensity increases, the total dose necessary to produce an acute reaction decreases. The more intensely the radiation dose is delivered, the more likely that acute reactions will develop and the more severe they will be. Fortunately, complications that arise in dividing tissues are manageable with supportive and symptomatic therapy, and rarely limit administration of the prescribed radiation dose or compromise quality of life.

Late responding tissues

Tissues that do not divide regularly, such as bone, brain, spinal cord and peripheral nerve, are classified as late responding tissues. Complications that occur in late responding tissues as a result of radiation therapy, such as necrosis and demyelination, develop months to years following completion of radiation therapy. As late responding tissues are not dividing, or are dividing only very slowly, the development of complications is not related to the time over which treatment is given, but rather is associated with the size of each individual dose fraction, the volume of tissue irradiated and the total dose. The larger the size of each fraction, the lower the total dose required to produce serious complications. Therefore, the probability that late complications may develop can be reduced by using small fraction sizes.

Unfortunately, because of the critical functions performed by most late responding tissues, especially the neural tissues, complications are serious and always adversely affect quality of life. In addition, these complications are not treatable, thus their development should be avoided if at all possible. Contemporary radiation time–dose prescriptions are designed with a key objective being the avoidance of complications in late responding tissues.

Radiation effects on the nervous system

Three clinical reactions specific to the nervous system have been recognized based on the time taken for signs to develop (New, 2001). These are:

- Acute reactions
- Early delayed reactions
- Late delayed reactions.

Acute reactions: Acute reactions occur days to weeks after the initiation of treatment. Patients may experience fatigue and an increase in neurological signs. Acute CNS radiation injury is thought to be secondary to oedema and disruption of the blood–brain barrier (Wong and Van der Kogel, 2004).

Early delayed reactions: Early delayed reactions occur within 2–4 months of completion of radiation therapy. The underlying mechanism is believed to be transient demyelination, which can result in exacerbation of neurological signs. As demyelination is transient, spontaneous recovery occurs. Two specific early delayed reactions that occur in humans are somnolence syndrome and Lhermitte's sign.

- Somnolence syndrome describes periods of drowsiness, lethargy and loss of appetite following radiation therapy to the head.
- Lhermitte's sign is an electrical sensation that runs down the back and into the limbs upon flexion of the neck and can occur following irradiation of the spine.

As with more general types of early delayed reactions, these specific syndromes also typically last for a few months and are followed by complete clinical recovery (New, 2001). Neither of these syndromes has been reported in dogs.

Late delayed reactions: Late delayed radiation injury is the most clinically significant CNS complication of radiation therapy because it is irreversible and the clinical effects can be devastating. Late delayed injuries likely involve damage to both the capillary endothelial cells and oligodendrocytes, and may occur 6 months to years following radiation therapy (New, 2001).

Reported histopathological changes associated with late radiation-induced CNS injury include glial cell atrophy, demyelination and white matter necrosis, as well as varying degrees of vasculopathy in both the white and grey matter. Changes in the CNS microvessels associated with late radiation-induced injury include telangiectasias, dilatation, and vessel wall hyalinization and thickening with fibrinoid necrosis (Wong and Van der Kogel, 2004). Late radiation effects on the canine brain have also been evaluated and a correlation between CT/MRI and histopathological changes has been noted. The clinical consequences of these late effects often depend on the size and location of the histological lesions (Fike *et al.*, 1984, 1988; Benczik *et al.*, 2002).

Radiation time–dose considerations

It is typical in the radiation treatment of most types of human cancer for the prescribed dose to be given in 30–40 fractions of 1.8–2.0 Gy per fraction, for a total dose of 60–72 Gy. This fractionation scheme, which requires approximately 7 weeks of treatment, was developed empirically and the relatively small fraction size is beneficial in minimizing the probability of complications arising in critical late responding tissues. Compared with other non-proliferating tissues such as bone or muscle, the brain and spinal cord are more sensitive to the effects of the size of the dose per fraction. Therefore, the total dose, in addition to the fraction size, needs to be reduced in order to avoid serious brain and spinal cord complications, especially if large volumes of these tissues are irradiated.

Mathematical models that incorporate the total dose of radiation and fraction size at which injury occurs are used to predict a 5% and 50% probability of injury within 5 years (TD 5/5, TD 5/50). The TD 5/5 for the whole brain is approximately 45 Gy and for one-third of the volume is approximately 60 Gy. The TD 5/5 for the spinal cord is approximately 47–50 Gy, depending on the total volume irradiated. The TD 5/5 values assume fraction sizes of 1.8–2.0 Gy per day. In human radiation therapy, fraction sizes rarely exceed 2.0 Gy per day in patients with primary brain tumours (Emami *et al.*, 1991). If larger fraction sizes are used, the total dose needs to be reduced to avoid increasing the risk of late complications to the brain and spinal cord.

Unfortunately, such protracted fractionation schemes are less feasible in veterinary radiation practice due to:

- The requirement for anaesthesia for the administration of each radiation fraction
- Prolonged hospitalization for patients where outpatient treatment is not possible
- The associated cost to the pet owner.

As a result, daily fraction sizes are typically increased to reduce overall time and expense. This necessitates a reduction in the total dose to avoid increased complications in late responding normal tissues, especially the brain and spinal cord.

At North Carolina State University, a fractionation scheme comprising 19 fractions of 3.0 Gy each, given daily Monday to Friday, has been used for many years for the treatment of most malignant tumours outside the nervous system. This dose prescription results in occasional moderate to severe acute reactions such as mucositis and desquamation, particularly when large tissue volumes are irradiated, but serious complications in late responding tissues are extremely rare. However, given the serious consequences of complications arising in the brain and spinal cord, and the more limited overall radiation tolerance of these tissues, the total dose is reduced to 48 Gy divided into 16 fractions (rather than 19) when the brain or spinal cord are in the treatment field. This fractionation scheme has been well tolerated with very few documented instances of radiation-induced complications (Heidner *et al.*, 1991; Spugnini *et al.*, 2000).

Another approach to avoiding overly protracted radiation time–dose prescriptions is to use larger fraction sizes, in the 4.0–4.5 Gy range, given 3 times a week rather than 5 times. Although this reduces the total number of radiation fractions, the larger fraction size imposes further limitations on the total dose tolerable by the late responding normal tissues.

Finally, the tolerable total dose delivered by use of either 3.0 Gy or larger fractions is inadequate to control most macroscopic tumours affecting the brain or spinal cord. More sophisticated treatment methods involving conformal administration of radiation or combined therapies using surgery or other approaches such as biological modification are necessary before tumour control at these sites is optimized.

Reported studies

The following paragraphs summarize clinical reports describing results obtained from irradiation of various tumours affecting the brain or spinal cord. Reports dealing with very small numbers of patients have not been discussed because of the probability that observed responses may not be typical of the patient population at risk. In addition, care must be taken when interpreting results derived from retrospective studies because of the lack of organized follow-up and the non-randomized treatment assignment. Absolute survival information from trials involving small patient numbers, or retrospective studies, must be viewed with caution and all such trials should be considered as hypothesis-generating exercises rather than the final word with regard to counselling pet owners.

Brain tumours

Intracranial mass lesions
There is probably less known about the response of canine and feline brain tumours to radiation than any other type of tumour in veterinary oncology practice. This uncertainty has resulted from the failure to obtain a definitive histopathological diagnosis in all patients with brain masses undergoing radiation therapy, a lack of information on the natural course of the disease if untreated, and the difficulty in ascertaining whether recurrent neurological signs following irradiation are due to tumour recurrence, radiation neuropathy or intercurrent disease.

It seems ill advised to administer radiation therapy to patients with a brain mass when the definitive histopathological diagnosis is unknown. However, given the potential morbidity and cost associated with obtaining a definitive diagnosis prior to treatment, patients are sometimes irradiated without definitive evidence that the brain mass is neoplastic. Although certain tumours have relatively specific imaging characteristics, an accurate diagnosis of tumour type based on these features is not possible because of the similarity in imaging appearance of some tumours (Kraft *et al.*, 1997; Sturges *et al.*, 2008) (Figure 24.1).

It is common practice for owners to be given the option to have a brain biopsy performed, although some may refuse when the morbidity and cost of the procedure are compared with those associated

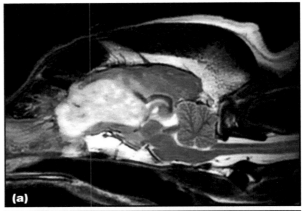

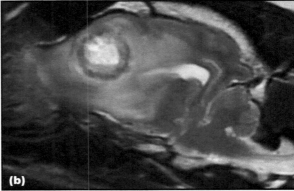

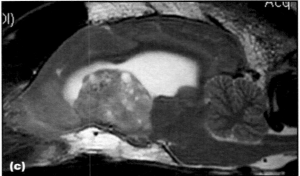

24.1 Sagittal T2-weighted MR images of three different brain tumours that have similar characteristics. The lesions are all reasonably well defined, isointense to hyperintense compared with the surrounding parenchyma, and mass like. **(a)** Grade 2 oligodendroglioma. **(b)** Meningioma. **(c)** Choroid plexus papilloma. (Courtesy of S Platt)

with radiation therapy. Stereotactic CT-guided biopsy frames have been adapted for veterinary use (Koblik *et al.*, 1999; Flegel *et al.*, 2002; Giroux *et al.*, 2002; Troxel and Vite, 2008) (see Chapter 6) and it is likely that as their use becomes more widespread, a higher proportion of patients with a brain mass will undergo a biopsy prior to treatment. However, caution should be exercised when basing the diagnosis of a brain mass on a sample obtained by needle aspiration. Fine-needle aspiration can be used to determine the presence of neoplasia in the brain, but it is not as definitive as Tru-cut biopsy for determining the specific tumour type (Platt *et al.*, 2002). A biopsy smear technique using a stereotactic frame is useful for the rapid accurate intraoperative diagnosis of many primary nervous system tumours (Vernau *et al.*, 2001). At this time, however, inclusion of patients without a definitive diagnosis in reports of treatment efficacy diminishes the ability to use response information to counsel owners.

Comparing therapies: Survival was analysed in 86 dogs with an intracranial mass treated with a variety of modalities, including surgery, cobalt irradiation, chemotherapy and hyperthermia, alone and in combination, as well as supportive care alone (Heidner *et al.*, 1991). Dogs undergoing radiation usually received 3.8 or 4.0 Gy fractions and a total dose of 46–48 Gy. Of the 86 dogs, 69 had histological confirmation of tumour type and 17 had CT evidence compatible with a tumour.

Factors associated with a more favourable outcome were: use of radiation *versus* surgery or supportive treatment; single *versus* multifocal brain lesions; mild initial neurological impairment; and meningioma *versus* other tumour types. Results of this study suggest that:

- Radiation may be of value for the treatment of intracranial tumours
- Initial clinical severity and number of brain regions involved are related to outcome
- Meningiomas may respond more favourably than tumours of the neuropil.

Radiation alone: Results from 29 dogs with intracranial signs and imaging findings suggestive of a tumour and irradiated with cobalt photons have been reported. Of these, 28 dogs received the same radiation time–dose prescription of 48 Gy divided into 3.0 Gy fractions, without surgery (Spugnini *et al.*, 2000). Although follow-up was sporadic, the median survival time was 250 days (range: 21–804); 22 dogs (76%) died with progressive neurological signs but it was not determined whether these were due to tumour progression or radiation necrosis. Based on the median survival time, the results of this study suggest a limitation of radiation alone for the treatment of gross intracranial tumours. The results also illustrate the problem of determining whether relapse following irradiation is due to tumour recurrence or radiation effects, unless a post-mortem examination is conducted.

In a retrospective study, 46 dogs with intracranial signs and imaging findings suggestive of a tumour were treated with radiation therapy alone (Bley *et al.*, 2005). The mean total dose of radiation was 40.9 Gy (range: 35–52.5 Gy) divided into 2.5–4 Gy fractions (mean 3.2 Gy). The median survival time was 699 days. Favourable prognostic factors (e.g. tumour size, tumour location and neurological signs) were not identified at presentation.

Hypofractionated radiation: Results from irradiation of intracranial masses in dogs using a hypofractionated fractionation scheme have been published (Brearley *et al.*, 1999). Dogs were treated once weekly and the total dose was 38 Gy. Although fraction size varied between dogs, the mean fractional dose was approximately 7.5 Gy. Results from a study evaluating postoperative radiation therapy in 17 dogs with meningiomas treated with a similar protocol have also been reported (Platt *et al.*, 2006). As mentioned above, the CNS is sensitive to such large doses of radiation per fraction. Using an accepted isoeffect formula (Withers *et al.*, 1983), a total dose of 38 Gy administered in 7.5 Gy fractions is biologically equivalent to approximately 90 Gy given in 2.0 Gy fractions. The probability of brain necrosis resulting from a dose of 90 Gy administered in 2.0 Gy fractions is nearly 100%. Interestingly, the median survival time was 44 weeks (range: 0.1–72 weeks) and 62 weeks (range: 12–185 weeks), respectively, for these retrospective studies. However, caution must be exercised when administering this coarsely fractionated protocol to patients in a definitive setting as the probability of serious complications is high.

Randomized trial: The only randomized trial of radiation therapy for canine intracranial masses was reported in 1999 (Thrall *et al.*, 1999). It involved evaluation of increased tumour temperature (hyperthermia) combined with irradiation as a means to enhance tumour response. A total of 45 dogs with neurological signs and imaging findings consistent with an intracranial tumour were studied. One advantage of this study was the rigorous follow-up imaging assessment of the response of the tumour to treatment. The radiation dose ranged from 44–60 Gy, given in daily 2.0 Gy fractions. Of the dogs, 24 had a meningioma and 5 had a glioma. The remaining 16 dogs were either alive at the end of the study (7), had other tumour types (4), had no tumour at necropsy examination (3) or did not have a necropsy examination (2).

Hyperthermia was ineffective at prolonging survival times. The 1-year and 2-year survival probabilities (reflecting the response to radiation therapy alone) were approximately 0.42 and 0.27, respectively. The overall median survival time was approximately 200 days. Thus, this study supports the suggestion that the mean survival time following irradiation of an intracranial mass in dogs is approximately 200 days. The range of radiation doses used and the toxicity associated with the hyperthermia procedure complicate interpretation of the results. Interestingly, in a Phase III trial of radiation and hyperthermia for the treatment of gliomas in humans, hyperthermia was shown to result in a statistically significant improvement in survival time when combined with radiation therapy compared with radiation therapy alone (Sneed *et al.*, 1998). Nevertheless, the radiation response of glioblastoma multiforme in humans remains one of the most dismal of all tumour types.

Meningiomas

As meningiomas are often located peripherally, surgical removal is more frequently attempted for this type of tumour than any other intracranial lesion.

Surgery alone: Long-term survival following surgical resection of meningioma has been documented in cats (Gordon *et al.*, 1994). In this study of 42 cats, although immediate perioperative mortality was relatively high (8 cats) and a further 10 cats had an unimproved or a worsened neurological status, overall survival was 71% at 6 months, 66% at 1 year and 50% at 2 years post-surgery.

In another study, 11 of 17 cats did not develop evidence of tumour recurrence within 18–47 months following surgery (median: 27 months) (Gallagher *et al.*, 1993). Thus, surgery alone may be curative in some cats with meningiomas; however repeated imaging studies are recommended to assess the margins of the excision because cats with residual macroscopic tumours would theoretically benefit from postoperative irradiation.

Long-term survival times have been reported for 33 dogs with meningiomas that underwent endoscopic-assisted surgical tumour removal (Klopp and Rao, 2009). These dogs had an unusually long median survival time of 2104 days for forebrain meningiomas and 702 days for caudal meningiomas. This approach appears to improve the ability of the surgeon to completely resect the tumour and has the potential to improve surgical outcomes in the future.

Postoperative irradiation: With regard to canine meningiomas, one study suggests that use of postoperative irradiation significantly improves survival times (Axlund *et al.*, 2002). Of a total of 26 dogs, 14 dogs were treated surgically and 12 dogs were treated surgically followed by postoperative irradiation. The mean survival times were 7.0 and 16.5 months, respectively (Figure 24.2). Irradiated dogs received a total radiation dose of 40–49.5 Gy, but the fraction size was not specified and post-mortem information on brain necrosis was not available. It is not clear how the decision was made with regard to which patients received postoperative irradiation and this non-random assignment of treatment may have biased the population of patients in each group and thus affected the survival times. Nevertheless, these results support the use of postoperative irradiation in dogs undergoing meningioma resection. What is not known with certainty is the median survival time of dogs with meningioma treated with radiation alone; this would aid in evaluating the need for surgical removal of a portion of the tumour.

Immunohistochemistry: There is great interest in assessing the microenvironmental characteristics of tumours to identify factors that may be used to counsel owners more accurately, or to identify tumours suitable for antineoplastic interventions. Tumour proliferation is one factor that has been studied in an attempt to identify tumours that may be at higher risk of treatment failure due to rapid tumour cell proliferation.

Using immunohistochemical detection of proliferating cell nuclear antigen (PCNA), an endo-

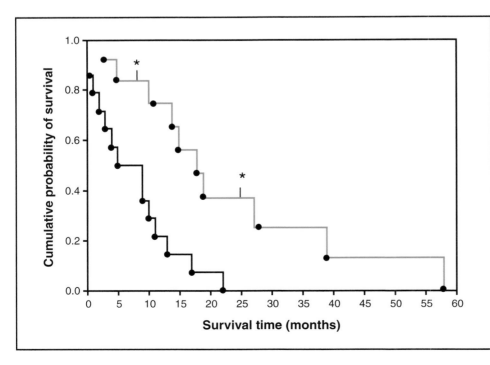

24.2 Cumulative probability of survival as a function of time after treatment for canine meningioma treated with surgery alone (black line) or surgery followed by irradiation (blue line). Median survival times are 7.0 and 16.5 months, respectively, suggesting a role for postoperative irradiation in canine meningioma patients. ★ = censored data point. (Reproduced from Axlund *et al.* (2002) with permission from the *Journal of the American Veterinary Medical Association*)

genous marker of tumour cell proliferation, one study demonstrated that dogs with rapidly proliferating meningiomas had significantly shorter progression-free survival (PFS) compared with dogs that had slowly proliferating tumours (Theon *et al.*, 2000). A total of 20 dogs received postoperative irradiation following meningioma resection. The overall median PFS was 30 months. After separating the dogs based on the median PCNA labelling fraction, the median PFS in dogs with rapidly proliferating tumours was approximately 20 months compared with >50 months in dogs with slowly proliferating tumours (Figure 24.3).

Another factor that may be associated with an increased risk of treatment failure is tumour angiogenesis. Shorter survival times have been associated with the expression of vascular endothelial growth factor (VEGF) in canine intracranial meningiomas (Platt *et al.*, 2006). Thus, assessment of PCNA labelling and VEGF expression in resected meningioma specimens is useful for owner counselling as well as the identification of dogs at higher risk of early treatment failure. These high risk dogs can then be considered for other more aggressive therapies, such as a higher radiation dose, accelerated administration of the radiation dose or combined radiation and chemotherapy.

Pituitary gland tumours

More detailed information is known about the response of canine pituitary macrotumours (masses >1 cm in diameter) to radiation than for all other types of intracranial mass. The anatomical location of pituitary gland tumours makes complete excision extremely difficult (Lantz *et al.*, 1988); thus, there is a clear indication for irradiation.

A highly informative description of factors associated with a favourable outcome following irradiation of pituitary macroadenomas has been published (Theon and Feldman, 1998). A total of 24 dogs with a pituitary macrotumour and associated neurological signs were studied. All dogs received the same radiation time–dose prescription of 48 Gy, given in 4.0 Gy fractions 3 times a week. There were significant positive associations between relative tumour size and both endogenous plasma adrenocorticotropic hormone (ACTH) concentration and the severity of the neurological signs. Overall median PFS was 13.1 months (± 8.3 months). Dogs with larger tumours (Figure 24.4) and endocrinologically inactive tumours (Figure 24.5) had shorter survival times than dogs with small or active tumours. These results support the use of irradiation in dogs with pituitary macrotumours.

Dogs with small and/or endocrinologically active tumours are likely to respond best to treatment. More aggressive therapy (such as a higher dose of radiation or conformal radiation techniques) should be considered for dogs with large and/or endocrinologically inactive tumours. The radiation time–dose prescription used in this study was suboptimal because of the large fraction size (which predisposes to radionecrosis) and the thrice-weekly fraction administration (which allows tumour repopulation during treatment). Significant radiation associated changes in normal brain tissue were found in a number of dogs from this study, especially those with large tumours necessitating large radiation fields.

Results from a study using a more finely fractionated protocol and comparing survival and prognostic factors in dogs with pituitary gland masses treated with radiation therapy and untreated dogs have been

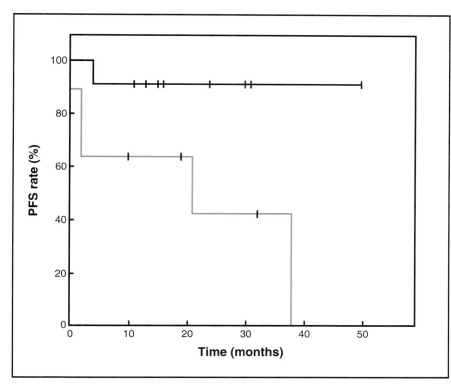

24.3 Progression-free survival (PFS) as a function of time after treatment for canine meningioma based on the proliferative capacity of the tumour. Survival times of dogs with rapidly proliferating tumours (blue line) are shorter than those of dogs with slowly proliferating tumours (black line). Proliferative capacity was based on immunohistochemical quantification of PCNA. (Reproduced from Theon *et al.* (2000) with permission from the *Journal of the American Veterinary Medical Association*)

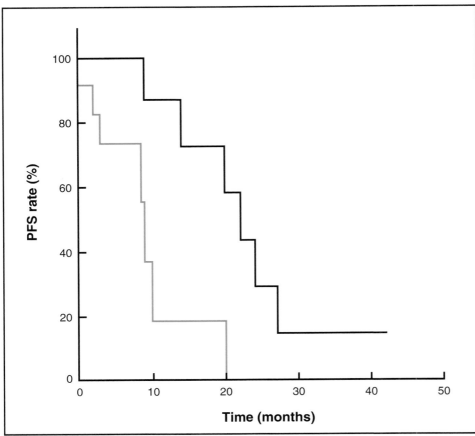

24.4 Progression-free survival (PFS) as a function of time after irradiation of canine pituitary macrotumours. Survival times are shorter in dogs with large tumours (blue line) than in dogs with small tumours (black line). Tumour size was characterized as relative tumour size, defined as the largest tumour area visible on CT or MRI, divided by the area of the cranial cavity at that level. (Reproduced from Theon and Feldman (1998) with permission from the *Journal of the American Veterinary Medical Association*)

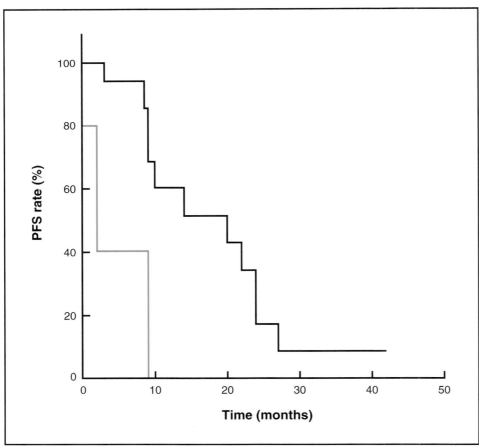

24.5 Progression-free survival (PFS) as a function of time after irradiation of canine pituitary macrotumours. Survival times are shorter in dogs with endocrinologically inactive tumours (blue line) than in dogs with active tumours (black line). (Reproduced from Theon and Feldman (1998) with permission from the *Journal of the American Veterinary Medical Association*)

published (Kent *et al.*, 2007). Of the 46 dogs studied, 19 were treated with radiation therapy and 27 were untreated control animals. All treated dogs received a total radiation dose of 48 Gy in daily (Monday to Friday) 3 Gy fractions. Dogs that received radiation therapy had significantly longer survival times than the untreated dogs (Figure 24.6). Median survival time was not reached in the treated group, but was >2000 days (mean survival time was 1405 days). The median survival time in the untreated group was 359 days (mean survival time was 551 days). As in the study by Theon and Feldman (1998), treated dogs with relatively smaller sized tumours lived longer than those animals with larger tumours.

The efficacy of lower doses of radiotherapy for the treatment of pituitary macroadenomas has also been evaluated (de Fornel *et al.*, 2007). A total of 12 dogs with pituitary gland tumours were treated with a radiation dose of 36 Gy given in 12 fractions of 3 Gy each over 4–6 weeks. Post-treatment CT images revealed a decrease in tumour size in 11 of the dogs, with a >50% reduction noted in 6 dogs. The median survival time was 17.7 months and 3 dogs were reirradiated with 18–27 Gy.

Occasionally, pituitary irradiation is considered for treatment of patients with macroadenomas and pituitary gland hyperfunction but without associated neurological dysfunction. In one study, six dogs with pituitary-dependent hyperadrenocorticism and a detectable pituitary mass, but no evidence of mass-associated neurological dysfunction, were treated using irradiation (Goossens *et al.*, 1998a). Each dog received a total dose of 44 Gy given in 11 fractions of 4.0 Gy each 3 times a week. The plasma ACTH concentration was measured before and at regular intervals after completion of radiation therapy. Imaging studies were repeated 1 year following irradiation. Radiotherapy did not result in adequate control of the clinical signs associated with hyperadrenocorticism in 5 dogs, but the size of the pituitary tumours had dramatically reduced. However, in a more recent study there was a slight improvement in the number of patients (5 of 14 dogs) in which clinical signs related to hyperadrenocorticism resolved following radiation therapy (Kent *et al.*, 2007). Thus, pituitary irradiation in dogs with macroadenomas and pituitary gland dysfunction, but not neurological deficits, may be useful in preventing the development of signs but is only effective in normalizing the endocrinopathy in a small percentage of dogs.

The results of irradiation of a pituitary gland tumour in 3 acromegalic cats have been reported (Goossens *et al.*, 1998b). The cats received a total radiation dose of 48 Gy given in 12 fractions of 4.0 Gy each 3 times a week. In 2 cats, growth hormone levels decreased slowly; in the third cat, no decrease was observed. The successful treatment of a further 5 cats using the same radiation protocol has also been reported (Kaser-Hotz *et al.*, 2002a). Two retrospective studies describing the treatment of cats with pituitary gland tumours have been published. In the first study, 12 cats (4 cats with neurological signs and 8 cats with insulin-resistant diabetes mellitus alone) received a total radiation dose of 37 Gy given in 7.4 Gy fractions once a week (Brearley *et al.*, 2006). Of the 4 cats with neurological signs, 3 improved. Of the 8 cats with diabetes mellitus, 5 no longer required insulin, 1 required a lower dose of insulin and 2 were considered stabilized. In the second study, 8 cats were treated with a total radiation dose of 45–54 Gy given in fractions of 2.7–3 Gy (Mayer *et al.*, 2006). The median survival time, regardless of the cause of death, was 17.4 months. Neurological signs (circling, head pressing, dullness and behavioural changes), in the 5 cats affected, improved within 2 months. Hyperadrenocorticism and acromegaly, in the 7 cats affected, improved within 1–5 months.

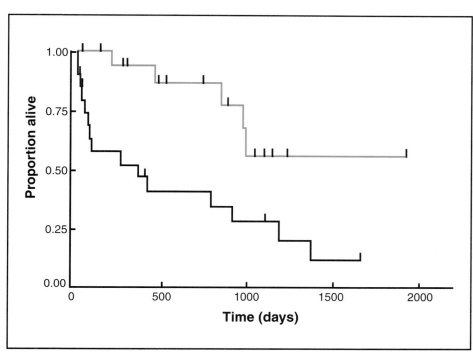

24.6 Survival times of dogs with pituitary masses treated with either radiation therapy (blue line) or left untreated (black line). Radiation treatment was given to 19 dogs and 27 dogs received no treatment. The lines are significantly different (log-rank test: P5 .0039). Censored dogs are indicated by vertical marks. (Reproduced from Kent *et al.* (2007) with permission from the *Journal of Veterinary Internal Medicine*)

Radiosurgery as treatment for pituitary tumours has been evaluated in 11 cats (Sellon *et al.*, 2009). Radiosurgery was performed by delivering a single large dose of radiation (15 or 20 Gy) whilst arcing a beam from a linear accelerator around the centre of the tumour mass. Of the 11 cats, 8 were treated once, 2 were treated twice and 1 was treated three times. Presenting clinical signs included poorly regulated diabetes mellitus (7 cats) and neurological signs, including abnormal behaviour and vision deficits (2 cats). Improvement in the clinical signs was noted in 7 of the 11 cats following treatment. The median survival time was 25 months. Thus, pituitary radiation may be effective at decreasing hyperfunction in some cats; and if there is improvement in the underlying endocrinopathy, the survival time following radiosurgery may be in the order of months to years.

Lymphoreticular tumours

There is essentially no information on the outcome of brain lymphomas treated with radiation. In general, lymphoid tumours are very responsive and irradiation of a solitary brain lymphoid mass is expected to be associated with a favourable outcome. In animals, it is not known whether it is beneficial to combine radiation therapy with chemotherapy for patients with brain lymphoma, but in humans a survival advantage has been reported from such an integrated approach (Ferreri *et al.*, 2002).

Although not technically a neoplastic process, granulomatous meningoencephalitis (GME) may result in lesions in the brain and/or spinal cord that are poorly responsive to chemotherapy and not amenable to surgery. Prognostic factors in 42 dogs with GME have been reviewed (Muñana and Luttgen, 1998). Signalment, clinical signs, cerebrospinal fluid (CSF) derangements, treatment and survival times were reviewed to identify factors associated with prolonged survival. A significant positive difference in survival time was demonstrated for focal versus multifocal clinical signs, neurolocalization of focal signs to the forebrain, and treatment with radiation. Although only 7 of the 42 dogs received radiation therapy, it was the only independent predictor of survival.

Spinal cord tumours

The spinal cord can be affected by primary neural tumours, tumours of the nerve roots, and primary or secondary tumours of the paraspinal structures. Little is known about the response of primary spinal cord tumours to irradiation. Reticuloendothelial tumours of the vertebral canal, such as lymphosarcoma, would be expected to be responsive to irradiation, but there is limited specific information available.

The results of postoperative irradiation of 9 dogs with tumours affecting the spinal cord have been reported (Siegel *et al.*, 1996). Of the 9 dogs, 1 had an intramedullary tumour and the other 8 dogs had either extramedullary or intradural–extramedullary tumours, which were most likely nerve root tumours. Surgical excision of the tumours had been performed on all dogs and all excisions were considered incomplete. Median survival time was 17 months (range: 12–70 months). The results of surgery with or without radiation therapy for the treatment of canine intraspinal meningiomas have also been reported (Peterson *et al.*, 2008). In this retrospective study, 10 dogs had surgery alone and 7 dogs had surgery followed by radiation therapy. The results of this study suggest that dogs with intraspinal meningiomas treated with postoperative radiation therapy had longer survival times (18–78 months). Thus, postoperative irradiation of incompletely resected nerve root tumours and meningiomas may result in a satisfactory outcome, but further studies are required to more precisely characterize the median survival time.

Results for the treatment of canine spinal nephroblastoma (thoracolumbar spinal tumour of young dogs) have recently been published (Brewer *et al.*, 2011; Liebel *et al.*, 2011). In one report, 11 dogs with canine spinal nephroblastoma were evaluated (Brewer *et al.*, 2011). Of the 11 dogs, 6 underwent surgery and 1 was treated with surgery, definitive radiation therapy and polyethylene glycol. The median survival time for the treated dogs was 70.5 days (range: 2–976). The dog treated with radiation therapy and polyethylene glycol in addition to surgery had no clinical evidence of disease >2.5 years post-therapy, suggesting that survival times may be improved with the use of radiation and/or polyethylene glycol. In another study, dogs treated with surgery (n=6) or radiotherapy (n=1) survived longer (median: 374 days) than dogs treated palliatively with prednisolone and pain medication (n=3; median: 55 days) (Liebel *et al.*, 2011). The results suggest that surgery and radiotherapy are effective at improving survival times in dogs with canine spinal nephroblastoma.

There is very little information on the radiation response of paraspinal tumours. The results following treatment of vertebral tumours in 20 dogs have been reported (Dernell *et al.*, 2000). Of the 20 dogs, 14 had osteosarcomas and 6 had fibrosarcomas (confirmed on histopathology). The tumours were treated with a variety of modalities: surgery alone (n=4), surgery and chemotherapy (n=2), radiation therapy and chemotherapy (n=6) and surgery, radiation and chemotherapy (n=8). The overall median survival time was 135 days (range: 15–600 days). Macroscopic paraspinal mesenchymal tumours (e.g. vertebral body oesteosarcomas) are unlikely to be controlled permanently by irradiation. Macroscopic solitary paraspinal reticuloendothelial tumours (e.g. vertebral body plasma cell tumours) have a much better prognosis and, if pathological vertebral fractures can be avoided, the chance for long-term remission is likely to be high.

Palliative irradiation

When permanent control of a primary tumour is unlikely but some temporary relief of clinical signs is desired, palliative irradiation may be useful. Palliative irradiation involves administration of a small number of radiation fractions with the sole intent being temporary resolution of clinical signs associated with pain or dysfunction, not prolongation of life (Thrall and LaRue, 1995).

In veterinary medicine, palliative radiotherapy was initially used for the treatment of osteosarcomas (Ramirez *et al.*, 1999) but it is now widely used for the treatment of non-resectable soft tissue tumours (Siegel and Cronin, 1997; Lawrence *et al.*, 2008; Buchholz *et al.*, 2009). Although there are no specific reports of the use of palliative radiation for CNS tumours, there is no reason why it should not be of value. Typically, palliative radiotherapy employs larger doses per fraction (often in the 4.0–10 Gy range). Although these large fractions are much more likely to result in brain necrosis or myelopathy, this is of less concern given the limited life expectancy of patients receiving radiation in a palliative setting. However, should unexpected long-term remission be encountered, it must be borne in mind that the patient is at higher risk of developing complications related to the irradiation, and retreatment becomes more risky.

There are many radiation time–dose prescriptions used for palliation, but these are not reviewed here. However, some prescriptions are designed to allow the course of palliation to be repeated should an initial favourable response be obtained but the clinical signs recur due to tumour relapse. Although this approach is suitable for tumours not involving the CNS, it is not clear whether repeat palliative radiotherapy of CNS lesions is feasible. It depends on the time–dose prescription used. However, recent reports suggest that retreatment may be more feasible than once thought. Using a formula for calculating the biologically effective dose (BED) of a radiation treatment protocol, different fractionation regimes can be compared (Hall and Giaccia, 2006). The results from two randomized trials evaluating reirradiation of human metastatic spinal cord lesions have been reported (Maranzano *et al.*, 2011). Myelopathy was not recorded. The reirradiation was given at different doses and fraction sizes with the cumulative BED in all cases ≤120 Gy2. A retrospective review of published clinical data suggests (with caution) that the risk of myelopathy appears small after a cumulative BED ≤135.5 Gy2 when the interval between treatment courses is not shorter than 6 months and the dose of each course has a BED ≤98 Gy2 (Nieder *et al.*, 2005).

Future directions

Technically, most brain masses are irradiated with two parallel opposed fields or four-field orthogonal arrangements. This results in a cuboidal volume of tissue receiving a relatively homogeneous dose. Although adequate in principle, the volume of normal brain tissue commonly included in the high-dose region limits the dose of radiation that can be given to the tumour. However, various technologies have been developed that allow a more conformal delivery of the radiation dose, providing (in principle)

a method to increase the dose to the tumour whilst decreasing the dose to the normal brain tissue.

Stereotactic dosing

The results of treatment of 3 canine brain tumours using radiosurgery and a stereotactic frame have been reported (Lester *et al.*, 2001). Radiosurgery involves the administration of a single relatively large dose of radiation (10–15 Gy) to the tumour in a highly conformal manner. A stereotactic frame is attached to the patient and the coordinates of the frame and visible tumour are recorded in three-dimensional (3D) space using CT. The multiple non-coplanar beams of radiation are then focused on the target using the image based computer system. The radiation source rotates in an arc around the tumour, with multiple non-coplanar arcs used for each isocentre. This results in a highly conformal distribution of the radiation dose to the tumour and a substantial reduction in the dose delivered to the adjacent normal brain tissue. The 3 dogs survived for a period of time comparable with reports of dogs with intracranial masses treated with conventional radiation techniques. One major advantage of this technique (other than the reduced radiation dose to the normal brain tissue) is that only one treatment is given and therefore anaesthesia is required only once. However, the technique is labour- and time-intensive, requiring sophisticated technology and high-level physics support. In addition, cross-sectional imaging is relied upon to precisely delineate the tumour margins and the accuracy of such determinations is still being debated.

Molecular targeting and dose painting

Modulating the biology of the tumour to sensitize tumour cells to radiation therapy using novel anti-cancer therapies directed at specific molecular targets is an exciting new development in veterinary oncology. Much work has been directed at developing molecular inhibitors of different components of the cell signal transduction pathways and angiogenesis. Inhibition of epidermal growth factor receptors and VEGF has been shown to be effective in increasing the radiation responsiveness of neoplastic cells both *in vitro* and in human trials.

There has also been interest in integrating biological information (factors that influence treatment outcome such as tumour proliferation and hypoxia) into radiation treatment planning for the purpose of targeting radiation resistant regions within the tumour. One strategy, termed dose painting, is biological image-guided dose escalation. It relies on non-invasive biological imaging such as positron emission tomography, functional MRI and MR spectroscopy to obtain a 3D distribution of tumour radiosensitivity. The information gained from the biological imaging is used to guide focal dose escalation to radioresistant regions within the tumour. Image-guided biological dose escalation may significantly increase the probability of being able to control the tumour and decrease toxicity in the normal tissues.

Proton radiotherapy

Another modality that has been used in veterinary radiation oncology but has not yet been applied to the treatment of canine brain tumours is proton radiotherapy. Protons (hydrogen nuclei) are characterized by enhanced ionization and cause biological damage when they come to rest in the tissues. It has been shown that use of pencil-beams of protons delivered from multiple angles results in a highly conformed radiation dose distribution in canine tumours (Kaser-Hotz *et al.*, 2002b). Thus, this method can also be used to increase the radiation dose to the tumour and decrease the probability of radionecrosis in the adjacent brain tissue.

It is highly likely that such innovations in radiation therapy technology will make their way into veterinary radiation oncology practice. However, it is highly unlikely that radiation therapy alone will ever be the first-line treatment for macroscopic brain masses. It is imperative that forward-thinking veterinary surgeons get involved in looking for more inventive methods to improve outcome other than simply giving a higher radiation dose. Effort must be directed at identifying molecular targets and introducing innovative adjunctive therapies such as the integration of functional imaging into radiation treatment planning.

Summary

Overall, compared with information regarding other tumour sites, there is little known about the radiation response of tumours affecting the brain and/or spinal column in animals. This results, in part, from the difficulty in obtaining a pre-treatment diagnosis of tumour type, particularly for brain tumours. In addition, the number of patients in each study is relatively small. Veterinary surgeons must organize their efforts and embark on more prospective assessment of the various approaches. Until this is accomplished, the quality of the available data will not become more robust.

The following conclusions can be drawn about the utility of radiation for treatment of tumours affecting the brain or spinal cord:

- We do not know the relative value of radiation therapy given alone or in combination with surgery for the treatment of tumours of glial cell origin
- Radiation combined with surgery is likely to be more effective than surgery alone for the treatment of canine meningioma, but the relative value of radiation alone is unknown. There are data suggesting that the proliferative and angiogenic capacity of meningiomas is related to outcome following treatment with surgery and radiation
- Some pituitary gland tumours respond well to irradiation and there are some data supporting the negative influence of tumour size and lack of endocrine activity on outcome
- There are no data on the response of reticuloendothelial tumours of the brain to radiation therapy. Based on the high radiocurability of solitary lymphoid tumours in humans, veterinary patients with a similar tumour may respond favourably. Dogs with GME also appear to have a favourable prognosis provided involvement is focal
- There are essentially no reliable data enabling accurate counselling of owners of animals with spinal/vertebral tumours. Some general principles, derived from other tumours in animals and human studies, are probably accurate. These include:
  - Macroscopic mesenchymal paraspinal or nerve root tumours are not likely to be controlled permanently with radiation
  - Postoperative radiation of microscopic mesenchymal paraspinal or nerve root tumours is expected to be superior to incomplete resection alone
  - Macroscopic paraspinal reticuloendothelial tumours are probably radiosensitive and definitive irradiation may be justifiable in a large percentage of patients.

References and further reading

Available on accompanying DVD

25

Rehabilitation of the neurological patient

John Sherman[†], Natasha Olby and Krista B. Halling

Physical rehabilitation plays an essential role in the management of human neurological diseases. It is recognized that although axonal regeneration can occur in the peripheral nervous system (PNS), regeneration in the central nervous system (CNS) is usually unsuccessful, and recovery in the CNS is largely due to the plasticity of the system (Jeffery and Blakemore, 1999). Plasticity refers to alterations in the role of the neuron caused by changes in synapse density and type, as well as the sprouting of axons to make contact with other local targets. This process allows surviving neurons to assume functions that they did not previously perform, and is enhanced by repeated stimulation of the tracts involved. Specific rehabilitative exercises can be designed to achieve this end.

It is also well recognized that disuse and immobilization of the limbs results in loss of muscle mass, muscle contractures, and deterioration in the joints and associated structures. Physical rehabilitation plays a critical role in limiting and reversing these effects during recovery from a neurological injury, and maximizes the extent of functional recovery.

To date, there have been few published studies on the use of physical rehabilitation in veterinary medicine and most of these focus on patients with orthopaedic disease (Marsolais *et al.*, 2002; Steiss, 2002; Gandini *et al.*, 2003). This is because, historically, it has been unusual for physical rehabilitation to be recommended routinely as part of a neurological treatment plan. However, the merit of rehabilitation is increasingly recognized, which has led to the establishment of continuing education courses in veterinary physical rehabilitation as well as dedicated veterinary rehabilitation centres. Methods of quantifying functional outcomes, such as the use of goniometry to measure range of motion (ROM) (Jaegger *et al.*, 2002), kinematic analysis of gait (McLaughlin, 2001; Hamilton *et al.*, 2007, 2008) and expanded gait scoring systems (Olby *et al.*, 2001), have also been developed. In humans, recovery of an acceptable quality of life is linked to those activities identified by an individual as essential to support physical, social and psychological wellbeing. In veterinary medicine, the needs of both the patient and the owner have to be considered in this assessment. A good functional outcome in the neurological patient is dependent not only on the integrity of the nervous system but also on the overall health of the animal. Preventing secondary disease in the organ systems of a neurological patient is much easier than treating it, and is an important aspect of rehabilitation.

Terminology

- Range of motion (ROM) – the maximum path of motion (distance or angle) a joint can move through in any one direction, usually measured in degrees.
  - Active range of motion (AROM) – range of motion at a given joint achieved by the patient using their own muscle strength.
  - Active-assisted range of motion (AAROM) – range of motion at a given joint achieved by the patient using their own muscle strength with assistance.
  - Passive range of motion (PROM) – range of motion at a given joint when moved by the therapist.
- Thermotherapy – the use of heat or cold for therapeutic purposes.
  - Cryotherapy – therapeutic application of cold on a body part (e.g. using ice).
  - Heat therapy – therapeutic application of heat on a body part.
- Massage techniques:
  - Effleurage – stroking of the skin; performed with the palm of the hand to stimulate deep tissues, or with the fingertips to stimulate sensory nerves
  - Friction – a method of massage in which force is applied perpendicular to the muscle fibre or scar tissue direction
  - Petrissage – a method of massage that involves lifting and kneading of the skin, subcutaneous tissues and muscle with the fingers or hand.
- Electrical stimulation:
  - Neuromuscular electric stimulation (NMES) – the use of electrical stimulation to stimulate a peripheral nerve and cause either a sensory, motor or noxious response
  - Interferential electrical stimulation (IES) – a type of NMES that uses two channels which interact and create a unique waveform to treat pain, improve circulation and increase cellular metabolism.
- Gait training – methods used to encourage correct patient ambulation.
  - Proprioceptive neuromuscular training – a form of therapeutic exercise in which accommodating resistance is applied to various patterns of movement for the purpose of strengthening and restraining the muscles guiding joint motion using proprioceptive input.
- Hydrotherapy – intervention using water.

Patient assessment

The clinician's overall assessment of the individual neurological patient is critical for the rehabilitation process. The evaluation should involve the patient, owner and supervising veterinary surgeon (if applicable). This helps to ensure that the clinician has a thorough understanding of the:

- Patient's previous and current ailments
- Patient's normal physical activities and psychological status
- Owner's desired and anticipated expectations of outcome
- Owner's ability to provide time and expertise
- Specific details of the presenting neurological problem.

The details that must be considered with respect to the presenting neurological condition include:

- Duration and progression of clinical signs
- Localization of the neurological lesion
- Type and severity of pathology
- Treatment – including surgical procedures performed
- Any changes in the neurological status since those procedures.

Initial assessment considerations for rehabilitation of patients with spinal disease

- Level of pain.
- Joint stiffness and ROM.
- Muscle mass.
- Proprioception.
- Integrity of spinal reflexes.
- Neuromuscular coordination/ataxia.
- Concurrent orthopaedic conditions.
- Decubital ulcers.
- Aspiration pneumonia.

In the case of common neurological diseases, such as thoracolumbar intervertebral disc herniations and caudal cervical spondylomyelopathy, published information about the typical time course and level of recovery can be referred to when determining the expectations for recovery (see Chapters 15 and 16).

Treatment plan

The treatment plan can be developed as a programme for:

- An owner, with guidance
- A combination of the owner and primary veterinary surgeon
- A dedicated facility for animal physical rehabilitation on an inpatient or outpatient basis.

Medical points to consider when deciding which programme would be most suitable include whether the animal is ambulatory, whether they are continent, and the presence of additional health problems. In addition, there must be adequate people available to enable the animal to perform exercises with no increased risk of injury. For example, before

an animal is placed in a water bath, there must be sufficient people available to get them out quickly in case of an emergency.

Regardless of the option chosen, the principles of treatment are the same:

- Appropriate supportive care must be provided (see below)
- Every effort should be made to decrease the progression of pathology within the nervous system and encourage an environment for healing to take place. Appropriate diagnosis and treatment of underlying problems should be sought if not already addressed
- Functional recovery should be enhanced by designing a treatment plan that focuses on preservation of muscle mass and ROM, maximizes the plasticity of the nervous system and includes proprioceptive neuromuscular training to promote recovery of a normal gait (Figure 25.1).

It is important to define the owner's expectations very clearly and to develop a realistic time line for reaching those goals. A sample homecare sheet is provided in Figure 25.2.

Supportive care

Bladder and bowel management

Urination

Animals that have spinal cord disease or primary autonomic dysfunction (e.g. dysautonomia) may be unable to urinate voluntarily or effectively (see Chapter 19 for details of innervation of the bladder and physiology of micturition). These animals are at risk of:

- Developing a urinary tract infection (UTI)
- Damaging their bladder wall by overstretching
- Damaging their upper urinary tract in severe cases.

It is prudent to assume that paraplegic animals are unable to urinate until proven otherwise. Such animals should have their bladders expressed manually 3–4 times a day. Drugs can facilitate manual expression in animals where this is difficult, by relaxing the external urethral sphincter (e.g. diazepam at 0.25–0.5 mg/kg orally 20 minutes prior to expression) and the internal urethral sphincter (e.g. phenoxybenzamine at 0.5 mg/kg orally q8–12h). As phenoxybenzamine is an alpha-adrenergic antagonist, hypotension can be an unwanted side effect at high doses.

In animals where manual expression is not possible, repeated aseptic catheterization may be necessary (see Chapter 19). This may not be possible in females and in these cases a soft Foley catheter should be placed and maintained in an aseptic manner. Routine placement of indwelling urinary catheters is not recommended, if it can be avoided,

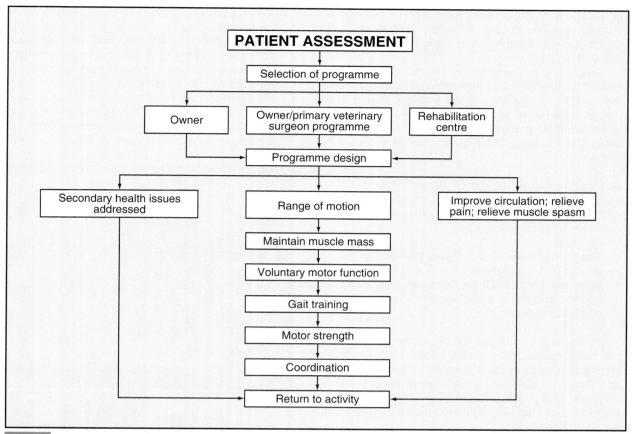

PATIENT ASSESSMENT

Selection of programme

Owner | Owner/primary veterinary surgeon programme | Rehabilitation centre

Programme design

Secondary health issues addressed | Range of motion | Improve circulation; relieve pain; relieve muscle spasm

Maintain muscle mass

Voluntary motor function

Gait training

Motor strength

Coordination

Return to activity

25.1 Developing a treatment plan for the neurological patient.

Physical rehabilitation home treatment plan									

Name: _____   Date: _____

Treatment	Frequency	Monday	Tuesday	Wednesday	Thursday	Friday	Saturday	Sunday
Example: Range of motion Short leash walk Stand and balance	5 min; 4/day 2 min; 2/day 30 sec; 4/day							

25.2 Sample physical rehabilitation home treatment plan.

as it increases the risk of an antibiotic-resistant UTI developing; however, short-term use (<4 days) is acceptable (Bubenik and Hosgood, 2008). An additional risk in male cats is iatrogenic trauma to the bladder wall. The authors have had to transfuse male cats that have had an indwelling tomcat catheter placed for >2 days, as a result of trauma-induced haematuria.

- Urine should be monitored daily for changes in odour and colour.
- Urine dipsticks can be used intermittently to check the protein content and for the presence of blood.

If a UTI develops, specific antibiotics should be administered based on the results of urine cultures.

In a recent study of dogs recovering from spinal cord injuries due to disc herniation, 38% of animals developed a UTI within 3 months following the injury (Olby *et al.*, 2010).

Animals with lower motor neuron (LMN) paralysis of the bladder may leak urine constantly, causing irritation to the skin in the perineal region and pelvic limbs (urine scald) (see Figure 25.4). These animals almost always have persistent UTIs and are difficult to manage, but regular bladder expression can help.

Defecation

The innervation of the gastrointestinal tract allows animals to defecate reflexively even when the spinal cord has been transected.

- The normal defecation reflex is initiated by stretch of the rectal wall.
- Voluntary control of the external anal sphincter and the abdominal muscles allows voluntary control of defecation.

In animals with upper motor neuron (UMN) spinal cord injuries, this reflex becomes overactive, such that a small amount of rectal distension results in initiation of defecation that cannot be prevented (Holmes *et al.*, 1998). Recumbent animals must be checked and cleaned regularly so that they are not lying in faeces.

- The defecation reflex can be initiated in recumbent animals by stimulating the perineal region with a gloved hand.
- Changing the diet to decrease stool volume and establishing a routine can also be helpful in controlling the frequency of defecation.

In animals that have lesions affecting the cauda equina, there can be constant leakage of stool. This is very difficult to deal with but can be addressed by:

- Feeding a low-residue diet that decreases stool volume
- Frequent cleaning of the animal
- Use of appropriate bedding (see below)
- Application of a waterproof barrier cream following drying of the perineal skin.

Toilet training is so imprinted on some dogs that they are extremely unlikely to urinate or defecate indoors. It is important that each animal is given the opportunity to perform these activities in a situation and on a surface to which it is accustomed.

Bedding

Suitable bedding depends on the circumstances.

- Animals that can maintain sternal recumbency should be placed on a grate or sling bed that allows drainage of urine away from the animal (Figure 25.3).
- Such flooring and beds do not always provide adequate padding for recumbent, thin, large-breed dogs. These animals should be placed on a well padded surface that is porous, so that the skin does not get moist and urine can drain away.
- If the animal is trying to rise, it is important that the floor is non-slip and that the area is confined to minimize the risk of falling.
- Multiple absorbent disposable pads can be placed under the animal's hind end and removed and disposed of easily whenever the animal urinates or defecates (Figure 25.3).

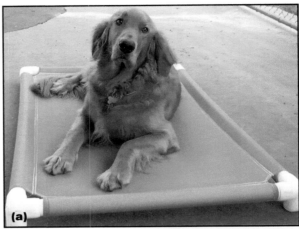
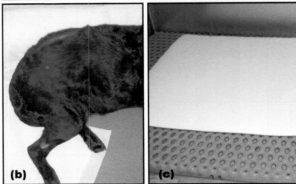

25.3 Various forms of bedding. **(a)** A sling bed made of netting to allow fluids to drain away from the animal. **(b)** This dog is lying on a thick rubber mat with easily removable nappies (diapers) underneath its hind end. **(c)** A grate with porous bedding material on it for recumbent animals.

Skin care

Animals with neurological disease develop skin problems as a result of recumbency, incontinence, sensory dysfunction and boredom (stereotypical behaviour). Problems range from mild skin irritation to decubital ulcers, severe urine scald and self-mutilation (Figure 25.4).

General skin care of the recumbent animal involves keeping the animal clean and dry. Incontinent animals with long hair coats should be clipped in the perineal and inguinal regions so that the underlying skin can be cared for appropriately. However, the coat should be left over the common pressure points, if possible, to provide some natural padding.

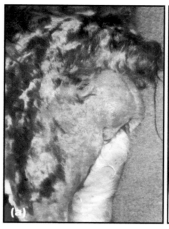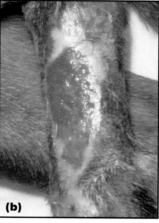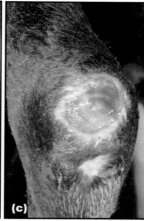

25.4 Dermatological consequences of neurological disease. **(a)** This dog has severe urine scalding from 2 days of recumbency and inability to urinate, combined with urine overflow and a UTI. **(b)** This chronically paraplegic dog has been licking the dorsal aspect of its tarsus. **(c)** A chronic decubital ulcer over the calcaneus.

Decubital ulcers

Decubital ulcers develop over pressure points such as the greater trochanter of the femur as a result of obstruction of local circulation over prolonged periods. Ulcers can develop in small as well as large dogs, but are unusual in cats. The affected tissue undergoes ischaemic necrosis and apparently inconsequential lesions can rapidly develop into large, deep ulcers as the dead tissue sloughs (see Figure 25.4). Prevention of ulcers is better than cure and this can be achieved by:

- The regular turning of recumbent animals (every 4–6 hours)
- Massage over pressure points to promote circulation every 4–6 hours
- Suitable bedding
- Hydrotherapy
- Elevation of 'at-risk' pressure points off the ground using 'doughnuts' of padding
- Daily sling-supported walking ('slinging') of recumbent animals so that they have a period when they are in a normal standing position.

'Doughnuts' can be made from bubble wrap that is rolled into a cylinder and then formed into a circle and covered with a conforming bandage. The 'doughnut' should be large enough to surround the area of concern and elevate it off the ground, whilst not compromising circulation to the margins of the ulcer.

- The use of slings, hoists and carts to get dogs into a normal standing position is important and should be attempted at least twice a day (Figure 25.5), although this may not be possible in animals that have suffered severe trauma.
- In general, dogs are placed in their cart for as long as they will tolerate it: this can range from as short a time as a minute to half an hour, depending on the stage of recovery and the individual.
- When the patient puts their entire bodyweight on the sling instead of supporting it themselves or shows signs of discomfort, they should be taken down from the sling.

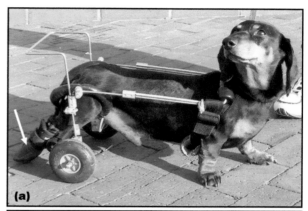

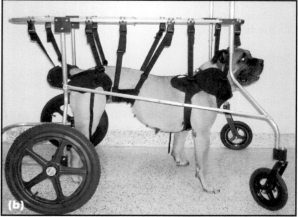

25.5 Carts for **(a)** paraparetic and **(b)** tetraparetic animals. Note that the paraparetic dog is wearing boots on its hindfeet (arrowed) to protect them from abrasions.

The ischial tuberosities represent a pressure point that needs to be carefully monitored in paraplegic dogs that sit upright and rock back on to these bones (Figure 25.6). Although a 'doughnut' can be made for such dogs to sit on, they will usually move off it very quickly. Anxiolytic drugs such as diazepam (0.25–0.5 mg/kg orally up to three times a day) can be tried in these animals in order to make them lie down. It is also important to sling these patients intermittently to get their weight off the affected area.

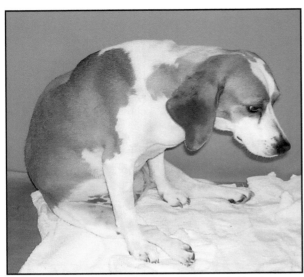

| 25.6 | Typical pose of a dog with a caudal lumbar lesion, causing it to sit on its ischial tuberosities. |

Treatment of decubital ulcers, beyond providing appropriate bedding and pressure relief, includes:

- Clipping of the hair to show the full extent of the problem
- Surgical debridement of ischaemic tissue
- The application of wound dressings to promote healing by second intention
- Massage of the surrounding area to encourage blood flow.

Provision of a balanced diet is also important for tissue healing.

Self-mutilation

Self-mutilation occurs in animals with a complete lack of sensation (i.e. nociception negative animals, due to spinal cord or peripheral nerve disease), as a result of paraesthesias, and in bored and stressed animals as a stereotypical behaviour. Self-mutilation has been described in animals with neuropathies as a result of lumbosacral disease, trauma and inherited sensory neuropathies (Tarvin and Prata, 1980; Cummings et al., 1983; Jacobson and Schrader, 1987).

If an animal starts to lick, or worse bite, a part of their body, this should be prevented by the use of an Elizabethan collar or bite collar. In addition the patient should be assessed for an obvious trigger (e.g. a decubital ulcer) and treated appropriately. The environment should be made as stimulating as possible in case the problem is a reflection of stress and boredom.

- Gabapentin can be used for both pain relief and behavioural modification at a dose of 5–10 mg/kg orally q8h–q12h.
- A multi-drug approach can be used in problematic cases, by adding in other classes of drug such as opioids or behaviour modifiers such as fluoxetine (Wynchank and Berk, 1998), trazodone or tricyclic antidepressants.

- Topical capsaicin has been used for a long time in humans and has been used successfully in dogs with atopic dermatitis as an anti-pruritic agent (Marsella et al., 2002).

The authors have had good success with topical capsaicin in combination with oral gabapentin (Flecknell and Waterman-Pearson, 2000).

Care of the respiratory system

Neurological, particularly recumbent, patients are at risk of:

- Hypoventilation
- Aspiration pneumonia
- Pulmonary atelectasis
- Non-cardiogenic pulmonary oedema.

Any tetraplegic animal is at risk of hypoventilation as a result of paralysis of the muscles of respiration (the diaphragm and intercostal muscles). This paralysis can be a result of LMN (e.g. botulism, polyradiculoneuritis) or UMN (e.g. cervical fracture, atlanto-axial subluxation, brainstem disease) problems.

Hypoventilation

Hypoventilation should be suspected in any tetraplegic animal and the respiratory pattern of all recumbent animals should be checked regularly. If hypoventilation is suspected, a blood gas analysis should be obtained; an arterial PCO_2 >45 mmHg is concerning and may indicate the need for a ventilator (see Chapter 21 for further details). It is also important that the body temperature of tetraplegic animals is monitored and kept within the normal range as hypothermia can exacerbate motor weakness, particularly in LMN animals. Hyperthermia can occur in animals that are unable to pant effectively.

Aspiration pneumonia

Animals with megaoesophagus, regurgitation and dysphagia (common with various LMN diseases) are particularly at risk of developing aspiration pneumonia. Aspiration of acidic stomach contents can cause severe pulmonary damage and secondary bacterial pneumonia.

The effect of aspiration can be reduced by decreasing the acidity of the stomach contents. This can be achieved with the administration of H2 antagonists, such as famotidine (0.5 mg/kg orally, i.v. q12–24h), or proton pump inhibitors such as omeprazole (0.5–1 mg/kg orally q24h) or pantoprazole (1 mg/kg i.v. q24h); stomach content acidity should be checked and the doses adjusted accordingly. As regurgitation of acidic stomach contents also causes a local oesophagitis that exacerbates megaoesophagus, acid neutralization has a two-fold benefit.

Oesophageal and pharyngeal dysfunction is often clearly apparent (in the form of regurgitation), but can sometimes be difficult to identify. It should be suspected in any animal with LMN disease that swallows repeatedly, drools saliva, and that coughs after eating or drinking. In animals with megaoesophagus, the risk of regurgitation and aspiration can be reduced by placing a naso-oesophageal tube.

- The oesophagus is kept empty by intermittent (every 2–6 hours) aspiration of the naso-oesophageal tube.
- The tube can be left *in situ* for only 2–4 days at most and is not well tolerated by some animals.
- Nothing should be given by mouth to animals that have recently regurgitated.
- If there has been no regurgitation for approximately 8 hours, a test feeding can be undertaken: the animal should be propped up so that the head is vertically above the stomach and the upright position maintained for at least 20 minutes following feeding.
- Some animals manage meatballs best, whilst others do better with gruel or a more liquid-type food.
- The oesophagus can be aspirated 1 hour later to ensure that the food has passed down into the stomach.
- It is important not to attempt any active exercise for approximately 4 hours after feeding.

Pulmonary atelactasis

Prolonged lateral recumbency causes atelectasis of the dependent lung and compromises respiratory function. Whenever possible, animals should be propped into sternal recumbency and their hips flipped from side to side every 4–6 hours, although extremely weak animals may not be able to maintain the sternal position.

Coupage of the entire lung fields should be performed every 4–6 hours as a routine measure in recumbent animals. To do this, the hand is made into a cup and used to percuss the thorax firmly with the aim of making the animal cough (Figure 25.7).

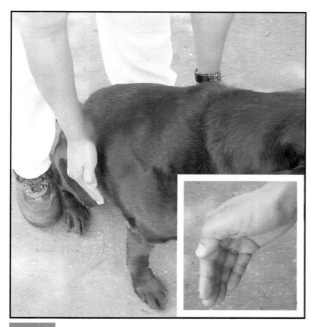

25.7 Correct hand position for coupage.

This is not possible in some animals immediately after spinal surgery, or in trauma victims, because it can cause pain. In patients with pneumonia, the animal should be nebulized with sterile saline for 5–10 minutes prior to coupage.

When performing hydrotherapy, it is important to remember that the hydrostatic force of water decreases the patient's tidal volume when fully submerged. The increased effort needed to breathe against the hydrostatic force is helpful in cases of pulmonary atelectasis, as it increases the functional tidal volume. However, caution should be used in patients with serious respiratory compromise. The additional effort may cause the patient to decompensate and have serious respiratory complications. In such patients, hydrotherapy should only be performed under experienced supervision (Figure 25.8).

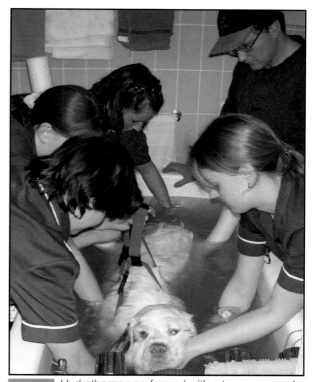

25.8 Hydrotherapy performed with a team approach to ensure that it is both safe and effective.

Behaviour

The recovery of neurological patients is greatly influenced by their mental status. Patients that either cannot move or are confined may become bored, the stress of which can cause depression and stereotypical behaviours such as self-mutilation. Added stresses include chronic pain and the inability to complete normal functions such as urination, defecation, eating and drinking.

To a certain extent, the response to injury is influenced by breed and varies with each individual. It is important to know the personality and routine of each individual animal and make their environment compatible with their emotional and physical needs (e.g. some dogs eat and drink better if they are placed in a sling or cart with elevated bowls).

Knowledge of the animal's personality also helps determine how best to motivate them when trying to perform physiotherapy. Some dogs respond to treats, some love toys and some dogs just have a willingness to please. Mental status should be evaluated daily, and the environment altered or an underlying cause sought if it worsens.

Regular contact with the owner is essential, both for the animal and for the owner so that they can learn how to care for their pet appropriately.

Nutrition

Providing adequate nutritional support is a very important aspect of the supportive care for neurological patients, as these animals have undergone significant physiological and psychological stress.

Metabolic response to injury

Nutritional intake is often reduced in neurological patients because they are unable or unwilling to eat, and the metabolic changes that then occur are drastically different to those seen in a healthy fasting dog. After glycogen stores are depleted, the body does not turn to fatty acids as the primary energy source but instead relies on protein catabolism. The term coined to describe this condition is 'complicated starvation'. The metabolic response to injury has been divided into three phases:

1. The shock phase – this occurs in conjunction with the injury and is a brief period during which the body is in a hypometabolic state.
2. The hypermetabolic phase – increases in the metabolic rate and protein catabolism appear to parallel the severity of the illness. During this phase, the clinician must be proactive in order to minimize the loss of lean body mass and provide the nutrients needed for recovery.
3. The convalescent phase – the time required by the body to replenish the lean body mass and fat stores, and return to a normal metabolic state.

Energy requirements

The daily energy requirements for each patient should be calculated and adjustments can then be made based on the response of the animal. Daily maintenance energy requirements can be calculated using the formula:

$$\text{Resting energy requirement (kcal/day)} = 70 \times \text{bodyweight (kg)}^{0.75}$$

This maintenance value can then be multiplied by an 'illness factor' of 1.2 to 1.6. The illness factor is determined by the severity of the illness, the phase of recovery, and an assessment of the patient's bodyweight, body condition and lean body mass.

The food sources used should be of high density, palatable and nutritionally balanced with the majority of calories being provided by high quality protein and fat (assuming that the patient does not have any other systemic disease that would be complicated by these ingredients). There are several prescription diets on the market that meet these requirements.

Nutritional intake

The final consideration with respect to nutrition is that the animal actually receives the prescribed nutrients. Feeding by the owner and hand-feeding can be extremely beneficial early in the rehabilitation process. If these suggestions fail to produce results, assisted enteral feeding must be employed. The specific techniques, management and complications of the various methods of assisted feeding are beyond the scope of this chapter but can be found elsewhere (see **References and further reading** on DVD).

Water requirements are estimated to be between 50 and 100 ml/kg bodyweight per day. Patients that are not eating and drinking on their own should be weighed on the same scales daily to ensure that their hydration status is adequate.

Physical rehabilitation

The physical therapy techniques used in rehabilitation are summarized in Figure 25.9.

Modality	Indications	Benefits	Contraindications
Range of motion (ROM)	Non-ambulatory; monoparesis, paraparesis or tetraparesis; spasticity	Maintains flexibility; maintains integrity of joints, muscles and tendons	Excessive pain; recent surgical repair
Cryotherapy	Recent surgical site; post-exercise	Pain relief; decreased metabolic demands; decreased haemorrhage/inflammation	Careful use in areas with decreased blood supply
Heat therapy	Subacute/chronic pain; chronic inflammatory conditions; muscle spasms; decreased ROM; excess scar tissue; pre-exercise	Pain relief; increased circulation; decreased inflammation; increased nerve conduction velocity; decreased muscle spasms	Acute inflammation; use with caution in areas with decreased blood supply or patients with circulatory compromise
Massage	Stress/pain; muscle spasms; decreased ROM; recumbency; contractures	Stress/pain relief; decreased muscle spasms; maintenance of tissue perfusion; sensory input to spinal cord	Excessive pain

25.9 An overview of the physical therapy modalities available and their indications, benefits and limitations. (continues) ▶

Modality	Indications	Benefits	Contraindications
Interferential electrical stimulation (IES)	Acute/chronic pain; poor circulation; muscle spasms	Pain relief; increased circulation; decreased muscle spasms	Seizures; neoplasia; sepsis; pacemakers; coagulopathies
Active muscle contraction	Paresis (monoparesis, paraparesis, hemiparesis, tetraparesis)	Increases muscle strength; counteracts muscle atrophy	Cannot perform if reflex arc is absent (LMN disease)
Neuromuscular electrical stimulation (NMES)	Lower motor neuron (LMN) paresis	Increases muscle strength; counteracts muscle atrophy	Some patients will not tolerate; not as effective as active muscle contraction
Treadmill (land or water)	Paresis (monoparesis, paraparesis, hemiparesis, tetraparesis)	Increases muscle strength; counteracts muscle atrophy; increased coordination; controlled environment	Accessibility; manpower needed
Swimming	Paresis (monoparesis, paraparesis, hemiparesis, tetraparesis)	Increases muscle strength; counteracts muscle atrophy; increased coordination; water provides weight support, cleans coat	Need appropriate swimming area; urinary tract infection
Proprioceptive training	Paresis (monoparesis, paraparesis, hemiparesis, tetraparesis)	Encourages accurate coordination; simple exercises can be done at home	Cannot perform in non-ambulatory animals

25.9 (continued) An overview of the physical therapy modalities available and their indications, benefits and limitations.

Range of motion

By definition, ROM is the angle (measured in degrees) through which a joint moves from the anatomical position to the extreme limit of its motion in a particular direction (Figure 25.10). This process can be achieved by three methods:

- Passive range of motion (PROM) – the clinician provides the force needed to drive the motion
- Active range of motion (AROM) – the muscles of the patient are responsible for the motion
- Active-assisted range of motion (AAROM) – the clinician provides manual assistance during a muscular contraction.

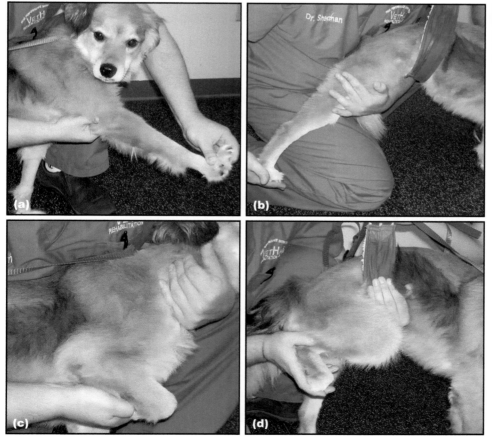

25.10 Full ROM in the thoracic and pelvic limbs. Note that the digits have also been extended and flexed.

Moving a body segment or joint through ROM influences the:

- Muscles
- Articular cartilage
- Joint capsule
- Ligaments
- Tendons
- Fascia
- Blood vessels
- Nerves.

Immobilization (regardless of cause) leads to changes in all of these tissues, and some of these changes can be irreversible if not addressed early in the rehabilitation process. Changes that have been described include: morphological and biochemical changes in the articular cartilage; joint capsular and pericapsular contractures; a decrease in the thickness and strength of the ligaments and tendons (especially at the bone interface); osteoporosis; loss of flexibility in the involved muscles, fascia, vessels and nerves; and, rarely, myopathic changes (Braund *et al.*, 1980).

PROM is used early in the rehabilitation process to maintain the integrity of all the tissues of the body segment involved and to counteract the effects of immobilization. It is also thought that joint movement provides sensory input into the spinal cord, even if the patient does not have voluntary motor function, thereby enhancing establishment of new neural pathways.

Each segment or joint must be taken through its full ROM (to patient tolerance) 15–20 times every 4–8 hours (see **Passive range of motion** clip on DVD). The ROM should be recorded once a week by the veterinary surgeon or trained physical therapy provider so that changes can be documented. PROM is an exercise that can easily be completed by educated owners and repeated as part of a homecare programme, as long as they understand not to persist if it appears to be painful for the animal. Contraindications to PROM include situations where motion will jeopardize a surgical repair, increase inflammation, increase pain or where the temperament of the patient precludes hands-on therapy.

Thermotherapy

Thermotherapy is defined as the application of heat or cold to a specific body region for the purpose of physical therapy.

Cryotherapy

Cryotherapy lowers the temperature of the target tissues by removing body heat via conduction, convection and evaporation. The degree of cooling is related to the:

- Temperature of the modality
- Duration of treatment
- Vascularization of the treatment area
- Surface area of the target tissue.

This treatment is most commonly delivered via ice packs, ice baths, ice massage and cold compression units. These methods penetrate tissues up to 1–4 cm deep and achieve a decrease in temperature of 1–4°C in the muscle and of 12°C at the level of the skin.

The local effects of cryotherapy include vasoconstriction and a decrease in cellular metabolism, cell waste, oedema and pain. These local effects result in pain relief, decreased demand for oxygen, decreased haemorrhage and inflammation, and inhibition of degradative enzymes. These properties make cryotherapy the treatment of choice for surgical incisions in the immediate (0–48 hours) postoperative period, to reduce swelling and pain, when they are repeated every 4 hours. It is often helpful to also treat the surgical area after the animal has undertaken exercise.

Care must be taken not to overcool an area whilst treating a patient. The treated areas often have decreased pain sensation and a compromised circulation, so the area will cool faster and for longer than normal tissue. The best way to ensure even cooling is to have even contact over the target surface. It is also recommended that a damp towel be placed between the ice packs and the skin, and that the duration of cooling is limited to <15 minutes. During cryotherapy application, the skin should be monitored intermittently and if it appears cyanotic, or the animal shows discomfort, treatment should be discontinued. Once the cold source has been removed, the affected tissues return to baseline temperature within 15–30 minutes.

Heat therapy

The application of heat to the body can be broken down into superficial and deep heating.

- Superficial heat is used most commonly in veterinary physical rehabilitation and is therefore the focus of discussion. It can be employed using simple methods, such as moist heat packs or towels (at 70–75°C) and warm whirlpools.
- The heating of deep tissue structures (3–5 cm underneath the skin) is better accomplished with therapeutic ultrasonography (set at 1 MHz on continuous mode).

The local effects of heat therapy include: vasodilation; an increase in cellular metabolism, extensibility of collagen, local blood flow and nerve conduction velocity; and decreased muscle spasms. These properties make heat therapy useful in the subacute and chronic phases when the animal is being prepared for therapeutic exercise, to improve the mobility of the connective tissues, or to provide relief from muscle spasms or pain.

Heat is transferred from the medium to the target tissue. The degree of heating depends upon the:

- Temperature of the modality used
- Time of exposure
- Area of tissue treated
- Vascularity of the target tissue.

As with cryotherapy, care should be taken when treating areas of reduced vascular supply and innervation to avoid overheating the tissues. In most cases moist hot packs (at 74°C) wrapped in a towel can heat target tissues to the desired temperature within 10–15 minutes. Whirlpools and hydrotherapy units should be maintained at 32–40°C to provide effective heating of tissues. However, if the patient is exercising in the water, the temperature should be maintained closer to 32°C to prevent overheating. Heat therapy is particularly useful in cases where ROM has become a problem (e.g. where scar tissue has become excessive and immobile), in animals with muscle spasms, and in patients that are just starting therapeutic exercise.

Massage

The benefits of massage fall into three categories: psychological, mechanical and physiological. Describing all of the different types of massage technique is beyond the scope of this chapter, but there are a few strokes that are basic to the delivery of massage (Starkey, 1999):

- Effleurage is the technique of stroking or gliding over the muscles with the hands. This technique is usually started with a light touch and gradually intensified as it is continued. It is suggested to follow the pattern of blood flow back to the heart
- Petrissage is a technique that uses a kneading action or pressure and release and is performed along the entire length of muscle groups
- Friction massage is a technique that uses pressure perpendicular to either the muscle fibre or the scar tissue direction.

If performed correctly, the animal should at least tolerate the massage and, ideally, appear to enjoy it.

- The psychological benefits are that massage is enjoyable for the animal; it is relaxing and creates a stronger bond with the patient. These factors contribute to stress relief.
- The mechanical benefits of massage include keeping the tissue planes mobile during the recovery process, breaking down adhesions formed by excess scar tissue (using the friction technique), and relieving muscle spasms.
- The reported physiological benefits of massage include providing sensory input into the nervous system, thereby stimulating the neural pathways, and increasing blood and lymphatic flow, which in turn speeds delivery of nutrients and expedites the removal of waste products and inflammatory mediators.

Massage is particularly beneficial in patients that are non-ambulatory, stressed, undergoing neurogenic atrophy, or are in the early stages of therapeutic exercise. Massage can be contraindicated in some situations (e.g. it should not be performed directly over a laminectomy site).

Interferential electrical stimulation

Interferential electrical stimulation (IES) is a specific type of stimulation that uses alternating currents on two separate channels (Starkey, 1999). The four electrodes are placed either on the skin or the sides of a specially designed pool (Figure 25.11) so that the treatment area is within the confines of the electrodes. When stimulation occurs, mild muscle fasciculations are seen but complete muscle contractions should not occur.

The purpose of using IES is to treat pain, improve the microcirculation and increase cellular metabolism. This technique is particularly useful in the acute postoperative phase and can be used as needed for pain relief. Contraindications for this type of therapy include cancer, infection, coagulopathies, pacemakers and seizure conditions. Specialized equipment is needed to perform IES; therefore, patients need to be referred to a dedicated rehabilitation clinic.

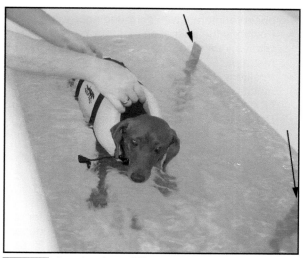

25.11 A patient in an IES unit. The metal strips on the sides of the bath are the electrodes (arrowed). The patient is wearing a life jacket for dogs.

Preserving muscle mass and increasing strength

Preservation of muscle mass is a very difficult aspect of physical rehabilitation in the neurological patient. Upon presentation, some patients have chronic conditions and significant muscle atrophy due to disuse, whilst dogs that have suffered significant injury (e.g. in road traffic accidents) or have LMN disorders develop rapid and dramatic muscle atrophy. An accurate assessment of the patient provides insight on how best to combat atrophy (e.g. providing adequate nutrition in the hypermetabolic phase of recovery following injury may prevent dramatic muscle atrophy).

Active and repetitive muscle contraction by the patient is the best way to maintain and strengthen muscle. Numerous experiments have demonstrated that neuromuscular electrical stimulation (NMES) cannot equal an active voluntary contraction in force, strength or endurance. However, patients that have severe LMN signs do not have intact reflex arcs (at least not at the level of the lesion) and NMES is the only therapeutic option for these patients.

Active muscle contraction

If the patient has an intact reflex arc, with or without voluntary motor function, active contraction is by far the best way to preserve muscle mass, and exercises should be started as soon as possible after injury. Patients can be placed in slings or carts several times a day in a manner that enables them to bear some weight at least for short periods of time (see Figure 25.5). The duration of 'slinging' is entirely dependent on each individual and varies from a few seconds to up to 30 minutes before the animal stops bearing weight and just hangs in the slings. This simple treatment plan can accomplish many goals:

- Prevention of decubital ulcers
- Prevention of atelectasis
- Places the animal in a normal position to eat and observe/interact with surroundings
- Positions the animal so that they can be treated with various modalities using fewer staff and less restraint
- Positions the animal so that a normal posture is maintained, ensuring that the gains made in ROM are not lost
- Partial weight bearing requires active muscle contraction by the weight-bearing muscle groups
- Partial weight bearing stimulates the other connective tissues in the body (i.e. bone, tendons, ligaments, articular cartilage) so that the effects of immobilization are minimized.

The patient can also be submerged in water up to its flank or greater trochanter of the femur, depending on the body style of the patient (Figure 25.12). If there is a surgical incision, this can be covered with sterile petroleum jelly to prevent complications in wound healing. Suspension provides support and weight reduction so that exercise is easier to perform. The goal is to have the limbs in a normal weight-bearing position but only bearing a fraction of the weight. Suspension in water also helps to keep the skin clean (although animals must be dried carefully after the procedure) and the hydrostatic force of the water helps minimize oedema in the extremities and increases tidal volume.

The exercises performed with each patient are determined by their neurological status. Withdrawal reflexes can be stimulated in animals that lack voluntary motor function. The clinician can provide additional resistance and change the degree of abduction of the limb in order to exercise different muscles as the patient improves. It is beneficial, occasionally, in paraplegic animals to exercise the non-affected limbs using swimming. Muscle groups that cannot be stimulated with reflexive action are treated with NMES. Patients that have regained voluntary motor function have more exercise options:

- Postural reactions can be performed while the patient is supported in either the cart or water
- Creating waves or rocking motions can help stimulate the same sensory and motor pathways as the postural reactions.

In animals where one limb is more severely affected than the others (e.g. brachial plexus avulsion or lateralized LMN signs as a result of fibrocartilaginous embolism), the strength of that limb can be increased by lifting the normal limb and forcing weight bearing by the severely affected limb (see **Weight shift** clip on DVD). Sit to stand exercises can help strengthen extensor muscles in particular (see **Sit to stand** clip on DVD). As the patient improves, the degree of support provided by either the cart or water is decreased and the duration of exercise is increased. Exercises can be performed to fatigue but, as a general rule, if the patient is too tired the day following exercise to perform at the same level, the amount of exercise should be cut back or dropped to every other day until strength and endurance have improved.

Neuromuscular electrical stimulation

NMES produces tetanic contraction of muscles via dermal electrodes placed over the muscles to be worked. It is indicated in animals that cannot produce an active contraction of a muscle (i.e. LMN paralysis) and helps to slow neurogenic muscle atrophy.

There are several types of unit on the market (Figure 25.13). Each unit has several different parameters, some of which can be adjusted. The

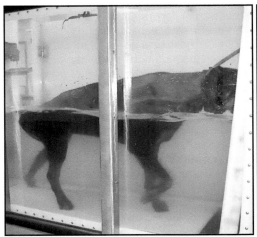
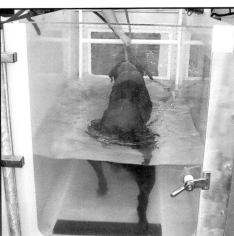

25.12 A dog walking in an underwater treadmill. This dog can now bear weight on its own with the water level coming up to its shoulder, and is completing 15 minutes of exercise.

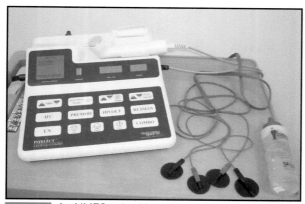

An NMES unit with carbon rubber electrodes attached.

authors' advice is to buy a unit that allows changes to the stimulation parameters in order to give greater flexibility in treatment. A unit that has multiple channels is also beneficial as more than one muscle group can be contracted simultaneously during the treatment, allowing co-contraction or alternating contraction of muscle groups.

The parameters that need to be considered include:

- Type of current – monophasic (DC), biphasic (AC), polyphasic (Russian). There is no demonstrated benefit of one current over another, but some animals will only tolerate one particular current
- Frequency – rate of oscillations in cycles per second (pulses per second, PPS)
- Phase/pulse duration – the length of time of a single phase or pulse (microseconds)
- Waveform – the visual shape of the waveform on a graph
- Amplitude – the intensity of the delivered pulse
- On/off time – the length of time the stimulator is on compared with the length of rest time between contractions; can be given as a ratio (i.e. 1:5 = 10 seconds on and 50 seconds off)
- Ramp – the time that the machine takes to go from 0 to the set amplitude
- Polarity – anode or cathode.

When treatment is being administered, the clinician needs to consider the following points:

- The hair over the muscle groups that are to be stimulated should be clipped and the skin cleaned
- The largest size electrodes that will fit on the muscle to be stimulated should be used – carbon rubber electrodes are excellent because they can be trimmed easily and reused
- Ultrasound gel can be used as a conduction medium
- An electrode should be placed at the origin and insertion of the muscle to be stimulated and moved around at a low setting to find the motor point of the muscle (area of best contraction; usually in the proximal third of the muscle)

- The muscles can be stimulated once a day for up to 15 minutes until the animal is able to produce an active contraction
- Some patients will not tolerate NMES and some will only tolerate it with sedation
- Handlers should always use caution with the patient, especially the first time this modality is used, as it is an unusual sensation for the animal.

Suggested protocol for NMES treatment

- Start with an on/off time of 1:3 and work up to a 1:2.
- Use a frequency between 30 and 50 PPS and a ramp time of 2–3 seconds.
- Amplitude is set to patient tolerance with the goal of obtaining good muscle contraction.

Low-level laser therapy

Low-level laser therapy (LLLT) is an emerging therapeutic modality in veterinary medicine, after having received widespread use in human medicine for patients with spinal cord trauma or disease. LLLT involves using a hand-held laser unit to deliver light energy directly to the affected tissues. The light energy used in LLLT can penetrate the patient's skin and stimulate the deeper tissues, such as muscle, bone and spinal cord. The light energy from the laser is transferred into biochemical energy (adenosine triphosphate, ATP) by the mitochondria of the target tissue cells. ATP is in turn used for tissue healing and regeneration.

LLLT is a non-invasive and potentially very effective method of decreasing local pain and increasing tissue healing when delivered in repeated short treatments. A typical treatment protocol would be 2–4 minutes per affected region of tissue once daily for 5–14 days. LLLT has anecdotally shown promising results for accelerating wound healing and decreasing the pain associated with osteoarthritis in dogs and cats; its efficacy in treating veterinary neurological patients remains to be determined.

Gait training

This term describes the methods used to encourage normal ambulation using the affected limbs correctly in a straight line at different speeds. The equipment needed to perform this type of exercise depends on the neurological status of the patient.

- If the patient has no voluntary motor function, they can be placed in an underwater treadmill at standing height (see Figure 25.12).
- The treadmill is started at a slow walking speed and the veterinary surgeon (who is in the tank with the patient) stimulates the withdrawal reflex by pinching over the bones of the digit, and then the extensor reflex by digital stimulation of the plantar/palmar aspect of the paw in each limb to produce stepping movements.

This process does take a little practice but is not hard to learn. The same exercise can be accomplished with a cart for support and a human land treadmill. The patient's paws should be protected because of the non-slip surface on the treadmill. This exercise can be performed for 5–10 minutes twice a day. As the patient begins to regain voluntary motor function, or in some cases learns to walk reflexively, the muscle groups will start to contract without external stimulation. At this point, assistance should be provided for correct movement and placement of the affected limbs.

As the patient progresses and their need for assistance decreases, the speed of the treadmill and the duration of the exercises can slowly be increased (see **Underwater treadmill** clip on DVD). Correct placement of the paws and limb coordination should be maintained at all times to ensure that the patient does not develop 'bad habits' (e.g. 'bunny hopping' with both hindlimbs together).

Once a fast walk is reached, the amount of support provided by the cart or water can be decreased whilst decreasing the speed of the treadmill. Correct cadence to the walk should always be encouraged. The patient should not be allowed to trot, pace or gallop until late in the rehabilitative process (i.e. well advanced in the proprioceptive neuromuscular training). Animals are masters at compensation and bad habits are easy to develop and hard to correct.

Hydrotherapy in the form of swimming can be a very effective means of enhancing strength and coordination in the recovering dog. In general, this is started between 7 and 14 days following surgery to allow time for the incision to heal. Life jackets for dogs can be purchased to provide extra support (see Figure 25.11) and owners can swim their dogs either in the bathtub (if a small animal) or in a swimming pool, lake or even the sea.

- When starting in the bathtub, the patient should be able to touch the bottom at first before progressing to swimming.
- The patient can be encouraged to swim the length of the tub by offering treats or playing with a ball.
- As for other exercises, the duration of swimming is dictated by each animal.
- When the animal appears fatigued, the exercise should be discontinued (if they are unable to perform to the same level the next day, the duration of exercise should be reduced or taken to every other day until endurance has improved).

It is important that owners only attempt to place their pet in water if they have the capability to get the animal in and out of the water safely. Thus, large non-ambulatory dogs need to undergo therapy at a specialized facility where adequate slings and lifts are available (Figure 25.14).

Proprioceptive neuromuscular training
This term describes the exercises used to enhance the patient's awareness and use of their limbs at rest and in motion (Figure 25.15). Typically, patients do not start these exercises until they are

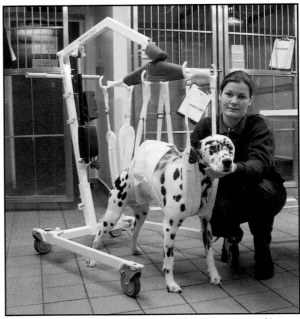

25.14 A mechanical hoist enables movement of large patients into and out of bathing facilities.

able to bear a significant portion of weight and can walk with some assistance. The author [JS] has had success introducing exercises in the following order:

1. Balance of weight in a stationary position.
2. Balance of weight in a stationary position with methods used to throw the patient off balance (i.e. wobble board, physical pressure, waves, closed cell foam mat on top of water).
3. Patient lifting limbs over obstacles whilst walking in a straight line (height of obstacles and distance between them can be increased and decreased, respectively, as the patient progresses) (see **Caveletti** clip on DVD).
4. Off-balance walking – patient walks in straight line whilst the clinician throws the patient off balance using pressure or a theraband sling.
5. Weaving in and out of cones – start with a distance between the cones at least equal to the distance between the thoracic and pelvic limbs (as the patient improves decrease the distance between the cones) (see **Weaving clip** on DVD).
6. Patient lifting limbs over obstacles in a circular fashion (similar to a wagon wheel) – start with four to six objects; make sure the patient performs the exercise in both clockwise and anticlockwise directions.
7. Patient performs previously mentioned drills with increased stimulation on affected limbs (e.g. boots, band around the ankle).
8. Patient performs the above exercises after a level of fatigue is reached with another type of exercise.

The aim of these exercises is to enhance correct paw placement and coordination. Many of these exercises can be supervised at home by the owner if they are shown what to do.

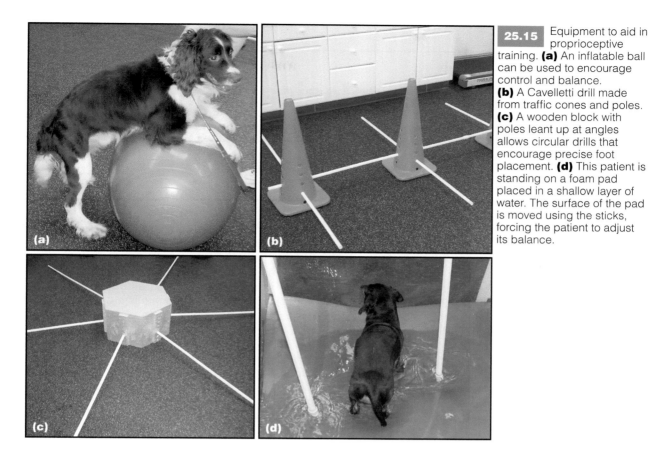

25.15 Equipment to aid in proprioceptive training. **(a)** An inflatable ball can be used to encourage control and balance. **(b)** A Cavelletti drill made from traffic cones and poles. **(c)** A wooden block with poles leant up at angles allows circular drills that encourage precise foot placement. **(d)** This patient is standing on a foam pad placed in a shallow layer of water. The surface of the pad is moved using the sticks, forcing the patient to adjust its balance.

Summary

Devising an appropriate plan for physical rehabilitation is a critical component of treating patients recovering from or with ongoing neurological disease. Animals with severe injuries (i.e. non-ambulatory animals) greatly benefit from rehabilitation at a dedicated centre, where their general management can be achieved more easily and they can benefit from the use of specialist equipment, such as underwater treadmills. However, exercises such as PROM, cone drills and swimming can be completed by the owner at home without difficulty. Appropriate care of the animal's overall health and wellbeing improves the response to therapy and it is important to understand that the rehabilitative process should start immediately after injury or surgery.

References and further reading

Available on accompanying DVD

DVD extras

- Caveletti
- Passive range of motion
- Sit to stand
- Underwater treadmill
- Weaving
- Weight shift

26

Treatment of neurological disorders with traditional Chinese veterinary medicine

Cheryl L. Chrisman

Traditional Chinese veterinary medicine (TCVM) includes acupuncture, Chinese herbal medicines, *Tui-na* (manual therapy) and food therapy. The primary effects of TCVM treatments in disease are to relieve clinical signs, restore normal physiological functions and promote recovery. These treatments can also be used to maintain normal homeostasis for disease prevention. The TCVM treatments are emerging therapies that may be integrated with conventional treatments or used alone for neurological disorders of animals. This discussion will focus on acupuncture and Chinese herbal medicines, because there is currently more scientific validation for these treatments in humans and animals.

Acupoints and channels

Acupuncture points (acupoints) are small areas, usually a few millimetres in size and located beneath the surface of the skin (Figures 26.1 to 26.3) (Xie and Preast, 2002, 2007). The acupoints can be located with an ohm-meter, as they have low electrical resistance compared to the surrounding areas. Anatomical structures around acupoints include free and specialized nerve endings, small arterioles, veins, connective tissue and tissue mast cells (Figure 26.4). Although all of these structures may play a role in the mechanism of action of acupuncture, the nervous system plays a predominant role. Activation of specific brain regions, unique to the particular acupoint, can be observed on magnetic resonance imaging (MRI) during acupoint stimulation (Xie and Preast, 2007). Acupoints are located at motor points (nerve endings within muscles), along superficial nerves and their branches, at bony foramen and fascial regions where nerves enter and exit (Kline *et al.*, 2001; Xie and Preast, 2007). Acupoint stimulation can alter the physiological functions and blood supply of local and distant tissues via spinal cord reflexes involving sensory afferents and somatic and visceral efferents, as well as ascending and descending pathways in the spinal cord and brain (Figure 26.4).

Approximately 361 acupoints have been transposed from humans and horses to dogs. Related

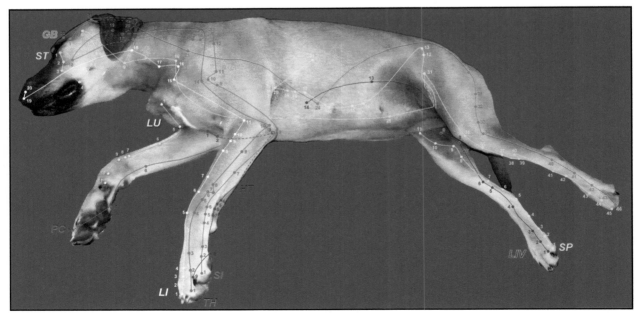

26.1 A ventrolateral view of the locations and commonly treated acupoints of the lung (LU), large intestine (LI), stomach (ST), spleen (SP), heart (HT), small intestine (SI), triple heater (TH) and gallbladder (GB) channels of a dog. Acupoints are numbered consecutively from the beginning of the channel to the end. All of these channels are bilateral. Chinese herbs produce their effects through one or more of these channels. LIV = liver; PC = pericardium. (Reprinted with permission from The Chi Institute, Reddick, FL, www.tcvm.com)

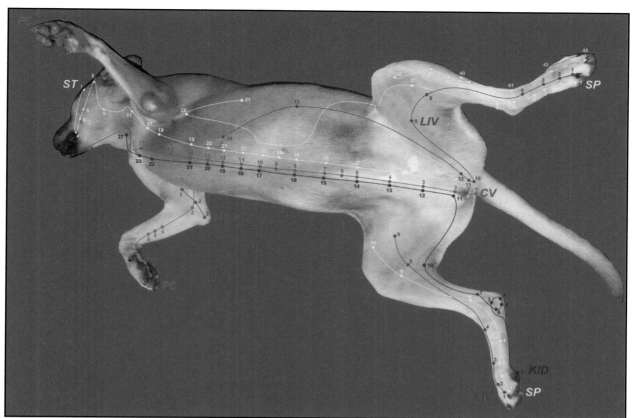

26.2 A ventral and medial view of the locations and commonly treated acupoints of the pericardium (PC), medial heart (HT), stomach (ST), spleen (SP), kidney (KID), liver (LIV) and conception vessel (CV) channels of a dog. Acupoints are numbered consecutively from the beginning of the channel to the end. All these channels are bilateral except for the conception vessel, which courses along the ventral midline. Chinese herbs produce their effects through one or more of these channels. (Reprinted with permission from The Chi Institute, Reddick, FL, www.tcvm.com)

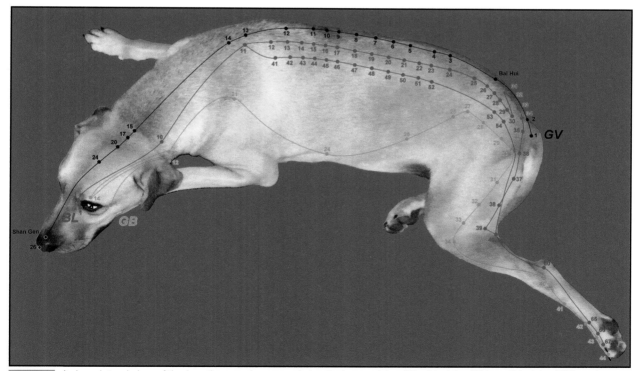

26.3 A dorsolateral view of the locations and commonly treated acupoints of the bladder (BL), gallbladder (GB) and governing vessel (GV) channels. Acupoints are numbered consecutively from the beginning of the channel to the end. Throughout the thoracolumbar region the bladder channel has two lines one more medial to the other. The bladder and gallbladder channels are bilateral and the governing vessel courses along the dorsal midline. Chinese herbs produce their effects through one or more of these channels. (Reprinted with permission from The Chi Institute, Reddick, FL, www.tcvm.com)

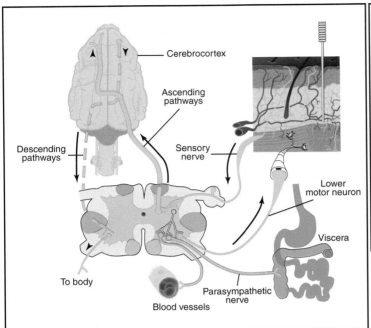
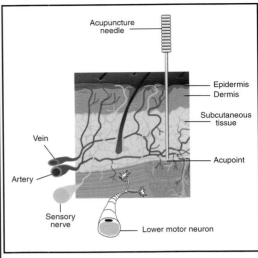

26.4 Most acupoints are located beneath the dermis and subcutaneous regions at the fascia and muscle interface near neurovascular connective tissue bundles or motor points. Some of the effects of acupuncture are associated with sensory nerve stimulation that evokes reflexes via somatic motor and autonomic (sympathetic and parasympathetic) nerves. Systemic effects are in part due to stimulation of ascending and descending pathways in the spinal cord and brain, which produce generalized neurohumoral effects.

transpositional acupoints follow lines referred to as channels (meridians) located along fascial and muscle planes near the surface of the body (see Figures 26.1 to 26.3). Twelve paired channels correspond to each of the 12 TCVM organ systems and contain different numbers of acupoints (Figure 26.5). These acupoints are named according to their channel and number (e.g. kidney 3 or KID-3 is the third acupoint on the kidney channel). Two other unpaired channels, the governing vessel on the dorsal midline and the conception vessel on the ventral midline, also contain acupoints commonly used for disease treatment and prevention (see Figures 26.2 and 26.5).

Channel	Abbreviation	Number of acupoints	Name of acupoints	Location
Lung	LU	9	LU-1 through LU-9	Begins in the superficial pectoral muscle, courses along the medial thoracic limb and ends on the medial aspect of the 1st digit nail bed
Large intestine	LI	20	LI-1 through LI-20	Begins on the medial aspect of the 3rd digit nail bed of the thoracic limb, courses along the lateral aspect of the limb, shoulder and neck and ends on the nose
Stomach	ST	45	ST-1 through ST-45	Begins on the orbital rim, ventral to the eye, courses along the ventral aspect of the body and the cranial lateral aspect of pelvic limb and ends on the lateral aspect of the 3rd digit nail bed
Spleen	SP	21	SP-1 through SP-21	Begins on the medial aspect of the 2nd digit nail bed of the pelvic limb, courses along the medial aspect of the limb and ends on the thorax at the seventh intercostal space level with the shoulder
Heart	HT	9	HT-1 through HT-9	Begins in the centre of the axillary space, courses along the medial aspect of the thoracic limb and ends on the medial aspect of the 5th digit nail bed
Small intestine	SI	19	SI-1 through SI-19	Begins on the lateral aspect of the 5th digit nail bed of the thoracic limb, courses along the lateral aspect of the thoracic limb and neck and ends just cranial to the tragus (auricular cartilage)
Bladder	BL	67	BL-1 through BL-67	Begins at the medial canthus of the eye, courses over the top of the head, along the dorsolateral aspect of the neck and body and the caudolateral aspect of the pelvic limb and ends on the lateral aspect of the 5th digit nail bed

26.5 The names, abbreviations, number of acupoints and basic location of the 14 traditional Chinese veterinary medicine channels in dogs and cats. (continues) ▶

Channel	Abbreviation	Number of acupoints	Name of acupoints	Location
Kidney	KID	27	KID-1 through KID-27	Begins under the large central pad of the pelvic limb paw, courses along the medial aspect of the pelvic limb, ventrolateral thorax and ends off the ventral midline between the sternum and 1st rib
Pericardium	PC	9	PC-1 through PC-9	Begins medial to the elbow in the 5th intercostal space, courses along the medial aspect of the thoracic limb and ends on the medial aspect of the 4th digit nail bed
Triple heater	TH	23	TH-1 through TH-23	Begins at the lateral aspect of the 4th digit nail bed of the thoracic limb, courses along the lateral aspect of the limb and neck and ends on the rim of the orbit at the end of the eyebrow, were it extended to the lateral canthus
Gallbladder	GB	44	GB-1 through GB-44	Begins at the lateral canthus of the eye, courses back and forth between the ear and eyebrow then along the ventrolateral aspect of the thorax and the lateral aspect of the pelvic limb and ends on the lateral aspect of the 4th digit nail bed
Liver	LIV	14	LIV-1 through LIV-14	Begins on the lateral side of the 2nd digit nail bed of the pelvic limb, courses along the medial aspect of the limb and the ventrolateral aspect of the thorax and ends at the 6th intercostal space at the costochondral junction
Governing vessel	GV	28	GV-1 through GV-28	Begins between the tail base and anus, courses along the dorsal midline and ends on the inside of the lip
Conception vessel	CV	24	CV-1 through CV-24	Begins between the anus and vulva or scrotum, courses along the ventral midline and ends at the lower lip margin

26.5 (continued) The names, abbreviations, number of acupoints and basic location of the 14 traditional Chinese veterinary medicine channels in dogs and cats.

There are 77 classical acupoints in dogs that are not associated with a specific channel but have Chinese names and specific locations and actions; they are often used during acupuncture treatment to achieve certain effects. For example, the classical acupoint *Da-feng-men* (Great Wind Gate) is located on the midline, level with the cranial edge of the ear bases, and is used to treat seizures (Figure 26.6).

The channels, containing the acupoints used for treatment, represent only the exterior portion of an intricate web of connecting channel branches that communicate with all organs, tissues and cells.

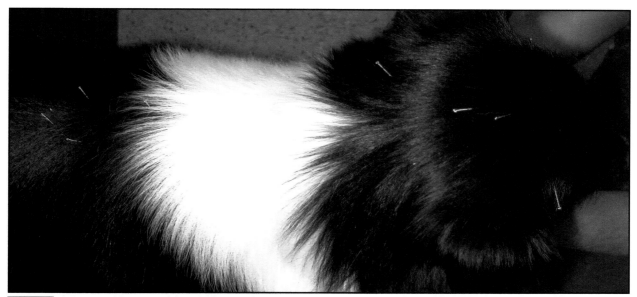

26.6 A 3-year-old neutered female Border Collie with intermittent uncontrollable seizures for the past year receiving dry needle acupuncture of acupoints known to control epilepsy and resolve her underlying TCVM pattern. Acupoints being treated that are visible in the picture (from cranial to caudal) are: the classical acupoints *Nao-shu* (bilateral, one-third of the distance along a line from the cranial edge of the ears and the lateral canthus of the eye), *Da-feng-men* (on the midline at the cranial edge of the ears) and transpositional acupoints GV-20 (midline), GB-20 (bilateral), GV-14 (midline) and bilateral BL-17 and BL-18. The dog also received the Chinese herbal medicines *di tang tong* and *yang yin xi feng*. Historically the dog was being treated with phenobarbital and potassium bromide at serum-confirmed therapeutic levels, but was still having partial seizures two or three times a month, lasting up to 30 minutes in duration. She was also sedated, ataxic and had lost her lust for life. The combination of acupuncture and Chinese herbal medicines improved the seizure control and allowed a reduction in her anticonvulsant medication. The sedation and ataxia resolved and she returned to her normal personality and activity level.

Since the 1970s, studies utilizing acoustic recordings, scintigraphy, electrical recordings, thermography, various tissue-specific dyes, confocal scanning and electron microscopy, computed tomography (CT) and MRI have provided insights into the structure and function of the channels and their network of collateral branches (*Jing Luo* system) in humans and animals (Chrisman and Xie, 2011). During an acupuncture treatment, acupoints may be stimulated with needles alone, needles with electrical stimulation, needles with heat or heat alone (moxibustion), low level impulse lasers, injections of substances such as vitamin B12 or implantation of substances (e.g. gold beads).

Chinese herbal medicines

Advanced training and experience in the use of Chinese herbal medicines for animals is essential prior to their use (Chi Institute, 2011; IVAS, 2011). Approximately 150 herbs with known actions are most commonly used in veterinary practice (Xie and Preast, 2010). Each Chinese herb affects one or more of the 12 paired channels (see Figures 26.1 to 26.3). Chinese herbs are usually combined, using specific regulations and guidelines for herb compatibility, to create formulas that enhance their individual effects and reduce potential toxicity. Chinese herbal medicines (specific herbal formulas) are then classified by the actions they produce from a TCVM perspective and prescribed for a specific TCVM pattern diagnosis (see below). There are approximately 200 Chinese herbal formulas used to treat different TCVM patterns in dogs and cats. These are usually administered orally as loose or encapsulated powder, concentrated extracts formulated into small pills (tea pills) or chewable biscuits (Xie and Preast, 2010). Chinese herbal medicines are often combined with acupuncture to achieve a longer lasting acupuncture effect or may be used alone (Xie and Preast, 2002). The effects of acupuncture usually occur within 1–48 hours of treatment, while many of the Chinese herbal medicines require 1–2 weeks to produce an effect. The combination of acupuncture and Chinese herbal medicines may lead to more rapid, longer-acting and synergistic effects than either treatment alone. For the long-term management of chronic conditions, fewer acupuncture treatments may be needed, if animals are also maintained on the appropriate Chinese herbal medicines.

Conventional and TCVM pattern diagnoses

To understand TCVM and use acupuncture and Chinese herbal medicines most effectively, veterinary surgeons must receive advanced training in the principles, diagnosis and treatment techniques of this paradigm of medicine. Besides a conventional diagnosis (e.g. intervertebral disc disease or epilepsy), the TCVM-trained veterinary surgeon also makes a pattern diagnosis or *Bian zheng*, applying five TCVM and traditional Chinese medicine (TCM) theories (Xie and Preast, 2002; Maciocia, 2005):

- Yin/Yang
- Eight Principles
- Five Elements
- Five Treasures
- *Zang Fu* physiology and pathology.

Applying these theories, a TCVM pattern diagnosis is made, based on the historical and physical examination findings and alterations in tongue and pulse parameters. The TCVM practitioner will then develop a treatment strategy to relieve the clinical signs associated with the conventional diagnosis and also treat the underlying pattern diagnosis ('root' cause) from a TCVM perspective. The acupoints, Chinese herbal medicines, *Tui-na* techniques and additional food selected are based on the TCVM pattern diagnoses (Xie and Preast, 2002, 2007, 2010; Xie *et al.*, 2007; Basko, 2009).

Some dogs with the same clinical signs and conventional diagnosis (e.g. paraparesis from intervertebral disc protrusion) have completely different underlying TCVM pattern diagnoses, which require treatment of different acupoints, Chinese herbal medicines, *Tui-na* techniques or types of food (Xie and Preast, 2002, 2007, 2010; Xie *et al.*, 2007; Basko, 2009).

If incorrect acupoints are treated, the animal is unlikely to be harmed but the treatment may not be effective. If the incorrect Chinese herbal medicine is prescribed, there may be adverse reactions. Initially many TCVM terms and concepts may be meaningless or confusing to veterinary surgeons with only conventional training, but with further study of the Chinese paradigm, a deeper and expanded understanding of disease prevention, the response of individual bodies to disease and the inter-relationships of organ systems in health and disease can be appreciated.

The evolution of TCVM

Like conventional medicine, TCM and TCVM have evolved over the past approximately 2500 years with increased experience, knowledge and scientific evaluation. Although used to treat diseases of royal horses for over a thousand years, acupuncture and Chinese herbal medicines have only been commonly used to treat small companion animal diseases since the 1950s. Clinical interest and research in TCM and TCVM treatments have increased exponentially, as novel treatments for untreatable diseases and treatments with less adverse side effects have been sought. In 1958, the Institute of Traditional Chinese Veterinary Medicine (ITCVM) was founded in Lanzhou, China, as a national research institution managed by the Chinese Academy of Agricultural Sciences and China's Ministry of Agriculture. Researchers at the ITCVM have published over 4200 scientific papers and 128 books, and some have been translated into English.

The International Veterinary Acupuncture Society (IVAS), currently located in Fort Collins, Colorado, was established in 1974 because of growing interest in acupuncture in the USA. As of late 2010, IVAS membership was 1900 veterinary surgeons, including members in a subsidiary group, the American Academy of Veterinary Acupuncture (AAVA). IVAS membership includes 635 veterinary surgeons outside the USA, including 45 members from the UK (IVAS, 2011). The Association of British Veterinary Acupuncturists (ABVA) was formed in 1987 and, as of late 2010, had 96 members. The Chi Institute of Chinese Medicine was established in Reddick, Florida, in 1998 for TCVM training in acupuncture, Chinese herbal medicine, Tui-na and food therapy, patterned after the TCVM curriculum of colleges in China. Conventional veterinary surgeons can find potential training programmes and the names and contact information for acupuncturists in various locations online. The American Association of Traditional Chinese Veterinary Medicine (AATCVM) was founded in Gainesville, Florida, in 2006, to provide a forum for TCVM practitioners to share case questions, promote, support and publish TCVM research and develop standardized evidence-based practices. *The American Journal of Traditional Chinese Veterinary Medicine* was also established in 2006 as a peer-reviewed scientific journal to publish TCVM research and further support the development of evidence-based TCVM.

The increasing worldwide interest in acupuncture and Chinese herbal medicine research in all species is reflected in PubMed, the US Library of Medicine database, which by mid 2011 had listed over 16,480 acupuncture references, mostly from the past 15 years. Research interest in Chinese herbal medicine has also increased and by mid 2011 there were over 11,500 Chinese herbal medicine references on the PubMed database. High quality veterinary research of TCVM treatments is still lagging far behind human TCM research, but much of the basic science research has been performed in laboratory animals, so may be applicable to the treatment of naturally occurring diseases of dogs and cats.

By 2010, approximately 4300 US veterinary surgeons had received training in acupuncture, which is 6% of the estimated number of practicing US veterinarians (Chrisman and Xie, 2010). Of the 28 American Veterinary Medical Association (AVMA) accredited US Colleges of Veterinary Medicine, 50% (14/28) have one or more faculty using acupuncture and other TCVM treatments integrated with conventional therapies or as sole therapy for the treatment of animal disease (Chrisman and Xie, 2010). More research of TCVM treatments for naturally occurring animal diseases should be forthcoming from these institutions and the increasing number of TCVM practitioners.

An in-depth discussion of the prevention, diagnosis and specific treatments of neurological disorders from a TCVM perspective is beyond the scope of this text. Instead an overview will be presented of some of the research that justifies referral of patients to TCVM practitioners and further research evaluation

of this paradigm of medicine. Conventional veterinary surgeons will then know what types of neurological disorders might benefit from referral to a veterinary surgeon who has training and expertise in acupuncture, Chinese herbal medicines and other TCVM treatments (Figure 26.7).

Clinical signs	Conventional diagnoses
Neck or back pain	Intervertebral disc disease Vertebral degeneration Discospondylitis Meningitis Vertebral and meningeal neoplasia
Acute tetraparesis, tetraplegia, paraparesis or paraplegia	Intervertebral disc disease Trauma Fibrocartilaginous embolism Meningomyelitis Atlantoaxial subluxation Acute polyradiculoneuritis Myasthenia gravis Polymyositis
Chronic progressive ataxia (spinal cord), tetraparesis, paraparesis, paraplegia	Intervertebral disc degeneration Caudal cervical spondylomyelopathy (Wobbler syndrome) Degenerative myelopathy Vertebral malformations Myelitis Spinal cord and vertebral neoplasia Polyneuropathies Polymyopathies
Monoparesis or monoplegia	Brachial plexus injury Sciatic nerve injury Brachial plexus neoplasia
Seizures	Idiopathic epilepsy Hydrocephalus Meningoencephalitis Hepatic encephalopathy Cerebrovascular disorders Brain tumours
Facial nerve paralysis	Idiopathic paralysis Otitis media/interna Trauma
Heat tilt, nystagmus and dysequilibrium	Otitis interna Idiopathic vestibular syndrome Trauma Iatrogenic from ear cleaning Ototoxicity Neoplasia
Deafness	Inner ear infection Senile degeneration Idiopathic deafness
Stupor or coma	Head injury Cerebrovascular accidents (stroke) Resuscitation Cognitive dysfunction Brain tumours Hydrocephalus Meningoencephalitis

26.7 The neurological disorders by clinical signs that might benefit from acupuncture and/or Chinese herbal medicines integrated with conventional treatments or as sole therapies.

TCVM treatment of neurological disorders

Cervical and thoracolumbar pain

Pain associated with intervertebral disc disease, vertebral degeneration (including osteophyte formation and synovial cysts), discospondylitis, spondylitis, meningitis and vertebral and meningeal neoplasia are common clinical complaints in small animal practice. Electro-acupuncture (EA) is the application of an electrical stimulus to the specialized needles inserted into the acupoints (Kline *et al.*, 2001; Xie and Preast, 2007). For pain relief, EA is more effective than acupuncture needles alone (Janssens, 2001; WHO, 2003; Xie and Preast, 2007; Fu *et al.*, 2009; Laim *et al.*, 2009; Cantwell, 2010; Horton and Macpherson, 2010; Kenney, 2010).

In a 2003 analysis of controlled human clinical trials, the World Health Organization (WHO) concluded that there was enough scientific support to recommend acupuncture for cervical, lumbar and postoperative pain (WHO, 2003). In a 2010 meta-analysis of human clinical randomized controlled trials (RCTs), EA was shown to be more effective than placebo controls for lumbar, knee and headache pain (Horton and Macpherson, 2010). The analgesic efficacy of acupuncture for cervical pain was again confirmed after another meta-analysis of human clinical RCTs (Fu *et al.*, 2009). Significant pain reduction was reported in two clinical RCTs of acupuncture and thoracolumbar pain of sport horses (Kenney, 2010).

Acupuncture, integrated with conventional treatments or as a sole therapy, has been reported to control pain associated with intervertebral disc disease in dogs (Janssens, 2001; Kline *et al.*, 2001; Xie and Preast, 2007). Conventional drug dosages may be reduced and adverse side effects of drugs and surgery avoided when EA is integrated into pain management strategies. A significant reduction in the severity of postoperative pain has been reported for humans receiving acupuncture before and after lumbar disc surgery (WHO, 2003; Horton and Macpherson, 2010). In a small study of 15 dogs undergoing hemilaminectomy, half received EA postoperatively (Laim *et al.*, 2009). The total dose of fentanyl administered was lower in the first 12 hours and pain scores were less at 36 hours for the EA group compared to the conventionally treated group. Clinical RCTs with larger numbers of animals are warranted to evaluate the effect of EA on postoperative pain.

The mechanisms of EA pain control primarily involve the stimulation of peripheral sensory afferent nerves that modulate the activity of nuclei in the central nervous system (see Figure 26.4) (Cantwell, 2010; Kenney, 2010). At the spinal cord level, inhibitory encephalinergic internuncial neurons are stimulated, which blocks incoming C fibre pain impulses and reduces substance P. There is also inhibition of neurons that transmit pain signals to higher brain centres. The effects of EA on the hypothalamic–pituitary axis can be visualized using MRI. Hypothalamic effects of EA result in increased circulating

β-endorphin. Midbrain periaqueductal grey matter effects include the release of β-endorphin, encephalin and dynorphin. Alterations in serotonergic descending inhibitory pain pathways are also an important part of the mechanism of EA analgesia (Cantwell, 2010; Kenney, 2010).

The effects of EA appear to be cumulative and after several EA treatments, depending on the diagnosis, conventional medication may be reduced or discontinued and only intermittent EA may be needed to control pain (Figure 26.8) (Kline *et al.*, 2001; Xie and Preast, 2002, 2007). In acute discospondylitis, spondylitis and meningitis, EA can be combined with antibiotics, non-steroidal anti-inflammatory drugs, corticosteroids or other conventional medications to control pain and treat the disorder (Kline *et al.*, 2001; Xie and Preast, 2002, 2007).

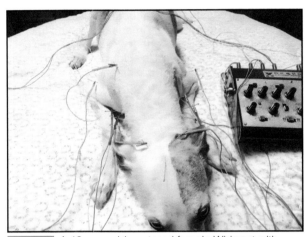

26.8 A 12-year-old neutered female Whippet with suspected cervical intervertebral disc disease receiving EA at GB-20/GB-21, SI-9/SI-16 and bilateral classical acupoints *Jing-jia-ji* (between the cervical vertebrae, above and below the transverse processes) to relieve neck pain, and dry needle acupuncture of other acupoints to treat the underlying TCVM pattern that has caused insidiously progressive ataxia and tetraparesis of approximately 6–9 months' duration. The dog also received the Chinese herbal medicines *Bu yang huan wu* and Cervical Formula (www.tcvm.com) orally twice daily and occasional *Shen tong zu yu tong* for pain if needed. The dog has never received corticosteroids, non-steroidal anti-inflammatory drugs or other conventional pain medication. With EA every 4–6 weeks and the Chinese herbal medicines, the pain is controlled and the neurological deficits have improved to a mild intermittent ataxia for the past year. The dog has an excellent quality of life and further diagnostic tests or surgical intervention have not been required. (See also **Acupuncture** clip on DVD)

TCVM practitioners often combine EA with Chinese herbal medicines and *Tui-na* for the long-term management of chronic pain (Xie and Preast, 2002, 2007, 2010). In a study of human patients with cervical pain, the Chinese herbal medicine *Bi tong xiao* was shown to increase encephalins significantly, as well as reducing substance P in the plasma; pain was also reduced compared with control patients (Li *et al.*, 2001). The Chinese herbal medicine *Qi shen wan* was shown to relieve cervical pain more effectively than a placebo in two human clinical trials of 680 patients with cervical intervertebral disc disease (Cui *et al.*, 2010). In another human clinical RCT of 60 patients with cervical pain from intervertebral disc disease, a Chinese herbal medicine containing *Huang qi* (Astragalus), *Dang shen* (Codonopsis), *San qi* (Notoginseng), *Chuan xiong* (Ligusticum), *Lu jiao jiao* (Cervus) and *Zhi mu* (Anemarrhena) relieved pain more effectively than meloxicam or mecobalamin (B12) (Cui *et al.*, 2010). *Shen tong zhu yu* and *Bu yang huan wu* are two commonly used Chinese herbal medicines reported to reduce cervical and thoracolumbar pain in dogs (see Figure 26.8), but further clinical RCTs are needed (Xie and Preast, 2002, 2007, 2010).

Prevention of progressive vertebral and intervertebral disc degeneration is a research priority in humans and preliminary studies indicate that Chinese herbal medicines may be useful to prevent or slow the progression in humans and laboratory animals (Liang *et al.*, 2010). Future research will focus on the effects of Chinese herbal medicines not only to reduce pain, but to enhance collagen synthesis in the intervertebral discs, inhibit disc degeneration, promote the resorption of herniated nucleus pulposus and epidural hemorrhage, prevent nerve cell apoptosis and promote nerve cell regeneration (Lin and Chen, 2007).

Although other disorders causing pain have been treated clinically there are no reports of outcomes for dogs and cats. In human and laboratory animal RCTs, acupuncture has been shown to reduce the pain and neurological deficits associated with diabetic polyneuropathy (Tong *et al.*, 2010). Many cats with diabetes mellitus exhibit signs of pain, appear to be irritated when touched and also develop tarsal weakness; investigation of the use of EA and Chinese herbal medicines to reduce this pain and paresis, and improve quality of life, is therefore warranted (Kline *et al.*, 2001; Xie and Preast, 2002, 2007, 2010).

Acute tetraparesis, tetraplegia, paraparesis and paraplegia

Acute tetraparesis, tetraplegia, paraparesis and paraplegia are associated with spinal cord insults from many different aetiologies (see Figure 26.7). Spinal cord injury from external trauma or acute intervertebral disc herniation is common in dogs and cats. A well known secondary cascade of neurodegenerative processes occurs within the first 72 hours following spinal cord trauma, and research of methods to inhibit or reduce this response has been the focus of attention for many decades (Choi *et al.*, 2010). The benefits and mechanisms of EA to reduce neuronal and glial cell death and axonal loss and improve functional recovery have been demonstrated in many laboratory animal RCTs (Shin *et al.*, 2009; Choi *et al.*, 2010). In five human clinical RCTs of recovery following acute spinal injury, patients receiving EA integrated with conventional drugs and rehabilitation had significantly increased recovery rates compared to those receiving only conventional drugs and rehabilitation (Shin *et al.*, 2009). Further well designed studies are needed to confirm these findings.

In an RCT of experimental spinal cord compression, 20 paraplegic dogs with preserved nociception were divided into four treatment groups to monitor recovery time using daily neurological examinations and somatosensory evoked potentials (Yang *et al.*, 2003). One group received only corticosteroids, one only EA, one a combination of corticosteroids and EA, and one no treatment. Groups receiving only corticosteroids or EA recovered significantly faster than the group receiving no treatment, but were not significantly different from each other. The group receiving a combination of corticosteroids and EA recovered significantly faster than all other groups. Evaluation of EA in larger numbers of dogs is needed to confirm the findings of this pilot study.

Neurological improvement of dogs and cats with spinal cord injury and fibrocartilaginous embolism, treated with acupuncture and Chinese herbal medicines, has been primarily anecdotal, but there have been three recent clinical trials involving a total of 170 dogs with intervertebral disc disease (Figure 26.9) (Kline *et al.*, 2001; Xie and Preast, 2002, 2007, 2010; Hayashi and Matera, 2007; Han *et al.*, 2010; Joaquim *et al.*, 2010). The effect of EA on recovery was evaluated in one clinical RCT of 50 dogs with neurological deficits from confirmed intervertebral disc disease (Hayashi and Matera, 2007). Neurological deficits were graded using a standard severity scale from 1 to 5 (e.g. grade 1= pain only, grade 2= ataxia and paraparesis, grade 3= non-ambulatory paraparesis, grade 4= paraplegia with nociception and grade 5= paraplegia with absent nociception). All dogs were treated with tapering doses of prednisone and one group also received EA weekly or bi-weekly (dogs with grade 5 neurological deficits). The time to recover ambulation in seven dogs with grade 3 and 4 deficits treated with EA was significantly less than that for nine similarly affected dogs not receiving EA. Nociception and the ability to ambulate without assistance was regained in 50% (3/6) of dogs, with grade 5 dysfunction, treated with EA and 12.5% (1/8) of dogs in the control group, although the difference was not statistically significant.

Recovery with and without EA was also compared in another study of 40 dogs with grade 4 or 5 neurological deficits associated with intervertebral disc herniation (Joaquim *et al.*, 2010). All dogs received conventional treatment with tapering doses of prednisone, but were also treated with surgery, surgery plus EA, or EA alone. Recovery rate (grade 4 or 5 becoming grade 1–2 within 6 months) was significantly higher for dogs treated with EA alone (15/19) and EA plus surgery (8/11) than for dogs that had only had surgery (4/10). The investigators concluded that if early surgical intervention was not possible, dogs with grade 4 or 5 neurological deficits might benefit from tapering doses of prednisone and EA.

The effects of EA and needles alone (dry needle acupuncture, AP) were compared in a retrospective study of 80 paraplegic dogs with intact nociception associated with intervertebral disc disease (Han *et al.*, 2010). The time to achieve back pain relief

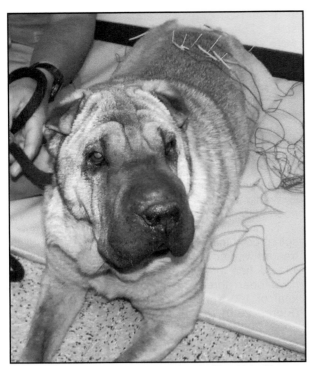

26.9 An 8-year-old neutered male Shar Pei with acute paraplegia from a suspected L1–L2 fibrocartilaginous embolism of the spinal cord, diagnosed with MRI, receiving EA. Acupoints visible in the picture include the classical acupoints *Bai-hui* (midline at the lumbosacral space) and *Hua-tuo-jia-ji* (in the intervertebral space just lateral to the midline) and transpositional acupoints BL-54 and BL-23. Other acupoints were treated with EA, dry needle acupuncture and aqua-acupuncture and *Tui-na* and physical therapy were also administered. The dog received a modification of the herbal formula *Da huo luo dan* (Double P II (www.tcvm.com)) orally twice daily. By 4 months after the onset of clinical signs, the dog was ambulatory with residual slightly decreased conscious proprioception greater on the left than right side. (Reprinted with permission from: Medina C (2010) An integrative approach for the treatment of suspected fibrocartilaginous embolism of the spinal cord in a dog. *American Journal of Traditional Chinese Veterinary Medicine* **5**(2), 55–60)

and recover (ambulation), along with recovery and relapse rates were compared for a group receiving prednisone alone (n=37) and a group receiving prednisone plus EA and AP (n=43). Dogs receiving prednisone plus EA and AP had a significantly shorter time to achieve pain relief and ambulation, a better overall recovery rate and fewer relapses than dogs treated with prednisone alone. The overall number of dogs in each group of the three studies was low and further studies with larger groups of dogs are needed (Hayashi and Matera, 2007; Han *et al.*, 2010; Joaquim *et al.*, 2010). However, there is enough evidence to support referral for TCVM treatment for larger clinical studies of the effects of EA, integrated with conventional treatments and rehabilitation, on the recovery of dogs and cats from spinal cord injury.

Stem cell transplantation to enhance spinal cord regeneration is currently being investigated (Sun *et al.*, 2009). Stem cell differentiation may be

affected by EA and the combination of EA and stem cell transplantation may prove to be superior to stem cell transplantation alone (Sun *et al.*, 2009; Yan *et al.*, 2010). In a recent laboratory animal spinal cord injury RCT, the group that had mesenchymal stem cell (MSC) implantation plus EA had significantly higher numbers of neuron-like cells, oligodendrocyte-like cells and 5-hydroxytryptophan-positive nerve fibres than groups receiving only MSC implantation, EA alone or no treatment (Yan *et al.*, 2010).

Acute and chronic bladder dysfunction is often associated with spinal cord injury in dogs and cats. In a spinal cord injury laboratory animal RCT, EA reduced detrusor hyperreflexia compared to controls (Yu *et al.*, 2010). Positive effects of EA on recovery of bladder function after spinal cord injury has been reported in two human clinical RCTs (Shin *et al.*, 2009). Improvement of faecal incontinence with EA has also been reported in humans (Scaglia *et al.*, 2009). The use of EA to manage bladder and bowel dysfunction of dogs and cats following spinal cord insults from intervertebral disc disease, external trauma, fibrocartilaginous emboli and other aetiologies should be further evaluated.

The effects of Chinese herbal medicines on spinal cord regeneration and functional recovery following injury have also been studied. The Chinese herbal medicine *Bu yang huan wu* has been used for hundreds of years in China to treat human paralysis and for approximately the past 25 years in dogs (see Figure 26.8) (Chen *et al.*, 2008). *Bu yang huan wu* has recently been shown to enhance neuronal regeneration and reduce damage from ischaemia/reperfusion in rat spinal cord trauma models (Chen *et al.*, 2008; Wang and Jiang, 2009). The Chinese herbal medicines *Sheng mai san* and *Sui fu kang* have been reported to reduce the size of spinal cord lesions and increase many biological parameters that indicate spinal cord regeneration and axonal regrowth in spinal injury laboratory animal RCTs (Huang *et al.*, 2007; Seo *et al.*, 2009). There is currently no other research on the use of EA and Chinese herbal medicines for the other aetiologies of acute tetraparesis, tetraplegia, paraparesis and paraplegia in animals, but anecdotal accounts of their positive effects justify further investigation (Kline *et al.*, 2001; Xie and Preast, 2002, 2007, 2010).

Chronic progressive ataxia, tetraparesis and paraparesis

Chronic progressive ataxia, paraparesis, paraplegia and tetraparesis with or without cervical or thoracolumbar pain, are associated with many disorders, but intervertebral disc disease and cervical spondylomyelopathy (Wobbler syndrome) are common in dogs (see Figure 26.7). Lumbosacral stenosis, which commonly occurs in large-breed dogs, usually does not cause paraparesis, but compresses L7, S1–3 and caudal nerve roots, causing lumbosacral pain and bladder, anal sphincter and tail paresis (Kline *et al.*, 2001). Although the mechanisms of disease, conventional treatments, underlying TCVM patterns and prognoses vary, acupuncture and

Chinese herbal medicines have been used alone or integrated with conventional treatments to reduce clinical signs, to enhance recovery, or to slow progression of these disorders (Figure 26.10; see also Figure 26.8 and **Acupuncture** clip on DVD) (Kline *et al.*, 2001; Xie and Preast, 2002, 2007, 2010).

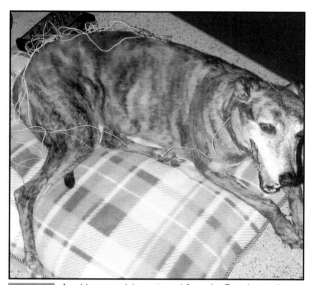

26.10 An 11-year-old neutered female Greyhound treated with EA for a chronic progressive upper motor neuron paraparesis from a T13–L1 type II intervertebral disc protrusion and lethargy. Visible acupoints treated included GV-20/*Bai-hui* (midline lumbosacral space), BL-21/BL-21, BL-22/BL-22, BL-23/23 and BL-62/KID3/BL-62/KID-3. Other acupoints were treated to resolve the underlying TCVM pattern. With monthly EA treatment, her paraparesis and attitude improved and conventional drug therapy and surgery were avoided.

In a clinical RCT of 40 dogs with Wobbler syndrome (cervical spondylomyelopathy), dogs were graded based on the severity of their neurological deficits and were then randomly assigned to one of two groups to ensure equal overall severity between groups (Sumano *et al.*, 2000). Group 1 consisted of 20 dogs that received surgery and conventional medicine and Group 2 consisted of 20 dogs that received EA with or without surgery and conventional medicine. The authors reported an overall success rate of 85% for dogs that received EA and 20% for dogs that received surgery and conventional medication alone. Although most investigators have a greater success rate than 20% with conventional treatments, further investigation of the treatment of Wobbler syndrome with EA alone or integrated with conventional medication and surgery is warranted. Further veterinary clinical RCTs of the effects of EA and Chinese herbal medicines integrated with conventional treatments for chronic progressive spinal cord injury and degeneration in animals are justified by the preliminary data.

There is currently no other research on the use of EA and Chinese herbal medicines for the other causes of chronic progressive ataxia, tetraparesis and paraparesis in dogs and cats but, based on anecdotal experiences, affected animals may

benefit from these treatments (Kline *et al.*, 2001; Xie and Preast, 2002, 2007, 2010).

Monoparesis and monoplegia

Injury of the brachial plexus or sciatic nerve is a common cause of monoparesis and monoplegia in dogs and cats, and these injuries have been treated with EA to enhance recovery (Kline *et al.*, 2001; Xie and Preast, 2002, 2007). There are many laboratory animal RCTs that investigate peripheral nerve injuries and report significant positive effects of Chinese herbal medicines and/or EA to reduce pain and self-mutilation and promote nerve regeneration, but no clinical RCTs have been performed in veterinary medicine (Hao *et al.*, 1995; Xiao *et al.*, 2007; Wei *et al.*, 2008; Kenney, 2010; Shu *et al.*, 2010). In one study of 54 humans with peripheral nerve injuries, the EA treatment group had significantly improved recovery compared to the control group (Hao *et al.*, 1995). In a human clinical RCT of 90 cases of peripheral nerve injury, the combination of EA and physical therapy resulted in significantly improved recovery and quality of life compared to either treatment alone (Xiao *et al.*, 2007). Further clinical RCTs of peripheral nerve injuries in dogs and cats could confirm the benefits of adding these TCVM treatments to currently recommended rehabilitation regimes.

Peripheral nerve neoplasia causes a painful progressive monoparesis; EA and Chinese herbal medicines may reduce the clinical signs and improve the quality of life of affected animals. No reports have been made or research done, but often there are limited conventional options for affected animals, especially if clinical signs return even after surgical resection.

Seizures

Seizures are associated with many aetiologies. A variety of short-term and long-term anticonvulsant drugs comprise standard therapy, but side effects include hepatotoxicity, drowsiness, hyperactivity and ataxia, so the lowest possible effective dose is often sought.

In TCVM and TCM, seizures are referred to as 'internal Wind' and acupoints on the head and other parts of the body, known to eliminate Wind, are treated along with acupoints to address the underlying TCVM pattern diagnosis (Kline *et al.*, 2001; Xie and Preast, 2002, 2007; Maciocia, 2005). Chinese herbal medicines known to eliminate Wind and treat the underlying TCVM pattern diagnosis may also be prescribed (Xie and Preast, 2002, 2007, 2010). Successful treatment of canine and feline seizure disorders with acupuncture and Chinese herbal medicines has been reported anecdotally (see Figure 26.6).

The most common acupuncture techniques used to treat seizures include needles with no electricity (dry needle acupuncture), aqua-acupuncture using B12, and implantation of gold beads or other substances into acupoints (Kline *et al.*, 2001; Xie and Preast, 2002, 2007). Seizures may be induced by EA in some dogs and, although used in laboratory animal RCTs evaluating seizures, EA is generally avoided in the clinical treatment of seizures in dogs and cats. Depending on the aetiology, frequency and severity of the seizures, acupuncture and/or Chinese herbal medicines may be used as a sole therapy or integrated with conventional anticonvulsant drugs to improve seizure control or reduce conventional drug dosages and side effects. Gold bead implantation at acupoints on the head may result in artefacts that can interfere with interpretation of future MRI and CT brain scans.

In a clinical trial of 15 dogs diagnosed with idiopathic epilepsy, the seizure frequency and severity and electroencephalogram (EEG) were recorded 15 weeks before and after gold bead implantation into acupoints (Goiz-Marquez *et al.*, 2009). After acupoint implantation, there was an overall significant reduction in seizure frequency (12/15) and severity (11/15). Seizure frequency was reduced by 50% or more in 9/15 dogs (60%). There was no significant change in the EEG before and after acupoint implantation.

A 75% or greater reduction in seizure frequency after dry needle acupuncture was reported in two human clinical RCTs comparing acupuncture and phenytoin (Cheuk and Wong, 2008). Three other human RCTs comparing catgut implantation at acupoints and valproate, reported a 75% or greater reduction in seizure frequency in the acupoint implantation groups (Cheuk and Wong, 2008). Reviewers of human clinical RCTs concluded that larger and better designed studies were needed before acupuncture recommendations for human epilepsy could be made.

Increased glycine, taurine and GABA and decreased somatostatin, aspartate and glutamine in the hippocampus are thought to contribute to the anti-epileptic properties of acupuncture (Shu *et al.*, 2004; Li *et al.*, 2005). A laboratory animal RCT comparing vagus nerve stimulation (VNS) and EA for seizure control showed equally inhibited cortical and thalamic epileptiform activities, and the authors suggested EA as an alternative to VNS (Zhang *et al.*, 2008).

In a systematic review of human clinical RCTs evaluating seizure control (Li *et al.*, 2009), the Chinese herbal medicine *Xia xing ci* and phenytoin were equally effective in two studies, and another study found *Dian xian ning* and valproate to be equally effective for different types of epilepsy. Three other studies reported a 50% or greater reduction in seizure frequency with other Chinese herbal medicines. After a review of the human clinical RCTs of acupuncture and epilepsy (Li *et al.*, 2009), it was concluded that larger numbers of patients were needed to ensure the effectiveness and safety of Chinese herbal medicines for treating epilepsy in humans. Veterinary clinical RCTs are warranted and may scientifically support the clinical impressions of the positive effects of acupuncture and Chinese herbal medicines for the management of seizure disorders of dogs and cats (Kline *et al.*, 2001; Xie and Preast, 2002, 2007, 2010).

Acute facial paralysis

Acute facial paralysis has several aetiologies, but is often idiopathic in dogs. Although dogs with facial paralysis have been treated with EA and Chinese herbal medicines, only one case report has been published and veterinary clinical RCTs are needed (Jeong *et al.*, 2001; Kline *et al.*, 2001; Xie and Preast, 2002, 2007, 2010). One systematic review of human clinical RCTs evaluating acupuncture treatment for facial nerve paralysis reported significantly positive effects with EA and recommended a standardized treatment regime (Zheng *et al.*, 2009). Another systematic review of several human clinical RCTs of acupuncture for idiopathic facial nerve paralysis (Bell's palsy) concluded that, although preliminary positive results had been reported, higher quality studies with larger numbers of patients were still needed before recommendations could be made (Chen *et al.*, 2010). Veterinary clinical RCTs of EA for facial paralysis are warranted.

Acute vestibular dysfunction

Acute onset of head tilt, nystagmus, circling and/or rolling associated with peripheral vestibular disease has many aetiologies, but is often idiopathic in dogs and cats. Although animals with acute vestibular disease have been treated with acupuncture and Chinese herbal medicines, no case reports or RCTs have been published (Kline *et al.*, 2001; Xie and Preast, 2002, 2007, 2010). Human case reports and clinical RCTs report successful treatment of acute idiopathic vestibular syndrome (Ménière's disease) with acupuncture (Long *et al.*, 2009). After a recent systematic review of human clinical RCTs, evaluating acupuncture for Ménière's disease, it was concluded that acupuncture was beneficial, but further human clinical RCTs were needed to clarify questions around the appropriate frequency and number of acupuncture treatments required (Long *et al.*, 2009). Based on the success reported in humans and anecdotally for animals, acupuncture and Chinese herbal medicine treatment of dogs and cats with vestibular dysfunction should be further investigated.

Acquired deafness

Deafness may be acquired from chronic middle and inner ear infections, toxicity, senile degeneration and idiopathic aetiologies. Although animals with acquired deafness have been treated with acupuncture and Chinese herbal medicines, no case reports or clinical RCTs are available (Kline *et al.*, 2001; Xie and Preast, 2002, 2007, 2010). In a laboratory animal RCT of acquired deafness, improvement in brainstem auditory evoked responses and hair cell morphology and increased mitochondrial succinate dehydrogenase activity were reported following EA (Liu *et al.*, 1999). Of 60 clinical reports (1994–2004), regarding the effectiveness of acupuncture for deafness in humans, 71.7% were descriptive studies and 28.3% were clinical trials (Liu and Du, 2005). Although improved hearing after acupuncture was reported, after a review of all the studies it was concluded that higher quality, larger clinical RCTs were needed before the efficacy of acupuncture for deafness could be confirmed. Since there are positive effects reported for humans and few other treatment options for dogs and cats with acquired deafness, further studies to explore the potential benefits of acupuncture and Chinese herbal medicines for deaf animals are warranted.

Stupor and coma

Many disorders can cause stupor and coma in dogs. Brain haemorrhage and ischaemia are commonly associated with head trauma and cerebrovascular accidents. WHO has recommended the integration of acupuncture with conventional treatments for the rehabilitation of humans with strokes (WHO, 2003). Although anecdotal success has been reported with the use of acupuncture and Chinese herbal medicines for dogs and cats with head injuries and strokes, there are no clinical RCTs to confirm these findings (Kline *et al.*, 2001; Xie and Preast, 2002, 2007, 2010). Specific acupoints are experientially known to have resuscitative effects and have been studied in humans, but further studies are needed before further recommendations can be made (Xie and Preast, 2002, 2007; Zhang, 2005). Cognitive dysfunction in elderly dogs has been treated with acupuncture and Chinese herbal medicines, and improvement in cognition and quality of life have been anecdotally reported, but veterinary RCTs are needed to support this clinical impression (Xie and Preast, 2002, 2007, 2010).

Neoplasia of varying types can affect the nervous system of animals and produce progressive stupor, seizures, ataxia, tetraparesis and paraparesis (see Figure 26.7). Current conventional treatments consist primarily of palliative drugs, surgery, radiation and/or chemotherapy. Studies of the effects of acupuncture and Chinese herbal medicines for the treatment of nervous system neoplasia are currently under way, but there are no clinical RCTs in humans or animals published in English (Armstrong and Gilbert, 2008; Feng *et al.*, 2010). Acupuncture may be effective to assist pain control or nausea associated with chemotherapy (Armstrong and Gilbert, 2008).

Many laboratory animal RCTs have reported that a variety of Chinese herbal medicines can inhibit tumour angiogenesis, cancer gene expression and tumour cell metabolism, proliferation and differentiation, as well as induce tumour cell death (Feng *et al.*, 2010). Chinese herbal medicines have also been shown to stimulate immune function, reduce immunosuppression from conventional cancer treatments, reverse drug resistance and enhance chemotherapeutic effects. Based on laboratory animal RCT findings, human and animal clinical RCTs for the integration of acupuncture and Chinese herbal medicines with conventional treatments of neoplasia are warranted. Treatment of hydrocephalus and meningoencephalitis with acupuncture and Chinese herbal medicines has been suggested, but no case studies or veterinary RCTs have been reported (Kline *et al.*, 2001; Xie and Preast, 2002, 2007, 2010).

Conclusions

Enough experimental data have been generated from human clinical and laboratory animal RCTs to justify further investigation of the effects of acupuncture and Chinese herbal medicines for the treatment of many different neurological disorders in small animals. In summary, animals with acute or chronic pain, intervertebral disc disease, brain and spinal cord trauma, Wobbler syndrome, peripheral nerve injuries, seizures, facial nerve paralysis, idiopathic vestibular syndrome, deafness, neoplasia and some neuromuscular disorders may benefit from referral to a veterinary surgeon trained in acupuncture, Chinese herbal medicines and other TCVM treatments. With the addition of TCVM treatments, individual dogs and cats may recover faster and more completely or maintain a higher quality of life for longer, and the veterinary scientific knowledge base can be expanded. Only in this way can it be determined which current experience-based TCVM treatments will also become evidence-based treatments for improved management of neurological disorders of small animals in the future.

References and further reading

Available on accompanying DVD

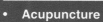

DVD extras
* **Acupuncture**

Appendix 1

Neurological disorders associated with cat and dog breeds

Carley J. Giovanella

This section lists neurological disorders that are likely to be encountered in practice. Some of these have proven modes of inheritance in a breed, others have a breed over-representation, and some have been reported in the breed but the exact prevalence is still unknown. Many of these disorders are 'diagnosed' only by elimination of other causes of neurological dysfunction or on post-mortem pathology; however, the diagnostic aids listed are tools that may assist in confirming a suspected disorder. Although every effort has been made to offer as much clinically useful information as possible, there can be no guarantee that this is a complete list of breed-related diseases at the time of publication. Figures A1.1 and A1.2 detail the idiopathic, inherited and breed-associated diseases in cats and dogs.

Breed	Disease	Clinical signs (including age of onset where known)	Diagnostic aids
Abyssinian	Myasthenia gravis	Generalized weakness	Anti-ACh receptor antibody; electrodiagnostics; edrophonium (Tensilon) test
Birman	Distal central–peripheral axonopathy	8–10 weeks; hypermetria; progressive paraparesis; plantigrade stance	Nerve biopsy
	Spongiform encephalopathy	7 weeks; hypermetria; paraparesis; depression	Pathology
Burmese	Hypokalaemia	2–6 months; intermittent muscle weakness; ventroflexion of neck	Hypokalaemia; elevated CK
	Congenital vestibular disease	Birth to 4 months; head tilt; ataxia; circling	Clinical signs; exclusion diagnosis; pathology
Devon Rex	Hereditary myopathy	1–6 months; muscle atrophy; megaoesophagus; cervical ventroflexion; progressive tetraparesis	Muscle biopsy
Domestic Shorthaired	Neuroaxonal dystrophy	5–6 weeks; head tremors; ataxia; hypermetria	Pathology
	X-linked (hypertrophic) muscular dystrophy	5–6 months; skeletal muscle hypertrophy; exercise intolerance; regurgitation; tongue protrusion; hypertrophic cardiomyopathy	Elevated CK; EMG abnormalities; pathology
	Cerebellar abiotrophy	Adult-onset; progressive cerebellar signs	Pathology
Egyptian Mau	Spongiform encephalopathy	7 weeks; hypermetria; paraparesis; depression	Pathology
Korat	Lissencephaly	Within 12 months; depression; behaviour change; seizures	Imaging (CT, MRI); pathology
Maine Coon	Spinal muscular atrophy	3–4 months; muscle weakness and atrophy	DNA [5,14,15]
Manx	Spina bifida/sacrocaudal dysgenesis	4 weeks to months; paraparesis; urinary and faecal incontinence; hypoalgesia in the pelvic limbs	Imaging (radiography, myelography, CT, MRI); pathology

A1.1 Idiopathic, inherited and breed-associated diseases in cats. ACh = acetylcholine; BAEP = brainstem auditory evoked potential; CK = creatine kinase; CT = computed tomography; EMG = electromyogram; MRI = magnetic resonance imaging. (continues) ▶

Breed	Disease	Clinical signs (including age of onset where known)	Diagnostic aids
Siamese	Congenital vestibular disease and deafness	Birth to 4 months; head tilt; ataxia; circling; deafness	Clinical signs; exclusion diagnosis; BAEP; pathology
	Cerebellar abiotrophy	Adult-onset; progressive cerebellar signs	Pathology
Sphynx	Muscular dystrophy	Birth; progressive general weakness	Muscle biopsy
Tonkinese	Congenital vestibular disease	Birth to 4 months; head tilt; ataxia; circling	Clinical signs; exclusion diagnosis; pathology

A1.1 (continued) Idiopathic, inherited and breed-associated diseases in cats. ACh = acetylcholine; BAEP = brainstem auditory evoked potential; CK = creatine kinase; CT = computed tomography; EMG = electromyogram; MRI = magnetic resonance imaging.

Breed	Disease	Clinical signs (including age of onset where known)	Diagnostic aids
Afghan Hound	Hereditary myelopathy	3–13 months; paraparesis; ataxia; progressive to tetraparesis and death from respiratory failure	Clinical signs; pathology
Airedale Terrier	Cerebellar degeneration	12 weeks; cerebellar syndrome	Pathology
Akita	Cerebellar degeneration	Cerebellar syndrome	Pathology
	Congenital vestibular disease	Up to 4 weeks; head tilt; circling; ataxia	Clinical signs
	Myasthenia gravis	Generalized weakness; megaoesophagus; laryngeal paralysis	Clinical signs; edrophonium (Tensilon) test; anti-ACh receptor antibody; electrodiagnostics; muscle biopsy
Alaskan Husky	Necrotizing encephalopathy (Leigh's disease)	7 months to 3 years; ataxia; seizures; behaviour changes; may stabilize with intermittent gait disorder and seizures	Pathology
Alaskan Malamute	Peripheral neuropathy	7–18 months; progressive tetraparesis; poor reflexes; muscle atrophy	Electrodiagnostics; nerve and muscle biopsy
Australian Cattle Dog	Polioencephalomyelopathy	Within 12 months; seizures followed by fatigue and progressive spastic tetraparesis	Pathology
Australian Kelpie	Cerebellar cortical degeneration	6–12 weeks; cerebellar syndrome; proprioceptive deficits	Pathology
Basset Hound	Cervical spondylomyelopathy	Progressive tetraparesis; neck pain	Imaging (CT, MRI, myelography)
Beagle	Congenital vestibular disease	Up to 4 weeks; head tilt; circling; ataxia	Clinical signs; exclusion diagnosis
	Cerebellar cortical degeneration	3 weeks; cerebellar syndrome	Pathology
	Idiopathic epilepsy	Up to 6 years; seizures	Exclusion diagnosis
	Steroid-responsive meningitis–arteritis	<12 months; recurrent fever and neck pain	Clinical signs; neutrophilic pleocytosis; serum and CSF IgA levels [17]
Belgian Tervuren	Idiopathic epilepsy	Up to 6 years; seizures	Exclusion diagnosis
	Muscular dystrophy	6 weeks; stiff gait; stunted growth; muscle atrophy	Elevated CK; muscle biopsy

A1.2 Idiopathic, inherited and breed-associated diseases in dogs. Degenerative myelopathy occurs in many breeds and can be diagnosed with DNA tests [6]. ACh = acetylcholine; BAEP = brainstem auditory evoked potential; CK = creatine kinase; CSF = cerebrospinal fluid; CT = computed tomography; EMG = electromyogram; MRI = magnetic resonance imaging. (continues) ▶

Appendix 1 Neurological disorders associated with cat and dog breeds

Breed	Disease	Clinical signs (including age of onset where known)	Diagnostic aids
Bernese Mountain Dog	Dysmyelination	2–8 weeks; fine tremor of head and limbs; weakness; stiffness; may improve with age	Clinical signs; pathology
	Steroid-responsive meningitis–arteritis	<12 months; recurrent fever and neck pain	Clinical signs; neutrophilic pleocytosis; serum and CSF IgA levels [17]
	Hepatocerebellar disease	4–6 weeks; progressive wide-based stance; spontaneous nystagmus; head bobbing; paresis	Raised bile acids; ammonia; pathology
Border Collie	Cerebellar cortical degeneration	6–8 weeks; cerebellar syndrome	Clinical signs; pathology
	Idiopathic epilepsy	Up to 6 years; seizures	Exclusion diagnosis
	Deafness	6–8 weeks	BAEP
	Peripheral sensory neuropathy	2–6 months; progressive ataxia; gait abnormality in all limbs with preservation of strength; self-mutilation	Clinical signs confirming sensory loss in limbs; electrodiagnostics; nerve biopsy
Borzoi	Cervical malformation (Wobbler syndrome)	Progressive tetraparesis; neck pain	Imaging (CT, MRI, myelography)
Boston Terrier	Hydrocephalus	Cerebral signs (seizures, depression)	Imaging (ultrasonography, CT, MRI)
	Hemivertebrae	Ataxia; spinal curvature; incontinence; paresis	Imaging (radiography, CT, MRI)
Bouvier des Flandres	Idiopathic laryngeal paralysis	4–6 months; inspiratory stridor; voice change; dyspnoea	Electrodiagnostics; laryngoscopy
	Myopathy	Within 2 years; generalized muscle weakness and atrophy; dysphagia; degeneration of pharyngeal and oesophageal muscles leading to regurgitation	Elevated CK; electrodiagnostics; muscle biopsy
Boxer	Progressive axonopathy	2 months; progressive ataxia and weakness; diminished proprioception, muscle tone, patellar reflexes; intact pain sensation	Electrodiagnostics; nerve biopsy; pathology
	Steroid-responsive meningitis–arteritis	<12 months; recurrent fever and neck pain	Clinical signs; neutrophilic pleocytosis; serum and CSF IgA levels [17]
	Immune-mediated polymyositis	Generalized muscle weakness; myalgia; possible dysphagia and/or megaoesophagus; muscle atrophy	Elevated CK; electrodiagnostics; muscle biopsy
	Degenerative myelopathy	>5 years (younger reported); progressive paraparesis	Exclusion diagnosis; pathology
Brittany Spaniel	Cerebellar degeneration	7–13 years; progressive spasticity; hypermetria and truncal ataxia	Pathology
	Spinal muscular atrophy (motor neuron disease)	Weakness; atrophy of proximal muscles. Accelerated form: 6–8 weeks, immobile by 3–4 months; intermediate form: 6–12 months, immobile by 3 years; chronic form: survive into adulthood	Clinical signs; EMG abnormalities; pathology
Brussels Griffon	Chiari-like malformation (caudal occipital malformation syndrome)	Often has accompanying hydrocephalus and syringomyelia; seizures; depression; ataxia; cerebellar syndrome; vestibular signs; other signs of syringomyelia (see below)	Imaging (MRI)
	Syringomyelia	Ataxia; depressed reflexes if in spinal cord intumescence; spinal curvature; paraesthesia of paraspinal dermal zone	Imaging (MRI)

A1.2 (continued) Idiopathic, inherited and breed-associated diseases in dogs. Degenerative myelopathy occurs in many breeds and can be diagnosed with DNA tests [6]. ACh = acetylcholine; BAEP = brainstem auditory evoked potential; CK = creatine kinase; CSF = cerebrospinal fluid; CT = computed tomography; EMG = electromyogram; MRI = magnetic resonance imaging. (continues) ▶

Breed	Disease	Clinical signs (including age of onset where known)	Diagnostic aids
Bull Terrier	Cerebellar degeneration	Cerebellar syndrome	Pathology
	Idiopathic laryngeal paralysis	Stridor; exercise intolerance	EMG abnormalities; laryngoscopy
Bullmastiff	Spongiosis of grey matter	6–9 weeks; ataxia; hypermetria; intention tremor; slow menace; visual deficits; poor proprioception	Pathology
Cairn Terrier	Cerebellar degeneration	Cerebellar syndrome	Pathology
	Multisystem neuronal degeneration	4–7 months; progressive tetraparesis; cataplexy; cerebellar dysfunction	Pathology
Cavalier King Charles Spaniel	Episodic hypertonicity	3–4 months; pelvic limb stiffness/collapse after exercise or stress; no loss of consciousness; progressive	Clinical signs; exclusion diagnosis; DNA [4]
	Chiari-like malformation (caudal occipital malformation syndrome)	Often has accompanying hydrocephalus and syringomyelia; seizures; depression; ataxia; cerebellar syndrome; vestibular signs; other signs of syringomyelia (see below)	Imaging (MRI)
	Syringomyelia	Ataxia; depressed reflexes if in spinal cord intumescence; spinal curvature; paraesthesia of paraspinal dermal zone	Imaging (MRI)
Chesapeake Bay Duck Tolling Retriever	Steroid-responsive meningitis–arteritis	<12 months; recurrent fever and neck pain	Clinical signs; neutrophilic pleocytosis; serum and CSF IgA levels [17]
	Degenerative myelopathy	>5 years (younger reported); progressive paraparesis	Exclusion diagnosis; pathology
Chihuahua	Hydrocephalus	Cerebral signs (seizures, depression)	Imaging (ultrasonography, CT, MRI)
	Necrotizing meningoencephalitis	6 months to 7 years; seizures; depression; circling; head pressing; central blindness	Signalment; CSF; imaging (MRI or CT); pathology
Chow Chow	Dysmyelination	2–4 weeks; intention tremors; dysmetria 'bunny-hopping'; improves after 1 year	Clinical signs; pathology
	Myotonia congenita	2–3 months; stiffness after rest that improves with exercise; possible dyspnoea	Clinical signs; EMG abnormalities; muscle biopsy
	Cerebellar hypoplasia	Cerebellar syndrome	Pathology
Cocker Spaniel	Congenital vestibular disease	Head tilt; ataxia; circling	Clinical signs
	Neuronal degeneration	10–14 months; behaviour and personality change; absent menace; variable hypermetria and falling	Pathology
Collies (Smooth and Rough-Coated)	Dermatomyositis	2–6 months; inflammation of muscle, skin, blood vessels; cyclical and self-limiting	Muscle and skin biopsy; EMG abnormalities
	Cerebellar cortical degeneration	1–2 months; cerebellar syndrome may stabilize by 12 months	Pathology
	Neuroaxonal dystrophy	2–4 months; hypermetria; ataxia; intention tremor	Clinical signs; pathology
Coton de Tulear Dog	Neonatal cerebellar ataxia	2 weeks; ataxia; 'swimming' movements (unable to stand); ocular saccadic dysmetria; head titubation; non-progressive until at least 4 months	Ultrastructural (electron microscopy) pathology; DNA [6]
	Cerebellar degeneration	2–3 months; cerebellar syndrome	Pathology
Cretan Hound	Spongiform leucoencephalopathy (hypomyelination/'shaker' pup)	2–3 weeks; generalized tremors worse with excitement	Pathology

A1.2 (continued) Idiopathic, inherited and breed-associated diseases in dogs. Degenerative myelopathy occurs in many breeds and can be diagnosed with DNA tests [6]. ACh = acetylcholine; BAEP = brainstem auditory evoked potential; CK = creatine kinase; CSF = cerebrospinal fluid; CT = computed tomography; EMG = electromyogram; MRI = magnetic resonance imaging. (continues) ▶

Breed	Disease	Clinical signs (including age of onset where known)	Diagnostic aids
Curly-Coated Retriever	Exercise-induced collapse	7 months to 2 years; mostly field-trial breeds; weakness and collapse after strenuous exercise; requires 10–20 minutes to recover; may be fatal	Clinical signs; DNA [3,9,12,13,14,15]
Dachshund	Narcolepsy–cataplexy	Sudden flaccid paralysis ± loss of consciousness	Clinical signs; DNA [7,15]
	Sensory neuropathy	Progressive loss of spinal reflexes; self-mutilation	Clinical signs; nerve biopsy
	Idiopathic epilepsy	Up to 6 years; seizures	Exclusion diagnosis
	Congenital myasthenia gravis	5–6 weeks; progressive episodic weakness resolves with age	Edrophonium (Tensilon) test; electrodiagnostics; muscle biopsy
Dalmatian	Laryngeal paralysis–polyneuropathy complex	4–6 months; inspiratory stridor; voice change; dyspnoea; generalized weakness; megaoesophagus	Electrodiagnostics; laryngoscopy; pathology
	Cerebral and spinal leucodystrophy	3–6 months; visual deficits; progressive ataxia and weakness	Pathology
	Congenital deafness	6–8 weeks	BAEP
Dobermann	Narcolepsy–cataplexy	Sudden flaccid paralysis ± loss of consciousness	Clinical signs; DNA [3,7,10,11,15]
	'Dancing Dobermann disease' (neuropathy/myopathy)	6 months to 7 years; progressive intermittent flexion of one, then both pelvic limbs	Clinical signs; muscle and nerve biopsy; EMG (especially gastrocnemius muscle)
	Cervical spondylomyelopathy (Wobbler syndrome)	>5 years; progressive tetraparesis ± neck pain	Imaging (CT, MRI, myelography)
	Congenital vestibular disease and deafness	Up to 4 weeks; head tilt; circling; ataxia; deafness	Clinical signs
English Bulldog	Cerebellar cortical degeneration	2 months; progressive cerebellar syndrome	Pathology
	Spina bifida	4 weeks to months; paraparesis; urinary and faecal incontinence; hypoalgesia in the pelvic limbs	Imaging (radiography, myelography, CT, MRI); pathology
	Hemivertebrae	Ataxia; spine curvature; incontinence	Imaging (radiography, CT, MRI)
English Pointer	Spinal muscular atrophy (motor neuron disease)	5 months; weakness; dysphonia; loss of spinal reflexes; progressive muscle atrophy over 3–4 months	Clinical signs; electrodiagnostics; nerve biopsy; pathology
	Sensory neuropathy	Loss of spinal reflexes with preservation of muscle strength; ataxia; hypoalgesia; self-mutilation	Clinical signs; nerve biopsy
Finnish Harrier	Cerebellar degeneration	Cerebellar syndrome	Pathology
French Bulldog	Hemivertebrae	Ataxia; spine curvature; incontinence	Imaging (radiography, CT, MRI)
Gammel Dansk Hønsehund (Old Danish Pointer)	Congenital myasthenia gravis (presynaptic)	Progressive episodic weakness	Edrophonium (Tensilon) test; electrodiagnostics; muscle biopsy
German Shepherd Dog	Congenital vestibular disease	3 months; head tilt; ataxia	Exclusion diagnosis
	Giant axonal neuropathy	14–16 months; progressive paresis; decreased proprioception; poor muscle tone; atrophy of distal limb muscles	Clinical signs; electrodiagnostics; nerve biopsy

A1.2 (continued) Idiopathic, inherited and breed-associated diseases in dogs. Degenerative myelopathy occurs in many breeds and can be diagnosed with DNA tests [6]. ACh = acetylcholine; BAEP = brainstem auditory evoked potential; CK = creatine kinase; CSF = cerebrospinal fluid; CT = computed tomography; EMG = electromyogram; MRI = magnetic resonance imaging. (continues) ▶

Breed	Disease	Clinical signs (including age of onset where known)	Diagnostic aids
German Shepherd Dog (continued)	Idiopathic epilepsy	Up to 6 years; seizures	Exclusion diagnosis
	Fibrotic myopathy	2–7 years; non-painful lameness in pelvic limb; palpable fibrous band in semitendinosus muscle	Clinical signs; electrodiagnostics; muscle biopsy
	Megaoesophagus	From birth; regurgitation	Clinical signs; imaging (radiography, oesophagram)
	Degenerative myelopathy	>5 years (younger reported); progressive paraparesis	Exclusion diagnosis; pathology
	Myasthenia gravis	Generalized weakness; megaoesophagus; laryngeal paralysis	Clinical signs; edrophonium (Tensilon) test; anti-ACh receptor antibody; electrodiagnostics
	Immune-mediated polymyositis	Generalized muscle weakness; myalgia; possible dysphagia and/or megaoesophagus; muscle atrophy	Elevated CK; electrodiagnostics; muscle biopsy
German Shorthaired Pointer	Steroid-responsive meningitis–arteritis	<12 months; recurrent fever and neck pain	Clinical signs; neutrophilic pleocytosis; serum and CSF IgA levels 17
	X-linked muscular dystrophy	<12 weeks; stunted growth, stiff/stilted gait; exercise intolerance; muscle atrophy and contractures; pharyngeal/laryngeal dysfunction	Elevated CK, electrodiagnostics, muscle biopsy
Golden Retriever	Idiopathic epilepsy	Up to 6 years; seizures	Exclusion diagnosis
	X-linked muscular dystrophy	6–9 weeks; stunted growth; stiff/stilted gait; exercise intolerance; muscle atrophy and contractures; pharyngeal/laryngeal dysfunction	Elevated CK; electrodiagnostics; muscle biopsy; DNA [3,10,15]
	Myasthenia gravis	Generalized weakness; megaoesophagus; laryngeal paralysis	Clinical signs; edrophonium (Tensilon) test; anti-ACh receptor antibody; electrodiagnostics
	Hypomyelinating polyneuropathy	5–7 weeks; hindlimb ataxia; crouched appearance; non-fatal	Nerve biopsy
Gordon Setter	Cerebellar cortical degeneration	6–30 months; slow progressive cerebellar and vestibular signs	Pathology; DNA [18]
Great Dane	Myotonic myopathy	2–3 months; stiffness after rest that resolves with exercise; possible dyspnoea	Clinical signs; EMG abnormalities; muscle biopsy
	Cervical spondylomyelopathy (Wobbler syndrome)	<2 years; progressive tetraparesis ± neck pain	Imaging (CT, MRI, myelography)
	Megaoesophagus	From birth; regurgitation	Clinical signs; imaging (radiography, oesophagram)
	Distal symmetrical polyneuropathy	1–5 years; paraparesis progressing to tetraparesis	Electrodiagnostics; nerve biopsy
	Inherited (core-like) myopathy of Great Danes	6 months; generalized weakness; exercise intolerance; mild proximal muscle atrophy	Electrodiagnostics; muscle biopsy
	Orthostatic tremor	Limb tremors associated with weight bearing	Electrodiagnostics
Greyhound	Megaoesophagus	Birth; regurgitation	Clinical signs; imaging (radiography, oesophagram)
	Steroid-responsive meningitis–arteritis	<12 months; recurrent fever and neck pain	Clinical signs; neutrophilic pleocytosis; serum and CSF IgA levels [17]
	Neuropathy	8–12 weeks; progressive muscle weakness; exercise intolerance; 'bunny-hopping'	DNA [7]

A1.2 (continued) Idiopathic, inherited and breed-associated diseases in dogs. Degenerative myelopathy occurs in many breeds and can be diagnosed with DNA tests [6]. ACh = acetylcholine; BAEP = brainstem auditory evoked potential; CK = creatine kinase; CSF = cerebrospinal fluid; CT = computed tomography; EMG = electromyogram; MRI = magnetic resonance imaging. (continues) ▶

Breed	Disease	Clinical signs (including age of onset where known)	Diagnostic aids
Irish Setter	Idiopathic epilepsy	Up to 6 years; seizures	Exclusion diagnosis
	Lissencephaly	Within 12 months; depression; behaviour change; seizures	Imaging (CT, MRI); pathology
	Megaoesophagus	From birth; regurgitation	Clinical signs; imaging (radiography, oesophagram)
	Cerebellar dysplasia	Cerebellar syndrome	Pathology
Irish Terrier	Muscular dystrophy	6 weeks; stiff gait; stunted growth; muscle atrophy	Elevated CK; muscle biopsy
Italian Spinone	Cerebellar cortical degeneration	Adult-onset; progressive cerebellar signs (UK)	Pathology; DNA [4]
Jack Russell Terrier (Parson Russell Terrier)	Congenital myasthenia gravis	6–9 weeks; progressive episodic weakness	Edrophonium (Tensilon) test; electrodiagnostics; muscle biopsy
	Spinocerebellar degeneration/hereditary ataxia	2–6 months; cerebellar ataxia; progressive dysmetria and spasticity; intention tremor	Pathology
Japanese Spitz	Muscular dystrophy	10–12 weeks; excessive salivation and dysphagia; progressive exercise intolerance; myalgia	Elevated CK; muscle biopsy
Keeshond	Idiopathic epilepsy	Up to 6 years; seizures	Exclusion diagnosis
Kerry Blue Terrier	Cerebellar cortical degeneration	8–16 weeks; pelvic limb stiffness and head tremors; then dysmetria	Pathology
Kooiker Hound (Dutch Decoy Dog)	Hereditary necrotizing myelopathy	3–12 months; hindlimb paresis; possible urinary incontinence	Pathology
Labrador Retriever	Narcolepsy–cataplexy	Sudden flaccid paralysis ± loss of consciousness	Clinical signs; DNA [9]
	Idiopathic epilepsy	Up to 6 years; seizures	Exclusion diagnosis
	Exercise-induced collapse	7 months to 2 years; mostly field-trial breeds; weakness and collapse after strenuous exercise; requires 10–20 minutes to recover; may be fatal	Clinical signs; DNA [9]
	Centronuclear myopathy	6 weeks to 7 months; recessive inheritance; stiff gait; 'bunny-hopping'; cervical ventroflexion; depressed spinal reflexes; stabilizes by 8–12 months	Clinical signs; muscle biopsy; DNA [4,8,12,13,15]
	Familial reflex myoclonus	3 weeks; intermittent muscle spasms; progressive stiffness	Clinical signs
	Cerebellar cortical degeneration	12 weeks; cerebellar syndrome	Pathology
	Axonopathy	From birth; crouched; short-strided gait; thoracic limb hypermetria; unable to stand by 5 months	Clinical signs; electrodiagnostics; nerve biopsy; pathology
Leonberger	Polyneuropathy	1–2 years; progressive tetraparesis; muscle atrophy; decreased spinal reflexes; dysphonia	Clinical signs; electrophysiology; muscle and nerve biopsy; DNA [9]
Lhasa Apso	Lissencephaly	Within 12 months; depression; behaviour change; seizures	Imaging (CT, MRI); pathology
Maltese	Shaker dog/idiopathic tremors	9 months to 2 years; generalized tremors; mild hypermetria	Clinical signs; exclusion diagnosis; treatment response
	Necrotizing meningoencephalitis	6 months to 7 years; seizures; depression; circling; head pressing; central blindness	Signalment; CSF; imaging (MRI or CT); pathology

A1.2 (continued) Idiopathic, inherited and breed-associated diseases in dogs. Degenerative myelopathy occurs in many breeds and can be diagnosed with DNA tests [6]. ACh = acetylcholine; BAEP = brainstem auditory evoked potential; CK = creatine kinase; CSF = cerebrospinal fluid; CT = computed tomography; EMG = electromyogram; MRI = magnetic resonance imaging. (continues) ▶

Breed	Disease	Clinical signs (including age of onset where known)	Diagnostic aids
Miniature Schnauzer	Myotonia congenita	Muscular stiffness; possible dyspnoea	Clinical signs; EMG; pathology; DNA [1,3,10,11,15]
	Megaoesophagus	From birth; regurgitation	Clinical signs; imaging (radiography, oesophagram)
	Muscular dystrophy	6–8 weeks; stiff gait; stunted growth; muscle atrophy	Elevated CK; electrodiagnostics; muscle biopsy
Newfoundland	Megaoesophagus	From birth; regurgitation	Clinical signs; imaging (radiography, oesophagram)
	Immune-mediated polymyositis	Generalized muscle weakness; myalgia; possible dysphagia and/or megaoesophagus; muscle atrophy	Elevated CK; electrodiagnostics; muscle biopsy
Old English Sheepdog	Cerebellar cortical degeneration	Progressive cerebellar syndrome	Clinical signs; pathology; DNA [18]
	Muscular dystrophy	6 weeks; stiff gait; stunted growth; muscle atrophy	Elevated CK; electrodiagnostics; muscle biopsy
Papillon	Neuroaxonal dystrophy (only one litter reported)	14 weeks; rapidly progressive ataxia and hypermetria; decreased postural reactions	Pathology
Pembroke Welsh Corgi	Degenerative myelopathy	>5 years; progressive paraparesis	Exclusion diagnosis; pathology
Pomeranian	Hydrocephalus	Cerebral signs (depression, seizures)	Imaging (ultrasonography, CT, MRI)
Poodle	Narcolepsy–cataplexy	Sudden flaccid paralysis without loss of consciousness	Clinical signs; exclusion diagnosis; CSF hypocretin levels
	Idiopathic epilepsy (Standard Poodle)	Up to 6 years; seizures	Exclusion diagnosis
	Neonatal encephalopathy	Soon after birth; cerebellar signs; seizures	DNA [3,6,8,15]
Pug	Necrotizing meningoencephalitis	6 months to 7 years; seizures; depression; circling; head pressing; central blindness	Signalment; CSF; imaging (MRI or CT); pathology; DNA for susceptibility [2]
	Hemivertebrae	Ataxia; spine curvature; incontinence	Imaging (radiography, CT, MRI)
Pyrenean Mountain Dog	Laryngeal paralysis–polyneuropathy complex	4–6 months; inspiratory stridor; voice change; dyspnoea; generalized weakness; megaoesophagus	Electrodiagnostics; laryngoscopy; pathology
Rhodesian Ridgeback	Cerebellar cortical abiotrophy and colour dilution	2 weeks; ataxia; lateral recumbency; opisthotonus; poor growth; affected pups have light hair coat and blue irises at birth	Pathology
Rottweiler	Progressive polyneuropathy	Adult-onset; progressive tetraparesis; hyporeflexia; hypotonia; appendicular muscle atrophy	Electrodiagnostics; nerve biopsy
	Spinal muscular atrophy (motor neuron disease)	4 weeks; pelvic limb ataxia progressing to tetraparesis	Clinical signs; EMG abnormalities; pathology
	Muscular dystrophy	6 weeks; stiff gait; stunted growth; muscle atrophy	Elevated CK; electrodiagnostics; muscle biopsy
	Spongiosis of grey matter	6–16 weeks; progressive ataxia and dysmetria; some behaviour change; laryngeal paralysis; microphthalmia	Imaging (MRI); pathology
	Leucoencephalomyelopathy	1–4 years; ataxia; tetraparesis; hypermetria; increased muscle tone/spinal reflexes; often more severe in thoracic limbs	Clinical signs; pathology

A1.2 (continued) Idiopathic, inherited and breed-associated diseases in dogs. Degenerative myelopathy occurs in many breeds and can be diagnosed with DNA tests [6]. ACh = acetylcholine; BAEP = brainstem auditory evoked potential; CK = creatine kinase; CSF = cerebrospinal fluid; CT = computed tomography; EMG = electromyogram; MRI = magnetic resonance imaging. (continues) ▶

Appendix 1 Neurological disorders associated with cat and dog breeds

Breed	Disease	Clinical signs (including age of onset where known)	Diagnostic aids
Rottweiler (continued)	Neuroaxonal dystrophy	Within 12 months; slowly progressive ataxia; hypermetria; wide-based stance; eventually intention tremors and nystagmus	Clinical signs; pathology
	Distal myopathy	Begins at time puppy starts walking; plantigrade/palmigrade stance; hypotonia; poor muscle mass	EMG abnormalities; muscle biopsy (distal)
	Spinal subarachnoid (pseudo) cyst	Progressive ataxia; often ambulatory tetraparesis	Imaging (myelography, CT, MRI); surgical pathology
	Laryngeal paralysis–polyneuropathy complex	4–6 months; inspiratory stridor; voice change; dyspnoea; generalized weakness; megaoesophagus	Electrodiagnostics; laryngoscopy; pathology
Saluki	Spongiosis of grey matter	Behaviour changes; seizures; aimless wandering	Imaging (MRI); pathology
Samoyed	Hypomyelination	3 weeks; generalized tremors; nystagmus; absent menace	Clinical signs; pathology
	Lissencephaly	Within 12 months; depression; behaviour change; seizures	Imaging (CT, MRI); pathology
	Cerebellar cortical abiotrophy	Cerebellar syndrome	Pathology
	Muscular dystrophy	6 weeks; stiff gait; stunted growth; muscle atrophy	Elevated CK; muscle biopsy
Scottish Terrier	Scotty cramp	Mostly <6 months at onset; progressive stiffness to collapse upon exercise	Clinical signs; methysergide test
	Cerebellar cortical degeneration	2–8 years; progressive cerebellar and vestibular signs	Pathology; cerebellar atrophy on MRI
Shar Pei	Megaoesophagus	From birth; regurgitation	Clinical signs; imaging (radiography, oesophagram)
Shetland Sheepdog	Dermatomyositis	2–6 months; inflammation of muscle, skin, blood vessels; cyclical and self-limiting	Muscle and skin biopsy; EMG abnormalities
	Dysmyelination	1–3 weeks; seizures; depression; lateral recumbency; intention tremors	Pathology
Siberian Husky	Laryngeal paralysis	4–6 months; inspiratory stridor; voice change; dyspnoea	EMG abnormalities; laryngoscopy; pathology
	Degenerative myelopathy	Progressive paraparesis	Exclusion diagnosis; pathology
Smooth-haired Fox Terrier	Congenital myasthenia gravis	6–9 weeks; progressive episodic weakness; megaoesophagus	Edrophonium (Tensilon) test; electrodiagnostics; muscle biopsy
	Congenital vestibular disease	3 months; head tilt; ataxia	Exclusion diagnosis
Springer Spaniel	Congenital myasthenia gravis	6–9 weeks; progressive episodic weakness	Edrophonium (Tensilon) test; electrodiagnostics; muscle biopsy
	Dysmyelination	2–4 weeks; severe tremors; difficulty standing; seizures; progressive debilitation	Pathology
St Bernard	Idiopathic epilepsy	Up to 6 years; seizures	Exclusion diagnosis
Staffordshire Bull Terrier	Myotonic myopathy	2–3 months; stiffness after rest that resolves with exercise; possible dyspnoea	Clinical signs; EMG abnormalities; muscle biopsy
Swedish Lapland Dog	Spinal muscular atrophy/multisystem neuronal abiotrophy	5–7 weeks; progressive tetraparesis; muscle wasting and deformation (distal limbs); loss of spinal reflexes	Clinical signs; EMG abnormalities; pathology

A1.2 (continued) Idiopathic, inherited and breed-associated diseases in dogs. Degenerative myelopathy occurs in many breeds and can be diagnosed with DNA tests [6]. ACh = acetylcholine; BAEP = brainstem auditory evoked potential; CK = creatine kinase; CSF = cerebrospinal fluid; CT = computed tomography; EMG = electromyogram; MRI = magnetic resonance imaging. (continues) ▶

Breed	Disease	Clinical signs (including age of onset where known)	Diagnostic aids
Tibetan Mastiff	Hypertrophic neuropathy	7–10 weeks; generalized weakness; poor reflexes; dysphonia; normal pain perception; may be recumbent within 3–4 weeks; muscle atrophy	Clinical signs; electrodiagnostics; nerve biopsy
Viszla (Hungarian)	Idiopathic epilepsy	Up to 6 years; seizures	Exclusion diagnosis
	Focal polymyositis	Masticatory muscle atrophy; dysphonia; dysphagia; salivation; regurgitation	Electrodiagnostics; muscle biopsy
Weimaraner	Hypomyelination	3 weeks; generalized tremors; dysmetria; several dogs normal by 12 months	Clinical signs; pathology
	Steroid-responsive meningitis–arteritis	<12 months; recurrent fever and neck pain	Clinical signs; neutrophilic pleocytosis; serum and CSF IgA levels[17]
West Highland White Terrier	Shaker dog/idiopathic tremors	9 months to 2 years; generalized tremors; mild hypermetria	Clinical signs; treatment response
Wirehaired Fox Terrier	Idiopathic epilepsy	Up to 6 years; seizures	Exclusion diagnosis
	Lissencephaly	Within 12 months; depression; behaviour change; seizures	Imaging (CT, MRI); pathology
	Cerebellar hypoplasia	Birth; cerebellar syndrome	Imaging (CT, MRI); pathology
	Megaoesophagus	Birth; regurgitation	Clinical signs; imaging (radiography, oesophagram)
Yorkshire Terrier	Necrotizing leucoencephalitis	Seizures; motor dysfunction; mental disorientation	CSF; imaging (MRI, CT); pathology
	Necrotizing encephalopathy (Leigh's disease)	4–12 months; seizures; progressive ataxia and dysmetria; central blindness; cranial nerve deficits	Imaging (CT, MRI); pathology; ultrastructural (electron microscopy) pathology

A1.2   (continued) Idiopathic, inherited and breed-associated diseases in dogs. Degenerative myelopathy occurs in many breeds and can be diagnosed with DNA tests [6]. ACh = acetylcholine; BAEP = brainstem auditory evoked potential; CK = creatine kinase; CSF = cerebrospinal fluid; CT = computed tomography; EMG = electromyogram; MRI = magnetic resonance imaging.

Inborn errors of metabolism

This section contains information on the inborn errors of metabolism that affect the central nervous system (CNS) in dogs and cats (Figures A1.3 and A1.4). These include storage diseases (metabolic errors that lead to a build-up of an intermediate product within the cell, see Chapters 9 and 13) and non-storage diseases (no gross accumulation of material within the cell, but lack of a final product or toxic levels of an intermediate product lead to malfunction of the cell).

These diseases all share the pathology of a metabolic enzyme abnormality, which is inherited – usually (but not always) as an autosomal recessive disorder. There are several laboratories that screen for these disorders, either via DNA testing or metabolite analysis of tissues or body fluids (e.g. urine or blood). A list of laboratories that currently offer these commercial services is given at the end of this section. Although every effort has been made to offer as much clinically useful information as possible, there can be no guarantee that this is a complete list of diseases, breed associations and laboratory services at the time of publication.

Breed	Disease	Clinical signs (including age of onset where known)	Diagnosis
Balinese	Niemann–Pick type A	Cerebellar/vestibular signs; depression; peripheral neuropathy	Enzyme assay in leucocytes and/or cultured fibroblasts
Burmese	GM2 gangliosidosis	Cerebellar/vestibular signs	DNA [1,2]

A1.3   Inborn errors of metabolism of the central nervous system in cats. GM = granulomatous meningoencephalitis; MPS = mucopolysaccharidosis. (continues) ▶

Appendix 1   Neurological disorders associated with cat and dog breeds

Domestic	Mannosidosis	<6 months at onset; connective tissue and skeletal malformation; possible peripheral nerve pathology	DNA [1]
	GM1 gangliosidosis	Young animals show cerebellar signs; may have dwarfism and facial dysmorphism	Oligosaccharide urinalysis [1,16]; enzyme assay in whole skin; cultured skin fibroblasts; liver; leucocytes
	GM2 gangliosidosis	Cerebellar/vestibular signs	Oligosaccharide urinalysis [1,16]; enzyme assay in whole skin; cultured skin fibroblasts; liver; leucocytes
	Globoid cell leucodystrophy (Krabbe disease)	Early cerebellar signs and ascending paralysis; cerebral signs later; may have peripheral neuropathy	Peripheral nerve biopsy is suggestive of diagnosis; enzyme assay in leucocytes; cultured fibroblasts
	Niemann–Pick type C	Ataxia; cerebellar/vestibular signs; peripheral neuropathy possible; hepatomegaly	Enzyme assay in leucocytes; cultured fibroblasts
	MPS VII	Progressive paraparesis	Urine metabolite screening [1]; DNA for related cats
	Mucolipidosis II (I-cell disease)	Dysmorphism; failure to thrive; delayed mineralization; skeletal abnormalities; retinal degeneration at 2.5 months of age	Inclusions in cultured fibroblasts; serum lysosomal enzyme assay [1,16]
Korat	GM2 gangliosidosis	Cerebellar/vestibular signs	DNA [2,3]
Norwegian Forest Cat	Glycogenosis IV	Incoordination; exercise intolerance	DNA [1,3,14,15]
Persian	Mannosidosis	8 weeks at onset; connective tissue and skeletal malformation; possible peripheral nerve pathology	DNA [1]
Siamese	GM1 gangliosidosis	Young animals show cerebellar signs; may have dwarfism and facial dysmorphism	DNA [1,3,15]
	Niemann–Pick type A	Cerebellar/vestibular signs; depression; peripheral neuropathy	Enzyme assay in leucocytes; cultured fibroblasts
	MPS VI	Dysmorphism; paraparesis	DNA [1]; urine metabolite screening [1,16]
	Ceroid lipofuscinosis	Adult and juvenile forms; ataxia; seizures; progressive blindness (central ± retinal)	Skin biopsy to look for lipopigment

A1.3 (continued) Inborn errors of metabolism of the central nervous system in cats. GM = granulomatous meningoencephalitis; MPS = mucopolysaccharidosis.

Breed	Disease	Clinical signs (including age of onset where known)	Diagnosis
Akita	Glycogenosis III	Muscular weakness; hepatomegaly	Liver; muscle; nervous system pathology
American Bulldog	Neuronal ceroid lipofuscinosis	1–4 years; progressive ataxia; wide-based stance	DNA [6,8,15]
American Staffordshire Terrier	Ceroid lipofuscinosis	2–8 years; progressive cerebellar and vestibular signs	Pathology; cerebellar atrophy on MRI; DNA [7,14,15]
Australian Cattle Dog	Ceroid lipofuscinosis	1 year; progressive visual loss; ataxia	Skin biopsy; brain pathology
Australian Kelpie	Globoid cell leucodystrophy (Krabbe disease)	3–4 months; progressive ataxia; tremors; paresis	Peripheral nerve biopsy is suggestive of diagnosis; enzyme assay in leucocytes; cultured fibroblasts

A1.4 Inborn errors of metabolism of the central nervous system in dogs. EMG = electromyogram; GM = granulomatous meningoencephalitis; MPS = mucopolysaccharidosis; PAS = periodic acid–Schiff (stain). (continues) ▶

Breed	Disease	Clinical signs (including age of onset where known)	Diagnosis
Basset Hound	Lafora disease	Myoclonic epilepsy	Muscle biopsy to look for intracytoplasmic PAS-positive inclusions
	Methylmalonic aciduria	3–6 months; failure to thrive; anaemia; encephalopathy	Urine organic acid screen [1]
Beagle	GM1 gangliosidosis	Young animals show cerebellar signs; may have dwarfism and facial dysmorphism	Oligosaccharide urinalysis [1]; enzyme assay in whole skin; cultured skin fibroblasts; liver; leucocytes
	Lafora disease	Myoclonic epilepsy	Muscle biopsy to look for intracytoplasmic PAS-positive inclusions
	Globoid cell leucodystrophy (Krabbe disease)	Early cerebellar signs and ascending paralysis; cerebral signs later; may have peripheral neuropathy	DNA [3,11]; peripheral nerve biopsy is suggestive of diagnosis; enzyme assay in leucocytes; cultured fibroblasts
Border Collie	Ceroid lipofuscinosis	Adult and juvenile forms; ataxia; seizures; progressive blindness (central ± retinal)	Skin biopsy; DNA [3,4,7,13,15]
	Methylmalonic aciduria	2–6 months; failure to thrive; anaemia; encephalopathy	Urine organic acid screen [1]
Boxer	Niemann–Pick type C	Ataxia; cerebellar/vestibular signs; peripheral neuropathy; possible hepatomegaly	Enzyme assay in leucocytes; cultured fibroblasts
Cairn Terrier	Globoid cell leucodystrophy (Krabbe disease)	Early cerebellar signs and ascending paralysis; cerebral signs later; may have peripheral neuropathy	DNA [3,10,11,15]; peripheral nerve biopsy is suggestive of diagnosis; enzyme assay in leucocytes; cultured fibroblasts
Chihuahua	Ceroid lipofuscinosis	Adult and juvenile forms; ataxia; seizures; progressive blindness (central ± retinal)	DNA [6]
Clumber Spaniel	Pyruvate dehydrogenase deficiency (metabolic myopathy)	3 months; progressive exercise intolerance and collapse	Enzyme assays using cultured fibro-blasts; organic acid analysis [1]; DNA [4,6]
Cocker Spaniel	Ceroid lipofuscinosis	1–6 years; progressive ataxia; aggression; vision impairment; seizures; tremors	Skin biopsy; pathology
Cross-breed dog	MPS VII	Pelvic limb weakness; joint laxity; atrioventricular valve incompetence seen in affected dogs	Urine metabolite screening [1,16]
Curly-Coated Retriever	Glycogen storage disease IIIa	Lethargy; exercise intolerance	DNA [3,5,15]
Dachshund	Lafora disease	Myoclonic epilepsy	Muscle biopsy to look for intracytoplasmic PAS-positive inclusions
	Ceroid lipofuscinosis	Adult and juvenile forms; ataxia; seizures; progressive blindness (central ± retinal)	DNA [6]
	MPS IIIA	Adult-onset; progressive spinocerebellar ataxia	Heparan sulphate urinary excretion; fibroblast and hepatic enzyme assay
Dalmatian	Ceroid lipofuscinosis	6 months to 1 year; visual impairment; tremors; aggression; seizures	Skin biopsy; pathology
English Setter	Ceroid lipofuscinosis	Adult and juvenile forms; ataxia; seizures; progressive blindness (central ± retinal)	Skin biopsy; DNA [6,8,13]

A1.4 (continued) Inborn errors of metabolism of the central nervous system in dogs. EMG = electromyogram; GM = granulomatous meningoencephalitis; MPS = mucopolysaccharidosis; PAS = periodic acid–Schiff (stain). (continues) ▶

Appendix 1 Neurological disorders associated with cat and dog breeds

Breed	Disease	Clinical signs (including age of onset where known)	Diagnosis
English Springer Spaniel	Fucosidosis	Adult-onset of cerebral signs (1–4 years)	DNA [1,4,6,13,15]
	GM1 gangliosidosis	Young animals show cerebellar signs; may have dwarfism and facial dysmorphism	Oligosaccharide urinalysis [1,16]; enzyme assay in whole skin; cultured skin fibroblasts; liver; leucocytes
German Shepherd Dog	Glycogenosis III	Muscular weakness; hepatomegaly	Liver; muscle; nervous system pathology
	MPS VII	Birth; progressive tetraparesis; visual impairment; dementia	Urine organic acid screening; DNA [1,3]
German Shorthaired Pointer	GM2 gangliosidosis	Cerebellar/vestibular signs	Oligosaccharide urinalysis [1,16]; enzyme assay in whole skin; cultured skin fibroblasts; liver; leucocytes
Giant Schnauzer	Methylmalonic aciduria	6–12 weeks; anaemia; failure to thrive; encephalopathy	Urine organic acid screening [1]
Husky	GM1 gangliosidosis	Birth; bone anomalies; encephalopathy	DNA [3,15]
Irish Setter	Globoid cell leucodystrophy (Krabbe disease)	Early cerebellar signs and ascending paralysis; cerebral signs later; may have peripheral neuropathy	DNA [11]; peripheral nerve biopsy is suggestive of diagnosis; enzyme assay in leucocytes; cultured fibroblasts
Japanese Spaniel (Chin)	GM2 gangliosidosis	Cerebellar/vestibular signs	Oligosaccharide urinalysis [1,16]; enzyme assay in whole skin; cultured skin fibroblasts; liver; leucocytes
Labrador Retriever	MPS II	Incoordination; exercise intolerance; visual deficits	Urine metabolic screening [1,16]
Lapland Dog	Glycogenosis II	Muscle weakness; vomiting; megaoesophagus; cardiac and respiratory abnormalities	Liver; muscle; nervous system pathology; EMG abnormalities
Maltese	Malonic aciduria	Seizures; stupor	Urine organic acid screening [1,16]
Miniature Pinscher	MPS VI	Dysmorphism; paraparesis (spinal abnormalities)	DNA 1; urine metabolite screening [1,16]
Miniature Schnauzer	Ceroid lipofuscinosis	2–4 years; visual impairment; disorientation; tremors	Skin biopsy; pathology
	MPS VI	Dysmorphism; paraparesis (spinal abnormalities)	Urine metabolic screening; DNA [1]
New Zealand Huntaway Dog	MPS IIIA	1–2 years; progressive ataxia; hypermetria	Lysosomal enzyme assay; urine metabolic screening
Old English Sheepdog	Cytochrome oxidase deficiency	3 months; exercise intolerance; generalized weakness	Pre- and post-exercise lactate and pyruvate; EMG abnormalities; muscle biopsy
Plotthound	MPS I	Dysmorphism; spinal abnormalities	Urine metabolic screening [1,16]
Polish Lowland Sheepdog	Ceroid lipofuscinosis	6 months to 5 years; progressive ataxia; visual impairment; behaviour changes	Skin biopsy; pathology
Poodle	Globoid cell leucodystrophy (Krabbe disease)	Early cerebellar signs and ascending paralysis; cerebral signs later; may have peripheral neuropathy	DNA [11]; peripheral nerve biopsy is suggestive of diagnosis; enzyme assay in leucocytes; cultured fibroblasts
Portuguese Water Dog	GM1 gangliosidosis	Young animals show cerebellar signs; may have dwarfism and facial dysmorphism	Oligosaccharide urinalysis [1,16]; enzyme assay in whole skin; cultured skin fibroblasts; liver; leucocytes; DNA [10,15]

A1.4 (continued) Inborn errors of metabolism of the central nervous system in dogs. EMG = electromyogram; GM = granulomatous meningoencephalitis; MPS = mucopolysaccharidosis; PAS = periodic acid–Schiff (stain).
(continues) ▶

Breed	Disease	Clinical signs (including age of onset where known)	Diagnosis
Rottweiler	MPS I	Young animals; ataxia	Urine metabolic screening [1]
Schipperke	MPS IIIB	≥3 years; progressive cerebellar signs	Urine metabolic screening [1,16]; enzyme assay in cultured fibroblasts; DNA [1]
Shar Pei	Methylmalonic aciduria	Failure to thrive; anaemia; disorientation	Urine metabolic screening [1]
Siberian Husky	GM1 gangliosidosis	Young animals show cerebellar signs; may have dwarfism and facial dysmorphism	Oligosaccharide urinalysis [1,16]; enzyme assay in whole skin; cultured skin fibroblasts; liver; leucocytes
Silky Terrier	Glucocerebrosidosis (Gaucher disease)	6–8 months; ataxia; hypermetria; cerebellar signs	Enzyme assay (beta-glucosidase) in leucocytes
Staffordshire Bull Terrier	L-2-hydroxyglutaric aciduria	4–10 months; ataxia; seizures; dementia	Urine organic acid screening [1]; DNA [3,4,6,14,15]
Sussex Spaniel	Pyruvate dehydrogenase deficiency (metabolic myopathy)	3 months; progressive exercise intolerance	Enzyme assay in cultured fibroblasts; organic acid analysis [11]; DNA [4,6]
Tibetan Terrier	Ceroid lipofuscinosis	Adult and juvenile forms; ataxia; seizures; progressive blindness (central ± retinal)	Skin biopsy; DNA [6]
Welsh Corgi	Ceroid lipofuscinosis	6–8 years; visual impairment; behaviour changes	Pathology
	MPS VI	Dysmorphism; paraparesis (spinal abnormalities)	Urine metabolic screening [1]
West Highland White Terrier	Globoid cell leukodystrophy (Krabbe disease)	Early cerebellar signs and ascending paralysis; cerebral signs later; may have peripheral neuropathy	DNA [3,10,11,15]; peripheral nerve biopsy is suggestive of diagnosis; enzyme assay in leucocytes; cultured fibroblasts
Wirehaired Dachshund	MPS III	Ataxia; intention tremors	Urine metabolite screening [1]
	Lafora disease	Myoclonic epilepsy	Muscle biopsy to look for intracytoplasmic PAS-positive inclusions

A1.4 (continued) Inborn errors of metabolism of the central nervous system in dogs. EMG = electromyogram; GM = granulomatous meningoencephalitis; MPS = mucopolysaccharidosis; PAS = periodic acid–Schiff (stain).

Veterinary genetic and molecular investigational centres

1. PennGenn Laboratories, Dr Giger/PennGen, School of Veterinary Medicine, University of Pennsylvania, 3900 Delancey Street, Room 4013, Philadelphia, PA 19104-6010, USA
   Phone: 001-215-898-8894
   Fax: 001-215-573-2162
   email: penngen@lists.upenn.edu
   http://www.research.vet.upenn.edu/Default.aspx?alias=research.vet.upenn.edu/penngen

2. UC Davis Veterinary Genetics Laboratory, One Shields Ave., Davis, CA 95616-8744, USA
   Phone: 001-530-752-2211
   Fax: 001-530-752-3556
   http://www.vgl.ucdavis.edu

3. Laboklin (UK), 61 Mouldsworth Avenue, Manchester M20 1GG, UK
   Phone: +44 (0)161-282-3066
   Fax: +44 (0)870-161-6981
   email: info@laboklin.co.uk
   http://laboklin.co.uk

   Laboklin (GMBH & Co. KG), SteubenstrauBe4, Post Box 1810, D-97688 Bad Kissingen, Germany
   Phone: 0049-971-72020
   Fax: 0049-971-68546
   email: info@laboklin.de
   http://www.laboklin.de

4. Animal Health Trust, Genetics Unit, Lanwades Park, Kentford, Newmarket, Suffolk CB8 7UU, UK
   Phone: +44 (0)8700-509169
   Fax: +44 (0)8700-502386
   http://www.aht.org.uk/

5. Dr John C. Fyfe, Laboratory of Comparative Medical Genetics, 2209 Biomedical Physical Sciences Building, Michigan State University, East Lansing, MI 48824-4320, USA
   Phone: 001-517-884-5348
   email: fyfe@cvm.msu.edu
   http://www.mmg.msu.edu/fyfe.html

6. Animal Molecular Genetic Diseases Laboratory, College of Veterinary Medicine, University of Missouri-Columbia, Columbia, MO 65211, USA
   Phone: 001-573-884-3712
   email: HansenL@missouri.edu
   http://caninegeneticdiseases.net
   (Test for US and international submission found on the main website. Many tests are now administered through the Orthopedic Foundation for Animals at http://www.offa.org/dnatesting/)

7. Optigen, 767 Warren Road, Suite 300, Ithaca, NY 14850, USA
   Phone: 001-607-257-0301
   Fax: 001-607-257-0353
   email: genetest@optigen.com or optigen@clarityconnect.com
   http://optigen.com

8. VetGen, 3728 Plaza Drive, Suite 1, Ann Arbor, MI 48108, USA
   Phone: 001-734-669-8440 or (USA & Canada) 1-800-483-8436
   Fax: 001-734-669-8441
   http://www.vetgen.com

9. Veterinary Diagnostic Laboratory,
   College of Veterinary Medicine, University of Minnesota,
   1333 Gortner Avenue, St. Paul, MN, 55108-1098, USA
   Phone: 001-612-625-8787 or (USA & Canada) 1-800-605-8787
   Fax: 001-612-624-8707
   email: vdl@umn.edu
   http://ww.bdl.umn.edu/ourservices/canineneuromuscular/home.html

10. HealthGene Corp, 2175 Keele Street, Toronto,
    Ontario M6M 3Z4, Canada
    Phone: 001-416-658-2040 or (USA & Canada) 1-877-371-1551
    Fax: 001-416-658-2042
    email: info@healthgene.com
    http://healthgene.com

11. Jefferson Medical College, Department of Neurology,
    1020 Locust Street, JAH 394, PA 19104-6010, USA
    Phone: 001-215-955-1666
    Fax: 001-215-955-9554
    http://www.tju.edu/jmc/home/index.cfm

12. DDC Veterinary, One DDC Way, Fairfield, OH 45014, USA
    Phone: 001-800-625-0874
    email: contact@vetdnacenter.com
    http://www.vetdnacenter.com

13. Animal Genetics Inc., 1336 Timberlane Road,
    Tallahassee, FL 32312-1766, USA
    Phone: 001-850-386-2973 or (USA) 1-866-922-6436
    Fax: 001-850-386-1146
    email: contact@animalgenetics.us
    http://animalgenetics.us

14. Antagene, Immeuble Le Meltem,
    2, alle 'e des Se'quoias,
    69760 Limonest, France
    Phone: 0033-04-37-49-90-03
    Fax: 0033-04-37-49-04-89
    email: contact@antagene.com
    http://www.antagene.com

15. Dr Van Haering Laboratorium b.v.,
    PO Box 408, 6700 AK Wageningen,
    The Netherlands
    Phone: 0031-317-416-402
    Fax: 0031-317-426-117
    email: info@vhlgenetics.com
    http://www.vhlgenetics.com

16. Comparative Neuromuscular Laboratory,
    Basic Science Building,
    Room 2095,
    University of California,
    San Diego, La Jolla,
    CA 92093-0612, USA
    Phone: 001-858-532-1537 or (USA) 001-858-534-1537
    Fax: 001-858-534-7319
    http://www.vetneuromuscular.ucsd.edu

17. University of Hannover,
    Department of Small Animal
    Medicine and Surgery,
    Veterinary Medical School,
    Hannover, Bischofsholder Damm 15,
    D-30173, Hannover, Germany

18. The Veterinary Genetics Laboratory,
    North Carolina State University,
    College of Veterinary Medicine,
    1052 William Moore Drive, Raleigh, NC27607, USA
    Phone: 001-919-513-3314
    http://www.cvm.ncsu.edu/vhc/csds/vcgl/index.html

DAMNITV classification of diseases

The 'mechanism' of disease responsible for a neurological disorder can be one of ten broad categories; each category describes a multitude of specific diseases listed in the table below. Consideration of each of these mechanisms, based on patient signalment, presenting complaint, clinical history and the neurological examination, should take place following localization of the neurological lesion(s). The ultimate aim is to develop a list of differential diagnoses for the patient.

Specific disorders are described in chapters based on presenting problems. As a result, many disorders are relevant to more than one chapter. The numbers in square brackets refer to the chapters in which the disease is considered in greatest detail.

Mechanism of disease	Specific diseases
Degenerative	Calcinosis circumscripta [14, 15, 16]; canine cognitive dysfunction [9]; cerebellar cortical degeneration [13]; cervical stenotic myelopathy (Wobbler syndrome) [15]; degenerative myelopathy [16]; degenerative lumbosacral stenosis (LSS) [19]; dural ossification [14, 16]; feline encephalomyelopathy [13]; foraminal stenosis [17]; intervertebral disc disease [14, 15, 16, 19]; Labrador Retriever myopathy and exercise-induced collapse [18]; Lafora's disease [13]; lysosomal storage diseases [11, 13]; mucopolysaccharidosis [16]; muscular dystrophy [18]; myotonia [18]; neurodegenerative brain diseases [9, 13]; peripheral neuropathy [15]; spinal synovial cysts [15, 16]; spondylosis deformans [14, 16]
Anomalous	Atlantoaxial instability [14, 15]; Chiari-like malformations [11, 14]; congenital abnormalities in eye position [10]; congenital deafness [12]; congenital vestibular disease [11]; dermoid sinus [15, 16]; dysmyelination/ hypomyelination [13]; feline cerebellar hypoplasia [13]; hydrocephalus [9]; intra-arachnoid cysts [11, 15, 16]; lissencephaly [10]; osteochondromatosis [15, 16]; scoliosis [14]; vertebral and spinal cord anomalies [14, 15, 16, 19]
Metabolic	Calcium abnormalities [8, 13]; diabetes mellitus [15]; endocrine neuropathies [15, 16]; hepatic encephalopathy [9]; hyperadrenocorticism [15, 18]; hypoglycaemia [9]; hypothyroidism [11, 15]; metabolic myopathies [18]; myxoedema coma [9]; potassium abnormalities [9]; sodium abnormalities [9]
Neoplastic	Brain tumours [9, 11]; chordomas [19]; choroid plexus tumours [9]; gliomas [9]; inner and middle ear tumours [11]; insulinoma [15]; lipomas [19]; lymphoma [17]; meningiomas [9]; nerve sheath tumours [12, 17]; paraneoplastic neuropathy [15]; pituitary gland tumours [9]; spinal lymphoma [16]; spinal neuroepithelioma [16]; vertebral body tumours [16]; vertebral plasma cell tumours [16]
Nutritional	Hypervitaminosis A [14]; thiamine deficiency [9, 11]
Inflammatory (immune-mediated and infectious)	Bacterial encephalitis [11]; canine distemper virus infection [11]; canine distemper viral myelitis [16]; chronic inflammatory demyelinating polyneuropathy [15]; cryptococcosis [11]; discospondylitis [14, 15]; empyema [14]; encephalitis [9, 11]; extraocular myositis [10]; feline encephalomyelitis [13]; feline cornavirus (which causes feline infectious peritonitis), myelitis and meningitis [11, 16]; feline leukaemia virus-associated myelopathy [16]; feline spongiform encephalopathy [13]; ganglioradiculitis [15]; generalized tremor syndrome in dogs [13]; granulomatous meningoencephalomyelitis (GME) [11, 14]; infectious meningitis [14]; infectious polymyositis [18]; inflammatory myopathies [18]; inflammatory spinal cord diseases [16]; masticatory myositis [12]; meningitis [9]; meningoencephalitis [11]; meningoencephalomyelitis [15]; myasthenia gravis [18]; nasopharyngeal polyps [11]; necrotizing meningoencephalomyelitis [11]; neosporosis [11]; optic neuritis [10]; osteomyelitis [14]; otitis media/ interna (OM/OI) [11]; parasitic diseases [9]; plexus neuritis [17]; polioencephalomyelitis [13]; polyarthritis [14]; polymyositis [14]; polyradiculoneuritis [15]; presumed immune-mediated cerebellar granulprival degeneration in Coton de Tulear dogs [13]; protozoal myelitis [16]; protozoal neuritis [15]; rabies; spinal empyema [15, 16]; steroid-responsive meningitis–arteritis (SRMA) [14, 15]; tail abscessation [19]; toxoplasmosis [11]; vertebral physitis [16]
Idiopathic	Canine and feline dysautonomia [19]; disseminated idiopathic skeletal hyperostosis [16]; distal denervating disease [15]; feline hyperaesthesia syndrome [13]; Horner's syndrome [10]; hypertonicity in Cavalier King Charles Spaniels [13]; idiopathic epilepsy [8]; idiopathic facial paresis [12]; idiopathic vestibular disease [11]; laryngeal paralysis [12]; megaoesophagus [12]; narcolepsy–cataplexy [17]; reflex myoclonus [13, 18]; Scottie cramp [13]

Appendix 2 DAMNITV classification of diseases

Mechanism of disease	Specific diseases
Toxic	Antiepileptic drugs [8, 16]; botulism [15]; drug-induced toxic neuropathy [15]; ivermectin [9]; lead [9]; metronidazole [11]; organophosphates/carbamates [13, 18]; ototoxicity [11]; tetanus [15, 17]; tick paralysis [15]
Traumatic	Brachial plexus avulsion [17]; caudal lumbar/lumbosacral trauma [17]; cervical vertebral fractures and luxations [15]; femoral nerve injury [17]; fractures and luxations of the caudal lumbar and sacral vertebrae [19]; fractures and luxations of the thoracolumbar spine [16]; head trauma [11]; inner ear trauma [11]; lumbosacral plexus trauma [17]; middle ear trauma [11]; pelvic trauma [17]; peroneal and tibial nerve injury [17]; proximal sciatic nerve injury [17]; radial nerve injury [17]; sacral fractures [19]; sacrococcygeal fracture/luxation and tail avulsions [19]; spinal cord contusion [15]; thoracolumbar fractures and luxations [16]; traumatic disc herniation [15]
Vascular	Aortic thrombosis [16]; brachial thrombosis [17]; canine cerebrovascular accidents [9, 11, 13]; cerebrovascular disease [11]; coccygeal muscle injury [19]; feline ischaemic encephalopathy [9]; fibrocartilaginous embolism (FCE) [15, 16, 19]; spinal haemorrhage [15]

Conversion tables

Biochemistry

	SI unit	Conversion factor	Conventional unit
Alanine aminotransferase	IU/l	1	IU/l
Albumin	g/l	0.1	g/dl
Alkaline phosphatase	IU/l	1	IU/l
Aspartate aminotransferase	IU/l	1	IU/l
Bilirubin	mmol/l	0.0584	mg/dl
Blood urea nitrogen (BUN)	mmol/l	2.8	mg/dl
Calcium	mmol/l	4	mg/dl
Carbon dioxide (total)	mmol/l	1	mEq/l
Cholesterol	mmol/l	38.61	mg/dl
Chloride	mmol/l	1	mEq/l
Cortisol	nmol/l	0.362	ng/ml
Creatine kinase	IU/l	1	IU/l
Creatinine	mmol/l	0.0113	mg/dl
Glucose	mmol/l	18.02	mg/dl
Insulin	pmol/l	0.1394	mIU/ml
Iron	µmol/l	5.587	mg/dl
Magnesium	mmol/l	2	mEq/l
Phosphorus	mmol/l	3.1	mg/dl
Potassium	mmol/l	1	mEq/l
Sodium	mmol/l	1	mEq/l
Total protein	g/l	0.1	g/dl
Thyroxine (T4) (free)	pmol/l	0.0775	ng/dl
Thyroxine (T4) (total)	nmol/l	0.0775	mg/dl
Tri-iodothyronine (T3)	nmol/l	65.1	ng/dl
Triglycerides	mmol/l	88.5	mg/dl

Haematology

	SI unit	Conversion factor	Conventional unit
Red blood cells	10^{12}/l	1	10^6/ml
Haemoglobin	g/l	0.1	g/dl
MCH	pg/cell	1	pg/cell
MCHC	g/l	0.1	g/dl
MCV	fl	1	mm^3
Platelet count	10^9/l	1	10^3/ml
White blood cells	10^9/l	1	10^3/ml

Serum drug levels

	SI unit	Conversion factor	Conventional unit
Bromide	mmol/l	8	mg/dl
Phenobarbital	µmol/l	0.232	mg/l

Temperature

SI unit	Conversion factor	Conventional unit
°C	(x9/5) + 32	°F

Index

Index